Biomedical Research, Medicine, and Disease

Biomedical research is the first step towards the creation of new medications and treatments that help to manage different types of health conditions and diseases. The prevention and cure of diseases would be practically impossible without such type of research. Although the drug discovery and development processes are far too costly, time-consuming, prone to failure, and have low success rate, today the term "translational research or medicine" seems to have become trendy, even though it is insufficient.

The present book is a sincere attempt by dedicated researchers to convey the importance of translational biomedical research, medicine, and disease, primarily, basic and clinical difficulties in the translation of diagnostic measures, pharmaceutical advances, biomarkers, diagnostics, and therapeutics.

This book is meant for researchers, scientists, healthcare professionals, industry, innovators, and students of biomedical sciences, as well as for those involved in the basic sciences, biochemistry, biotechnology, biophysics, and life sciences in general.

The volume comprehensively covers:

i.   Emerging technologies for healthcare,
ii. Various aspects of biomedical research toward understanding of pathophysiology of the diseases,
iii. Advances in improvement in diagnostic procedures and therapeutic tools, and
iv. The fundamental role of biomedical research in the development of new medicinal products.

Translating Animal Science Research

Series Editor

R.C. Sobti, Department of Biotechnology, Panjab University, Chandigarh, India

Biodiversity: Threats and Conservation
R.C. Sobti

Environmental Studies and Climate Change
R.C. Sobti, S.K. Malhotra, Kamal Jaiswal, and Sanjeev Puri

Genomics, Proteomics and Biotechnology
R.C. Sobti, Manishi Mukesh, and Aastha Sobti

Biomedical Research, Medicine, and Disease
R.C. Sobti and Aastha Sobti

For more information, visit webpage: www.routledge.com/Translating-Animal-Science-Research/book-series/TASR

Biomedical Research, Medicine, and Disease

Edited by
R.C. Sobti and Aastha Sobti

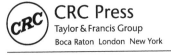

CRC Press
Taylor & Francis Group
Boca Raton London New York

CRC Press is an imprint of the
Taylor & Francis Group, an **informa** business

First edition published 2023
by CRC Press
6000 Broken Sound Parkway NW, Suite 300, Boca Raton, FL 33487-2742

and by CRC Press
4 Park Square, Milton Park, Abingdon, Oxon, OX14 4RN

CRC Press is an imprint of Taylor & Francis Group, LLC

Library of Congress Cataloging-in-Publication Data
Names: Sobti, R. C., editor. | Sobti, Aastha, editor.
Title: Biomedical research, medicine and disease / edited by RC Sobti and Aastha Sobti.
Other titles: Translating animal science research (Series)
Description: First edition. | Boca Raton : CRC Press, 2023. |
Series: Translating animal science research | Includes bibliographical references and index.
Identifiers: LCCN 2022030531 (print) | LCCN 2022030532 (ebook) |
ISBN 9781032115498 (hardback) | ISBN 9781032115504 (paperback) |
ISBN 9781003220404 (ebook)
Subjects: MESH: Translational Research, Biomedical
Classification: LCC R852 (print) | LCC R852 (ebook) |
NLM W 20.55.T7 | DDC 610.72/4–dc23/eng/20221110
LC record available at https://lccn.loc.gov/2022030531
LC ebook record available at https://lccn.loc.gov/2022030532

ISBN: 9781032115498 (hbk)
ISBN: 9781032115504 (pbk)
ISBN: 9781003220404 (ebk)

DOI: 10.1201/9781003220404

Typeset in Times New Roman
by Newgen Publishing UK

Contents

Section I Advancement in Techniques in Biomedical Science

23 Human Papillomavirus (HPV): Molecular Epidemiology of Infection and its Associated Diseases 337
Abhishek Pandeya, Raj Kumar Khalko, Bharti Kotarya, Hema, Jitendra Kumar Yadav, Sudipta Saha, Sunil Babu Gosipatala, and R.C. Sobti

24 Challenges of Multidrug-Resistant Microbes on Public Health 363
Ram Krishan Negi, Himani Khurana, Monika Sharma, Meghali Bharti, Tarana Negi and Sonakshi Modeel

25 Role of Probiotics in the Prevention and Management of Obesity: What Have We Learned So Far? 377
Tajpreet Kaur, Ashwani Kumar Sharma, Balbir Singh, Harpal S. Buttar, and Amrit Pal Singh

Section III Therapeutics and Novel Approaches

26 Protease Inhibitors of Marine Origin: Promising Anticancer and HIV Therapies 397
Maushmi S. Kumar, Yashodhara Dalal, Sahil Khan, and Harpal S. Buttar

Section IV   Drugs and Delivery Systems

35 Therapeutic Translational Potential of Surface-Decorated Nanoparticles 547
Nidhi Mishra, Raquibun Nisha, Ravi Raj, Pal Alka, Priya Singh, Neelu Singh, and Shubhini Saraf

Section V   Nutra-Chemistry

36 Towards Developing Biofortified Food Crops for Enhancing Nutritional Aspects and Human Health.. 571
Manu Priya and Harsh Nayyar

Preface

In the last few decades there have been remarkable conceptual and practical technological advances in molecular biology as well as biomedical sciences that are continuing at a fast pace, thereby giving rise to emerging areas of molecular medicine and personalized drug therapies. There now exists comprehensive and detailed understanding about the underlying mechanisms that underscore the development and normal functions of the human body during health and disease. Most of our comprehensive knowledge in biomedical sciences has been gained through in vitro and in vivo studies carried out with microorganisms, cell lines, and laboratory animals, including primates and marine organisms. The insights into the physiological and pathophysiological mechanisms are helping us to delineate health and disease processes. Attempts are being made to understand the integrated functions of the human body organs and lower organisms by using a combination of molecular, computational, and structural biology, as well as imaging technologies. These new technologies and molecular concepts about many acquired and inheritable diseases have enabled us to gain in-depth knowledge about the underlying mechanisms of diseases.

The aftermath of the genome project and molecular developments, involving next-generation sequencing (NGS) and gene-editing technologies, have provided new knowledge to understand the mechanistic occurrence of acute and chronic diseases and to develop strategies for their prevention.

The primary and clinical workforces linked by biomedical scientists are now termed as "translational" researchers, who are trained to be knowledgeable in the primary and clinical biomedical sciences and proficient in the bedside quality of care of patients. Biotechnological innovations are helping to develop targeted medicines for patients of cancer and other diseases, and to help people live longer and enjoy healthier lives. Novel molecular techniques have helped to produce prophylactic vaccines as well as other diagnostic tools to prevent and contain epidemics, and to detect and diagnose conditions sooner with greater accuracy and precision.

At present, parasitic infectious diseases such as malaria, as well as acquired immunodeficiency syndrome (AIDS) and tuberculosis (TB), can be diagnosed rapidly at relatively lower cost with molecular diagnostic tools, including polymerase chain reaction (PCR), recombinant antigens, and monoclonal antibodies.

Modern diagnostic test kits for rickettsial, bacterial, and viral diseases, along with radiolabeled biological therapeutics for imaging and analysis have been developed. Vaccines have almost eliminated globally small pox, polio, cholera, and some other deadly diseases for the last hundred years. Advancements have been made in making recombinant vaccines that have the potential to eradicate non-communicable diseases (NCDs) like cancer. Naked DNA vaccines, viral vector vaccines, and plant-derived vaccines have been found to be most effective against a number of bacterial and viral disorders. Therapeutic proteins, polyunsaturated fatty acids (PUFA), and dietary interventions have had a large impact in the prevention of NCDs responsible for more than 60 percent of deaths in developing countries. Immunotherapy, which uses the body's own immune system, has enabled us to fight pathogenic organisms and to develop a vaccine to keep disease symptoms in check. Biotechnology therapies and vaccines have reduced the spread of infectious diseases and have assisted in the containment of epidemics and pandemics.

Antiretroviral (ARV) techniques are bound to increase the longevity of HIV/AIDS patients. In the "London Patient" case, for example, by targeting CCR5 gene mutation through stem-cell transplants, the patient was successfully cured of the disease. Biotechnology companies are working to deliver high-impact health technologies to countries across the globe to reduce the inequities in healthcare results, and determine on-the-spot treatment and develop biopharmaceutical products, which would help to reduce healthcare costs, create healthier workforces, and boost economic development.

Transgenic bacteria, yeasts, medicinal plants, and animals used in experimentation have been utilized as a factory for producing recombinant therapeutic proteins and other products. Novel gene therapies are being used in these systems to produce therapeutic proteins of interest in large quantities that are then purified as therapeutic agents. The most important recombinant therapeutic proteins include: erythropoietin for anemia treatment. Interferon alpha against leukemia, viral diseases and insulin against type-1 diabetes mellitus have been produced with new technologies. Other therapeutic agents include: growth hormones, cytokines, recombinant blood products, monoclonal antibodies, gene therapy products, molecular pharmaceutical agents, and bioengineered tissue products. Xenografts, bone grafts, collagen, and heart valves have been successfully engineered. New technologies offer relatively cost-effective and affordabledrugs and vaccine-delivery tools and eliminate the blood-borne infections caused by re-use of needles. Drugs and vaccines are efficiently delivered in a controlled manner. This avoids the use of injections. Drugs can be propelled into the body speedily by gas jets and can also be inhaled through nasal sprays. Drugs are efficiently delivered into the body using nano-particle solutions and emulsions. Recent advances in biotechnology and nanotechnology have helped to reduce drug dosages required for a particular treatment. Stem cell therapy is still in its infancy stages, but it has promising therapeutic applications.

Genetically modified crops fulfill the requirement of essential micronutrients (vitamins and minerals) required in physiological functions. They are helpful in the physical growth and cognitive development of children. Novel and desired genes are introduced into genetically modified crops which become nutritionally enriched to cope with the growing nutritional needs of people worldwide. For example, iron-rich rice fulfills the dietary requirement of iron and helps to prevent anemia. Golden rice, rich in vitamin A, prevents blindness among a lot of children in developing countries. Potatoes and tomatoes containing a number of vitamins/minerals have proven satisfactory to fulfill the nutritional needs of people globally. Thus, nutritional needs and quality of life can be improved with the use of genetically modified foods. They can become a part of staple foods. Flax seeds, corn, maize, tomatoes, papaya, squash, soybeans, sugar beets, canola, and cottonseeds are the other genetically engineered food plants.

While there has been an explosion of information in all the above mentioned areas, it has been difficult to collate and translate all that knowledge under one umbrella for practical purposes. Thus, there exists a wide gap in our gained knowledge and its applications for human use. To mitigate the challenges faced by humanity, this gap must be bridged with multidisciplinary therapeutic choices. The synthesis of knowledge will help to accelerate our understanding about the pathophysiology of human diseases and develop new strategies to prevent, diagnose, and treat human illnesses. The route of our journey to discovering new therapies may pass through different experimental and validation stages in lower organisms and higher animal species, cell-free systems, and pharmacometabolomics. To improve disease outcomes in numerous fields of medicine, researchers strive to predict how younger, middle-aged, and elderly patients will react to certain medications. Using pharmacogenomic methods, scientists can identify genetic markers that predict drug responses, and consequently use that information to customize patient treatment plans.

The present book is an attempt to update this knowledge in the application of biomedical sciences in disease and medicine. The authors made sincere efforts to elucidate the major elements of a dense chain of actions that contribute to a seamless and consistent translation of experimental evidence into clinical outcomes. These dedicated researchers had in mind an ideology to cover the importance of translational biomedical research into medicine and disease.

This book is intended for researchers, scientists, healthcare professionals, industry, innovators, and students of biomedical sciences (as well as basic sciences, biochemistry, biotechnology, biophysics, and life sciences in general).

Acknowledgments

The editors are thankful to Dr. Vipin Sobti, Er. Aditi Sobti, Er. Vineet and Er. Ankit for their forbearance and encouragement in the preparation of this volume. They take pleasure in thanking Irene for her support through inspiring words. Thanks to Sh. Ashok Kumar for his help with typographical work.

Dr. R.C. Sobti gratefully acknowledges the Indian National Science Academy and Panjab University Chandigarh for providing him with platforms as Senior Scientist and Emeritus Professor respectively to continue the work in this direction.

Editor Biographies

Ranbir Chander Sobti, former Vice-Chancellor Panjab University, Chandigarh & Babasaheb Bhimrao Ambedkar University (Central University), Lucknow is a scientist, an able administrator, and dynamic institution builder.

He has published more than 350 papers in journals of national and international repute such as *Mutation Research, Carcinogenesis, Archives of Toxicology, Cancer Genetics and Cytogenetics, Molecular Cell Biochemistry,* and *PLOS One* to name a few. He has also published more than 50 books by international publishers such as Springer, Academic Press, CRC, Elsevier, and others.

He is Fellow of the Third World Academy of Sciences, National Academy of Sciences India, Indian National Science Academy, National Academy of Medical Sciences, National Academy of Agricultural Sciences, Canadian Academy of Cardiovascular Diseases, and a few others. He was the General President of the Indian Science Congress Association for the 102nd session, held at University of Jammu in 2013. He is the recipient of many prestigious awards, such as the INSA Young Scientist Medal, UGC Career Award, Punjab Rattan Award, JC Bose Oration and Sriram Oration Awards, and Lifetime Achievement Awards of the Punjab Academy of Sciences, Zoological Society of India, and the Environment Academy of India, besides many other medals and awards of national and international levels. He was awarded Padmashri, the third highest civilian award by the Government of India in 2009 for his contributions to the cause of education. He has widely travelled across the globe.

Dr. Sobti, an active researcher, is also steadfastly committed to the popularization of science in the community through popular lectures and community engagement programs.

Aastha Sobti has a master's degree in clinical dentistry and oro-facial surgery (UK) and works in the field of head and neck cancers using her intellect and her background in oral and maxillofacial surgery to bring reforms that are required in the present multifarious surgical and research areas.

She has seven years of teaching and research experience and has published a number of papers in reputed journals. She has been awarded a number of prizes and medals for her exceptional work. She has attended and presented papers in international conferences in Croatia, Brazil, Canada, USA, Japan, Switzerland, and other countries.

Contributors

Alka Agrawal
Department of Information Technology,
   Babasaheb Bhimrao Ambedkar University,
   Lucknow, India

Masood Ahmad
Department of Information Technology,
   Babasaheb Bhimrao Ambedkar University,
   Lucknow, India

Aitizaz Ahsan
Department of Zoology, Panjab University,
   Chandigarh, India

Sneha Anand
Department of Pharmaceutical Sciences,
   Babasaheb Bhimrao Ambedkar University,
   Lucknow, India

Kumari Anupam
Department of Biochemistry, Panjab University,
   Chandigarh, India

Dilip Kumar Arya
Department of Pharmaceutical Sciences,
   Babasaheb Bhimrao Ambedkar University,
   Lucknow, India

Reena Badhwar
Delhi Pharmaceutical Science and Research
   University, New Delhi, India

Savita Bains
Department of Biotechnology, Panjab University,
   Chandigarh, India

Vijay Bhalla
Shree Guru Gobind Singh Tricentenary
   University, Gurugram, India

A.J.S. Bhanwer
Department of Human Genetics, Guru Nanak Dev
   University, Amritsar, India

Shiv Bharadwaj
Department of Biotechnology,
   Yeungnam University, College of Life
   and Applied Sciences, Gyeongsan-si,
   Republic of Korea

Meena Bharti
School of Life and Environmental Sciences,
   Deakin University, Warrnambool, Australia

Meghali Bharti
Department of Zoology, University of Delhi,
   Delhi, India

Archana Bhatnagar
Department of Biochemistry, Panjab University,
   Chandigarh, India

Jagat Bhushan
Department of Conservative Dentistry and
   Endodontics, Dr. Harvansh Singh Judge
   Institute of Dental Sciences, Panjab University,
   Chandigarh, India

Harpal S. Buttar
Department of Pathology and Laboratory
   Medicine, University of Ottawa,
   Ottawa, Canada

Ekta Chaudhary
Department of Biochemistry, Panjab University,
   Chandigarh, India

Ganga Ram Chaudhary
Department of Chemistry and Centre of Advanced
   Studies in Chemistry, Panjab University,
   Chandigarh, India

Kratika Chauhan
Department of Conservative Dentistry and
   Endodontics, Dr. Harvansh Singh Judge
   Institute of Dental Sciences, Panjab University,
   Chandigarh, India

Mani Chopra
Department of Zoology, Panjab University,
  Chandigarh, India

Yashodhara Dalal
School of Pharmacy and Technology
  Management, SVKM's NMIMS,
  Mumbai, India

Jagdeep S. Deep
IISER Mohali, India

Payal Deepak
Department of Pharmaceutical Sciences,
  Babasaheb Bhimrao Ambedkar University,
  Lucknow, India

Preeti Garg
Department of Chemistry and Centre of
  Advanced Studies in Chemistry, Panjab
  University, Chandigarh, India

Shreya Ghosh
Indian Institute of Technology, Kanpur, India

Sunil Babu Gosipatala
Department of Biotechnology, Babasaheb
  Bhimrao Ambedkar University,
  Lucknow, India

Mostafa Gouda
Department of Nutrition and Food Science,
  National Research Centre, Giza, Egypt

Parul Chawla Gupta
Department of Opthalmology, Post Graduate
  Institute of Medical and Research,
  Chandigarh, India

Hema
Department of Biotechnology, Babasaheb
  Bhimrao Ambedkar University,
  Lucknow, India

Laila Hussein
Department of Nutrition and Food Science,
  National Research Centre, Giza, Egypt

Shweta Jaiswal
Department of Pharmaceutical Sciences,
  Babasaheb Bhimrao Ambedkar University,
  Lucknow, India

Priya Joon
University Institute of Pharmaceutical Sciences,
  Panjab University, Chandigarh, India

Swaty Jhamb
H S Judge Institute of Dental Sciences,
  Panjab University, Chandigarh, India

Jyoti Joshi
Department of Zoology, Panjab University,
  Chandigarh, India

Deepak Jugran
Department of Ophthalmology, Post Graduate
  Institute of Medical Education and Research,
  Chandigarh, India

Gurpreet Kaur
Department of Chemistry and Centre of Advanced
  Studies in Chemistry, Panjab University,
  Chandigarh, India

Harjot Kaur
Department of Zoology, Panjab University,
  Chandigarh, India

Ravneet Kaur
Department of Biotechnology, Panjab University,
  Chandigarh, India

Rupinder Kaur
Department of Zoology, Panjab University,
  Chandigarh, India

Sukhbir Kaur
Department of Zoology, Panjab University,
  Chandigarh, India

Surjeet Kaur
IISER Mohali, India

Tajpreet Kaur
Department of Pharmaceutics, Khalsa College of
  Pharmacy, Amritsar, India

Jyotsana Kaushal
Department of Biochemistry, Panjab University,
  Chandigarh, India

Raj Kumar Khalko
Department of Biotechnology, Babasaheb
  Bhimrao Ambedkar University, Lucknow, India

Raees Ahmad Khan
Department of Information Technology,
Babasaheb Bhimrao Ambedkar University,
Lucknow, India

Sahil Khan
Shobhaben Pratapbhai Patel School of Pharmacy
and Technology Management, SVKM's
NMIMS, Mumbai, India

Dibbendhu Khanra
Indian Institute of Technology Kanpur, India

Himani Khurana
Department of Zoology, University of Delhi,
Delhi, India

Sanchita Khurana
Department of Zoology, Panjab University,
Chandigarh, India

Surbhi Khurana
Department of Ophthalmology, Post Graduate
Institute of Medical Education and Research,
Chandigarh, India

Nikhil Kirtipal
Department of Science, MIT, Rishikesh, India

Shweta Kishen
Department of Biochemistry, Panjab University,
Chandigarh, India

Bharti Kotarya
Department of Biotechnology, School of Life
Sciences, Babasaheb Bhimrao Ambedkar
University, Lucknow, India

Anil Kumar
University Institute of Pharmaceutical Sciences
(UIPS), Panjab University, Chandigarh, India

Maushmi S. Kumar
School of Pharmacy and Technology
Management, SVKM's NMIMS,
Mumbai, India

Rajeev Kumar
Department of Computer Applications,
Shri Ramswaroop Memorial University,
Barabanki, India

Ravinder Kumar
Department of Zoology, Panjab University,
Chandigarh, India

Surendra Kumar
Department of Biotechnology, Babasaheb
Bhimrao Ambedkar University, Lucknow, India

Vijay Kumar
Department of Zoology, Panjab University,
Chandigarh, India

Vikas Kushwaha
Department of Biotechnology, Panjab University,
Chandigarh, India

Rajni Lasyal
Department of Science, MIT, Rishikesh, India

Zosia Maciorowski
University of France, Paris, France

Samir Mehndiratta
Faculty of Engineering and Information
Technology, University of Technology Sydney,
Sydney, NSW, Australia
Department of Pathology, Faculty of Medicine,
Dalhousie University, Halifax, Nova Scotia,
Canada

Sweety Mehra
Department of Zoology, Panjab University,
Chandigarh, India

Avshesh Mishra
Department of Biotechnology, Babasaheb
Bhimrao Ambedkar University, Lucknow, India

Nidhi Mishra
Department of Pharmaceutical Sciences,
Babasaheb Bhimrao Ambedkar University,
Lucknow, India

Balraj Mittal
Department of Biotechnology, Babasaheb
Bhimrao Ambedkar University, Lucknow, India

Rama Mittal
Department of Biotechnology, Babasaheb
Bhimrao Ambedkar University,
Lucknow, India

Sonakshi Modeel
Department of Zoology, University of Delhi,
Delhi, India

Harsh Nayyar
Department of Botany, Panjab University,
Chandigarh, India

Ram Krishan Negi
Department of Zoology, University of Delhi,
Delhi, India

Tarana Negi
Department of Zoology, Government College,
Bahadurgarh, India

Raquibun Nisha
Department of Pharmaceutical Sciences,
Babasaheb Bhimrao Ambedkar University,
Lucknow, India

Alka Pal
Department of Pharmaceutical Sciences,
Babasaheb Bhimrao Ambedkar University,
Lucknow, India

Prashant Pandey
Department of Pharmaceutical Sciences,
Babasaheb Bhimrao Ambedkar University,
Lucknow, India

Abhishek Pandeya
Department of Biotechnology, Babasaheb
Bhimrao Ambedkar University,
Lucknow, India

Milind Parle
Department of Pharmaceutical Sciences, Guru
Jambheshwar University of Science and
Technology, Hisar (Haryana), India

Davinder Parsad
Department of Dermatology, PGIMER,
Chandigarh, India

Naveed Pervaiz
Department of Zoology, Panjab University,
Chandigarh, India

Harvinder Popli
Delhi Pharmaceutical Science and Research
University, New Delhi, India

Anand Prakash
M G Central University, Motihari, India

Mukesh Prasad
Faculty of Engineering and Information
Technology, University of Technology Sydney,
Sydney, NSW, Australia

Manu Priya
Department of Botany, Panjab University,
Chandigarh, India

Deepak K. Rahi
Department of Biochemistry Panjab University,
Chandigarh, India

Sonu Rahi
Department of Biochemistry Panjab University,
Chandigarh, India

Ekta Rai
School of Biotechnology, Shri Mata Vaishno Devi
University, Katra, India

Seemha Rai
Centre for Stem Cell and Tissue Engineering,
Panjab University, Chandigarh, India

Priyanka Raina
Integrative Genomics of Ageing Group,
Institute of Ageing and Chronic Disease,
University of Liverpool, Liverpool, UK

Ravi Raj
Department of Pharmaceutical Sciences,
Babasaheb Bhimrao Ambedkar University,
Lucknow, India

P.S. Rajinikanth
Department of Pharmaceutical Sciences,
Babasaheb Bhimrao Ambedkar University,
Lucknow, India

Jagat Ram
Department of Ophthalmology, Post Graduate
Institute of Medical and Research,
Chandigarh, India

Sudipta Saha
Department of Pharmaceutical Sciences,
Babasaheb Bhimrao Ambedkar University,
Lucknow, India

Dipti Sareen
Department of Biochemistry, Panjab University,
  Chandigarh, India

Vijay Laxmi Saxena
Department of Zoology, D.G. (P.G.) College
  Kanpur, India

Era Seth
Department of Zoology, Panjab University,
  Chandigarh, India

Ankita Sethia
Department of Zoology, D.G. (P.G.) College
  Kanpur, India

Anuradha Sharma
Department of Zoology, Panjab University,
  Chandigarh, India

Ashwani Kumar Sharma
Department of Zoology, D.G. (P.G.) College
  Kanpur, India

Indu Sharma
Department of Zoology Panjab University,
  Chandigarh, India

Monika Sharma
Department of Zoology, University of Delhi,
  Delhi, India

Reena Sharma
Brookhaven National Laboratory, Department of
  Biology, Upton, NY, USA

Sukesh Chander Sharma
Department of Biochemistry, Panjab University,
  Chandigarh, India

Swarkar Sharma
School of Biotechnology, Shri Mata Vaishno
  Devi University, Katra, India

Saraf Shubhini
Department of Pharmaceutical Sciences,
  Babasaheb Bhimrao Ambedkar University,
  Lucknow, India

Pragya Shukla
Centre for Stem Cell and Tissue Engineering,
  Panjab University, Chandigarh, India

Sukhjeet Sidhu
IISER Mohali, India

Amrit Pal Singh
Department of Pharmacology, Khalsa
  College of Pharmacy, Amritsar, India

Balbir Singh
Department of Pharmacology, Khalsa
  College of Pharmacy, Amritsar, India

Gurvinder Singh
Department of Human Genetics, Guru Nanak Dev
  University, Amritsar, India

Kashmir Singh
Department of Biotechnology, Panjab University,
  Chandigarh, India

Mangal Singh
Department of Biochemistry, Panjab University,
  Chandigarh, India

Neelu Singh
Department of Pharmaceutical Sciences,
  Babasaheb Bhimrao Ambedkar University,
  Lucknow, India

Priya Singh
Department of Pharmaceutical Sciences,
  Babasaheb Bhimrao Ambedkar University,
  Lucknow, India

Ruchi Singla
Department of Conservative Dentistry and
  Endodontics, Dr. Harvansh Singh Judge
  Institute of Dental Sciences, Panjab University,
  Chandigarh, India

Aastha Sobti
Department of Immunogenetics, Lund
  University, Sweden

R.C. Sobti
Department of Biotechnology, Panjab University,
  Chandigarh, India

Anshika Srivastava
Department of Biotechnology, Babasaheb
  Bhimrao Ambedkar University,
  Lucknow, India

Swati Srivastava
Department of Bioscience, Integral University,
  Lucknow, India

Ankit Tandon
Department of Biochemistry, Panjab University,
  Chandigarh, India

Istvan G. Telessy
Department of Pathology and Laboratory
  Medicine, University of Ottawa,
  Ottawa, Canada

William Telford
NCI Flow Cytometry Core Laboratory, National
  Cancer Institute, National Institutes of Health,
  Washington, USA

Ashwani Kumar Thakur
Indian Institute of Technology Kanpur,
  Kanpur, India

Sunita Thakur
Department of Pharmaceutical Sciences,
  Babasaheb Bhimrao Ambedkar University,
  Lucknow, India

Vasundhara Thakur
Department of Biotechnology, Panjab University,
  Chandigarh, India

Yogesh Thapen
Department of Zoology, Panjab University,
  Chandigarh, India

Sukanya Tripathy
M G Central University, Motihari, India

Douglas W. Wilson
School of Medicine, Pharmacy
  and Health, Durham University,
  Durham, UK
College of Biosystems Engineering
  and Food Science, Zhejiang University,
  China

Jitendra Kumar Yadav
Department of Biotechnology, Babasaheb
  Bhimrao Ambedkar University,
  Lucknow, India

Section I

Advancement in Techniques in Biomedical Science

1

Recent Advancements in Biomedical Sciences and Their Healthcare Applications

Reena Sharma
Brookhaven National Laboratory, Department of Biology, Upton, NY, USA

Mukesh Prasad
Faculty of Engineering and Information Technology, University of Technology Sydney, Sydney, NSW, Australia

Samir Mehndiratta
Faculty of Engineering and Information Technology, University of Technology Sydney, Sydney, NSW, Australia
Department of Pathology, Faculty of Medicine, Dalhousie University, Halifax, Nova Scotia, Canada

1.1 Introduction

The significant transformation in biomedical, public health, and healthcare system approaches has been recognized by multiple organizations. There is an overwhelming requirement for the integration between informatics, artificial intelligence, and machine learning and biomedical research to improve the public health conditions (Mak and Pichika, 2019).

Recent developments in biomedical science come from the significant advances in artificial intelligence (AI), machine learning (ML), cloud computing, and high performance computing resources for AI. These developments have transformed the conduct of large-and small-scale biological and biomedical research in rather dramatic ways (Mitra, 2019).

AI is a system capable of perceiving and understanding its surroundings and taking appropriate action to maximize its chances of achieving its goals. AI has a significant influence on genetics, biotechnology, and medicine in general, and can be applied in real-world applications using techniques such as machine learning, neural computing, genetic algorithms, etc. Artificial Intelligence Applications in Biomedicine (AIAB) brings together five cutting-edge research approaches on machine learning methodologies: AI support systems for patient tracking, genetic algorithms, optimization techniques, and semantics (Chan, Shan et al., 2019). AI assists in problem solving by learning and analyzing in a similar fashion to humans. ML is another term for artificial intelligence.

The most pressing need for AI and ML in biomedical science is in disease diagnosis, elucidating signaling pathways and understanding gene editing technologies. In this area, there have been a number of notable breakthroughs. AI enables doctors to have earlier and more precise diagnoses for a variety of diseases. Precise diagnosis is based on in vitro diagnostics using biosensors or biochips, which is one of the most common types of diagnosis (Gussow, Park et al., 2020). Gene expression study is an effective diagnostic method that can be analyzed using ML, which uses AI to interpret microarray or transcriptomic data to identify and diagnose abnormalities. In biomedical sciences ML can be used to enhance diagnosis and care.

The aim of this chapter is to detail recent scientific achievements, recognize technology availability, discuss the enormous potential of AI and ML in biomedicine, and provide inspiration to researchers in

DOI: 10.1201/9781003220404-2

related fields. It is fair to say that, like AI itself, AI's application in biomedicine is still in its infancy. New breakthroughs and improvements will continue to be made. In this chapter we present a vision for how AI and ML can transform three major areas of biomedical science – clinical diagnostics, precision therapies, and health monitoring – with the aim of maintaining health in the face of disease detection.

1.2 AI and ML in Disease Diagnostics and Prediction

With the emergence of modern AI and ML techniques, the practice of medicine is evolving. AI-based systems are now improving the precision and reliability of diagnosis and care across different specializations, thanks to rapid advances in computer processing. The most pressing need for AI in bio-medicine is in disease diagnosis. In this area, there have been a number of notable breakthroughs (Paul, Sanap et al., 2021). AI enables doctors to have earlier and more precise diagnoses for a variety of diseases. In addition to diagnosis, AI may aid in the prediction of cancer patient survival rates, such as for colon cancer patients (Vlamos et al., 2013). Researchers have also established some of ML's shortcomings in biomedical diagnosis, as well as measures to mitigate these disadvantages. As a result, AI in diagnostics and prognostics still has a lot of room to develop.

Years of medical training are required to correctly diagnose diseases. Even so, diagnostics can be a lengthy and time-consuming operation. The market for experts in many fields far outnumbers the available supply. This puts doctors under a lot of pressure, and it frequently causes life-saving patient diagnoses to be delayed. ML algorithms, especially deep learning algorithms, have recently made significant progress in automatically diagnosing diseases (Xue, Li et al., 2018).

1.3 AI in Drug Development

Drug development is a notoriously costly operation. ML can improve the efficiency of many of the analytical processes used in drug production. This will save years of work and hundreds of millions of dollars in investments. AI is involved in improving various stages of drug design (i.e., identifying action goals, potential drug candidates screening, clinical trials, and identification of biomarkers for early disease detection). Understanding the biological origins of a disease (signaling pathways) as well as its resistance mechanisms is the first step in drug production (Merk, Friedrich et al., 2018), followed by determining the target proteins to be analyzed and used to treat the disease. High-throughput methods, such as short hairpin RNA (shRNA) screening and deep sequencing, are now widely available.

The next step is to find a compound that has the desired interaction with the specified target molecule. This entails testing a large number of possible compounds – sometimes tens of thousands or even millions – for their effect on the target (affinity), as well as any off-target side effects (toxicity) (Zeng, Zhu et al., 2020). Actual, synthetic, or bioengineered compounds are all possibilities. ML can help speed up the design of clinical trials by automatically selecting appropriate candidates and ensuring that groups of trial participants are distributed correctly. Algorithms may assist in identifying patterns that distinguish one individual from another. Figure 1.1 represents some of the examples of AI and ML in drug discovery and development.

1.3.1 AI in Drug Design

During the process of development of a novel/new drug molecule, assigning the right target is important for a successful treatment outcome. Various proteins are involved in on-setting a disease when they are either downregulated or upregulated. Therefore, to selectively targetany particular disease, it is important to know the proteins involved and to accurately predict the 2D/3D structure of the target proteins to design a successful drug molecule (Zeng, Zhu et al., 2020). AI can play an important role by assisting in structure-based drug discovery to predict the effect of a drug molecule on the target protein and also the safety considerations before actually synthesizing drug molecules, thus saving time and cost. Table 1.1, illustrates some examples of the use of AI in effective drug design.

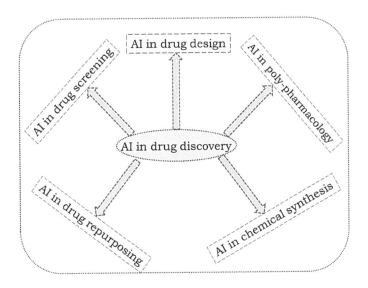

FIGURE 1.1 Roles of AI and ML in drug discovery and development.

TABLE 1.1

Illustrates Examples of Some Important Implementations of AI in Drug Design

Approach	Forecast
3D Target Protein Structure Prediction (Zeng, Zhu et al., 2020)	Used an AI-based tool, AlphaFoldto predict 3D target protein structure by analyzing distance between the adjacent amino acids and the corresponding angles of the peptide bonds
Recurrent Neural Network (AlQuraishi, 2019)	Used a recurrent neural network (RNN)-based approach to analyze 3D structure of proteins
Prediction of Secondary Protein Structure Using CB513 Database (Zikrija et al., 2009)	Used MATLAB to predict 2D structures of protein with 62.72% accuracy
Support Vector Machine (Sugaya, 2013)	Support Vector Machine (SVM) imply training based on ligand efficiency to improves prediction of bioactivities for drug target proteins
Random Rorest (RF) Models to Predict Possible Drug-Protein Interactions (Yu, Chen et al., 2012)	Integrated chemical and pharmacological data using two random forest (RF) models to predict possible drug-protein interactions and validate them for high sensitivity and specificity against known platforms, such as SVM. They were capable of predicting drug-target associations that could be used to determine associations between target-target and target-disease, thus speeding up the drug discovery process.

1.3.2 AI in Polypharmacology

The study of drug–protein interactions is helping researchers to see the potential of polypharmacology. Polypharmacology is the affinity of a drug molecule to interact with targets/receptors other than the desired target, thus displaying off-target adverse effects. AI and machine learning can help design new molecules based on the rationale of polypharmacology and thus can facilitate the development of drugs with better safety profile. Table 1.2 illustrates some examples of the use of AI in polypharmacology.

1.3.3 AI in Chemical Synthesis

These days, the traditional approach of *de novo* drug design is getting replaced by evolving deep learning (DL) methods. Traditional approaches generally have complicated synthesis routes and lack bioactivity

TABLE 1.2

Role of AI in Polypharmacology

Approach	Forecast
KinomeX & Deep Neural Networks (Li, Li et al., 2019)	An online medium based on AI, which uses deep neural networks (DNNs) for the detection of polypharmacology of kinases according to their chemical structures. KinomeX uses DNNs equipped with approximately 14,000 bioactivity data points developed based on more than 300 kinases and assist to study overall selectivity of a lead compound towards the kinase family and particular subfamilies of kinases (Li, Li et al., 2019). Studied NVP-BHG712 with reasonable accuracy in predicting its primary as well as off-targets.
Cyclica Launches Ligand Express™, a Disruptive Cloud-Based Platform to Revolutionize Drug Discovery (Paul, Sanap et al., 2021)	Cyclica's recently launched cloud-based proteome-screening AI platform, Ligand Express, is useful to find receptors that can interact with a particular small molecule to understandon and off-target interactions, thus helping to understand the possible adverse effects.

TABLE 1.3

Some Applications of AI in Drug Repurposing

Approach	Forecast
Cellular Network-Based Deep Learning Technology (Zeng, Zhu et al., 2020)	Used cellular network-based deep learning technology (deepDTnet) for predicting repurposing of topotecan, a topoisomerase inhibitor, as a treatment of multiple sclerosis by inhibiting human retinoic acid receptor-related orphan receptor-gamma t (ROR-γt)
Deep Neural Networks (Ke, Peng et al., 2020)	Used deep neural networks (DNN) to repurpose existing drugs with proven efficacy against SARS-CoV, influenza virus, HIV, and the drugs that can target 3C-like protease to fight COVID-19 pandemic.
	An octanol-water partition coefficient (ALogP_count), functional-class fingerprints (FCFPs), and extended connectivity fingerprint (ECFP) were considered to train the AI platform.
	As conclusion of this study, 13 of the screened drugs were reported for further development based on their cytotoxicity and viral inhibition

prediction of newly synthesized molecules (Vlamos et al., 2013). Computer-aided synthesis planning can generate many structures with optimal physio-chemical/biological properties that can be easily synthesized along with predicting several synthesis routes for them. Table 1.3 illustrates some examples of use of AI in *de novo* drug design.

1.3.4 AI in Drug Repurposing

Drug repurposing has emerged as a useful tool especially during the COVID 19 pandemic, which has underscored the efficacy of this method for finding new cures. Moreover, drug repurposing qualifies a drug directly for Phase II clinical trials (Mak and Pichika, 2019). It is also a cost-effective strategy since it significantly reduces expenditure of approximately US\$41.3 million on launching a new drug into market to approximately US\$8.4 million on drug relaunch (Zikrija et al., 2009). The 'guilt by association' approach is generally used to foresee the association between a drug and disease, which is either a knowledge-based or computationally driven network (Koromina, Pandi et al., 2019). Table 1.3 illustrates some examples of the use of AI-based drug repurposing.

1.3.5 AI in Drug Screening

AI in drug design plays an important role in terms of prediction of toxicity, prediction of bioactivity, prediction of physio-chemical properties, etc. AI has been successfully utilized by various researchers for effective drug screening (Vlamos et al., 2013). Moreover, many pharmaceutical companies such as Roche, Bayer, and Pfizer, etc., are working along with IT companies for the discovery of effective therapies in areas of cardiovascular diseases, mmune-oncology, etc. (Ke, Peng et al., 2020).

1.4 Conclusion

For years, there has been a lot of interest in learning more about our genetic makeup because genetics plays such a significant role in the illnesses people face during their lives. Our development was hampered by the complexity and scale of the data that needed to be analyzed. Artificial intelligence and machine learning applications have improved researchers' ability to interpret data.

Whole genome sequencing, for example, is a very costly process that requires complex lab equipment and specialized expertise. Biomarkers are compounds present in body fluids (typically human blood) that can determine whether a patient has a disease or not. They make diagnosing easier. A diagnostic biomarker detects the existence of a disease as soon as possible and indicates the likelihood of a patient contracting the disease. A prognostic biomarker indicates how likely a disease will progress and is a predictive biomarker for determining if a patient will react to a medication. Similarly, CRISPR (Clustered Regularly Interspaced Short Palindromic Repeats), specifically the CRISPR-Cas9 gene editing technique, is a huge step forward in our ability to edit DNA cheaply and precisely, like a surgeon. Short-guide RNAs (sgRNA) are used in this technique to target and modify a particular position on DNA. However, the guide RNA can match several DNA locations, which can lead to unintended consequences (Gussow, Park et al., 2020). All these processes are time consuming and still very costly with a lot of variability in results. This is where AI and machine learning are helping researchers.

Artificial intelligence and machine learning can help make gene editing more precise, less expensive, and simpler. Pharmacogenomics, genetic screening methods for newborns, agricultural improvements, and other applications of AI and gene technology are anticipated in the future.

REFERENCES

AlQuraishi, M. (2019). "End-to-End Differentiable Learning of Protein Structure." *Cell Syst* 8(4): 292–301 e293.

Chan, H. C. S. et al. (2019). "Advancing Drug Discovery via Artificial Intelligence." *Trends Pharmacol Sci* 40(8): 592–604.

Grzybowski, B. A. et al. (2018). "Chematica: A Story of Computer Code That Started to Think like a Chemist." *Chem* 4(3): 390–398.

Gussow, A. B. et al. (2020). "Machine-Learning Approach Expands the Repertoire of Anti-CRISPR Protein Families." *Nat Commun* 11(1): 3784.

Ke, Y. Y. et al. (2020). "Artificial Intelligence Approach Fighting COVID-19 with Repurposing Drugs." *Biomed J* 43(4): 355–362.

Koromina, M. et al. (2019). "Rethinking Drug Repositioning and Development with Artificial Intelligence, Machine Learning, and Omics." *OMICS* 23(11): 539–548.

Li, Z. et al. (2019). "KinomeX: A Web Application for Predicting Kinome-Wide Polypharmacology Effect of Small Molecules." *Bioinformatics* 35(24): 5354–5356.

Mak, K. K. and M. R. Pichika (2019). "Artificial Intelligence in Drug Development: Present Status and Future Prospects." *Drug Discov Today* 24(3): 773–780.

Merk, D. et al. (2018). "De Novo Design of Bioactive Small Molecules by Artificial Intelligence." *Mol Inform* 37(1–2).

Mitra, M. (2019). "Artificial Intelligence in Biomedical Science." *Advances in Bioengineering and Biomedical Science Research* 2(4).

Paul, D. et al. (2021). "Artificial Intelligence in Drug Discovery and Development." *Drug Discov Today* 26(1): 80–93.

Sugaya, N. (2013). "Training Based on Ligand Efficiency Improves Prediction of Bioactivities of Ligands and Drug Target Proteins in a Machine Learning Approach." *J Chem Inf Model* 53(10): 2525–2537.

Vlamos, P. et al. (2013). "Artificial Intelligence Applications in Biomedicine." *Advances in Artificial Intelligence* 2013: 1–2.

Xue, H. et al. (2018). "Review of Drug Repositioning Approaches and Resources." *Int J Biol Sci* 14(10): 1232–1244.

Yu, H. et al. (2012). "A Systematic Prediction of Multiple Drug-Target Interactions from Chemical, Genomic, and Pharmacological Data." *PLoS One* 7(5): e37608.

Zeng, X. et al. (2020). "Target Identification Among Known Drugs by Deep Learning from Heterogeneous Networks." *Chemical Science* 11(7): 1775–1797.

Zikrija A. et al. (2009). "Artificial Intelligence in Prediction of Secondary Protein Structure Using CB513 Database." *Summit on Translational Bioinformatics* 1–5.

2

Nanotechnology in Medicine: A Promising Future

Rajni Lasyal
Department of Chemistry, Rajkiya Mahavidyalaya, Chinyalisaur, India

Nikhil Kirtipal
Department of Science, Modern Institute of Technology, Rishikesh, India

R.C. Sobti
Department of Biotechnology, Panjab University, Chandigarh, India

2.1 Introduction

Nanotechnology is one of the most important emerging fields in medical sciences. In a broader sense, it is a field where the diverse fields of physics, chemistry, biology, materials science, and engineering converge at a scale ranging from 1 to 100 nanometers, essentially known as the nanoscale[1]. Nanotechnology is the science of understanding and controlling atoms and molecules at nanoscale using a procedure called nano-manufacturing. The art of nano-manufacturing has brought about a revolution in the field of biomedical engineering where the nano-materials and devices are designed to interact with the body at sub-cellular level [1]. A wide range of biomedical applications have been benefiting from nanotechnology, such as biosensors, drug and gene delivery, artificial cells, nanorobots for surgery, and many more. The most significant property of nanoparticles is the carbon strength, which is so tough that recently carbon nanotube bulletproof T-shirt/vests were manufactured.[2]

The medical application of nanotechnology is widely termed as nanomedicine. It ranges from medical applications of nanomaterials to nanoelectronics biosensors. The research and development of nanomedicine is broadly divided into three stages. The first impact of nanoscience on medicine is evolutionary. A second development is explicit and revolutionary, emphasizing great advances to be gained by radical new nanotechnology approaches. A third source of nanotechnology on medicine is indirect through the development and application of ever-improving nanotools and devices based on smaller and more precise technologies. These technologies impact research, diagnostics, and therapeutics.[1] Most of the nanotechnology applications in medicine are widespread. It starts with identification and validation and is extended up to the treatment.

2.2 Reviewing Nanotechnology in Biomedical Applications

Many medical nanotechnology applications are still in their infancy. However, an increasing number of products is currently under clinical investigation and some products are already commercially available, such as surgical blades and suture needles, contrast-enhancing agents for magnetic resonance imaging, bone replacement materials, wound dressings, anti-microbial textiles, chips for in vitro molecular diagnostics, microcantilevers, and microneedles.[3] Here are some of the key technologies and trending imapcts of medical nanotechnology.

DOI: 10.1201/9781003220404-3

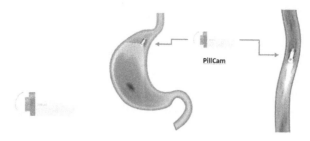

a. A PillCam   b. PillCam view inside the body in the stomach and colon

FIGURE 2.1   Pill cam view inside the body.[5]

The PillCam is ideal for use in the passageways of the gastrointestinal system since it can be swallowed.

2.2.1 PillCam

With the introduction of PillCam by "GIVEN IMAGING" in 2001, the first step towards application of nanotechnology in medicine was taken.[4] The PillCam is a capsule, ideally the size of a normal pill, that contains a light and camera that is swallowed by the patient (Figure 2.1).[5] Images beamed wirelessly from the capsule can be analyzed and used for diagnostic purposes, thus replacing procedures like the traditional endoscopy, in which a flexible tube containing a flashlight and camera is inserted into the digestive tract.

2.2.2 Drug Delivery

Since 1960, researchers have been developing drug delivery systems that can directly target the affected regions. Due to the small size of nanoparticles, they are proving to be suitable for such drug delivery systems. Based on the type of particle, the active nanoparticle ingredient can be encapsulated or attached to the surface. This means that even if they dissolve poorly in water, they can be transported in an aqueous solution, such as blood, and are better protected against degradation by enzymes (e.g., a suitable coating on the nanoparticle can prevent identification and removal by the immune system.[6] The nanoparticles Dendrimers (nano-sized, radially symmetric molecules) are commonly used for drug delivery system due to their well-defined size, shape, molecular weight, and monodispersity.[7] Although they are complicated to synthesize, the advantage of dendrimers is that their synthesis results in a single molecular weight rather than a distribution of sizes.[7]

2.2.3 Biomarkers

Nanoparticles can be used for both quantitative and qualitative in vitro detection of tumor cells. They enhance the detection process by concentrating and protecting a marker from degradation, in order to render the analysis more sensitive. The research results have shown that the fluorescent nanospheres provided a sensitivity of 25 times more than that of the conjugate streptavidin-fluorescein.[8] Many kinds of nanomaterials are used to help researchers develop prototype nanotechnology-based sensors for measurement of biomarkers. Materials like metal nanoparticles (gold, silver), semiconductor nanoparticles, and enzyme-loaded carbon nanotubes (CNTs) may be used to amplify biomarker signals.

2.2.4 Microbots

Microbots are extremely small devices that can work inside the human body to help fight diseases. One of the microbots being developed resembles the flagella – a spiral-shaped tail that helps bacterium to swim. These artificial bacterial flagella (ABFs) are about half the diameter of a human hair and are made using computer chip technology. These small robots are called nanobots, and are much smaller than bacteria. A magnetic head is attached to the ABF, so that, through a magnetic field, it can be made to rotate and move forward and backward. Once it is directed to a precise location, the robot can deliver medicine that destroys tumors.[7] In addition to cancer treatment, microbots are also being considered potentially useful for other medical purposes. Diabetes patients have to test their blood multiple times daily to ensure that their glucose levels are stable. Using nanobots would enable doctors to receive data from many different locations simultaneously throughout the body and allow for more continuous monitoring of blood sugar levels without the pain and inconvenience of selftesting.[7]

2.3 Cancer Detection and Treatment

The NCI Alliance for Nanotechnology in Cancer states notes that in the fight against cancer, half the battle is won by early detection. Nanotechnology research is contributing to improved cancer survival rates through advances in screening, diagnosis, monitoring, and treatment. In the traditional methods of chemotherapy, it was found that 99% of the time the drug did not reach the target cell. Nanotechnology has proved its efficiency in early detection of cancerous cells as well as treatment of cancer. Nanoparticles also carry the potential for targeted and time-release drugs. A potent dose of drugs could be delivered to a specific area but engineered to release over a planned period to ensure maximum effectiveness and the patient's safety. These treatments aim to take advantage of the power of nanotechnology and the voracious tendencies of cancer cells, which feast on everything in sight, including drug-laden nanoparticles. One experiment of this type used modified bacteria cells that were 20% the size of normal cells. These cells were equipped with antibodies that latched onto cancer cells before releasing the anticancer drugs they contained. Another use of nanoparticles is as a companion to other treatments. These particles were sucked up by cancer cells and the cells were then heated with a magnetic field to weaken them. The weakened cancer cells were then much more susceptible to chemotherapy.[7]

2.3.1 Multiplexing and Immunoassays

Highlighting the issue of inter-and intra-tumor heterogeneity, many single-cell analysis techniques, such as cell-based, nucleic acid-based, protein-based, metabolite-based, and lipid-based, emerged over the last decade as an important approach to detecting variations in morphology, genetic or proteomic expression within the tumor niche.[9] The demand for parallel, multiplex analysis of protein biomarkers from very small biospecimens obtained at time of surgery, or through blood/CSF samples during follow-up, represented for years an increasing trend, mostly aimed at creating spatially encoded microarrays able to capture multiple proteins of interest in a cell lysate all at once.[10] For instance, in one of the articles identified by this systematic review, the gene expression levels of NANOG, a key regulator of pluripotency, and therefore a marker of stem cell-like behavior, was quantitatively tested along with other proteins (i.e., SOX2, OCT4, KLF4, ABCG2, CMYC, MSI1, CD44, NOTCH1, NES, SALL4B, TP53, and EPAS1) using Real Time-quantitative PCR (RT-qPCR) in 33 surgical specimens of low-(WHO grade I) as well as in high-grade (WHO grade II/III) meningiomas.[11] Additionally, immunofluorescence co-localization analysis following confocal fluorescence microscopy for NANOG, OCT4, SOX2, Nestin, KI-67, and CD44 was also performed. These techniques made it possible to support the research theory that overexpression of NANOG and other markers of pluripotency and stemness in meningiomas, such as SOX2 and OCT4, could be exploited to target potentially pluripotent "stem cell-like" cells.[11] Those NANOG-positive cells seem to be only 1% in low-grade, and 2% in grade II/III meningiomas; nonetheless, in this study and in other literature, they have demonstrated their remarkable impact on tumorigenesis and progression in human meningiomas and high-grade gliomas, being correlated with the overall clinical and surgical prognosis.[11,12,13,14]

2.4 Extracellular Cancer Biomarkers

2.4.1 Detection by mRNA and microRNA

microRNAs are involved in the crucial processes of development and diseases and have emerged as a new class of biomarkers in cancer diagnosis. A two-step sensing platform for sensitive detection of miR-141, a promising biomarker for prostate cancer, has been reported by Jou AF. The first step of the sensing platform used CdSe/ZnS quantum dots (QDs) modified with FRET quencher-functionalized nucleic acids, which contain a telomerase primer sequence together with a recognition sequence for the miR-141 recognition sequence. The FRET quencher exhibited covalent binding to the nucleic acid-functionalized CdSe/ZnS QDs. When miR-141 hybridized with the probe, a duplex was formed, which would be cleaved by duplex-specific nuclease (DSN). The cleavage released the quencher unit and activated the fluorescence of the QDs. This cleavage also led to exposure of the telomerase primer sequence. The next step involved the primer unit elongation stimulated by telomerase/dNTPs, incorporation of hemin, and chemiluminescence generated with the help of luminol/H_2O_2. This platform was helpful in detecting miR-141 in a serum sample and discriminated healthy individuals from prostate cancer carriers.[15,16]

Meanwhile, researchers have developed nanoflares for simultaneous intracellular detection of various mRNA transcripts. In these multiplexed nanoflare studies, AuNPs functionalized with 2–3 DNA recognition strands and later hybridized with short complementary reporter strands were generated as nanoflares. For example, the use of multiplexed nanoflares to detect survivin in addition to actin has been investigated for normalizing nanoflare fluorescence differences in cellular uptake. Therefore, the technique is comparable with conventional qRT-PCR for quantification of intracellular mRNA but can be performed at the single live cell level.

In some cases, the nanoflare platform was expanded to quantify intracellular RNA and detect spatiotemporal localization in living cells.[17]

2.4.2 DNA Methylation Detection

The genome methylation landscape (Methylscape) was recently reported as a common characteristic of most types and cancers and therefore could be a common cancer biomarker.[18] In this study, the authors observed differences between cancer genomes and normal genomes based on DNA-gold affinity and DNA solvation and developed simple, quick, selective, and sensitive electrochemical or colorimetric one-step assays to detect cancer.[15]

2.5 Nanotechnology for In Vivo Imaging

In addition to cancer diagnosis through ex vivo detection of cancer cells and biomarkers in liquid biopsy samples, identifying cancerous tissues in the body has many advantages in diagnosing and treating cancer. A proper nanoparticle probe for detecting cancer tissue should exhibit a long circulation time, be specific to tumor tissue, and present low toxicity to nearby healthy tissue.[19] Current related studies have focused on nanoparticle probe accumulation in tumor tissue for diagnosing cancer in animal models, generally mouse models.

Nanoparticle probes can preferentially accumulate in tumor tissues through active or positive targeting, thereby allowing imaging and diagnosis of cancer in vivo.[20] Interactions between nanoparticles and blood proteins, uptake, and clearance by the reticuloendothelial system (RES), penetration into solid tumors, and optimized active (vs. passive) targeting for diagnosis of cancer constitute the main clinical application barriers. Fortunately, many developments related to these aspects have been achieved.

2.5.1 Challenges in Clinical Translation

Although there has been much promising progress in nanotechnology-based cancer diagnosis, only a few examples have advanced to clinical trials.[21] There are a number of factors that can impose significant obstacles to their clinical translation, irrespective of whether they are therapeutically beneficial or not. Therefore, to accelerate the translation of nanotechnology into clinical applications, many challenges need to be addressed. Reliability is the first challenge in nanotechnology-based cancer diagnosis. It is essential to obtain reliable and quantitative detection results for clinical application. There are many factors that can affect NP-based detection signals, including nonspecific binding of NP probes, aggregation, and unfit detection conditions.[22] Fluctuations in the signals can also be attributed to complicated body fluid compositions. From a clinical validation perspective, assay reliability and reproducibility need to be extensively investigated in large clinical sample pools before NP-based assays can reach the clinical application.

The large-scale production of nanoprobes that are highly sensitive, highly reproducible, and have long-term storage stability at an acceptable cost is one of the key challenges in this field.[23] The production of most of the current nanoprobes is performed under highly optimized conditions in laboratories; however, it is still a big challenge to produce these probes in batches. Because of variation in the shape, size, composition, charge, and surface coating of nanoprobes, the variation is also observed in the detection results.

The production of most of the current nanoprobes is performed under highly optimized conditions in labs; however, it is still a big challenge to produce these probes in batches.[15]

The third challenge is to develop NP-based devices with high sensitivity and that are easy to handle and cost-efficient. Most NP-based assays are prepared in academic laboratories, and many assays are unrealistic for clinical translation. For example, complicated confocal Raman microscopes were used to implement most studies based on SERS but are rarely present in hospitals or clinical laboratories. Successful development of NP-based POC (point-of-care) devices will greatly facilitate clinical application of nanotechnology in cancer diagnosis.[15]

The possible toxicity of nanoparticles induced by their systemic administration is the fourth and one of the major concerns faced by medical nanotechnology. This challenge is mostly related to NP-based imaging in vivo. For the application of novel nanoparticle probes to in vivo imaging, the possible toxicity of these nanoparticles should be assessed. The properties of nanoparticles (such as shape, size, charge, surface chemistry, targeting ligands, and composition) can also influence their toxicity. One should also account the biodistribution, biodegradability, and pharmacokinetic properties of nanoparticles for better results.[15]

2.6 Discussion

The field of biomedical nanotechnology is a boon since extremely small devices such as the nanobots or the PillCam can be created to help and cure people faster and without the side effects of traditional drugs. Traditional drugs have a drawback that they dissolve poorly in water; however, the drugs developed with the help of nanotechnology have the ability to transport easily in an aqueous solution, such as blood. You will also find that the research of nanotechnology in medicine is now focusing on areas like tissue regeneration, bone repair, immunity, and even cures for such ailments like cancer, diabetes, and other life-threatening diseases. Although today nanotechnology is a fast growing field, there are some challenges associated with using nanotechnology in biomedical engineering that need to be taken care of. Since these particles are very small, problems can actually arise from the inhalation of these minute particles, much like the problems associated with inhaling minute asbestos particles.[24,25] If we change the structure of material on the nanolevel without understanding the potential impact on the nanoscale, we risk creating a whole world of materials that have atoms that actually do not fit together cohesively.[24] Presently, nanotechnology is very expensive and developing it can cost a lot of money. It is also pretty difficult to manufacture, which is probably why products made with nanotechnology are more expensive.[24,25]

2.7 Conclusion

No doubt, nanotechnology in medicine holds promising potential in improving the diagnosis and treatment of a wide variety of diseases. The use of nanotechnology in the field of medicine could revolutionize the way we detect and treat damage to the human body and disease in the future, and many techniques that were only imagined a few years ago are making remarkable progress towards becoming realities. We can now conclude that with such a wide range of applications, nanotechnology in medicine does have an endless scope. However, with its limitations, this technology should be tested on more realistic grounds to obtain better and safe results. Thus, it is required to go for a situational approach while assessing the pros and cons of using nanoparticles for medical diagnosis as well as treatment.

REFERENCES

1. Kalangutkar, P. K. In *The Evolution of Nanomedicine with the Re-Evolution of Nanotechnology*, 2014.
2. Singh, S., Nanostructures: Enhancing Potential Applications in Biomedicals. *Journal of Biomaterials and Nanobiotechnology* 2013, *04*, 12–16.
3. Roszek, B.; De Jong, W. H.; Geertsma, R. E., Nanotechnology in medical applications: state-of-the-art in materials and devices. 2005.
4. Internet resource, Microbots using nanotechnology in medicine. *YaleScientific* 2013.
5. Suresh, C.; Vidhya, V.; Shamli, E.; Muthulakshmi, R.; Mahalakshmi, P., PILL Camera. *International Journal of Engineering Trends and Applications (IJETA)* 2016, *3* (1), 1–10.
6. Mohanraj, V. J.; Chen, Y., Nanoparticles-a review. *Tropical journal of pharmaceutical research* 2006, *5* (1), 561–573.
7. Kalangutkar, P. K., Nanotechnology – advancing the field of biomedical engineering. *International Journal of Current Research and Review* 2015, *7* (9), 66.
8. Ernest, H.; Shetty, R., Impact of Nanotechnology on Biomedical Sciences: Review of Current Concepts on Convergence of Nanotechnology With Biology. *AZojono* 2005, *1*.
9. Ganau, L.; Paris, M.; Ligarotti, G. K.; Ganau, M., Management of gliomas: overview of the latest technological advancements and related behavioral drawbacks. *Behavioural neurology* 2015, *2015*.
10. Ganau, M.; Bosco, A.; Palma, A.; Corvaglia, S.; Parisse, P.; Fruk, L.; Beltrami, A. P.; Cesselli, D.; Casalis, L.; Scoles, G., A DNA-based nano-immunoassay for the label-free detection of glial fibrillary acidic protein in multicell lysates. *Nanomedicine: Nanotechnology, Biology and Medicine* 2015, *11* (2), 293–300.
11. Freitag, D.; McLean, A. L.; Simon, M.; Koch, A.; Grube, S.; Walter, J.; Kalff, R.; Ewald, C., NANOG overexpression and its correlation with stem cell and differentiation markers in meningiomas of different WHO grades. *Molecular carcinogenesis* 2017, *56* (8), 1953–1964.
12. Ben-Porath, I.; Thomson, M. W.; Carey, V. J.; Ge, R.; Bell, G. W.; Regev, A.; Weinberg, R. A., An embryonic stem cell–like gene expression signature in poorly differentiated aggressive human tumors. *Nature genetics* 2008, *40* (5), 499–507.
13. Niu, C.-S.; Li, D.-X.; Liu, Y.-H.; Fu, X.-M.; Tang, S.-F.; Li, J., Expression of NANOG in human gliomas and its relationship with undifferentiated glioma cells. *Oncology reports* 2011, *26* (3), 593–601.
14. Soni, P.; Qayoom, S.; Husain, N.; Kumar, P.; Chandra, A.; Ojha, B. K.; Gupta, R. K., CD24 and nanog expression in stem cells in glioblastoma: correlation with response to chemoradiation and overall survival. *Asian Pacific journal of cancer prevention: APJCP* 2017, *18* (8), 2215.
15. Zhang, Y.; Li, M.; Gao, X.; Chen, Y.; Liu, T., Nanotechnology in cancer diagnosis: progress, challenges and opportunities. *Journal of Hematology & Oncology* 2019, *12* (1), 137.
16. Jou, A. F.-j.; Lu, C.-H.; Ou, Y.-C.; Wang, S.-S.; Hsu, S.-L.; Willner, I.; Ho, J.-a. A., Diagnosing the miR-141 prostate cancer biomarker using nucleic acid-functionalized CdSe/ZnS QDs and telomerase. *Chemical science* 2015, *6* (1), 659–665.
17. Briley, W. E.; Bondy, M. H.; Randeria, P. S.; Dupper, T. J.; Mirkin, C. A., Quantification and real-time tracking of RNA in live cells using Sticky-flares. *Proceedings of the National Academy of Sciences* 2015, *112* (31), 9591–9595.
18. Sina, A. A. I.; Carrascosa, L. G.; Liang, Z.; Grewal, Y. S.; Wardiana, A.; Shiddiky, M. J. A.; Gardiner, R. A.; Samaratunga, H.; Gandhi, M. K.; Scott, R. J., Epigenetically reprogrammed methylation landscape drives the DNA self-assembly and serves as a universal cancer biomarker. *Nature communications* 2018, *9* (1), 1–13.
19. Chinen, A. B.; Guan, C. M.; Ferrer, J. R.; Barnaby, S. N.; Merkel, T. J.; Mirkin, C. A., Nanoparticle probes for the detection of cancer biomarkers, cells, and tissues by fluorescence. *Chemical reviews* 2015, *115* (19), 10530–10574.

20. Bertrand, N.; Wu, J.; Xu, X.; Kamaly, N.; Farokhzad, O. C., Cancer nanotechnology: the impact of passive and active targeting in the era of modern cancer biology. *Advanced drug delivery reviews* 2014, *66*, 2–25.

21. Muthu, M. S.; Leong, D. T.; Mei, L.; Feng, S.-S., Nanotheranostics- application and further development of nanomedicine strategies for advanced theranostics. *Theranostics* 2014, *4* (6), 660.

22. Lin, Y.-W.; Huang, C.-C.; Chang, H.-T., Gold nanoparticle probes for the detection of mercury, lead and copper ions. *Analyst* 2011, *136* (5), 863–871.

23. Kim, H.-M.; Jeong, S.; Hahm, E.; Kim, J.; Cha, M. G.; Kim, K.-M.; Kang, H.; Kyeong, S.; Pham, X.-H.; Lee, Y.-S., Large scale synthesis of surface-enhanced Raman scattering nanoprobes with high reproducibility and long-term stability. *Journal of Industrial and Engineering Chemistry* 2016, *33*, 22–27.

24. Internet resource, Advantages and disadvantages of nanotechnology. https://nanogloss.com/nanotechnology/advantages-and-disadvantages-of-nanotechnology

25. Tonk, R., The science and technology of using nano-materials in engine oil as a lubricant additives. *Materials Today: Proceedings* 2021, *37*, 3475–3479.

3

How Flow Cytometers Work: An Introduction for Biomedical Scientists

William Telford
NCI Flow Cytometry Core Laboratory, National Cancer Institute, National Institutes of Health, Bethesda, MD, USA

3.1 Introduction

Flow cytometers employ sophisticated fluidic control, lasers, sensitive detectors, optics, electronics, and software to analyze individual cells prepared in a single-cell suspension. The basic elements of a flow cytometer are shown in Figure 3.1a. Cells prepared as a single-cell suspension are injected in a liquid stream (cell or core stream) into the path of a light source, almost always a laser on modern instrumentation. The cell stream for cell injection is hydrodynamically focused within an outer sheath stream to generate a narrow fluid path, allowing single-cell analysis within the stream. One or more lasers intercept the stream. Laser light scattered by the cells is detected in detectors opposite and at angles to the laser source and provide information about cell size and optical density. The lasers also excite fluorescent markers that have been incorporated into the cells. These markers can be tagged to antibodies directed against extracellular or intracellular protein targets. Fluorescent markers can also label cellular structures (such as DNA) or detect physiological states in cells such as plasma membrane or mitochondrial electrical potential among many others. Both light scattering and fluorescence is detected using sensitive light detectors, usually photomultiplier tubes (PMTs) or photodiodes (PDs). Coated optics including bandpass filters and dichroic mirrors are used to separate different wavelengths of the fluorescent markers prior to reaching the detectors, allowing multiple fluorescent probe emission wavelengths to be detected simultaneously (Melamed et al., 1990). The resulting signals are processed using preamplifiers and amplifiers and digitized using analog-to-digital conversion electronics. Data for all collected scatter and fluorescence parameters is then displayed as single or multi-dimensional plots on computer using specialized analytical software (Shapiro, 2003). These elements are visible in the interior of the flow cytometer shown in Figure 3.1b (an ACEA Biosciences/Agilent NovoCyte™, a typical commercial instrument).

The key feature that distinguishes flow cytometry from other techniques is its ability to perform rapid analysis of many parameters in large numbers of individual cells. All analyzed parameter data is correlated, allowing many subpopulations (often rare) to be characterized in complex cell populations. In this chapter, we will "walk through" the operation of a flow cytometer and focus on each step in the process from initial cell delivery to final analysis.

3.2 Instrument Fluidics

3.2.1 Flow Cells and Hydrodynamic Focusing

Flow cytometric analysis needs to start with a single-cell suspension, since each cell will be "interrogated" by the cytometer individually. Immune cells from blood and solid immune organs can be readily prepared in single-cell suspension; however, many cell types including solid tissues and tumors have been analyzed by flow cytometry using mechanical and enzymatic disaggregation and filtering to remove aggregates and producing a single-cell suspension.

DOI: 10.1201/9781003220404-4

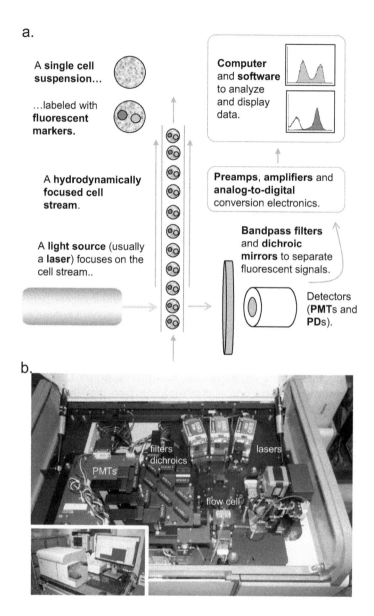

FIGURE 3.1 *a,* basic elements of a flow cytometer. *b,* interior of a representative flow cytometer with multiple laser and photomultiplier tube (PMT) detectors (ACEA Biosciences NovoCyte, Agilent/ACEA Biosciences San Diego, CA USA).

The cells are then injected into a quartz flow cell, with a narrow square or rectangular capillary (typically ~200 microns in width) aligned to a laser source. This sample injection an be achieved using air pressure, a syringe pump, or a peristaltic pump. However, simply injecting the cells into the capillary will not generate the highly focused cell stream required for accurate cell analysis; the cells will flow through the entire capillary and not be confined to a narrow path. Flow cytometers almost always employ hydrodynamic focusing to generate a single-cell stream. In hydrodynamic focusing, the cells are injected into an outer cylinder of moving liquid (the sheath stream). The laminar flow effect of the sheath stream pushes horizontally on the sample or core stream and focuses it to a very narrow path in the center of the sheath flow. The sheath flow also exerts a vertical force on sample stream, exerting control its forward motion. By carefully controlling the ratio between sheath and sample flow pressure, a very narrow sample stream (less than 100 microns in diameter) with high stability can be generated, allowing the contained cells to be efficiently and precisely aligned to and excited by the laser source (Melamed et al., 1990).

A typical flow cell is shown in Figure 3.2a, with the quartz cuvette indicated with an arrow. This flow cell has a 200-micron capillary space running through it vertically, shown magnified in Figure 3.2b. Cells are injected into the capillary from the bottom of the flow cell assembly. Sheath buffer is introduced through the conical reservoir under the cuvette, where it merges with the sample stream. Figure 3.2c shows how the sample stream is focused within the cylindrical sheath flow, with sheath buffer exerting a horizontal focusing effect.

Magnified images of the cuvette are shown in Figures 3.2c-f. The quartz cuvette (rectangular in cross-section) is shown in Figure 3.2d. The vertical walls of the cuvette are visible in the light of the instrument laser illuminating the flow cells. In Figure 3.2e, bright fluorescent beads are being run as a sample, and the laser light has been blocked with a notch filter. Only the fluorescent beads are visible. The hydrodynamically focused bead stream is clearly visible and is confined to the center of the flow cell. Without sheath flow, the beads would not be confined to the center of the flow cell; they would not be uniformly excited by the laser, and many would arrive at the laser intercept simultaneously and unevenly, making single-cell analysis impossible. This is shown in Figure 3.2f, where the sheath flow has been shut off while continuing to inject sample; the fluorescent bead stream fills the entire flow cell. Hydrodynamic focusing is essential to flow cytometry, and virtually all flow cytometers employ it.

A high numerical aperture light collection optic is coupled to the back of the flow cell using an optically matched gel. This optic efficiently transmits scatter and fluorescence signals from the flow cell capillary to the downstream optical detectors (3.5).

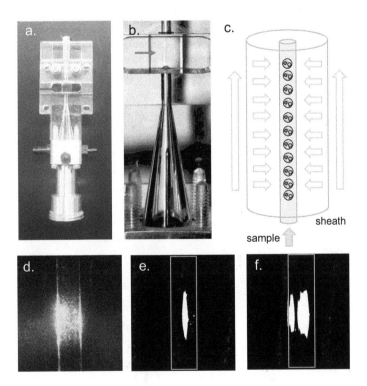

FIGURE 3.2 **Flow cell.** *a,* quartz cuvette flow cell (BD Biosciences). Cuvette and capillary are indicated by the arrow. *b,* hydrodynamic focusing. Sample (core) stream is indicated in gray. Sheath stream exerts horizontal force to focus the sample stream, and vertical force to affect forward movement. *c,* magnified image of flow cell cuvette capillary, no fluorescent particles, laser light only. *d,* magnified image of capillary, laser light blocked with filter, fluorescent beads running and subjected to hydrodynamic focusing. *e,* magnified image of capillary, laser light blocked with filter, fluorescent beads running with sheath pressure off (no hydrodynamic focusing).

3.2.2 Instrument Fluidics

The sheath and sample (core) streams described above are generated by the instrument fluidics, which push sheath buffer and sample into the flow cell. There are many ways do this this, using air pumps, syringe pumps, peristaltic pumps, or a combination. Hydrostatic (positive pressure) systems are the simplest and are historically the most common. A typical positive pressure system is shown in Figure 3.3. These systems use a sheath buffer tank, which is pressurized with an air pump. Sheath buffer is pushed into the flow cell and capillary. This pressure can be controlled and adjusted. The same air pump also pressurizes a sample tube, pushing sample into the capillary and the sheath flow. By controlling the ratio between sheath and sample pressure, a narrow sample or core stream can be achieved. Sample pressure must be slightly higher than sheath pressure, allowing sample to successfully push against the sample flow and enter the capillary. After passing through the capillary, both sheath and sample are ejected into a waste container.

Most commercial analyzers use a fixed sheath pressure and allow adjustment of the sample pressure to increase or decrease the flow rate of the cell suspension. Increasing sample pressure does *not* increase the velocity of cells through the capillary; rather, increases the diameter of the sample stream as it pushes more strongly on the sheath stream. This has important implications for analysis; a wider sample stream will increase the probability that two cells will arrive at the laser intercept together. Such coincident events can be misinterpreted as a single event or must discarded as uninterpretable. The laser beam might not also uniformly illuminate a wide sample stream. Maintaining a low sample pressure is therefore desirable in flow cytometry to maximize the precision of analysis.

Flow analyzers (which do not sort cells) typically operate at low sheath pressures, in the range of 3 to 6 psi. Cell sorters, which physically separate cells following analysis, often operate at much higher sheath pressures, from 20 to 80 psi. While sample pressure dictates the diameter of the sample stream but not its velocity, increase sheath pressure does increase overall stream velocity. This increase reduces the time cells spend in the laser beam and can decrease overall fluorescence sensitivity. The high cell flow rates often required in cell sorting as opposed to analysis-only are often a necessary compromise for the needs of high-speed cell separation.

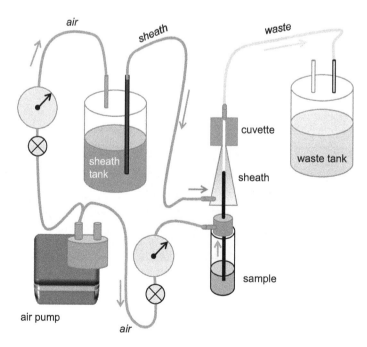

FIGURE 3.3   Fluidics. Fluidic diagram for a hydrostatic (positive pressure) flow cytometry system. Included sheath and waste tanks, air pump, regulators (dials with gauge), pressure switches (X symbol), sample tube, and flow cell.

While positive pressure systems are historically the most wide-spread mechanism for delivering cells in a flow cytometer, many other systems exist. Negative air pressure (vacuum) systems are becoming more common. Many cytometers use syringe and peristaltic pumps to deliver sheath buffer and/or sample. These systems have more precise volume control and allow absolute cell counts to be calculated based on the flow rate of the pump mechanism.

3.3 Instrument Optics

3.3.1 Lasers, Laser Optics, and the Laser Intercept

Once the sample stream enters the flow cell capillary, it is intercepted by one or more laser beams. Flow cytometers usually employs single-mode continuous wave (CW) lasers with power levels ranging from a few to several hundred milliwatts. While a few early flow cytometers used other light sources, the coherent nature of laser light is uniquely suited to the need of flow cytometers for the projection of a concentrated light source on a very small area.

Early flow cytometers used the large water-cooled gas lasers available at the time, making the instruments large as well. These lasers gradually became smaller and air-cooled, allowing instrument size to decrease. Recent advances in solid-state laser technology have had further beneficial effects on cytometer design. Figure 3.4a shows several laser types, ranging from air-cooled argon-ion laser at the top to a recent solid-state laser at the bottom. Solid-state lasers are smaller, easier to operate, and last longer than their earlier gas counterparts and are now the dominant laser type on commercial instruments. Their small size (Figure 3.4b) and low heat output allows the design of very small instruments and permits many lasers and wavelengths to be incorporated into a single instrument (Shapiro, 2003; Shapiro, 2018).

The primary laser wavelength for flow cytometry is blue-green or cyan 488 nm. This is due both to its easy availability from argon-ion lasers in the early days of flow cytometry, and its ability to excite many fluorochromes used in flow cytometric analysis, including the low molecular weight fluorophore fluorescein, and natural product fluorochromes like phycoerythrin. The somewhat arbitrary designation of cyan

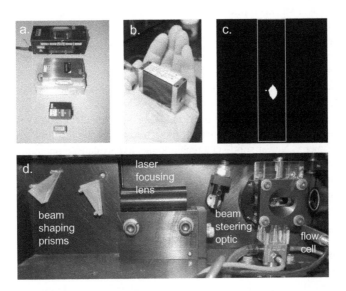

FIGURE 3.4   Lasers *a*, a progression of cyan 488 nm lasers in flow cytometry, including (from top to bottom) an air-cooled gas laser, large and medium sized solid state DPSS lasers, and a small direct diode laser (JDS Uniphase, Coherent, CVI Melles Griot and Vortran Laser Technology, respectively). *b*, a small direct diode solid-state cyan 488 nm laser typical of these now used in flow cytometry (Vortran Laser Technology). *c*, the same magnified image of capillary shown in Figure 2d with laser beam focusing. *e*, laser beam processing optics, including anamorphic beam shaping prisms, focusing lens, and steering prism (BD FACScan, BD Biosciences).

488 nm as the primary laser wavelength makes it the usual wavelength for light scattering measurements. However, most modern flow cytometers utilize multiple laser wavelengths to take advantage of the many fluorescent probes now available for flow cytometry. Red and violet lasers are common on most instruments, and five or more wavelengths can be found on high-end analyzers. This variety of available excitation wavelengths has pushed the total number of simultaneous available fluorescent parameters to over forty (Shapiro, 2018).

The laser beam is aligned to the center of flow cell, allowing it to intercept the cell stream and excite the target cells. The beam needs to be optically modified to prior to cell stream interception to maximize excitation. A laser focusing optic is usually used to focus the beam to a diameter slightly larger than the stream diameter, maximizing laser energy on the cell stream. On simple cytometers this is usually a plano-convex lens. On multi-laser instrument, a more complex achromatic lens is required to focus several laser wavelengths simultaneously. A beam steering mechanism is used to translate the laser beam and move it to the center of the cell stream. Laser beam shaping optics such as anamorphic prism pairs can be used to modify the beam shape; an elliptical beam spot is usually most efficient at completely eclipsing the cell intercept with minimal vertical spillover for multi-laser systems. All of these devices are shown in Figure 3.4d and are installed prior to the flow cell. The same magnified flow cell image shown in Figure 3.2 is shown in Figure 3.4c with proper laser focusing. This allows both high-resolution scatter measurement and maximal fluorochrome excitation. For systems using multiple lasers, the beads are usually arranged with spatial separation, and the detector electronics configured to collect cell data from each laser and combine the results into single-cell measurements.

3.3.2 Light Collection and Detectors

Once the intercepts the cell, the resulting signals must be collected by downstream detectors. The quartz flow cell is usually coupled to a high-numerical aperture light collection optic, which focuses the scatter and fluorescence signals into the instrument optical path.

Cell signals differ in strength; the laser scatter signals can be very strong, while fluorescence signals excited by the laser can be very weak. Different technologies are required to detect these signals. Very strong signals are typically detected using conventional photodiodes (PDs), either passive (unpowered) or with a low voltage bias. Weaker signals typically require far more sensitive photon detectors. Photomultiplier tubes (PMTs) are historically the detectors of choice for fluorescent signals. PMTs are extremely sensitive photon detectors; some PMTs can detect a single photon of light. The PMTs on flow cytometers, while not this sensitive, can detect as few as a few thousand molecules of some fluorescent probes.

A typical flow cytometer PMT is shown in Figure 3.5a. PMTs require high voltage for signal amplification; adjustment of the PMTs sensitivity and dynamic range are made by controlling the voltage flowing to the PMT. While older PMTs are relatively large, smaller ones shown in Figure 3.5b are now available and have contributed to the recent decrease in instrument size. Until recently, PMTs were the only practical light detection technology sensitive enough to detect the low levels of fluorescence often required for flow cytometry. Newer solid-state technologies like avalanche photodiodes (APDs) and silicone photomultipliers (SiPMs) are starting to achieve similar sensitivities and are now being incorporated into commercial instrumentation (Figure 3.5c). Their durability, small size, and low cost are also contributing to improved instrument designs.

3.3.3 Detection Optics

Detection of laser light scatter and multiple fluorescent probes requires additional optics to separate different emission wavelengths simultaneously. Dichroic mirrors are coated mirrors than allow light transmission above or below a certain wavelength, while reflecting light below or above. The dichroic mirror in Figure 3.4d is a 560 nm long pass (LP), transmitting light greater than 560 nm (orange) and reflecting light less than 560 nm (blue green). Dichroic mirrors are used to separate emission wavelengths. Bandpass filters allow a certain bandwidth of light to pass through the optic, while blocking light above or below the range. The bandpass filter in Figure 3.4e is a 535/45 nm filter, transmitting light centered at 535 nm with a 45 nm window. Most flow cytometers make extensive use of both dichroic mirrors and bandpass filters to separate and filter emission light from any fluorochromes simultaneously.

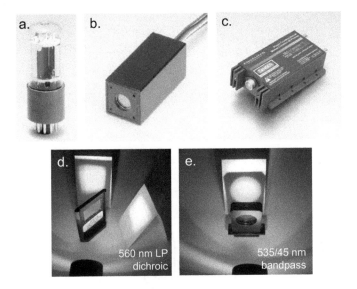

FIGURE 3.5   Detectors. *a,* a photomultiplier tube (PMT) (Hamamatsu, Japan). *b,* a small front-end photomultiplier tube (PMT) (Hamamatsu, Japan). *c,* an avalanche photodiode (APD) (Excelitas, Waltham, MA, USA). *d,* a 560 nm longpass dichroic mirror, showing transmission of light above 560 nm (orange) and reflection of light below 560 nm (blue-green). *e,* a 535/45 nm bandpass filter, showing transmission of light centered at 535 nm with a 45 nm window (green).

3.4 Electronics, Computers, and Software

The resulting signals are then processed by the instrument electronics and digitized for transmission to the system's computer. Early cytometers relied heavily on signal processing in analog electronics, converting the data to digital only as a last step (Melamed et al., 1990). Modern systems use integrated digital electronics for initial signal processing, allowing faster and more accurate data analysis. Modern systems also make use of conventional computers for data acquisition. All commercial cytometers have proprietary software packages that allow control of the instrument, including detector sensitivity adjustment, as well as data acquisition and display. There are also a variety of third-party software packages that allow analysis of previously acquired data. While not able to initially acquire data, these software packages are often more powerful for post-acquisition data analysis and are often preferred for this purpose.

3.5 Flow Cytometric Data Acquisition and Analysis

3.5.1 Forward and Side Scatter

What do flow cytometers measure? Two critical measurements made by flow cytometers are forward scatter (or 180-degree light scatter) and side scatter (or 90-degree light scatter). The optical mechanisms for both measurements are shown in Figure 3.6a. Both measurements are made with scattered laser light, usually the primary cyan 488 nm wavelength. In forward scatter, laser light scattered 180 degrees opposite the laser source is analyzed (with a blocking bar to exclude direct laser light, and a 488/10 nm bandpass filter). Forward scatter is a rough measure of cell size, with larger cells scattering more laser light and producing a stronger signal. In mixed cell populations such as blood, smaller cells like platelets and erythrocytes will have a lower forward scatter signal; larger cells like lymphocytes and myeloid cells will have a stronger signal. Forward signal is relatively strong and is usually collected with a lower sensitivity like a photodiode (although forward scatter from submicron objects may require a PMT).

Side scatter is collected at a 90-degree angle to the incoming laser light. It is a rough measure of cell optical density; cells with simple interior structure like erythrocytes and lymphocytes will have a low side scatter signal, while more granular cells like macrophages and granulocytes will have a stronger side scatter signal. Side scatter is usually detected with a PMT.

a.

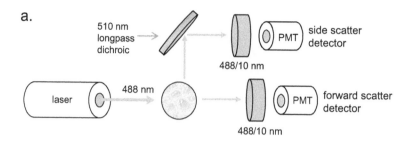

b.

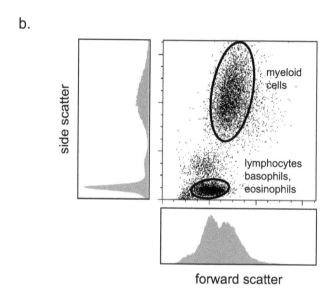

FIGURE 3.6 Forward and side scatter. *a,* optical layout of forward and side scatter detectors on a flow cytometer. *b,* two-parameter scatter or dot plots of forward versus side scatter for human peripheral blood, with one-parameter histograms for each characteristic shown. Each pixel represents a single cell.

Forward and side scatter measurements are the primary means of initially analyzing complex cell mixtures, particularly blood and immune cell tissues like bone marrow. While they can be analyzed separately, they are most often used together, with the resulting data displayed in a scatter or dot plot. Figure 3.6b shows both one-and two-parameter for human peripheral blood with forward and side scatter on and x-and y-axes. Recall that flow cytometer collects and displays data in an inter-relational manner; all data parameters can be displayed relative to one another. The on-parameter plots of forward and side scatter shown in Figure 3.6b are useful, but viewing both parameters in a two-dimensional format is more informative. This powerful analysis characteristic allows multiple cell types to be displayed in this scatterplot, distinguishing the erythrocytes, lymphocytes, and myeloid cells based on both of these light scattering characteristics. Two-dimensional plots are therefore considered more useful for multiparametric analysis.

3.5.2 Fluorescence Detection and Multicolor Analysis

Fluorescence measurements can be collected simultaneously with laser light scattering, allowing both size/optical density and cell markers to be analyzed at the same time. Fluorescent signals are almost always collected with PMTs or specialized sensitive photodiodes. An optical layout for a simple flow cytometer is shown in Figure 3.7a. This instrument has the same forward and side scatter detectors as in Figure 3.6, but with the addition of three fluorescence detectors on the same 90-degree axis as the

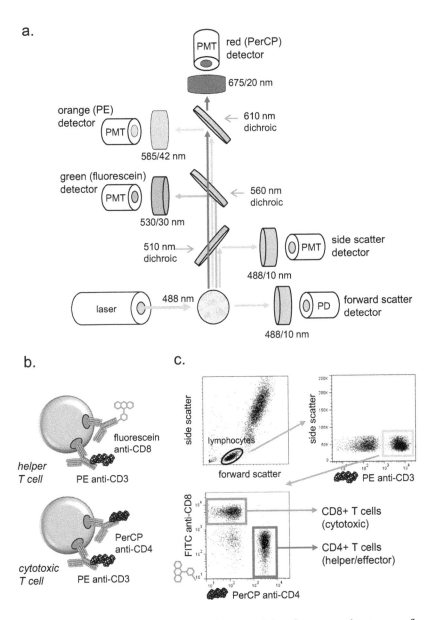

FIGURE 3.7 **Fluorescence detection.** *a,* Optical layout of scatter and three fluorescence detectors on a flow cytometer. Note the location and function of bandpass filters and dichroic mirrors. *b,* Fluorochrome conjugated labeling scheme for T cells. CD3 (PerCP) is expressed on both helper and cytotoxic T cells, but CD4 (PE) and CD8 (fluorescein) are expressed only on helper and cytotoxic T cells, respectively and exclusively. *c,* Flow cytometric analysis of T cells. Cells are gated for scatter (all lymphocytes), CD3 expression (all T cells) and displayed for CD4 and CD8 (helper and cytotoxic T cells).

side scatter detector. A 510 nm longpass dichroic mirror is used to reflect the side scatter signal into its detector and transmit longer green, orange, and red wavelengths to additional downstream detectors. Additional dichroic mirrors (560 and 610 nm long pass) is used to separate the fluorescence signals of fluorescein, phycoerythrin (PE), and PerCP, three fluorescent probes with emission wavelengths of roughly 530, 580, and 670 nm, respectively. Bandpass filters (488/10 nm, 530/30 nm, 585/42 nm, and 675/20 nm) further filter the individual scatter and fluorescent signals and allow them to be distinguished from one another.

While necessary to distinguish multiple fluorochromes, dichroic mirrors and bandpass filters are not sufficient to completely distinguish fluorescent probes with overlapping emission ranges. Fluorescent compensation is required to subtract unwanted fluorescent overlaps from other fluorescent markers into the probe of interest. This compensation can be calculated in the instrument electronics (typically found on older analog instrument), or in the instrument acquisition software. An unlabeled autofluorescence control sample and single-color control samples are required to generate a compensation or spillover matrix that, when applied to multicolor data, separate each fluorescent probe, and allow multiple cell markers to be analyzed simultaneously and inter-relationally (Mahnke & Roederer, 2007; Maciorowski et al., 2017).

Typical multicolor data from the instrument shown in Figure 3.7a is shown in Figure 3.7b and 3.7c. A peripheral blood sample was labeled with antibodies coupled to the three fluorescent probes detected by this instrument: anti-human CD8 coupled to fluorescein (green), anti-human CD4 coupled to PE (orange), and anti-human CD3 couples to PerCP (red). CD3, CD4, and CD8 are all markers for T cells, an important leukocyte subset. The CD3 target protein identifies all T cells; CD4 and CD8 identify subsets of T cells within the CD3-positive population and are markers for helper and cytotoxic T cells, respectively (Figure 3.7b).

The cells were then analyzed for these three T cell markers as well as forward and side scatter (Figure 3.7c). The first scatterplot displayed is for forward vs. side scatter (size vs. optical density). An elliptical region is drawn around the lymphocyte subset, which will contain the T cells. Another scatter plot is displayed, this time showing side scatter versus anti-CD3 PerCP, one of our fluorescent markers. This plot was gated on the lymphocyte subset, showing only events in this region. Gating is a critical tool in flow cytometry, allowing selective analysis of different cell populations. This plot shows cell populations that are both positive and negative for CD3 expression based on their PerCP fluorescence. A second gate was drawn around the CD3 positive (PerCP bright) cells, and a third plot displayed showing the fluorescence of the markers for CD4 and CD8 expression. The single positive populations expressing CD4 or CD8 represent the helper and cytotoxic T cell subsets, respectively. Note that there were no cells positive for both markers; CD4 and CD8 are usually expressed on different cell populations in healthy donors.

There are several key points that should be emphasized:

- First, we are analyzing multiple cell characteristics simultaneously, and are able to display them all relative to each other. The multiparametric nature of flow cytometry data allows complex cell mixtures to be analyzed and different cell types identified, since all characteristics can be seen relative to all other characteristics.
- Second, we can distinguish multiple fluorescent probes simultaneously and use them together to do these analyses. As stated previously, instrument optics alone are not sufficient to fully separate the fluorescence emissions of these probes; additional mathematical compensation must be used as well. The data shown in Figure 3.7 was compensated using single-color control samples for each marker. This spectral separation (expressed as a compensation or spillover matrix) can become complex as more probes are added and is normally done using an automated computer algorithm.
- Third, we followed a logical progression in analyzing this data, initially viewing forward and side scatter, then our total T cell marker, then our T cell subset markers. This so-called gating logic is a critical element of multiparametric flow cytometry, and again can become very complex for larger experiments.

3.6 The Limits of Multicolor Flow Cytometry

The flow cytometer in Figure 3.7 is a very simple instrument, with only one laser and three fluorescent parameters. Modern flow cytometers are typically equipped with at least three laser wavelengths. Synthetic fluorescent probe development has resulted in large arrays of spectrally distinguishable dyes excited at most wavelengths in the visible spectrum, particularly with violet and ultraviolet laser sources. So-called high-dimensional flow cytometers are capable of detecting from twenty to forty fluorochromes simultaneously (Chattopadhyay et al., 2012). One such instrument (a BD Biosciences Influx™) is shown in Figure 3.8; this instrument has five spatially separate laser sources (ultraviolet, violet, cyan, yellow, and red) and 22 fluorescent detectors. However, the overall optical design is not very different from the simple cytometer in Figure 3.7; we have simply added more lasers, detectors, and optics. High-dimensional flow cytometry has allowed deep profiling of the immune system, detecting and correlating many extracellular, and intracellular protein markers and identifying dozens of distinct leukocyte subsets (Cossarizza et al., 2019). At the time of this writing, high-dimensional flow cytometric analysis using traditional optics has allowed the analysis of over thirty distinct markers simultaneously. This is probably the upper limit of traditional systems.

Improvements in fluidic and optical technology are pushing the limits of flow cytometry even further. Spectral flow cytometry collects the entire spectra of multiple fluorescent probes rather than simple bandwidths. Spectral deconvolution instead of compensation is used to separate fluorochrome signals from one another. This technology allows fluorochrome groups with similar spectral characteristics to be used together with less overlap than with traditional optical methods. Mass cytometry used atomic mass spectroscopy and stable transition metal and lanthanide probes instead of fluorescence to achieve simultaneous labeling panels of up to fifty cell markers. This non-optical technology is not appropriate for all studies (the cells are destroyed upon analysis) but has achieved very high levels of deep profiling immune cell analysis. Spectral cytometry has exceeded forty simultaneous markers, and mass cytometry should be able to reach 60 markers and beyond (Cossarizza et al., 2019).

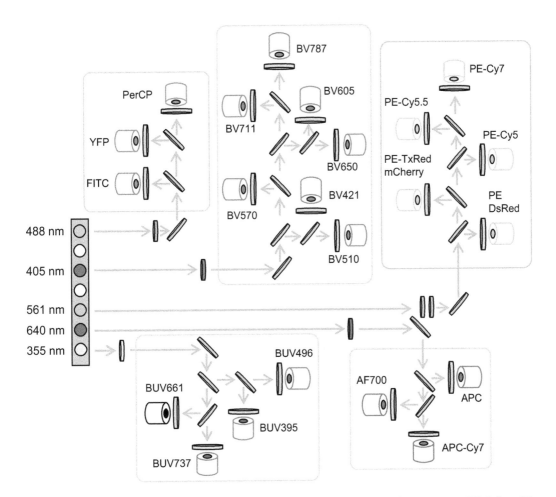

FIGURE 3.8 Forward and side scatter. *a*, Optical layout for a high-dimensional flow cytometer (BD Influx, BD Biosciences), equipped with 5 laser sources and 22 fluorescence detectors. Labels on each detector refer to a fluorescent probe.

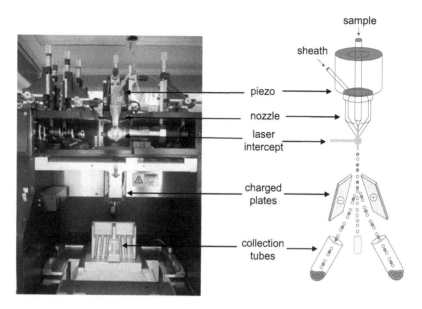

FIGURE 3.9 Fluorescence-activated cell sorting. Image and diagram of a cell sorter (BD Influx, BD Biosciences) with nozzle, piezo, laser intercept, electrostatic plates, and collection tubes indicated.

3.7 Cell Sorting

Fluorescence-activated cell sorters (FACS) are flow analyzers with the capability to physically sort cell populations, a powerful adjunct to flow cytometry allowing the isolation and purification of often rare cell subpoulations. Most cell sorters use an electrostatic plate system to separate cells for collection. Rather than a quartz cuvette, most cell sorters use a stream-in air nozzle system, where the sheath/sample stream is ejected into the open air for laser interrogation. The nozzle is equipped with a piezo that oscillates at a very high frequency to break the sample stream into droplets. Upon identification of a cell type of interest, the stream is electrically charged immediately prior to breakoff of the liquid droplet containing the desired cell. Upon breakoff, that droplet is then deflected into a collection tube using a charged metal plate (Figure 3.9). Flow cytometric analysis is therefore almost immediately translated into physical separation of the population of interest. The resulting cells can be recultured, transplanted into a laboratory animal, or subjected to genomic or proteomic analysis. Cell sorting has been crucial in identifying leukocyte phylogeny and ontogeny, and in the isolation and characterization of rare cell types such as stem cells.

3.8 Other Applications for Flow Cytometry

Leukocyte immunophenotyping is only one application of many for flow cytometry. Any cell type that can be rendered into a single-cell suspension can be analyzed by flow. Tumor cells, hepatocytes, neurons, and cells from virtually all tissues have all been analyzed by flow cytometry. Bacteria, protozoa, plant cells, aquatic and marine prokaryotes and eukaryotes have all been analyzed by flow, often using instrumentation specially modified for their size. Submicron objects including viruses, cellular organelles, microvesicles, and exosomes have all been analyzed by cytometry using specially designed instruments, making flow cytometry an important technology for this emerging field.

Flow cytometry is also not limited to antibody-based immunofluorescence. Fluorescent DNA binding dyes can be used to measure cell cycle progression based on DNA fluorescence in labeled cells. Fluorescent assays for cell proliferation, apoptosis, senescence, cellular ion flux, plasma membrane and mitochondrial membrane potential, and other cell physiological conditions are widely used in flow cytometry. Expressible fluorescent proteins such as Green Fluorescent Protein (GFP) have seen extensive use in flow cytometry. Any fluorescence-based cell assay can be adapted for flow cytometry, making it a research tool with vast applications.

REFERENCES

Chattopadhyay PK, Gaylord, B, Palmer A, Jiang N, Raven MA, Lewis G, Reuter MA, Nur-ur Rahman AK, Price DA, Betts MR, Roederer M (2012) Brilliant violet fluorophores: a new class of ultrabright fluorescent compounds for immunofluorescence experiments. *Cytometry A* 81, 456–466. *An example of the new polymer fluorochromes allowing expansion of high-dimensional flow cytometry.*

Cossarizza A et al (2019) Guidelines for the use of flow cytometry and cell sorting in immunological studies (second edition). *Eur J Immunol* 49: 1457–1973. https://doi-org.proxy.insermbiblio.inist.fr/10.1002/eji.201970107. *An extensive review of flow cytometry techniques, frequently updated.*

Maciorowski Z, Chattopadhyay PK, Jain P (2017) Basic multicolor flow cytometry. *Curr Protoc Immunol*, 117, 5.4.1–5.4.38. doi: 10.1002/cpim.26. *A good introduction to multicolor flow cytometry.*

Mahnke Y, Roederer M. (2007) Optimizing a multicolor immunophenotyping assay. *Clin Lab Med*, 27: 469–485, v. doi:10.1016/j.cll.2007.05.002. *Critical parameters for multi-color analysis.*

Melamed MR, Lindmo T, Mendelsohn MI (1990) Flow cytometry and sorting, 2nd edition, John Wiley and Sons, New York, NY. *A comprehensive review of the underlying technology of flow cytometry.*

Shapiro HM, Telford WG (2018) Lasers for flow cytometry: current and future trends. In *Current Protocols in Cytometry*, Robinson JP, Darzynkiewicz Z, Dobrucki J, Hoffman RA, Nolan JP, Orfao A, Rabinovitch PS, Telford WG, eds., John Wiley and Sons, New York, NY, 86, 1.9.1–11.9.21, doi: 10.1002/cpcy.30. *A comprehensive overview of lasers in flow cytometry.*

Shapiro HM (2003) Practical flow cytometry, 4th edition, John Wiley and Sons, New York, NY. *A wonderful introduction to flow cytometry both past and present, including many technical details of instrument operation. Out of print but available for free online.*

4

Multicolor Flow Cytometry and Panel Design

Zosia Maciorowski
Institut Curie, Paris, France, retired

4.1 Introduction

A wide range of fluorochromes are available for use in flow cytometry and optimization of the antibody/fluorochrome combinations used for the different cellular markers is essential. The fluorochromes used in these multicolor assays must be carefully chosen to maximize the sensitivity of the assays, particularly for the detection of rare antigens or very small cell populations. Poorly designed multicolor panels can severely compromise discrimination of the subpopulations of interest.

Individual fluorochrome characteristics, brightness, spectral overlap, spillover, and spread all impact on how fluorochromes are used and combined in multicolor panels. In addition, individual instrument characteristics, cellular antigen density, and coexpression are essential elements in multicolor panel design. The panel design tools and procedures needed to tailor fluorochrome combinations to best identify the desired populations will be elaborated on here.

4.2 The Basics: Light, Fluorochromes, and Fluorescence

Flow cytometry uses light primarily in the visible range, from 350 up to 800 nm wavelengths, as seen in Figure 4.1 A. The shorter wavelengths are higher energy, longer wavelengths are lower energy.

Fluorochromes are molecules that can absorb light at one wavelength, and then re-emit that light energy at a longer wavelength with lower energy. This process is called fluorescence. Figure 4.1B shows the chemical structure of two fluorochromes commonly used in flow cytometry: fluorescein (FITC) and phycoerytherin (PE). The schema in Figure 4.1C illustrates how fluorescence occurs: a fluorochrome electron, which is at a resting energy level, absorbs energy from the light source, in this case blue 488 nm laser light, and jumps up to a higher unstable energy level ("excitation"). A little of this energy is then lost as heat or non-radiatively, and the rest of the energy emitted as fluorescence at a higher wavelength, in this case a green fluorescence at about 520 nm ("emission"). This is a very simplified schema; it is the fluorochrome's electron cloud that excites and emits.

The excitation and emission wavelengths are specific to each fluorochrome (Figure 4.2). A fluorochrome can absorb light all across its specific excitation spectral curve, but excites most efficiently at its excitation maximum. Figure 2A shows the excitation spectra for FITC with an excitation maximum at around 495 nm. The excitation spectra can be used to determine which laser excitation wavelength is optimal for that fluorochrome.

Similarly for the emission spectra, a fluorochrome can emit light all across its emission spectral curve, but most efficiently at its emission maximum. Figure 2B shows the emission spectra for FITC with an emission maximum at around 520 nm. Note the width of the emission spectra, with less efficient emission into the higher wavelengths. The emission spectra will determine which optical filter will best capture the emission for that fluorochrome.

These excitation and emission spectra are essential considerations in fluorochrome selection. The spectral information for any fluorochrome can be easily found using the multiple spectral viewer websites available online (see the Internet Resources on Spectral Viewers).

DOI: 10.1201/9781003220404-5

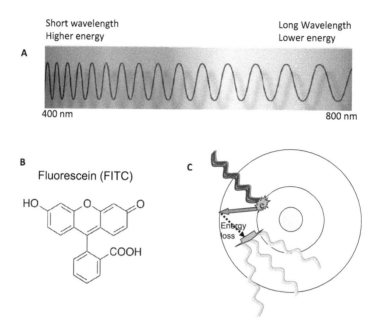

FIGURE 4.1 A. Light: The spectrum of light wavelengths utilized in flow cytometry range from about 350 nm to 800 nm. Short wavelengths have higher energy, long wavelengths have lower energy. B. Fluorochrome structure: Chemical structure of two widely used fluorochromes: FITC (fluorescein) and PE (phycoerytherin). C. The process of fluorescence: A fluorochrome electron in resting state is excited by light energy and jumps to an unstable higher energy level. It loses some energy as heat or non-radiatively, then re-emits the rest of the energy as fluorescence at a higher wavelength. This is a very simplified schema: it is actually the electron cloud of the fluorochrome molecule's conjugated double-bond system that excites and fluoresces.

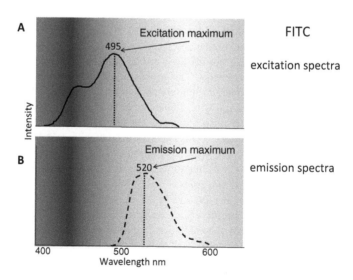

FIGURE 4.2 A. Excitation spectra: Each fluorochrome is capable of absorbing light energy over a specific range of wavelengths, but most efficiently at its excitation maximum. Here, FITC can absorb energy at all these wavelengths, but best at 495 nm. Examination of the excitation spectra allows determination of which laser wavelengths are likely to most efficiently excite the fluorochrome. B. Emission spectra: Similarly, each fluorochrome is capable of emitting light energy over a specific range of wavelengths, but most efficiently at its emission maximum. FITC will fluoresce at all these wavelengths but highest at 520 nm. Note the width of the spectra, showing that some emission from that fluorochrome at non-optimal wavelengths is to be expected.

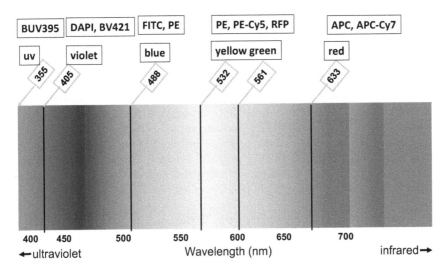

FIGURE 4.3 Laser wavelengths: Shown here are laser wavelengths commonly found on standard cytometers, with examples of a few of the fluorochromes that are excited by each laser. Most cytometers now come equipped with a blue 488 nm, a red 640 nm, and violet 405 nm laser, with additional options of yellow-green 532 or 561 and UV 355 nm lasers.

Lasers emit a stable uniform beam of light at a specific wavelength and are used as sources of excitation light for the fluorochromes. The laser wavelengths currently found on standard flow cytometers are shown in Figure 4.3, along with examples of some of the fluorochromes excited by each laser. A standard three laser configuration has a blue 488 nm, a red 640 nm, and a violet 405 nm. Yellow-green 560 nm and/or UV 365 nm lasers are often added for a four-or five-laser instrument configuration. It is essential to know which laser wavelengths and filter configurations are available on the cytometer that will be used for the assays in order to select appropriate fluorochromes. Fluorochromes are chosen so that they are excitable by the lasers available on the instrument and have emission spectra that are different from each other.

Tandem fluorochromes are also used in flow cytometry and are composed of two fluorochromes tightly coupled together. The emission spectra of the base or donor fluorochrome must overlap the excitation spectra of the second or acceptor fluorochrome. The base fluorochrome is excited by the laser light, and transfers this energy non-radiatively to the second fluorochrome, which then emits fluorescence at its own higher emission spectra wavelengths. An example would be PE-Cy5, where PE is the base fluorochrome, which excites at 560 nm, and transfers energy to Cy5 the acceptor fluorochrome, which then emits fluorescence around 670 nm. If the fluorochromes are not coupled tightly or degrade over time, there can be loss of energy transfer, thus some leakage or "spill" of fluorescent emission from the base fluorochrome at its own emission wavelengths.

Fluorochromes are commonly used coupled to antibodies specific for an antigen or marker of interest on the surface or inside the cell. The amount of fluorescence measured on the cell is thus proportional to the amount of marker expressed on that cell. Other fluorochromes are specific for different physiological states of the cell (e.g., pH, calcium flux, and membrane potential). Fluorochromes that attach to DNA can be used for quantitation of cell cycle status or proliferation, or often for discrimination of live/dead cells. This plethora of fluorochromes contributes to the multiparameter capability of flow cytometry to simultaneously measure many cellular characteristics.

4.3 Spectral Spillover and Compensation

Refer to Chapter 3, Basic Principles of Flow Cytometer Operation for Biomedical Scientists in this volume for an explanation of how the optical filters and detectors function in a flow cytometer. In brief, specific optical filters are placed in front of each light detector to ensure that the detector only sees the wavelengths of light corresponding to the maximal emission of the desired fluorochrome, and that this "primary detector" correctly measures light emission from only that fluorochrome.

As we have seen, fluorochrome emission spectra are quite wide, with emission generally tailing off to the right into the longer wavelengths. This lesser emission at wavelengths outside of the emission maximum can pass through, or "spillover," into the optical filters in front of the light detectors targeted to measure other fluorochromes. Figure 4.4 shows the emission spectra of two fluorochromes, FITC and PE, and the optical filters through which each are usually measured. As can be seen, there is some emission by FITC at wavelengths that will pass through the filters targeted for PE. This means that some FITC emission will be measured in the PE detector. It is necessary, however, to measure only FITC in the FITC "primary" detector. This problem of spectral overlap and spillover into other detectors is solved by applying a mathematical correction factor, called compensation, to remove the contribution of FITC spillover into the PE detector (Bagwell and Adams, 1993; Roederer, 2001).

Figure 4.5 shows the effect of this spectral overlap before and after compensation. This is a FITC single-color control: cells stained only with a FITC coupled antibody. In Figure 4.5A, looking at the

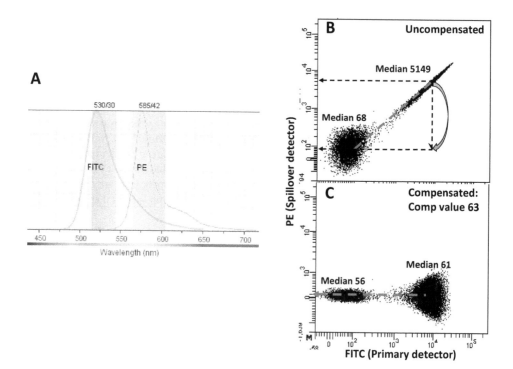

FIGURE 4.4   A. Spectral overlap: This figure shows the overlap of the emission spectra of two fluorochromes, FITC and PE, and the optical filters through which each fluorochrome is collected. It can be seen that there is some FITC emission at the wavelengths measured through the PE filter. B. Spectral spillover:

Here we can see the result of this FITC spillover into the PE detector. This is a FITC stained single-color control, with FITC positive and negative cells. FITC fluorescence is shown on the X axis, PE fluorescence on the Y axis. On the FITC axis, there is one FITC positive and one negative population, as would be expected. The FITC positive popluation also appears to be positive in the PE channel, with a median intensity of 5149 compared to the negative peak at 68. This is due solely to spillover of FITC emission at the higher wavelengths measured in the PE detector. C. Compensation: To calculate compensation, the median intensities of the positive and negative populations in each channel are first measured. The compensation calculation is based on the slope of the line between the medians of the positive and negative populations. The single-color control has now been correctly compensated, and the median of the FITC positive (61) is now the same as the median of the FITC negative (56) in the PE channel. Application of this compensation correction to an experimental double-stained sample would now allow correct identification of true double-positive cells.

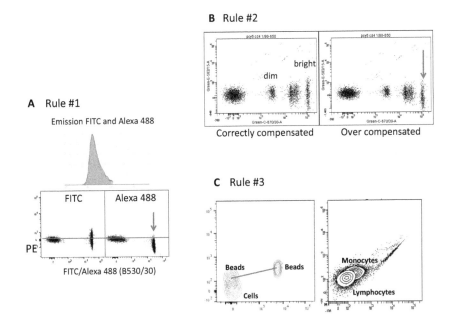

FIGURE 4.5 Compensation rules: A. Rule #1: The antibody in the single-color control must have exactly the same spectral characteristics as the one in the mix. The spectra of the green emission fluorochromes FITC and Alexa 488 appear to be very similar, but it can be seen that the compensation value against PE, calculated using a single-color FITC control, results in overcompensation when applied to a single-color Alexa 488. B. Rule #2: The single color must be as bright or brighter than the positive cells in the mix. On the left, the compensation has been calculated using the bright population as the positive and is correct for all the populations. On the right, compensation has been calculated using the dim population as the positive: the compensation is adequate for the dim population, but the brighter population is overcompensated (arrow). C. Rule #3: The autofluorescence of the negative must match the autofluorescence of the positive population. It can be seen that the slope of the line used to calculate compensation would be quite different, depending on which negative autofluorescent population is used. On the left, negative beads must be used, not negative cells. On the right, negative lymphocytes must be used for positive lymphocytes, not monocytes; the difference in autofluorescence is visible. Using a mismatched negative will generate an erroneous compensation correction.

dot plot of FITC fluorescence on the X axis vs. PE fluorescence on the Y axis, it can be seen that on the FITC axis, the population that is positive for FITC, is nicely separated from the negative population. Looking at the PE axis, however, it appears that FITC positive population is also positive for PE, with a median PE channel number of 5149, compared to the negative cells at 68. We know that there is no PE in the tube; it has only FITC, thus that positivity seen in the PE channel is due solely to FITC spillover into the PE detector. In Figure 4.5B, a compensation correction has been applied, so that now the FITC positive population single color has a median channel number of 61 that is the same as the negative population at 56.

The compensation correction is calculated by running a series of single-color stained controls, where we are sure that any fluorescence measured in any detector is due only to the single fluorochrome present in the control tube. Software compensation algorithms are then used to calculate and apply the compensation necessary, so that each detector is measuring only the fluorochrome for which it is targeted.

Note, however, the width or "spread" of the compensated FITC postive population in the spillover PE channel compared to the FITC negative population. This spread due to spillover is not reduced after compensation, and will make the distinction of a double-positive population more difficult. The amount of spread depends on the fluorochrome combination and intensity of staining, and varies greatly between pairs of fluorochrome. Careful fluorochrome choices in multicolor panel design are neccessary to avoid high-spread situations.

4.3.1 Practical Rules for Good Compensation

Compensation must be accurately calculated, then applied to the multistained experimental samples in order to correctly measure each fluorochrome/marker in its dedicated detector. Incorrect compensation will lead to errors in identification and quantification of cell populations.

To do this, single-color control tubes must be run for each color in the panel, and each tube must contain only one fluorochrome.

The following are three rules that must be adhered in order to correctly calculate the compensation corrections:

Rule #1: The single-color control must use the same fluorochrome as that used in the mix (Figure 4.5A). What appear to be similar or even identical emission spectra between fluorochomes that emit in roughly the same wavelength range, such as green FITC, GFP, and Alexa 488, are seen as quite different by the cytometer and have different spillover. Single color controls for each of these will give very different compensation values. Thus, compensation values calculated using a FITC single color applied to a tube that contains Alexa 488 or GFP will generate erroneous data.

It is particularly important when ing tandem dyes that the antibody/fluorochrome in the single-color control is exactly the same as the mix. Different lots of tandems have different coupling efficiency and thus more or less spillover into the base emission channel. Tandem breakdown over time can also give different spillover values, particularly if left out in the heat or light.

Rule #2: The positive population in the single-color control must be as bright or brighter than the most positive population in the experimental samples (Figure 4.5B). Small errors in compensation calculated on dim positive populations can lead to large errors when applied to bright populations.

Rule #3: For each single-color control, the autofluorescence of the negative population must be the same as that of the positive population (Figure 5C). Cells or beads can be used, but negative beads must be used as the control for positive beads and negative cells for positive cells. Further, negative cells of the same autofluorescence as the positive cells must be used, such as lymphocytes with lymphocytes, or monocytes with monocytes.

Good quality single-color controls are crucial for good compensation calculations, and should be run with each experiment. Either cells or antibody capture compensation beads can be used as single-color controls but must have bright well-defined positive and negative populations. Cells are ideal, but are often not available, contain very few positive cells, or have dim staining. Beads give reliable brightly stained single colors, but can occasionally give different compensation values.

Compensation is easily and accurately calculated using the automated software compensation algorithms, which are generally more accurate than compensation performed manually. Figure 4.6 shows the necessity for good compensation. The uncompensated sample shows three apparently double-positive populations. After compensation, it can be seen that two of these populations were in reality single positives that would have been misclassified.

4.3.2 Sources of Spectral Spillover

There are three main sources of spectral spillover, all of which will require compensation. The first is adjacent spectra overlap, which we've just seen in the example of FITC into PE (Figure 7A). The second and third, discussed below, are due to tandem fluorochrome to base spillover or to cross-laser excitation.

Tandem to base spillover (Figure 7B): As discussed above, fluorochrome tandem dyes, if not tightly coupled or if the coupling has degraded, will leak fluorescence directly from the base fluorochrome at its emission wavelength. Here we see spillover from the PE base moiety of the PE-Cy5 tandem into the detector dedicated to PE alone.

Cross-laser excitation (Figure 7C): The wide excitation spectra of many fluorochromes means that while the fluorochrome is best excited at the high point of the spectra by a laser that is close to that maximum, it can often be excited to a lesser degree by lasers at another wavelength. This is called cross-laser excitation. That fluorochrome will then emit into the detector dedicated to a fluorochrome, which has a

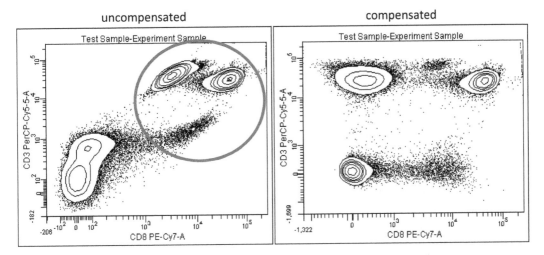

FIGURE 4.6 The value of correct compensation: The uncompensated multicolor stained sample on the left appears to show three double-positive populations. When correctly compensated, it can be seen that two of those populations are really single-positive and the true double-positive population is now visible.

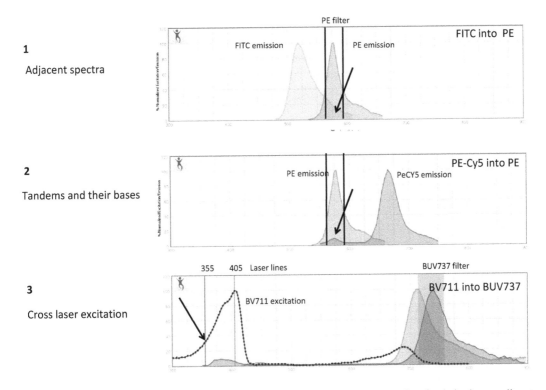

FIGURE 4.7 Three sources of spillover: A. Adjacent emission curves: spillover due to overlap of emission into an adjacent detector. Here FITC spills into the PE detector. B. Tandem to base: Spillover from a tandem dye into the detector for its base fluorochrome. Here PE-Cy5 spills into the PE detector. C. Cross-laser excitation: Fluorochromes excited by different lasers, but with similar emission spectra, will show spillover if there is some excitation by the other laser; here BV711 spills into BUV780 detector.

Spectra taken from the BioLegend Spectral Viewer website (Internet Resources).

similar emission spectra but that is maximally excited by the other laser. Here BV711, best excited by the 405 laser but also excited by 355nm UV laser, will spill over into the detector for BUV737 detector.

Spillover is additive: the more colors, the more spillover into each detector channel. Compensation can accurately correct for the spillover from all of other fluorochromes into each detector, but cannot change the amount of spread of the compensated populations. Careful fluorochrome choice is needed to avoid such problems. The amount of spread to be expected for all possible fluorochrome pairs, the "spillover spread matrix," can be easily calculated using single-color compensation controls (Nguyen et al., 2013) with third-party software such as Flowjo or FCS Express. The spillover spread matrix generated is specific for each instrument and a very useful tool in panel design.

4.4 Resolution and Background: Distinguishing Positive from Negative

Crucial in multicolor flow ctometry is the ability to resolve cell populations: the degree to which positive cells can be distinguished from negative. Figure 4.8 shows three populations: negative, dimly stained, and brightly stained cells. In Figure 4.8A the negatives are seen as a low narrow background peak, with good separation from the dimly stained positive cells. However, in Figure 4.8B the background negative peak has a wide spread and the negative cells overlap with the dim positives, making resolution more difficult. Thus, resolution is a function not only of the brightness of the positive cells, but of both the position and spread of the background negative peak (Wood, 1995; Wood, 1998; Wood and Hoffman, 1998). The width of the negative peak is dependent on electronic and optical properties of the cytometer, but also on reagent concentration, instrument settings, and spillover from other fluorochromes.

Stain Index is a practical tool that quantifies the separation of positive and negative cells (Bigos, 2007). As seen in Figure 4.9, the Stain Index is generated using a single-color control with positive and negative populations and takes into account the separation between the positive and negative peaks as well as the width of the negative peak. Stain Index can be used to determine optimal experimental conditions, as in

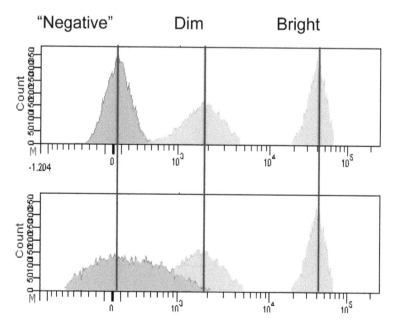

FIGURE 4.8   Resolution: Three populations or peaks are seen here: negative (background) cells, dimly stained, and brighty stained cells. In the upper panel, both the bright and dim positive populations are easily distinguished from the negative peak, which is low and narrow. In the lower panel, the position of background negative peak has widened or "spread" to a point where it overlaps with the dim peak, making discrimination of dim from negative difficult.

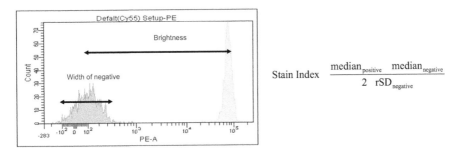

FIGURE 4.9 Stain index: Stain index calculates the resolution of positive and negative peaks using a single-color control: the distance between the medians of the positive and negative peaks divided by width (2xSD) of the negative peak.

antibody titration or voltration/gain settings described below, and to compare resolution and sensitivity between different fluorochromes on one cytometer or between cytometers.

Antibody titration: Titration of fluorochrome-labeled antibodies is essential to determine the optimal reagent concentration to maximize positivity and minimize background spread (Hulspas, 2010; Stewart and Stewart, 2001). Calculation of the Stain Index over a range of antibody concentrations will allow determination of the best antibody titer and should be performed for each new lot of antibody.

Instrument characteristics: Individual instrument characteristics are an important variable that must be taken into consideration in the design of multicolor experiments, even between instruments that are supposedly identical. Laser wavelength, laser power, instrument alignment, filter choices, and detector sensitivity all affect the accuracy and sensitivity of the different fluorochrome measurements from instrument to instrument.

Voltration: Instrument detector setup is another important factor affecting resolution and is instrument and detector specific (Maecker and Trotter, 2006; Perfetto et al., 2006, Perfetto et al., 2012; Steen, 1992). At too low a voltage or gain setting, the detector will not have the sensitivity to resolve dim positive staining. At too high a voltage or gain, the background peak will spread and overlap with dimly stained cells. Calculation of Stain Index over a range of voltages will allow determination of the best setting for each detector.

Detailed explanations and laboratory protocols for Stain Index calculation, antibody titration, and voltration can be found in Maciorowski et al. (2017).

4.5 Elements to Consider when Designing a Multicolor Panel

A number of factors (Mahnke and Roederer, 2007) should be considered in the design of a multicolor panel that impact resolution of desired populations of cells.

Fluorochrome brightness: Fluorochromes vary greatly in their intrinsic brightness, which is dependant on the amount of light energy the fluorochrome is capable of absorbing (Extinction Coefficient) and the amount of that energy it can re-emit as fluorescence (Quantum Yield). Fluorochrome choice is in large part based on brightness level. Fluorochrome comparative brightness tables can found on the web (see Internet Resources), and while these fluorochrome classifications of very bright, bright, moderate, and dim generally hold true, they are based on averages across different cytometers. Figure 4.10 lists the average relative brightness categories of some commonly used fluorochromes. You may find the relative brightness to be different on your cytometer. Comparative brightness levels for your instrument can be calculated by comparing the Stain Index generated on a series of controls stained with the same antibody clone coupled to different fluorochromes. Antibody/fluorochrome kits to do this are available commercially.

Spillover and spread: As we have seen above, spectral spillover and the ensuing spread of the compensated positive populations can cause problems in distinguishing dim double-positive cells. The spread cannot be eliminated, thus the fluorochrome combinations must be carefully chosen to avoid

Relative Fluorochrome Brightness

Very Bright	Bright	Moderate	Dim
PE	PE-Cy7	Alexa 488	FITC
BV421	PerCP-Cy5.5	BUV395	Alexa 700
PE-Cy5	BV605	BV785	APC-Cy7
APC	BV711	BV510	
PE-CF594	BUV737		
	BUV661		
	Alexa 647		

FIGURE 4.10 Fluorochrome brightness levels: Fluorochromes are grouped into brightness categories averaged across cytometers. Stain Index using single-color controls can be used to calculate fluorochrome brightness levels on your own cytometer.

situations. A spillover spread matrix (Nguyen et al., 2013) calculated for each instrument can be used to determine which combinations to avoid, which fluorochromes spill into numerous detector channels, and which channels receive a lot of spillover.

Instrument characteristics: Individual instrument characteristics will affect the fluorochrome brightness and resolution, depending on laser wavelength, laser power, alignment, collection optics and detectors, even instruments, which are supposedly identical. This can result in variations in the efficiency of excitation and emission of the fluorochromes. Know your instrument, the optimized voltage/gain settings that give you the best results, and your spillover spread matrix.

Antigen expression and density: Antigen expression patterns and levels are an important determinant in assigning fluorochromes to antigens (Mahnke and Roederer, 2007). Generally, if antigen expression is high, a weak intensity fluorochrome can be used, and if antigen expression is low, it will need a bright flurourochrome to be detected. High antigen density will increase the brightness of the positive populations as well, since more fluorochrome/antibody will be attached to the cell. A bright population will have, however, increased spillover spread into other channels compared to a dimly stained population.

Information on the expression levels of all the antigens in the desired panel should be researched in the literature. Reference articles (Kalina et al., 2019) and websites (Internet Resources: CD Maps) are available that give estimated antigen density of many commonly used antigens on multiple cell types. If the antigen of interest is rare or unknown, staining cells with the antibody coupled to a bright fluorochrome like PE can give an idea of expression level.

Antigen Coexpression: The spillover due to spread becomes problematic when there is antigen coexpression (i.e., cells are expressing two or more antigens). It is crucial to evaluate the expected expression and coexpression patterns. If coexpression exists, fluorochrome brightness, spillover, and spread must be carefully evaluated to avoid situations where spread from one fluorochrome compromises the ability to distiguish dim double positive cells. An experimental tree schema such as seen in Figure 4.11 will help identify which markers are expected to be coexpressed on the same cell and for which care must be taken.

To illustrate the importance of fluorochrome choices, Figure 4.12 shows three different fluorochrome pairs and the effect the intensity and spread has on the resolution of a dimly stained population of cells.

4.6 Multicolor Panel Design Summary

1. Know your instrument, laser, and filter configuration. Verify that the fluorochromes you are choosing are excitable by the lasers available, have appropriate optical filters for light collection, and have minimum spillover. The optical filters on an instrument can often be swapped out for a more appropriate one if necessary.

2. Optimize your instrument settings for the highest sensitivity. Know which fluorochromes are brightest on your instrument, and which combinations cause spread problems making use of a

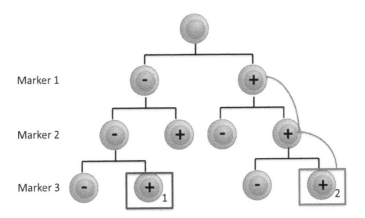

FIGURE 4.11 Antigen coexpression: Biological marker expression should be evaluated to determine how much coexpression is expected to occur on the cell populations of interest. Here, cell #1 on the left is positive only for marker 3, thus has no coexpression issues. Cell #2 on the right, however, coexpresses all of the markers, so great care must be taken in fluorochrome choice to ensure resolution if some of the markers are dim.

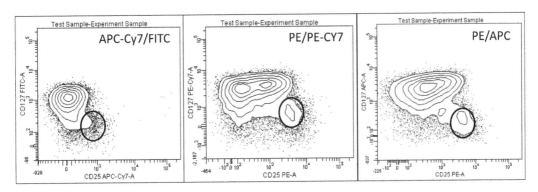

FIGURE 4.12 Fluorochrome choice effect on treg detection: Three different fluorochrome combinations to identify Tregs are seen here that show the improvement in resolution that can be gained with careful fluorochrome selection. The need to reduce background due to spillover spread is particularly important in the detection of low-density antigens such as CD25 in coexpression situations.

spillover spread matrix specific to your instrument. If you have many lasers, choosing fluorochromes spread across multiple lasers helps to reduce spillover problems.

3. Know the antigen expression levels on your cells of interest. Choose bright fluorochromes for weakly expressed antigens and dim fluorochromes for highly expressed fluorochromes.

4. Evaluate antigen coexpression. If there is no coexpression, fluorochromes can be assigned based on antigen density. If there is coexpression, evaluate which antigen is more weakly expressed and which is more highy expressed. Choose a bright fluorochrome for the weakly expressed antigen, and a dim fluorochrome for the higher expression antigen, preferably one that does not cause any spread into the weak antigen detector. Several iterations may be necessary to find the best combinations.

5. Initial panel evaluation should include many controls:
   Instrument controls: Quality control beads should be run at least once a day.
   Compensation controls: Run single-color controls with cells and beads in parallel to see which work best for each fluorochrome and determine which will be used in your experimental runs.

Gating controls to identify populations of interest.

FMO (fluorescence minus one) controls, described below, for each fluorochrome to evaluate potential artifacts.

Controls with positive and negative cells.

A test series of controls and experimental samples to evaluate potential problems or artifacts.

6. Fully test the panel to make sure the cell populations of interest are well resolved. Several iterations may be necessary to find a good working multicolor panel.

4.6.1 Experimental Controls

Once the panel has been set up and fully evaluated, controls (Hulspas et al., 2009; Maecker and Trotter, 2006) for each experiment will be necessary to ensure that the data and conclusions generated are valid and consistently reliable over time.

Instrument quality control using appropriate beads according to instrument manufacturer's recommendations must be run and recorded at least once a day, and sometimes more often if instrument problems are encountered or data looks aberrant.

Good quality compensation controls, as discussed above, are essential and should be run with each experiment, with either beads or cells as determined during panel development.

Fluorescence Minus One controls (FMO) (Perfetto et al., 2004) are the currently preferred control for identifying positive vs. negative cells. Isotype controls, even matched isotypes, are not considered acceptable, as they do not take into account spread of negative populations due to spillover from other fluorochromes. Indeed, there has been much controversy over the utility of isotype controls in flow cytometry (Keeney et al., 1998; O'Gorman and Thomas, 1999). An FMO control is stained with all of the antibodies except the one of interest for setting the gate. While it is recommended that FMOs for each color be run when developing the panel, only the markers that pose difficult (e.g., dimly stained or very small populations) may require that particular FMO for each experiment.

Biological positive and negative controls or stimulated vs. unstimulated controls may be needed (Maecker and Trotter, 2006; Cossarizza et al., 2019). Frozen aliquots of known standard or normal cells are recommended as controls for each run.

Potential artifacts should be considered and eliminated if possible. Time gating of data files will show if there are artifacts due to fluidics problems during data acquisition. Dead cell markers are recommended to eliminate false-positive dead cells. Doublet discrimination will eliminate most of the aggregates, which can mask as false positive. Fc blocks should be used in cases where cells with Fc receptors may be present. Sources and solutions for these common artifacts are covered in more detail in Maciorowski et al., 2017 and Brummelman et al., 2019. Recommendations for how to correctly display data and for publication of flow cytometry data can be found in Herzenberg et al., 2006 and Spidlen et al., 2012.

4.7 Conclusions

Multicolor flow cytometry is rapidly evolving and is now an essential technology for many disciplines, both research and clinical. Fluorochromes choices can make or break the sensitivity and accuracy of these assays. Several panel design softwares to help automate these choices are also available and evolving (Internet Resources, Panel Design Programs). They can be very helpful, but at this point are not yet capable of reliably and automatically generating a fully optimized multicolor panel. Their wide capabilities for searching commercially available antibody/fluorochrome combinations are very useful. This chapter laid out the basic theory needed to understand the elements of panel design and the steps to follow in order to develop and validate the panels. These panel design criteria apply to the current classical flow cytometers using standard optical filters to direct the fluorescence to the detectors, but also to the new full spectrum "spectral" flow cytometers now available, which offer exciting new possibilities.

REFERENCES

Bagwell, C. B., & Adams, E. G. (1993). Fluorescence spectral overlap compensation for any number of flow cytometry parameters. Ann N Y Acad Sci, 677, 167–184.

Bigos, M. (2007). Separation index: an easy-to-use metric for evaluation of different configurations on the same flow cytometer. Curr Protoc Cytom, Chapter 1, Unit1 21. doi:10.1002/0471142956.cy0121s40

Brummelman, J., Haftmann, C., Núñez, N.G. et al., 2019 Development, application and computational analysis of high-dimensional fluorescent antibody panels for single-cell flow cytometry. *Nat Protoc* 14, 1946–1969 (2019). doi:10.1038/s41596-019-0166-2

Cossarizza, A. et al (2019), Guidelines for the use of flow cytometry and cell sorting in immunological studies (second edition). Eur. J. Immunol., 49: 1457–1973. doi:10.1002/eji.201970107

Herzenberg, L. A., Tung, J., Moore, W. A., Herzenberg, L. A., & Parks, D. R. (2006). Interpreting flow cytometry data: a guide for the perplexed. Nat Immunol, 7(7), 681–685. doi:10.1038/ni0706-681

Hulspas, R. (2010). Titration of fluorochrome-conjugated antibodies for labeling cell surface markers on live cells. Curr Protoc Cytom, Chapter 6, Unit 6 29. doi:10.1002/0471142956.cy0629s54

Hulspas, R., O'Gorman, M. R., Wood, B. L., Gratama, J. W., & Sutherland, D. R. (2009). Considerations for the control of background fluorescence in clinical flow cytometry. Cytometry B Clin Cytom, 76(6), 355–364. doi:10.1002/cyto.b.20485

Kalina T., Fišer K., Pérez-Andrés M., Kuzílková D., Cuenca M., Bartol S. J. W., Blanco E., Engel P., van Zelm M. C. CD Maps-Dynamic Profiling of CD1-CD100 Surface Expression on Human Leukocyte and Lymphocyte Subsets. Front Immunol. 2019 Oct 23;10:2434. doi:10.3389/fimmu.2019.02434. PMID: 31708916; PMCID: PMC6820661.

Keeney, M., Gratama, J. W., Chin-Yee, I. H., & Sutherland, Ð. R. (1998). Isotype controls in the analysis of lymphocytes and CD34+ stem and progenitor cells by flow cytometry--time to let go! Cytometry, 34(6), 280–283.

Maciorowski, Z., Chattopadhyay, P. K., & Jain, P. (2017). Basic multicolor flow cytometry. *Current Protocols in Immunology*, 117, 5.4.1–5.4.38. doi:10.1002/cpim.26

Maecker, H. T., & Trotter, J. (2006). Flow cytometry controls, instrument setup, and the determination of positivity. Cytometry A, 69(9), 1037–1042. doi:10.1002/cyto.a.20333

Mahnke, Y. D., & Roederer, M. (2007). Optimizing a multicolor immunophenotyping assay. Clin Lab Med, 27(3), 469–485, v. doi:10.1016/j.cll.2007.05.002

Nguyen, R., Perfetto, S., Mahnke, Y. D., Chattopadhyay, P., & Roederer, M. (2013). Quantifying spillover spreading for comparing instrument performance and aiding in multicolor panel design. Cytometry A, 83(3), 306–315. doi:10.1002/cyto.a.22251

O'Gorman, M. R., & Thomas, J. (1999). Isotype controls--time to let go? Cytometry, 38(2), 78–80.

Perfetto, S. P., Ambrozak, D., Nguyen, R., Chattopadhyay, P., & Roederer, M. (2006). Quality assurance for polychromatic flow cytometry. Nat Protoc, 1(3), 1522–1530. doi:10.1038/nprot.2006.250

Perfetto, S. P., Ambrozak, D., Nguyen, R., Chattopadhyay, P. K., & Roederer, M. (2012). Quality assurance for polychromatic flow cytometry using a suite of calibration beads. Nat Protoc, 7(12), 2067–2079. doi:10.1038/nprot.2012.126

Perfetto, S. P., Chattopadhyay, P. K., & Roederer, M. (2004). Seventeen-colour flow cytometry: unravelling the immune system. Nat Rev Immunol, 4(8), 648–655. doi:10.1038/nri1416

Roederer, M. (2001). Spectral compensation for flow cytometry: visualization artifacts, limitations, and caveats. Cytometry, 45(3), 194–205. doi:10.1002/1097-0320(20011101)45:3<194::AID-CYTO1163>3.0.CO;2-C

Spidlen, J., Breuer, K., & Brinkman, R. (2012). Preparing a Minimum Information about a Flow Cytometry Experiment (MIFlowCyt) compliant manuscript using the International Society for Advancement of Cytometry (ISAC) FCS file repository (FlowRepository.org). Curr Protoc Cytom, Chapter 10, Unit 10 18. doi:10.1002/0471142956.cy1018s61

Steen, H. B. (1992). Noise, sensitivity, and resolution of flow cytometers. Cytometry, 13(8), 822–830. doi:10.1002/cyto.990130804

Stewart, C. C., & Stewart, S. J. (2001). Titering antibodies. Curr Protoc Cytom, Chapter 4, Unit 4 1. doi:10.1002/0471142956.cy0401s14

Wood, J. C. (1995). Flow cytometer performance: fluorochrome dependent sensitivity and instrument configuration. Cytometry, 22(4), 331–332. doi:10.1002/cyto.990220412

Wood, J. C. (1998). Fundamental flow cytometer properties governing sensitivity and resolution. Cytometry, 33(2), 260–266.

Wood, J. C., & Hoffman, R. A. (1998). Evaluating fluorescence sensitivity on flow cytometers: an overview. Cytometry, 33(2), 256–259.

Internet Resources

Spectral Viewers
www.biolegend.com/spectraanalyzer

BioLegend Spectral Viewer
www.bdbiosciences.com/br/research/multicolor/spectrum_viewer/index.jsp

BD Biosciences Spectral Viewer
www.thermofisher.com/fr/fr/home/life-science/cell-analysis/labeling-chemistry/fluorescence-spectravie
wer.html#

Thermofisher spectral viewer
Panel Design Programs
www.fluorish.com/

Fluorish panel design program
https://fluorofinder.com/

Fluorofinder panel design program
www.bdbiosciences.com/sg/paneldesigner/index.jsp

BD Biosciences panel design program
Fluorochrome Brightness
www.biolegend.com/brightness_index

Biolegend brightness index
http://static.bdbiosciences.com/documents/multicolor_fluorochrome_laser_chart.pdf?_ga=1.193693357.144
7862526.1480066966

BD Biosciences fluorochrome relative brightness
CD Maps: antigen expression
http://bioinformin.cesnet.cz/CDmaps/

General
The International Society for the Advancement of Cytometry (ISAC) CYTOU web site has a wealth of free
webinars on many aspect of flow and image cytometry
http://cytou.peachnewmedia.com/store/provider/custompage.php?pageid=7

5

Digital Watermarking Techniques for Medical Image Security Using the Fuzzy Analytical Hierarchy Process

Masood Ahmad, Alka Agrawal, and Raees Ahmad Khan
Department of Information Technology, Babasaheb Bhimrao Ambedkar University, Lucknow, India

Rajeev Kumar
Department of Computer Science and Engineering, Babu Banarasi Das University, Lucknow, India

5.1 Introduction

Medical image and patient data security is a strong issue at present. Network-connected devices that are accessed by doctors for the diagnosis of the patients' diseases are being trespassed by attackers. In order to diagnose a patient's disease, the data is shared over the network or is sent to the cloud-based image de-noising or processing system. Medical images contain patient information that is useful for medical analysis. If there is any alteration in the medical images, wrong diagnostics and wrong diagnosis can result and maybe even death. Hence, ensuring utmost security of medical images and maintaining the integrity, authenticity, robustness, availability, and confidentiality at the time of image sharing is a significant focus (Allaf, A. H., & Kbir, M. A., 2019). Watermarking techniques are used for providing the security of medical image. A digital watermark is a type of marker that is subtly incorporated into a signal that can tolerate noise, such as audio, video, or image data. It is often used to establish who owns the copyright to a certain signal. Digital information is "watermarked" by being concealed within a carrier signal; the concealed data should, but does not need to be, related to the carrier signal. The legitimacy or integrity of the carrier signal may be confirmed using digital watermarks, and their owners' identities may also be revealed. It is frequently used for banknote authentication and for tracking copyright violations. Different types of watermark techniques are available, such as simple watermark, joint watermark, double watermark, reversible watermark, and many more (Saini, L. K., & Shrivastava, V., 2014).

Watermark technique selection is based on different criteria. Depending on the weights of the criteria, the alternatives (e.g., various watermarking techniques) are basically represented by the linguistic values. The fuzzy AHP approach is good for determining the most appropriate watermarked technique. Moreover, this method can also help in accurate selection of the watermarked technique. Fuzzy set theory can be applied to set up Multi-based Criteria Decision Making (MCDM) problems. In this chapter, the authors used the fuzzy AHP technique for watermarking technique selection for use in medical image security. Here the different alternative ranks and weights for the alternatives are presented in fuzzy numbers.

Medical image security is imperative for every hospital and healthcare organization as the exact treatment of patients depends on patient data. In the present digital era, electronic records of patients have become easy to manage online. This also includes sharing of the data or medical images across the world for diagnosis services (e.g., telemedicine, telediagnosis, and teleconsultation) (Verma, U., & Sharma, N., 2019). The critical issues that arise at the time of image handling are security and privacy of patient data

DOI: 10.1201/9781003220404-6

against any altering through the unauthorised access of information. To maintain the privacy, authenticity, and integrity of the medical images or information, watermark techniques are used. A watermark is inserted in the hosting image and this watermark confirms that the image comes from the original source, while maintaining the integrity of the image. Classification of watermark techniques is based on the view, the embedded information, or the spatial or transform domain. A watermark is applied on the host image in the pixels in the spatial domain. This technique is easy and fast and good for embedding watermarks in images. However, watermarks can be altered easily by attackers. On the other hand, in the transform domain, a watermark is imposed on the transform conversion of the host image. Mostly people's perception is that the watermarking techniques are categorized as visible or invisible watermarks. But this is an illusion, because visible and invisible watermarks are used simultaneously. In the dual watermarked data, the invisible watermark is used as a backup for the visible watermark. All these watermarking techniques are used for medical image security and privacy. Selection of a better watermarking technique for medical image security is a difficult task for a human. However, using the MCDM methods, selection of a better watermark technique becomes easy and efficient (Alosaimi, W. et al., 2021). Selection of the techniques becomes easy using experts' opinion or the Decision Support System (DSS) designed with the aid of Fuzzy AHP (Kumar, R. et al., 2016). Fuzzy AHP is very important to evaluate the algorithm. Security algorithms have multiple criteria that affect the algorithm's performance, and it may be very difficult to choose the algorithms and rankings of the algorithms. In this chapter, we use the Fuzzy AHP method for the selection of the watermark technique.

5.2 Fuzzy Sets

Zadeh developed fuzzy set theory to correlate the ambiguities in the behaviour of humans (Alosaimi, W. et al., 2021). Fuzzy set theory allows for gradual evaluation of an element's membership in a set. This is done using a membership function with a value in the real unit range [0, 1]. Crisp set is a type of set theory in which the value is either one or zero, i.e. yes or no, whereas fuzzy set defines the value as between zero and one inclusive. Defining whether a value belongs to the set is called membership function. Traditional mathematical models cannot apply simple analysis because traditional methods cannot gives approximation results. Fuzzy set theory is widely used in place of classical theory. Fuzzy sets have the ability to reflect the real world in the results (Sahu, K. et al., 2021). Fuzzy set theory is an effective way to formulate a multi-decision making problem where the data available is subjective and imprecise.

5.2.1 Linguistic Variable

A linguistic variable is a linguistic term and general language sentence. For example, temperature is a linguistic variable if the temperature is assumed in fuzzy concept as being very hot, hot and cold, etc. (Sahu, K. et al., 2020). In place of numbers 1, 2, and 3, etc., linguistic variables provide the approximation characterization of events that are unsolved and complex. For instance, the NP-complete problems that have no solutions can be approximated by the use of linguistic variables. Linguistic approaches are used in artificial intelligence, decision support system, pattern and voice recognition, economics analysis, and medical or biomedical imaging.

5.2.2 Fuzzy Number

A fuzzy number is a generalisation of a regular, real number in that it refers to a connected collection of potential values, each of which has a weight between 0 and 1, rather than referring to a single, discrete value. These values are called the membership values. Depending on the type of problem, different fuzzy membership functions can be used. Triangular Fuzzy Numbers (TFNs) are useful in data transforming in fuzzy situations (Sahu, K. et al., 2021). In Sahu, K. et al., 2020, TFNs are used with the fuzzy AHP method. Triangular numbers can be represented as (lo, mi, up) where lo indicates the lower values, mi is the most promising value, and up is the upper (large) value in fuzzy sets as shown in Figure 1. Other operations are defined in the next section in detail.

5.2.3 Fuzzy AHP

The Analytic Hierarchy Process (AHP) was proposed by the Thomas L. Saaty. This method is used in MCDM (Zadeh, L. A. et al., 1975). The traditional AHP method does not mimic the expert's behaviour or thinking. Traditional AHP is used with crisp values to define the opinions of the experts in place of alternatives. This method creates ambiguities In the case of variant and multiple opinions and is not able to handle uncertainty In the case of pair-to-pair comparison (Sahu, K, et al., 2020). By removing these challenges, the Fuzzy Analytic Hierarchy Process (FAHP) is enlisted to remove the hierarchy issues. Fuzzy AHP gives the solution in place of a fixed solution found by decision makers. This is possible due to the fuzzy nature of the comparison procedure. Fuzzy AHP is based on membership functions. Different researchers have used different membership factions for criteria. Buckley used trapezoidal membership functions for conveying the experts' assessment of alternatives based on each criterion. Chang proposed a new methodology to tackle the fuzzy AHP by the use of triangular membership function for pair-wise testing of fuzzy AHP. this process used the degree method for counterfeit degree values of pair-wise comparison matrix (Sahu, K, et al., 2020). The methodology of fuzzy AHP can be enumerated as:

- Goal in the hierarchy should be divided in different levels of the criteria and alternative. A criterion is followed by the alternative. In this manner a hierarchy of the problem is created.
- Relationship of each criterion should be analyzed with the other criteria at the same level. Comparisons between each criterion should be made in order to make the pair-wise comparison matrix.
- Weight of each criterion is calculated.

For estimating the priority of the criterion, the first level is calculated by the weight of the criterion. Firstly, the AHP is applied to get the weights of criteria of the hierarchy.

Step 1: In this step, we converted the linguistic values into the real numbers and TFNs. In our study, we used TFN, for which the value lies between the 0 and 1 interval. The main purpose of choosing the TFN is that it is easy to calculate TFN and thus easier to achieve the fuzzy data. A fuzzy set a in the universe of information x is described by $\mu_a(x)$: X [0,1], where every component of X is mapped at interval 0 and 1. This interval is called the membership value in the X to fuzzy set a. The linguistic variables are described as: Equally needed, weakly needed, etc., and the real values are described as 1, 2,...........9. In inclusion, a TFN membership function can be calculated by Eq. (1):

$$\mu_a(x) = \{\frac{x}{mi - lo} - \frac{lo}{mi - lo} x \in [lo, mi] \frac{x}{mi - up} - \frac{u}{mi - up} x \in [mi, up] \tag{5.1}$$

In Eq. (5.1), lo represents the lower limit, mi represents the middle limit, and up is the upper limit with respect to triangular membership function as depicted in Figure 5.1.

Experts assign the numbers to the factors that affect the assessments numerically through the Saaty scale, which is represented in Table 5.1.

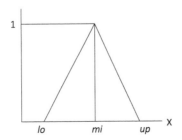

FIGURE 5.1 Triangular fuzzy numbers.

TABLE 5.1

TFN Value

Saaty value	Fuzzy Triangle value	
1	Equally needed	(1,1, 1)
3	Weakly needed	(2,3, 4)
5	Fairly needed	(4,5, 6)
7	Strongly needed	(6,7, 8)
9	Absolutely needed	(9,9, 9)
2		(1,2, 3)
4	Intermittent values between	(3,4, 5)
6	two adjacent values	(5,6, 7)
8		(7,8, 9)

From Eqs. (5.2-5.5), numeric values are converted into TFN in which loij denotes the lower limit, miij is the middle limit, and upij is the upper limit. Jijd represents the equivalent level of the numbers at interval of the two factors, which is described by experts; e, and i, j represent the pair of aspects determined by the experts. TFN [ŋij] can be calculated by:

$$\Phi_{ij} = \left(lo_{ij},\ mi_{ij},\ up_{ij}\right) \tag{5.2}$$

$$where \quad lo_{ij} \le mi_{ij} \le up_{ij}$$

$$lo_{ij} = min\left(J_{ije}\right) \tag{5.3}$$

$$mi_{ij} = \left(J_{ij1}, J_{ij2}, J_{ij3}\right)^{\frac{1}{x}} \tag{5.4}$$

$$and \quad up_{ij} = max\left(J_{ije}\right) \tag{5.5}$$

The geometric mean of the criteria is evaluated by adding and multiplying by two fuzzy sets. By the Eqs. (5.6-5.8), we have evaluated the geometric mean. Two TFN sets are as A1= (lo1, mi1, up1) and A2= (lo2, mi2, up2). The calculations on them are:

$$\left(lo_1, mi_1, up_1\right) + \left(lo_2, mi_2, up_2\right) = \left(lo_1 + lo_2, mi_1 + mi_2, up_2 + up_2\right) \tag{5.6}$$

$$\left(lo_1, mi_1, up_1\right) \times \left(lo_2, mi_2, up_2\right) = \left(lo_1 \times lo_2, mi_1 \times mi_2, up_1 \times up_2\right) \tag{5.7}$$

$$\left(lo_1, mi_{1,} up_1\right)^{-1} = \left(\frac{1}{up_1}, \frac{1}{mi_1}, \frac{1}{lo_1}\right) \tag{5.8}$$

Step 2: After getting the geometric means values for each pair of comparisons, a fuzzy pair-wise n x n matrix is designed by dividing the row and column elements by Eq. (5.9).

$$\widetilde{F^d} = \left[M_{11}^d M_{12}^d \ldots \tilde{M}_{1n}^d \tilde{M}_{21}^d \tilde{M}_{22}^d \ldots M_{2n}^d \cdots\cdots\cdots M\tilde{C}_{n2}^d \ldots \tilde{M}_{nn}^d\right] \tag{5.9}$$

In Eq. (9), $\widetilde{M_{ij}^k}$ – the eth experts promotes the ith criteria over the jth criteria. If in a given team, more than one expert is available, then the mean of the preferences of the experts are planned by the help of Eq. (5.10).

$$\tilde{M}_{ij} = \sum_{e=1}^{e} \tilde{\mathrm{M}}_{ij}^{e} \tag{5.10}$$

Step 3: In this step, we converted the pair-wise matrix to all criteria in the system by Eq. (5.11).

$$\tilde{\mathrm{F}} = \left[\widetilde{M_{11}} \dots \widetilde{M_{1n}} \cdots \ddots \cdots \tilde{\mathrm{M}} \cdots \mathrm{M}_{nn} \right] \tag{5.11}$$

After changing the pair-wise matrix, we calculated the fuzzy weights of the criteria through Eq. (5.12).

$$\tilde{p}_i = \left(\prod_{j=1}^{n} \tilde{M}_{ij} \right)^{\frac{1}{n}}, \ i = 1, 2, 3 \dots \mathrm{n} \tag{5.12}$$

Step 4: In this step, the normalized fuzzy weight of the each criteria by Eq. (13).

$$\tilde{w}_i = \tilde{p}_i \otimes \left(\tilde{p}_1 \oplus \tilde{p}_2 \oplus \tilde{p}_3 \dots \oplus \tilde{p}_n \right)^{-1} \tag{5.13}$$

Step 5: In the last stage, we calculated the defuzzification weights of the fuzzy weights by Eq. (14), and totalled the defuzzify weight. If the weight is greater than 1, then it is normalized with the help of Eq. (15). Thereafter, the weights are assigned to the rank the criteria.

$$COA(M)_i = \frac{\tilde{w}_1 \oplus \tilde{w}_2 \dots \oplus \tilde{w}_n}{n} \tag{5.14}$$

$$Nr_i = \frac{M_i}{M_1 \oplus M_2 \oplus \dots \oplus M_n} \tag{5.15}$$

5.3 The Empirical Framework

5.3.1 Criteria Selection

The first step involves the selection of the criteria. The ranking order is determined by the criteria. The most valuable step of the framework is to find the criteria and their relation with the variables used in decision making. Opting for the most relevant criterion or the attribute is also an integral aspect of the process because it through the choice of the right criteria list that the goal can be reached with accuracy. Both the selection criteria and the alternatives are based on the opinions of the experts. Here, we chose chosen five elemental attributes (IN, RO, AU, CO, COM) for algorithms in medical image security. The criteria are discussed in Figure 5.2 and are denoted as:

- IN= Integrity
- RO= Robustness
- AU= Authentication
- CO= Confidentiality
- COM= Complexity
- *Integrity* -In the data, the integrity process assures the users that information cannot be changed and modified in the entire lifecycle of the data. The conclusion is that the information cannot be altered in an undetectable way.
- *Robustness* – Robustness is the system's ability to resist against the change without changing its original shape.
- *Authentication* – Authentication is a process of verifying the users and validating if the input is arriving from the trusted source and user. This process validates the incoming data that is coming from the trusted users and valid transmission and network.

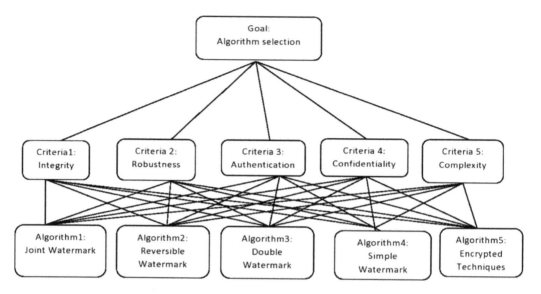

FIGURE 5.2   Medical image security algorithm and attributes.

- *Confidentiality* -Confidentiality is the process of preventing the sensitive information from unauthorized users. It enables the system to ascertain that the information can only be accessed by the authorized source.
- *Complexity* -Complexity alludes to the data size of the inputs and the necessary steps counted in completion of any operation.

All these criteria directly affect the medical image security. Each criterion affects each alternative (e.g. Integrity, Robustness, Authentication, Confidentiality, and Complexity). As mapped in Figure 2, it is evident that Integrity, Robustness, Authentication, Confidentiality, and Complexity are directly attached to each and every alternative and affect them. On the basis of criterion, we can select the best alternative that fulfils the goal and achieves the best results.

5.3.2 Results Analysis

Qualitative analysis is suitable for medical image security algorithm selection. Medical image and patient data security are of the utmost importance in the healthcare industry. Watermark techniques are used for the protection of medical images and patient data. Watermark techniques ensure the images and data remain confidential, while ensuring its integrity, authentication, and robustness. Watermark techniques are imposed on the source image and other data like video and audio without disturbing the visual quality of the image and data. Watermark techniques are classified based on time and types of watermark techniques. For the watermark algorithm selection, we used the fuzzy AHP for medical image security algorithm selection. Fuzzy AHP is a decision-based method.

5.4 Empirical Analysis

In the first step, we selected the criteria and alternatives that affect the security of the medical image. For medical image security selection algorithm, we enlisted the opinions of 10 experts from academia, hospitals, or healthcare and the industry. Experts' opinions form the input that was used to measure the security of the medical image algorithm. With the help of Eqs. (5.1-5.5), we evaluated the fuzzy triangular numbers. Through the linguistic variables, the decision makers calculate the rankings of alternatives

TABLE 5.2

Fuzzy Pair-wise Matrix

Criteria	IN	RO	AU	CO	COM
IN	1	5	4	9	7
RO	1/5	1	2	½	5
AU	¼	1/2	1	1/3	3
CO	1/9	2	3	1	3
COM	1/7	1/5	1/3	1/3	1

TABLE 5.3

Converted into TFN Matrix Form

Criteria	IN	RO	AU	CO	COM
IN	(1,1,1)	(4,5,6)	(3,4,5)	(9,9,9)	(6,7,8)
RO	(1/6,1/5,1/4)	(1,1,1)	(1,2,3)	(3,2,1)	(4,5,6)
AU	(1/5,1/41/3)	(3,2,1)	(1,1,1)	(2,3,4)	(3,4,5)
CO	(1/9,1/9,1/9)	(1,2,3)	(2,3,4)	(1,1,1)	(2,3,4)
COM	(1/8,1/7,1/6)	(1/6,1/5,1/4)	(1/4,1/3,1/2)	(1/4,1/3,1/2)	(1,1,1)

TABLE 5.4

Calculating the Geometric Mean

Criteria	Fuzzy geometric means
IN	3.650, 4.521, 4.3643
RO	1.148, 1.319, 1.350
AU	1.291, 1.430, 1.461
CO	.850, 1.148, 1.397
COM	.251, .321, .398

through the criteria and convert it into TFNs. By using the Saaty scale, Table 1 prepares the pair-wise comparison. Table 5.2 and Table 5.3 represent the pair-wise matrix and triangular pair-wise matrix.

5.4.1 Fuzzy Pair-Wise Matrix

When we get the importance of the level 1 criterion, we match i, j at the same hierarchy level and the order is assigned through the decision makers. With the help of AHP, we calculate the importance between criteria in numeric form through the scale and the scale lies between 1-9. The comparison matrix is C=Cij, if there are n criteria at the level. By using Eqs. 1-5, the pair-wise matrix is prepared as shown in Table 2.

After converting the value in matrix form, the geometric means is calculated by the Eqs. (5.6-5.8) and the normalized geometric values are obtained. Eqs. 5.6-5.8 represent the multiplication of the lower values with lower values and middle values with middle values and upper with upper. The geometric mean calculation results are given in Table 5.4.

After multiplying the inverse values of the lower middle and upper values with the geometric mean values, we get the fuzzy weights, and construct the fuzzy weights matrix by Eq. (5.9). Fuzzy weights' calculation results are tabulated in Table 5.5.

After calculating the fuzzy weights, we did the defuzzification by Centre of Area (COA) and calculated the performance values of the fuzzy weights. The defuzzification values are listed in Table 5.6.

TABLE 5.5

Calculating the Fuzzy Weights

Criteria	Fuzzy weights
IN	.394, .517, .645
RO	.124, .151, .187
AU	.139, .163, .203
CO	.091, .131, .194
COM	.027, .035, .055

TABLE 5.6

Calculating the Defuzzification Values

Criteria	Fuzzy weights	Defuzzification	Ranking
IN	.394, .517, .645	.518	1
RO	.124, .151, .187	.154	3
AU	.139, .163, .203	.168	2
CO	.091, .131, .194	.138	4
COM	.027, .035, .055	.039	5

TABLE 5.7

Normalized the Defuzzification Value

Criteria	Fuzzy weights	Defuzzification normalized values	Ranking	Medical image security Algorithms
IN	.394, .517,.645	.509	1	Joint watermark techniques
AU	.139, .163,.203	.165	2	Reversible watermark techniques
RO	.124, .151,.187	.151	3	Double watermark techniques
CO	.091, .131,.194	.135	4	Simple Watermark techniques
COM	.027,.035, .055	.038	5	Encrypted techniques

If the sum of the total weights after defuzzification is > 1, it is not acceptable and again the process is followed for the normalized defuzzification weights.

We provided the rank according to the obtained weights of the algorithm. The overall results and ranking of the algorithms are shown in Table 5.7. Integrity has the highest weight. (.509), as compared to the other criteria. The weight of the other criteria being: Authentication (.165), Robustness (.151), Confidentiality (.135), and Complexity (.038). Thus in terms of ranking, Integrity gets the highest priority among the five criteria or the attributes. In this chapter, we used only five attributes that affect the security of image and watermark technique. This method is a quantitative assessment of the security of the medical image algorithm. If it is applied on the security algorithm of the image, then the data may produce the best results.

5.5 Conclusion

The proposed fuzzy AHP method is a highly effective decision support system that eliminates all ambiguities that might occur in a MCDM process through varying opinions of the experts. The fuzzy AHP has been used here for the selection of medical image security algorithm. In fuzzy AHP, we used the linguistic variables for the empirical analysis of the criteria. Linguistic variables were converted in TFNs to form the pair-wise matrix. Thereafter, the best alternative was determined according to the obtained weights of criteria. Researchers can use this method for algorithm selection for medical image security. For further study, different multi-criteria techniques can be applied for the algorithm selection.

Acknowledgement

This work is sponsored by Council of Science & Technology, Uttar Pradesh, India under F. No. CST/D-2408.

REFERENCES

Allaf, A. H., & Kbir, M. A. (2018, October). A review of digital watermarking applications for medical image exchange security. In *The Proceedings of the Third International Conference on Smart City Applications* (pp. 472–480). Springer, Cham.

Alosaimi, W., Alharbi, A., Alyami, H., Ahmad, M., Pandey, A. K., Kumar, R., & Khan, R. A. (2021). Impact of tools and techniques for securing consultancy services. *Computer Systems Science and Engineering*, *37*(3), 347–360.

Kumar, R., Khan, S. A., & Khan, R. A. (2016). Analytical network process for software security: a design perspective. *CSI transactions on ICT*, *4*(2–4), 255–258.

Sahu, K., Alzahrani, F. A., Srivastava, R. K., & Kumar, R. (2021). Evaluating the impact of prediction techniques: software reliability perspective. *CMC-Computers Materials & Continua*, *67*(2), 1471–1488.

Sahu, K., Alzahrani, F. A., Srivastava, R. K., & Kumar, R. (2020). Hesitant fuzzy sets based symmetrical model of decision-making for estimating the durability of Web application. *Symmetry*, *12*(11), 1770.

Saini, L. K., & Shrivastava, V. (2014). A survey of digital watermarking techniques and its applications. *arXiv preprint arXiv:1407.4735*.

Verma, U., & Sharma, N. (2019). Hybrid mode of medical image watermarking to enhance robustness and imperceptibility. *Int J Innov Technol Explor Eng*, *9*(1), 351–359.

Zadeh, L. A. (1975). The concept of a linguistic variable and its application to approximate reasoning—I. *Information Sciences*, *8*(3), 199–249.

6

Limbal Stem Cell Deficiency: Concurrent Approaches and Scope of Regenerative Stem Cell Therapy and Blood Derivatives

Pragya Shukla and Seemha Rai
Centre for Stem Cell and Tissue Engineering, Panjab University, Chandigarh, India

6.1 Introduction

The cornea is our window to the world and it takes the dependency of vision by maintaining the corneal integrity and clarity (**1,58**). The cornea contains a reservoir of self-regenerating epithelial cells that are necessary for maintaining its transparency and proper vision. The study of stem cells in this functionally important organ has grown in the modern era, Partly due to the ease with which this tissue is visualized, its accessibility with minimally invasive instruction, and the fact that its stem cells are segregated within a transitional zone between two functionally diverse epithelia (**1,2,58**).

The epithelium represents one of the most rapidly regenerating mammalian tissues with full turnover over approximately 1 or 2 weeks. This robust regenerative capacity is dependent on the function of stem cells residing in the limbus, a structure that marks the border between conjunctiva and cornea (**1,58**). Limbal stem cells (LSCs) maintain the normal homeostasis and wound healing of cornea (**3**). These remain as a quiescent population with a proliferative capacity in a cell niche that in addition to LSCs contains various populations of cells (limbal stromal fibroblasts, melanocytes, and immune cells), extracellular matrix (ECM), and signalling molecules (growth factors and cytokines), which are essential for LSC maintenance, LSC-driven regeneration, and proliferation (**1,2,12,58**). The niche components are of diverse origin with a capacity of retaining the LSC population for long term and corneal restoration (**1,3,5,6,58**).

A reduction in the number of LSCs or limbal stem cell deficiency (LSCD) is a pathological condition that leads to corneal dysfunction and further opacification resulting from several extrinsic factors (chemical or thermal injuries) and intrinsic factors (reduction by clinical conditions like diabetes, dry eye disease, or persistent epithelial defects) (**1,3,4,5,6**). Thus this chapter provides a focus on updates of the current and emerging treatment strategies, the future directions in which both basic science and clinical research in this field is headed by regenerative cell therapy and blood derivatives for treating LSCD.

6.2 The Limbus and the Limbal Stem Cell Niche

6.2.1 Structural Anatomy

The human ocular surface serves the unique function of forming a resilient barrier to pathogens and environmental factors, providing metabolic requirements to the underlying stroma, and maintaining a smooth transparent optical surface. It is composed of two main tissues: the cornea and the conjunctiva (**7,62**). The anterior ocular surface is a continuous sheet of tissue that consists of the transparent cornea and the more peripherallylocated conjunctiva overlying the opaque, whitesclera. The cornea transitions into the sclera at the zone known as the corneoscleral junction or the limbus. The corneal limbus, the in

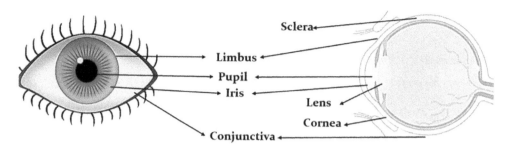

FIGURE 6.1   General parts of the eye and their locations (outer and inner).

vivo location of corneal epithelialstem cells, is the transitional region between the cornea and conjunctiva/sclera **(8,62)**. The normal corneal epithelium is composed of superficial cells, wing cells, and basal cells **(10)**. The basal layer of the limbal epithelium appears corrugated because it is arranged in rete pegs (finger-like projections of the epithelium into the stroma below), also named interpalisade rete ridges, with the upward projections of the stroma termed the palisades of Vogt **(8)**.

Stem cells are generally located in a "niche," a specific environment that provides the factors necessary to maintain the cell in its "stemness." The palisades of Vogt are the "niche" for limbal stem cells **(11)**. The palisades of Vogtare radial projections of fibrovascular tissue in spoke-like fashion around the corneal periphery **(31)**. They are concentrated in the superior and inferior limbus and contain nerves, blood vessels, and lymphatics. On biomicroscopy these projections appear as thin, gray pegs approximately 0.04 mm wide and 0.36 mm long. The surface of the limbal area where the palisades of Vogt arise remains flat **(11)**. The longstanding view has been that these rete ridges/pegs harbor the cells for corneal maintenance. **(7,16)**. A population of cells residing in the basal epithelial layer in this area has been identified as possessing the characteristics of stem cells; that is. (1) a cell with self-renewal properties (i.e., after cell division one of the daughter cells remains a stem cell); (2) the cell is undifferentiated but has differentiation ability; and (3) the cell is in an arrested state most of the time but can be stimulated to divide **(11)**. In this anatomically protected region, LESC and their progenitors, the transient amplifying cells, are clustered at the bottom of the epithelial crypts, where they maintain close contact with various supporting cell types including melanocytes and mesenchymal stromal cells (MSCs), vascular cells, and nerves across a fenestrated epithelial basement membrane **(12)**.

The epithelial crypt is a solid cord of cells that extends from the peripheral aspect of the undersurface of interpalisade rete ridges of limbal palisades of Vogt into the limbal stroma. There are up to 6 or 7 such LEC (limbal epithelial cells), variably distributed along the limbus in each human eye. The limbal stroma is an integral part of this microenvironmentas limbal epithelial SCs closely interact with cells in the underlying limbal stroma **(8,13,14)**. Limbal niche cells are another source of local mesenchymal stem cells located in the limbal Palisades of Vogt, next to limbal basal epithelial cells **(15,17,18)**.

6.2.2 Microenvironment (ECM) and Putative Biomarkers

LESCs are the smallest cells in the basal layer with a high nucleus-cytoplasm ratio **(20)**, and they express a panel of putative stem cell markers including the transporter ABCG2 **(21)**, transcription factors such as p63 **(22)** and its ΔNp63α isoform cell adhesion molecules such as integrin α9 **(21)** and N-cadherin and have a high proliferative potential in culture **(19)**. However, in prolonged limbal explant cultures cultivated on plastic plates without any scaffolds, the LMC (limbal mesenchymal cell) and putative SC (stem cell) population was determined with the simultaneous co-expression of ISCT-determined positive markers CD73/CD90/CD105 and a negative marker CD45 **(18,17)**. The limbal stem cell niche is a specialized protective anatomical location that regulates stem cell function through its interactions with extracellular matrix components and neighbouring cells via direct contact or soluble growth and signaling factors **(12)** including aquaporin 1 and vimentin **(27)**, nestin, SDF-1/CXCR4 **(28)**, and BMP/Wnt **(25,26)** and IL-6/STAT3 **(29)**. Vimentin-positive sphere-forming cells isolated from peripheral cornea expressed

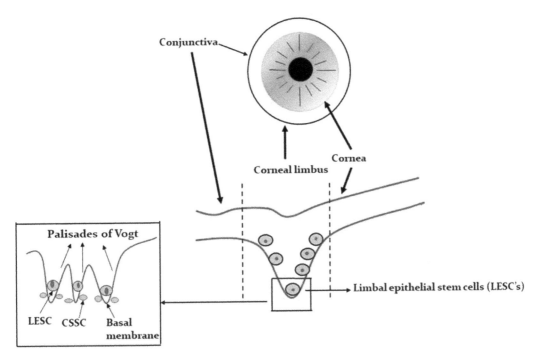

FIGURE 6.2   Location of limbus and limbal stem cells in their stem cell niche.

a potential use as transplantable elements for limbal stem cell repopulation by methods like immunocyto-chemistry (**2**).

Despite its small size, the limbus excites our interest because it maintains nourishment of the peripheral cornea; it contains the pathways of aqueous humor outflow, and it is the site of surgical incisions into the anterior chamber for cataract and glaucoma (**9**).

6.3 Etiology

Full regeneration of the entire corneal epithelium is expected when limbal SCs are intact and healthy (**32**). Dysfunction or deficiency of these LESCs either due to inherited (aniridia, congenital erythrokeratodermia) or acquired (thermal/chemical injury or chronic inflammatory) diseases disrupt corneal epithelial homeo-stasis, leading to conjunctivalisation, neovascularization, and eventually to blindness. As a result, the barrier function of the limbus is compromisedl This condition is known as limbal stem cell deficiency (LSCD) (**10,30**). Earlier, LSCD diagnosis rested primarily on history and clinical signs, with confirm-ation by histology and impression cytology (**10,30**). With the advent of in vivo laser scanning confocal microscopy (IVCM), live imaging of the corneo-limbal epithelial architecture in healthy individuals and diagnosing LSCD patients became possible (**30,33**).

6.4 Common Surgical Methods for Treating LSCD

6.4.1 Mechanical Debridement/Keratectomy and Phototherapeutic Keratectomy

Mechanical debridement, also known as superficial keratectomy/keratoepthelioplasty, is a procedure performed in a private room or an office of the clinic or hospital setting under topical anaesthesia (**34**). This can be achieved by mechanically scraping the advancing conjunctival epithelial sheet and may have to be repeated two or three times because the conjunctival epithelium migrates rapidly compared

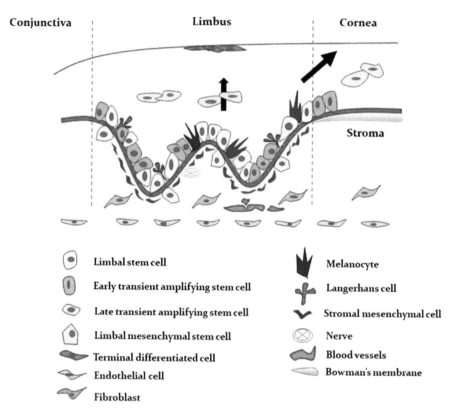

Conjunctiva   **Limbus**   **Cornea**

Stroma

- ⊙ Limbal stem cell   ❧ Melanocyte
- ◐ Early transient amplifying stem cell   ⚕ Langerhans cell
- ◒ Late transient amplifying stem cell   ⌄ Stromal mesenchymal cell
- ⬠ Limbal mesenchymal stem cell   ⊗ Nerve
- ⌒ Terminal differentiated cell   ⌒ Blood vessels
- ⌒ Endothelial cell   ⌒ Bowman's membrane
- ⌒ Fibroblast

FIGURE 6.3   Types of cells and their arrangement in limbal stem cell niche (limbal microenvironment).

TABLE 6.1

Ocular Conditions Causing Limbal Stem Cell Deficiency

Traumatic and malignant causes	Inflammatory and hereditary causes
1. Chemical or thermal burns	1. Diabetes
2. Radiation exposure	2. Aniridia
3. Multiple surgeries	3. Herpes: Simplex and zoster
4. Contact lens wear infection	4. Steven-Johnsons syndrome
5. Neoplasia	5. Mucous membrane pemphigoid
	6. Chronic limbitis

to the limbal sheets **(35)**. Mechanical debridement may be useful in conjunction with other treatment modalities, such as lubrication and topical steroids **(34)** like prednisolone acetate **(36)**. If the total corneal and limbal epithelium is lost and replaced by conjunctival epithelium, limbal (auto)transplants or keratoepithelioplasty should be considered **(35)**.

Phototherapeutic keratectomy is a safe and effective procedure in the management of superficial corneal diseases such as corneal scars, degenerations, and dystrophies **(23)**. Phototherapeutic keratectomy (PTK) using an excimer laser has been shown to remove anterior corneal scars, including those due to LSCD **(34,38)**.

6.4.2 Amniotic Membrane Transplantation

Amniotic membrane transplantation (AMT) for LSCD was first described by Kim and Tseng in 1995 (**34,37**). AMT is a safe and effective procedure to restore the corneal epithelial surface in patients with partial LSCD (**37**). Transplantation of cryo-preserved amniotic membrane has been shown to exert antiinflammatory, antiscarring, and antiangiogenic actions and to promote epithelial wound healing in ocular surface reconstruction (**38**). Several studies show that a novel matrix component termed heavy chain-hyaluronan/pentraxin 3 (HC-HA/PTX3) purified from cryopreserved AM is the active component responsible for the aforementioned AM's biological properties (**38,39,40**). HC-HA/PTX3 is formed by the tight association between pentraxin 3 (PTX3) and HC-HA, which consists of high molecular weight hyaluronic acid (HA) covalently linked to heavy chain 1 (HC1) of inter-a-trypsin inhibitor (IaI) through the catalytic action of tumor necrosis factor-stimulated gene-6 (**38,41,42**). HC-HA/PTX3 upregulates BMP signalling and downregulates Wnt signalling in LNCs to promote the quiescence of LEPCs (**38**). The main advantages of AMT are reduced risk of rejection and avoidance of donor eye complications and systemic immunosuppression. AMT requires at least partial preservation of LSCs and thus should not be utilized as the sole treatment for complete LSCD (**37**).

6.4.3 Autologous and Allograft Limbal Stem Cell Transplantation

The first successful reports of autologous limbal transplantation were by Kenyon and Tseng in 1989 (**34**). The procedure is used for unilateral LSCD, with donor limbus being harvested from the patient's healthy contralateral eye and transplanted onto the diseased eye (**34,44**). SLET is a single-stage procedure that eliminates the need for an expensive ex vivo cultivation of cells (**45**).In a SLET surgery, a small strip of donor limbal tissue (e.g., 2 × 2 mm) is divided into several smaller pieces and are spread over a HAM placed on the cornea. The long-term effectiveness of the technique has yet to be proven (**44**).

For bilateral disease, allogeneic tissues are needed as stem cell sources (**46**). The options include living-related conjunctival limbal allografts (lr-CLAL), cadaveric KLAL, combined lr-CLAL and KLAL, and ex vivo expanded limbal allograft (**46**). In this method of limbal transplantation, donor tissue is taken from either a cadaver (keratolimbal allograft, KLAL) or a living relative (HLA-matched living-related conjunctival limbal allograft, lr-CLAL), and thus may be used in patients with bilateral disease (**34**). Cadaver allograft limbal transplantation eliminates the risk of inducing LSCD in a relative's donor eye (**34**). Liang et al. (**47**) demonstrated the prevalence and threat of surface deficits and the augmentation

TABLE 6.2
Common Surgical Treatment Options for LSCD

Surgical treatment	Use for LSCD
Mechanical Debridement/keratectomy & Photographic keratectomy	1.Removes corneal conjunctivalisation. (**34,35,36**) 2. Laser therapy to improve stromal scars. (**23,34,38**)
Amniotic membrane transplant (AMT)	Surgical treatment for partial LSCD and as an adjuvant substrate for total LSCD. (**34,37,38,39,40,41,42**)
Autologous limbal stem cell transplantation	Simple limbal epithelial transplantation (SLET) for unilateral LSCD that harvests less donor tissue. (**34,43,44,45**)
Allograft limbal stem cell transplantation	lr-CLAL and KLAL for bilateral LSCD where donor tissue is taken from a living relative or cadaver. (**34,46,47**)
Cultivated limbal stem cell transplantation	Expansion of donor epithelial cells in vitro in a culture either in suspension or via biological or synthetic substrate. (**18,34,49,50,51,52,53,54,55**)

of the long-term success of KLAL for eyes with total LSCD through the application of corrective measures (46).

6.4.4 Cultivated Limbal Epithelial Stem Cells

In 1997, Pellegrini et al. described the use of autologous cultured limbal epithelial cells (CLET) for the treatment of unilateral LSCD (57,58,34). In this method, a limbal biopsy of approximately 1 x 2 mm in size is obtained from the donor eye and transferred for culturing in laboratories (52). There are two main culture methods: cell suspension culture and explant culture.

   a. **Suspension culture:** The biopsy sample taken from the limbal area is dissociated into individual cells using enzymes such as dispase, trypsin, and collagenase. These individual cells are grown in culture medium (49,50,52).
   b. **Explant culture:** The explant tissue is placed on a substrate, allowing the proliferation and growth of cells onto the substrate surface (51). These substrates include mitomycin-treated murine 3T3 cells (53,54), HAM (18), and synthetic biomaterials such as collagen and fibrin (55).

6.5 Regenerative Cell-Based Therapy by Stem Cells: The Emerging Hope

Corneal transplantation is the most frequent type of transplantation worldwide and millions of transplants are performed on a regular basis. As the population grows and people live much longer, the demand for corneal transplants will undoubtedly increase, particularly if there is a non-disruptive and steady treatment technology. This problem will be further exacerbated by the global prevalence of an increase in autoimmune diseases like diabetes and other systemic diseases, which can contribute to immune rejection and failure of the transplant.The cornea is an immune-privilege and an avascular ideal organ that is suitable for regenerative cell therapy. Hence, alternative solutions such as regenerative cell-based therapy are being explored.

6.5.1 Dental Pulp Stem Cells

Dental MSCs are unique adult MSCs, derived from the ectomesenchyme's neural cells (59). Dental pulp stem cells (DPSCs) can be found within the "cell-rich zone" of the dental pulp. Their embryonic origin derived from neural crests explains their multipotency (60). Thus, the multipotent nature of these DPSCs may be utilized in both dental and medical applications (60). Also due to their easy accessibility, high plasticity, and minimal ethical issues, they have received much attention in regenerative medicine (93,94,61). At present, the mesenchymal stem cell populations with a high proliferative capacity and multi-lineage differentiation have been isolated from dental tissues (95,96). Various sources of stem cells are derived from dental pulp cells, which are periodontal ligament stem cells (PDLSCs), human exfoliated deciduous teeth (SHEDs), dental follicle progenitor stem cells (DFPSCs), and stem cells from apical papilla (SCAPs) (60). Human immature dental pulp cells (IDPSCs) can also be diverged to corneal like epithelial cells (98).

In an animal study by Gomes et. al (60,63,64) a tissue-engineered sheet of DPSC was transplanted on the corneal bed and de-epithelialized human amniotic membrane covering was done. A healthy uniform corneal epithelium was formed after three months of healing (60).

In addition to cornea reconstruction, human PDLSCs may also be directed towards retinal progenitors having competence for photoreceptor differentiation (97,63). Adult dental pulp cells (DPCs) isolated from third molars have the capability to differentiate into keratocytes, cells of the corneal stoma. After inducing differentiation in vitro, DPCs expressed molecules characteristic of keratocytes, keratocan, and keratan sulfate proteoglycans at both the gene and the protein levels (63). In this regard, dental stem cells may represent a good alternative to BMSCs due to the ease with which they can be obtained and lack of morbidity at the donor site (63).

6.5.2 Hair Follicle Stem Cells

The mesenchymal stem cells of the dermal papilla and the connective tissue of the hair follicle are the most easily and most abundant source of cells that can differentiate to several cell lineages in vitro and in vivo if provided with appropriate conditions (**66**). The location of this original population of stem cells is termed the "bulge" and is found in the "permanent" compartment of the follicle. It is a small cluster of cells located in the basal layer of the follicle, beneath the sebaceous gland (**66**). This bulge-derived keratinocyte population is characterized by expression of a wide spectrum of cytokeratins, that is, Krt5, Krt15, Krt17, and Krt19 (**99,100,101,67**). Krt15 has been reported to be a specific SC and progenitor cell marker and has been successfully used for purification and enrichment of SC employing clonal growth on a 3T3 feeder cell layer (**102,67**). Bulge cells maintain their stem cell characteristics after propagation in vitro, thus they may ultimately be useful for tissue engineering applications (**68**).

Investigators have demonstrated the transdifferentiation potential of murine vibrissal hair follicle bulge-derived stem cells as a potential autologous stem cell source for ocular surface repair, based on their ability to assume corneal epithelial-like properties when exposed to a corneal limbus-specific microenvironment in vitro (**69**). In a study, it was shown that transdifferentiation of HFSCs (hair follicle stem cells) into cells assuming a corneal epithelial phenotype is possible when the cells are cultured in limbal fibroblast-derived conditioned medium (**102,67**). These show that hair follicle bulge-derived stem cells have the potential to reconstruct the corneal surface in a limbal stem cell-deficient murine model (**69**).

Their low immunogenicity, ease of access, and efficient differentiation all support the exploration of their potential. Thus, hair follicles are a truly unique source of cells and materials for regenerative medicine (**66**).

6.5.3 Adipose-Derived Stem Cells and Conditioned Medium

Adipose-derived stromal/stem cells (ASCs) seem to be a promising regenerative therapeutic agent due to the minimally invasive approach of their harvest and multi-lineage differentiation potential. ASCs have been reported for their pluripotency/plasticity into various cells, such as chondrocytes, osteoblasts, myocytes, adipocytes, neural cells, and epithelial cells (**121,122,123**). Therefore, their regenerative potential has been explored in the treatment of various diseases (**75**).

In a pilot clinical trial, stromal cell therapy using autologous adipose MSC was reported in treating patients with advanced keratoconus (**76**). This study evaluated a six-month safety outcome of autologous adipose MSC injection with minimal intraoperative or postoperative complications. The manifest refraction and topographic keratometry remained stable and the keratoconic eyes had improved visual function, central corneal thickness, and corneal clarity, along with new stromal collagen production (**61**). In a recent study of 2020, human ADSC-derived mesenchymal-epithelial transition (MET) progenitors generated tissue-engineered TE-MET-Epi constructs, which significantly improved the corneal epithelium recovery with efficient re-epithelialization and a more stable corneal surface, compared to other treatment arms, in a rat alkali-induced LSCD model (**77**). In another study, human corneal endothelial cells (HCECs) were isolated and cultured using a conditioned medium obtained from orbital adipose-derived stem cells (OASC-CM) in vitro. The cultured HCECs were then transplanted into rabbit and monkey corneal endothelial dysfunction models by cell injection. Findings showed that HCECs could maintain quite a good proliferative and cell-based therapeutic capacity even after 10 passages & the use of the OASC-CM not only stimulated the proliferation of HCECs in vitro but also effectively promoted their repair capacity (**78**).

Later, it was observed that a non-invasive method involving the delivery of topical administration of orbital-derived fat stem cells (OFSCs) helps in the reconstruction of ocular surface (**79**).

6.5.4 Embryonic Stem Cells and Conditioned Medium

Totipotent cells or the embryonic stem cells can be successfully linearized to corneal epithelial-like cells as they are derived during gastrulation from the inner cell mass of the blastocyst. Human embryonic stem cells (hESCs) possess the features of unlimited proliferation paired with an ability to differentiate into cells of all three embryonic germ layers (74,104,105,106,24). Embryonic stem cells (ESCs) are regarded as an attractive source of donor cells due to their pluripotency and unlimited expansion capacity in vitro and have been widely researched for retinal lineage differentiation in mice and humans (110–114,52). Transplantation of these ESC-derived cells in animal models with the degenerative retinal disease has proven to be a realistic approach to rescue visual function (107, 108, 115, 116,52).

In Ref. (24) an effective and feasible strategy for the differentiation of CEPCs from hESCs in vitro under defined conditions was established. The sorted cells expressed the LSC markers ABCG2, p63, and CK14 and formed stratified epithelioid cell sheets. These findings suggested that the differentiated cells have similar features to primary cultured hLSCs. FACS indicated that an average of 27.41% of the cells were ABCG2-positive (24). In another study, in particular, human ESC-derived retinal pigmented epithelial cells (RPE) were recently tested to treat patients suffering from degenerative retinal diseases and the visual acuities were improved in 10 out of 18 transplanted patients (107,52).

Liu et al. (118) found that treating hCECs with mouse embryonic stem cell-conditioned medium (ESC-CM) significantly enhanced the proliferation of rabbit corneal epithelial cells, rabbit conjunctival epithelial cells. In a study, findings demonstrated that 25% ESC-CM significantly enhanced the proliferative capacity of HCECs and also maintained the morphology, cell size, and biologic functions of these cells (70).

Despite these findings, human embryonic stem cells are quite a controversial source due to the ethical and religious issues and immune response they elicit (117).

6.5.5 Umbilical Cord Stem Cells

Umbilical cord-derived mesenchymal stem cells (UMSCs) from newborns are presumably young and therefore are likely to have a more potent proliferation and differentiation capability (71,72). These cells have numerous advantages over other stem cell sources as they are less immunogenic and less tumerogenic and free of ethical and religious issues. Human UMSCs, similar to other MSCs, have been shown to differentiate into chondrocytes, adipocytes, and osteocytes (119,120,73).

In a study it was found that umbilical mucin-expressing cord lining cell (CLECs) sheets planted on a HAM (human amniotic membrane) scaffold and their engraftment to rabbits expressed cells populations like that of corneal stem cells. In a recent study, it was observed that UMSC transplantation into $Col5a1^{\Delta st/\Delta st}$ mice reduced corneal opacity by re-establishing collagen fibril arrangement through the production of collagen V. Collagen V expression as a result of UMSCs reduced corneal opacity 14 days post-transplantation. Improvement in corneal opacity occurred more quickly in the control mice (post 7 days) (73).

In another study, intrastromal injection of UMSCs in lumican null mice($Lum^{-/-}$) increased corneal thickness, and reduced the corneal opacity, due to the production of keratan sulfate proteoglycans, which re-established the organization of the collagen fibrils (71,73). The advantages to the use of UMSCs is that the availability of umbilical cords from newborn babies is almost unlimited and the cells can be expanded and stored in liquid nitrogen in a tissue bank and thawed for use. However, the utilization of human UMSCs in treating disease is surprisingly rare in comparison to the use of bone marrow MSCs (71).

6.5.6 Epidermal/Epithelial Stem Cells

Concerning the epidermis, the cells are generated through proliferation that occurs only in the basal layer; therefore, stem cells must be located there. Self-renewing tissues, such as the epidermis and hair follicle, continuously generate new cells to replenish the dead squames and hairs, which are sloughed into the environment (80,65). The field of epithelial stem cells is progressing rapidly largely because of technical advances in molecular and cellular biology (80).

A cultured sheet of LSCs taken from the healthy eye can restore the corneal epithelium and a clear cornea (57,81). Focus has recently turned to the investigation of other epithelial cell types to provide an alternative source of autologous cells. There are many similarities between corneal and skin epithelia, such as a typical stratified epithelial morphology and expression of SC marker p63 (**124,82**). While both epithelia are derived from ectoderm, the eye master control gene, PAX6, initiates lens placode invagination during development, delineating ocular epithelial cells from skin epidermal keratinocytes (**81**).

An animal study indicated that skin EPSCs can partially or even fully restore a clear cornea, and the reconstructed corneal epithelium expresses the eye-specific markers KRT3, KRT12, and paired box (PAX)6 but does not express skin-specific KRT10 (**126,81,82**). The PAX6 gene is a master control gene involved in retinal development and eye formation during the embryonic development itself. Also, CEAs (cultured epidermal autografts) with prior genetic modification, such as PAX6, can re-establish a clear cornea, even after repeated corneal scraping (**125,82**). In another approach, Ouyang et al. (**125**) showed that PAX6-transduced CES (cultured epithelial sheets) can maintain a clear cornea in an animal model of LSCD, even after repeated corneal scraping over a long-term period (**81**). The above research suggests that the plasticity and regenerative capacity of EPSCs enable regeneration of epithelium in other organs (**81**).

Moreover epidermal cells are extremely easy to access and take less time and a less painful procedure for their extraction making them an excellent source to treat LSCD in humans.

6.5.7 Bone Marrow-Derived Mesenchymal Stem Cells

Studies in previous times have already shown the multi-lineage potential of bone marrow-derived mesenchymal stem cells, which have been used for treating several cardiac and neural diseases by providing them conditions to differentiate into cardiac progenitor cells or neural stem cells. These are also found to have less immune rejection in human and mice. Mesenchymal stem cells (MSCs) with regenerative and differentiation capabilities have received much attention among ophthalmologists and visual scientists as an alternative modality in the management of corneal diseases (**61**). The role of BM-MSCs has also been observed in corneal tissue regeneration (**130,131,132,133,137**).

In a study, transplantation of human bone marrow MSCs tissue-engineered on human amnion onto chemically injured rat corneas did not show any CK3-expressing human cells (**85**). The application of rabbit bone marrow MSCs, mixed in fibrin gel to rabbit corneal surface injured by alkali-burn, showed epithelial healing and CK3 expression (**138,61**). The therapeutic efficacy of transplantation of human MSCs was evaluated by systematic comparison with LSCs in a rat model. Transplantation of human MSCs on an amniotic membrane, like LSCs on an amniotic membrane, could reconstruct severely damaged rat corneal surface. Due to their easy isolation from patients and relatively easy expansion, MSCs have been tried to treat a variety of human diseases based on the idea that MSCs could become functional cells in host tissues. In this experiment, however, the expression of human keratin 3 and keratin-pan was not detected in the rat cornea transplanted with MSCs on the amniotic membrane by immunofluorescent staining (**85**). Therefore, this suggests that transdifferentiation is probably not the main mechanism of the healing effect of MSCs (**135,144**). A more important role is represented by the production of numerous trophic and growth factors that can support the growth of residual corneal epithelial cells and LSCs (**141-143**), and by the ability of MSCs to suppress the local inflammatory reaction that could impede the healing process (**140,145,84**) It is speculated that the favourable effect of bone marrow-derived MSCs may be mediated by the intercellular signalling of epidermal growth factor (EGF) (**129**). It has been suggested that EGF may be one of the most important mitogens of corneal epithelial cells (**138,139,65**). Trosan et al. showed that mice BM-MSCs cultured in corneal extracts and insulin-like growth factor-I (IGF-I) efficiently differentiate into corneal-like cells withexpression of corneal-specific markers, such as cytokeratin 12, keratocan, and lumican (**146,83**). Di et al. assayed *subconjunctival injections* of BM-MSCs in diabetic mice and reported an increased corneal epithelial cell proliferation as well as an attenuated inflammatory response mediated by tumor necrosis factor-α-stimulated gene 6 (TSG6) (**147,83**).

Demirayak et al. reported that BM-MSCs and ADASCs suspended in phosphate-buffered solution (PBS) and injected into the anterior chamber after a penetrating corneal injury in a mouse model can colonize the corneal stroma and increase the expression of keratocyte-specific markers such as keratocan, with a demonstrated increase in keratocyte density by confocal microscopy (**148,83**). By intravenous injection, MSCs have also been tested. Intravenous injection of BM-MSCs in mice after an allograft corneal transplant was able to colonize the transplanted cornea and conjunctiva (**84**). More recently, it has been discovered that bone marrow-derived MSCs are capable of differentiating into corneal epithelial-like cells, when cultured in specialized DMEM-medium (**149,43**). These findings together suggest that that BM-MSCs and tissue-specific LSCs had similar therapeutic effects. Clinical characterization of the healing process, as well as the evaluation of corneal thickness, re-epithelialization, neovascularization, and the suppression of a local inflammatory reaction, were comparable in the BM-MSC-and LSC-treated eyes (**64**).

6.6 Blood-Derived Factors for Corneal Regeneration: The Budding Potential

Blood or hemo-derived factors have been found to have great therapeutic potential for ocular surface regeneration. Serum or derived eye drops have been found as an excelling alternative. One common treatment for dry eye is artificial tears, which provide lubrication to the surface of the eye. However, artificial tears lack the biologically active components found in natural tears that are critical to the maintenance of the tear film (**86,84**). Autologous serum application for the treatment of ocular surface disease has been dated back at least to 1975 when it was used via a mobile perfusion pump to treat ocular alkali injuries (**150,87,88**). Later, in 1984, Fox et al. first described the successful use of autologous serum as an eye drop in patients with dry eye (**151,87**). The rationale for the use of autologous serum arises from its strong similarity to tears, which contains growth factors, cytokines, vitamins, and bactericidal components that provide the necessary nutritional factors to maintain cellular tropism and reduce the risk of contamination and infection during epithelial repair processes (**159**). Human serum contains substances such as epithelial growth factor (EGF), which speeds epithelial cell migration and has antiapoptotic effects (**160**) transforming growth factor β (TGF-β), which is involved in the epithelial and stromal repair process (**161,153**). Ready-made ABO-identical allogeneic serum eye drops were straightforwardly produced, quality-assured, and registered as a safe standard blood product for the treatment of certain cases of severe dry eye disease (**152**). Although most published studies reported the use of 20% autologous serum eye drops for treating many ocular surface conditions, some demonstrated good results in terms of both efficacy and safety at higher concentrations of 50–100% as well (**155,156,157,87**). Undiluted serum eye drops are also asserted to provide a higher concentration of growth factors as well as avoid possible toxicity of diluents and any contamination during the dilution process (**88,87**). In a study, it was concluded that although cord blood may have some drawbacks compared to other blood components, EGF and TGF-β content may be significantly higher in cord blood serum (**89**).

Platelets are critically important in the wound-healing process. They translocate rapidly to the wound site and adhere to the damaged tissue, initiating a healing reaction that includes the release of a variety of cytokines and growth factors (**91,84**). Platelet preparations have also been found as a therapeutic totreat corneal surfaces. Platelet alfa granules are a major source of GFs and are rich in platelet-derived growth factor (PDGF), which plays an important role in the maintenance of ocular surface and tear film stability. PDGF promotes the chemotaxis of fibroblasts, monocytes, and macrophages and stimulates the expression of TGF-β that inhibits metalloproteases and decreases inflammation (**153,90,84**). These findings prompted the use of platelet-rich plasma (PRP), platelet-rich plasma in growth factors (PRGF), and autologous plasma rich in PDGFs eye drops (PRGD) (**90,84**). PRP contains more concentrated platelets than whole blood and can be obtained via centrifugation from whole blood mixed with anticoagulant (**91**). Alio et al. (**154**) concluded that autologous PRP promoted healing of dormant corneal ulcers and was accompanied by a reduction in pain and inflammation (**91**). In a study, it was concluded that PRP eye drops are an effective, novel treatment option for chronic ocular surface disease (**91**). Autologous platelet lysate eye drops are effective on both subjective symptoms and objective findings, in the treatment of significant dry eye, in patients with primary Sjögren syndrome (**90**).

A pilot study provides evidence in favour of the use of fingerpricked autologous blood (FAB) in the treatment of severe dry eye syndrome (DES) refractory to conventional treatment. FAB presents a cheap, practical, and effective therapy that avoids the need for blood donation and specialist processing (**92**). Though potential complications of FAB therapy need to be explored further in future studies (**92**).

6.7 Discussion and Future Perspectives

Limbal stem cell deficiency (LSCD) is a widely prevalent disease identified by damage of cornea and the limbal stem cells resulting in the deterioration of corneal epithelium turnover and invasiveness of the cornea by the conjunctival epithelium. These limbal stem cells are responsible for generating a constant and unending supply of corneal epithelial cells throughout life, thus maintaining a stable and uniformly refractive corneal surface. Thesestem cells exist in an optimal micro-environment, which promotes their maintenance in an undifferentiated manner. The corneal stem cell niche is located at the limbus, in the palisades of vogt. Loss of limbal stem cell function allows colonization of the corneal surface by conjunctival epithelium. Several ocular surface disruptions with intrinsic or extrinsic insults hamper LESCs and can lead to LSCD. Millions of people worldwide are affected by corneal blindness and LSCD is one of the main causes. Current techniques allow for the harvesting of cells from the healthy donor eye to restore the ocular surface of the diseased eye with gentle acceptable risks. Stem cells are obtained from the autologous sources to treat unilateral LSCD.

Even though significant progress has been made to improve the prognosis of patients with bilateral LSCD with the currently available surgical techniques, still these patients require a regimen of systemic immunosuppression. Even when adequate therapy is selected for the right patient, there are some patients where the regenerated epithelium does well long term while in others it only survives for a few years. Hence, why transplanted LSC cells fail to maintain a clear epithelium over the long term is a question that remains unanswered. For this reason, regenerative stem cell therapy and new culturing techniques are bound to play a significant role in the future. Over the past years, several stem cell sources have been suggested for the treatment of ocular surface disorders.

The facts and studies that prove that LSCD can be treated by several stem cell types are giving clinical success. More stem cell sources and factors particularly being involved in reconstruction of corneal surface can be identified in future and this is an exciting avenue for researchers.

Blood-derived factors for treating corneal surface regeneration are the upcoming and emerging alternatives. Eye drops prepared from these factors are now becoming a well-liked and a publicly accepted source to treat ocular surface diseases. These have been found to be rich in growth factors, cytokines, vitamins, and minerals, which are vital for maintaining corneal epithelial homeostasis. Such recent signs of progress lead us to the conclusion that the quest of understanding limbal epithelial stem cell biology and therapy has built foundations for novel therapies.

However, despite the successful repopulation and rehabilitation that has been observed with these emerging methods they do come with their drawbacks inclusive of no standardized manufacturing and application protocols. The need of the hour is to generate safe and stable methods for the use of regenerative stem cell therapy and the use of hemoderivatives to develop non-immunogenic tissues eliminating the need for systemic immunosuppression.

REFERENCES

1. Ahmad S. (2012). Concise review: limbal stem cell deficiency, dysfunction, and distress. *Stem Cells Translational Medicine, 1*(2), 110–115. https://doi.org/10.5966/sctm.2011-0037
2. Li, W., Hayashida, Y., Chen, Y. T., & Tseng, S. C. (2007). Niche regulation of corneal epithelial stem cells at the limbus. *Cell Research, 17*(1), 26–36. https://doi.org/10.1038/sj.cr.7310137
3. Medical Advisory Secretariat (2008). Limbal stem cell transplantation: an evidence-based analysis. *Ontario Health Technology Assessment Series, 8*(7), 1–58.
4. Bakhtiari, P., & Djalilian, A. (2010). Update on limbal stem cell transplantation. *Middle East African Journal of Ophthalmology, 17*(1), 9–14. https://doi.org/10.4103/0974-9233.61211
5. Ebrahimi, M., Taghi-Abadi, E., & Baharvand, H. (2009). Limbal stem cells in review. *Journal of Ophthalmic & Vision Research, 4*(1), 40–58.
6. Sangwan, V. S. (2001). Limbal stem cells in health and disease. *Bioscience Reports, 21*(4), 385–405. https://doi.org/10.1023/a:1017935624867
7. Amescua, G., Atallah, M., Palioura, S., & Perez, V. (2016). Limbal stem cell transplantation: current perspectives. *Clinical Ophthalmology*, 593. https://doi.org/10.2147/opth.s83676

8. Mathan, J., Ismail, S., McGhee, J., McGhee, C., & Sherwin, T. (2016). Sphere-forming cells from peripheral cornea demonstrate the ability to repopulate the ocular surface. *Stem Cell Research & Therapy*, *7*(1). https://doi.org/10.1186/s13287-016-0339-7

9. Van Buskirk, E. (1989). The anatomy of the limbus. *Eye*, *3*(2), 101–108. https://doi.org/10.1038/eye.1989.16

10. Le, Q., Xu, J., Deng, S.X. The diagnosis of limbal stem cell deficiency. *Ocul Surf.* 2018;16(1):58-69. https://doi.org/10.1016/j.jtos.2017.11.002

11. Remington, L.A. *Clinical Anatomy and Physiology of the Visual System.* St. Louis: Butterworth-Heineman, 2012.

12. Polisetti, N., Zenkel, M., Menzel-Severing, J., Kruse, F., & Schlötzer-Schrehardt, U. (2015). Cell adhesion molecules and stem cell-niche-interactions in the limbal stem cell niche. *Stem Cells*, *34*(1), 203–219. https://doi.org/10.1002/stem.2191

13. Xie, H., Chen, S., Li, G., & Tseng, S. (2012). Isolation and expansion of human limbal stromal niche cells. *Investigative Opthalmology & Visual Science*, *53*(1), 279. https://doi.org/10.1167/iovs.11-8441

14. Kulkarni, B., Tighe, P., Mohammed, I., Yeung, A., Powe, D., & Hopkinson, A. et al. (2010). Comparative transcriptional profiling of the limbal epithelial crypt demonstrates its putative stem cell niche characteristics. *BMC Genomics*, *11*(1), 526. https://doi.org/10.1186/1471-2164-11-526

15. Dua, H. (2005). Limbal epithelial crypts: a novel anatomical structure and a putative limbal stem cell niche. *British Journal of Ophthalmology*, *89*(5), 529–532. https://doi.org/10.1136/bjo.2004.049742

16. Mariappan, I., Kacham, S., Purushotham, J., Maddileti, S., Siamwala, J., & Sangwan, V. (2014). Spatial Distribution of Niche and Stem Cells in Ex Vivo Human Limbal Cultures. *Stem Cells Translational Medicine*, *3*(11), 1331–1341 https://doi.org/10.5966/sctm.2014-0120

17. Guo, P., Sun, H., Zhang, Y., Tighe, S., Chen, S., & Su, C. et al. (2018). Limbal niche cells are a potent resource of adult mesenchymal progenitors. *Journal of Cellular and Molecular Medicine*, *22*(7), 3315–3322. https://doi.org/10.1111/jcmm.13635

18. Lužnik, Z., Hawlina, M., Maličev, E., Bertolin, M., Kopitar, A., & Ihan, A. et al. (2016). Effect of cryopreserved amniotic membrane orientation on the expression of limbal mesenchymal and epithelial stem cell markers in prolonged limbal explant cultures. *PLOS ONE*, *11*(10), e0164408. https://doi.org/10.1371/journal.pone.0164408

19. Dziasko, M., Armer, H., Levis, H., Shortt, A., Tuft, S., & Daniels, J. (2014). Localisation of epithelial cells capable of holoclone formation in vitro and direct interaction with stromal cells in the native human limbal crypt. *PLOS ONE*, *9*(4), e94283. https://doi.org/10.1371/journal.pone.0094283

20. Romano, A. C., Espana, E. M., Yoo, S. H., Budak, M. T., Wolosin, J. M., & Tseng, S. C. (2003). Different cell sizes in human limbal and central corneal basal epithelia measured by confocal microscopy and flow cytometry. *Investigative Ophthalmology & Visual Science*, *44*(12), 5125–5129. https://doi.org/10.1167/iovs.03-0628

21. Chen, Z., de Paiva, C. S., Luo, L., Kretzer, F. L., Pflugfelder, S. C., & Li, D. Q. (2004). Characterization of putative stem cell phenotype in human limbal epithelia. *Stem Cells (Dayton, Ohio)*, *22*(3), 355–366. https://doi.org/10.1634/stemcells.22-3-355

22. Cotsarelis, G., Kaur, P., Dhouailly, D., Hengge, U., & Bickenbach, J. (1999). Epithelial stem cells in the skin: definition, markers, localization and functions. *Experimental Dermatology*, *8*(1), 80–88. https://doi.org/10.1111/j.1600-0625.1999.tb00351.x

23. Rathi, V. M., Vyas, S. P., & Sangwan, V. S. (2012). Phototherapeutic keratectomy. *Indian Journal of Ophthalmology*, *60*(1), 5–14. https://doi.org/10.4103/0301-4738.91335

24. Zhang, C., Du, L., Pang, K., & Wu, X. (2017). Differentiation of human embryonic stem cells into corneal epithelial progenitor cells under defined conditions. *PLOS ONE*, *12*(8), e0183303. https://doi.org/10.1371/journal.pone.0183303

25. Han, B., Chen, S. Y., Zhu, Y. T., & Tseng, S. C. (2014). Integration of BMP/Wnt signaling to control clonal growth of limbal epithelial progenitor cells by niche cells. *Stem Cell Research*, *12*(2), 562–573. https://doi.org/10.1016/j.scr.2014.01.003

26. Chen, S. Y., Han, B., Zhu, Y. T., Mahabole, M., Huang, J., Beebe, D. C., & Tseng, S. C. (2015). HC-HA/PTX3 purified from amniotic membrane promotes BMP signaling in limbal niche cells to maintain quiescence of limbal epithelial progenitor/stem cells. *Stem Cells (Dayton, Ohio)*, *33*(11), 3341–3355. https://doi.org/10.1002/stem.2091

27. Higa, K., Kato, N., Yoshida, S., Ogawa, Y., Shimazaki, J., Tsubota, K., & Shimmura, S. (2013). Aquaporin 1-positive stromal niche-like cells directly interact with N-cadherin-positive clusters in the basal limbal epithelium. *Stem Cell Research, 10*(2), 147–155. https://doi.org/10.1016/j.scr.2012.11.001

28. Xie, H. T., Chen, S. Y., Li, G. G., & Tseng, S. C. (2011). Limbal epithelial stem/progenitor cells attract stromal niche cells by SDF-1/CXCR4 signaling to prevent differentiation. *Stem Cells (Dayton, Ohio), 29*(11), 1874–1885. https://doi.org/10.1002/stem.743

29. Notara, M., Shortt, A. J., Galatowicz, G., Calder, V., & Daniels, J. T. (2010). IL6 and the human limbal stem cell niche: a mediator of epithelial-stromal interaction. *Stem Cell Research, 5*(3), 188–200. https://doi.org/10.1016/j.scr.2010.07.002

30. Guo, Z. H., Zhang, W., Jia, Y., Liu, Q. X., Li, Z. F., & Lin, J. S. (2018). An insight into the difficulties in the discovery of specific biomarkers of limbal stem cells. *International Journal of Molecular Sciences, 19*(7), 1982. https://doi.org/10.3390/ijms19071982

31. Castro-Muñozledo F. (2013). Review: corneal epithelial stem cells, their niche and wound healing. *Molecular Vision, 19*, 1600–1613.

32. Tseng, S. C., He, H., Zhang, S., & Chen, S. Y. (2016). Niche regulation of limbal epithelial stem cells: Relationship between inflammation and regeneration. *The Ocular Surface, 14*(2), 100–112. https://doi.org/10.1016/j.jtos.2015.12.002

33. Mathews, S., Chidambaram, J. D., Lanjewar, S., Mascarenhas, J., Prajna, N. V., Muthukkaruppan, V., & Chidambaranathan, G. P. (2015). In vivo confocal microscopic analysis of normal human anterior limbal stroma. *Cornea, 34*(4), 464–470. https://doi.org/10.1097/ICO.0000000000000369

34. Rossen, J., Amram, A., Milani, B., Park, D., Harthan, J., Joslin, C., McMahon, T., & Djalilian, A. (2016). Contact lens-induced limbal stem cell deficiency. *The Ocular Surface, 14*(4), 419–434. https://doi.org/10.1016/j.jtos.2016.06.003

35. Dua H. S. (1998). The conjunctiva in corneal epithelial wound healing. *The British Journal of Ophthalmology, 82*(12), 1407–1411. https://doi.org/10.1136/bjo.82.12.1407

36. Aras, C., Ozdamar, A., Aktunç, R., & Erçikan, C. (1998). The effects of topical steroids on refractive outcome and corneal haze, thickness, and curvature after photorefractive keratectomy with a 6.0-mm ablation diameter. *Ophthalmic Surgery and Lasers, 29*(8), 621–627.

37. Anderson, D. F., Ellies, P., Pires, R. T., & Tseng, S. C. (2001). Amniotic membrane transplantation for partial limbal stem cell deficiency. *The British Journal of Ophthalmology, 85*(5), 567–575. https://doi.org/10.1136/bjo.85.5.567

38. Stem, M. S., & Hood, C. T. (2015). Salzmann nodular degeneration associated with epithelial ingrowth after LASIK treated with superficial keratectomy. *BMJ Case Reports, 2015*, bcr2014207776. https://doi.org/10.1136/bcr-2014-207776

39. Le, Q., & Deng, S. X. (2019). The application of human amniotic membrane in the surgical management of limbal stem cell deficiency. *The Ocular Surface, 17*(2), 221–229. https://doi.org/10.1016/j.jtos.2019.01.003

40. Tseng S. C. (2016). HC-HA/PTX3 Purified from amniotic membrane as novel regenerative matrix: Insight into relationship between inflammation and regeneration. *Investigative Ophthalmology & Visual Science, 57*(5), ORSFh1–ORSFh8. https://doi.org/10.1167/iovs.15-17637

41. He, H., Li, W., Tseng, D. Y., Zhang, S., Chen, S. Y., Day, A. J., & Tseng, S. C. (2009). Biochemical characterization and function of complexes formed by hyaluronan and the heavy chains of inter-alpha-inhibitor (HC*HA) purified from extracts of human amniotic membrane. *The Journal of Biological Chemistry, 284*(30), 20136–20146. https://doi.org/10.1074/jbc.M109.021881

42. Zhang, S., Zhu, Y. T., Chen, S. Y., He, H., & Tseng, S. C. (2014). Constitutive expression of pentraxin 3 (PTX3) protein by human amniotic membrane cells leads to formation of the heavy chain (HC)-hyaluronan (HA)-PTX3 complex. *The Journal of Biological Chemistry, 289*(19), 13531–13542. https://doi.org/10.1074/jbc.M113.525287

43. Haagdorens, M., Van Acker, S. I., Van Gerwen, V., Ní Dhubhghaill, S., Koppen, C., Tassignon, M. J., & Zakaria, N. (2016). Limbal stem cell deficiency: Current treatment options and emerging therapies. *Stem Cells International, 2016*, 9798374. https://doi.org/10.1155/2016/9798374

44. Jackson, C. J., Myklebust Ernø, I. T., Ringstad, H., Tønseth, K. A., Dartt, D. A., & Utheim, T. P. (2020). Simple limbal epithelial transplantation: Current status and future perspectives. *Stem Cells Translational Medicine, 9*(3), 316–327. https://doi.org/10.1002/sctm.19-0203

45. Vazirani, J., Basu, S., & Sangwan, V. (2013). Successful simple limbal epithelial transplantation (SLET) in lime injury-induced limbal stem cell deficiency with ocular surface granuloma. *BMJ Case Reports*, *2013*, bcr2013009405. https://doi.org/10.1136/bcr-2013-009405

46. Krysik, K., Dobrowolski, D., Tarnawska, D., Wylegala, E., & Lyssek-Boroń, A. (2020). Long-term outcomes of allogeneic ocular surface reconstruction: Keratolimbal allograft (KLAL) followed by penetrating keratoplasty (PK). *Journal of Ophthalmology*, *2020*, 5189179. https://doi.org/10.1155/2020/5189179

47. Liang, L., Sheha, H., & Tseng, S. C. (2009). Long-term outcomes of keratolimbal allograft for total limbal stem cell deficiency using combined immunosuppressive agents and correction of ocular surface deficits. *Archives of Ophthalmology (Chicago, Ill.: 1960)*, *127*(11), 1428–1434. https://doi.org/10.1001/archophthalmol.2009.263

48. Chew H. F. (2011). Limbal stem cell disease: Treatment and advances in technology. *Saudi Journal of Ophthalmology: Official Journal of the Saudi Ophthalmological Society*, *25*(3), 213–218. https://doi.org/10.1016/j.sjopt.2011.04.012

49. Koizumi, N., Cooper, L. J., Fullwood, N. J., Nakamura, T., Inoki, K., Tsuzuki, M., & Kinoshita, S. (2002). An evaluation of cultivated corneal limbal epithelial cells, using cell-suspension culture. *Investigative Ophthalmology & Visual Science*, *43*(7), 2114–2121.

50. Zhang, X., Sun, H., Tang, X., Ji, J., Li, X., Sun, J., Ma, Z., Yuan, J., & Han, Z. C. (2005). Comparison of cell-suspension and explant culture of rabbit limbal epithelial cells. *Experimental Eye Research*, *80*(2), 227–233. https://doi.org/10.1016/j.exer.2004.09.005

51. Selver, O. B., Barash, A., Ahmed, M., & Wolosin, J. M. (2011). ABCG2-dependent dye exclusion activity and clonal potential in epithelial cells continuously growing for 1 month from limbal explants. *Investigative Ophthalmology & Visual Science*, *52*(7), 4330–4337. https://doi.org/10.1167/iovs.10-5897

52. Qu, Z., Guan, Y., Cui, L., Song, J., Gu, J., Zhao, H., Xu, L., Lu, L., Jin, Y., & Xu, G. T. (2015). Transplantation of rat embryonic stem cell-derived retinal progenitor cells preserves the retinal structure and function in rat retinal degeneration. *Stem Cell Research & Therapy*, *6*, 219. https://doi.org/10.1186/s13287-015-0207-x

53. Sharma, S. M., Fuchsluger, T., Ahmad, S., Katikireddy, K. R., Armant, M., Dana, R., & Jurkunas, U. V. (2012). Comparative analysis of human-derived feeder layers with 3T3 fibroblasts for the ex vivo expansion of human limbal and oral epithelium. *Stem Cell Reviews and Reports*, *8*(3), 696–705. https://doi.org/10.1007/s12015-011-9319-6

54. Schwab, I. R., Johnson, N. T., & Harkin, D. G. (2006). Inherent risks associated with manufacture of bioengineered ocular surface tissue. *Archives of Ophthalmology (Chicago, Ill.: 1960)*, *124*(12), 1734–1740. https://doi.org/10.1001/archopht.124.12.1734

55. Sasamoto, Y., Ksander, B. R., Frank, M. H., & Frank, N. Y. (2018). Repairing the corneal epithelium using limbal stem cells or alternative cell-based therapies. *Expert Opinion on Biological Therapy*, *18*(5), 505–513. https://doi.org/10.1080/14712598.2018.1443442

56. Barut Selver, Ö., Yağcı, A., Eğrilmez, S., Gürdal, M., Palamar, M., Çavuşoğlu, T., Ateş, U., Veral, A., Güven, Ç., & Wolosin, J. M. (2017). Limbal Stem Cell Deficiency and Treatment with Stem Cell Transplantation. *Turkish Journal of Ophthalmology*, *47*(5), 285–291. https://doi.org/10.4274/tjo.72593

57. Pellegrini, G., Traverso, C. E., Franzi, A. T., Zingirian, M., Cancedda, R., & De Luca, M. (1997). Long-term restoration of damaged corneal surfaces with autologous cultivated corneal epithelium. *Lancet (London, England)*, *349*(9057), 990–993. https://doi.org/10.1016/S0140-6736(96)11188-0

58. Gonzalez, G., Sasamoto, Y., Ksander, B. R., Frank, M. H., & Frank, N. Y. (2018). Limbal stem cells: identity, developmental origin, and therapeutic potential. *Wiley Interdisciplinary Reviews. Developmental Biology*, *7*(2), 10.1002/wdev.303. https://doi.org/10.1002/wdev.303

59. El Moshy, S., Radwan, I. A., Rady, D., Abbass, M., El-Rashidy, A. A., Sadek, K. M., Dörfer, C. E., & Fawzy El-Sayed, K. M. (2020). Dental stem cell-derived secretome/conditioned medium: The future for regenerative therapeutic applications. *Stem Cells International*, *2020*, 7593402. https://doi.org/10.1155/2020/7593402

60. Kabir, R., Gupta, M., Aggarwal, A., Sharma, D., Sarin, A., & Kola, M. Z. (2014). Imperative role of dental pulp stem cells in regenerative therapies: A systematic review. *Nigerian Journal of Surgery: Official Publication of the Nigerian Surgical Research Society*, *20*(1), 1–8. https://doi.org/10.4103/1117-6806.127092

61. Mansoor, H., Ong, H. S., Riau, A. K., Stanzel, T. P., Mehta, J. S., & Yam, G. H. (2019). Current trends and future perspective of mesenchymal stem cells and exosomes in corneal diseases. *International Journal of Molecular Sciences*, *20*(12), 2853. https://doi.org/10.3390/ijms20122853

62. Barrera, V., Troughton, L. D., Iorio, V., Liu, S., Oyewole, O., Sheridan, C. M., & Hamill, K. J. (2018). Differential distribution of laminin n-terminus α31 across the ocular surface: Implications for corneal wound repair. *Investigative Ophthalmology & Visual Science*, *59*(10), 4082–4093. https://doi.org/10.1167/iovs.18-24037

63. Park, Y. J., Cha, S., & Park, Y. S. (2016). Regenerative applications using tooth derived stem cells in other than tooth regeneration: A literature review. *Stem Cells International*, *2016*, 9305986. https://doi.org/10.1155/2016/9305986

64. Holan, V., Trosan, P., Cejka, C., Javorkova, E., Zajicova, A., Hermankova, B., Chudickova, M., & Cejkova, J. (2015). A comparative study of the therapeutic potential of mesenchymal stem cells and limbal epithelial stem cells for ocular surface reconstruction. *Stem Cells Translational Medicine*, *4*(9), 1052–1063. https://doi.org/10.5966/sctm.2015-0039

65. Sehic, A., Utheim, Ø. A., Ommundsen, K., & Utheim, T. P. (2015). Pre-clinical cell-based therapy for limbal stem cell deficiency. *Journal of Functional Biomaterials*, *6*(3), 863–888. https://doi.org/10.3390/jfb6030863

66. Kiani, M. T., Higgins, C. A., & Almquist, B. D. (2018). The hair follicle: An underutilized source of cells and materials for regenerative medicine. *ACS Biomaterials Science & Engineering*, *4*(4), 1193–1207. https://doi.org/10.1021/acsbiomaterials.7b00072

67. Meyer-Blazejewska, E. A., Call, M. K., Yamanaka, O., Liu, H., Schlötzer-Schrehardt, U., Kruse, F. E., & Kao, W. W. (2011). From hair to cornea: toward the therapeutic use of hair follicle-derived stem cells in the treatment of limbal stem cell deficiency. *Stem Cells (Dayton, Ohio)*, *29*(1), 57–66. https://doi.org/10.1002/stem.550

68. Richardson, G. D., Arnott, E. C., Whitehouse, C. J., Lawrence, C. M., Reynolds, A. J., Hole, N., & Jahoda, C. A. (2005). Plasticity of rodent and human hair follicle dermal cells: implications for cell therapy and tissue engineering. *The Journal of Investigative Dermatology. Symposium Proceedings*, *10*(3), 180–183. https://doi.org/10.1111/j.1087-0024.2005.10101.x

69. Bains, K. K., Fukuoka, H., Hammond, G. M., Sotozono, C., & Quantock, A. J. (2019). Recovering vision in corneal epithelial stem cell deficient eyes. *Contact Lens & Anterior Eye: The Journal of the British Contact Lens Association*, *42*(4), 350–358. https://doi.org/10.1016/j.clae.2019.04.006

70. Lu, X., Chen, D., Liu, Z., Li, C., Liu, Y., Zhou, J., Wan, P., Mou, Y. G., & Wang, Z. (2010). Enhanced survival in vitro of human corneal endothelial cells using mouse embryonic stem cell conditioned medium. *Molecular Vision*, *16*, 611–622. https://doi.org/10.1167/2.7.611

71. Liu, H., Zhang, J., Liu, C. Y., Wang, I. J., Sieber, M., Chang, J., Jester, J. V., & Kao, W. W. (2010). Cell therapy of congenital corneal diseases with umbilical mesenchymal stem cells: lumican null mice. *PLOS ONE*, *5*(5), e10707. https://doi.org/10.1371/journal.pone.0010707

72. Saleh, R., & Reza, H. M. (2017). Short review on human umbilical cord lining epithelial cells and their potential clinical applications. *Stem Cell Research & Therapy*, *8*(1), 222. https://doi.org/10.1186/s13287-017-0679-y

73. Call, M., Elzarka, M., Kunesh, M., Hura, N., Birk, D. E., & Kao, W. W. (2019). Therapeutic efficacy of mesenchymal stem cells for the treatment of congenital and acquired corneal opacity. *Molecular Vision*, *25*, 415–426.

74. Garzón, I., Martín-Piedra, M. A., Alfonso-Rodríguez, C., González-Andrades, M., Carriel, V., Martínez-Gómez, C., Campos, A., & Alaminos, M. (2014). Generation of a biomimetic human artificial cornea model using Wharton's jelly mesenchymal stem cells. *Investigative Ophthalmology & Visual Science*, *55*(7), 4073–4083. https://doi.org/10.1167/iovs.14-14304

75. Dubey, N. K., Mishra, V. K., Dubey, R., Deng, Y. H., Tsai, F. C., & Deng, W. P. (2018). Revisiting the advances in isolation, characterization and secretome of adipose-derived stromal/stem cells. *International Journal of Molecular Sciences*, *19*(8), 2200. https://doi.org/10.3390/ijms19082200

76. Alió Del Barrio, J. L., El Zarif, M., de Miguel, M. P., Azaar, A., Makdissy, N., Harb, W., El Achkar, I., Arnalich-Montiel, F., & Alió, J. L. (2017). Cellular therapy with human autologous adipose-derived adult stem cells for advanced keratoconus. *Cornea*, *36*(8), 952–960. https://doi.org/10.1097/ICO.0000000000001228

77. Bandeira, F., Goh, T. W., Setiawan, M., Yam, G. H., & Mehta, J. S. (2020). Cellular therapy of corneal epithelial defect by adipose mesenchymal stem cell-derived epithelial progenitors. *Stem Cell Research & Therapy*, *11*(1), 14. https://doi.org/10.1186/s13287-019-1533-1

78. Sun, P., Shen, L., Zhang, C., Du, L., & Wu, X. (2017). Promoting the expansion and function of human corneal endothelial cells with an orbital adipose-derived stem cell-conditioned medium. *Stem Cell Research & Therapy*, *8*(1), 287. https://doi.org/10.1186/s13287-017-0737-5

79. Lin, K. J., Loi, M. X., Lien, G. S., Cheng, C. F., Pao, H. Y., Chang, Y. C., Ji, A. T., & Ho, J. H. (2013). Topical administration of orbital fat-derived stem cells promotes corneal tissue regeneration. *Stem Cell Research & Therapy*, *4*(3), 72. https://doi.org/10.1186/scrt223

80. Cotsarelis G. (2006). Epithelial stem cells: a folliculocentric view. *The Journal of Investigative Dermatology*, *126*(7), 1459–1468. https://doi.org/10.1038/sj.jid.5700376

81. Jackson, C. J., Tønseth, K. A., & Utheim, T. P. (2017). Cultured epidermal stem cells in regenerative medicine. *Stem Cell Research & Therapy*, *8*(1), 155. https://doi.org/10.1186/s13287-017-0587-1

82. Yang, R., Liu, F., Wang, J., Chen, X., Xie, J., & Xiong, K. (2019). Epidermal stem cells in wound healing and their clinical applications. *Stem Cell Research & Therapy*, *10*(1), 229. https://doi.org/10.1186/s13287-019-1312-z

83. Alió Del Barrio, J. L., & Alió, J. L. (2018). Cellular therapy of the corneal stroma: a new type of corneal surgery for keratoconus and corneal dystrophies. *Eye and Vision (London, England)*, *5*, 28. https://doi.org/10.1186/s40662-018-0122-1

84. Liu, L., Hartwig, D., Harloff, S., Herminghaus, P., Wedel, T., Kasper, K., & Geerling, G. (2006). Corneal epitheliotrophic capacity of three different blood-derived preparations. *Investigative Ophthalmology & Visual Science*, *47*(6), 2438–2444. https://doi.org/10.1167/iovs.05-0876

85. Ma, Y., Xu, Y., Xiao, Z., Yang, W., Zhang, C., Song, E., Du, Y., & Li, L. (2006). Reconstruction of chemically burned rat corneal surface by bone marrow-derived human mesenchymal stem cells. *Stem Cells (Dayton, Ohio)*, *24*(2), 315–321. https://doi.org/10.1634/stemcells.2005-0046

86. Rauz, S., Koay, S. Y., Foot, B., Kaye, S. B., Figueiredo, F., Burdon, M. A., Dancey, E., Chandrasekar, A., & Lomas, R. (2018). The Royal College of Ophthalmologists guidelines on serum eye drops for the treatment of severe ocular surface disease: executive summary. *Eye (London, England)*, *32*(1), 44–48. https://doi.org/10.1038/eye.2017.208

87. Lekhanont, K., Jongkhajornpong, P., Choubtum, L., & Chuckpaiwong, V. (2013). Topical 100% serum eye drops for treating corneal epithelial defect after ocular surgery. *BioMed Research International*, *2013*, 521315. https://doi.org/10.1155/2013/521315

88. Lekhanont, K., Jongkhajornpong, P., Anothaisintawee, T., & Chuckpaiwong, V. (2016). Undiluted serum eye drops for the treatment of persistent corneal epitheilal defects. *Scientific Reports*, *6*, 38143. https://doi.org/10.1038/srep38143

89. Versura, P., Buzzi, M., Giannaccare, G., Terzi, A., Fresina, M., Velati, C., & Campos, E. C. (2016). Targeting growth factor supply in keratopathy treatment: comparison between maternal peripheral blood and cord blood as sources for the preparation of topical eye drops. *Blood Transfusion = Trasfusione Del Sangue*, *14*(2), 145–151. https://doi.org/10.2450/2015.0020-15

90. Fea, A. M., Aragno, V., Testa, V., Machetta, F., Parisi, S., D'Antico, S., Spinetta, R., Fusaro, E., & Grignolo, F. M. (2016). The effect of autologous platelet lysate eye drops: An in vivo confocal microscopy study. *BioMed Research International*, *2016*, 8406832. https://doi.org/10.1155/2016/8406832

91. Lee, J. H., Kim, M. J., Ha, S. W., & Kim, H. K. (2016). Autologous platelet-rich plasma eye drops in the treatment of recurrent corneal erosions. *Korean Journal of Ophthalmology: KJO*, *30*(2), 101–107. https://doi.org/10.3341/kjo.2016.30.2.101

92. Than, J., Balal, S., Wawrzynski, J., Nesaratnam, N., Saleh, G. M., Moore, J., Patel, A., Shah, S., Sharma, B., Kumar, B., Smith, J., & Sharma, A. (2017). Fingerprick autologous blood: A novel treatment for dry eye syndrome. *Eye (London, England)*, *31*(12), 1655–1663. https://doi.org/10.1038/eye.2017.118

93. Huang, G. T., Gronthos, S., & Shi, S. (2009). Mesenchymal stem cells derived from dental tissues vs. those from other sources: Their biology and role in regenerative medicine. *Journal of Dental Research*, *88*(9), 792–806. https://doi.org/10.1177/0022034509340867

94. Yam, G. H., Peh, G. S., Singhal, S., Goh, B. T., & Mehta, J. S. (2015). Dental stem cells: a future asset of ocular cell therapy. *Expert Reviews in Molecular Medicine*, *17*, e20. https://doi.org/10.1017/erm.2015.16

95. Young, C. S., Terada, S., Vacanti, J. P., Honda, M., Bartlett, J. D., & Yelick, P. C. (2002). Tissue engineering of complex tooth structures on biodegradable polymer scaffolds. *Journal of Dental Research, 81*(10), 695–700. https://doi.org/10.1177/154405910208101008

96. Hao, J., Ramachandran, A., & George, A. (2009). Temporal and spatial localization of the dentin matrix proteins during dentin biomineralization. *The Journal of Histochemistry and Cytochemistry: Official Journal of the Histochemistry Society, 57*(3), 227–237. https://doi.org/10.1369/jhc.2008.952119

97. Huang, H., Wang, Y., Pan, B., Yang, X., Wang, L., Chen, J., Ma, D., & Yang, C. (2013). Simple bipolar hosts with high glass transition temperatures based on 1,8-disubstituted carbazole for efficient blue and green electrophosphorescent devices with "ideal" turn-on voltage. *Chemistry (Weinheim an der Bergstrasse, Germany), 19*(5), 1828–1834. https://doi.org/10.1002/chem.201202329

98. Monteiro, B. G., Serafim, R. C., Melo, G. B., Silva, M. C., Lizier, N. F., Maranduba, C. M., Smith, R. L., Kerkis, A., Cerruti, H., Gomes, J. A., & Kerkis, I. (2009). Human immature dental pulp stem cells share key characteristic features with limbal stem cells. *Cell Proliferation, 42*(5), 587–594. https://doi.org/10.1111/j.1365-2184.2009.00623.x

99. Kloepper, J. E., Tiede, S., Brinckmann, J., Reinhardt, D. P., Meyer, W., Faessler, R., & Paus, R. (2008). Immunophenotyping of the human bulge region: the quest to define useful in situ markers for human epithelial hair follicle stem cells and their niche. *Experimental Dermatology, 17*(7), 592–609. https://doi.org/10.1111/j.1600-0625.2008.00720.x

100. Tiede, S., Kloepper, J. E., Bodò, E., Tiwari, S., Kruse, C., & Paus, R. (2007). Hair follicle stem cells: walking the maze. *European Journal of Cell Biology, 86*(7), 355–376. https://doi.org/10.1016/j.ejcb.2007.03.006

101. Larouche, D., Tong, X., Fradette, J., Coulombe, P. A., & Germain, L. (2008). Vibrissa hair bulge houses two populations of skin epithelial stem cells distinct by their keratin profile. *FASEB Journal: Official Publication of the Federation of American Societies for Experimental Biology, 22*(5), 1404–1415. https://doi.org/10.1096/fj.07-8109com

102. Blazejewska, E. A., Schlötzer-Schrehardt, U., Zenkel, M., Bachmann, B., Chankiewitz, E., Jacobi, C., & Kruse, F. E. (2009). Corneal limbal microenvironment can induce transdifferentiation of hair follicle stem cells into corneal epithelial-like cells. *Stem Cells (Dayton, Ohio), 27*(3), 642–652. https://doi.org/10.1634/stemcells.2008-0721

103. Ali, N. N., Edgar, A. J., Samadikuchaksaraei, A., Timson, C. M., Romanska, H. M., Polak, J. M., & Bishop, A. E. (2002). Derivation of type II alveolar epithelial cells from murine embryonic stem cells. *Tissue Engineering, 8*(4), 541–550. https://doi.org/10.1089/107632702760240463

104. Rodewald, H. R., Paul, S., Haller, C., Bluethmann, H., & Blum, C. (2001). Thymus medulla consisting of epithelial islets each derived from a single progenitor. *Nature, 414*(6865), 763–768. https://doi.org/10.1038/414763a

105. Thomson, J. A., Itskovitz-Eldor, J., Shapiro, S. S., Waknitz, M. A., Swiergiel, J. J., Marshall, V. S., & Jones, J. M. (1998). Embryonic stem cell lines derived from human blastocysts. *Science (New York, N.Y.), 282*(5391), 1145–1147. https://doi.org/10.1126/science.282.5391.1145

106. Takahashi, K., Tanabe, K., Ohnuki, M., Narita, M., Ichisaka, T., Tomoda, K., & Yamanaka, S. (2007). Induction of pluripotent stem cells from adult human fibroblasts by defined factors. *Cell, 131*(5), 861–872. https://doi.org/10.1016/j.cell.2007.11.019

107. Schwartz, S. D., Regillo, C. D., Lam, B. L., Eliott, D., Rosenfeld, P. J., Gregori, N. Z., Hubschman, J. P., Davis, J. L., Heilwell, G., Spirn, M., Maguire, J., Gay, R., Bateman, J., Ostrick, R. M., Morris, D., Vincent, M., Anglade, E., Del Priore, L. V., & Lanza, R. (2015). Human embryonic stem cell-derived retinal pigment epithelium in patients with age-related macular degeneration and Stargardt's macular dystrophy: follow-up of two open-label phase 1/2 studies. *Lancet (London, England), 385*(9967), 509–516. https://doi.org/10.1016/S0140-6736(14)61376-3

108. Cui, L., Guan, Y., Qu, Z., Zhang, J., Liao, B., Ma, B., Qian, J., Li, D., Li, W., Xu, G. T., & Jin, Y. (2016). WNT signaling determines tumorigenicity and function of ESC-derived retinal progenitors. *The Journal of Clinical Investigation, 126*(10), 4061. https://doi.org/10.1172/JCI89436

109. Decembrini, S., Koch, U., Radtke, F., Moulin, A., & Arsenijevic, Y. (2014). Derivation of traceable and transplantable photoreceptors from mouse embryonic Stem Cells. *Stem Cell Reports, 2*(6), 853–865. https://doi.org/10.1016/j.stemcr.2014.04.010

110. Nakano, T., Ando, S., Takata, N., Kawada, M., Muguruma, K., Sekiguchi, K., Saito, K., Yonemura, S., Eiraku, M., & Sasai, Y. (2012). Self-formation of optic cups and storable stratified neural retina from human ESCs. *Cell Stem Cell, 10*(6), 771–785. https://doi.org/10.1016/j.stem.2012.05.009

111. Eiraku, M., Takata, N., Ishibashi, H., Kawada, M., Sakakura, E., Okuda, S., Sekiguchi, K., Adachi, T., & Sasai, Y. (2011). Self-organizing optic-cup morphogenesis in three-dimensional culture. *Nature, 472*(7341), 51–56. https://doi.org/10.1038/nature09941

112. Osakada, F., Ikeda, H., Sasai, Y., & Takahashi, M. (2009). Stepwise differentiation of pluripotent stem cells into retinal cells. *Nature Protocols, 4*(6), 811–824. https://doi.org/10.1038/nprot.2009.51

113. Meyer, J. S., Shearer, R. L., Capowski, E. E., Wright, L. S., Wallace, K. A., McMillan, E. L., Zhang, S. C., & Gamm, D. M. (2009). Modeling early retinal development with human embryonic and induced pluripotent stem cells. *Proceedings of the National Academy of Sciences of the United States of America, 106*(39), 16698–16703. https://doi.org/10.1073/pnas.0905245106

114. Meyer, J. S., Howden, S. E., Wallace, K. A., Verhoeven, A. D., Wright, L. S., Capowski, E. E., Pinilla, I., Martin, J. M., Tian, S., Stewart, R., Pattnaik, B., Thomson, J. A., & Gamm, D. M. (2011). Optic vesicle-like structures derived from human pluripotent stem cells facilitate a customized approach to retinal disease treatment. *Stem Cells (Dayton, Ohio), 29*(8), 1206–1218. https://doi.org/10.1002/stem.674

115. Lamba, D. A., Gust, J., & Reh, T. A. (2009). Transplantation of human embryonic stem cell-derived photoreceptors restores some visual function in Crx-deficient mice. *Cell Stem Cell, 4*(1), 73–79. https://doi.org/10.1016/j.stem.2008.10.015

116. Gonzalez-Cordero, A., West, E. L., Pearson, R. A., Duran, Y., Carvalho, L. S., Chu, C. J., Naeem, A., Blackford, S., Georgiadis, A., Lakowski, J., Hubank, M., Smith, A. J., Bainbridge, J., Sowden, J. C., & Ali, R. R. (2013). Photoreceptor precursors derived from three-dimensional embryonic stem cell cultures integrate and mature within adult degenerate retina. *Nature Biotechnology, 31*(8), 741–747. https://doi.org/10.1038/nbt.2643

117. Zhu, J., Zhang, K., Sun, Y., Gao, X., Li, Y., Chen, Z., & Wu, X. (2013). Reconstruction of functional ocular surface by acellular porcine cornea matrix scaffold and limbal stem cells derived from human embryonic stem cells. *Tissue Engineering. Part A, 19*(21-22), 2412–2425. https://doi.org/10.1089/ten.TEA.2013.0097

118. Liu, Y., Ding, Y., Ma, P., Wu, Z., Duan, H., Liu, Z., Wan, P., Lu, X., Xiang, P., Ge, J., & Wang, Z. (2010). Enhancement of long-term proliferative capacity of rabbit corneal epithelial cells by embryonic stem cell conditioned medium. *Tissue Engineering. Part C, Methods, 16*(4), 793–802. https://doi.org/10.1089/ten.TEC.2009.0380

119. Weiss, M. L., & Troyer, D. L. (2006). Stem cells in the umbilical cord. *Stem Cell Reviews, 2*(2), 155–162. https://doi.org/10.1007/s12015-006-0022-y

120. Weiss, M. L., Medicetty, S., Bledsoe, A. R., Rachakatla, R. S., Choi, M., Merchav, S., Luo, Y., Rao, M. S., Velagaleti, G., & Troyer, D. (2006). Human umbilical cord matrix stem cells: preliminary characterization and effect of transplantation in a rodent model of Parkinson's disease. *Stem cells (Dayton, Ohio), 24*(3), 781–792. https://doi.org/10.1634/stemcells.2005-0330

121. Liu, H. Y., Chiou, J. F., Wu, A. T., Tsai, C. Y., Leu, J. D., Ting, L. L., Wang, M. F., Chen, H. Y., Lin, C. T., Williams, D. F., & Deng, W. P. (2012). The effect of diminished osteogenic signals on reduced osteoporosis recovery in aged mice and the potential therapeutic use of adipose-derived stem cells. *Biomaterials, 33*(26), 6105–6112. https://doi.org/10.1016/j.biomaterials.2012.05.024

122. Brzoska, M., Geiger, H., Gauer, S., & Baer, P. (2005). Epithelial differentiation of human adipose tissue-derived adult stem cells. *Biochemical and Biophysical Research Communications, 330*(1), 142–150. https://doi.org/10.1016/j.bbrc.2005.02.141

123. Gao, S., Zhao, P., Lin, C., Sun, Y., Wang, Y., Zhou, Z., Yang, D., Wang, X., Xu, H., Zhou, F., Cao, L., Zhou, W., Ning, K., Chen, X., & Xu, J. (2014). Differentiation of human adipose-derived stem cells into neuron-like cells which are compatible with photocurable three-dimensional scaffolds. *Tissue Engineering. Part A, 20*(7-8), 1271–1284. https://doi.org/10.1089/ten.TEA.2012.0773

124. Pellegrini, G., Dellambra, E., Golisano, O., Martinelli, E., Fantozzi, I., Bondanza, S., Ponzin, D., McKeon, F., & De Luca, M. (2001). p63 identifies keratinocyte stem cells. *Proceedings of the National Academy of Sciences of the United States of America, 98*(6), 3156–3161. https://doi.org/10.1073/pnas.061032098

125. Ouyang, H., Xue, Y., Lin, Y., Zhang, X., Xi, L., Patel, S., Cai, H., Luo, J., Zhang, M., Zhang, M., Yang, Y., Li, G., Li, H., Jiang, W., Yeh, E., Lin, J., Pei, M., Zhu, J., Cao, G., Zhang, L., Zhang, K, et al. (2014). WNT7A and PAX6 define corneal epithelium homeostasis and pathogenesis. *Nature, 511*(7509), 358–361. https://doi.org/10.1038/nature13465

126. Gao, N., Wang, Z., Huang, B., Ge, J., Lu, R., Zhang, K., Fan, Z., Lu, L., Peng, Z., & Cui, G. (2007). Putative epidermal stem cell convert into corneal epithelium-like cell under corneal tissue in vitro. *Science in China. Series C, Life Sciences, 50*(1), 101–110. https://doi.org/10.1007/s11427-007-0006-4

127. Tsonis, P. A., & Fuentes, E. J. (2006). Focus on molecules: Pax-6, the eye master. *Experimental Eye Research, 83*(2), 233–234. https://doi.org/10.1016/j.exer.2005.11.019

128. Treisman J. E. (2004). How to make an eye. *Development (Cambridge, England), 131*(16), 3823–3827. https://doi.org/10.1242/dev.01319

129. Hu, N., Zhang, Y. Y., Gu, H. W., & Guan, H. J. (2012). Effects of bone marrow mesenchymal stem cells on cell proliferation and growth factor expression of limbal epithelial cells in vitro. *Ophthalmic Research, 48*(2), 82–88. https://doi.org/10.1159/000331006

130. Zappia, E., Casazza, S., Pedemonte, E., Benvenuto, F., Bonanni, I., Gerdoni, E., Giunti, D., Ceravolo, A., Cazzanti, F., Frassoni, F., Mancardi, G., & Uccelli, A. (2005). Mesenchymal stem cells ameliorate experimental autoimmune encephalomyelitis inducing T-cell anergy. *Blood, 106*(5), 1755–1761. https://doi.org/10.1182/blood-2005-04-1496

131. Le Blanc, K., Rasmusson, I., Sundberg, B., Götherström, C., Hassan, M., Uzunel, M., & Ringdén, O. (2004). Treatment of severe acute graft-versus-host disease with third party haploidentical mesenchymal stem cells. *Lancet (London, England), 363*(9419), 1439–1441. https://doi.org/10.1016/S0140-6736(04)16104-7

132. Lazarus, H. M., Koc, O. N., Devine, S. M., Curtin, P., Maziarz, R. T., Holland, H. K., Shpall, E. J., McCarthy, P., Atkinson, K., Cooper, B. W., Gerson, S. L., Laughlin, M. J., Loberiza, F. R., Jr, Moseley, A. B., & Bacigalupo, A. (2005). Cotransplantation of HLA-identical sibling culture-expanded mesenchymal stem cells and hematopoietic stem cells in hematologic malignancy patients. *Biology of Blood and Marrow Transplantation: Journal of the American Society for Blood and Marrow Transplantation, 11*(5), 389–398. https://doi.org/10.1016/j.bbmt.2005.02.001

133. Wang, J., Ding, F., Gu, Y., Liu, J., & Gu, X. (2009). Bone marrow mesenchymal stem cells promote cell proliferation and neurotrophic function of Schwann cells in vitro and in vivo. *Brain Research, 1262*, 7–15. https://doi.org/10.1016/j.brainres.2009.01.056

134. Deng, Y. B., Ye, W. B., Hu, Z. Z., Yan, Y., Wang, Y., Takon, B. F., Zhou, G. Q., & Zhou, Y. F. (2010). Intravenously administered BMSCs reduce neuronal apoptosis and promote neuronal proliferation through the release of VEGF after stroke in rats. *Neurological Research, 32*(2), 148–156. https://doi.org/10.1179/174313209X414434

135. Yoo, S. W., Kim, S. S., Lee, S. Y., Lee, H. S., Kim, H. S., Lee, Y. D., & Suh-Kim, H. (2008). Mesenchymal stem cells promote proliferation of endogenous neural stem cells and survival of newborn cells in a rat stroke model. *Experimental & Molecular Medicine, 40*(4), 387–397. https://doi.org/10.3858/emm.2008.40.4.387

136. Nakanishi, C., Yamagishi, M., Yamahara, K., Hagino, I., Mori, H., Sawa, Y., Yagihara, T., Kitamura, S., & Nagaya, N. (2008). Activation of cardiac progenitor cells through paracrine effects of mesenchymal stem cells. *Biochemical and Biophysical Research Communications, 374*(1), 11–16. https://doi.org/10.1016/j.bbrc.2008.06.074

137. Pittenger, M. F., Mackay, A. M., Beck, S. C., Jaiswal, R. K., Douglas, R., Mosca, J. D., Moorman, M. A., Simonetti, D. W., Craig, S., & Marshak, D. R. (1999). Multilineage potential of adult human mesenchymal stem cells. *Science (New York, N.Y.), 284*(5411), 143–147. https://doi.org/10.1126/science.284.5411.143

138. Gu, S., Xing, C., Han, J., Tso, M. O., & Hong, J. (2009). Differentiation of rabbit bone marrow mesenchymal stem cells into corneal epithelial cells in vivo and ex vivo. *Molecular Vision, 15*, 99–107.

139. Jiang, T. S., Cai, L., Ji, W. Y., Hui, Y. N., Wang, Y. S., Hu, D., & Zhu, J. (2010). Reconstruction of the corneal epithelium with induced marrow mesenchymal stem cells in rats. *Molecular Vision, 16*, 1304–1316.

140. Cejkova, J., Trosan, P., Cejka, C., Lencova, A., Zajicova, A., Javorkova, E., Kubinova, S., Sykova, E., & Holan, V. (2013). Suppression of alkali-induced oxidative injury in the cornea by mesenchymal stem cells growing on nanofiber scaffolds and transferred onto the damaged corneal surface. *Experimental Eye Research, 116*, 312–323. https://doi.org/10.1016/j.exer.2013.10.002

141. Oh, J. Y., Kim, M. K., Shin, M. S., Wee, W. R., & Lee, J. H. (2009). Cytokine secretion by human mesenchymal stem cells cocultured with damaged corneal epithelial cells. *Cytokine, 46*(1), 100–103. https://doi.org/10.1016/j.cyto.2008.12.011

142. Di Nicola, M., Carlo-Stella, C., Magni, M., Milanesi, M., Longoni, P. D., Matteucci, P., Grisanti, S., & Gianni, A. M. (2002). Human bone marrow stromal cells suppress T-lymphocyte proliferation induced by cellular or nonspecific mitogenic stimuli. *Blood*, *99*(10), 3838–3843. https://doi.org/10.1182/blood.v99.10.3838

143. Najar, M., Raicevic, G., Fayyad-Kazan, H., De Bruyn, C., Bron, D., Toungouz, M., & Lagneaux, L. (2012). Immune-related antigens, surface molecules and regulatory factors in human-derived mesenchymal stromal cells: the expression and impact of inflammatory priming. *Stem Cell Reviews and Reports*, *8*(4), 1188–1198. https://doi.org/10.1007/s12015-012-9408-1

144. Harkin, D. G., Foyn, L., Bray, L. J., Sutherland, A. J., Li, F. J., & Cronin, B. G. (2015). Concise reviews: can mesenchymal stromal cells differentiate into corneal cells? A systematic review of published data. *Stem Cells (Dayton, Ohio)*, *33*(3), 785–791. https://doi.org/10.1002/stem.1895

145. Abumaree, M., Al Jumah, M., Pace, R. A., & Kalionis, B. (2012). Immunosuppressive properties of mesenchymal stem cells. *Stem Cell Reviews and Reports*, *8*(2), 375–392. https://doi.org/10.1007/s12015-011-9312-0

146. Trosan, P., Javorkova, E., Zajicova, A., Hajkova, M., Hermankova, B., Kossl, J., Krulova, M., & Holan, V. (2016). The supportive role of insulin-like growth factor-I in the differentiation of murine mesenchymal stem cells into corneal-like cells. *Stem Cells and Development*, *25*(11), 874–881. https://doi.org/10.1089/scd.2016.0030

147. Di, G., Du, X., Qi, X., Zhao, X., Duan, H., Li, S., Xie, L., & Zhou, Q. (2017). Mesenchymal stem cells promote diabetic corneal epithelial wound healing through TSG-6-dependent stem cell activation and macrophage switch. *Investigative Ophthalmology & Visual Science*, *58*(10), 4344–4354. https://doi.org/10.1167/iovs.17-21506

148. Demirayak, B., Yüksel, N., Çelik, O. S., Subaşı, C., Duruksu, G., Unal, Z. S., Yıldız, D. K., & Karaöz, E. (2016). Effect of bone marrow and adipose tissue-derived mesenchymal stem cells on the natural course of corneal scarring after penetrating injury. *Experimental Eye Research*, *151*, 227–235. https://doi.org/10.1016/j.exer.2016.08.011

149. Rohaina, C. M., Then, K. Y., Ng, A. M., Wan Abdul Halim, W. H., Zahidin, A. Z., Saim, A., & Idrus, R. B. (2014). Reconstruction of limbal stem cell deficient corneal surface with induced human bone marrow mesenchymal stem cells on amniotic membrane. *Translational Research: The Journal of Laboratory and Clinical Medicine*, *163*(3), 200–210. https://doi.org/10.1016/j.trsl.2013.11.004

150. Ralph, R. A., Doane, M. G., & Dohlman, C. H. (1975). Clinical experience with a mobile ocular perfusion pump. *Archives of Ophthalmology (Chicago, Ill.: 1960)*, *93*(10), 1039–1043. https://doi.org/10.1001/archopht.1975.01010020815015

151. Fox, R. I., Chan, R., Michelson, J. B., Belmont, J. B., & Michelson, P. E. (1984). Beneficial effect of artificial tears made with autologous serum in patients with keratoconjunctivitis sicca. *Arthritis and Rheumatism*, *27*(4), 459–461. https://doi.org/10.1002/art.1780270415

152. Harritshøj, L. H., Nielsen, C., Ullum, H., Hansen, M. B., & Julian, H. O. (2014). Ready-made allogeneic ABO-specific serum eye drops: production from regular male blood donors, clinical routine, safety and efficacy. *Acta ophthalmologica*, *92*(8), 783–786. https://doi.org/10.1111/aos.12386

153. Anitua, E., Muruzabal, F., Tayebba, A., Riestra, A., Perez, V. L., Merayo-Lloves, J., & Orive, G. (2015). Autologous serum and plasma rich in growth factors in ophthalmology: preclinical and clinical studies. *Acta ophthalmologica*, *93*(8), e605–e614. https://doi.org/10.1111/aos.12710

154. Alio, J. L., Abad, M., Artola, A., Rodriguez-Prats, J. L., Pastor, S., & Ruiz-Colecha, J. (2007). Use of autologous platelet-rich plasma in the treatment of dormant corneal ulcers. *Ophthalmology*, *114*(7), 1286–1293.e1. https://doi.org/10.1016/j.ophtha.2006.10.044

155. Poon, A. C., Geerling, G., Dart, J. K., Fraenkel, G. E., & Daniels, J. T. (2001). Autologous serum eyedrops for dry eyes and epithelial defects: clinical and in vitro toxicity studies. *The British Journal of Ophthalmology*, *85*(10), 1188–1197. https://doi.org/10.1136/bjo.85.10.1188

156. Jover Botella, A., Márquez Peiró, J. F., Márques, K., Monts Cambero, N., & Selva Otaolaurruchi, J. (2011). Effectiveness of 100% autologous serum drops in ocular surface disorders. *Farmacia hospitalaria: organo oficial de expresion cientifica de la Sociedad Espanola de Farmacia Hospitalaria*, *35*(1), 8–13. https://doi.org/10.1016/j.farma.2010.02.004

157. Jeng, B. H., & Dupps, W. J., Jr (2009). Autologous serum 50% eyedrops in the treatment of persistent corneal epithelial defects. *Cornea*, *28*(10), 1104–1108. https://doi.org/10.1097/ICO.0b013e3181a2a7f6

158. Semeraro, F., Forbice, E., Braga, O., Bova, A., Di Salvatore, A., & Azzolini, C. (2014). Evaluation of the efficacy of 50% autologous serum eye drops in different ocular surface pathologies. *BioMed Research International, 2014,* 826970. https://doi.org/10.1155/2014/826970

159. Quinto, G. G., Campos, M., & Behrens, A. (2008). Autologous serum for ocular surface diseases. *Arquivos brasileiros de oftalmologia, 71*(6 Suppl), 47–54.

160. Wilson, S. E., Chen, L., Mohan, R. R., Liang, Q., & Liu, J. (1999). Expression of HGF, KGF, EGF and receptor messenger RNAs following corneal epithelial wounding. *Experimental Eye Research, 68*(4), 377–397. https://doi.org/10.1006/exer.1998.0603

161. Kokawa, N., Sotozono, C., Nishida, K., & Kinoshita, S. (1996). High total TGF-beta 2 levels in normal human tears. *Current Eye Research, 15*(3), 341–343. https://doi.org/10.3109/0271368960 9007630

7

White Rot Exopolysaccharide: Avenues to Biomedical Applications

Deepak K. Rahi and Ekta Chaudhary
Department of Microbiology, Panjab University, Chandigarh, India

Sonu Rahi
Department of Botany, Government Girls College, A.P.S. University, Rewa, India

7.1 Introduction

Polysaccharides are vital polymeric carbohydrate molecules that are composed of tens to thousands of monosaccharide units bound together by glycosidic linkages. All the polysaccharides existing in nature are formed by the same process wherein the monosaccharide units are connected together by glycosidic bonds. The polysaccharides have slight modification of the repeating units and thus can have distinct properties from their individual building blocks. During the formation of glycosidic bond condensation reaction occurs wherein one molecule of water is released along with linking of a sugar molecule to another molecule via an ether bond. Polysaccharides are considered to be the most abundant carbohydrates in nature and are found in various parts of plants, animals, fungi, bacteria, and seaweed (Zhong et al., 2012). The polysaccharides range in structure from linear to highly branched and can be amorphous and even insoluble in water (Varki et al., 1999). These polysaccharides function either as storage polysaccharide or structural polysaccharide. Storage polysaccharides serve as food reserve that at the time of need hydrolyse into constituent sugars that become available to the living cells. The two main storage polysaccharides include starch and glycogen. Structural polysaccharides on the other hand are involved in forming the structural framework of both plant and microbial cell walls. Commonly occurring structural polysaccharides include chitin and cellulose.

7.2 Sources of Polysaccharides

Polysaccharides are usually classified as those derived from animals, plants, bacteria, lichen, fungi, and algae (Figure 7.1).

7.2.1 Microbial Polysaccharides

Microbial polysaccharides comprise a large number of versatile biopolymers produced by several bacteria, yeast, and fungi (Giavasis 2003). The forms of polysaccharides produced by organisms can be subdivided into bound polysaccharides that are closely bound to the cell (sheaths, capsular polymers, condensed gels, loosely bound polymers, and attached organic materials) and soluble polysaccharides (exopolysaccharides) that are weakly bound or are dissolved into the solution (soluble macromolecules, colloids, and slimes) (Nielsen and Jahn 1999; Laspidou and Rittmann 2002) (Figure 7.2).

DOI: 10.1201/9781003220404-8

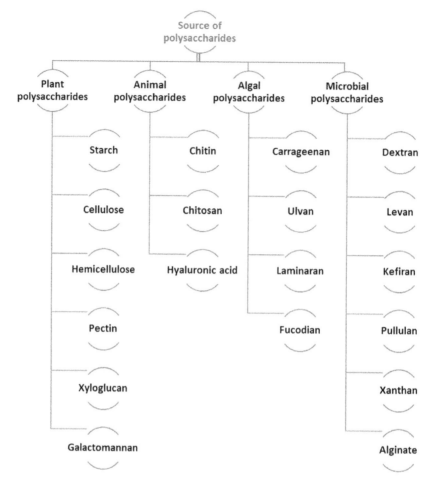

FIGURE 7.1   Different sources of polysaccharides.

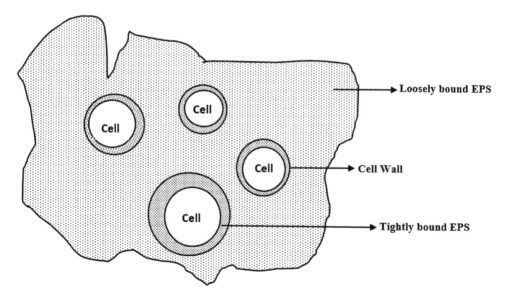

FIGURE 7.2   Types of polysaccharide produced by micro-organisms.

7.2.2 Exopolysaccharides

Exopolysaccharides (EPSs) can be defined as the high-molecular-weight heterogeneous polymers that are secreted into the surrounding environment by organisms. The EPS production by microbes was first reported in 1861 as a "viscous fermentation" by Pasteur and the term exopolysaccharide was first used by Sutherland in 1972 to describe high-molecular-weight carbohydrate polymers produced by marine bacteria. The production of EPS is a general property of microorganisms and occurs both in prokaryotic (bacteria, archea) and eukaryotic (algae, fungi) microbes under nonlimited oxygen conditions. EPSs are acidic in nature and usually contain branched, repeating units of sugars or sugar derivatives such as glucose, fructose, mannose, galactose, etc. (Ismail and Nampoothiri, 2010) and a variety of negatively charged functional groups (e.g., carboxyl, phosphoric, sulfate, and hydroxyl), as well as positively charged (e.g., amino) groups (Majumdar et al., 1999). EPSs consist of macromolecules such as polysaccharides, proteins, nucleic acids, humic substances, lipids, and other nonpolymeric constituents of low molecular weight. Carbohydrates and proteins are usually found to be the major and best investigated components of EPS (Frolund et al., 1995; 1996). In addition, some organic matters from medium can also be adsorbed to the EPS matrix (Nielsen and Jahn 1999; Liu and Fang 2003).

7.3 Composition and Linkages

EPSs can be either homopolysaccharides or heteropolysaccharides (Vuyst et al., 1999).

Homopolysaccharides are composed of only one type of monosaccharide: D-glucose or L-fructose. These polysaccharides belong to three distinct groups:

1) α-D-glucans: These compounds contain mostly α (1→6) linked D-glucosyl units. The degree of branching involves α (1→3) linkages, seldom α (1→2) and α (1→4) linkages.
2) β-D-glucans: These are synthesized by *Pediococcus spp.* and *Streptococcus spp.* The molecules are composed of β (1→3) linked D-glucosyl units with branching involving β (1→2) linkages.
3) Fructans: They are produced by *Streptococcus salivarius* containing β (2→6) linked fructosyl units (Branda et al., 2005).

Heteropolysaccharides are composed of repeating units, varying in size from disaccharides to heptasaccharides such as D-glucose, D-galactose, L-fructose, L-rhamnose, D-glucuronic acid, L-guluronic acid, and D-mannuronic acid. The type of both the linkages between monosaccharide units and the branching of the chain determine the physical properties of microbial heteropolysaccharides. Most heteropolysaccharides also possess substituents of pyruvates, succinates, and formates (Monsan et al., 2001; Branda et al., 2005).

A number of microbial exopolysaccharide have been reported over the last decade. These polysaccharides display a variety of structural combinations, which confers them with unique structural and chemical properties. Microbial production shows several advantages over plant- or macroalgae-derived products. Microbes can be cultivated at a large scale in bioreactors for the production of various biopolymers in an energy-efficient manner. However, algae requires large amounts of water and significant fertilizer use to be productive. The production of polysaccharides from algae has regional suitability issues causing variations in the final product reaching the market and is not always an energy-efficient process. However, plant-based gums are being commercially produced on a large scale and the yield as compared to other microbial polysaccharides is much greater, but plant-based gums face seasonal variation and the entire process is highly time consuming.

Microbial EPSs are known to possess remarkable medical applications. A number of microbial polysaccharides such as dextran, pullulan, xanthan, hyaluronic acid, and many more have found wide applicability in the medical field. The first ever microbial polysaccharide to reach clinical trials was dextran, which was used as a plasma expander. Other EPSs used include xanthan (suspension stabilizer); pullulan (capsules and oral care products); alginates (used as antireflux, dental impressions, or as matrix for tablets); hyaluronic acid and derivatives (used in surgery, arthritis treatment, or wound healing); and bacterial cellulose (wound dressings or scaffolds for tissue engineering). Other potential applications such as immunomodulation, antitumor, antimicrobial, antioxidant, etc., are related to the bioactive nature of the polysaccharide produced. However, numerous potential applications still wait to be explored and developed into commercial appliactions.

7.4 White Rot Fungi

White rot fungi constitutes a group of ecophysiological basidiomycetes/litter–decomposing fungi, which are able to decompose wood fractions, including lignin leaving the wood with a white, fibrous appearance. These are ubiquitous in nature and mostly grow on hardwoods (e.g, birch and aspen). However, certain species on softwoods such as spruce and pine also harbor white rots (Blanchette et al., 1990). White rot fungi are well known for the production of various extracellular enzymes, which play an important role in a variety of industrial applications (Bains et al., 2006; Rahi et al., 2009). Some of the prominent white rot fungal species include *Ganoderma* sp., *Pleurotus* sp., *Trametes* sp., *Phanerochaete* sp., and *Schizophyllum* sp.

7.4.1 Taxonomic Classification

The white rot fungi taxonomically represent the phylum basidiomycotina, and are distributed among four orders in the class agaricomycetes and fourteen families (Figure 3,4).

7.4.2 General Characteristics of White Rot Fungi

* **Agaricales:** Basidiocarp: Fleshy, fan-shaped, or broadly convex; irregular surface, with wavy margins; Presence or absence of stipe varies with the family; Gills: white, decurrently arranged, 3-4 per cm, thick texture and fimbriate margin. Hyphal system: mostly monomitic, clamp connection present; Spores: smooth, elongated. Habitat: Dead hardwood or conifers.

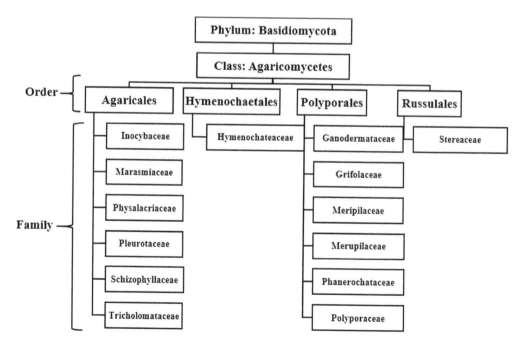

FIGURE 7.3   Taxonomic classification of white rot fungi.

Relative distribution of white rots on the basis of number of species in each family

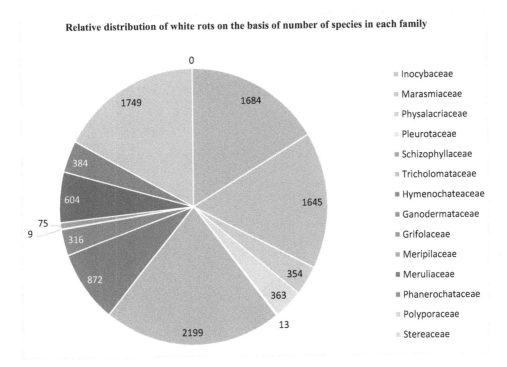

FIGURE 7.4   Relative distribution of white rots on the basis of number of species in each family.

- **Hymenochaetales:** Basidiocarp: Annual, effuse-reflexed, or pileated, turns black in the presence of an alkali; Hyphal system: generative hyphae, lacks clamp connections; Thick-walled thorn-shaped cystidia present; Basidiospore: Cylindrical or allantoid, hyaline, thin walled, smooth. Habitat: Dead wood and living tree.
- **Polyporales: Gilled fungi**: Basidiocarp: broady convex with navel-like depression, dry, fibrillose scaly surface, incurved margin; Gills: running down the stem, crowded, serrated edges, white to creamy in color, covered with partial veil; stipe: 4-5 cm long, slightly tapered, scaly; Spores: ellipsoid, smooth, hyaline, inamyloid, thick-walled hyhae with clamp connections.
- **Porous fungi:** Basidiocarp: hoof or disc shapes attached directly to the substrate with no stipe, Color ranges from gray to black, concentric rings may be present; Pore surface: Pale brown, with numerous pores and brown pore tubes; Hyphae: dimitic/trimitic, which can be generative, skeletal, or binding type, clamp connections present: Spores: cylindrical, large, hyaline, smooth. Habitat: Decaying wood.
- **Russulales: Basidiocarp:** Shelf-like, fused, white to grayish in color, surface covered by coarse, stiff hair; Lower surface: Smooth, reddish to yellow in color, lacks gills or tubes; Clamp connections absent and produce amyloid basidiospores. Habitat: Decaying wood.

7.5 Biomedical Applications

The white rot mushrooms contain approximately 400 different bioactive compounds, which mainly include triterpenoids, polysaccharides, nucleotides, sterols, steroids, fatty acids, proteins/peptides, and trace elements. Of all these compounds polysaccharides are considered to be an important group that possesses remarkable bioactive properties. The mushroom polysaccharide is considered to be a high value macromolecule (Rahi, 2015). A number of polysaccharide-producing white rots have been studied but only few of them produce polysaccharides of medical importance (Figure 7.5).

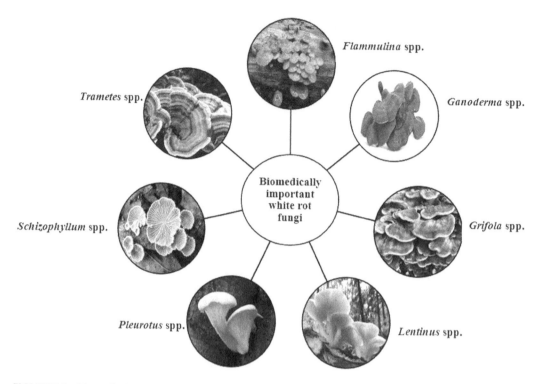

FIGURE 7.5   Bio-medically important white rot fungal species.

The polysaccharides produced by mushrooms have been reported to have a number of pharmacological effects including immunomodulation, antiatherosclerotic, antiinflammatory, analgesic, chemopreventive, antitumor, chemo- and radioprotective, sleep promoting, antibacterial, antiviral (including anti-HIV), hypolipidemic, antifibrotic, hepatoprotective, antidiabetic, antiandrogenic, antiangiogenic, antiherpetic, antioxidative and radical-scavenging, antiaging, hypoglycemic, estrogenic activity, and antiulcer properties (Sanodiya et al., 2009). Some of the important biomedical applications of these polysaccharides are discussed below (Figure 7.6).

7.5.1   Immunomodulating and Antitumor Activity

Immunomodulating and antitumor activity is one of the widely studied properties of fungal polysaccharides. The immunomodulating activity of these polysaccharides is mainly affected by various physical and chemical properties such as the chemical composition of the molecule, the degree of branching, the type of glycosidic bonds, conformation, or molecular weight. These properties in turn affect the antitumor activity of the polysaccharides (Methacanon et al., 2005). Of all the white rot fungal polysaccharides described so far, β-glucans containing β 1,3-glycosidic bonds with side chains linked via β 1,6-glycosidic bonds are considered to be the most active (Chen and Seviour, 2007). The structural features of these glucans are considered to be the reason behind their immuno-modulatory activity.

Conformation: Different studies suggest that the triple helical structure of these glucans confers the immunostimulatory activity to these glucans by promoting the release of TNF-α by monocyte or macrophage cells (Falch et al., 2000; Satitmanwiwatetal, 2012). The importance of this triple helical structure has also been demonstrated by various other studies (Wang et al., 2009b; Wang & Zhang 2009).

Molecular weight: Different studies have shown that the immunomodulatory effect of the glucans depend on their conformation rather than on their molecular weight. Glucans ranging in weight from

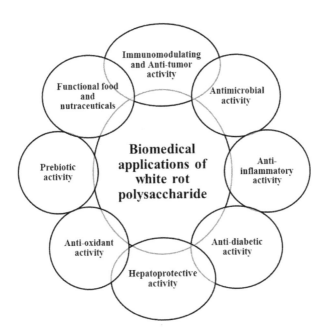

FIGURE 7.6 Biomedical applications of white rot polysaccharide.

8 KDa to 1100 KDa have all been found capable of stimulating the immune cells. Thus the molecular weight of a glucan cannot be considered as a parameter to determine its immunostimulationg activity (Falch et al., 2000; Mueller et al., 2000; Jamois et al., 2005; Guo et al., 2009; Descroix et al., 2010).

Functional groups: The glucans isolated from natural sources generally lack functional groups. Bao et al., 2001 reported that when these glucans are chemically functionalized in order to form their sulfated derivatives it results in increasing the solubility of these glucans that in turn enhances their immunostimulating properties. The enhanced effect is considered to be because of the impact of these functional groups on the intramolecular and intermolecular hydrogen bonding. They also strengthen the effect of electrostatic repulsion and enable the adoption of a certain structure (Bao et al., 2001; Wang et al., 2009b).

Various clinical trials have shown that the glucans produced by white rots such as *Grifola frondosa* and *Trametes versicolor* are found capable of increasing the survival rate and time of patients suffereing from different forms of cancer (Lindequist et al., 2005; Stachowiak and Regula, 2012).

The inhibition of tumor cell growth is considered to be a result of β-glucan-dependent stimulation of macrophages and dendritic cells, which is followed by secretion of various cytokines including TNF-α, IFN-γ, and IL-1β, and stimulation of natural killer cells, T and B cells (Lindequist et al., 2005; Li et al., 2014). Moreover, the stimulation of immune cells β-glucans inhibit the tumor development by cutting off the nutrient supply to tumor cells (Shenbhagaraman et al., 2012). Lentinan and Schizophyllan are the most studied immunomodulating polysaccharides, which are known to stimulate the secretion of tumor necrosis factor-α by human monocytes and activation of macrophages.

Various studies have also reported that these bioactive polysaccharides effectively prevent metastasis and minimize the side effects of drugs when given in combination with the conventional antitumor drugs or chemotherapy (Ikekawa, 2001; Lo et al., 2011; Chang and Wasser, 2012; Stachowiak and Regula, 2012; Giavasi,s 2013). Ganoderan is one such white rot polysaccharide produced by *Ganoderma* sp., which when used as an adjuvant in cancer therapy effectively increases the cytotoxic effect of chemotheraphy and also enhances the immune response (Yuen and Gohel, 2005; Mahajna et al., 2008; Vannucci et al., 2013). The immune-modulating and antitumor effect of polysaccharide produced by different white rot fungi has been summarized in Table 7.1.

TABLE 7.1

Exopolysaccharide-Producing White Rot Species and Their Immune-Modulatory Effect

Organism	Nature of polysaccharide	Immunomodulatory effect	Reference
Amauroderma rugosum	Glucan	Stimulate cytokine production and activate the iNOS, PLA2-AA, and MAPK pathways	Zhang 2017
Ganoderma lucidium	Glucan	Stimulate TNF-a, IL-1, IFN-g production, activate NF-kB.	Zhu et al., 2007; Xu et al., 2011
Grifola frondosa	Grifolan	Macrophage activation, induction of IL-1, IL-6, and TNF-a secretion	Yang et al., 2007
Inonotus obliquus	Glucan	Enhance expression of IL-1b, IL-6, TNF-a, and iNOS in macrophages	Zhang et al., 2007; Won et al., 2011; Zheng et al., 2011
Lentinus edodes	Lentinan	Potently stimulated cytokine production, stimulate phagocytosis	Bisen et al., 2010; Kojima et al., 2010
Phellinus linteus	Acidic polysaccharides	Activation of murine B cells, Induce IL-12 and IFN-g production Block NF-kB, TNF-a, IL-1a, IL-1b, and IL-4 production	Wu et al., 2013
Pleurotus albidus	Glucan	Enhanced production of tumor necrosis factor alpha (TNF-α) and nitric oxide (NO)	Castro-Alves et al., 2017
Pleurotus eryngii	Glucan	Enhanced production of tumor necrosis factor-α, interleukin-1β, and interleukin-6, upregulation of expression levels of nuclear factor-κB and toll-like receptor signaling genes in cells	Ma et al., 2015
Pleurotus florida	Glucan	Immunoenhancing, stimulates macrophages, splenocytes, and thymocytes	Roy et al., 2009; Latha and Bhaskar 2014
Pleurotus ostreatus	Heteropolysaccharide	Stimulates macrophages, splenocytes, and thymocytes	Maity et al., 2011
Schizophyllum commune	Schizophyllan	Activation of T cell, increase interleukin, and TNF-a production	Hobbs 2005
Trametes versicolor	Polysaccharide-Krestin (PSK); Polysaccharopeptide (PSP)	Stimulate cytokine production	Stachowiak and Reguła 2012; Sugiyama 2016; Friedmann 2016

7.5.2 Antimicrobial Activity

Mushroom polysaccharides are known to possess antimicrobial properties and are found to be active against many bacterial and viral infections both in vitro and in vivo. The antimicrobial activity of these polysaccharides is considered due to their ability to stimulate phagocytosis by macrophages and neutrophils (Giavasis, 2014). Various studies have suggested that the polysaccharides produced by white rots such as *Pleurotus eryngii, Ganoderma lucidium, Lentinus edodes,* and *Schizophyllum commune* are found capable of inhibiting pathogens such as *E. coli, Pseudomonas aeruginosa, Salmonella enteritidis, Salmonella,* and *S. epidermidis* (Zhu et al., *2012; Li and Shah, 2014; Wan-Mohtar et al., 2016). Moreover, the polysaccharie produced by these white rots is also known to exhibit antiviral activity against the herpes virus, influenza virus, and polio virus (Eo et al., 1999; Kakumu et al., 1991, Sasidhara and Thirunalasundari, 2012).* It has been reported that the exopolysaccharide produced by *Pleurotus ostreatus* when given as a part of daily water intake was able to impart prevention against the infectious bursal

TABLE 7.2

Antimicrobial Activity of White Rot Polysaccharides

Organism	Susceptible bacterial/viral strains	Reference
Ganoderma lucidum	*E. coli, Pseudomonas aeruginosa, Salmonella enteritidis, Salmonella, Listeria monocytogenes, Shigella sonnei, Staphylococcus aureus, S. epidermidis, and methicillin-susceptible- S. aureus* ATCC 292123	Wan-Mohtar et al., 2016
Grifola frondosa	Enterovirus 71	Zhao et al., 2016
Lentinus edodes	*Streptococcus mutans, Prevotella intermedia, E. coli, S. aureus, and Sarcina lutea*	Zhu et al., 2012; Signoretto et al., 2014
Pleurotus eryngii	*E. coli* and *Staphylococcus aureus*	Li et al., 2014
Pleurotus ostreatus	Bursal disease virus	Giavasis and Biliaderi 2006
Trametes versicolor	HIV	Markova et al., 2002; Lindequist et al., 2005; Giavasis and Biliaderis. 2006; Sasidhara and Thirunalasundari, 2012

disease virus in young broilers (Selegean et al., 2009). Another polysaccharide produced by *Grifola frondosa* was reported to possess antiviral activity against enterovirus 71. The polysaccharide produced by Grifola frondosa suppresses viral VP1 protein (immunodominant capsid protein) expression, genomic RNA synthesis, *and also blocks the* viral replication (Zhao et al., 2016). Another possible mechanism for their antiviral activity is considered to be the increased release of IFN-γ and enhanced proliferation of peripheral blood mononuclear cells (PBMC) (Lindequist et al., 2005; Markova et al., 2002; Sasidhara and Thirunalasundari, 2012). Different studies have reported that the lentinan produced by *Lentinus edodes* and a glucans from *G. lucidum, G. frondosa,* and *T. versicolor* can enhance resistance to HIV virus and can also limit the toxicity of synthetic anti-HIV drugs and thus they have been used as an adjunct therapy with conventional anti-HIV drugs (Giavasis and Biliaderis, 2006; Lindequist et al., 2005, Markova et al., 2002; Sasidhara and Thirunalasundari, 2012). Table 7.2 summarizes the antimicrobial activity of the white rot polysaccharides.

7.5.3 Antiinflammatory Activity

Inflammation is a complex biological process characterized by heat, pain, redness, and tumor (Wilgus et al., 2013; Tracy, 2006). Inflammation usually occurs in response to remove injury or harmful pathogens (Elsayed et al., 2014). Nonsteroidal antiinflammatory drugs are the most common drugs used to reduce inflammation, but they are associated with potential side effects such as mucosal lesions, ulcers, intestinal perforations, acute renal failure, hypertension, nephrotic syndrome, etc. (Dugowson and Gnanashanmugam, 2006; Fosbol et al., 2009; Meek et al., 2010; Sinha et al., 2013). Therefore, there is a need for potential natural alternates to existing antiinflammatory drugs with no harmful side effects.

Studies suggest that the β-glucans produced by mushrooms are capable of influencing the production of both proinflammatory (IL-1β, IL-6, and TNF-α) as well as antiinflammatory (IL-10) cytokines. They also show high affinity towards the immune cell surface receptors with pattern recognition receptors (PRRs) and activate the proliferation and maturation of immune cells and also stimulate activation of macrophages and natural killer cells (Akramiene et al., 2010; Masuda et al., 2015; Muszyńska et al., 2018).

The polysaccharides produced by white rots have been widely investigated for their antiinflammatory properties. Studies show that the glucans extracted from *Pleurotus pulmonarius* exhibit antiinflammatory properties (Lavi et al., 2010; 2012; Schwartz et al., 2013). In vitro studies suggested that the glucans were found capable of inhibiting the TNF-α-dependent activation of NF-κB in human intestinal cells (Lavi et al., 2012). Similar antiinflammatory properties are also reported from the α-and β-D-glucans produced by *Pleurotus albidus*. (Castro-Alves et al., 2018). In another study it was reported that the α- and β-glucans from *Lentinus edodes* were found capable of suppressing LPS-induced dependent activation of TNF-α, IL-6, and IL-12 in RAW 264.7 murine macrophage cells and inhibiting LPS-induced production of prostaglandin E2 (PGE2) and nitric oxide (NO) due to the downregulation of COX-2 and iNOS expression, respectively (Jedinak et al., 2011). Another report suggests antiinflammatory activity of the polysaccharide produced by the golden needle mushroom (*Flammulina velutipes*). It was found that the polysaccharide was capable of significantly decreasing CD4+ CD8+, ICAM-1, and MPO in both the serum and colon of normal and burned rats (Wu et al., 2010). The glucans from *Inonotus obliquus* were found capable of inhibiting the signaling pathway of nuclear factor-κB (NF-κB), COX-2, and iNOS inflammatory property in RAW 264.7 cells (Ma et al., 2013).

7.5.4 Antidiabetic Activity

Diabetes mellitus is a chronic, metabolic disease and is considered a major health concern around the world. Antidiabetic medications currently in use have several side effects such as high cost, nephrotoxicity, and drug resistance (Scheen, 2005). Therefore, there is a need to explore nontoxic, more efficient alternatives for the treatment of diabetes. Polysaccharides can be considered one such alternative since they have wide range of sources and possess a number of biological activities.

Mushroom polysaccharides are not readily digested in the intestine and thus the indigestible polysaccharide binds to the intestinal epithelium leading to reduced glucose absorption (Giavasis, 2013; Lakhanpal and Rana, 2005). Another possible mechanism for the hypolipidemic activity of these bioactive polysaccharides could be the modulation of carbohydrate metabolism and insulin synthesis (Lakhanpal and Rana, 2005). Various animal and human studies suggest that the glucans obtained from various white rots such as *L. edodes, G. lucidum, S. commune, P. ostreatus,* and *G. frondosa* are able to reduce blood sugar and serum cholesterol level (Chen et al., 2013; Lakhanpal and Rana, 2005: Lindequist et al., 2005). Different studies have reported that the polysaccharide produced by *Pleurotus ostreatus* and *Pleurotus ferulae* are known to prevent the beta pancreatic cell damage as well as reduce the levels of LDL-C in animal models (Choi et al., 2016; Wahyuni et al., 2017). Due to their remarkable hypolipidemic properties the National Mushroom Development and Extension Centre in Bangladesh has recommended a daily dose of *Pleurotus* sp., which ranges from 5 to 10 g of dried mushroom for healthy individuals to 20 g for patients with diabetes, hypertension, cardiovascular complications, or cancer. The β-glucans extracted from *Lentinula edodes* and *Ganoderma atrum* are known to reduce the levels of BGL and also red alanine transaminase (ALT), hepatic glycogen, and aspartate aminotransferase (AST) (Zhu et al., 2016; Afiati et al., 2019). The hypolipidemic effect of the white rot polysaccharide has been summarized in Table 7.3.

7.5.5 Hepatoprotective Activity

Liver is a key organ and plays an important role in many metabolic processes occurring inside the body. Any injury to the liver on exposure to any drug (paracetamol or acetaminophen), noninfectious agents (ethanol), or toxins (thioacetamide, carbon tetrachloride, diethylnitrosamine, N-galactosamine) along with impaired liver function is referred to as hepatotoxicity (Navarro and Senior, 2006). These hepatotoxic agents react with the basic cellular components of liver and induce lesions that in turn results in increased levels of aspartate aminotransferase (AST) and alanine aminotransferase (ALT) in serum. Recently, polysaccharides derived from mushrooms are considered to be the new functional medicines that can be used for preventing the hepatic damage with minimal side effects (Liu et al., 2014; Zeng et al., 2016; Fan et al., 2014). Different in vitro and in vivo studies have reported that the polysaccharides produced by various white rot mushrooms such as *Ganoderma lucidium* and *Phellinus rimosus* exhibit hepato-protective activity. In another study it was reported that the polysaccharide produced by *Pleurotus eryngii* var. *tuoliensis exhibit hepatoprotctive properties (Zhou* et al*., 2002; Joseph* et al*., 2012; Xu* et al*., 2017).* In a study carried out by Zhu et al., 2019 the hepatoprotective activity of the polysaccharide produced by *Pleurotus ostraetus* was evaluated and it was found that the polysaccharide was capable of decreasing the levels of alanine transaminase and aspartate transaminase levels in blood and was also found to increase superoxide dismutase, catalase, and glutathione peroxidase levels, and decreased malondialdehyde levels in blood and liver.

TABLE 7.3

Hypolipidemic Effect of Polysaccharide Produced by White Rot Fungi

Organism	Hypolipidemic effect	Reference
Ganoderma atrum	Reduce fasting blood glucose and serum insulin levels	Zhu et al., 2016
Ganoderma lucidium	Increased insulin sensitivity and reduced hepatic glucose output	Gulati et al., 2019
Grifola frondosa	Reduce the serum levels of fasting blood glucose (FBG), oral glucose tolerance (OGT), cholesterol (TC), triglyceride (TG), and low-density lipoprotein cholesterol (LDL-C), and significantly decrease the hepatic levels of TC, TG and free fatty acids (FFA)	Guo et al., 2020
Inonotus obliquus	Suppresses DPP4 enzymes and induce GLUT4 translocation	Gulati et al., 2019
Lentinus edodes	Increase plasma insulin and reduce BGL	Gulati et al., 2019
Phellinus rimosus	Decrease serum triglyceride, total cholesterol, low-density lipoprotein, with elevating the high-density lipoprotein	Rony et al., 2014
Pleurotus ferulae	Reduce plasma total cholesterol, triglyceride, low-density lipoprotein (LDL), total lipid, phospholipids, and LDL/high-density lipoprotein ratio	Alam et al., 2011
Pleurotus pulmonaris	Reduce plasma fasting glucose	Gulati et al., 2019
Pleurotus tuber-regium	serum TC, TG, and LDL concentrations	Huang et al., 2014
Pleurotus sajor-caju	Improve glucose tolerance, attenuate hyperglycemia and insulin resistance by upregulating the expression of glucose transporter protein 4 (GLUT-4) and adiponectin genes, and down-regulates the expression of inflammatory markers (IL-6, TNF-α, SAA2, CRP and MCP-1) via the attenuation of NF-κB pathway	Kanagasabapathy et al., 2012
Pleurotus florida	Lower blood glucose, serum cholesterol, triglycerides, as well as urine glucose and ketones. Restores anti-oxidant enzymes SOD, CAT.	Ganeshpurkar et al., 2014

The possible mechanism for the hepatoprotective activity is considered to be the ability of the white rot polysaccharide to reduce the hepatic lipid levels by moderating the serum enzyme activities and serum lipid levels, enhancing the antioxidant enzymes and reducing lipid peroxidation (Gao et al., 2003). The studies on hepatoprotective effect of white rot polysaccharide are scarce and only a few genera of white rots (*Ganoderma, Phellinus,* and *Pleurotus*) have been studied so far (Table 7.4).

7.5.6 Antioxidant Potential

The normal functioning of biological processes require energy that is obtained via various oxidation reactions occurring inside the body. These oxidation reactions are often coupled with the production of oxygen free and nonoxygen free radicals as by products (Liu et al., 2016). Uncontrolled production of these free radicals causes damage to cells and their functions, including interference and manipulation of proteins, peroxidation of membrane lipids, genetic damage, induction of disease and inflammation, promotion of aging, and tissue loosening (Kan et al., 2015). In order to reduce the associated health risks and to scavenge these radicals from the body there is a need to supplement food items with antioxidants (Huang et al., 2012). There is a high demand from consumers for food ingredients containing natural antioxidants as synthetic antioxidants are associated with potential health hazards such as liver damage and carcinogenesis (Aug et al., 2014) and only a limited number of natural antioxidants are available.

Thus, there is a need to look for effective alternatives to already existing synthetic stabilizers. Fruits, whole grains, vegetables, spices, and herbs are considered to be a good natural source containing appreciable amounts of antioxidants. However, mushrooms, particularly the white rots, have been widely

TABLE 7.4

Hepatoprotective Activity of White Rot Polysaccharide

Organism	Hepato-protective effect	Reference
Ganoderma lucidum	Decrease the levels of ALT (alanine aminotransferase), AST (aspartate aminotransferase), and MDA (malonialdehyde) and significantly increased the levels of SOD (superoxide dismutase) and CAT (catalase)	Susilo et al., 2019
Phellinus gilvus	Decrease hepatic malondialdehyde and elevate the levels of hepatic antioxidant enzymes (superoxide dismutase, catalase, and glutathione peroxidase)	Park et al., 2009
Phellinus linteus	Increase serum aminotransferase levels, promote oxidative stress by increasing lipid peroxidation and decreasing antioxidant enzyme activities	Chen et al., 2020
Phellinus rimosus	Increase the levels of serum glutamate pyruvate transaminase (SGPT), serum glutamate oxaloacetate transaminase (SGOT) and serum alkaline phosphatase (ALP)	Ajith and Janardhan 2002
Pleurotus djamor	Remarkably increase the levels of TC, TG and ALB, and prominently restored the activities of SOD, GSH-Px, CAT and T-AOC in serum/liver homogenate	Zhang et al., 2015
Pleurotus eryngii SI-04	Increase the serum enzyme activities and bilirubin (BIL) levels, decrease the serum albumin (ALB) and triglyceride (TG) levels, improve the hepatic antioxidant status, and ameliorate the hepatic structure damage.	Zhang et al., 2016
Pleurotus geesteranus	Increase the activity of hepatic enzymes (superoxide dismutase, glutathione peroxidase and catalase) and reduce lipid peroxidation	Song et al., 2018
Pleurotus ostreatus	Decrease alanine transaminase and aspartate transaminase levels in blood, increase superoxide dismutase, catalase, and glutathione peroxidase levels, and decrease malondialdehyde levels in blood and liver	Zhu et al., 2019

studied for their antioxidant effect. White rots produce a variety of bioactive compounds that possess antioxidant activity. One of these bioactive compounds is exopolysaccharide, which has been proven to be effective in scavenging the reactive radicals such as superoxide, hydrogen peroxide, and hydroxyl radicals (Rahi et al., 2018a). Various studies have reported that the antioxidant activity of polysaccharides extracted from white rot fungi such as *Ganoderma lucidium, Lentinus edodes, Pleurotus linteus,* and *Trametes versicolor* is mainly due to their ability to efficiently reduce and chelate the free radicals. Moreover, some white rot polysaccharides such as Ganoderan (produced by *Ganoderma* sp.) are known to limit the production of oxygen-free radicals and enhance the activity of antioxidant enzymes in the serum (You and Lin, 2002; XiaoPing et al., 2009). The antioxidant effect of the polysaccharide produced by white rot fungi has been summarized in Table 7.5.

7.5.7 Prebiotic Activity

Prebiotics represent one of the category of functional foods that have gained importance lately due to their health benefits (Rahi et al., 2018b). Prebiotics are crucial for human health as they are capable of regulating the structure and number of intestinal flora (Singhdevsachan et al., 2016). The bioactive polysaccharides produced by white rots cannot be digested easily in the human intestine and thus are

TABLE 7.5

Exopolysaccharide-Producing White Rot Species with Antioxidant Properties

Organism	Nature of polysaccharide	Antioxidant activity	Reference
Amauroderma rugosum	Glucan	Inhibition of NO production and NO scavenging activity	Chan et al., 2013; Zhang et al., 2017
Cerrena unicolor	Glucan	Free radical scavenging activity	Jaszek et al., 2013
Flammulina velutipes	Glucan	Scavenge superoxide anion radicals, inhibition of MDA production	Wu et al., 2014; Dong et al., 2017
Ganoderma lucidium	Glucan	Superoxide and hydroxyl radical scavenging activities, lipid peroxidation- inhibiting activity	Cherian et al., 2009; Si et al., 2019
Inonotus obliquus		Increased radical scavenging,	De Silva et al., 2012
Lentinus edodes	Lentinan	Free radical scavenging activity	Mattila et al., 2000; Ina et al., 2013; Giavasis 2014; Sugiyama 2016
Phellinus vaninii		Ferric reducing antioxidant power (FRAP), hydroxyl radical scavenging activity (HSA), and DPPH radical scavenging	Li et al., 2019
Pleurotus ostreatus	Pleurotan	Radical scavenging activity, ferric ion reducing power, chelating transition metal ions, lipid peroxidation inhibition, and fluorescence quenching	Barakat and Sadik 2014
Pleurotus pulmonarius RDM9	Glucan	Radical scavenging and reducing activity	Malik et al., 2019
Schizophyllum commune	Schizophyllan	Radical scavenging activity, ferric ion reducing power	Zong et al., 2012; Zhang et al., 2013

known to serve as potential dietary fibers (Giavasis, 2013). These polysaccharides significantly modify the intestinal flora by promoting the growth of beneficial microbes and by inhibiting the proliferation of harmful pathogenic bacteria (Zhou et al., 2011). Different mushroom polysaccharides like pleuran (Pleurotus sp.), lentinan (Lentinus sp.), schizophyllan (Schizophyllum sp.), and β- and α-glucans are known to possess remarkable prebiotic properties. Currently β-glucans isolated from *Pleurotus ostreatus* (Pleuran) and *Lentinus edodes (Lentinan)* are the most frequently used glucans as prebiotics showing positive effect on the intestinal flora. They also increase the resistance of intestine mucosa to inflammation and also inhibit development of gastric ulcers (Zeman et al., 2001). The β-1,3-1,6-glucan and linear α-1,3-glucan from *P. ostreatus* and *P. eryngii* have been reported to enhance the growth of prebiotic strains *Lactobacillus, Bifidobacterium,* and *Enterococcus* (Synytsya et al., 2009). β-glucans obtained from the sclerotia of *P. tuber-regium* is also reported to enhance the growth of *Bifidobacterium infantis, Bifidobacterium longum*, and *Bifidobacterium adolescentis* in liquid cultures (Zhao and Cheung, 2011). Moreover, these glucans are also known to enhance absorption of calcium and magnesium from the gut. In a study carried out by Chou et al. (2013) it was found that the polysaccharides from *Flammulina velutipes, Lentinula edodes*, and *Pleurotus eryngii* were found to enhance the survival rate of probiotics (*Lactobacillus acidophilus, Lactobacillus casei*, and *Bifidobacterium longum* subsp. *longum*) during cold storage. In another study it was reported that the polysaccharide produced by *G. lucidum* was capable of reducing the pathogenic bacteria while augmenting the beneficial strains (Khan et al., 2018). Yamin et al., 2012 also reported a positive effect of *Ganoderma lucidium* polysaccharide on the growth of *Bifidobacterium* sp. and *Lactobacillus* sp. and a negative effect on the growth of *Salmonella* sp.

TABLE 7.6

Nutraceuticals vs. Functional Foods and Pharmaceuticals

Nutraceuticals	Functional food	Pharmaceuticals
Nutraceuticals are generally defined as food or a component of food that provides health benefits, along with the prevention or treatment of a disease	Functional foods are the fortified/enriched foods that besides providing the body with essential nutrients also confer positive health benefits when consumed at sufficient level as a part of regular diet.	Pharmaceuticals are the drugs manufactured for treating a specific disease
Nutraceuticals can be from plant, animal, and mineral source	Naturally derived	Pharmaceuticals are mainly derived from a synthetic source
As per Section 22 of the FSS Act license is needed for the manufacturing, sale, distribution of nutraceutical product.	As per Section 22 of the FSS Act license is needed for the manufacturing, sale, distribution of functional foods.	License is needed from regulatory body for selling the pharmaceutical product (other than OTC products)
No prescription is required for purchasing nutraceutical products	No prescription is required for purchasing nutraceutical products	Pharmaceutical products can be purchased only by prescriptions (other than OTC products)

7.5.8 Nutraceutical Potential and Functional Foods

7.5.8.1 Nutraceutical versus Functional Foods and Pharmaceuticals

The term nutraceutical was coined in 1989 by Stephen DeFelice, MD, founder and chairman of the Foundation for Innovation in Medicine (FIM), Cranford, NJ from the terms "nutrition" and "pharmaceutical." A nutraceutical is generally defined as a food or a component of food that provides health benefits, along with the prevention or treatment of a disease (Brower, 1998). Nutraceutical is mainly a refined extract that is consumed either in the form of capsules or tablets as a supplement (Rahi et al., 2005). A functional food on the other hand reduce the risk of chronic disease by providing the body with the required amount of vitamins, fats, proteins, carbohydrates, etc., needed for its healthy survival.

A pharmaceutical is any kind of drug that is manufactured for medicinal purposes. The major difference between a nutraceutical and pharmaceutical is that pharmaceuticals are designed specifically for medical use under a physician's supervision, and are subjected to the Food and Drug Administration approval. Due to their high cost and associated side effects consumers are now turning towards nutraceuticals since they are naturally derived and possess almost no side effects (Table 7.6).

7.5.8.2 Potential of white rot polysaccharide as nutraceuticals and functional food

Mushrooms are the only fungi that knowingly are consumed by humans since they complement and supplement the human diet. The flavor and texture of mushrooms have been devoured by mankind for a long time. They have been reported to be the most valuable ones for humans and research on their therapeutic and nutritional aspects is underway throughout the world (Rahi et al., 2005). Mushrooms have been used as nutraceuticals for a very long time (Rahi et al., 2004). The white rot mushrooms with remarkable nutraceutical properties include *Lentinus* sp., *Grifola* sp., *Pleurotus* sp., and *Ganoderma* sp. The biological activity of mushrooms is attributed to a number of bioactive compounds such as alkaloids, steroids, polyphenols, polysaccharides, fatty acids, etc., produced by them (Souilem et al., 2017; Sánchez 2017). Mushroom glucans are considered to be one of the most promising nutraceutical compounds with excellent nutritional and therapeutic properties (Ren et al., 2018a; Wang et al., 2017e). Mushroom polysaccharides are being incorporated into various food items to obtain fortified functional foods. One such example is the addition of polysaccharides from *Lentinula edodes*, *Pleurotus eryngii*, and *Flammulina velutipes in order* to improve the survival rate of probiotics in yogurt. Other studies have reported that the glucan isolated from *Lentinus edodes* can be used to produce a novel functional food with low calories and high fiber content by using it as a replacement for wheat flour (Kim et al., 2011). These glucans can also be used as partial flour replacement in noodles to increase their fiber content and enhance quality characteristics (Kim et al., 2008; 2009). Various other studies have reported that the glucans from *Ganoderma* sp., *Flammulina* spp., and *Lentinus* sp. have notable antioxidant potential and thus can be used as natural antioxidants for fortification of food items (Kozarski et al., 2011; Giavasis, 2014). Cultures of *Schizophyllum commune* can be used to ferment lactose to produce beta glucan cheese, which is known to have significant antithrombotic effect (Okamura-Matsui et al., 2001). The polysaccharide produced by *Pleurotus ostreatus* has been added to an Indian papad snack to improve its fiber content. A potential advantage of using these polysaccharides is that they contain monosodium glutamate-like components and savory taste, which helps in improving the flavor of the final product.

7.6 Conclusion

White rot fungi are the heterogeneous group of fungi belonging to basidiomycetes and comprise 90% of the total wood-rotting fungi. The white rots are known to possess immense pharmaceutical potential as they are capable of producing a variety of bioactive compounds such as the polysaccharides, sterols, terpenoids, phenolic compounds, etc. Of these metabolites, polysaccharide is considered to be a major group, and has been extensively studied in the recent past. The polysaccharides produced by white rot fungi are of great medical importance and have been extensively used in food and pharmaceutical industries. The unique properties of these polysaccharides render them suitable for applicability in various fields. The polysaccharides produced by them can serve as immune-modulating agents, have antioxidant, anti-inflammatory, hypolipidemic, hepatoprotective, antitumor properties, can act as prebiotics, and also serve for the development of novel functional foods. In spite of their remarkable bioactivities, so far only a handful of white rots have been explored for their ability to produce bioactive polysaccharides. A comprehensive exploration of white rot fungi and their properties is thus required in this field to fully utilize their potential in order to open new avenues towards various biomedical applications.

REFERENCES

Afiati F, Firza SF, Kusmiati, Aliya LS (2019) The effectiveness β-glucan of shiitake mushrooms and Saccharomyces cerevisiae as antidiabetic and antioxidant in mice Sprague Dawley induced alloxan. In *AIP Conference Proceedings* 2120 (1): 070006

Ajith TA, Janardhanan KK (2002) Antioxidant and antihepatotoxic activities of *Phellinus rimosus* (Berk) Pilat. J Ethnopharmacol 81(3): 387–391

Akramiene D, Aleksandraviciene C, Grazeliene G, Zalinkevicius R, Suziedelis K, Didziapetriene J, Kevelaitis E (2010) Potentiating effect of β-glucans on photodynamic therapy of implanted cancer cells in mice. Tohoku J Exp Med 220(4): 299–306

Alam N, Yoon KN, Lee TS (2011) Antihyperlipidemic activities of *Pleurotus ferulae* on biochemical and histological function in hypercholesterolemic rats. J Res Med Sci 16(6): 776

Aug A, Altraja A, Altraja S, Laaniste L, Mahlapuu R, Soomets U, Kilk K (2014) Alterations of Bronchial Epithelial Metabolome by Cigarette Smoke Are Reversible by an Antioxidant, O-Methyl-l-Tyrosinyl-γ-l-Glutamyl-l-Cysteinylglycine. Am J Resp Cell Mol 51(4): 586–594

Bains RK, Rahi DK, Hoondal GS (2006) Evaluation of wood degradation enzymes of some indigenous white rot fungi. J Mycol Pl Pathol 36: 161–164

Bao X, Liu C, Fang J, Li X (2001) Structural and immunological studies of a major polysaccharide from spores of *Ganoderma lucidum* (Fr.) Karst. Carbohydr Res 332(1): 67–74

Barakat OS, Sadik MW (2014) Mycelial growth and bioactive substance production of pleurotusostreatusin submerged culture. Int J Curr Microbiol Appl Sci 3(4): 1073–1085

Bisen PS, Baghel RK, Sanodiya BS, Thakur GS, Prasad GBKS (2010) *Lentinus edodes*: a macrofungus with pharmacological activities. Curr Med Chem 17(22): 2419–2430

Blanchette RA, Farrell RL, Iverson S (1995) Pitch degradation with white rot fungi. U.S. Patent # 5,476,790

Branda SS, Vik A, Friedman L, Kolter R (2005). Biofilm: the matrix revisited. Trends Microbiol 13: 20–26

Brower V (1998) Nutraceuticals: poised for a healthy slice of the healthcare market? Nat Biotechnol 16(8): 728–731

Castro-Alves VC, Gomes D, Menolli Jr N, Sforça M L, do Nascimento JRO (2017) Characterization and immunomodulatory effects of glucans from *Pleurotus albidus*, a promising species of mushroom for farming and biomass production. Int J Biol macromol 95: 215–223

Chan PM, Kanagasabapathy G, Tan YS, Sabaratnam V, Kuppusamy UR (2013) *Amauroderma rugosum* (Blume & T. Nees) Torrend: nutritional composition and antioxidant and potential antiinflammatory properties. Evid Based Complement Alternat Med 1–10

Chang ST, Wasser SP (2012) The role of culinary-medicinal mushrooms on human welfare with a pyramid model for human health. Int J Med Mushrooms 14(2): 95–134

Chen C, Liu X, Qi S, Dias AC, Yan J, Zhang X (2020) Hepatoprotective effect of *Phellinus linteus* mycelia polysaccharide (PL-N1) against acetaminophen-induced liver injury in mouse. Int J Biol macromol 154: 1276–1284

Chen F, Long X, Yu M, Liu Z, Liu L, Shao H (2013) Phenolics and antifungal activities analysis in industrial crop Jerusalem artichoke (*Helianthus tuberosus* L.) leaves. Ind Crop Prod 47: 339–345

Chen J, Seviour R (2007). Medicinal importance of fungal β-(1→ 3),(1→ 6)-glucans. Mycol Res, 111(6): 635–652

Cherian E, Sudheesh NP, Janardhanan KK, Patani G (2009) Free radical scavenging and mitochondrial antioxidant activities of Reishi-*Ganoderma lucidum* (Curt: Fr) P. Karst and Arogyapacha-Trichopus zeylanicus Gaertn extracts. J Basic Clin Physiol Pharmacol 20(4): 289–308

Choi D. Piao Y, Yu SJ, Lee YW, Lim DH, Chang YC, Cho H (2016) Antihyperglycemic and antioxidant activities of polysaccharide produced from *Pleurotus ferulae* in streptozotocin-induced diabetic rats. Korean J Chem Eng 33(6): 1872–1882

Chou WT, Sheih IC, Fang TJ (2013) The applications of polysaccharides from various mushroom wastes as prebiotics in different systems. J Food Sci *78*(7): 1041–1048

De Silva DD, Rapior S, Hyde KD, Bahkali AH (2012). Medicinal mushrooms in prevention and control of diabetes mellitus Fungal Divers 56(1): 1–29

Descroix K, Větvička V, Laurent I, Jamois F, Yvin JC, Ferrières V (2010) New oligo-β-(1, 3)-glucan derivatives as immunostimulating agents. Bioorg Med Chem, 18(1): 348–357

Dong YR, Cheng SJ, Qi GH, Yang ZP, Yin SY, Chen GT (2017) Antimicrobial and antioxidant activities of Flammulina velutipes polysacchrides and polysacchride-iron (III) complex. Carbohydr polym 161: 26–32

Dugowson CE, Gnanashanmugam P (2006) Nonsteroidal anti-inflammatory drugs. Phys Med Rehabil Clin 17(2): 347–354

Elsayed EA, El Enshasy H, Wadaan MA, Aziz R (2014) Mushrooms: a potential natural source of anti-inflammatory compounds for medical applications. Mediators of inflamm 805841

Falch BH, Espevik T, Ryan L, Stokke BT (2000) Thecytokine stimulating activity of(1→3)-d-glucans is dependent on the triple helix conformation. Carbohyde Res 329: 587–596

Fan J, Wu Z, Zhao T, Sun Y, Ye H, Xu R, Zeng X (2014). Characterization, antioxidant and hepatoprotective activities of polysaccharides from *Ilex latifolia* Thunb. Carbohydr polym 101: 990–997

Fosbøl EL, Gislason GH, Jacobsen S, Folke F, Hansen ML, Schramm TK, Torp-Pedersen C (2009) Risk of myocardial infarction and death associated with the use of nonsteroidal anti-inflammatory drugs (NSAIDs) among healthy individuals: a nationwide cohort study. Clin Pharmacol Ther 85(2): 190–197

Friedman M (2016) Mushroom polysaccharides: Chemistry and antiobesity, anti-diabetes, anticancer, and antibiotic properties in cells, rodents and humans. Foods 5(4): 80

Frolund B, Griebe T, Nielsen PH (1995) Enzymatic activity in the activated-sludge floc matrix. Appl Microbiol Biotechnol 43: 755–761.

Frolund B, Palmgren R, Keiding K, Nielsen PH (1996) Extraction of extracellular polymers from activated sludge using a cation exchange resin. Water Res 30: 1749–1758

Ganeshpurkar A, Kohli S, Rai G (2014) Antidiabetic potential of polysaccharides from the white oyster culinary-medicinal mushroom *Pleurotus florida* (higher Basidiomycetes). Int J Med Mushrooms 6(3)

Gao YH, Huang M, Lin ZB, Zhou SF (2003) Hepatoprotective activity and the mechanisms of action of *Ganoderma lucidum* (Curt:Fr) P. Karst. (Ling Zhi, Reishi Mushroom) (Aphyllophoromycetidae). Int J Med Mushrooms 5: 111–131

Giavasis I (2003) Physiological studies on the production of gellan gum by *Sphingomonas paucimobilis* (Doctoral dissertation, University of Strathclyde)

Giavasis I (2013) Production of microbial polysaccharides for use in food. pp. 413–468. In: McNeil, B., Archer, D., Giavasis, I. and Harvey, L. (eds.). Microbial production of food ingredients, enzymes and nutraceuticals, Woodhead Publishing

Giavasis I (2014) Bioactive fungal polysaccharides as potential functional ingredients in food and nutraceuticals. Curr Opin Biotechnol 26: 162–173

Giavasis I, Biliaderis C (2006) Microbial polysaccharides. In Functional Food Carbohydrates, ed. C. Biliaderis, and M. Izydorczyk, pp. 167–214. Boca Raton: CRC Press

Gulati V, Singh MD, Gulati P (2019) Role of mushrooms in gestational diabetes mellitus. AIMS Med Sci 6(1): 49–66

Guo L, Xie J, Ruan Y, Zhou L, Zhu H, Yun X, Gu J (2009) Characterization and immunostimulatory activity of a polysaccharide from the spores of *Ganoderma lucidum*. Int immunopharmacol 9(10): 1175–1182

Guo WL, Deng JC, Pan YY, Xu JX, Hong JL, Shi FF, Lv XC (2020). Hypoglycemic and hypolipidemic activities of *Grifola frondosa* polysaccharides and their relationships with the modulation of intestinal microflora in diabetic mice induced by high-fat diet and streptozotocin. Int J Biol macromol 153: 1231–1240

Hobbs C (2005) The chemistry, nutritional value, immunopharmacology, and safety of the traditional food of medicinal split-gill fugus *Schizophyllum commune* Fr.: Fr.(Schizophyllaceae). A literature review. Int J Med Mushrooms 7(1,2)

Huang HY, Korivi M, Yang HT, Huang CC, Chaing YY, Tsai YC (2014) Effect of *Pleurotus tuber-regium* polysaccharides supplementation on the progression of diabetes complications in obese-diabetic rats. Chin J Physiol 57(4): 198–208

Huang SQ, Ding S, Fan L (2012) Antioxidant activities of five polysaccharides from *Inonotus obliquus*. Int J Biol Macromol 50(5): 1183–1187

Ikekawa T (2001) Beneficial effects of edible and medicinal mushrooms on health care. Int J Med Mushrooms 3(2–3)

Ina K, Kataoka T, Ando T (2013) The use of lentinan for treating gastric cancer. Anti-Canc Ag Med Chem 13(5): 681–688

Ismail B, Nampoothiri KM (2010) Production, purification and structural characterization of an exopolysaccharide produced by a probiotic *Lactobacillus plantarum* MTCC 9510. Arch Microbiol 192: 1049–1057

Jamois F, Ferrières V, Guégan JP, Yvin JC, Plusquellec D, Vetvicka V (2005) Glucan-like synthetic oligosaccharides: iterative synthesis of linear oligo-β-(1, 3)-glucans and immunostimulatory effects. Glycobiol 15(4): 393–407

Jaszek M, Osińska-Jaroszuk M, Janusz G, Matuszewska A, Stefaniuk D (2013) New bioactive fungal molecules with high antioxidant and antimicrobial capacity isolated from *Cerrena unicolor* idiophasic cultures. BioMed Res Int 497492: 1–11

Jedinak A, Dudhgaonkar S, Wu QL, Simon J, Sliva D (2011) Anti-inflammatory activity of edible oyster mushroom is mediated through the inhibition of NF-κB and AP-1 signaling. Nutr. J., 10(1): 52

Joseph MM, Aravind SR, Varghese S, Mini S, Sreelekha TT (2012) Evaluation of antioxidant, antitumor and immunomodulatory properties of polysaccharide isolated from fruit rind of *Punica granatum*. Mol Med Rep 5(2): 489–496

Kakumu S, Ishikawa T, Wakita T, Yoshioka K, Ito Y, Shinagawa T (1991) Effect of sizofiran, a polysaccharide, on interferon gamma, antibody production and lymphocyte proliferation specific for hepatitis B virus antigen in patients with chronic hepatitis B. Int Immunopharmacol 13(7): 969–975

Kan Y, Chen T, Wu Y, Wu J (2015) Antioxidant activity of polysaccharide extracted from *Ganoderma lucidum* using response surface methodology. Int J Biol Macromol 72: 151–157

Kanagasabapathy G, Kuppusamy UR, Abd Malek SN, Abdulla MA, Chua KH, Sabaratnam V (2012) Glucan-rich polysaccharides from *Pleurotus sajor-caju* (Fr.) Singer prevents glucose intolerance, insulin resistance and inflammation in C57BL/6J mice fed a high-fat diet. BMC Compl Alternative Med 12(1): 261

Khan I, Huang G, Li X, Leong W, Xia W, Hsiao WW (2018) Mushroom polysaccharides from *Ganoderma lucidum* and *Poria cocos* reveal prebiotic functions. J func foods 41: 191–201

Kim J, Lee SM, Bae IY, Park HG, Lee HG, Lee S (2011) (1–3)(1–6)-β-Glucan-enriched materials from *Lentinus edodes* mushroom as a high-fibre and low-calorie flour substitute for baked foods. J Sci Food Agric 91(10): 1915–1919

Kim SY, Chung SI, Nam SH, Kang MY (2009) Cholesterol lowering action and antioxidant status improving efficacy of noodles made from unmarketable oak mushroom (*Lentinus edodes*) in high cholesterol fed rats. J Kor Soc Appl Biol Chem 52(3): 207–212

Kim SY, Kang MY, Kim MH (2008) Quality characteristics of noodle added with browned oak mushroom (*Lentinus edodes*). Korean J Food Cook Sci 24(5): 665–671

Kojima H, Akaki J, Nakajima S, Kamei K, Tamesada M (2010) Structural analysis of glycogen-like polysaccharides having macrophage-activating activity in extracts of *Lentinula edodes* mycelia. J Nat Med 64(1): 16–23

Kozarski M, Klaus A, Niksic M, Jakovljevic D, Helsper JP, Van Griensven LJ (2011) Antioxidative and immunomodulating activities of polysaccharide extracts of the medicinal mushrooms *Agaricus bisporus, Agaricus brasiliensis, Ganoderma lucidum* and *Phellinus linteus*. Food Chem 129(4): 1667–1675

Lakhanpal TN, Rana M (2005) Medicinal and nutraceutical genetic resources of mushrooms. Plant Genet Resour 3(2): 288–303

Laspidou CS, Rittmann BE (2002) A unified theory for extracellular polymeric substances, soluble microbial products, and active and inert biomass. Water Res 36: 2711–2720

Latha K, Baskar R (2014) Comparative study on the production, purification and characterization of exopolysaccharides from oyster mushrooms, *Pleurotus florida* and *Hypsizygus ulmarius* and their applications. Proc 8th Int Conf Mush Biol Mush Prod 192–198

Lavi I, Levinson D, Peri I, Nimri L, Hadar Y, Schwartz B (2010) Orally administered glucans from the edible mushroom *Pleurotus pulmonarius* reduce acute inflammation in dextran sulfate sodium-induced experimental colitis. Br J Nutr 103(3): 393–402

Lavi I, Nimri L, Levinson D, Peri I, Hadar Y, Schwartz B (2012) Glucans from the edible mushroom *Pleurotus pulmonarius* inhibit colitis-associated colon carcinogenesis in mice. J. gastroentero 47(5): 504–518

Li J, Jia X, Yao Y, Bai Y (2019) Characterization of exopolysaccharide produced by *Phellinus vaninii* (Agaricomycetes) and antioxidant potential for meat batter. Int J Med. Mushrooms 21(5)

Li S, Shah NP (2014) Antioxidant and antibacterial activities of sulphated polysaccharides from *Pleurotus eryngii* and *Streptococcus thermophilus* ASCC 1275. Food chem 165: 262–270

Lindequist U, Niedermeyer TH, Jülich WD (2005) The pharmacological potential of mushrooms. Evid Based Complementary Altern Med 2

Liu Q, Tian G, Yan H, Geng X, Cao Q, Wang H, Ng TB (2014) Characterization of polysaccharides with antioxidant and hepatoprotective activities from the wild edible mushroom *Russula vinos*a Lindblad. J agric food chem 62(35): 8858–8866

Liu Y, Fang HHP (2003) Influence of extracellular polymeric substances (EPS) on flocculation, settling, and dewatering of activated sludge. Crit Rev Environ Sci Technol. 33: 237–273

Liu Y, Zhang B, Ibrahim SA, Gao SS, Yang H, Huang W (2016) Purification, characterization and antioxidant activity of polysaccharides from *Flammulina velutipes* residue. Carbohydr Polym 145: 71–77.

Lo TCT, Hsu FM, Chang CA, Cheng JCH (2011) Branched α-(1, 4) glucans from *Lentinula edodes* (L10) in combination with radiation enhance cytotoxic effect on human lung adenocarcinoma through the toll-like receptor 4 mediated induction of THP-1 differentiation/activation. J Agric Food Chem 59(22): 11997–12005

Ma K, Ruan Z (2015) Production of a lignocellulolytic enzyme system for simultaneous bio-delignification and saccharification of corn stover employing co-culture of fungi. Bioresour Technol 175: 586–593

Ma L, Chen H, Zhu W, Wang Z (2013) Effect of different drying methods on physicochemical properties and antioxidant activities of polysaccharides extracted from mushroom *Inonotus obliquus*. Food Res Int 50(2): 633–640

Mahajna J, Dotan, N, Zaidman, BZ, Petrova, RD, Wasser SP (2008) Pharmacological values of medicinal mushrooms for prostate cancer therapy: the case of *Ganoderma lucidum*. Nutr Canc 61(1): 16–26

Maiti S, Mallick SK, Bhutia SK, Behera B, Mandal M, Maiti TK (2011) Antitumor effect of culinary-medicinal oyster mushroom, *Pleurotus ostreatus* (Jacq.: Fr.) P. Kumm., derived protein fraction on tumor-bearing mice models. Int J Med Mushrooms 13(5)

Majumdar I, D'Souza F, Bhosle NB (1999) Microbial exopolysaccharides: effect on corrosion and partial chemical characterization. J Ind Inst Sci 79: 539–550.

Malik D, Rahi DK, Prabha V (2019) Safety Evaluation and In vitro Antioxidant Activity of Exopolysaccharide Produced by an Indigenous Species of *Pleurotus pulmonarius* RDM9. Toxicol Int 25(1): 40–47

Markova NV, Kussovski T, Radoucheva K, Dilova, Georgieva N (2002) Effects of intraperitoneal and intranasal application of Lentinan on cellular response in rats. Int Immunopharm 2: 1641–1645

Masuda Y, Nawa D, Nakayama Y, Konishi M, Nanba H (2015) Soluble β-glucan from *Grifola frondosa* induces tumor regression in synergy with TLR9 agonist via dendritic cell-mediated immunity. J Leukoc Biol 98(6): 1015–1025

Mattila P, Suonpää K, Piironen V (2000) Functional properties of edible mushrooms. Nutrition 16(7–8): 694–696

Meek IL, Van de Laar MA, E Vonkeman H (2010) Non-steroidal anti-inflammatory drugs: an overview of cardiovascular risks. Pharmaceuticals 3(7): 2146–2162

Methacanon P, Madla S, Kirtikara K, Prasitsil M (2005) Structural elucidation of bioactive fungi-derived polymers. Carbohydr Polym 60(2): 199–203

Monsan P, Bozonnet S, Albenne C, Joucla G, Willemot RM and Remaud M (2001) Homopolysaccharides from lactic acid bacteria. Int Dairy J 11: 675–685

Mueller A, Raptis J, Rice PJ, Kalbfleisch JH, Stout RD, Ensley HE, Williams DL (2000) The influence of glucan polymer structure and solution conformation on binding to (1→ 3)-β-D-glucan receptors in a human monocyte-like cell line. Glycobiol 10(4): 339–346

Muszyńska B, Grzywacz-Kisielewska A, Kała K, Gdula-Argasińska J (2018) Anti-inflammatory properties of edible mushrooms: A review. Food Chem 243: 373–381

Navarro VJ, Senior JR (2006) Drug-related Hepatotoxicity. New England J Med 354: 731–739

Nielsen PH, Jahn A (1999) Extraction of EPS. In Wingender J, Neu TR, Flemming HC (Ed.), Microbial extracellular polymeric substances: characterization, structure and function. pp. 43-72.

Okamura-Matsui T, Takemura K, Sera M, Takeno T, Noda H (2001) Characteristics of a cheese-like food produced by fermentation of the mushroom *Schizophyllum commune*. J Biosci Bioeng 92(1): 30–32

Park SC, Cheon YP, Son WY, Rhee MH, Kim TW, Song JC and Kim KS (2009) Hepatoprotective effects of polysaccharides isolated from *Phellinus gilvus* against carbon tetrachloride-induced liver injury in rats. Toxicol Res 25(1): 29–33

Rahi DK, Chaudhary E, Malik D (2018a) Production of Exopolysaccharide by *Enterobacter cloacae,* a root nodule isolate from *Phaseolus vulgaris*: Parameter optimization for yield enhancement under submerged fermentation. Int J Basic Appl Res 8(9): 936–948

Rahi DK, Rajak RC, Pandey AK (2005) Mushroom Nutriceuticals: An Emerging Health Care Aid. Front Plant Sci 481–496

Rahi DK, Rahi S, Pandey AK, Rajak RC (2009) Enzymes from Mushrooms and their Industrial Applications. pp. 136–184. In: Rai, M. (ed.). Advances in Fungal Biotechnology, I.K. International Publishing House Pvt. Ltd., New Delhi

Rahi DK, Richa, Kaur M (2018b) Production of xylooligosaccharide from corn cob xylan by xylanase obtained from *Aureobasidium Pullulans*. Int J Sci Res Sci En Technol 4(4): 1142–1448

Rahi DK, Shukla KK, Rajak RC, Pandey AK (2004) Mushrooms and their sustainable utilization. Everyman Sci 38: 357–365

Rahi DK (2015) Fungal Production of Exopolysaccharides: Applications & Perspectives. pp.195–221. *In:* Sobti, R.C., Sharma, P. and Puri, S. (eds.). Emerging Trends in Microbial Biotechnology Energy and Environment, Narendra Publishing House, Delhi, India.

Ren Y, Geng Y, Du Y, Li W, Lu ZM, Xu HY, Xu ZH (2018) Polysaccharide of *Hericium erinaceus* attenuates colitis in C57BL/6 mice via regulation of oxidative stress, inflammation-related signaling pathways and modulating the composition of the gut microbiota. J Nutr Biochem 57: 67–76

Rony KA, Ajith TA, Nima N, Janardhanan KK (2014) Hypolipidemic activity of *Phellinus rimosus* against triton WR-1339 and high cholesterol diet induced hyperlipidemic rats. Environ Toxicol Pharmacol 37(2): 482–492

Roy SK, Das D, Mondal S, Maiti D, Bhunia B, Maiti TK, Islam SS (2009) Structural studies of an immunoenhancing water-soluble glucan isolated from hot water extract of an edible mushroom, i, cultivar Assam Florida. Carbohydr Res 344(18): 2596–2601

Satitmanwiwat S, Ratanakhanokchai K, Laohakunjit N, Chao LK, Chen ST, Pason P, Kyu KL (2012) Improved purity and immunostimulatory activity of β-(1→ 3)(1→ 6)-glucan from *Pleurotus sajor-caju* using cell wall-degrading enzymes. J Agric Food Chem 60(21): 5423–5430

Sánchez C (2017) Reactive oxygen species and antioxidant properties from mushrooms. Synth syst biotechnol 2(1): 3–22

Sanodiya BS, Thakur GS, Baghel RK, Prasad GBKS, Bisen PS (2009) *Ganodermalucidum*: a potent pharmacological macrofungus. Curr pharm biotechnol 10(8): 717–742

Sasidhara R, Thirunalasundari T (2012) Antimicrobial activity of mushrooms. Acta Pharmacol Sin 23(9): 787–791

Scheen AJ (2005) Diabetes mellitus in the elderly: insulin resistance and/or impaired insulin secretion. Diabetes Metab J, 31: 27–34

Schwartz B, Hadar Y, Sliva D (2013) The use of edible mushroom water soluble polysaccharides in the treatment and prevention of chronic diseases: a mechanistic approach. In Antitumor Potential and other Emerging Medicinal Properties of Natural Compounds. Springer, Dordrecht. pp. 263–283.

Selegean M, Putz MV, Rugea T (2009) Effect of the polysaccharide extract from the edible mushroom *Pleurotus ostreatus* against infectious Bursal disease virus. Int J Mol Sci 10: 3616–3634.

Shenbhagaraman R, Jagadish LK, Premalatha K, Kaviyarasan V (2012) Optimization of extracellular glucan production from Pleurotus eryngii and its impact on angiogenesis. Int. J biol. Macromol., 50(4): 957–964.

Si J, Meng G, Wu Y, Ma HF, Cui BK, Dai YC (2019) Medium composition optimization, structural characterization, and antioxidant activity of exopolysaccharides from the medicinal mushroom *Ganoderma lingzhi*. Int J biol Macromol 124: 1186–1196

Signoretto C, Marchi A, Bertoncelli A, Burlacchini G, Papetti A, Pruzzo C, Canepari P (2014) The anti-adhesive mode of action of a purified mushroom (*Lentinus edodes*) extract with anticaries and antigingivitis properties in two oral bacterial pathogens. BMC Compl Alternative Med 14(1): 1–9

Singdevsachan SK, Auroshree P, Mishra J, Baliyarsingh B, Tayung K, Thatoi H (2016) Mushroom polysaccharides as potential prebiotics with their antitumor and immunomodulating properties: A review. Bioact Carbohydr Diet 7(1): 1–14.

Sinha M, Gautam L, Shukla PK, Kaur P, Sharma S, Singh TP (2013) Current perspectives in NSAID-induced gastropathy. Mediators inflamm 2013: 258209

Song X, Liu Z, Zhang J, Yang Q, Ren Z, Zhang C, Jia L (2018) Anti-inflammatory and hepatoprotective effects of exopolysaccharides isolated from *Pleurotus geesteranus* on alcohol-induced liver injury. Sci Rep 8(1): 1–13

Souilem F, Fernandes Â, Calhelha RC, Barreira JC, Barros L, Skhiri F, Ferreira IC (2017) Wild mushrooms and their mycelia as sources of bioactive compounds: Antioxidant, anti-inflammatory and cytotoxic properties. Food chem 230: 40–48

Stachowiak B, Reguła J (2012) Health-promoting potential of edible macromycetes under special consideration of polysaccharides: a review. Eur Food Res Technol 234(3): 369–380.

Sugiyama Y (2016) Polysaccharides. pp. 37–50. In: Yamaguchi, Y. (ed.). Immunotherapy of cancer, Springer, Berlin

Susilo RJK, Winarni D, Husen SA, Hayaza S, Punnapayak H, Wahyuningsih SPA, Darmanto W (2019) Hepatoprotective effect of crude polysaccharides extracted from *Ganoderma lucidum* against carbon tetrachloride-induced liver injury in mice. Vet. World 12(12): 1987

Sutherland IW (1972) Biosynthesis of microbial polysaccharides. Adv Microb Physiol 23: 79–150

Synytsya A, Míčková K, Synytsya A, Jablonský I, Spěváček J, Erban V, Čopíková J (2009) Glucans from fruit bodies of cultivated mushrooms *Pleurotus ostreatus* and *Pleurotus eryngii:* Structure and potential prebiotic activity. Carbohydr polym 76(4): 548–556

Tracy RP (2006) The five cardinal signs of inflammation: calor, dolor, rubor, tumor and penuria. J Gerontol A-biol 61(10): 1051–1052

Vannucci L, Krizan J, Sima P, Stakheev D, Caja F, Rajsiglova L, Saieh, M (2013) Immunostimulatory properties and antitumor activities of glucans. Int J Oncol 43(2): 357–364

Varki A, Cummings R, Esko J, Freeze H, Hart G, Marth J (1999) Essentials of Glycobiology Cold Spring.

Vuyst L, Degeest B (1999) Heteropolysaccharides from lactic acid bacteria. FEMS Microbiol Rev 23: 153–177

Wahyuni N, Ilyas S, Fitrie AA (2017) Effect of *Pleurotus Ostreatus* on Pancreatic Beta Cells of Diabetes Mellitus Mice Model. J K L 15(2): 155–159

Wang J, Xu X, Zheng H, Li J, Deng C, Xu Z, Chen J (2009) Structural characterization, chain conformation, and morphology of a β-(1→ 3)-d-glucan isolated from the fruiting body of Dictyophora indusiata. J Agric Food Chem 57(13): 5918–5924

Wang X, Zhang L (2009) Physicochemical properties and antitumor activities for sulfated derivatives of lentinan. Carbohydr Res 344(16): 2209–2216

Wang Y, Liu Y, Yu H, Zhou S, Zhang Z, Wu D (2017e) Structural characterization and immuno-enhancing activity of a highly branched water-soluble betaglucan from the spores of *Ganoderma lucidum*. Carbohydr Polym 167: 337–344

Wan-Mohtar WAAQI, Young L, Abbott GM, Clements C, Harvey LM, Kothari D (2018) Biomed. Pharmacother 105: 377–394

Wilgus TA, Roy S, McDaniel JC (2013) Neutrophils and wound repair: positive actions and negative reactions. Adv wound care 2(7): 379–388

Won DP, Lee JS, Kwon DS, Lee KE, Shin WC, Hong EK (2011) Immunostimulating activity by polysaccharides isolated from fruiting body of *Inonotus obliquus*. Mol Cells 31(2): 165–173

Wu DM, Duan WQ, Liu Y, Cen Y (2010) Anti-inflammatory effect of the polysaccharides of Golden needle mushroom in burned rats. Int J biol macromol 46(1): 100–103

Wu M, Luo X, Xu X, Wei W, Yu M (2014) Antioxidant and immunomodulatory activities of a polysaccharide from *Flammulina velutipes*. J Tradit Chin Med 34(6): 733–740

Wu SJ, Liaw CC, Pan SZ, Yang HC, Ng LT (2013) *Phellinus linteus* polysaccharides and their immunomodulatory properties in human monocytic cells. J Func Foods 5(2): 679–688

XiaoPing C, Yan C, ShuiBing L, YouGuo C, JianYun L, LanPing L (2009) Free radical scavenging of *Ganoderma lucidum* polysaccharides and its effect on antioxidant enzymes and immunity activities in cervical carcinoma rats. Carbohydr Res 77(2): 389–393

Xu Z, Chen X, Zhong Z, Chen L, Wang Y (2011) *Ganoderma lucidum* polysaccharides: immunomodulation and potential anti-tumor activities. AJCMB 39(01): 15–27

Yamin S, Shuhaimi M, Arbakariya A, Fatimah AB, Khalilah AK, Anas O, Yazid AM (2012) Effect of *Ganoderma lucidum* polysaccharides on the growth of *Bifidobacterium* spp. as assessed using Real-time PCR. Int Food Res J 19(3): 1199

Yang BK, Gu YA, Jeong YT, Jeong H, Song CH (2007) Chemical characteristics and immuno-modulating activities of exo-biopolymers produced by *Grifola frondosa* during submerged fermentation process. Int J Biol Macromol 41(3): 227–233

You YH, Lin ZB (2002) Protective effects of *Ganoderma lucidum* polysaccharides peptide on injury of macrophages induced by reactive oxygen species. Acta Pharmacol Sin 23(9): 787–791

Yuen JW, Gohel MDI (2005) Anticancer effects of *Ganoderma lucidum*: a review of scientific evidence. Nutr Canc 53(1): 11–17

Zeman M, Nosal ova V, Bobek P, Zakálová M, Cerna S (2001) Changes of endogenous melatonin and protective effect of diet containing pleuran and extract of black elder in colonic inflammation in rats. Biolgia-Bratisl 57(6): 695–702

Zeng B, Su M, Chen Q, Chang Q, Wang W, Li H (2016) Antioxidant and hepatoprotective activities of polysaccharides from *Anoectochilus roxburghii*. Carbohydr polym, 153: 391–398

Zhang C, Li S, Zhang J, Hu C, Che G, Zhou M, Jia, L (2016) Antioxidant and hepatoprotective activities of intracellular polysaccharide from *Pleurotus eryngii* SI-04. Int J Biol macromol 91: 568–577

Zhang J, Meng G, Zhang C, Lin L, Xu N, Liu M, Jia L (2015) The antioxidative effects of acidic-, alkalic-, and enzymatic-extractable mycelium zinc polysaccharides by *Pleurotus djamor* on liver and kidney of streptozocin-induced diabetic mice. BMC Complement Altern Med 15(1): 1–12

Zhang L, Khoo C, Koyyalamudi SR, Pedro ND, Reddy N (2017) Antioxidant, anti-inflammatory and anticancer activities of ethanol soluble organics from water extracts of selected medicinal herbs and their relation with flavonoid and phenolic contents. Pharmacologia 8(2): 59–72

Zhang M, Cui SW, Cheung PCK, Wang Q (2007) Antitumor polysaccharides from mushrooms: a review on their isolation process, structural characteristics and antitumor activity. Tr Food Sci Technol 18(1): 4–19

Zhang Y, Kong H, Fang Y, Nishinari K, Phillips GO (2013) Schizophyllan: A review on its structure, properties, bioactivities and recent developments. Bioact Carbohyd Diet Fibre 1(1): 53–71

Zhao C, Gao L, Wang C, Liu B, Jin Y, Xing Z (2016) Structural characterization and antiviral activity of a novel heteropolysaccharide isolated from *Grifola frondosa* against enterovirus 71. Carbohydr Polym 144: 382–389

Zhao J, Cheung PC (2011) Fermentation of β-glucans derived from different sources by bifidobacteria: evaluation of their bifidogenic effect. J Agric Food Chem 59(11): 5986–5992.

Zheng W, Zhao Y, Zheng X, Liu Y, Pan S (2011) Production of antioxidant and antitumor metabolites by submerged cultures of *Inonotus obliquus* cocultured with *Phellinus punctatus*. Appl Microbial Biotechnol 89(1): 157–167

Zhong K, Lin W, Wang Q, Zhou S (2012) Extraction and radicals scavenging activity of polysaccharides with microwave extraction from mung bean hulls. Int J biol macromol, 51(4): 612–617

Zhou BL, Liang Q, Zou Y, Ming J, Zhao GH (2011) Research progress in prebiotic properties of edible mushroom. Food Sci 2(15): 303–307

Zhu B, Li Y, Hu T, Zhang Y (2019) The hepatoprotective effect of polysaccharides from Pleurotus ostreatus on carbon tetrachloride-induced acute liver injury rats. Int J Biol macromol 131: 1–9

Zhu H, Sheng K, Yan E, Qiao J, Lv F (2012) Extraction, purification and antibacterial activities of a polysaccharide from spent mushroom substrate. Int J biol macromol *50*(3): 840–843

Zhu KX, Nie SP, Tan LH, Li C, Gong DM, Xie MY (2016) A polysaccharide from *Ganoderma atrum* improves liver function in type 2 diabetic rats via antioxidant action and short-chain fatty acids excretion. J Agric Food Chem 64(9): 1938–1944

Zhu XL, Chen AF, Lin ZB (2007) *Ganoderma lucidum* polysaccharides enhance the function of immunological effector cells in immunosuppressed mice. J ethnopharmacol 111(2): 219–226.

Zong A, Cao H, Wang F (2012) Anticancer polysaccharides from natural resources: A review of recent research. Carbohyd Polym 90(4): 1395–1410

Section II

Health, Disease, and Management

8

Membrane Lipids from Cellular Barriers to Health and Homeostasis

Sukesh Chander Sharma
Department of Biochemistry, Panjab University Chandigarh, India

8.1 Introduction

The plasma membrane represents a perfect example of self organisation in biology. Living cells are essential components comprising an aqueous system as a result amphipathic nature of phospholipids leading to the formation of bilayers. The interface between the living cells and their surroundings plays tremendous roles in the biological processes. One of the key hallmarks of eukaryotic cells is an array of intracellular organelles that carry out specialized functions. The differences between lipid composition among different organelles has been a conundrum whereby components of biological membranes are assemblages of mature structures. Studies on the lipid bilayers have focused on the factors on the acyl-chain length, unsaturation, and sterol content (Singer, 2004). Lipids have also been classified as annular and bulk ones where the former are responsible for the function of membrane proteins acting as glue after the emergence of the lipid polymorphism concept at various physiological conditions (Cullis and de Kruijff, 1979). Lipids play a role in limiting lateral mobility of several membrane proteins and play the role of cholesterol in making of caveolae; structurally unique invaginations in the plasma membrane later are also rich in glycosyl-phosphatidylinositol (GPI)-linked proteins, a class of complex metabolically and most expensive class of posttranslational lipid modification (Lee and Jacobson, 1994). Furthermore, GPI anchor is known as a promoter of lipid rafts rich in sphingolipids and cholesterol and paving the way for functional association of proteins; about 65% of the membranes are in nonraft phase (Edidin, 2003; Simon and Sampaio, 2011). Lipid rafts/microdomains have been known as detergent-resistant membranes (Malinsky et al., 2013. Later progress was made regarding molecular conformation and dynamics in the polar head group region, about polar interaction between lipid molecules across the plane of bilayer, and between lipids, water, and other solutes in the polar environment. The early insights that specific lipids can regulate membrane protein functions were largely ignored. Also in the field of signal transduction, important role(s) for potential allosteric regulator of signal transduction were no longer desired. However, a dead lock was recently busted with studies by newer analytical techniques like cellular lipidome being successfully analyzed by high-resolution mass spectrometry and NMR to understand various physico-chemical properties of phospholipids and their in situ roles too. In contrast to protein components of biological membranes lipids do not undergo chemical modifications. It was worthwhile to focus on lipids when raft hypothesis of membrane had its value. Recently phospholipids have been reported to be involved in the regulation of innate immunity and respiratory viral infections (Voelker and Nurata, 2019).

8.2 Phospholipids as a Backbone to Membrane Formation

Phospholipids are derivatives of phosphatidic acid (PA) or phosphatidate and the common alcohol moieties are choline, ethanolamine, inositol, serine, and glycerol, making them phosphatidylcholine (PC), phosphatidylethanolamine (PE), phosphatidylinositol (PI), phosphatidylserine (PS),

DOI: 10.1201/9781003220404-10

TABLE 8.1

Structures of Various Phospholipids and Their Physical Features: Z: zwitterionic, L: lamellar, and H: hexagonal

GLYCEROPHOSPHOLIPIDS	NAME	SHAPES		CHARGE
		L	H	
(structure)	Diacylglycerol			Nil
(structure)	Phosphatidic acid	+	-	2⁻
(structure)	Phosphatidylcholine	+	-	Z
(structure)	Phosphatidylethanolamine	+	+	Z
(structure)	Phosphatidylserine	+	+	-
(structure)	Phosphatidylinositol	+	-	-
(structure)	Cardiolipin	+	+	2⁻

and phosphatidylglycerol (PG), respectively, the structures of which are given in Table 8.1. Such phospholipids are the major backbone of basic eukaryotic bilayer structure. Interestingly, the role of PA has been reported as a biosensor that critically links membrane biogenesis to metabolism (Young et al., 2010). Bisphosphatidylglycerol (cardiolipins) are unique lipids, and are exclusively restricted to the inner mitochondrial membranes (Voelker, 1991). Cardiolipin in addition to being an important mitochondrial constituent has also been reported as acting as a selective barrier to toll-like receptor (Coats et al., 2016). Details about such lipids will be taken up later in this review.

The emergence of non-lamellar conformation adopted by various lipids to balance dynamics and stability cells use various lipid species in their membranes. The transformation of lipid bilayer into non-bilayer conformations is the manifestation of their chemico-physical properties.

This phenomenon not only provided adjustment to proteins but also assisted in the self regulation of lipid hypothesis (Garab et al., 2000). In the absence of proteins at the physiological pHs and ionic

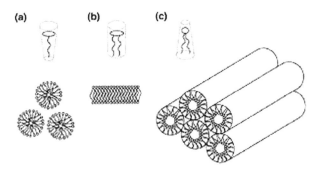

FIGURE 8.1 Various conformations adopted by phospholipids in the membranes at different physiological conditions: (a) Micellar. (b) lamellar. (c) hexagonal.

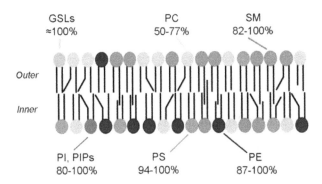

FIGURE 8.2 Trans-bilayer asymmetric distribution of phospholipids across various cellular membranes. (Adopted from Pomorski et al., 2004 doi 10.3389/fcell.2016.001155).

strengths lipid mixtures contain sufficient amount of non-bilayer lipids that cannot be forced to attain lamellar structures; this is clearly indicated by the involvement of proteins in forcing the former to form bilayer shapes.

8.3 Lipid Transbilayer Asymmetry

Most of the eukaryotic cellular membranes contain PC, PE, PS, PI, and PA as their structural constituents. The unequal transbilayer distribution of PC, PE, and PS across both leaflets creates a non-zero potential at both faces of membranes, which governs the lateral segregation of proteins and lipids (Grossman et al., 2007). This lipid asymmetry is an important feature for various cellular activities, such as apoptosis, vesicular trafficking, and cell division (Devaux, 1991; Fadok et al., 1992; Chen et al., 1999; Emoto and Umeda, 2000). Most of the PC is found in the outer leaflet whereas PE and PS are preferentially in the inner monolayer (Devaux, 1991). During apoptosis PS asymmetry is lost, and its externalization leading to physiological alterations, recognition, and removal of apoptotic cells by phagocytes occurs (Fadok et al., 1998).

The amount of PS in cancer cells in the external face is increased and makes the cells a suitable target for host defense peptides. Transbilayer asymmetry is regulated and maintained by the enzymatic activity of adenosine triphosphate (ATP) dependent flippases, later identified as P4 type ATPases and floppases facilitating outward- and inward-directed flow of aminophospholipids within membranes (Tang et al., 1996; Pomorski and Menon, 2006; van Meer, 2011).

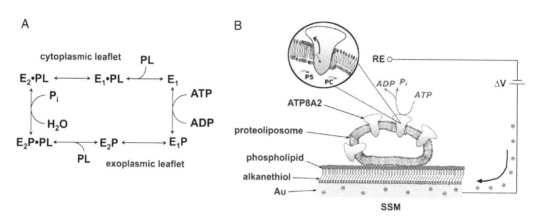

FIGURE 8.3 Aminophospholipid transport scheme (A) mediated by Flippase (B). (Adopted from Tadini-Bononsegni F, et al. doi10.1073/PNAS1919211116).

The movement of PE both laterally and across the bilayer is essential for membrane reorganization and trafficking. In normal resting mammalian cells, PE is retained on the cytosolic side of the plasma membrane by phospholipid translocases in an energy-dependent fashion.

8.4 Aminophospholipids in Health and Diseases

PE and PS are two important examples of such lipids. PE is a unique lipid that not only provides a precursor for PC but also functions as a chaperone for maintaining the proper conformation and function of transmembrane proteins. PE is a non-bilayer forming phospholipid containing a small polar head group diameter in proportion to its fatty-acid chains. The PE is the donor of ethanolamine moiety for GPI anchored to proteins (Menon and Stevens, 1992). A decrease in PE level has been associated with cytokinesis, Alzheimer's and Parkinson's diseases (Wang et al., 2014). It has been reported that being a multifunctional phospholipid PE is required for mammalian development that is essential for a variety of cellular processes. The intrinsic biophysical properties of this cone-shaped lipid induce the formation of hexagonal phases within the membrane and thereby promote membrane fusion and fission events, protein integration into membranes, and conformational changes in protein structure (Dowhan et al., 2019). A broad range of cyclotides isolated from plants belonging to families of Rubiaceae and Violaceae based bioactive compounds specifically interact with phosphatidylethanolamines on various targets such as RBCs, bacteria and HIV particles (Henriques and Craik, 2012). In addition, the role of PE in autophagy is an evolutionary conserved pathway for degradation of cytosolic proteins and posttranslational modification of various proteins. In addition to PE, in vitro conjugation experiments using liposomes showed that PS is also a target for ubiquitylation, a key process needed for the autophagy.

8.5 Cardiolipins as Unique Lipids and Their Functions in Mitochondria

The key and dynamic organelle mitochondria, usually called the powerhouse of cells, is also bestowed with crucial cellular functions such as metabolism, regulation of apoptosis, Ca homeostasis, and others (Mamaev and Zvyagilskaya, 2019). In addition mitochondria have a dual-membrane structure reminiscent of bacterial membranes. The dynamic membranes of mitochondria possess discrete lipid compositions that display bilayer and lateral asymmetry. Some of their lipids are synthesized within mitochondria, while others are imported or transported into mitochondria as precursor lipids. Between the membranes of mitochondria is an inter-membrane space, and inside the inner membrane is the mitochondrial matrix compartment. The inner mitochondrial membrane (MIM) is the most metabolically active membrane of mitochondria. It has highly complex structure that is freely permeable to oxygen, carbon dioxide, and water. Embedded in the MIM are the four respiratory-chain complexes, plus ATP synthase (complex V), ubiquinone, and carnitine-palmitoyl-transferase II, most of which makes up the electron transport chain (ETC). Mitochondria use oxidative phosphorylation via the ETC to produce energy, using reducing equivalents from the TCA cycle. The ETC accounts for about 90% of cellular oxygen consumption and provides more than 80% of cellular energy. It can be summed up that cardiolipin puts the seal on ATP synthase and regulate mitophagy through protein kinase C pathway (Mehdipour and Hummer, 2016; Shen et al., 2016). Mitochondria provide other critical functions for cells, including the modulation of calcium signaling, regulation of cell death, the maintenance of cellular redox balance, and innate immune signalling. Mitochondria also contain important biosynthetic pathways, especially for certain lipids. Because of their role in apoptosis, it is reasonable to assume that mitochondria function as gatekeepers of cell life and death. The key event leading to releasing of cytochrome c from mitochondria into cytoplasm and exposure of PS "eat me signal" for phagocytes. Apoptosis usually develops as a consequence of loss of barrier function of mitochondrial membranes (Vladimirov et al., 2020). Mitochondria contain a signature lipid molecule, an important one, tetra-acyl phospholipid, commonly called cardiolipin (CL), and also known as bis-phosphatidylglycerol, which is unique to mitochondria and essential for their function. CL constitutes approximately 15 to 20% of the total mitochondrial phospholipid. PE and CL are non-bilayer-forming phospholipids, best explained by their conical shapes. This allows the formation of hexagonal phases, depending on the pH and ionic strength. They are essential for cell survival, whereas CL is exclusively found in the MIM where it is required for oxidative phosphorylation, ATP synthesis, and mitochondrial bioenergetics. Overall, CL is functionally indispensable for MIM structure and function as well as for maintaining MIM trans-membrane potential.

8.6 Phosphatidylinositol Phosphates (PIP) and Signalling Molecules

PIP2 is an important phosphoinositide that is present in around 1% of the plasma membrane. It is also involved in signal transduction of intracellular and extracellular components. One of the most essential pathways of intracellular transduction involves the PIP2 molecule. The muscarinic receptor is a G-protein-coupled receptor that stimulates an enzyme known as phospholipase C. Hydrolysis of PIP2 by phospholipase C produces intracellular mediators such as IP3 (inositol triphosphate) and DAG (diacylglycerol). These intracellular enzymes produce downstream signaling components that generate and amplify the signals originated from the binding of ligand molecules. The targets of this intracellular signaling pathway include transcription factors that help in the control of gene expression. Inositol triphosphate is a second messenger that helps in transmission of chemical signals such as growth factors, neurotransmitters, hypertrophic stimuli called Angiotensin-II, and hormones for the transduction networks of the cell.

The basic structure of the IP3 receptor is comprised of three domains: an IP3 binding domain near the amino terminus, a coupling domain in the center of the molecule, and a transmembrane domain near the carboxyl terminus. IP3 is a negatively charged water-soluble molecule that can rapidly diffuse into cytosol to bind with IP3 receptor; it is opened to release Ca^{2+} out of endoplasmic reticulum. The production of IP3 is therefore capable of coupling the activated receptor in the plasma membrane to the Ca^{2+} ions released from an intracellular store. Various cellular responses can depend on this pathway, which includes contraction of smooth muscle and secretion of enzymes by the acinar cells of the pancreas. Additionally, calcium ions are capable of initiating or inhibiting signalling pathways in the cells. Hence, stimulation of IP3 signaling cascade controls the enzymatic activity within eukaryotic cells. Hydrolysis of PIP2 produces a hydrophobic molecule known as diacylglycerol (DAG). The concentration of DAGs get altered in diabetes, cancer, and several other diseased states (Li et al., 2007). After IP3 is formed, DAG is retained in the cell membrane. The DAG pathway is a message-generating pathway that is involved in the activation of enzymes and in turn produces various biological events, including transcription of DNA. Similar to other lipids, DAG also diffuses through the membrane surface where it can interact with another enzyme called protein kinase C and hence activating it. There is a wide range of transmembrane receptors that transduce extracellular signals through the activation of Bruton's tyrosine kinase. This mechanism activates phospholipase C-gamma 2 (PLCg2) that results in the generation of DAG and IP3.

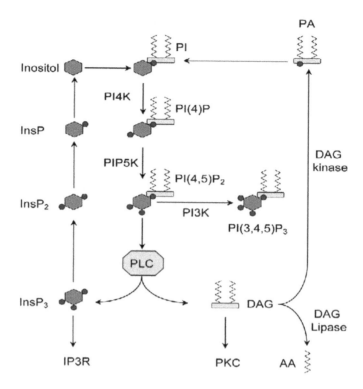

FIGURE 8.4 A general phosphatidylinositol signalling scheme. (Adopted from Bennet et al., 2006 doi 10.1007/ s00018-005-5446-z).

Ligation taking place outside the cell can activate the receptors, leading to phosphorylation and cross-phosphorylation of PLCg2, which is then active.

8.7 Lipid–Protein Interactions as Unique Fingerprints

Lipid-protein interactions are key factors in understanding the functional nature of cell membranes. Membrane proteins are approximately 30% constituted by human genome crucial for various cellular functions. The membrane is not simply a hydrophobic "sea" within which membrane proteins are distributed, but specific interactions occur between certain lipids and proteins, which regulate the function of many membrane proteins. The close relationship between number of lipid molecules surrounding a membrane protein (hydrophobic domain) and circumference of the latter is strong evidence for the presence of a distinct annular shell of lipids around the protein (Jost, et al., 1973; Lee, 2003). Lipids not only provide the matrix where proteins are embedded but can actively participate in the protein activity, trafficking. and target site. The lipid-dependent versatility and dynamic organization of membrane proteins are expected to provide a novel means of regulating protein functions (Dowhan et al., 2019). Several experimental techniques are available for studying this binding; such as fluorescence spectroscopy, X-ray crystallography, and mass spectrometry (Corradi et al., 2018).

8.8 Membrane Lipids Regulate Virus Entry and Replication

Viruses interact with cellular membrane to gain entry through lipid raft or endosomal membrane system. The pathogenesis of Respiratory Syncytial Virus (RSV) and Influenza A Virus (IAV) have

TABLE 8.2

Examples of Lipids or Their Derivatives and Their Roles in Signalling

Precursor	Signaling molecule	Function
Phosphatidyl choline	Phosphatidic acid	Phagocytic respiratory burst
Phosphatidic acid	Diacylglycerol	Protein kinase C regulation
Phosphatidyl inositol-4,5 *bis* phosphate	Diacylglycerol;inositol-1,4,5-*tris* phosphate	Protein kinase C regulation; calmodulin kinase control
Sphingomyelin	Ceramide	Apoptosis
Ceramide	Sphingosine;sphingosine-1-phosphate	Protein phosphorylation; release Ca^{2+}
PI phosphate	InP3	Ca^{2+}

been linked to TLR4 activation. Voelker and Nurata (2019) examined the action of palmitoyl oleoyl phospahtidylglycerol (POPG) and PI as potential antagonists of the pathology of these viruses. Surprisingly, POPG and PI dramatically curtail infection, in addition to inhibiting inflammatory sequelae associated with RSV and IAV infections. Studies suggested that lipid interactions, including invagination, fusion, and remodelling are important for successful replication of various viruses. Most cellular receptors are surface proteins of various functions like sialic acid for influenza virus and PS for vesicular stomatitis virus. Entry of many viruses is through lipid rafts where virus receptors reside. Recently the anti-malarial drug chloroquine and its derivative, which are weakly basic compounds that accumulate in acidic organelles due to pH partitioning and interaction with negatively charged phospholipids, have shown antiviral activities against many viruses. The accumulation of endosomal lipid bis (mono-acylglycero) phosphate is a key player as a mechanism of action of chloroquine against SARS-CoV-2 (Carriere et al., 2020). Analysis of lipid components of HIV revealed strong enrichment of lipid component rafts, and the inner leaflet of viral membranes rich in PS and the lipid composition of HIV strongly resemble that of detergent-resistant membrane (DRM) isolated from producer cells. Understanding the multiple roles of lipids in viral replication should also lead to the discovery of lipid active molecules as potential anti-virals in the future.

8.9 Lipid Therapy as a Natural Medicine

Recently, membrane lipid replacement (MLR) therapy has been proposed in which the use of functional oral supplements of membrane phospholipids and antioxidants with fructo-oligsaccharides has been highlighted to counter chronic illness, aging, cancer, and others by in cell membranes, cells, organelles, and tissues (Nicolson and Ash, 2017). Several neuro-degenerative diseases like Parkinson's, Alzheimer's Huntington's, Friedeich ataxia, and cardiovascular ailments are characterized by loss of efficiency of electron transport chain and reduction in ATP yield. Also such changes have been documented by increased oxidative stress and supplementation of various natural herbal products containing vitamins, antioxidants, cofactors (e.g., CoQ10, lipoic acid, NADH), and membrane phospholipids that can naturally restore these functions (Nicolson, 2014; Escriba, 2017). Incubation of human sperm with micelles prepared from glycerphospholipids have been shown to restore their functions of increased motility by decreasing oxidative stress when sperm was exposed to hydrogen peroxide as a result of their incorporation in the mitochondrial membranes (Ferriera et al., 2018). MLR components are prescribed to be taken orally and are absorbed by intestinal tract as such or as their individual molecular constituents as small micelles or globules or liposome as shown in Figure 8.5.

Indeed, clinical trials have shown positive results in MLR phospholipids in recovery of worn-out mitochondrial functions in aged people, as evidenced by amelioration of their fatigue and also in people characterized by loss of mitochondrial functions.

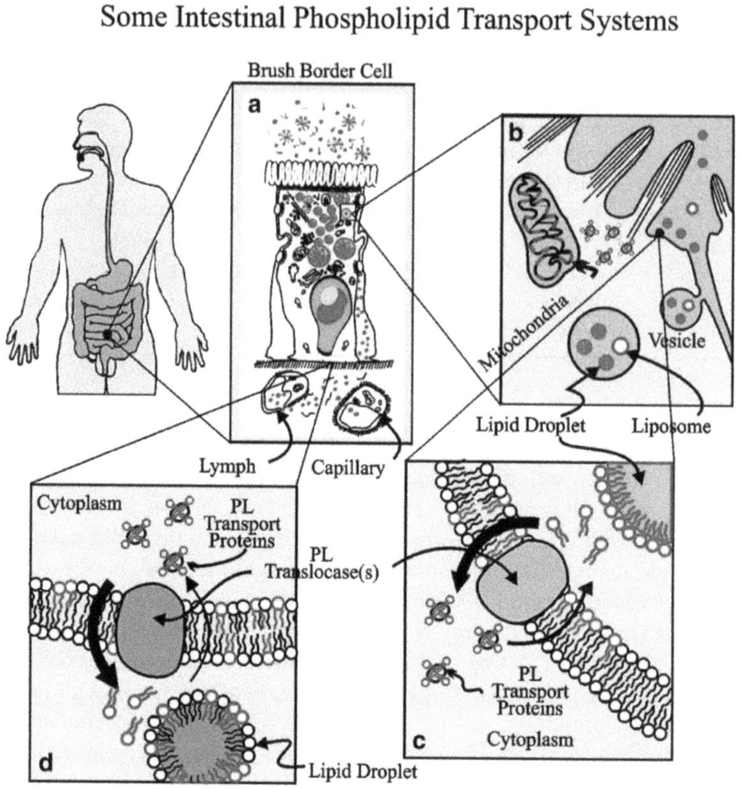

Some Intestinal Phospholipid Transport Systems

FIGURE 8.5 Some phospholipid transport systems used in delivery of MLR phospholipid therapy in the human system. (From Nicolson and Ash, 2017 doi 10.1016/jbbamemb 2013.11010).

8.10 Conclusions

Novel technological approaches have revealed that a vast number of lipid classes and species have implications in the various heterogeneous phases in addition to their bilayer nature. A particular lipid has a specific purpose in cellular functions. Lipid protein interaction and asymmetric distribution of lipids have shed more light on the molecular and physiological far-reaching implications for our understanding of the living cell membranes. Lipids act as cofactors and interact with pathogens to take care of them and provide a homeostatic mechanism. Lipid-dependent versatility and dynamic organization of membrane proteins are expected to provide a novel means of regulating protein functions. Some attempts are being made to therapeutically correct certain errors of metabolism by the use of oral supplements from cell membranes and antioxidants. Lipids are considered as structural components and barriers of cellular structures. However, they are more than spatial organizational units of metabolic compartments of living cells. Phospholipids have specific functions in many physiological functions in various stages of cellular life. The application of lipids for therapeutic purposes is now being explored.

Acknowledgements

The author thanks DST New Delhi for the purse grant for the laboratory, Mr. Lakhvinder Singh for helping in making figures, as well as Prof. Akhtar for reading the manuscript and providing suggestion therein.

REFERENCES

Bennet M, Onnebo SMN, Azevedo C, Saiardi A. 2006. Inositol pyrophosphates: metabolism and signalling. Cell Mol Life Sci 63: 552–564. doi: 10.1007/s00018-005-5446-z

Carriere F, Longhi S, Record M. 2020. Endosomal lipid bis (monoacylglycero) phosphate as a potential key player in the mechanism of action of chloroquine against SARS-COV2 and other enveloped viruses hijacking the endocytic pathway. Biochemie 179: 237–246. doi: 10.1016/j.Bionchi.2020.05.013

Chen CY, Ingram MF, Rosal PH, Graham TR. 1999. Roe for Drs2p, Ptype ATPAse and potential animophospholipid translocase, in yeast and golgi funations. J Cell Biol 147: 1223–1236.

Coats SR, Hashim A, Paramanov NA, To, TT, Curtis, MA, Darveau, RP. 2016. Cardiolipins act as a selective barrier to toll like receptor 4 activation in the intestine. App Envir Microbiol 82: 4264–4278. doi: 10.1128/AEM.00463-16

Corradi V, Mendez-Viluendas E, Ingolfsson HI, et al. 2018. Lipid–protein interactions are unique finger prints for membrane proteins. ACS central Sci 4: 709–717. doi: 10.1021.acscentsci8b00143

Cullis PR, de Kruijff B. 1979. Lipid polymorphism and the functional roles of lipids in biological membranes. Biochim Biophys Acta 559: 399–352.

Devaux, PF. 1991. Static and dynamic lipid asymmetry in cell membranes. Biochemistry 30: 1163–173.

Dowhan W, Vitrac H, Bogdanov M. 2019. Lipid-assisted membrane protein folding and topogenesis. Protein J 38: 274–288. doi: 10.1007/s10930-019-09826-7. PMID: 30937648. PMCID: PMC6589379.

Edidin M. 2003. The state of lipid rafts: From model membranes to cells. Ann Rev Biophys Biomol Struct 32: 257–283. doi: 10.1146/annrev.biophys.32.110601.142439

Emoto K, Umeda M. 2000. An essential role for a membrane lipid in cytokinesis regulation of contractile ring disassembly by redistribution of phosphatidylethanolamine. J Cell Biol 149: 1215–1224. doi: 10.1083/jcb.149.6.1215

Escriba PV. 2017. Membrane-lipid therapy: A historical perspective of membrane-targeted therapies-from bilayer structure to the pathophysiological regulation of cells. Biochim Biophyc Acta 1859: 1493–150. doi: 10.1016/jbbamem.2017.05.017

Fadok VA, Voelker DR, Campbell PA, Cohen JJ, Bratton DL Hensson PM. 1992. Exposure of phosphatidylserine on the surface apptotic lymphocytes triggers specific recognisition and removal by macrophages. J Immnunol 148:2207–2216.

Fadok VA, Bratton DL, Konowal A, Freed PW, Westcott JW, Hanson PM. 1998. Macrophages that ingested apoptotoic cells in vitro inhibit pro-inflammatory cytokines production through autocrine/paracrine mechanisms involving TGF-beta, PGE2, PAF. J Clin Invest 101: 890–898. doi: 10.1172/JCI1112

Ferriera G, Costa C, Bassaizteguy V, Santos M, Cardozo R, Montes J, Settineri R, Nicolson GL. 2018. Incubation of human sperm with micelles made from glycerophospholipids mixtures increases sperm motility and resistance to oxidative stress. PLOS one 13: e0197897. doi: 10.1371/journal.pone.0197897

Garab G Lohner K, Lagger P, Farkas T. 2000. Self-regulation of lipid bilayer content of membranes by non-bilayer lipids: a hypothesis. Trends Plant Sci 5: 489–494.

Grossmann G, Opekarová M, Malinsky J, Weig-Meckl I, Tanner W. 2007. Membrane potential governs lateral segregation of plasma membrane proteins and lipids in yeast. EMBO J. 26(1): 1–8. doi: 10.1038/sj.emboj.7601466. Epub 2006 Dec 14. PMID: 17170709; PMCID: PMC1782361.

Henriques ST, Craik DJ. 2012. Importance of cell membranes on the mechanism of action of cyclotides. ACS Chemical Biol 7: 626–636. doi: 10.1021/cb200395f

Jost PC, Griffith OH Capaldi RA, Vanderkooi G. 1973. Evidence for boundary lipids in membranes. Proc Natl Acad Sci USA 70: 480–484.

Lee AG. 2003. Lipid protein interactiuons in biological membranes: a structural perspectives. Biochimica Biophys Acta 1612: 1–40. doi: 10.106S00052736(03) 00056-7

Lee GM, Jacobson K. 1994. Lateral mobility of lipids in membranes. Curr Topics Membr 40: 111–142.

Li YL, Su X, Stahl PD, Gross ML. 2007 Quantification of diacylglycerol molecular species in biological samples by electrospray ionization mass spectrometry after one step derivatization. Anal Chem 79: 1569–1574. doi: 10.1021/ac0615910

Malinsky J, Operkarova M, Grossmann G, Tanner W. 2013. Membranes,micro-domains, rafts, and detergent resistant membranes in plants and fungi. Ann Rev Plant Biol 64: 501–529.

Mamaev DV, Zvyagilskaya RA. 2019. Mitophagy in yeast. Biochemistry (Moscow) 84: 225–232. doi: 10.1134/S000629791914013X

Mehdipour AR, Hummer G. 2016. Cardiolipin puts seal on ATPase synthase. Proc Natl Acad Sci USA 113: 8568–8570. doi: 10.1073/pnas.1609806113

Menon AK, Stevens VL. 1992. Phosphatidylethanolamine is the donor of the ethanolamine residue linking a glycosylphosphatidylinositol anchor to protein. J Biol Chem 267: 15277–15280.

Nicolson GL. 2014. Mitochondrial dysfunction and chronic disease: treatment with natural supplements. Integrative Medicine 13: 35–43.

Nicolson GL, Ash ME. 2014. Lipid replacement therapy: A natural medicine approach to replacing damaged lipids in cellular membranes and organelles and restoring function. Biochim Biophys Acta 1838(6):1657–1679. doi: 10.1016/j.bbamem.2013.11.010. Epub 2013 Nov 21. PMID: 24269541.

Pomprski T, Holthuis JCM, Herrmann A, van Meer G. 2004. Tracking down lipid flippases and their biological functions. J Cell Sci 117: 805–813. doi: 10.1242/jcs.01.055

Pomorski T, Menon AK. 2006. Lipid flippase and their biological functions. Cell Mol Life Sci 63: 2908–2921. doi.10.1007/s00018-006-6167-7

Shen Z, Li Z, Gasparski AN, Abeliovich H, Greenberg ML. 2016. Cardiolipin regulate mitophagy through protein kinase C pathway. J Biol Chem 292: 2916–2923. doi: 10.1074/jbcM116.753574

Simon K, Sampaio JL. 2011. Membrane organization and lipid rafts. Cold Spring Harbor Persp Biol 3(10): 1–18. doi: 10.1101/cshperspect.a004697

Singer SJ. 2004. Some early history of membrane molecular biology. Ann Rev Physiol 66: 1–27. doi: 10.1146/annrev.physiol.66.032902.131835

Tang X, Hallack MS, Schegal RA, Williamson P. 1996. A subfamily of P-type ATPases with aminophospholipid transporting activity. Science 272: 1495–1497.

Van Meer G. 2011. Dynamic transbilayer asymmetry. Cold Spring Harbor Persp Biol 3 (10) 137–147. doi: 10.1101/cshperspect.a004697

Voelker DR. 1991. Organelle biogenesis and intracellular lipid transport in eukaryotes. Microbiol Rev 55: 543–560.

Vladimirov GK, Nesterova AM, Levkina AA, Osipov AN, Teseelkin MV, Vladimirov YU. 2020. The dynamics of formation of cytochrome c complexes with anioniclipids and the mechanism of production of lipid radicals catalyzed by these complexes. Biochemistry (Moscow) 14: 232–241. doi: 10.1134/S1990747820030137

Voelker DR, Nurata M. 2019. Phospholipid regulation of innate and respiratory virus infection. J Biol Chem 294: 4282–4289. doi: 10.1074/jbcAW118.003229

Wang S, Zhang S, Liou LC, Ren Q, Zhang Z, Caldwell GA, Caldwell KA, Witt SN. 2014. Phosphatidylethanolamine deficiency disrupts α-synuclein homeostasis in yeast and worm models of Parkinson disease. Proc Natl Acad Sci USA 111(38):E3976-85. doi: 10.1073/pnas.1411694111. Epub 2014 Sep 8. PMID: 25201965; PMCID: PMC4183298.

Young BP, Shin JJ, Orij B, et al. 2010. Phosphatic acid is a pH biosensor that link membrane biogenesis to metabolism. Science 329: 1085–1088.

9

Childhood Cataract: A Clinico-Social Profile

Deepak Jugran, Surbhi Khurana, Parul Chawla Gupta, and Jagat Ram
*Department of Ophthalmology, Post Graduate Institute of Medical and Research,
Chandigarh, India*

9.1 Introduction

The visual system is one of the most important sensory organs of the human body.[1] As per the estimates almost 1.4 million children are blind in the world, with a majority living with socio-economic deprivation and inaccessibility to proper nutritional and medical care. As a result, they are more likely to have infectious diseases and malnutrition, leading to delayed cognitive development, frequent hospitalization and death within the first year of their birth.[2] Nearly 20% of childhood blindness is caused by childhood cataract, with almost 60% of blind children dying within the first year of their birth and the rest of them living about 40 years without vision.[3,4] Cataract is one of the major causes of childhood blindness and causes more disability in children, compared to any other form of preventable blindness. Blindness in children can have devastating effects on their quality of life and on the socio-economic condition of the family and society. Childhood cataract, if left untreated, can result in severe visual impairment, including blindness.[5]

Examination and diagnosis are difficult in children due to their inability to distinguish between clear and hazy vision and also because of their inability to communicate the same to their guardians/parents. At present, ophthalmologists evaluate childhood cataracts and decide the management plan according to the opacities present on the lens of the eye. After a detailed clinical examination, the decision to surgically intervene is taken in dense, unilateral, and central cataracts. Since all cataracts do not require surgical intervention, periodic evaluation and documentation is required to observe the progression of the opacity. Poor compliance to follow-up remains a major challenge in developing countries in the treatment of pediatric cataract.[4] Childhood cataract is more damaging than adult cataract, as its onset in developmental years can cause delayed neural development, delayed milestones, severe visual impairment, amblyopia, and even blindness. In the past, childhood cataracts were reported in association with genetic, infective, and metabolic diseases. It may be present at birth or can develop later due to a variety of reasons. The World Health Organization (WHO) has categorized childhood blindness from cataract as a priority area and has urged all countries to develop institutionalized mechanisms to tackle this threat, especially in low- and middle-income countries.[6] In developed countries, institutional mechanisms are in place for infantile screening for the detection of congenital diseases that include childhood cataract and retinopathy of prematurity (ROP). All over the world, midwives, primary healthcare workers, and pediatricians remain the first contact with the child, but due to a limited number of ophthalmologists in developing countries, the reporting and presentation of childhood cataract often gets delayed. All these diverse factors not only affect the early presentation, but also makes the detection and treatment of childhood cataract a challenging task. Hence, it is essential to study risk factors, clinical features, treatment, and visual rehabilitation to minimize disability among children.[3] Since the detection and surgical management of childhood cataract is difficult and requires specialization, there is an urgent need to develop artificial intelligence-based systems for paramedical staff, primary healthcare physicians, and midwives to look for childhood cataract in their routine screening of children after birth. It is therefore important for us to sensitize parents, primary care physicians, community healthcare workers, anesthesiologists, ophthalmic technicians, and

DOI: 10.1201/9781003220404-11

low vision rehabilitation technicians to closely coordinate with all stakeholders to minimize the extent of childhood blindness resulting from pediatric cataracts.

The early "biological embedding" process can have a huge impact on the adult life of a child. In developmental years, children need to have a sound physical, mental, and emotional state to achieve optimum physical strength and avoid physical disabilities, including visual impairment and blindness. Physical disabilities not only affect the child physically but can also have cascading effects on mental and emotional well-being. Children also face mental, emotional, and social stress during and after treatments. Children may recover positively from surgical treatment, but the painful and intriguing "sick role" might affect their overall mental and emotional health, especially during the treatment-seeking process. The long waiting hours in the hospital, mode of transportation, distance from the hospital, interactions with doctors and healthcare personnel, and uncertainty of the treatment may play a significant role, especially during developmental years. The sustained stress children face during illness has not been studied enough, taking the child as a standalone "unit of study."

9.2 Classification of Childhood Cataracts

The lens in the human eye has unique properties as the addition of new cells is continuous throughout the lifetime of an individual. The growth of the human lens takes place in two phases: the asymptotic phase and linear growth phase. The asymptotic growth starts during the gestational period and lasts up to 3 months after birth and the linear growth phase starts soon after. Due to this biphasic lens growth, two different and distinct compartments are formed within the lens. The lens nucleus is formed during the prenatal period followed by an ever-expanding cortex with unique physical and biochemical properties during the linear growth phase.[5]

The classification and pattern of childhood cataract can provide better insights for management and surgical plan. It is therefore desirable to describe the location, layer, density, and pattern of the lens opacities. Once the morphology is determined, then ophthalmologists can describe its etiology and associations. Broadly, the childhood cataract can be classified using three categories: based on age, etiology, and morphology (Table **9.**1).[6]

TABLE 9.1

Classification of Childhood Cataract Based on Age of Onset, Etiology, and Morphology)

Classification of childhood cataracts		
Age of onset	**Etiology**	**Morphology**
Congenital Cataract	Genetic/hereditary	Diffuse/Total Cataract
Secondary cataract	Secondary	Nuclear Cataract
	- Inflammation/Uveitis	
	- Traumatic	
	- Intrauterine	
	- Iatrogenic	
		Polar Cataract
		- Anterior polar cataract
		- Posterior polar cataract
		Lamellar Cataract
		Nuclear Combined with cortical
		- Coral like
		- Dust like
		- Blue dot
		Cortical Cataract
		Y-suture Cataract

9.2.1 Age of Onset

As per the definition, a cataract present at birth, or developing after birth but before 16 years of age is termed as a childhood cataract.[5] The lens in the human eye is composed of avascular transplant tissue with unique protein composition and cellular structure. The function of this lens, in combination with the cornea, is to focus the image on the retina. Its ability to change shape and transparency are the key factors in the production of a clear and focused image on the retina. It can further be divided into two categories based on age.

9.2.1.1 Congenital Cataract

The presence of lens opacity at the time of birth indicates its congenital onset. However, its diagnosis even at a later stage does not rule out its congenital onset. Detailed examination of the lens opacity, its etiology, and systemic associations may prove beneficial before the cataract extraction. Anterior polar, persistent hyperplastic primary vitreous (PHPV), central nuclear, and posterior polar cataract suggest a congenital onset.[7]

9.2.1.2 Developmental Cataract

These cataracts are mostly acquired after birth. All cataracts with onset in childhood, after infancy, irrespective of their underlying etiology, can be classified as "developmental cataract."[8]

9.2.2 Etiology

The transparent fibers in the lens are known as crystallin and the nucleus of the lens is layered with fibers, resembling the layers around the onion. As a result of continuous expansion during the lifetime of an individual, the lens becomes rigid and loses its innate ability to change shape, causing visual problems.

9.2.2.1 Genetic/Hereditary

In the majority of cases, etiology of the cataract is not known and is classified as "idiopathic."[5] However, congenital cataract has also been linked to mutation in genes linked with lens development. While most of these genes are dominantly inherited, cases with autosomal recessive or x-linked inheritance have also been reported.[7] With recent advancements such as next-generation sequencing, researchers are trying to find out the exact cause of congenital cataracts, but it is still in its preliminary stages and will require more time and validation before it can be used for diagnostic purposes.

9.2.2.2 Secondary

The opacity in different parts of the lens depends on the etiology of the cataract, and compared to congenital cataracts, the etiology of secondary cataracts are mostly known, including:

Inflammation or Uveitis: Due to persistent inflammation and steroids used in the treatment of uveitis, children may develop cataract, most commonly posterior sub-capsular cataract. Hence, ruling out active inflammation is essential before surgical intervention in these children. Many patients may also develop a pupillary membrane, making the surgery challenging. Juvenile idiopathic arthritis is one of the major causes of uveitis with cataract in children. In recent years, the use of systemic antimetabolites has helped to control the inflammation in these cases.[8,9]

9.2.2.3 Traumatic Cataract

Traumatic cataract remains a major challenge in low- and middle-income countries (Figure 9.1). The traumatic cataracts are not uncommon in boys due to their exposure to hazardous working conditions,

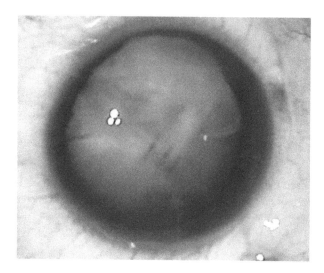

FIGURE 9.1   In traumatic cataract, there is usually a clouding of the lens due to blunt/penetrating trauma.

unhygienic living conditions, playing unconventional games, cracker burning, and fights with fellow friends.

9.2.2.4 Intrauterine Infections

Among many reasons, intrauterine infections such as toxoplasmosis, rubella, cytomegalovirus, and herpes (TORCH) are some of the major causes in low- and middle-income countries due to their high prevalence and require strict vaccination programs for mother and child.[10]

9.2.2.5 Iatrogenic

In the last few years, we have seen increased prevalence of cataract after laser treatment of ROP and other intraocular diseases requiring prolonged use of steroid therapy.[3]

9.2.3 Morphology

The lens opacities in childhood cataract can have multiple phenotypes and it is perhaps the most challenging task for ophthalmologists to list the precise morphology of the childhood cataract. Diagnosis of cataract can be made by an ophthalmologist under torch-light examination or slit-lamp examination (Figure 9.2). The morphology can guide the ophthalmologists to link its etiology, systemic association, and surgical plan. Based on morphology, childhood cataract can be classified based on the opacity of lens structure (Table 9.2).[7,8,11]

The opacity in the central part of the lens can be nuclear or lamellar (zonular) cataract. Zonular or lamellar cataract is the most common morphology seen in pediatric cataract (Figure 9.3).[8] The embryological defects in apoptosis and tissue migration may lead to an anterior polar cataract (Figure 9.4). Similarly, the opacity in the posterior part of the lens denotes failure of the embryological hyaloid artery to regress and can cause PHPV or posterior polar cataract.[8] Moreover, there are other abnormalities in the eye such as microphthalmia (abnormally small eye) or aniridia (rudimentary or absent iris), which can be associated with cataract.[3]

Cataracts with mild density or eccentrically placed cataracts can be kept under observation and operated on when required; however, dense and total cataracts (Figure 9.5) require immediate removal. Zonular and polar cataract has been reported as the most common type of bilateral and unilateral childhood cataract, respectively.[7,8]

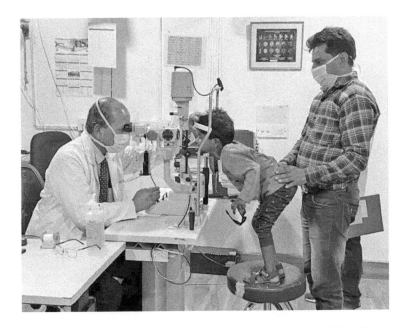

FIGURE 9.2 The ocular examination is being done on slit lamp by Prof. Jagat Ram, an ophthalmologist.

TABLE 9.2

Childhood Cataract Classification Based on Morphology

Whole lens	Total	Congenital	Morganian	Membranous	Partially	
Central	Lamellar	Zonular	Nuclear	Central	Sutural	Cortical
Anterior	Anterior polar • Dot like • Plaque like • Anterior pyramidal	Anterior subcapsular	Anterior lenticonus			
Posterior	Posterior polar	Posterior subcapsular	Posterior lenticonous			
Misc.	Linear opacities	Wedge-shaped/ Crystalline	Coralliform /Floriform	Dandelion like/ Starry sky cataract/Stud button	Reduplicated cataract/ Nodular stem of cactus	Barbed fence-like/ Oil droplet

9.3 Maternal Malnutrition and Intrauterine Infections

The role of micronutrients for a pregnant mother is essential for balanced fetal growth and ample studies have established the link between maternal malnutrition and intrauterine growth retardation, increased perinatal morbidity, and even mortality.[5]

9.3.1 Maternal Malnutrition

The incidence of idiopathic cataract is highest in low- and middle-income countries suggesting the role of low birth weight, malnutrition, and infectious causes in the development of idiopathic cataract. Also, low birth weight indicates poor fetal growth and maternal malnutrition can be one of the factors causing altered physiology of the fetal lens. A possible link has been suggested between maternal malnutrition,

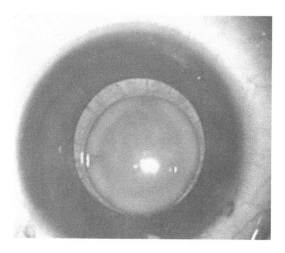

FIGURE 9.3   A classic picture of Zonular.

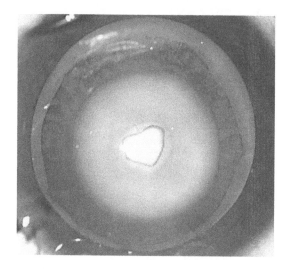

FIGURE 9.4   Anterior Polar Cataract / Lamellar Cataract. It is common in children.

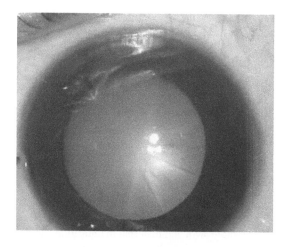

FIGURE 9.5   Total or Dense Cataract. This type of cataract requires immediate cataract surgery.

low birth weight, and the development of childhood cataract.[11] While exploring the existing literature on pathways delivering nutrients to the adult lens, the authors presented a cellular mechanism by which oxidative stress caused due to maternal malnutrition can impact the development of antioxidant defense pathways in the embryonic lens, thus accelerating the onset of nuclear cataract in childhood.[5]

Low birth weight indicates poor fetal growth and maternal malnutrition. Children with a birth weight of 2500 gms or less are 3.8 times more susceptible to the development of idiopathic cataract than those born above this birth weight.[5] Among several causes of low birth weight, maternal malnutrition remains a primary cause. Studies have shown a close association between low birth weight and oxidative stress caused during pregnancy. The cord blood of low-birth-weight babies revealed lower levels of superoxide dismutase catalase and glutathione. Moreover, animal studies also suggested that maternal malnutrition may impact fetal lens growth.[5] However, the lens damage was also reversed with prolonged nutritional rehabilitation. Taken together, these studies strongly suggest the impact of maternal malnutrition on fetal lens growth due to altered antioxidant pathways and increased oxidative stress.[5]

9.3.2 Intrauterine Infections

In the developing world, intrauterine infections are major causes of childhood blindness.[8] The mnemonic TORCH symbolizes the most common congenital intrauterine infections, which include toxoplasma gondii, others, rubella, cytomegalovirus, and herpes. The "others" include varicella-zoster, treponema pallidum, Epstein-Barr, HIV, lymphocytic choriomeningitis, and West Nile virus. Though they manifest relatively mild symptoms and illness in the mother, they can severely impact fetus growth. The more virulent forms of these viruses may also result in abortion and stillbirth, and can have direct toxic effects on the fetus. In these cases, the fetus is unable to eliminate these viruses, which can lead to chronic infections and elevated levels of IgM and IgA. In 1941, Sir, Norman Mcalister Gregg, an ophthalmologist from Australia, described the association of rubella with congenital cataract, congenital heart disease, and deafness. It was the first-ever demonstration of teratogenicity secondary to a virus.[10] Rubella is still a major cause of congenital cataracts and blindness across developing countries. If the lens development during the first trimester gets affected due to virus infection, it can lead to cataract formation. The most common types are nuclear and total cataracts. Since the virus can stay in the eye for years due precaution is required during cataract extraction to minimize exposure to the cortical material. Systemic steroids may be administered post-surgery to contain inflammatory reaction in these kinds of cataract surgeries.[8]

9.4 Symptoms, Diagnosis, and Treatment

9.4.1 Symptoms and Diagnosis

The ultimate goal of diagnosis and treatment of childhood cataract is successful visual rehabilitation. At present, ophthalmologists use a slit-lamp examination to diagnose childhood cataract. The decision to operate depends upon the density of lens opacity, evaluated with the help of a red-reflex test, retinoscopy, and EUA (examination under anaesthesia). Decreased vision, leukocoria, and strabismus are the most common symptoms seen in pediatric cataract.[7,8,12]

In general, ophthalmologists look for the following features to confirm the presence of cataract:

- White reflex in the eye (leukocoria)
- Misaligned eyes
- Rhythmic and uncontrolled movements of the eye (nystagmus)
- Cloudy or blurry vision
- Glare in the eye on the application of light (photophobia)

Moreover, the diagnosis of childhood cataract is also done using a visual acuity test. In a visual acuity test, ophthalmologists check the vision of the child from different distances wherein the pupil is dilated to get a closer view of the lens, retina, and optic nerve.

9.4.2 Treatment for Childhood Cataract

The treatment of childhood cataract depends on the density of the cataract. Generally, if the lens opacity is central and more than 3 mm in diameter, it should be removed. The ideal time to perform surgery is as early as possible, after the first 4 weeks of life. Primary intraocular lens implantation is favoured by most ophthalmologists in childhood cataract in developing countries, as aphakia require the use of glasses and contact lens for visual rehabilitation, which becomes difficult in low- and middle-income countries. Childhood cataract without the risk of amblyopia is generally avoided for surgery. However, ophthalmologists may continue to prescribe glasses or contact lenses. But there are certain categories of cataracts such as dense and total cataracts that require immediate surgical intervention to avoid visual impairment. Posterior capsular opacification (PCO) is the most common complication in childhood cataract surgery.[8]

Unlike an adult cataract, a childhood cataract is very soft and does not require ultrasonic phacoemulsification. Generally, in eyes with microphthalmia and microcornea, only the cataract is removed and the eyes are left aphakic. In aphakia, thick glasses or contact lenses are prescribed until the intraocular lens (IOL) can be implanted. In some cases, further surgeries may also be required due to anatomical changes during the development years. In young children, post-operative inflammation, PCO, risk of developing glaucoma, and retinal detachment are major complications and can be managed with medication or repeated surgery.[7,8,11] Regular monitoring and strict amblyopia therapy are required after surgery. Almost 50% of childhood cataracts are bilateral and visual outcome often remains poor in eyes with unilateral cataract. The development of red-eye with photophobia is also a sign of sight-threatening infection following cataract surgery.[3]

9.5 Prevalence and Epidemiology of Childhood Cataract

Despite significant improvements in health services over the last century, health inequalities persist among various population groups. The socio-economically disadvantaged areas of the world experience higher morbidity, mortality, and disability rates. In addition, even within developed and developing countries, inequalities exist based on the socio-economic status of the population. The definition of "health inequalities" refers to the health status of how worse off the disadvantaged group is from the privileged group. India, China, and Africa share almost 75% of the global burden of blindness. The data also indicate a disproportionate burden of blindness in developing countries compared to developed countries.[13,14]

The epidemiology of childhood blindness due to cataract corresponds to socio-economic development, demographic change, public health intervention for child-care, accessibility, and the availability of eye care services within a geographical area. Though there is a decline in the absolute number of blind children from 1.4 million in the 1990s to 1.14 million in 2014, this is attributed primarily to the improved performance of developed countries. In the past two decades, blindness due to corneal scarring has also reduced in low-income countries and cataract has emerged as the most common cause of avoidable blindness. In a major systematic review, the ratio of girls accessing bilateral cataract surgery was found lower especially in Asian countries. The possible reason for this may be a gender difference in birth rates reported from China and India. In 2015, the United Nations Population Division reported 12.1 and 13.4 million fewer girls than boys (0-9 years) in China and India, respectively.[15] The gender bias was reported in almost all categories of child healthcare including rates of immunization and nutritional values.

The studies further suggest huge variations in the causes of vision loss across different parts of the world. While low-income countries still face a shortage of healthcare infrastructure, malnourishment, and infectious diseases (rubella, measles), the causes in middle-income countries include congenital cataract and retinopathy of prematurity (ROP) as major causes of childhood blindness. However, in developed countries, hereditary or genetic causes are the primary causes of childhood blindness.[16] Almost 75% of the world's blind children live in Asia and Africa. In these countries, a majority of them live in extreme poverty and childhood cataracts and corneal diseases are the major causes of childhood blindness.

However, in one of the major systemic reviews published in 2016, the findings did not agree with the earlier reported results and suggested higher prevalence even in high-income countries. Overall, there is a substantial gap in the epidemiological knowledge of childhood cataract and the yearly figure, which is reflected in the yearly figure for new childhood cataract cases, which varies from 1,91,000 cases to 3,14,000.[16] The prevalence of childhood cataract was also reported with a wide range from 1-15/10000. One possible reason for this huge variation is different methodologies, age groups, and case definitions being used by the researchers in the past. In one of the studies, reports suggest that with a 2% birth rate in developed countries, the prevalence of bilateral cataract could be 4 children/million; however, the same may increase to 10 children/million in developing countries due to higher birth rate.[17]

9.6 Social Factors Affecting Health-Seeking Behaviour

The cultural, economical, and social conditions of the individual and family can have a substantial influence on the health-seeking behaviour of the individual and family, and remain the most significant determinants of the health-seeking behaviour in low- and middle-income countries.[15] Moreover, lower educational level of mother and gender disparities were also reported as major reasons in accessing healthcare services. In low- and middle-income countries, girls from families with higher socio-economic status are more likely to undergo treatment than girls from lower socio-economic status. There is a fear of surgeries in parents from lower socio-economic areas. In the studies conducted in Asia and Africa, the parents of a girl child from a lower socio-economic background were more likely to delay the presentation of their ailing girl child to hospitals, as they believed that it would be detrimental to her marriage prospects. Moreover, the lack of understanding of medical treatment and surgery and fear of visiting urban cities for treatment were also reported as major reasons for delayed presentation.[15] Though there are no studies available for out-of-pocket expenditure in cataract surgeries, the most reasonable justification for lower access to surgery by girls with bilateral cataract seems to be the complex interplay of social, economical, and behavioural factors. In addition, lower levels of maternal education, poverty, and cultural beliefs in low- and middle-income countries also play significant roles in health-seeking behaviour.

9.7 Economic Burden of Childhood Bindness

As per global estimates, childhood blindness contributes to an enormous loss in earning capacity of US$ 6000-27000 million. With extrapolation, if we assume a 3% growth rate in the global population, the economic loss over a period of 10 years resulting from childhood cataract varies from US$ 1000-6000 million. The Indian estimates suggest a loss of US$ 3500 million in earning capacity, considering an average of 33 blind years due to cataract.[18,19]

However, with early detection and timely management in cases of childhood cataract, a substantial share of this loss can be minimized. The latest estimates from Orbis India show that India can incur an economic loss of Rs. 88,000 crore in 2020, even though almost 35% of cases of blindness are preventable and curable. It has been reported that with this trend, the country can incur a loss of Rs. 3,31,000 crore in national GDP considering 40 lost working years.[19]

9.8 Psychosocial Impact on Children and Family

Unlike cataract in adults, where the results are highly encouraging after surgery, cataracts in children can have detrimental effects on their overall psychology and their families.[20] In childhood cataract, parents play a crucial role in the care of the child and it has been reported in two inductive studies that uncertainty can become a major barrier in self-efficacy. However, to balance the ability or inability of a child, parents generally use a process comprised of four main categories: mastering, collaborating, facilitating, and adapting.[20] Their painful journey starts from birth and continues for years with frequent visits to the eye clinics. The parents are also expected to be vigilant in reporting the complications. It has been seen that strict compliance during the treatment such as administering eye drops, handling contact lens, patching and motivating the child for treatment, and visiting the hospital can be extremely challenging.[21] Fatigue and physical and mental exhaustion can become barriers for parents as fatigue contributes significantly among parents with children having bilateral cataract. Fatigue can also diminish the meaningfulness and can negatively impact the willingness of the parents to handle contact lenses, eye drops, and patching.[21] It has been observed that the mothers are more likely to be affected than fathers during the care of the child, with mental fatigue and lack of motivation jointly contributing as significant barriers for loss in follow-up.

During treatment, most children began to feel self-conscious, embarrassed, and ashamed. In cases of amblyopia, children experience felt and enacted stigma. Felt stigma refers to the emotions of shame during one's illness. Children also feel that they draw adverse attention from others during and after treatment. They often feel interrogated and being stared at, with these concerns particularly dominant in children with an eye patch and glasses. However, some children respond positively as they think they look "smarter" and "faster" with glasses. Most children also adopt secrecy to minimize feelings of stigma, prevent breakdown, and maintain positivety. They often conceal treatment details from their friends and peers. Though the psychosocial impact may differ for each child and family, the level of perceived stigma and social support plays a significant role during and after the treatment.[22]

9.9 Conclusion

It is difficult to imagine life without vision as it provides rich and immediate details about objects and facilitates communication in combination with the neurological network. Without vision gathering, information becomes instinctive with conscious attention and is based on the information received by other senses. Psychosocial development in children may also be compromised in the absence of social input that vision offers. Visual impairments often leave the child in a state where they experience the world differently from their sighted peers and often relegate them to live in hopelessness and dependence.[23]

Over the years, tremendous progress has been made by medical sciences and rehabilitation, including advances in the field of optics and technology. Over the past century, rapid strides have been made in that have not only minimized the impact of childhood blindness but also given newer insights for research to look into the emerging causes of avoidable and preventable blindness. With change in time and environment, demographic-centric strategies will be required to maximize the efforts for sensitization of pregnant mothers to adopt a healthier lifestyle, with emphasis on the role of nutrition and intrauterine infections like rubella and measles. In addition, synchronized efforts are needed for early detection and management of avoidable causes of childhood blindness such as childhood cataract.

REFERENCES

1. Rogow SM. The Impact of Visual Impairments on Psychosocial Development. In: Schwean V.L., Saklofske D.H. (eds) Handbook of Psychosocial Characteristics of Exceptional Children. Springer Series on Human Exceptionality. Springer, Boston, MA, 1999. doi: 10.1007/978-1-4757-5375
2. Solebo AL, Teoh L, Rahi J. Epidemiology of blindness in children. Arch Dis Child. 2017. Sep;102(9):853–857. doi: 10.1136/archdischild-2016-310532
3. Allen EL. Childhood cataract. Symposium: Eyes and ENT. 2020. 30(1):28–32.
4. Long E, Lin Z, Chen J, et al. Monitoring and morphologic classification of pediatric cataract using slit-lamp-adapted photography. Transl Vis Sci Technol. 2017. 6(6):2. doi: 10.1167/tvst.6.6.2
5. Kumar D, Lim JC, Donaldson PJ. A link between maternal malnutrition and depletion of glutathione in the developing lens: a possible explanation for idiopathic childhood cataract? Clin Exp Optom. 2013. 96(6):523–528.
6. Sheeladevi S, Lawrenson JG, Fielder AR, Suttle CM. The global prevalence of childhood cataract: a systematic review. Eye (Lond). 2016. 30(9):1160–1169.

7.   Khokhar SK, Pillay G, Dhull C, Agarwal E, Mahabir M, Aggarwal P. Pediatric cataract. Indian J Ophthalmol. 2017. 65:1340–1349

8.   Ram J, Agarwal A. The challenge of childhood cataract blindness. Indian J Med Res. 2014. 140:472–474

9.   Wilson ME, Pandey SK, Thakur J. Paediatric cataract blindness in the developing world: surgical techniques and intraocular lenses in the new millennium. Br J Ophthalmol. 2003;87(1):14–19. doi: 10.1136/bjo.87.1.14

10. Mets MB, Chhabra MS. Eye manifestations of intrauterine infections and their impact on childhood blindness. Surv Ophthalmol. 2008. 53(2):95–111. doi: 10.1016/j.survophthal.2007.12.003. PMID: 18348876.

11. Khurana S, Ram J, Singh R, Gupta PC, Gupta R, Yangzes S, Sukhija J, Dogra MR. Surgical outcomes of cataract surgery in anterior and combined persistent fetal vasculature using a novel surgical technique: a single center, prospective study. Graefes Arch Clin Exp Ophthalmol. 2021. Jan; 259(1):213–221. doi: 10.1007/s00417-020-04883-6

12. Long E, Lin Z, Chen J, et al. Monitoring and morphologic classification of pediatric cataract using slit-lamp-adapted photography. Transl Vis Sci Technol. 2017. 6(6):2. doi: 10.1167/tvst.6.6.2

13. Dohvoma AV. Epidemiological and clinical profiles of childhood cataract seen at the Yaounde Central Hospital. Journal of Ophthalmology & Clinical Research. 2020. 7:1–5.

14. Dandona R, Dandona L. Socioeconomic status and blindness. British Journal of Ophthalmology. 2001. 85:1484–1488.

15. Gilbert CE, Lepvrier-Chomette N. Gender inequalities in surgery for bilateral cataract among children in low-income countries: a systematic review. Ophthalmology. 2016. 123(6):1245–1251.

16. Gupta VB, Rajagopala M, Ravishankar B. Etiopathogenesis of cataract: an appraisal. Indian Journal Of Ophthalmology. 2014. 62(2):103–110. doi: 10.4103/0301-4738.121141

17. Foster A, Gilbert C, Rahi J. Epidemiology of cataract in childhood: a global perspective. J Cataract Refract Surg. 1997. 23 Suppl 1:601–604.

18. Shamanna BR. Childhood cataract: magnitude, management, economics and impact. Community Eye Health. 2004. 17(50):17–18.

19. Orbis Report. www.newindianexpress.com/nation/2020/oct/11/blindness-to-cost-india-rs-88k-crore-in-2020-report-2208735.html

20. Tailor V, Abou-Rayyah Y, Brookes J, et al. Quality of life and functional vision in children treated for cataract—a cross-sectional study. Eye. 2017. 31:856–864.

21. Gyllén J, Magnusson G, Forsberg A. Parents' reported experiences when having a child with cataract-important aspects of self-management obtained from the paediatric cataract register (PECARE). International Journal of Environmental Research and Public Health. 2020. 17(17):6329.

22. Koklanis K, Abel LA, Aroni R. Psychosocial impact of amblyopia and its treatment: a multidisciplinary study. Clin Exp Ophthalmol. 2006. 34(8):743–750.

23. Schinazi VR. The psychosocial implication of blindness and low vision. Centre for Advanced Spatial Analysis. Paper Series 114. 2007. ISSN 1467-1298. University College, London.

10

Evidence-Based Practice in Neurodegenerative Disorders: Approaches and Challenges

Mani Chopra, Sweety Mehra, Era Seth, and Aitizaz Ul Ahsan
Department of Zoology, Panjab University, Chandigarh, India

R.C. Sobti
Department of Biotechnology, Panjab University, Chandigarh, India

10.1 Introduction

Evidence-based medicine (EBM) systematically reviews, evaluates, and integrates available clinical research evidence to deliver optimum clinical care (Rosenberg, 1995). This course of action is the need of the hour, the decision to provide appropriate healthcare to a patient/population that should be driven on the evidence of clinical findings and subsequent health outcomes that certainly differ in individuals.

EBM originated in the second half of the 19th century and earlier when Professor Archie Cochrane, director of the Medical Research Council Epidemiology Research Unit in Cardiff, expressed what later came to be known as evidence-based medicine in his book entitled *Effectiveness and Efficiency: Random Reflections on Health Services* (Cochrane, 1999). These concepts were then developed, expanded with further international collaborations, and turned into a specific practical methodology used as a conscious and reasonable use of the available scientific data for making decisions of a particular treatment.

Formerly, access to the latest published biomedical research was not that conveniently accessible to clinicians. They always worked to the best of their knowledge and judgment, which is not the best way to practice medicine. When researchers investigate a particular condition, they usually collect and corroborate data from many more patients than a clinician would. Considering, reviewing, and implementing all the evidence in the latest data available via researchers worldwide is called practicing EBM (Sackettet al., 1996).

The three key components of EBM are:

a) **Research-Based Evidence:** Application of precise medicine via healthcare workers means assimilating individual clinical signs, experience, and outcomes collectively with the best scientific data on a particular disease (Masic et al., 2008).
b) **The clinical expertise:** Modern-day application of EBM requires following a systematic approach to a clinical problem – the clinical accumulated experience, their knowledge, and clinical skills doctors have gained throughout years of practice – is an indispensable tool in EBM (Sackett et al., 1996).
c) **The patient values and practices:** The practice of EBM is lifelong development of self-directed, problem-based knowledge. Providing dedicated care to each patient builds the need for clinically important information about the diagnosis, prognosis, therapy, and other clinical and healthcare issues (Sackett et al., 2000).

Observing EBM as a tool in contemporary medicine paves the way for clinicians to achieve improved quality, upgraded patient satisfaction, and reduced treatment costs. To understand, let us consider an example of neurodegenerative disease treatment. With EBM's implementation, a provider/clinician can

DOI: 10.1201/9781003220404-12

assess the evidence's strength by reviewing the research database for a particular condition. Thus, he can weigh the risks and benefits of using specific diagnostic assay tests and treatments for each patient. Such a collaborative approach that includes providers' clinical experience, latest research evidence, and patient concerns enables a clinician to better predict a particular treatment's pros and cons. Moreover, EBM may help physicians to provide more rational care with better outcomes.

10.2 Need for Evidence-Based Medicine in Neurodegenerative Disorders

EBM is the amalgamation of best research evidence worldwide with years of clinical expertise and specific patient values. One of the main challenges for healthcare systems is the increasing prevalence of neurodegenerative pathologies and rapidly aging populations. EBM is an interdisciplinary approach that uses science, engineering, biostatistics, and epidemiology such as meta-analysis, decision analysis, risk-benefit analysis, and randomized controlled trials to deliver "the right care at the right time to the right patient" (Masic et al., 2008). The enormous progress made in biomedical research and informatics has been crucial for improving our understanding of how genes, epigenetic modifications, aging, nutrition, drugs, and microbiome have an impact on health and disease. The availability of high technology and computational facilities for large-scale analysis has enabled a more in-depth investigation of neurodegenerative disorders, providing a more comprehensive overview of the disease and encouraging the development of a precision medicine approach for these pathologies.

10.3 Evidence-Oriented Approach in the Case of Neurodegenerative Diseases

Evidence-based research (EBR) is a multidisciplinary approach that is used not only in designing the treatment plans but also in encouraging the clinicians and patients to make decisions. This systematic approach works to gain the momentums Health, Care, and Cost at the same time. An evidence-based approach in neurodegenerative diseases improves transparency, accountability, value, and plausibility of favorable outcomes. Reviewing the best available evidence improves the quality of efficacious research utilization and helps incorporate it in cost-effective clinical practices. Thus, the critical analysis of the divergent research findings could help design treatment strategies for the disorders (Chiappelli et al., 2006).

Evidence-based research in neurodegenerative disorders helps in:

Identification of the early diagnostic markers for neurodegenerative disorders (Robey & Panegyres, 2019)

Establishing the diagnostic assays for investigating the development and evolution of neurodegenerative disorders (Hussain et al., 2018)

Creating complementary non-harming methodologies for analyzing the dysfunctionality of the brain (Mariotti et al., 2010)

Identifying the genetics, environmental factors, and their inter-relationship with the disorder (Castillo et al., 2019; Pang et al., 2017; Bertram &Tanzi, 2005)

Investigating the molecular targets for treatments aimed at attenuating the impairments caused due to the neuronal degeneration (Rasool et al., 2014; Gupta et al., 2018; Seth et al., 2018)

Improving symptomatic treatments (Kiaei, 2013; Chiappelli et al., 2006)

Identifying the drugs/complementary non-pharma logical medicines that can help in preventing the progression of ND (Chiappelli et al., 2006; Rasool et al., 2014; Ahsan et al., 2020)

Identify risk factors that can elevate the prevalence of onset of neurodegenerative diseases (Brown et al., 2005; Emard et al., 1995).

Evidence-based research is a stepwise process (Figure 10.1):

    I.   Screening and identification of the problem

   II.   Accessing sources of information

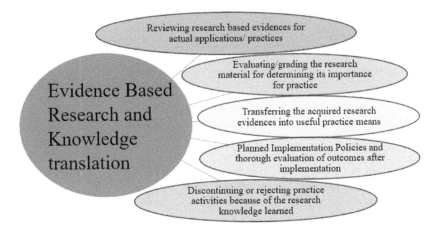

FIGURE 10.1 Framework of research utilization and knowledge translation to EBM practice.

III. Analyzing information/evaluation of information
IV. Information implementation to the patient
 V. Efficacy evaluation of this application on a patient

10.3.1 Screening and Identification of the Problem

The first step of the EBM practice is the identification of the problem and categorizing it. For this, clinicians need to design medical questionnaires for investigating the patient's situation (Kianifar et al., 2010). Thus, it is necessary to identify the type of problems associated with the patient, relevant history regarding the disorder, and the disorder's severity score. This can be done by following the **PICO** Approach in the questionnaire section (Kianifar et al., 2010). The questionnaires are divided into four parts:

1. **P**atients, Problem, or Population is referred to as the cohort the patient belongs to and the type of problem associated with the patient.
2. **I**ntervention is referred to as diagnostic, treatment, and management strategies that can help investigate the patient's problem.
3. A **C**omparison of interventions is referred to as comparing diagnostic, treatment, and management strategies.
4. The **O**utcome is referred to as the patient-relevant expected outcome we are interested in.

PICO elements vary according to the question type. Table 10.1 illustrates the PICO variation according to the type of question in neurodegenerative disorders.

For proper identification of the problem, a good clinician must formulate well-structured, exact questions directly focusing on the problem, which can be answerable by searching the literature.

10.3.2 Accessing Sources of Information

After identifying the problem, the next step is to access the available sources of information regarding the disorder. It is not easy in the case of neurodegenerative disorders, especially in poorly defined problems. To answer the clinical questions associated with the problem, we need reliable information/data regarding the associated problem. Several resources (mostly web-based) can be very useful in searching for the best available evidence. Some sources of information include:

- Publication sources (government publications, semi-government publications, international publications, reports of committees and commissions, newspaper, magazines, journals, research articles)

TABLE 10.1

PICO Variation According to the Type of Question in Neurodegenerative Disorders

Type of question	Patient problem or population	Intervention	Comparison of control	Outcome measures
Therapy/treatment for the disease	Patient's disease/condition/ severity score/duration of stage	Therapeutic intervention, (e.g., medication, change in lifestyle)	Care, medication intervention, or a placebo.	Consequences on quality of life, stress thresholds, physical strength mobility, etc.
Prevention of disease	Patient's disease/patient's risk factors/general health condition	Preventive intervention. (e.g., a lifestyle change or medication)	Another preventative measure, preventive medication Or maybe not applicable in severe conditions.	Mortality rate, consequences on quality of life, disease incidence, etc.
Diagnosis of specific disease	Specific disease or condition	Diagnostic test/ procedure	Reference standard test for specific disease or condition.	Measures of the test utility (i.e., sensitivity, specificity, odds ratio).
The prognosis (prediction) of disease	Duration/severity of main prognostic factors or disease	Watchful waiting approach/wait and watch strategy/ observational strategy	not applicable.	Survival rates, mortality rates, rates of disease progression.
Etiology of the disease (causation)	Causes/patient's risk factors, current disorders, general health situation, Comorbidity	Exposure interventions/ The dose of the risk factor/ The duration of the exposure	Not applicable.	Survival rates, mortality rates, rates of disease progression.

- Online electronic databases (Cochrane Collaboration and Cochrane Library; clinical evidence; Centre for Reviews and Dissemination Databases (CRD database; Joanna Briggs Institute EBP database (via Ovid); PubMed Clinical Queries; CINAHL Complete (via EBSCOhost); TRIP Database; SUMSearch; Australian New Zealand Clinical Trials Registry (ANZCTR); ClinicalTrials.gov) (Masic et al., 2008)
- Research studies (meta-analytic studies, randomized controlled research (RCR), well-designed controlled research, one quasi-experimental research, non-experimental studies, comparative research, case study, case series, and case reports) (Burns et al., 2011)
- Clinically applicable shreds of evidence from experts and clinical practices (Hake, 2002; De la Garza, 2003)
- Authenticated clinical, preclinical, non-pharm logical data (Reisberg et al., 2003; Tariot et al., 2004)
- S5 strategic data (studies, syntheses, synopses, summaries, and systems (Hyanes, 2007)

Ideal information sources should contain interdisciplinary, reliable, clinically applicable, easily accessible, and high-quality data.

10.3.3 Analyzing Information / Evaluation of Information

Innumerable clinically applicable pharmacology experiments in the case of neurodegenerative disorders are conducted, generating valid scientific data duly published. Therefore, critical evaluation of the available

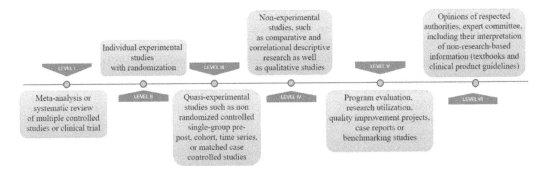

FIGURE 10.2 Levels of evidence and type of shreds of evidence (OCEBM, 2009).

and acquired information is indispensable (Bhandari et al., 2000; Poolman et al., 2006). It is necessary to investigate reproducibility, replicability, and validity of available information in neurodegenerative diseases. Rating the data's quality and interpreting the evidence level is an important step to evaluate the available information (Jadad et al., 1996; Burns et al., 2011; Moralejo et al., 2017). Various grading systems provide a comprehensible methodology for analyzing the risks of publication biases and inconsistent and inaccurate data. A collaborative working group, popularly referred as GRADE (**G**rading of **R**ecommendations, **A**ssessment, **D**evelopment, and **E**valuations), helps in rating the evidence's quality and making recommendations in the context of scientific integrity (Figure 10.2). **O**xford **C**entre for **E**vidence-**B**ased **M**edicine levels of evidence (OCEBM) and **S**trength **o**f **R**ecommendation **T**axonomy (SORT) are recommendation-based grading firms (Daramola and Rhee, 2011).

10.3.4 Information Implementation to the Patient

After evaluating the sources of information, the implementation of the information to the patients is the crucial step. After rating the articles, only scientifically integral, high-quality, and clinically safe evidence should be applied to the patients (Sadeghi et al., 2009). This defining step is intertwined with many issues, including socio-economical, religious, and ethical ones (Melnyk and Fineout-Overholt, 2005; Kianifar et al., 2010). Along with these issues, the success of the step is based on the

- Clinical applicability of the acquired pieces of evidence
- Permission from health systems for implementation
- Availability of the desired number of volunteers for application of pieces of evidence
- Whether the available pieces of evidence concerned with the treatment would be fruitful or have any side effects

10.3.5 Efficacy Evaluation of This Application on a Patient

After implementing the information to patients, it is highly recommended to precisely evaluate the patients' applied evidence-oriented approach. A complete evaluation of the results obtained from the trials of the evidence should be done. The proper investigation of obtained responses from the patients will help design treatment strategies. This process of assessing and measuring the outcomes of the conducted trials is the deciding factor for ensuring the applicability, accountability, and value of the pieces of evidence used.

10.3.5.1 Research Outcome Utilization or Response Scale

A research Outcome Utilization or Response Scale developed by Larsen (1982) ranks the stages of all information providing pieces of evidence (including research finding studies, syntheses, synopses, summaries, suggestions, or recommendations). This ordinal scale of ranking the value of pieces of evidence considers the reliability, applicability, accountability, and validity of used or non-used information (Sudsawad, 2007). According to this, information obtained is divided into utilization and non-utilization. Following are the seven stages of rank value-based scale with definitions (Larsen,1982):

1. **Considered and rejected**: Information has been rejected after a discussion.
2. **Nothing was done**: No action has been taken, not even any discussion has been taken.
3. **Under consideration**: Unused Information that is being used in discussion and under consideration.
4. **Steps toward implementation**: The decision is pending whether the information would be implemented or not; some initial planning steps toward the implementation are in process.
5. **Partially implemented**: Only some portion of the information has been used.
6. **Implemented as presented**: Presented information initially has been accepted and implemented.
7. **Implemented and adapted**: Before implementation, the information has been modified to fit in the scenario.

This Larsen model of analyzing information utilization or non-utilization could help in evaluating the efficacy of the evidence.

10.4 Difficulties and Challenges for Evidence-Based-Oriented Approach Against Neurodegenerative Diseases

In the case of neurodegenerative diseases, there are many practical hurdles for clinicians to practice EBM and deliver the best care to patients. Furthermore, translating the results of EBM research into everyday practice is a major challenge. Here are some challenges that clinicians face in practising evidence-based-oriented approaches against neurodegenerative diseases.

10.4.1 Heterogeneity in Population

The genotype of an individual is the responsible factor behind the structural and functional integrity of the individual. Understanding the relationship between genetics and traits helps to understand the anatomy, physiology, and biochemistry (Kumar, 2007). The relation of specific genes to several traits and characteristics defines the morbid variations shown by a particular disease. Due to heterogeneity, both in clinical features produced by the disease and genetic causes behind the diseases, the clinical diagnosis remains difficult even in hereditary diseases with a clear genetic contribution (Pang et al., 2017) For instance, tri-genic (*APP*, *PSEN1*, and *PSEN2*) fully penetrant autosomal dominant mutations are responsible for causing the Alzheimer's Disease (AD), and ε4 in *APOE* incompletely penetrant susceptibility variant is found responsible for increasing the risk of AD. Identifying responsible genes that make smaller overall contributions to the disease's genetic spectrum requires efficient analytic tools. This creates a challenge for clinicians to use evidence-based research in designing EBM.

10.4.2 Lack of Etiological Studies

Along with aging, some genetic and environmental factors are suspected of causing neurodegeneration. The comorbid contribution of genes and environmental factors has been debated in the case of neurodegeneration (Tan et al., 2015). Since the onset of neurodegeneration, suspected etiology has emerged as an unmet challenge for EBM clinicians to design effective neurodegeneration therapy. Lack of adequate experimental (animal) models to study the etiology and further study it in human systems emerged as a barrier to investigating effective medicine for neurodegeneration. Together, these facts limit the therapeutic potential to treat the symptoms rather than the causes (Castillo et al., 2019). Lack of defined etiological studies limits EBM clinicians in translating the knowledge obtained to therapeutically valuable outcomes.

10.4.3 Insufficient Data

Appropriate and leading studies could help in designing medicine for the disease. For appreciable outcomes, studies must be conducted with proper sample size, appropriate matching of the diseased cases with the control ones, and selection of adequate analysis strategies. But poorly characterized study participants, insufficiently sized samples, inadequate data collection using inappropriate matching of cases against the controls, inappropriate statistical analysis, etc., are the major barriers in the way of the designing EBM in the case of neurodegenerative diseases (Cohen-Mansfield, 2001; Snowden et al., 2003; Verkaik et al., 2005).

10.4.4 Publication Bias

Favouring the publication of positive findings and avoiding the false/negative/harmful findings produce unreliable data. This kind of publication bias makes it extremely challenging for EBM clinicians to reach firm conclusions. The reliability only on the published data and ignoring the negative/harmful findings disturbs a balance between the risks and benefits. To investigate a drug's effectiveness, companies should also provide detailed harm reports (Livingston, 2005).

10.4.5 Discordant Reviews

A systematic review of randomized controlled trials (RCTs) offers EBM clinicians one platform that can summarize past studies, investigate the studies by sample size and variability, and rate their quality. Systematic reviews help early clinicians to determine the efficacy and precaution measures of the medicine. Nevertheless, not all reviews are reliable. For instance, preferred drugs like donepezil, rivastigmine, or galantamine for AD treatment are questionable because of low methodological available trials (Kaduszkiewicz et al., 2005). Therefore, without a thorough understanding of the valid scientific methodology and the review of many other systematic reviews, it would be extremely challenging for clinicians to reach firm conclusions for designing treatment interventions.

10.5 Concluding Remarks

Evidence-based medicine is a young discipline and evolving with time. Despite research efforts, most designed strategies to manage neurodegenerative disorders are alleviative but not curative. Over the last few decades, evidence-based research is fundamental research providing pieces of evidence evaluating the effectiveness of traditional and new improved modes of treatment intervention in neurodegenerative disorders. Evidence-based medicine practices for neurodegenerative disorders require a holistic approach that integrates the best available epidemiological, biomedical, and clinical evidence. The use of valid and reliable research-generated knowledge in designing treatment strategies for brain degeneration is the main aim of the relevant field's EBM practices. A thorough understanding of evidence-based research can help in balancing the benefits and side effects produced due to the particular medicine against the disease.

REFERENCES

Ahsan AU, Sharma VL, Wani A, Chopra M (2020). Naringenin upregulates AMPK-mediated autophagy to rescue neuronal cells from β-amyloid (1–42) evoked neurotoxicity. *Mol Neurobiol* 57: 3589–3602.

Bertram L, Tanzi RE (2005). The genetic epidemiology of neurodegenerative disease. *J Clin Investig* 115: 1449–1457.

Bhandari M, Richards RR, Sprague S, Schemitsch EH (2000). The quality of reporting of randomized trials in the Journal of Bone and Joint Surgery from 1988 through. *J Bone Joint Surg Am* (84-A): 388–396.

Brown RC, Lockwood AH, Sonawane BR (2005). Neurodegenerative diseases: an overview of environmental risk factors. *Environ Health Perspect* 113: 1250–1256.

Burns MPH, Rohrich RJ, Chung KC (2011). The levels of evidence and their role in evidence-based medicine. *Plast Reconstr Surg* 128: 305–310.

Castillo X et al.,(2019). Re-thinking the etiological framework of neurodegeneration. *Front Neurosci* 13: 728.

Chiappelli F, Navarro1 AM, Moradi1 DR, Manfrini E, Prolo P (2006). Evidence-based research in complementary and alternative medicine III: treatment of patients with Alzheimer's disease. *Advance Access Publication. eCAM* 3: 411–424.

Cochrane AL (1999). *Effectiveness and Efficiency: Random Reflections on Health Services.* London: Royal Society of Medicine Press.

Cohen-Mansfield J (2001). Nonpharmacologic interventions for inappropriate behaviors in dementia: a review, summary, and critique. *Am J Geriatr Psychiatry* 9: 361–381.

Daramola OO, Rhee JS (2011). Rating evidence in medical literature. *Virtual Mentor* 13: 46–51.

De La G arza VW (2003). Pharmacologic treatment of Alzheimer's disease. An update. *Am Fam Physician* 68: 1365–1372.

Emard JF, Thouez JP, GauvreauD (1995). Neurodegenerative diseases and risk factors: A literature review. *Soc Sci Med* (40): 847–858.

Gupta M, Wani A, Ahsan AU, Chopra M, Vishwakarma RA, Singh G, Kumar A (2018). Soluble Aβ1-42 suppresses TNF-α and activates NLRP3 inflammasome in THP-1 macrophages. *Cytokine* 111: 84–87.

Hake AM (2002). The treatment of Alzheimer's disease: The approach from clinical specialist in the trenches. *Semin Neurol* 22: 71–74.

Haynes B (2007). Of studies, syntheses, synopses, summaries, and systems: the "5S" evolution of information services for evidence-based healthcare decisions. *Evid Based Nurs* 10: 6–7.

Hussain R, Zubair H, Pursell S, Shahab M (2018). Neurodegenerative diseases: Regenerative mechanisms and novel therapeutic approaches. *Brain Sci* 8: 177.

Jadad AR et al. (1996). Assessing the quality of reports of randomized clinical trials: Is blinding necessary? *Control Clin Trials* 17: 1–12.

Kaduszkiewicz H et al. (2005). Cholinesterase inhibitors for patients with Alzheimer's disease: Systematic review of randomised clinical trials. *BMJ* 331: 321–327.

Kiaei M (2013). New hopes and challenges for treatment of neurodegenerative disorders: Great opportunities for young neuroscientists. *Basic Clin Neurosci* 4: 3–4.

Kianifar HR, Akhondian MDJ, Najafi Sani MDN, Sadeghi R (2010). Evidence based medicine in pediatric practice: Brief review. *I Iran J Pediatr* 20: 261–268.

Kumar D (2007). From evidence-based medicine to genomic medicine. *HUGO J* 1: 95–104.

Larsen JK (1982). *Information Utilization and Non-Utilization.* Palo Alto, CA: American Institutes for Research in the Behavioral Sciences.

Livingston G, Johnston K, Katona C, Paton J, Lyketsos CG, Old Age Task Force of the World Federation of Biological Psychiatry (2005). Systematic review of psychological approaches to the management of neuropsychiatric symptoms of dementia. *Am Psychiatry* 162: 1996–2021.

Mariotti C et al. (2010). Predictive genetic tests in neurodegenerative disorders: A methodological approach integrating psychological counseling for at-risk individuals and referring clinicians. *Eur Neurol* 64: 33–41.

Masic I, Miokovic M, Muhamedagic B (2008). Evidence based medicine-new approaches and challenges. *Acta Inform Med* 16: 219–225.

Melnyk BM, Fineout-Overholt E (2005). Rapid critical appraisal of randomized controlled trials (RCTs): an essential skill for evidence-based practice (EBP). *Pediatr Nurs* 31: 50–52.

Moralejo D, Ogunremi MT, Dunn K (2017).Critical Appraisal Toolkit (CAT) for assessing multiple types of evidence. *Can Commun Dis Rep* 43: 176–181.

Oxford Levels of Evidence for Therapeutic Study Designs (2009).

Pang SYY, Teo1 KC, Hsu JS, Chang RSK, Miaoxin Li, Sham PC, Ho SL (2017). The role of gene variants in the pathogenesis of neurodegenerative disorders as revealed by next generation sequencing studies: a review. *Transl Neurodegener* 6: 27.

Poolman RW, Struijs PA, Krips R, Sierevelt IN, Lutz KH, Bhandari M (2006). Does a "Level I Evidence" rating imply high quality of reporting in orthopaedic randomised controlled trials? *BMC Med Res Methodol* 6: 44.

Rasool M et al. (2014). Recent updates in the treatment of neurodegenerative disorders using natural compounds. *Evid Based Complement Alternat Med* 2014: 979730.

Reisberg B, Doody R, Stoffler A, Schmitt F, Ferris S, Mobius HJ (2003). Memantine study group memantine in moderate-to-severe Alzheimer's disease. *N Engl J Med* 348: 1333–1341.

Robey TT, Panegyres PK (2019). Cerebrospinal fluid biomarkers in neurodegenerative disorders. *Future Neurology* 14.

Rosenberg W, Donald A (1995). Evidence based medicine: an approach to clinical problem-solving. *BMJ* 310: 122–1126.

Sackett DL, Richardson WS, Rosenberg W, Haynes RB (2000). *Evidence-Based Medicine: How to Practice and Teach*, 2nd Ed. Edinburgh: Churchill-Livingstone.

Sackett DL, Rosenberg WM, Gray JA, Richardson WS (1996). Evidence based medicine: what it is and what it isn't. *BMJ* 312: 71–72.

Sadeghi R, Zakavi SR, Dabbagh Kakhki VR (2009). How to apply evidence based medicine concept to the nuclear medicine diagnostic studies: A review. *Nucl Med Rev Cent East Eur* 12: 59–64.

Seth E, Kaushal S, Ahsan AU, Sharma VL, Chopra M (2018). Neuroprotective effects of Aegle marmelos (L.) Correa against cadmium toxicity by reducing oxidative stress and maintaining the histoarchitecture of neural tissue in BALB/c mice. *IJBB* 55: 95–104.

Snowden M, Sato K, Roy-Byrne P (2003). Assessment and treatment of nursing home residents with depression or behavioral symptoms associated with dementia: a review of the literature. *J Am Geriatr Soc* 51: 1305–1317.

Sudsawad P (2007). *Knowledge Translation: Introduction to Models, Strategies, and Measures*. Austin, TX: Southwest Educational Development Laboratory, National Center for the Dissemination of Disability Research.

Tan EK, Srivastava AK, Arnold WD, Singh MP, Zhang Y (2015). Neurodegeneration: Etiologies and new therapies. *Biomed Res Int* 2016: 8363179.

Tariot PN, Farlow MR, Grossberg GT, Graham SM, McDonald S, Gergel I (2004). Memantine study group. Memantine treatment in patients with moderate to severe Alzheimer disease already receiving donepezil: a randomized controlled trial. *JAMA* 291: 317–324.

Verkaik R, van Weert JC, Francke AL (2005). The effects of psychosocial methods on depressed, aggressive and apathetic behaviors of people with dementia: a systematic review. *Int J Geriatr Psychiatry* 20: 301–314.

11

Pragmatic Utilization of Technology in Dentistry: Current Status and Future Perspectives

Jagat Bhushan, Ruchi Singla, Swaty Jhamb, and Kratika Chauhan
H S Judge Institute of Dental Sciences, Panjab University, Chandigarh, India

Aastha Sobti
Department of Immunogenetics, Lund University, Sweden

11.1 Introduction

Science infuses the process of understanding problems and serves as fuel for development in any field. During the last century, biomedical sciences have undergone a sea change and have undergone diversification as well as mergers to adopt a thoroughly multi-disciplinary approach. There has been a convergence of distant fields and collaborative research is being done to achieve targets that were earlier thought to be unrealistic. This philosophy has also percolated down into the dental sciences. Over the course of time dentistry has evolved from being a primitive subsidiary of contemporary medicine to a discipline that can boast of a large number of specialist domain areas. From being an arena ruled by barber-surgeons, as they were referred to in the 13th century in Europe, dentistry is now the subject field of experts who are delivering state-of-the-art oral healthcare, which incidentally has a huge impact on the systematic health of the individual. From being a radical 'Drill, Fill And Bill' approach, now dental clinical services are targeting the regenerative repair process and reconstruction to halt and reverse damage. Currently, the most promising research outcomes are being documented in areas of stem cells, gene therapy, and nanotechnology. These areas will be deliberated upon in the following discussion.

11.2 Stem Cells

The term "stem cell" was used in 1868 by German biologist Haeckel (Yamaizumi et al., 1978). Russian histologist, Alexander Maksimov, in 1908 at the Congress of the Hematologic Society in Berlin postulated the existence of hematopoietic stem cells (Maximow, 1909). Possessing vast potential for widespread applications, stem cells have led to the establishment of regenerative medicine. A major breakthrough in the dental field was achieved in the year 2000 when Gronthos et al. identified and isolated odontogenic progenitor population in adult dental pulp (Gronthos et al., 2000). These cells were referred to as dental pulp stem cells (DPSCs). After that, a variety of dental stem cells have been identified. Stem cells are also known as "progenitor or precursor" cells and are defined as clonogenic cells capable of both self-renewal and multi-lineage differentiation. They are immature, undifferentiated cells that can divide and multiply for an extended period, differentiating into specific types of cells and tissues.

11.2.1 The Three Main Categories

The three main categories of stems cells are: embryonic stem cells (ES), adult stem cells that are naturally present in the human body, and induced pluripotent stem cells (iPS), which are generated artificially via genetic manipulation of somatic cells.

DOI: 10.1201/9781003220404-13

ES and iPS are collectively referred to as pluripotent stem cells because they can develop into all types of cells from all three germinal layers whereas most adult stem cells are multipotent (i.e., they can only differentiate into a limited number of all types).

Adult stem cells have been isolated from various tissues:

    i) Bone marrow-derived mesenchymal stem cells from the iliac crest and orofacial bones
    ii) Dental tissue-derived stem cells
    iii) Oral mucosa-derived stem cells
    iv) Periosteum-derived stem/progenitor cells
    v) Salivary gland-derived stem cells
    vi) Adipose tissue-derived stem cells

Dental Tissue Mesenchymal Stem Cells (MSCs) include:

    a) Stem cells from human pulp tissue (DPSCs, post-natal dental pulp stem cells)
    b) Stem cells from human exfoliated deciduous teeth (SHED)
    c) Periodontal ligament stem cells (PDLSC)
    d) Stem cells of apical papilla (SCAP)
    e) Dental follicle precursors cells (DFPC)

A brief description of these follows.

11.2.1.1 Dental Pulp Stem Cells (DPSCs)

Dental pulp contains a population of stem cells, called pulp stem cells. DPSCs were first isolated from human permanent third molars in 2000. Gronthos et al. characterized the self-renewal capability, multi-lineage differentiation capacity, and clonogenic efficiency of human dental pulp stem cells (Gronthos et al., 2000). DPSCs were capable of forming ectopic dentin and associated pulp tissue in vivo. Stromal-like cells were re-established in culture from primary DPSC transplants and re-transplanted into immune-compromised mice to generate a dentin-pulp-like tissue, demonstrating their self-renewal capability (Gronthos et al., 2000). Sometimes pulp stem cells are called odontoblastoid cells. Laino et al. described these cells as multi-potential cells that were able to give rise to a variety of cell types and tissues including osteoblasts, adipocytes, myoblasts, endotheliocytes, and melanocytes, as well as neural cell progenitors (neurons and glia), being of neural crest origin (d'Aquino et al., 2009).

Methods used for the isolation of dental pulp stem cells are:

    i) Explant method (DPSC-OG)
    ii) Enzymatic digestion method of the pulp tissue (DPSC-EZ)

11.2.1.2 Stem Cells from Human Exfoliated Deciduous Teeth (SHED)

SHED were isolated for the first time in 2003 by Miura et al., and it was reported that these cells have the potential to differentiate into various cell types like-neural cells, adipose cells, odontoblast-like, and osteoblast-like cells. In vivo transplantation showed that SHED were able to induce bone formation, regenerate dentin, and survive in the mouse brain along with the expression of neural markers. SHED demonstrated a strong capacity to induce recipient cell-mediated bone formation in vivo. SHED induced new bone formation by forming an osteoinductive template to recruit murine host osteogenic cells, but they themselves were not able to differentiate into osteoblasts (Miura et al., 2003). Sakai et al. (2010) reported that stem cells from exfoliated deciduous teeth (SHED) differentiate into endothelial cells and functional odontoblast capable of generating tubular dentin (Sakai et al., 2010).

11.2.1.3 Periodontal Ligament Stem Cells (PDLSCs)

The periodontal ligament has been found to be a source of a novel population of dental stem cells (PDLSC – periodontal ligament stem cell). These were isolated from the periodontal ligament of human third molars by Seo BM et al. in 2004. Under defined culture conditions, PDLSCs differentiate into cementoblast-like cells, adipocytes, and collagen-forming cells. When transplanted into immunocompromised rodents, PDLSCs show the capability of periodontal tissue repair by regeneration of cementum/periodontal ligament-like structure (Seo et al., 2004).

11.2.1.4 Stem Cells from Apical Papillae (SCAP)

A unique population of mesenchymal stem cells (MSCs) reside in the apical papilla of permanent immature teeth, known as stem cells from the apical papilla. SCAP cells were first isolated from extracted human third molars. SCAP are capable of forming odontoblast-like cells, producing dentin in vivo, and are likely to be the cell source of primary odontoblasts for root dentin formation. These cells are clonogenic and can undergo odontoblastic/osteogenic, adipogenic, or neurogenic differentiation (Sonoyama et al., 2008).

11.2.1.5 Dental Follicle Precursor Cells (DFPCs)

Dental follicle precursor cells were isolated from dental follicle by Morsczeck et al. in 2005, and these cells can be differentiated as cementoblasts, PDLcells, and osteoblasts.
The advantages of dental stem cells include:

- The easy surgical access to the site of extraction and also the low morbidity at the donor site make the dental stem cells a more putative candidate for dental tissue engineering.
- They can be easily amplified and cryopreserved for a long time without affecting their viability.
- They show good interaction with scaffold and growth factors.

11.2.2 Applications of Stem Cell Therapy in Dentistry

11.2.2.1 Regeneration of the Periodontal Ligament

Stem cells have the potential to regenerate into periodontal structures like periodontal ligament and other supporting structures. The complex structure of periodontium requires multi-potent cells for its complete regeneration. A study by Yu et al. (2013) showed regeneration of new cementum, alveolar bone, and periodontal ligament by transplantation ex vivo expanded autologous mesenchymal stem cell in dogs (Yu et al., 2013).

11.2.2.2 Regeneration of the Dentin and Pulp

The dentin pulp contains progenitor/stem cells that can proliferate and differentiate into dentin-forming odontoblasts (Nakashima et al., 1994). Damaged odontoblasts can be replaced by newly generated populations of odontoblasts derived from stem cells of pulp. Tissue engineering with the triad of dental pulp progenitor/stem cells, morphogens, and scaffolds provide a useful alternative method for pulp capping and root canal treatment (Tziafas et al., 2000).

11.2.2.3 Regeneration of the Oromaxillofacial Structure Craniofacial Defects

Adipose tissue-derived stem cells from the gluteal region along with the iliac crest are successful in treating head injuries and show promising results in treating difficult reconstructive procedures (San-Marina et al., 2017).

11.2.2.4 Soft Tissue Reconstruction

Soft tissues can be reconstructed from human MSCs, which can turn into adipose cells. SHED promotes wound healing and therefore deciduous teeth can be used for the treatment of wounds (Bansal et al., 2015).

11.2.2.5 Apexification and Apxogenesis

Stem cells isolated from pulp tissue, apical papilla, periodontal ligament, and alveolar bone have the potential to regenerate into the apex of an immature permanent tooth (Tziafas et al., 2000).

11.2.2.6 Tooth Regeneration

Development of fully functional bioengineered teeth that can replace lost teeth is the ultimate goal of tooth regeneration. Sonoyama et al. demonstrated that PDL stem cells (PDLSCs), stem cells of apical papilla (SCAP), and HA/TCP (Hydroxiapetite/Tricalcium Phosphate) scaffold are capable of constructing root/periodontal complex, which can support an artificial crown to provide normal tooth function in a swine model (Sonoyama et al., 2006). Many types of stem cells isolated from rats, mice, and pigs can be engineered to form dental structures. Though enormous successful results in tooth regeneration were achieved in various studies like Ikeda et al., there were some hurdles in the application of tooth regeneration technology in the identification of an appropriate autologous stem cell source in humans. iPS cell proved to be promising in this regard as they can differentiate to dental epithelial and mesenchymal cells and can prepare from patient's own somatic cells.

11.2.3 Future Perspectives

Regenerative medicine is gaining interest to treat several irreversible medical conditions that cannot be reversed with present treatment strategies. Most promising of these are Cancer Stem Cells.

> **Cancer Stem Cells (CSC):** These cells act as potentially important targets for the therapy of Oral Squamous Cell Carcinoma (SCC). These are the only cells of the human body that are capable of long-term self-renewal and generation of phenotypically diverse tumour cell populations. However, the lack of reliable markers for the identification of CSCs hinders the development of target-specific strategies in the treatment of SCC.
> **Stem Cell Banks:** Dental stem cells are a valuable source of stem cells and are found in teeth with healthy pulp. Dental stem cell banking is the process of isolating and storing stem cells from patients' deciduous and wisdom teeth. Presently, these teeth are discarded as medical waste. These stem cells containing tissues can be be cryopreserved for regenerative therapies in the future.

11.3 Gene Therapy

The first gene therapy in humans was performed in 1990 for treating severe combined immunodeficiency, which worked for only a few months (Prabhakar et al., 2011). In dentistry gene therapy was introduced in 1995 (Karthikeyan and Pradeep, 2006). In recent years, this therapy has developed by leaps and bounds including several areas applicable to dental practice.

Gene therapy deals with replacing the defective genes with their correct analogues to produce functional proteins. Evidence suggests that gene therapy can be used to prevent, alleviate, or cure cancers, infectious diseases, genetic, and autoimmune disorders (Misra, 2013). It is based on the principle that a normal gene is inserted to compensate for a non-functional gene and an abnormal gene can be repaired through selective reverse mutation.

11.3.1 Gene Therapy is a Two-Step Procedure

The first step includes the insertion of human genetic coding of therapeutic protein into the genome of an attenuated virus, which acts as a vector or carrier. The second step includes the entry of the construct into the cell resulting in the release of the DNA sequence that becomes integrated within the chromosome and thus allowing the production of genetically identical cells containing the DNA sequence introduced by the vector (Egusa et al., 2012).

Gene therapy can be classified into two distinct stages: somatic and germ line therapy.

Somatic gene therapy involves changes in the target cells but that are not transferred to the next generation. In contrast with germline therapy, the modified genes are transferred to the next generation. However, to date, only somatic gene therapy is allowed and germline therapy is limited to animal models due to ethical issues and the risk of unexpected damage to the developing fetus.

11.3.1.1 There are Two Methods of Delivery of the Vector: In Vivo or Ex Vivo

In vivo gene transfer involves the direct injection of foreign gene into the patient by either viral or non-viral methods.

Ex vivo gene transfer involves a foreign gene transduced into the cells of a tissue biopsy, outside the body, and then resulting genetically modified cells are transplanted back into the patient.

11.3.1.2 Vectors

There can be viral and non-viral vectors. Viral vectors cannot replicate or cause infections. These viruses are attenuated to transfer genes. Viral vectors used in experiments are retrovirus, adenovirus, lentivirus, vaccinia virus, and herpes simplex virus. Adenoviruses are the most commonly used vectors.

Non-viral vectors are electroporation, polymers, microinjection, calcium vectors, lipid vectors, and protein complexes.

The ideal vector should have characteristics like high efficiency, high specificity, and less virulence.

11.3.2 Applications of Gene Therapy in Dentistry

11.3.2.1 Gene Therapy for Bone Repair

Regeneration of bone is one of the most clinically important long-term research in tissue engineering. In cases of pathological fracture or massive bone defects, bone healing and repair is challenging. The ideal goal of gene therapy for bone repair is the regeneration of bone at the required area, and this requires the presence of at least four crucial elements: osteoinduction, differentiation of osteoblast leading to the production of an osteoid matrix, osteoconduction, and mechanical stimulation (Prabhakar et al., 2011).

The transforming growth factor (TGF) superfamily such as Platelet-derived Growth Factors (PDGFs), Bone Morphogenic Proteins (BMPs), Insulin-like Growth Factors (IGFs), and Transforming Growth Factor-β (TGF-βs) have been employed widely for tissue engineering purposes.

In vivo research has shown that different cell types such as non-osteogenic fibroblasts (from human gingiva and dental pulp) and myoblast, as well as osteoblast, can express BMP 7 gene after infected with an adenoviral vector (Baum and O'Connell, 1995).

11.3.2.2 Gene Therapy for Salivary Glands

Salivary gland destruction can occur due to various pathological conditions, treatment of head and neck cancer by radiotherapy, and autoimmune disorders like Sjögren's syndrome (Kagami et al., 2008). Salivary glands are an excellent site for gene transfer. As salivary glands excrete a large number of proteins in the bloodstream salivary gene therapy can be used to secrete particular substances and to overcome single-protein deficiencies (Ayllón Barbellido et al., 2008).

11.3.2.3 Gene Therapy for Cancer

The sixth most common cancer in the world is Squamous Cell Carcinoma (SCC) of the head and neck, which includes cancer of the oral cavity, pharynx, larynx, and paranasal sinuses. In contrast to cancer in other parts of the body, head and neck cancer is a target for local gene therapy because of its anatomical location. This allows the delivery of vectors directly to the desired sites with only small degrees of toxicity.

Various strategies and types of gene therapy approaches used for cancer treatment include:

i.   Corrective gene therapy involves the correction of the underlying genetic defect to control the unrestricted multiplications of the tumour cells. Inactivation of oncogenes or replacement of mutated tumour suppressor gene is done.

ii. Immunomodulatory gene therapy involves the injection of new and modified T cells and NK cells or upregulation of antigens on tumour cells.

iii. Cytoreductive gene therapy involves the destruction of tumour cells by inclusion of suicide genes and use of oncolytic viruses. Suicide genes convert a prodrug into an active drug that is toxic for target cells. Oncolytic virus therapy selectively kills tumour cells but not normal cells.

11.3.2.4 Gene Therapy for Autoimmune Diseases

In Sjögren's syndrome (SS) there is destruction of glandular tissue that involves salivary and lacrimal tissue or accompanied by secondary autoimmune diseases such as rheumatoid arthritis. Potential target genes in gene therapy for SS-damaged hypo salivation include inflammatory mediators cytokine inhibitors, apoptotic molecules, and cell interaction of intracellular molecules. Thus the main target for gene therapy in autoimmune diseases is gene coding for anti-inflammatory cytokines, and this has been achieved utilizing a recombinant adenovirus rAAV2h vasoactive intestinal peptide (VIP), encoding the human – VIP gene (Fox, 2007).

11.3.2.5 Gene Therapy for Pain Management

Pain management is the most essential part of dental practice. Promising gene therapy results in animal models hold the key to solving these conditions. Researchers at the Mount Sinai School of Medicine engineered a virus carrying a gene for an endogenous opioid, which is injected directly into the spinal fluid adjacent to the dorsal root ganglia. The dorsal root ganglia act as a gateway to higher pain centres and opioids block this pain gateway, and results lasting for three months have been achieved (Stein et al., 2009).

11.3.2.6 Gene Therapy for Orthodontic Tooth Movement

Remodelling of PDL alveolar bone leads to orthodontic tooth movement by action of osteoclasts and osteoblasts. Osteoblasts originate from stromal cells while haematopoietic cells are precursors for osteoclasts. Cells from the osteoblastic lineage, after due process, result in the activation and maturation of osteoclasts. Molecules like receptor activator of nuclear factor kappa B (RANK) or receptor activator of nuclear factor kappa β-Ligand (RANKL) mediates such interactions. OPG (osteoprotegerin) produced by osteoblasts is a soluble receptor that competes with RANK receptors in binding to RANKL. Researchers have reported acceleration and inhibition of orthodontic tooth movement in a rat model using gene therapy with OPG and RANKL (Kanzaki et al, 2004).

11.3.2.7 Gene Therapy for DNA Vaccinations

Researchers have made many attempts to produce a vaccine for the prevention of caries or periodontal disease, but they only achieved mixed success. In contrast to delivering an attenuated microbe or isolated protein to salivary tissues as was done earlier experiments have been performed to transfer DNA of specific genes of selected microbes to salivary tissues.

11.3.2.8 Gene Therapy for Growth of New Teeth

Research for the development of new teeth that are similar to human teeth but devoid of any nerves and vessels is going on that can be implanted in patients who have lost their natural teeth.

11.3.3 Challenges in Gene Therapy

Proper selection of appropriate vascular cells and scaffold materials. Scaffolds should provide support for the proper formation of vascular tissue and should possess mechanical properties that can match those of native arteries. The synthetic vessel must withstand the fluid shear stress and strain from blood flow and have adequate burst strength to withstand physiological blood pressures. Finally, incompatibilities between synthetic engineered grafts and native blood vessels must be quantified and evaluated.

11.4 Nanotechnology

The concept of nanotechnology was brought into the limelight by physicist Richard Feynman in his lecture titled 'There's Plenty of Room at the Bottom' delivered at Caltech in 1959. The term 'nanotechnology' was coined by Prof. Kerie.E. Drexler who emphasized the technological importance of nanoscale phenomena. The US government in 2000 launched the national nanotechnology initiative and paved the way for the research and development in the field of nanotechnology (Das and Nasim, 2017).

The term nanotechnology is defined as the science and engineering performed on a nanoscale, which is 1 to 100 nanometres (nm). These particles exhibit a notably large surface area that is ideal for biocompatibility, drug delivery, and strengthening of the material (Mookhtiar et al., 2020).

11.4.1 Various Types of Nanostructures

a) Nanofibers – Nanofibers have a diameter below 100 nm, have high surface area and porosity and because of these properties, and find applications in nanocatalysis, tissue scaffolds, filtration, and optical electronics. In dentistry, nanofibers are added to dental cements to reinforce them and improve the properties of cements.

b) Dendrimers – Dendrimers are macromolecules of polymers used to improve the efficacy of dental restorative materials (Viljanen et al., 2007).

c) Nanopores – Osteoblastic differentiation and osseointegration of implants have been shown by the titanium implants containing nanopores of 30 nm size (Lavenus et al., 2011).

d) Nanoshells – Nanoshellsare miniature beads having a gold coating that can absorb the near-infrared rays creating intense heat, which is lethal to cancer cells (Kanaparthy and Kanaparthy, 2011).

e) Nanotubes – In vitro, titanium oxide nanotubes have been used to accelerate the kinetics of hydroxyapatite formation, which in turn accelerate bone growth when coated over implants.

f) Nanorods– An artificial approximation of enamel rods that exhibit self-assembly properties (Chen et al., 2005).

g) Nanoparticles – Nanoparticles size range from 0.1–100 nm. They are the most extensively used particles in dentistry among nanoscale units.

11.4.2 Applications in Dentistry

11.4.2.1 Diagnosis

Nanobiosensors have high sensitivity and are useful in the diagnosis of cancer as they detect cancer cell molecules at a very early stage and in very low concentrations. Gold nanoparticle-modified DNA bioreceptor can detect an analyte at a concentration as low as 0.05 nm. Carbon nanotubules can detect circulating cancer cells (Foster, 2005).

11.4.2.2 Preventive Dentistry

- Nanotechnology in the prevention of dental caries: calcium nanoparticle carbonate and 3% nanosized sodium trimetaphosphate have shown remineralizaton of early carious lesions (Danelon, 2015). The antimicrobial activity of *Streptococcus mutans* is significantly lowered by the silver, zinc oxide, and gold nanoparticles (Hernández-Sierra et al., 2008).
- Nanorobotic dentifrice: Nanorobotic dentifrice (mouthwashes or toothpaste) cleans supra & subgingival surfaces, metabolizes trapped organic matter into harmless and odourless vapours, kills pathogenic bacteria, provides a continuous barrier to halitosis, and prevents tooth decay and gingival diseases (Kumar and Vijayalakshmi, 2006).

11.4.2.3 Restorative Dentistry

- Nanocomposites: Nanoparticles in the form of nanofillers are evenly distributed in composite resins and exhibit superior physical properties leading to excellent clinical outcome (Saunders, 2009).
- Nanosolutions: Nanosolutions used in bonding agents produce dispersible nanoparticles. This ensures uniformity in the bonding agent and ensures that the adhesive is perfectly mixed every time.

11.4.2.4 Prosthodontics

- Prosthetic implants: Through nanotechnology implant surfaces with definite topography and chemical composition were developed leading to predictable tissue integration (Le Guéhennec et al., 2007).
- Denture base: The addition of titanium oxide nanoparticle and zirconium oxide nanoparticle modify the physical properties of the denture base.
- Impression material: Vinyl polysiloxanes incorporated with nanofillers provide better flow and detailed precision. It is marketed as Nanotech Elite HD.

11.4.2.5 Endodontics

- Bioceramic nanoparticles such as bioglass, glass ceramics, and zirconia incorporated in endodontic sealer enhances the adaptation of adhesive to nanoirregularities and decreases setting time and solubility in tissue fluids (Utneja et al., 2015).
- Silver nanoparticles incorporated in calcium hydroxide intracanal medicament showed more effectiveness against E.faecalis than calcium hydroxide alone (Afkhami et al., 2015).

11.4.2.6 Orthodontics

Nano-orthodontics: Complete orthodontic realignment of a tooth (rotation and vertical repositioning) can be achieved in a single visit through orthodontic nanorobots.

11.4.2.7 Oral Surgery

- Local anaesthesia: A colloidal suspension of thousands of active analgesic nanorobots can be delivered on the patient's gingiva. They reach the pulp via the gingival sulcus, lamina propria, and dentinal tubules. Sensitivity in the required tooth is reduced on the command of the dentist and when the procedure is completed, normal sensation can be restored.
- Nanoneedles: Suture needles incorporating nanosized stainless steel crystals have been developed. Nanotweezers are also under development that will make cell surgery possible in the near future (Verma et al., 2010).

11.4.2.8 Periodontics

For periodontal drug delivery nanoparticles impregnated with triclosan can be used. Futuristic technology is also being used in Arestin, in which microspheres containing tetracycline are placed into periodontal pockets, and tetracycline is administered locally (Kong et al., 2000).

11.4.2.9 Dental Nanorobots

A pre-programmed computer that can control the movement and function of teeth and surrounding tissues. Any desired function can be achieved and can be deactivated when required by dental nanorobots (Drexler, 1992).

11.4.3 Challenges Faced by Nanodentistry

- Design cost is very high.
- Electrical systems can create stray fields that may activate bioelectric-based molecular recognition systems in biology.
- Simultaneous coordination of the activities of a large number of independent microscale nanorobots.
- Social challenges of ethics, public acceptance, regulation, and human safety.
- Precise positioning and assembly of molecular scale part.
- Biocompatibility.

11.5 Conclusion

Although there has been substantial progress in research on dental tissues, many challenges are still present for the application of this research clinically. Many pieces of research are still limited to animal models and their clinical application is still awaited. Recent developments in stem cells, gene therapy, and nanotechnology in different specialities of dentistry will play a growing role in the enhancement of the dental field. Although not currently available these may be applied clinically in the future.

REFERENCES

Afkhami, F., S. J. Pourhashemi, M. Sadegh, Y. Salehi, and M. J. K. Fard. "Antibiofilm efficacy of silver nanoparticles as a vehicle for calcium hydroxide medicament against Enterococcus faecalis." Journal of Dentistry 43, no. 12 (2015): 1573–1579.

Ayllón Barbellido, S., J. Campo Trapero, J. Cano Sánchez, M. A. Perea García, N. Escudero Castaño, A. Bascones Martínez. "Gene therapy in the management of oral cancer: review of the literature." Med Oral Patol Oral Cir Bucal. 2008:13:E15–21.

Bansal, R., and A. Jain. "Current overview on dental stem cells applications in regenerative dentistry." Journal of Natural Science, Biology, and Medicine 6, no. 1 (2015): 29–34.

Baum, B. J., and B. C. O'Connell. "The impact of gene therapy on dentistry." The Journal of the American Dental Association 126, no. 2 (1995): 179–189.

Chen, H., B. H. Clarkson, K. Sun, and J. F. Mansfield. "Self-assembly of synthetic hydroxyapatite nanorods into an enamel prism-like structure." Journal of Colloid and Interface Science 288, no. 1 (2005): 97–103.

d'Aquino, R., A. De Rosa, G. Laino, F. Caruso, L. Guida, R. Rullo, V. Checchi, L. Laino, V. Tirino, and G. Papaccio. "Human dental pulp stem cells: from biology to clinical applications." Journal of Experimental Zoology Part B: Molecular and Developmental Evolution 312, no. 5 (2009): 408–415.

Danelon, M., J. P. Pessan, F. N. S. Neto, E. R. de Camargo, and A. C. Botazzo. "Effect of toothpaste with nano-sized trimetaphosphate on dental caries: in situ study." Journal of Dentistry 43, no. 7 (2015): 806–813.

Das, A., I. Nasim. "Nanotechnology in dentistry: a review." J. Adv. Pharm. Edu. Res. 2017;7 (2):43–45.

Drexler. K. E., F. Erdman, and R. Berge. Nanosystems: Molecular Machinery, Manufacturing, and Computation. New York: John Wiley & Sons, 1992.

Egusa, H., W. Sonoyama, M. Nishimura, I. Atsuta, and K. Akiyama. "Stem cells in dentistry–part I: stem cell sources." Journal of Prosthodontic Research 56, no. 3 (2012): 151–165.

Foster, L. E. Nanotechnology: Science, Innovation and Opportunity. Prentice-Hall PTR, 2005.

Fox, P. C. "Autoimmune diseases and Sjögren's syndrome: an autoimmune exocrinopathy." Annals of the New York Academy of Sciences 1098, no. 1 (2007): 15–21.

Gronthos, S., M. Mankani, J. Brahim, P. G. Robey, and S. Shi. "Postnatal human dental pulp stem cells (DPSCs) in vitro and in vivo." Proceedings of the National Academy of Sciences 97, no. 25 (2000): 13625–13630.

Hernández-Sierra, J. F., F. Ruiz, D. C. C. Pena, F. Martínez-Gutiérrez, A. E. Martínez, A. D. P. Guillén, H. Tapia-Pérez, and G. M. Castañón. "The antimicrobial sensitivity of Streptococcus mutans to nanoparticles of silver, zinc oxide, and gold." Nanomedicine: Nanotechnology, Biology and Medicine 4, no. 3 (2008): 237–240.

Kagami, H., S. Wang, and B. Hai. "Restoring the function of salivary glands." Oral Siseases 14, no. 1 (2008): 15–24.

Kanaparthy R. and A. Kanaparthy. "The changing face of dentistry: nanotechnology." Int J Nanomedicine 2011:6,2799–804.

Karthikeyan, B. V., and A. R. Pradeep. "Gene therapy in periodontics: a review and future implications." J Contemp Dent Pract 7, no. 3 (2006): 83–91.

Kong, L. X., Z. Peng, S-D. Li, and P. M. Bartold. "Nanotechnology and its role in the management of periodontal diseases." Periodontology 2000 40, no. 1 (2006): 184–196.

Lavenus, S., M. Berreur, V. Trichet, P. Pilet, G. Louarn, and P. Layrolle. "Adhesion and osteogenic differentiation of human mesenchymal stem cells on titanium nanopores." Eur Cell Mater 22, no. 1 (2011): 84–96.

Le Guéhennec, L., A. Soueidan, P. Layrolle, and Y. Amouriq. "Surface treatments of titanium dental implants for rapid osseointegration." Dental Materials 23, no. 7 (2007): 844–854.

Maximow, A. "The lymphocyte as a stem cell, common to different blood elements in embryonic development and during the post-fetal life of mammals." Folia Haematologica 8, no. 3 (1909): 125–134.

Misra, S. "Human gene therapy: a brief overview of the genetic revolution." J Assoc Physicians India 61, no. 2 (2013): 127–33.

Miura, M., S. Gronthos, M. Zhao, B. Lu, L. W. Fisher, P. G. Robey, and S. Shi. "SHED: stem cells from human exfoliated deciduous teeth." Proceedings of the National Academy of Sciences 100, no. 10 (2003): 5807–5812.

Mookhtiar H., V. Hegde, K. Memon. "Nanotechnology in interdisciplinary dentistry." International Journal of Scientific Research. 2020 Jan 22:8 (12).

Morsczeck C. W. Götz, J. Schierholz, F. Zeilhofer, U. Kühn, C. Möhl, C. Sippel, and K. H. Hoffmann. "Isolation of precursor cells (PCs) from human dental follicle of wisdom teeth." Matrix Biol. 2005;24(2):155–165.

Nakashima, M. "Induction of dentin formation on canine amputated pulp by recombinant human bone morphogenetic proteins (BMP)-2 and-4." Journal of Dental Research 73, no. 9 (1994): 1515–1522.

Prabhakar, A. R., J. M. Paul, and N. Basappa. "Gene therapy and its implications in dentistry." International Journal of Clinical Pediatric Dentistry 4, no. 2 (2011): 85–92.

Sakai, V. T., Z. Zhang, Z. Dong, K. G. Neiva, M. A. A. M. Machado, S. Shi, C. F. Santos, and J. E. Nör. "SHED differentiate into functional odontoblasts and endothelium." Journal of Dental Research 89, no. 8 (2010): 791–796.

San-Marina, S., A. Sharma, S. G. Voss, J. R. Janus, and G. S. Hamilton. "Assessment of scaffolding properties for chondrogenic differentiation of adipose-derived mesenchymal stem cells in nasal reconstruction." JAMA Facial Plastic Surgery 19, no. 2 (2017): 108–114.

Saunders, S. A. (2009). "Current practicality of nanotechnology in dentistry. Part 1: Focus on nanocomposite restoratives and biomimetics. " Clinical, Cosmetic and Investigational Dentistry, 1, 47–61.

Seo, B-M., M. Miura, S. Gronthos, P. M. Bartold, S. Batouli, J.. Brahim, M. Young, P. G. Robey, C. Y. Wang, and S. Shi. "Investigation of multipotent postnatal stem cells from human periodontal ligament." The Lancet 364, no. 9429 (2004): 149–155.

Sonoyama, W., Y. Liu, D. Fang, T. Yamaza, B-M. Seo, C. Zhang, H. Liu et al., "Mesenchymal stem cell-mediated functional tooth regeneration in swine." PloS One 1, no. 1 (2006): e79.

Sonoyama, W., Y. Liu, T. Yamaza, R. S. Tuan, S. Wang, S. Shi, and G. T-J. Huang. "Characterization of the apical papilla and its residing stem cells from human immature permanent teeth: a pilot study." Journal of Endodontics 34, no. 2 (2008): 166–171.

Stein, C., J. D. Clark, U. Oh, M. R. Vasko, G. L. Wilcox, A. C. Overland, T. W. Vanderah, and R. H. Spencer. "Peripheral mechanisms of pain and analgesia." Brain Research Reviews 60, no. 1 (2009): 90–113.

Tziafas, D., A. J. Smith, and H. Lesot. "Designing new treatment strategies in vital pulp therapy." Journal of Dentistry 28, no. 2 (2000): 77–92.

Utneja, S., R. R. Nawal, S. Talwar, M. Verma. "Current perspectives of bio-ceramic technology in endodontics: calcium enriched mixture cement – review of its composition, properties, and applications." Restor Dent Endod. 2015 Feb;40 (1):1–13.

Verma, S. K., K. C. Prabhat, L. Goyal, M. Rani, and A. Jain. (2010). "A critical review of the implication of nanotechnology in modern dental practice. " National Journal of Maxillofacial Surgery, 1 (1), 41–44.

Viljanen, E. K., M. Skrifvars, and P. K. Vallittu. "Dendritic copolymers and particulate filler composites for dental applications: degree of conversion and thermal properties." Dental Materials 23, no. 11 (2007): 1420–1427.

Yamaizumi, M., E. Mekada, T. Uchida, and Y. Okada. "One molecule of diphtheria toxin fragment A introduced into a cell can kill the cell." Cell 15, no. 1 (1978): 245–250.

Yu, X., G. Shaohua, S. Chen, Q. Xu, J. Zhang, H. Guo, and P. Yang. "Human gingiva-derived mesenchymal stromal cells contribute to periodontal regeneration in beagle dogs." Cells Tissues Organs 198, no. 6 (2013): 428–437.

12

Stress Deregulates Memory Consolidation Through Epigentic Modifications

Sukanya Tripathy
Department of Biotechnology, Babasaheb Bhimrao Ambedkar University, Lucknow, India

Anand Prakash
Department of Biotechnology, M G Central University, Motihari, India

12.1 Introduction

Stress is an assignable process, arising from internal or external factors called stressors (Joëls et al., 2007). Exposure to various stressors leads to the arousal of various responses termed stress response that include activation of the nervous system (i.e., central, peripheral, and autonomic nervous system). However, in some situations it may lead to pathological conditions like PTSD and other stress- and fear-related disorders. Stress can be categorized as acute or chronic on the basis of timing and exposure of stressors. It has been shown through various studies that stress modulates memory formation, depending on the timing of exposure. It can enhance memory (Domes et al., 2002; Smeets et al., 2007; Schwabe et al., 2008) or impair it (Diamond et al., 2006). Acute stress leads to the memory consolidation, which may create a basis for post-traumatic stress disorder (PTSD) (Cahill et al., 2003) whereas chronic stress has been shown to contribute to impairment of memory formation (Pearson-Leary et al., 2015). Stress leads to the initiation and development of cognitive and mood disturbance in humans (Hammen, 2005). It has been found that exposure to stress induces remodeling of neuronal architecture within the amygdala, hippocampus, and prefrontal cortex (PFC). The neuroanatomical regions and circuits of fear memory and stress are linked, thus these two paradigms are interrelated (Table 12.1). The non-reinforced recovery of consolidated memory renews the previous engrams of those memories and produces an imbalanced state. Memories reportedly undergo two similar but opposite protein synthesis-dependent processes: extinction or new inhibitory learning (McGaugh, 2000; Izquierdo et al., 2008) and reconsolidation (Sara, 2000; Quirk et al., 2010, Bevilaqua et al., 2010).

   PTSD is a common type of neuropsychiatric disorder related to trauma and stress. This disorder affects the mental health of individuals and may lead to an economic burden on society. Several paradigms involving psychological and neurobiological mechanisms have been developed for the improvement of this disorder (Liberzon et al., 2007; Mahan et al., 2012; Pitman et al., 2012; Goswami et al., 2013; Rau et al., 2005), and many studies have been conducted to determine the neural circuits involved in consolidation of fear and extinction memory (Ehrlich et al., 2009; Pape et al., 2010; Milad et al., 2012; Duvarci et al., 2014). The circuitries involved in hard wiring of memory are an important therapeutic target for treatment of disorders like PTSD and anxiety-related disorders (Yehuda et al., 2007; Singewald et al., 2015).

DOI: 10.1201/9781003220404-14

TABLE 12.1

Relative analysis of neuroanatomical regions involved in fear memory and stress-induced anxiety disorders. The table represents antagonistic behavior in amygdala, dorsolateral prefrontal cortex (dlPFC), and locus coeruleus (LC) during stress and fear memory. Altered level of catecholamines can also be visualized in stress-induced anxiety disorders

Alert Safe and Interested	Under Stress
Moderate levels of catecholamine	High levels of catecholamine release
Dorsolateral prefrontal cortex (dlPFC) is strengthened	dlPFC is weakened.
Amygdala is weakened	Amygdala and striatum are strengthened
Reduced level of locus coeruleus (LC) firing. The LC is a nucleus in the pons of the brainstem involved with physiological responses to stress and panic.	Increased tonic firing of LC

12.2 Neurocircuitry of Memory Consolidation and Extinction

As we know, humans have an enormous ability to learn, and this is affected by the type of environment, stressors, and the changes occurring at the molecular level in the brain and other body parts. It has been shown through studies that during fear memory formation sub-regions of the brain like the amygdala, PFC, and hippocampus play a significant role and are regulated by levels of hormones and by the corticosterone released during stress (Srinivasan et al., 2013). During stress glucocorticoids have also been shown to play an important role in regulation of basal and stress-related homeostasis. Glucocorticoids impose a broad spectrum effect on various sets of genes located in organs and tissues, thus making it best suited to promote or prevent stress. The amygdala is a complex nuclei and a key brain region where processing of fear memory and stress-related signals takes place. It was found that amygdala and hippocampus along with PFC go hand in hand to cope up with stressful conditions. Amongst all the stress-related factors it was found that brain-derived neurotrophic factor (BDNF) mediates the stress-induced variations in these regions and its level is significantly increased in the basolateral amygdala (BLA) (Lakshminarasimhan et al., 2012).

Genetic deletion of glucocorticoid receptors (GRs) results in decreased fear response and leads to memory impairment (Kolber et al., 2008). The BLA has been shown to be involved in consolidation of stressful experiences. The neural approach of goal-oriented actions can be disrupted by the interactions between noradrenergic activity and glucocorticoid stress hormones (Schwabe et al., 2012).

The context also plays an important role in consolidation of memory under stressful conditions. It has been found that the dentategyrus (DG) region of the hippocampus plays a critical role in the regulation of its functions (Gould et al., 1999; Bruel-Jungerman et al., 2005). The neurons of DG are influenced by various factors like endocrine, neural, or physiological conditions either positively or negatively. For example, it was found that adrenal steroids suppress the neuronal proliferation in the rodent hippocampus through an NMDA-receptor pathway (N-methyl-D-aspartate-receptor pathway) (Cameron et al., 1995). GRsin the hippocampus play different roles in different conditions. For example, in healthy situations, they maintain homeostasis and during stressful conditions play a role in plasticity (Gourley et al., 2013; Lehmann et al., 2013). Hippocampal GRs also play a role in the formation of long-term inhibitory avoidance memory in rats by inducing the CaMKIIa-BDNF-CREB-dependent (CREB is cAMP response element-binding protein) neural plasticity pathways (Chen et al., 2012).

Similar to the amygdala and hippocampus, the PFC also plays a key role in converting stressful information to action. Studies performed in humans have suggested role of the ventral PFC in different stress-related psychopathologies like mood-related disorders and PTSD while similar studies in rodents show that prelimbic and infra-limbic cortex have analogous functions in memory processing of stress and regulating the magnitude of physiologic responses to adversity by the secretion of glucocorticoids (McKlveen et al., 2013). The prelimbic-PFC innervates in nucleus accumbens and BLA, thus regulating the inhibition and reward of stress. The second part of the v-PFC, the IL-PFC, is connected to visceral/emotional effector systems (e.g., central amygdaloid nucleus, hindbrain cardiovascular regulatory pathways) and

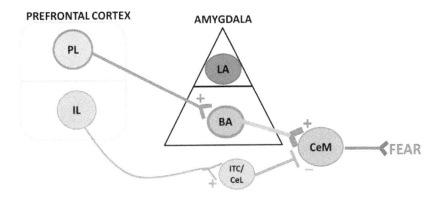

FIGURE 12.1   Neurocircuitry of stress and memory.

controls emotional responses of stress effector pathways (Vertes et al., 2004). In a study it was found that the infralimbic cortex is responsible for retention of extinction memory (Singh et al., 2018).

Figure 12.1 shows the innervations of PL-PFC and IL-PFC in the amygdala responsible for fear and stress memory formation and suppression. PL-PFC has its innervations in BLA, which activates the centromedial (CeM) amygdala generating fear consolidation. The IL-PFC innervates intercalated neurons and inhibits CeM, thus potentiating the extinction memory (+ represents activation; – represents suppression).

12.3 Memory Consolidation and Stress

Memory being a highly labile engram and a dynamic entity has been shown to be modified by the presence of stressor either intrinsic or extrinsic. After a number of elaborate studies performed on the molecular circuitry involved in consolidation of memory during fear and stress, the question of "how" has become the major focus. It has been found that the three regions, amygdala, PFC, and hippocampus, hand in hand facilitate stress-related issues. As discussed in the previous section, the amygdala plays a key role in fear learning and stress. Glucocorticoids are regulated during acute stress in the amygdala by noradrenergic release. The hypothalamus-pitutary axis (HPA) plays a role in fear acquisition in the amygdala due to exposure of stressors and thus stimulates the release of adrenocorticotropic hormone (ACTH). ACTH in turn activates the synthesis and secretion of glucocorticoid hormones, which further bind to mineralocorticoid receptors (MRs) and glucocorticoids located throughout the brain and body.

During stress glucocorticoids bind to receptors leading to consolidation of memory (Joëls et al., 2008). In acute stress conditions the release of norepinephrine increases in the lateral and basal amygdala. A study performed by infusion of β-adrenergic receptor antagonist atenolol into the BLA in the presence of corticosterone showed inhibitory effect on consolidation of memory, which indicates the necessary role of norepinephrine in the amygdala (Roozendaal et al., 2009), while a similar study in the absence of corticosterone showed no effect on consolidation of a conditioned fear memory (Bush et al., 2010). Thus, it appears that norepinephrine only affects fear memory consolidation when the stress response is activated within a short duration after learning.

The effect of stress on the PFC is through activation of both GRs and mineralocorticoid receptors. These receptors located in PFC impose feedback control of hypothalamic-pituitary adrenocortical (HPA) axis activity (Radley et al., 2006). GR signaling and PFC dysfunction in stress is primarily caused by glucocorticoid dyshomeostasis (Price et al., 2012). The PFC, which is mainly subdivided into two parts, IL and PL, has been shown to have a property of division of labor (i.e., the IL plays a significant role during extinction training while the PL has been shown to have a more significant effect during consolidation). Thus, any deregulation in PFC may lead to disturbance in fear acquisition and extinction, thus leading to conditions like PTSD. Along with brain regions and stressors, the timing of stress exposure also affects memory processes. Stress when induced before training causes increased consolidation of memory (Rau et al., 2009) while delayed inhibition causes decreased memory consolidation, thus showing the effect of time on stress consolidation.

12.4 Stress Effects on Extinction Learning

Figure 12.2 illustrates that the threats perceived by the LA and its innervations in the BA cause upregulation of adrenocorticotropic hormone, thus releasing cortisol. This cortisol further causes consolidation of memory and deficit of extinction memory.

Extinction learning follows a similar pathway as consolidation of memory but it is a newer form of training rather than the suppression of consolidated memory. It was found that the limbic system is involved in the extinction of traumatic memory (i.e., PFC, hippocampus, and amygdala). The difference in consolidation and extinction training is in the innervations to the subregions of the PFC. Unlike consolidation, which is dependent on the the dorsolateral prefrontal cortex (dlPFC) the extinction depends on the IL-PFC. The IL is known to inhibit the output of the fear response generated by the amygdaloid nucleus. As depicted in Figure 12.2, the IL projects to a group of inhibitory interneuron masses (i.e., intercalated cells (ITCs) of amygdala further shutting down the downstream output of amygdala). Inhibiting the IL prevents formation of extinction memory, indicating the cruciality of this region in formation of extinction memory. Therapeutic approaches targeting IL could have long-term implications in treatment of anxiety disorders.

Attenuation in extinction has been found when it is correlated to stress as shown by behavioral studies that include forced swim or restraint stress (Miracle et al., 2006). The loss of extinction may occur due to various acute and chronic stressors like early separation of pups from mother, exposure to predators, social isolation, restraint movement, tail flick, and elevated platform exposure (Yamamoto et al., 2009; Zhang et al., 2013; Zheng et al., 2013; Skelly et al., 2015). Restraint stress during which movement of animals is restricted for 6 hours is one of the most common procedures for studying changes associated with impairments in extinction and auditory conditioned stimulus (Knox et al., 2012). It leads to symptoms that are similar to the diagnostic features of PTSD patients. The major cause here is the deregulation of the hypothalamic–pituitary–adrenal (HPA) axis. As found for consolidation, extinction training also predicts the effect by the timing of stressor exposure. It was also found that decrease in stress occurs when it takes place immediately after consolidation of traumatic memory (Maren, 2014). When performed on human models the results were found to be affected by an additional factor (i.e., sex of the subject under consideration). For example, chronic (restraint) stress that causes impaired extinction training in males facilitates extinction in females (Baran et al., 2009; Xiong et al., 2014). Apart from this a lot more has to be studied in the sex dependence of stress.

Further, dendritic hypertrophy was found to take place due to chronic restraint stress in the BLA region (Mitra et al., 2005; Padival et al., 2015; Vyas et al., 2006; Vyas et al., 2002). While exposed to

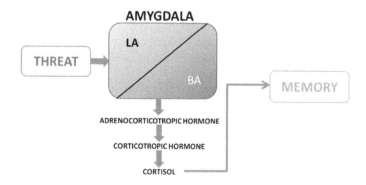

FIGURE 12.2   Stress affects the memory formation in amygdala through ACTH and CRH.

acute and chronic stress it was found that there is an upregulation in BLA spinogenesis, which may occur either immediately or after a certain period of incubation (Maroun et al., 2013). The higher level of spine development causes excitability in neurons, which is accompanied by NMDAR-mediated synaptic responsivity and long-term potentiation (LTP), along with upregulated levels of BDNF (Chauveau et al., 2012; Maroun et al., 2003; Rosenkranz et al., 2010; Suvrathan et al., 2013). A decrease in extinction learning in stress is also associated with increased expression of hippocampal immediate-early gene (c-Fos) activity and metabolism (2-deoxyglucose) (Hoffman et al., 2014; Toledo-Rodriguez et al., 2012). Hence, it can be inferred from the above studies that the excitability in the BLA may lead to consistent fear and reduced extinction. Dendrites also show varied types of effects in the BLA and PFC. In the BLA the number of dendritic branches increases after stress while in the PFC the number decreases significantly (Leuner et al., 2010). Minor exposure of a stressor shows a considerable dendrirtic retraction in IL neurons, thus causing decreased extinction learning (Holmes et al., 2009).The plasticity when restored by the BDNF gene promotes the extinction and thus rescuing the effect of stress (Graybeal et al., 2011; Peters et al., 2010). Similarly when the lesion studies are performed in the IL (infralimbic cortex), it prevents the impairing effects of stress (Farrell et al., 2010), thus suggesting that the IL must not be ruptured at the time of stress. These studies suggest a potential causal role of amygdala and PFC in stress-impaired extinction. Recent findings show that amygdala hyperexcitability is interrelated with the loss of input from the hippocampus and prefrontal areas during impairment of extinction in stressed animals.

12.5 Epigenetics, Memory, and Stress

Epigenetics is the study of heritable changes without involvement of underlying DNA sequence. The mechanism involves histone modifications like methylation, acetylation, phosphorylation, and sumoylation. It provides precise and bidirectional control of gene expression required during memory formation and stress leading to long-term changes in the behavior of an organism. Major epigenetic changes are incorporated in chromatin, which is an assembly of histone protein, DNA, and RNA. It is bounded by DNA, thus organizing it into a compact structure that fits to the nucleus of the cell. DNA and histones can both be modified through different a tagging pattern that is either open or restricts access to DNA and thus facilitates or impairs the gene expression to environmental contingencies. During learning events the genes responsible for suppression of memory are turned off while those for formation of memory are turned on with observational behavioral alterations required by the cell. Different types of epigenetic modifications include methylation, acetylation, phosphorylation, sumoylation, ubiquitination, etc. To perform the specific alterations there are three sets of enzymes that work in follow-up: readers, writers, and erasers. The mechanisms involved are dynamic rather than static and are specific for the particular tissue. Recent research in the field of behavioral neurosciences has focused on the epigenetic basis of gene regulation and emphasized molecular neural adaptations underlying behavioral changes in order to explore possible therapeutic measures to treat behavioral disorders. Nearly all traumatic disorders occur due to alteration in memory formation, which governs the behavior of chromatin structure responsible for epigenetic regulation of synaptic plasticity. Histone acetylation and deacetylation is an important regulatory process used by the epigenetic machinery to modify chromatin. Histone acetyltransferases (HAT) acetylate conserves lysine amino acids on histone proteins, which results in memory consolidation and LTP (long-term potentiation) (Monsey et al., 2011; Blouin et al., 2016; Siddiqui et al., 2017). Activity of HATs is kept in check by the HDACs (histone deacetylases), enzymes that remove acetyl groups, thus causing the repression of acquired memory. It is generally understood that histone acetylation facilitates gene expression and inhibition of HAT activity results in impairment of memory, whereas loss in the HDAC activity enhances synaptic plasticity and memory (Sharma, 2012). The epigenetic changes are similar in all respects in every region of the brain, but during stress they are modulated in a region-specific manner. The DNA methylation and histone modifications are the operative in the hippocampus, amygdala, and PFC during stress (Hunter et al., 2009). Apart from being pathological some of them are adaptive like DNA methylation, which plays a role in consolidation of fear memory that occurs during training in the hippocampus region (Miller et al., 2007).

Several studies have proved acute and chronic stress alter methylation of histone H3 in rat hippocampus. H3 lysine 4 trimethylation is found to be increased in chronic restraint stress. In acute stress H3K27 trimethylation decreases 50% whereas H3K9 trimethylation (H3K9me3) increases in hippocampus. The epigenetic changes occurring either in early or later phases of life may cause stress response. Methylation of genes for GRs and BDNF are associated with early-life trauma (McGowan et al., 2009; Roth et al., 2009). Trauma in the early phase of life occurs due to increased methylation on the promoter region of the neuron-specific exon 17 GR (*NR3C1*) gene, which causes reduced levels of glucocorticoids. The chronically increased level of cortisol in mice had epigenetic modifications in genes *Fkbp5, Nr3c1, Hsp90, Crh,* and *Crhr1* of the HPA axis (Lee et al., 2010). Increased levels of FKBP5 were correlated with the decreased level of HPA sensitivity and negative feedback (Binder, 2009). Such alterations cause long-term dysregulation of the HPA axis resulting in increased rates of response to stressful stimuli. These changes can be compensated by environmental or pharmacological means. Changes in DNA methylation and HPA response can be reversed using HDAC inhibitors TSA (trichostatin A) (Weaver et al., 2004). These changes can be reversed in adulthood using regulators of epigenetics and may also normalize HPA activity and behavioral responses to stress. Thus, epigenetic studies show the major impact on stress-based memory consolidation. Still a lot more has to be performed in future stress-related epigenetic studies.

12.6 Conclusion

The above review focused on the effect of stress on memory consolidation and extinction. It focused on how region-specific structural and molecular changes in the amygdala and PFC due to stress may result in the impairment of memory. Both acute and chronic stress have varied effects on memory due to the altered level of corticosteroids. Acute stress modulates the working memory while chronic stress modulates the remote memories. These alterations are due to deregulations in hormone and structural plasticity at neuronal and epigenetic levels. Epigenetic changes, which could be reversed using specific HDAC/HAT inhibitors, could be potential targets for both behavioral and therapeutic interventions of stress-related modulations of memory.

REFERENCES

Baran SE, Armstrong CE, Niren DC (2009) Chronic stress and sex differences on the recall of fear conditioning and extinction. Neurobiol Learn Mem 91:323–332.

Bevilaqua LRM, Cammarota M, Medina JH and Izquierdo I (2010) Neurobiology of Posttraumatic Stress Disorder. New York: Nova Publishers, pp. 309–330.

Binder EB (2009) The role of FKBP5, a co-chaperone of the glucocorticoid receptor in the pathogenesis and therapy of affective and anxiety disorders. Psychoneuroendocrinology 34:S186–S195.

Blouin AM, Sillivan SE, Joseph NF, Miller CA (2016) The potential of epigenetics in stress-enhanced fear learning models of PTSD. Learn Mem. 23(10):576–586.

Bruel-Jungerman E, Laroche S, Rampon C (2005) New neurons in the dentate gyrus are involved in the expression of enhanced long-term memory following environmental enrichment. Eur J Neurosci 21:513–521.

Bush DEA, Caparosa EM, Gekker A, LeDoux J (2010) Beta-adrenergic receptors in the lateral nucleus of the amygdala contribute to the acquisition but not the consolidation of auditory fear conditioning. Front Behav Neurosci 4:154.

Cahill L, Gorski L, Le K (2003) Enhanced human memory consolidation with postlearning stress: interaction with the degree of arousal at encoding. Learn Mem 10:270–274.

Cameron HA, McEwen BS, Gould E (1995) Regulation of adult neurogenesis by excitatory input and NMDA receptor activation in the dentate gyrus. J Neurosci 15:4687–4692.

Chauveau F, Lange MD, Jüngling K (2012) Prevention of stress-impaired fear extinction through neuropeptide S action in the lateral amygdala. Neuropsychopharmacology 37:1588–1599.

Chen DY, Bambah-Mukku D, Pollonini G, Alberini CM (2012) Glucocorticoid receptors recruit the CaMKIIα-BDNF-CREB pathways to mediate memory consolidation. NatNeurosci 15:1707–1714.

Diamond DM, Campbell AM, Park CR (2006) Influence of predator stress on the consolidation versus retrieval of long-term spatial memory and hippocampal spinogenesis. Hippocampus 16:571–576.

Domes G, Heinrichs M, Reichwald U, Hautzinger M (2002) Hypothalamic-pituitary adrenal axis reactivity to psychological stress and memory in middle-aged women: high responders exhibit enhanced declarative memory performance. Psychoneuroendocrinology 27:843–853.

Duvarci S, Pare D (2014) Amygdala microcircuits controlling learned fear. Neuron 82:966–980.

Ehrlich I, Humeau Y, Grenier F (2009) Amygdala inhibitory circuits and the control of fear memory. Neuron 62:757–771.

Farrell MR, Sayed JA, Underwood AR, Wellman CL (2010) Lesion of infralimbic cortex occludes stress effects on retrieval of extinction but not fear conditioning. Neurobiol Learn Mem 94:240–246.

Goswami S, Rodríguez-Sierra O, Cascardi M, Paré D (2013) Animal models of posttraumatic stress disorder: face validity. Front Neurosci 7:89.

Gould E, Tanapat P (1999) Stress and hippocampal neurogenesis. Biol Psychiatry 46:1472–1479.

Gourley SL, Swanson AM, Koleske AJ (2013) Corticosteroid-induced neural remodeling predicts behavioral vulnerability and resilience. J Neurosci 33:3107–3112.

Graybeal C, Feyder M, Schulman E (2011) Paradoxical reversal learning enhancement by stress or prefrontal cortical damage: rescue with BDNF. Nat Neurosci 14:1507–1509.

Hammen C (2005) Stress and depression. Annu Rev Clin Psychol 1:293–319.

Hoffman AN, Lorson NG, Sanabria F (2014) Chronic stress disrupts fear extinction and enhances amygdala and hippocampal Fos expression in an animal model of posttraumatic stress disorder. Neurobiol Learn Mem 112:139–147.

Holmes A, Wellman CL (2009) Stress-induced prefrontal reorganization and executive dysfunction in rodents. Neurosci Biobehav Rev 33:773–783.

Hunter RG, McCarthy KJ, Milne TA (2009) Regulation of hippocampal H3 histone methylation by acute and chronic stress. Proc Natl Acad Sci U S A 106:20912–20917.

Izquierdo I, Bevilaqua LR, Lima RH, et al (2008) Extinction learning: neurological features, therapeutic applications and the effect of aging. Future Neurol 3:133–140.

Joëls M, Karst H, DeRijk R, de Kloet ER (2008) The coming out of the brain mineralocorticoid receptor. Trends Neurosci 31:1–7.

Joëls M, Karst H, Krugers HJ, Lucassen PJ (2007) Chronic stress: implications for neuronal morphology, function and neurogenesis. Front Neuroendocrinol 28:72–96.

Knox D, George SA, Fitzpatrick CJ (2012) Single prolonged stress disrupts retention of extinguished fear in rats. Learn Mem 19:43–49.

Kolber BJ, Wieczorek L, Muglia LJ (2008) Hypothalamic–pituitary–adrenal axis dysregulation and behavioral analysis of mouse mutants with altered glucocorticoid or mineralocorticoid receptor function. Stress 11:321–338.

Lakshminarasimhan H, Chattarji S, Luine V (2012) Stress leads to contrasting effects on the levels of brain derived neurotrophic factor in the hippocampus andamygdala. PLoS One 7:e30481.

Lee RS, Tamashiro KLK, Yang X (2010) Chronic corticosterone exposure increases expression and decreases deoxyribonucleic acid methylation of *fkbp5* in mice. Endocrinology 151:4332–4343.

Lehmann ML, Brachman RA, Martinowich K, Schloesser RJ, Herkenham M (2013) Glucocorticoids orchestrate divergent effects on mood through adult neurogenesis. JNeurosci 33:2961–2972.

Leuner B, Gould E (2010) Structural plasticity and hippocampal function. Annu RevPsychol 61:111–140.

Liberzon I, Sripada CS (2007) The functional neuroanatomy of PTSD: a critical review. Prog. Brain Res 151–169.

Mahan AL, Ressler KJ (2012) Fear conditioning, synaptic plasticity and the amygdala: implications for post-traumatic stress disorder. Trends Neurosci 35:24–35.

Maren S (2014) Nature and causes of the immediate extinction deficit: A brief review. Neurobiol Learn Mem 113:19–24.

Maroun M, Ioannides PJ, Bergman KL (2013) Fear extinction deficits following acute stress associate with increased spine density and dendritic retraction in basolateral amygdala neurons. Eur J Neurosci 38: 2611–2620.

Maroun M, Richter-Levin G (2003) Exposure to acute stress blocks the induction of longterm potentiation of the amygdala-prefrontal cortex pathway in vivo. J Neurosci 23:4406–4409

McKlveen JM, Myers B, Flak JN (2013) Role of prefrontal cortex glucocorticoid receptors in stress and emotion. Biol Psychiatry 74:672–679.

McGaugh JL (2000) Memory - a century of consolidation. Science 287:248–251.

McGowan PO, Sasaki A, D'Alessio AC (2009) Epigenetic regulation of the glucocorticoid receptor in human brain associates with childhood abuse. Nat Neurosci 12:342–348.

Milad MR, Quirk GJ (2012) Fear extinction as a model for translational neuroscience: ten years of progress. Annu Rev Psychol 63:129–151.

Miller CA, Sweatt JD (2007) Covalent modification of DNA regulates memory formation. Neuron 53:857–869.

Miracle A, Brace M, Huyck K (2006) Chronic stress impairs recall of extinction of conditioned fear. Neurobiol Learn Mem 85:213–218.

Mitra R, Jadhav S, McEwen BS (2005) Stress duration modulates the spatiotemporal patterns of spine formation in the basolateral amygdala. Proc Natl AcadSci USA 102:9371–9376.

Padival MA, Blume SR, Rosenkranz JA (2013) Repeated restraint stress exerts different impact on structure of neurons in the lateral and basal nuclei of the amygdala. Neuroscience 246:230–242.

Pape HC, Pare D (2010) Plastic synaptic networks of the amygdala for the acquisition, expression, and extinction of conditioned fear. Physiol Rev 90:419–463.

Pearson-Leary J, Osborne DM, McNay EC (2015) Role of glia in stress-induced enhancement and impairment of memory. Front Integr Neurosci 9:63.

Peters J, Dieppa-Perea LM, Melendez LM, Quirk GJ (2010) Induction of fear extinction with hippocampal-infralimbic BDNF. Science 328:1288–1290.

Pitman RK, Rasmusson AM, Koenen KC (2012) Biological studies of posttraumatic stress disorder. Nat Rev Neurosci 13:769–787.

Price JL, Drevets WC (2012) Neural circuits underlying the pathophysiology of mood disorders. Trends Cogn Sci 16:61–71.

Quirk GJ, Pare D, Richardson R (2010) Erasing Fear Memories with Extinction Training. 30:14993–14997.

Radley JJ, Arias CM, Sawchenko PE (2006) Regional differentiation of the medial prefrontal cortex in regulating adaptive responses to acute emotional stress. J Neurosci 26:12967–12976.

Rau V, DeCola JP, Fanselow MS (2005) Stress-induced enhancement of fear learning: an animal model of posttraumatic stress disorder. Neurosci Biobehav Rev 29:1207–1223.

Rau V, Fanselow MS (2009) Exposure to a stressor produces a long lasting enhancement of fear learning in rats. Stress 12:125–133.

Roozendaal B, McEwen BS, Chattarji S (2009) Stress, memory and the amygdala. NatRev Neurosci 10:423–433.

Rosenkranz JA, Venheim ER, Padival M (2010) Chronic stress causes amygdala hyperexcitability in rodents. Biol Psychiatry 67:1128–1136.

Roth TL, Lubin FD, Funk AJ, Sweatt JD (2009) Lasting epigenetic influence of early life adversity on the BDNF gene. Biol Psychiatry 65:760–769.

Sara SJ (2000) Retrieval and reconsolidation: toward a neurobiology of remembering. Learn Mem 7:73–84.

Schwabe L, Bohringer A, Chatterjee M, Schachinger H (2008) Effects of pre-learning stress on memory for neutral, positive and negative words: different roles of cortisol and autonomic arousal. Neurobiol Learn Mem 90:44–53.

Schwabe L, Joëls M, Roozendaal B (2012) Stress effects on memory: an update and integration. Neurosci Biobehav Rev 36:1740–1749.

Sharma SK (2010) Protein acetylation in synaptic plasticity and memory. NeurosciBiobehav Rev 34:1234–1240.

Siddiqui SA, Singh S, Ugale R, Ranjan V, Kanojia R, Saha S, Tripathy S, Kumar S, Mehrotra S, Modi DR, Prakash A (2019) Regulation of HDAC1 and HDAC2 during consolidation and extinction of fear memory. Brain Res Bull. 150:86–101.

Singewald N, Schmuckermair C, Whittle N (2015) Pharmacology of cognitive enhancers for exposure-based therapy of fear, anxiety and trauma-related disorders. Pharmacol Ther 149:150–190.

Singh S, Siddiqui SA, Tripathy S, Kumar S, Saha S, Ugale R, Modi DR, Prakash A (2018) Decreased level of histone acetylation in the infralimbic prefrontal cortex following immediate extinction may result in deficit of extinction memory. Brain Res Bull 140:355–364.

Skelly MJ, Chappell AE, Carter E, Weiner JL (2015) Adolescent social isolation increases anxiety-like behavior and ethanol intake and impairs fear extinction inadulthood: Possible role of disrupted noradrenergic signaling. Neuropharmacology 97:149–159.

Smeets T, Giesbrecht T, Jelicic M, Merckelbach H (2007) Context-dependent enhancement of declarative memory performance following acute psychosocial stress. Biol Psychol 76:116–123.

Srinivasan S, Shariff M, Bartlett SE (2013) The role of the glucocorticoids in developing resilience to stress and addiction. Front Psychiatry 4:68.

Suvrathan A, Bennur S, Ghosh S (2013) Stress enhances fear by forming new synapses with greater capacity for long-term potentiation in the amygdala. Philos. Trans.R. Soc. London B Biol. Sci. 369.

Toledo-Rodriguez M, Pitiot A, Paus T, Sandi C (2012) Stress during puberty boosts metabolic activation associated with fear-extinction learning in hippocampus, basal amygdala and cingulate cortex. Neurobiol Learn Mem 98:93–101.

Vertes RP (2004) Differential projections of the infralimbic and prelimbic cortex in the rat. Synapse 51:32–58.

Vyas A, Jadhav S, Chattarji S (2006) Prolonged behavioral stress enhances synaptic connectivity in the basolateral amygdala. Neuroscience 143:387–393.

Vyas A, Mitra R, Shankaranarayana Rao BS, Chattarji S (2002) Chronic stress induces contrasting patterns of dendritic remodeling in hippocampal and amygdaloid neurons. JNeurosci 22:6810–8.

Weaver ICG, Cervoni N, Champagne FA (2004) Epigenetic programming by maternal behavior. Nat Neurosci 7:847–854.

Xiong G-J, Yang Y, Wang L-P (2014) Maternal separation exaggerates spontaneous recovery of extinguished contextual fear in adult female rats. Behav Brain Res 269:75–80.

Yamamoto S, Morinobu S, Takei S (2009) Single prolonged stress: toward ananimal model of posttraumatic stress disorder. Depress Anxiety 26:1110–1117.

Yehuda R, LeDoux J (2007) Response Variation following Trauma: A TranslationalNeuroscience Approach to Understanding PTSD. Neuron 56:19–32.

Zhang W, Rosenkranz JA (2013) Repeated restraint stress enhances cue-elicitedconditioned freezing and impairs acquisition of extinction in an age-dependent manner.Behav Brain Res 248:12–24.

Zheng X, Deschaux O, Lavigne J (2013) Prefrontal high-frequency stimulationprevents sub-conditioning procedure-provoked, but not acute stress-provoked,reemergence of extinguished fear. Neurobiol Learn Mem 101:33–38.

13

The Management of Autism Spectrum Disorder: Challenges Ahead

Priya Joon and Anil Kumar
Pharmacology Division, University Institute of Pharmaceutical Sciences (UIPS), Panjab University, Chandigarh, India

Milind Parle
Department of Pharmaceutical Sciences, Guru Jambheshwar University of Science and Technology, Hisar (Haryana), India

13.1 Introduction

Research in Autism Spectrum Disorder (ASD) was once focused primarily on infants and toddlers, since ASD was initially thought to be a rare disorder of childhood. As per *DSM-5*, ASD is a combined phrase for a family spectrum of developmental disabilities inclusive of "Autistic Disorder, Pervasive Developmental Disorder not Otherwise Specified (PDD-NOS), and Asperger's disorder." ASD is a complex heterogeneous, multifactorial developmental disorder with a wide variety of clinical manifestations, thereby requiring evaluation and intervention by a range of professionals working in coordination. ASD being a lifelong neurodevelopmental disability exhibits an unusual pattern of development producing a disturbing impact on the functioning of adults and senior citizens (Joon et al., 2021c). Although early ASD research focused primarily on children, there is increasing recognition that ASD is a lifelong neurodevelopmental disorder. Previously, it was thought that autism spectrum disorder is a rare childhood disorder. However, with the arrival of the DSM-5, the concept of ASD has evolved. The patients suffering from ASD are diagnosed during infancy, up to toddler years (8 years). This disorder doesn't occur in adults or elderly individuals, as per DSM-5. Since there is no cure for ASD, this disability continues into old age through adulthood. Now, it has become clear that ASD is a lifelong developmental disability with transition of symptoms from childhood to adolescence to adulthood and from adulthood to old age. Physicians and healthcare providers have acknowledged this expanding aspect of ASD and research is now being carried out to better understand the needs of children as well as adults with ASD. In the past two decades, the estimated prevalence of ASD has increased steadily and dramatically, affecting ~1% of both the child and adult population (Murphy et al., 2016). This worldwide rise in prevalence is thought to be a result of the complex combination of several factors, including broader diagnostic criteria and increased recognition and knowledge of the disorder. There are several reports available in the literature indicating that the incidence of ASD is much higher in males as compared to females. This heterogeneity is currently little studied and therefore poorly understood (Joon et al., 2021c). There is insufficient documentation of female cases suffering from autism because ASDs may go unnoticed, misdiagnosed, or diagnosed at a later stage in girls (Van Wijngaarden-Cremers et al., 2014). While health and education services for children with ASD are relatively well established, service provision for adults with ASD is in its infancy (Murphy et al., 2016). Therefore, there is an urgent need for extensive research focusing on Autism in adults and senior citizens along with careful handling of the transition phase involved in maturing of a toddler into an adult and adult into an aged individual. Although clinical features change with age and outcomes vary, the core symptoms such as social deficits, abnormal behavior, and impaired communication may continue into adulthood. A significant proportion of individuals with ASD continue to experience challenges with social relationships, independent living, and

DOI: 10.1201/9781003220404-15

mental health (Sengupta et al., 2017). Furthermore, other factors such as the influence of sex differences, life skills, acceptance in society, cost, and efficiency of health support also need to be adequately addressed. Likewise, the after-effects of recent international legislative efforts (such as the Autism Act) on service provision to aged patients suffering from Autism need to be determined. Future comparison of different international legislative approaches and strategies for raising awareness of ASD, service development, and measurement of outcomes may contribute to the development of evidence-based care for people with ASD. (Murphy et al., 2016). Due to high clinical and genetic heterogeneity, the pathogenesis of ASD continues to be a mystery making the treatment aspect of ASD a tough challenge (Joon et al., 2021b). Additionally, co-occurring conditions are common in children with ASD and may have great effects on child and family functioning and clinical management. The co-occurrence of different disorders in ASD seems to be a normal phenomenon rather than an exception. ASD perhaps is not a single disorder, but a blend of common core symptoms accompanied by large variable secondary symptoms characteristic of other co-morbidities (Joon et al., 2021b). Nevertheless, to date, there are no good approved medicines for treating the core symptoms of ASD, and the usefulness of complementary therapies is debatable. Hence, there is an immediate need for a better understanding of the neurobiology and prognosis of ASD across the lifespan of affected individuals. Parental cooperation is imperative during integrated interventions to sustain therapeutic gains. In India, families very often express their first concerns about their children to pediatricians and primary care physicians, who form a common source of referral for further evaluation and services. However, the role of the pediatrician goes much beyond recognizing the signs and symptoms of ASD and referring for a diagnostic evaluation (Sengupta et al., 2017). This picture may also be present in other developing countries. Pediatricians are often a trusted source of medical information that families adhere to for ongoing support. The existing autism literature in India is richer than in other low- and middle-income countries. However, literature that focuses on interventions in the pediatric and adult-age groups is still limited. In light of the above, we have made a humble attempt to outline various challenges involved with the aid of a flow chart in this book chapter to improve the present scenario of therapeutic management of ASD.

13.2 Management of Autism Spectrum Disorder

Patients suffering from ASD face challenges in finding adequate treatment as therapeutic management targets co- morbid conditions and ASD-associated symptoms only. Since there is no perfect cure available for ASD, thousands of options are being experimented with. The goals of treatment of children with ASD are to (i) minimize core deficits; (ii) build cognitive, communication, and social skills; (iii) maximize functional independence by promoting adaptive skills; (iv) eliminate maladaptive behaviors; (v) treat the co-morbid condition; (vi) counsel parents; (vii) prepare individuals and families for adolescence and adulthood; (viii) provide support to families; and (ix) enhance the quality of life of the entire family (Hyman et al., 2020; Mukherjee, 2017). The treatment strategy should be planned by a multi-disciplinary team comprising: 1) a clinician for holistic evaluation and pharmacotherapy; 2) a developmental pediatrician or clinical psychologist for evaluation of core symptoms, cognitive function, and adaptive function; 3) a speech-language pathologist for providing speech therapy; 4) an occupational therapist for streamlining activities of daily living; 5) a behavior analyst for behavior improvement; 6) a special educator for designing an Individualized Educational Plan; 7) a child & adolescent neurologist or psychiatrist; and 9) a community service providers for providing family support (Mukherjee, 2017). Treatment strategies for autism depend on the child's chronological age, developmental level, specific strengths, and family needs (Hyman et al., 2020).

The authors propose a **"Five-Fingers-Approach"** for both the management of ASD and improvement in life quality: Behavioral therapy, Educational Therapy, Focused interventions, Complementary therapy, and Pharmacotherapy (Figure 13.1).

13.3 "Five-Fingers-Approach" for Management of ASD

13.3.1 Behavioral Therapy

Behavioral interventions are based on the principles of behavior modification (Sengupta et al., 2017). Research has consistently shown that early intensive behavioral interventions can help young children with

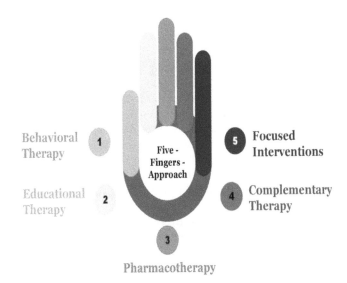

FIGURE 13.1 "Five-Fingers-Approach" for management of ASD.

ASD gain skills and improve long-term outcomes (Baumer and Spence, 2018). The goal of Behavioral therapy is positive reinforcement of desired behavior and breaking down tasks into simple achievable steps with frequent rewards and corrections (Joon et al., 2021a).

Applied behavior analysis (ABA): Applied behavior analysis adopts a methodology based on learning theory principles that teach skills and decrease maladaptive behaviors through repetition and reinforcement. ABA is currently considered the gold standard treatment for ASD (Baumer and Spence, 2018). The use of ABA methods to treat symptoms of ASD suggests that behaviors exhibited can be altered by programmed reinforcing skills related to communication and other skill acquisition. Thus, ABA treatments may target the development of new skills (e.g., social engagement) and minimize behaviors (e.g., aggression) that may interfere with a child's progress. ABA programs are typically designed and supervised by professionals certified in behavior analysis (Hyman et al., 2020).

Naturalistic developmental behavioral interventions (NDBIs): Naturalistic developmental behavioral interventions (NDBIs) incorporate elements of ABA and developmental principles such as emphasis on developmentally based learning targets and foundational social learning skills (Hyman et al., 2020; Schreibman et al., 2015). Naturalistic behavioral strategies are forms of ABA in which the child's interests or behavior initiate the instruction and lead to a reinforcing event ("natural reinforcer"). These approaches are more child-centered and the intervention is delivered in natural environments (Sengupta et al., 2017).

Cognitive-behavioral therapy (CBT): Cognitive-behavioral therapy (CBT) is a type of psychotherapeutic intervention that helps patients learn how to identify and change destructive/disturbing thought patterns that have a negative influence on behavior and emotions. The goal of CBT is on improving the concentration and behavioral patterns of the patient (Joon et al., 2021a).

13.3.2 Educational Therapy

The education of children and their caregivers is currently a popular form of treatment for autism. Education for individuals with ASD is defined as the fostering of the acquisition of skills or knowledge. It includes socialization, adaptive skills, language and communication, academic learning, and reduction of challenging behaviors to maximize functional independence, improve quality of life, and alleviate family stress (Sengupta et al., 2017). Educational programs for school-aged children with ASD should promote language, academic, adaptive, and social skills development and prepare them for postsecondary education or employment. Children with symptoms of ASD show substantial benefits with educational therapies (Hyman et al., 2020).

Classroom-based models: Many students with ASD are educated in inclusive classrooms with supports. Other school-aged children and youth benefit from disorder-specific approaches (Hyman et al., 2020).

Education in open/pleasant environment: Educating students with ASD in the open environment typically requires an individualized program that is modified to meet the Individualized Education Program goals set by the family, student, and school team (Hyman et al., 2020).

Social skills instruction: Social skill deficits may present differently depending on language abilities, developmental level, and age. Interventions may be divided into adult-mediated (skill building with the individual child), peer-mediated (skill building with the child and typically developing classmates), and mixed approaches. Child-directed social skill interventions are often delivered individually or in small groups with other children with similar needs. Interventions addressing social skills may increase the child's knowledge of social behavior and teach strategies for reciprocal social interaction (Hyman et al., 2020).

Parent-mediated treatment: Increasing evidence reveals that focused interventions delivered by trained parents or other caregivers can be an important part of a therapeutic program. Parent management training is divided into two categories: Parent support interventions and parent-mediated interventions. Parent support interventions are knowledge-focused and provide an indirect benefit to the child, including care coordination and psycho-education. Parent-mediated interventions are technique-focused and provide direct benefit to the child, and may target core symptoms of ASD or other behaviors or skills and may be built on ABA approaches in natural settings. Including parents in the intervention process is critically important (Hyman et al., 2020). Parent-mediated interventions are cost-effective and increase the sense of empowerment on the part of caregivers (Dalwai et al., 2017). Parent-mediated interventions are effective in helping parents to be more responsive and engaged with helping children to acquire communication skills or manage challenging behaviors (Angie et al., 2019).

13.3.3 Focused Interventions and Therapies

Alongside behavioral and educational therapies, children with ASD often need specific support services to address ASD-associated challenges. Focused intervention practices include one or a few instructional strategies that are designed to address a single or limited skill such as increasing social communication or learning a specific task, and may be delivered over a short period. Focused interventions practices target specific learner outcomes, and are effective for promoting skill development, speech, and communication (Hyman et al., 2020; Wong et al., 2015).

Speech-language therapy is the most commonly identified intervention provided for children with ASD. Speech-language therapy may be required to improve verbal, nonverbal, and social communication skills. A speech therapist or speech-language pathologist can offer alternative and augmentative communication aids, such as picture-based communication systems, communication boards, visual supports, signs, and gestures, or specialized devices and software to support functional communication in children who are nonverbal or whose language skills are impaired (Angie et al., 2019). Speech therapy helps in improving aphasia, speech apraxia, speech delays, difficulty with narrations & conversations, dysarthria, expressive disorder, language disorder, fluency disorder, and articulation disorder (Joon et al., 2021a).

Occupational therapy addresses functional challenges in the activities of daily living, including specific interventions to improve fine motor or sensory processing impairments and adaptive skills. An occupational therapist can help children acquire self-care, play skills, toy use, and handwriting (Hyman et al., 2020; Angie et al., 2019). Sensory Integration therapy is used alone or most often as a part of a broader program of occupational therapy for children with ASD (Sengupta et al., 2017).

Counseling or psychotherapy: In those with average intelligence and typical language skills, counseling methodologies can be successfully employed for core symptoms of rigidity and inflexibility as well as comorbid psychiatric disorders (e.g., depression, anxiety) and behavioral dysregulation (Baumer and Spence, 2018). A psychologist can perform a psychological assessment to evaluate for cognitive, adaptive, and learning skills as well as co-morbid conditions (e.g., anxiety, ADHD). Psychotherapy when administered by a professional therapist/psychologist has the potential to counter psychiatric symptoms such as obsessions, anxiety, minor or major depression, intellectual disability, and aphasia (Joon et al.,

2021a; Angie et al., 2019). However, the use of psychotherapy is limited for individuals with language and cognitive impairment.

Motor therapies: Children with ASD may have low muscle tone or a developmental coordination disorder. Both fine and gross motor skills may be impaired, which further decreases opportunities for social skill development and active learning in children with ASD. Therapeutic interventions focused on building strength, coordination, motor planning, or skill acquisition may be facilitated by promoting outdoor activities in children with ASD (Hyman et al., 2020).

13.3.4 Complementary and Alternative Therapies

Despite the advances in the understanding of the neurobiology of ASD, many unanswered questions remain about why ASD occurs in the first place and how best to treat it. Families often consider nutritional interventions and nonmedical therapies without a scientific evidence base to address the symptoms that conventional interventions cannot rapidly address, or there is limited access to conventional services in their community (Hyman et al., 2020). To date, there is insufficient scientific evidence for the benefits of various complementary therapy approaches (Baumer and Spence, 2018). Complementary therapies used for ASD can be grouped into two general areas: (a) natural products including diet, herbs, vitamins, minerals, probiotics, and (b) mind and body practices including music therapy, yoga, chiropractic, massage, acupuncture, physiotherapy, hydrotherapy, physical exercise, equine-assisted therapy, other types of animal or pet therapy, energy therapy, Reiki, dance therapy, drama therapy, and progressive relaxation (Joon et al., 2021a; Hyman et al., 2020). Although some complementary therapies are considered safe with appropriate monitoring, many therapies lack scientific supporting evidence. Researchers have described complementary therapies in detail (Joon et al., 2021a). Complementary approaches like supplementing the diet with vitamins B6, B9, B12, C, D, folate, magnesium, zinc, or omega-3 fatty acids, probiotics, or dietary interventions such as gluten-or casein-free diets and a ketogenic diet (KD) are found to be effective in ameliorating ASD-associated symptoms (Joon et al., 2021a; Angie et al., 2019). There has been conflicting evidence regarding the effect of massage therapy, music and expressive therapies, equine-assisted therapy, yoga, and energy therapies on the symptoms of ASD in children, but the evidence does not support these therapies for the treatment of the core deficits of ASD (Hyman et al., 2020; Angie et al., 2019). Therapies that are considered risky and ineffective for children with ASD include hyperbaric oxygen therapy, immunotherapy, chelation therapy, secretin, and the use of certain herbal products, antibiotics, antifungal agents, and facilitated communication strategies (Angie et al., 2019). Recent studies using medicinal herbs like Asparagus racemosus (Shatavari) (Joon et al., 2019; 2020), Ginkgo biloba, and Panax ginseng showed promising anti-autistic potential in animals without any serious adverse effects (Joon et al., 2021a).

13.3.5 Pharmacotherapy

Despite the increasing prevalence of ASD, associated costs, and the urgent need for a satisfactory remedy, there are no US-FDA-approved medicines that ameliorate the core symptoms of ASD, particularly the deficits in reciprocal conversation and social skills (Joon et al., 2021 a, c). Pharmacological treatment of basic symptoms of ASD is by and large intricate, owing to the complexity in the appearance of ASD, co-morbid conditions, and age-related response variability. Since a satisfactory therapeutic regimen is not available for the treatment of core symptoms of ASD, co-morbid conditions and ASD-associated symptoms are targeted (Joon et al., 2021a; Lamy et al., 2020). To date, aripiprazole and risperidone are the only medicines approved by the US-FDA, for controlling ASD-associated behavioral disturbances, such as aggression, self-harm, severe tantrums, agitation, irritability, and outbursts of ASD subjects (Joon et al., 2021a; Pistollato et al., 2020). Other medications are used to treat commonly occurring symptoms, such as anxiety or OCD (selective serotonin reuptake inhibitors (SSRIs), antidepressants); ADHD symptoms of impulsivity, hyperactivity, and inattention (alpha agonists, stimulants); sleep dysfunction (melatonin or sedatives); abnormal behaviors (antipsychotics) and mood disorders (SSRIs, atypical antipsychotics, and mood stabilizers) (Joon et al., 2021a; Baumer and Spence, 2018). Clinicians should carefully weigh potential risks and benefits before prescribing medication for behavior and use psychotropic medications as part of a comprehensive treatment approach. Several substances targeting immune dysfunction, neuroinflammation, glutamate/GABA imbalance, NMDA receptors, and neuropeptides are undergoing clinical trials with variable success (Joon et al., 2021a). Ketamine, a noncompetitive NMDA receptor agonist, has been found to be successful in reducing aggressive and suicidal behavioral episodes and social impairment. The NMDA glutamate receptor antagonists, Amantadine and Memantine, have been shown to improve memory and reduce maladaptive behavior in children with ASD. Acamprosate, a GABA-analog and NMDA receptor modulator has been shown to produce substantial benefits in social interaction and ADHD-related symptoms in adolescents with ASD (see Table 13.1) (Joon et al., 2021a; Lamy et al., 2020). The latest clinical studies suggest bumetanide, a loop diuretic acting via inhibition of Na–K–Ca co-transporter-1 chloride-importer and facilitation of GABA-ergic transmission, to be a promising remedy for improving the core symptoms of repetitive behavior and reciprocal social interaction in ASD subjects aged 3–11 years old (Kassem S and Oroszi, 2019). A clinical trial showed that intranasal oxytocin significantly improved social interaction in ASD children below 8 years of age (Yatawara et al., 2016). Balovaptan, a selective vasopressin 1a (V1a) receptor antagonist, has been found to manage social interaction deficits in children suffering from ASD (Joon et al., 2021a). Pharmacotherapy for the management of ASD-associated symptoms has been summarized in Table 13.1.

TABLE 13.1

Pharmacotherapy for Management of ASD

Medication	ASD Symptoms Targeted
Atypical Antipsychotics (e.g., Aripiprazole, Risperidone, Clozapine, etc]	Beneficial to treat aggressive episodes or self-injurious behaviors, irritability, outbursts, improvement in speech, and hyperactivity
Selective Serotonin Reuptake Inhibitors (SSRIs) (e.g., Fluoxetine, Fluvoxamine, etc.)	For the treatment of anxiety disorders and depression, improvement in social difficulties, maladaptive and repetitive behaviors
Anti-Convulsants (e.g., Divalproex, Oxcarbazepine)	Improvement in irritability, aggression and repetitive behaviors
Tricyclic Antidepressants (e.g., Clomipramine)	Improvement in social relatedness, obsessive compulsive and aggressive behaviors
Mood stabilizing agent (e.g., Lithium)	Treatment of mood swings
Psycho-Stimulant (e.g., Methylphenidate)	Improves hyperactivity, impulsivity, and attention deficits
Norepinephrine Reuptake inhibitor (e.g., Atomoxetine)	Improvement in hyperactivity
Alpha 2A Receptor Agonists (e.g., Clonidine, Guanfacine)	Improvements in hyperactivity, impulsivity, sleep onset and decreased night-time awakening
Melatonin	Reduction of sleep-related issues, improving sleep patterns; beneficial effects on anxiety, depression, pain, and GI dysfunctions
Oxytocin	Reduction in repetitive behaviors and improving social interaction
Acetylcholinesterase inhibitors (e.g., Donepezil, Rivastigmine, Galantamine)	Improvement in behavior and language, reduction of irritability and hyperactivity
N-methyl-D-Aspartate (NMDA) glutamate receptor agonist (e.g., Ketamine)	Decrease symptoms of depression and suicidality, reduction in aggressive behaviors
NMDA glutamate receptor antagonist (e.g., Amantadine, Memantine)	Improvement in hyperactivity, inappropriate speech, lethargy and irritability, beneficial in memory functioning
Na–K–Ca co-transporter-1 (NKCC1) chloride-importer inhibitor (Bumetanide)	Improvement in repetitive behavior and participatory social interaction
γ-Aminobutyric Acid (GABA) Analogue (Acamprosate)	Improvement in social behavior along with reductions in ADHD symptoms
Vasopressin 1a (V1a) Receptor Antagonist (Balovaptan)	Improvement in social behaviors

(Source: Joon et al., 2021a)

Physicians are advised to follow certain well-accepted guidelines (cited below) when prescribing and monitoring psychotropic medications.

13.4 General Guidelines

- All treatments should be individualized, developmentally appropriate, and intensive, with performance data relevant to treatment goals.
- All interventions should be specific and based on sound theoretical constructs, rigorous methodologies, targeting core as well as secondary features of autism.
- One constant guiding principle is that behavioral interventions for children at risk for ASD should be initiated **as early as possible,** ideally even before the diagnosis is confirmed.
- Interventions should be implemented in a stepwise fashion so that proper attribution of effect is possible and confounding factors can be identified.
- Families should be advised that complementary therapies should not replace proven drug therapies.
- Behavioral and educational interventions are the key to optimal outcomes, in conjunction with medications for specific symptoms.
- Co-occurring behavioral or psychiatric disorders along with ASD seem to be **normal rather than an exception.** Hence, medications used in other psychiatric disorders can be effective in individuals with ASD as well.
- Clinicians should carefully **weigh potential risks and benefits** before prescribing any medication for behavior and use psychotropic medications as part of a comprehensive treatment approach.
- Children with ASD experience more medication side effects than those without ASD.
- The dosing schedule should **"start low and go slow."**
- The prescribing clinician should understand the indications, contraindications, dosing schedule, potential adverse effects, drug-drug interactions, and monitoring requirements of the medications they prescribe.
- Most importantly **compassionate care** coupled with assurance and reassurance by parents and friends is crucial.

However, along with the integrated application of various therapies, the cooperation of family members backed by society is necessary for enhancing the quality of life of a child suffering from ASD.

13.5 Challenges Ahead

All parents hope their children will excel in personal and professional life. However, this becomes difficult for families in which a child with autism is born facing several challenges in their lives. Autism is a disorder for which there is no cure in allopathy and "where there is no cure, one hundred treatments appear to work" (Joon et al., 2021a). The challenges faced by individuals suffering from ASD and their families that need immediate consideration are as follows (Figure 13.2).

Inconsistent brain development across the lifespan in ASD: ASD is a lifelong neurodevelopmental disorder. Brain imaging studies offer the opportunity for a greater understanding of brain development and associated behavioral difficulties across the lifespan of people with ASD, which may contribute to the development of age-appropriate treatments (Lainhart, 2015). There is accumulating longitudinal evidence of abnormal, age-related changes in the brain anatomy of individuals with ASD in comparison to typically developing individuals, particularly in frontotemporal and striatal regions in early childhood and adolescence. Furthermore, there is increasing cross-sectional evidence of region-specific and age-related changes in the brain structure of people with ASD from childhood to adulthood across several areas associated with ASD symptoms, including parameters of volume (e.g., cerebellum, amygdala, and striatum) and surface-based measures of cortical thickness and surface area (e.g., medial frontotemporal and parietal regions) (Murphy et al., 2016). However, to date, there is a limited longitudinal investigation of brain maturation in people with ASD from childhood through adulthood. It is anticipated that the

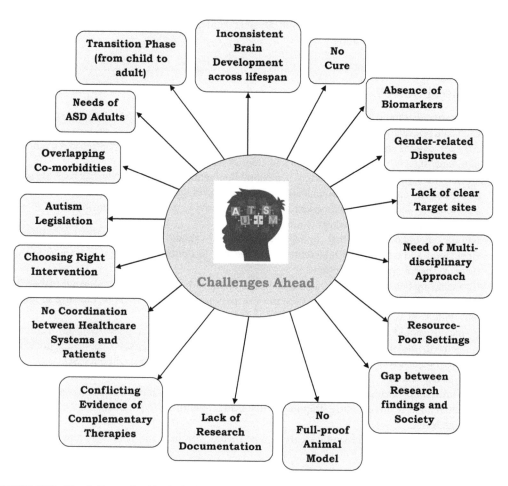

FIGURE 13.2 The challenges faced by the individuals suffering from ASD.

crucial advances in the area of high-risk genes and aberrant neuronal circuitry would lead to innovative breakthroughs (Joon et al., 2022). Future developmental investigations are warranted to enable better understanding of brain, cognition, and behavior in people with ASD across the lifespan to develop effective age-appropriate, personalized treatments (Murphy et al., 2016).

Absence of biomarkers: To date, no biomarker has been identified to have a direct link with Autism. ASD continues to be diagnosed based on the symptoms and behavior of the patient. However, the behavioral assessment of ASD can be time-consuming, expensive, and, in the absence of biomarkers, relies on an expert clinical assessment that is not usually available (Joon et al., 2021a; 2022). Biomarkers of ASD could potentially be used to predict ASD risk, enhance screening, and permit pre-symptomatic detection. Their use could improve the reliability and validity of clinical diagnosis, identify mechanisms for developing treatment, and confirm the need for a specific intervention (Hyman et al., 2020). Autism is currently one of the most visible and widely discussed developmental human conditions with no understanding of the biomarkers. The etiology and neurochemistry of this disorder are still a matter of speculation. Accelerated research into the neurobiology of ASD may result in the identification of valid biomarkers. Some potentially important lines of research involve medications that modulate the metabolism of excitatory neurotransmitters (such as glutamate and g-aminobutyric acid), block acetylcholinesterase, and/ or nicotinic acid receptors and act as hormones that naturally promote social affiliation (such as oxytocin and vasopressin) (Joon et al., 2021a; Hyman et al., 2020). A better understanding of the neurobiology responsible for the symptoms of ASD will allow for the identification of targeted psychopharmacologic interventions that will better manage co-occurring symptoms and/or address core deficits.

Lack of clear target sites: The promising remedies for ASD core symptoms are still lacking (Joon et al., 2021a). As a whole, we believe that the existing data support the hypothesis that the mechanisms underlying ASD etiology result from the effects of diverse gene-environment interactions, with possible cumulative or even multiplicative effects not only at the individual level but also through generations (Joon et al., 2021b). Medical classifications that are based on etiology and biomarkers have important advantages such as clear targets for intervention. In the case of mental disorders, this is not possible because the etiology of mental disorders is not only multi-dimensional but also incompletely understood (Joon et al., 2022). Nevertheless, the authors opine that recent developments in the understanding of gene-environment interactions are opening up new research vistas, which might eventually lead to a leap forward in our comprehension and treatment of this disorder. Large and heterogeneous sample sizes are needed to identify the interconnection between the effects of adverse environmental exposure during critical developmental periods of an embryo within the uterus and the dynamic role of protective factors. These well-designed investigations would offer new avenues to disentangle the mystery of the development of ASD (Joon et al., 2022).

Overlapping comorbidities: Comorbid mental health difficulties persist from childhood to adulthood and occur in both males and females with ASD (Joon et al., 2021b). Moreover, people with ASD can have specific cognitive anomalies, including poor planning, weak decision making, and sickly motor skills, which may adversely impact their everyday living skills and ability to access health services. Childhood neurodevelopmental disorders such as attention deficit hyperactivity disorder (ADHD), Autism spectrum disorder (ASD), childhood schizophrenia, and intellectual disability (ID) typically are complicated comorbid conditions that not only show considerable clinical overlap but often coexist. Furthermore, there is a debate regarding whether people with ASD, ADHD, or combined ASD and ADHD have shared or different neurobiology (Joon et al., 2022). This is important, as an increased understanding of the causal mechanisms underlying specific symptoms may contribute to the future development of individually tailored treatments (Joon et al., 2021a,b). Affective disorders including depression, anxiety, and OCD are common in adults with ASD (across both sexes). Despite high rates of anxiety in ASD adults, including generalized anxiety, social anxiety, phobias, and OCD, anxiety is often overlooked and assumed to be a part of an ASD profile, rather than warranting a separate diagnosis, which can limit access to treatment. Despite the increasing prevalence of ASD and associated costs, no medication is approved for the treatment of either core symptoms or comorbid mental health difficulties in adults with ASD (Murphy et al., 2016). Overall, the authors recommend an open and flexible approach in clinical practice, while dealing with these disorders, since the child's entire future life is at stake.

Autism legislation: The Autism Act has been introduced internationally to raise awareness about ASD recently, to highlight the consequences of mental disorders, and make support available for research. Yet, considerable geographic variation in services offered continues to exist along with an overall paucity of ASD services for adult and old patients suffering from Autism in different countries worldwide. The requirements of the Autism Act include i) improved training of frontline staff and ii) development of local ASD healthcare teams and development of service sector across social services. The general practitioners (GPs) are the gatekeepers of access to care for patients. It is assumed that GPs have an awareness of ASD and know how to access clinical and social care for their patients with ASD. To facilitate this, the Royal College of General Practitioners (RCGP) in the UK designated autism a clinical priority in 2014 and appointed an Autism Champion to provide clinical leadership and deliver innovative clinical programs. The outcomes of the RCGP autism initiative are not yet available. However, the RCGP plans that it will enable GPs to access high-quality training that will lead to the delivery of the best possible community services, including 1) development of ASD friendly services with appropriate referral, 2) timely diagnosis, 3) appropriate support for people with ASD (and their families), and 4) improved health and well-being outcomes (Murphy et al., 2016). However, there is an urgent need for research to determine the impact of ASD legislation on people with ASD and their families globally.

Needs of ASD adults: Overall, there is a dearth of research regarding the physical and mental health of adults with ASD. However, it is challenging to provide community health and social resources for adults and aged individuals with ASD. Despite having common and treatable health conditions, adults with ASD report difficulty in accessing healthcare. In particular, research is required to determine a better understanding of the needs of adults with ASD, including health, aging, service development, transition, treatment options across the lifespan, sex differences, and the views of people with ASD (Murphy et al., 2016). Significant legislative efforts have been put in place in some countries to increase community and professional awareness of ASD in adults. However, the outcomes of this legislation remain to be determined. Furthermore, focused research is required to identify evidence-based and cost-effective models of care and to enable adults with ASD to easily access coordinated, high-quality local health and social services. Additionally, future work is warranted at both ends of adulthood in ASD. This would facilitate the improved transition from youth to adult healthcare and increase understanding of aging and health in older adults with ASD (Murphy et al., 2016).

Transition phase (from child to adult): There is increasing recognition of the need for young people with neurodevelopmental disorders to have a planned transition from child to adult health services (NICE, 2012), but very limited research in this respect. Furthermore, successful transition requires adaptive skills that can be learned and adapted for use across future transitions. For example, in addition to moving from child to adult services, transitions occur naturally across many life events: adult relationships, parenthood, employment, and death of a parent (Murphy et al., 2016). Moreover, forethought is imperative for developmental change associated with the child's growth, maturity, middle-age, and old age, while finalizing the treatment schedule.

Gender-related disputes: There is insufficient documentation of females suffering from autism because ASDs may go unnoticed, misdiagnosed, or diagnosed at a later stage in girls. However, there is some evidence that the clinical presentation is different in males and females, and it is argued that phenotypic gender differences might lead to delayed diagnosis or even missed diagnosis in girls and women with autism (Van Wijngaarden-Cremers et al., 2014). The incidence of ASD is much higher in males as compared to females. However, ASD male: female proportion shows substantial variation within the range of 8:1 to 2:1 (Loomes et al., 2017). This substantial sex dimorphism in male: female preponderance of ASD prompted researchers to conduct ASD studies predominantly on male patients (Joon et al., 2021c). Studies have indicated that there could be disparity in prevalence because females disguise their clinical signs. A "female protective effect" is being supported by recent studies as an explanation for the higher prevalence of ASD in males as compared to females (Joon et al., 2021c; Tubío-Fungueiriño et al., 2020). This heterogeneity is currently little studied and therefore poorly understood. In addition, age may influence potential gender-related differences in the symptoms of ASD, as there is some evidence that age has a gender-specific role in symptom severity. More research is needed on the female phenotype of ASD with the development of appropriate instruments to detect and ascertain those (Van Wijngaarden-Cremers et al., 2014).

Lack of research documentation: Currently, despite various limitations, many government hospitals, private organizations, and NGOs across the country are doing stellar work in the field of autism intervention and supporting children with ASD and their families. However, comparatively little has been done in the area of evaluation and documentation of different indigenous intervention models. There is a considerable gap in research findings and evaluation of culturally appropriate models of intervention (Sengupta et al., 2017). The authors are hopeful that this challenge will have more interest and progress in the years ahead. Pediatricians and physicians need to become familiar with locally available therapy options and resources including hospitals and organizations working in this sphere to be able to help affected families and improve quality of life (Hyman et al., 2020).

Gaps between research findings and society: Gaps between the latest research findings in the area of ASD and clinical practice need to be bridged (Joon et al., 2021a; 2022).

Need of multi-Disciplinary/integrative approach: Experts from a wide range of disciplines (e.g., child psychiatrists, psychologists, pediatricians, neurologists, gynecologists, speech and language therapists, occupational therapists, etc.) need to be consulted for accurate diagnosis and treatment of children suffering from ASD and associated baffling disorders. Multi-disciplinary professional expertise and combined diagnostic facilities for children facing developmental disorders in general and ASD in particular at a multi-specialty center can help ensure precise assessment and intervention across all neurodevelopmental domains to explicitly recognize the overlaps (Joon et al., 2022). It is hoped that recent international multi-disciplinary collaborations will enable the development of bench-to-bedside novel therapeutic options that may include consideration of both genetic and neurobiological causes of ASD, co-morbid difficulties, and response to treatment (Murphy et al., 2016).

Choosing right intervention: Families and sometimes pediatricians too find it overwhelmingly difficult to assess which interventions/program would be a good fit for their child or patient given the wide array of individual variation, organizations, and approaches available. It would be helpful to keep in mind that irrespective of orientation (e.g., behavioral, naturalistic, or developmental) and specific training (e.g., psychologist, speech pathologist, occupational therapist, parent, therapist, etc.), all interventionists should follow certain principles to yield fruitful results (Sengupta et al., 2017).

Resource-poor settings: In developing countries like India, most resources for ASD are still clustered in the major cities. Even in the metros, therapeutic options for the poor are limited. In the rest of the country, resources are extremely scarce. One of the ways to address this challenge is to train community-level workers who have access to children in their natural settings, like primary school teachers, crèche, and daycare workers, etc. (Sengupta et al., 2017). This approach could be beneficial in other countries as well.

Conflicting evidence for complementary therapies: Despite advances in understanding the neurobiology of ASD, many unanswered questions remain such as "Why does ASD occur in the first place and how best to treat it?." Families often consider nutritional interventions and non-medical therapies without sufficient scientific evidence for addressing the symptoms of ASD (Hyman et al., 2020). There has been conflicting evidence regarding the effect of complementary therapies such as music therapy, dance therapy, drama therapy, chiropractic therapy, yoga, massage, and equine-assisted therapy on the symptoms of ASD in children (Ip Angie et al., 2019).

No coordination between healthcare systems and patients: Despite the positive role played by the organizations supporting ASD patients and awareness attempts of media, there are persisting needs for better coordination between healthcare systems, service providers, special training schools, residential and employment facilities for gifted individuals, and support measures available for disabled ASD patients (Joon et al., 2022).

No full-proof animal model: There is no satisfactory animal model to study ASD pathogenesis and new drugs for the management of ASD.

Future challenges include how to better understand the influence of sex differences, how to learn from these differences, and how to apply best what we know about the dimensions that significantly impact the lives of ASD patients in different countries, cultures, and populations. There is a dire need to explore "autistic voices" and feedback from youths and adults suffering from Autism and their families. Furthermore, amendments based on newer versions of the DSM and ICD would surely go a long way in improving the quality of life of the ASD community. We believe that although a good job has been done over the last one hundred years, there is ample scope in marching ahead in the light of the challenges highlighted above.

REFERENCES

Baumer N, Spence SJ. Evaluation and management of the child with autism spectrum disorder. Continuum: Lifelong Learning in Neurology. 2018; 24(1):248–275.

Dalwai S, Ahmed S, Udani V, Mundkur N, Kamath SS, Nair MK. Consensus statement of the Indian academy of pediatrics on evaluation and management of autism spectrum disorder. Indian Pediatrics. 2017; 54(5):385–393.

DSM-5: Diagnostic and Statistical Manual of Mental Disorders. Fifth edition. American Psychiatric Association. 2013; 21.

Hyman SL, Levy SE, Myers SM. Identification, evaluation, and management of children with autism spectrum disorder. Pediatrics. 2020; 145(1), e20193447

Ip Angie, Zwaigenbaum L, Brian JA. Post-diagnostic management and follow-up care for autism spectrum disorder. Paediatrics & Child Health. 2019; 24(7):461–468.

Joon P, Dhingra D, Parle M. Shatavari: A nature's gift for autism. Asian Journal of Bio Sciences. 2019; 14(1&2):12–21.

Joon P, Dhingra D, Parle, M. Biochemical evidence for anti-autistic potential of asparagus racemosus. International Journal of Plant Sciences. 2020; 15(1):42–51.

Joon P, Kumar A and Parle M: Strategic management of autism spectrum disorder. EC Neurology. 2021a; 13(6):9–22.

Joon P, Kumar A and Parle M: The interplay of protective and risk factors linked to autism. Journal of Clinical Images and Medical Case Reports. 2021b; 2(2):1070.

Joon P, Kumar A and Parle M: Unraveling the mystery of autism. International Journal of Pharmaceutical Sciences & Research. 2022; 13(10): 3864–3882. DOI: 10.13040/IJPSR.0975-8232.13(5).1000-19

Joon P, Kumar A and Parle M: What is autism. Pharmacological Reports. 2021c; 1–10. DOI: 10.1007/s43440-021-00244-0.

Kassem S, Oroszi T. Possible therapeutic use of bumetanide in the treatment of autism spectrum disorder. Journal of Biosciences and Medicines. 2019; 7(12):58.

Lainhart JE. Brain imaging research in autism spectrum disorders: in search of neuropathology and health across the lifespan. Current Opinion in Psychiatry. 2015; 28(2):76.

Lamy M, Pedapati EV, Dominick KL, Wink LK, Erickson CA. Recent advances in the pharmacological management of behavioral disturbances associated with autism spectrum disorder in children and adolescents. Pediatric Drugs. 2020; 20:1–11.

Loomes R, Hull L, Mandy WP. What is the male-to-female ratio in autism spectrum disorder? A systematic review and meta-analysis. Journal of the American Academy of Child & Adolescent Psychiatry. 2017; 56(6):466–474.

Mukherjee SB. Autism spectrum disorders—diagnosis and management. The Indian Journal of Pediatrics. 2017; 84(4):307–314.

Murphy CM, Wilson CE, Robertson DM, Ecker C, Daly EM, Hammond N, Galanopoulos A, Dud I, Murphy DG, McAlonan GM. Autism spectrum disorder in adults: diagnosis, management, and health services development. Neuropsychiatric Disease and Treatment. 2016; 12:1669–1686.

NICE. Guidelines Including Transition Recommendations. Available from: www.nice.org.uk/guidance/cg170/resources/guidance-autism NICE 2012.

Pistollato F, Forbes-Hernández TY, Iglesias RC, Ruiz R, Zabaleta ME, Cianciosi D, Giampieri F, Battino M. Pharmacological, non-pharmacological and stem cell therapies for the management of autism spectrum disorders: A focus on human studies. Pharmacological Research. 2020; 152:104579.

Schreibman L, Dawson G, Stahmer AC, Landa R, Rogers SJ, McGee GG, Kasari C, Ingersoll B, Kaiser AP, Bruinsma Y, McNerney E. Naturalistic developmental behavioral interventions: Empirically validated treatments for autism spectrum disorder. Journal of Autism and Developmental Disorders. 2015; 45(8):2411–2428.

Sengupta K, Lobo L, Krishnamurthy V. Educational and behavioral interventions in management of autism spectrum disorder. The Indian Journal of Pediatrics. 2017; 84(1):61–67.

Tubío-Fungueiriño M, Cruz S, Sampaio A, Carracedo A, Fernández-Prieto M. Social camouflaging in females with autism spectrum disorder: A systematic review. Journal of Autism and Developmental Disorders. 2021; 51(7):2190–2199.

Van Wijngaarden-Cremers PJ, van Eeten E, Groen WB, Van Deurzen PA, Oosterling IJ, Van der Gaag RJ. Gender and age differences in the core triad of impairments in autism spectrum disorders: a systematic review and meta-analysis. J Autism Dev Disord. 2014; 44(3):627–635.

Wong C, Odom SL, Hume KA, Cox AW, Fettig A, Kucharczyk S, Brock ME, Plavnick JB, Fleury VP, Schultz TR. Evidence-based practices for children, youth, and young adults with autism spectrum disorder: A comprehensive review. Journal of Autism and Developmental Disorders. 2015; 45(7):1951–1966.

Yatawara CJ, Einfeld SL, Hickie IB, Davenport TA, Guastella AJ. The effect of oxytocin nasal spray on social interaction deficits observed in young children with autism: a randomized clinical crossover trial. Molecular Psychiatry. 2016; 21(9):1225–1231.

14

Genetics of Left Ventricular Dysfunction in Coronary Artery Disease

Surendra Kumar
Department of Anatomy, All India Institute of Medical Sciences, New Delhi, India

Avshesh Mishra
Department of Genetics, Modern Diagnostic and Research Centre, Gurugram, India

Anshika Srivastava
Department of Genetics, Sanjay Gandhi Postgraduate Institute of Medical Sciences, Lucknow, India

Rama Mittal
Department of Urology, Sanjay Gandhi Postgraduate Institute of Medical Sciences, Lucknow, India

Balraj Mittal
Department of Biotechnology, Babasaheb Bhimrao Ambedkar University, Lucknow, India

14.1 Introduction

Cardiovascular diseases (CVDs) are major killers of human adults in both developing and developed countries. Despite considerable technological advances, coronary artery disease (CAD) and associated complications, which lead to heart failure, remain serious unsolved problems. CAD results from accumulation of atheromatous plaques (Ross, 1993) within the walls of the coronary arteries that supply oxygen-rich blood and nutrients to the heart muscle. Although the clinical signs and symptoms of CAD are noted in advanced state of disease, most individuals remain asymptomatic for decades. However, a major complication that some CAD patients face over time is the development of left ventricular dysfunction (LVD). LVD is a condition where the left ventricle pumps a lower fraction of ejected blood as compared to a healthy heart. LVD can involve the entire left ventricle (overall LVD) or only part of it (regional LVD). The latter is particularly common in CAD and can evolve into more severe overall LVD and dilatation (LV remodeling). Traditional risk factors for LVD are poorly developed collaterals, extensive atherosclerotic disease, and a large myocardial infarction (MI). However, it has been observed in clinical practice that since CAD patients who never had such complications still develop LVD, whereas others with well-defined predictors do not develop LVD.

Over the past few years, remarkable progress has been made in the understanding of the genetic etiology of LVD. LVD is a progressively debilitating condition and significant heterogeneity exists in individual subjects. Earlier genetic studies correlated LVD with dilated cardiomyopathy (DCM) (Takai et al., 2002). To date, two genes for X-linked FDCM (familial dystrophin, G4.5) have been identified and four genes for the autosomal dominant form (i.e., actin, desmin, lamin A/C, δ-sarcoglycan) have been described. In one form of inflammatory heart disease, coxsackievirus myocarditis, inflammatory mediators, and dystrophin cleavage play a role in the development of LVD (Towbin and Bowles, 2001).

DOI: 10.1201/9781003220404-16

However, mendelian forms of LVD are rare. In fact, clinical heterogeneity and racial differences in survival outcomes point toward multifactorial inheritance in the progression of LVD. The vast majority of CAD generally occurs in the background of polygenic susceptibility with potentially hundreds of genes playing a role (Lusis, 2003). In fact, CAD is a time-dependent, multistep process involving the interaction of many different key biochemical pathways including lipoprotein metabolism, coagulation, and inflammation. As can be expected, gene variations in any of these pathways may lead to altered function of key proteins thereby disrupting homeostasis. Intermediate phenotypes such as diabetes, hypertension, and obesity are polygenic traits that interact to modulate risk. Gene–gene interactions are also likely to be important, although little is understood with respect to CAD. Thus, the development of LVD in CAD patients involves a number of factors and hence seems to be a multifactorial and multigenic process. It is unlikely that any single gene would have a dramatic effect on LVD risk. Therefore, combinations of gene variants may improve the predictive ability and could be used as biomarkers for predicting susceptibility to LVD.

Based on pathophysiology of LVD, many different pathways may be involved in development of LVD. Some of the prominent ones are

1. Inflammatory pathways
2. Sarcomeric genes
3. Signalling pathway
4. Myocardial remodelling

14.2 Inflammatory Pathways

14.2.1 Inflammation

Any kind of damage in tissue resulting in an acute response with characteristic symptoms is known as inflammation. Usually it is resolves naturally. However, in the development of degenerative disease and loss of functions, chronic inflammation is believed to be a main factor. Chronic inflammation can be originated by cellular stress and cellular dysfunction, and can be triggered by high calorie consumption, oxidative stress, and high blood sugar levels. It is now well known that the destructive capacity of chronic inflammation is exceptional among physiologic processes (Karin, Lawrence & Nizet, 2006). Out of the ten top causes of death in the United States, a minimum of seven were contributed by inflammation to pathogenesis, including cardiovascular disease, cancer, chronic lower respiratory disease, nephritis, diabetes, Alzheimer's disease, and stroke (Bastard et al., 2006; Cao et al., 2011; Jha et al., 2009; Ferrucci et al., 2010; Singh and Newman, 2011; Kundu and Surh, 2008; Glorieux et al., 2009).

14.2.2 The Role of Inflammation in Heart Failure

In 1956 Elster SK et al. recorded a relation between inflammation and heart failure (HF) for the first time when they found a positive correlation between levels of C-reactive protein (CRP) and the severity of congestive HF (Elster, Braunwald & Wood, 1956). Later on, Levine et al. (1990) reported a positive correlation between tumour necrosis factor alpha (TNF α) and chronic HF (Levine et al., 1990). Research carried out since then has produced new data concerning the relation between many cytokines and HF. It seems that the HF syndrome is in large part due to an imbalance between increases in inflammatory and anti-inflammatory mediators.

14.2.3 Inflammatory Cytokines and HF

Numerous studies have reported the patho-genetic role of inflammation in HF, particularly the role of inflammatory cytokines. As per cytokine hypothesis (Figure 14.1), the development of HF is due to the damaging action of these factors and many of the pathogenetic consequences of HF are due to these inflammatory cytokines.

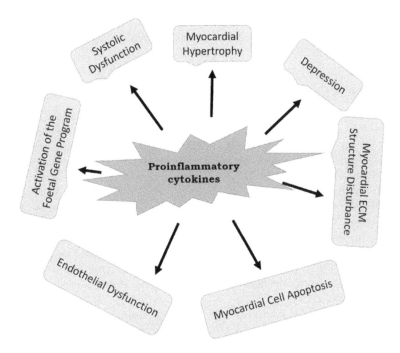

FIGURE 14.1 Pro-inflammatory cytokines: Pro-inflammatory cytokines participate in the pathogenesis and progression of HF by their action on cardiac and extra-cardiac tissues.

So far, two main classes of these cytokines have been identified in HF: (a) vasodepressor "pro-inflammatory" cytokines, such as TNF-α, IL-1, and IL-6 and (b) vasoconstrictor cytokines, such as endothelin-1 and big endothelin (Wei et al., 1994; Lerman et al., 1991; Seta et al., 1996). There is ample proof that overexpression of endothelin-1 in the heart may lead to progressive cardiac decompensation through myocytolysis, replacement fibrosis, and peripheral vasoconstriction, but the potential role for vasodepressor cytokines such as TNF-α, IL-1, and IL-6 has remained largely hypothetical, in large measure because of the lack of appropriate model systems to study the sustained effects of these cytokines on LV structure and function (Sakai et al., 1996; Kiowski et al., 1995).

14.2.4 Effect of Cytokines on LV Function

Recent studies indicate that inflammatory cytokines such as TNF-α, TNFR1, and IL-6 are related to echocardiographic indexes of both diastolic and systolic LV function (Chrysohoou et al., 2009; Valgimigli et al., 2005). A decrease of inflammatory cytokine effects on the myocardium prevents the progression to HF. Thus, blocking the action of nuclear factor-kappa B, a major agent that regulates inflammatory processes, appears to improve their LV systolic and diastolic function after the induction of MI in animals (Frantz et al., 2006; Kawano et al., 2006).

14.2.5 Effect of Cytokines on LV Remodelling

"Remodelling" is defined as the changes that happen in the composition, size, and shape of the heart wall (myocardium) in response to harmful injuries. In the process of ventricular remodeling, inflammatory cytokines exert significant effects.

Experimental evidence suggests that the deficiency of IL-1β and IL-18 reduces ventricular dilation after MI (Frantz et al., 2003). Also, it was observed that in animals that overexpress TNF-α, there is ventricular dilation and changes in collagen composition occurs (Diwan et al., 2004). Finally, the administration of IL-10 to animals caused a reduction in inflammatory processes and a reduction in ventricular remodelling after the induction of MI (Krishnamurthy et al., 2009). Similar action happens after blockage of nuclear factor-kappa B, when there is a relative inhibition of remodelling after experimentally induced MI (Frantz et al., 2006).

14.2.6 Association of Cytokine Gene Polymorphism with LVD

TNF-α G-308A Polymorphism: The TNF-α G-308A polymorphism is a single base pair polymorphism located at position 308 upstream of the TNF-α gene initiation site, resulting in substitution of the nucleotide adenine (A) for guanine (G) (Wilson et al., 1992). The TNF-308A allele is a more powerful transcriptional activator than the TNF-308G allele and results in a seven-fold increase in induced TNF-α gene transcription (Wilson et al., 1997). The TNF-308A allele also increases the sensitivity of white blood cells to endotoxin-stimulated white cell TNF-α production, which may be a significant source of TNF-α in more severe HF (Niebauer et al., 1999). Although there are data to suggest that the TNF-α G-308A polymorphism is not associated with TNF-α concentrations in HF (Ito et al., 2000; Kubota et al., 1998), the impact of the gene variant could still occur at a tissue level and subsequently modify cardiac effects.

NFKB1-94 ATTG ins/del Polymorphism: NFkB is a central integrator of stress response and cell survival pathways (Pahl, 1999). Its activation is observed in themyocardial tissue from HF patients of various etiologies suggesting that inflammatory pathways play an important role in the development of HF (Valen, Yan & Hansson, 2001).

Recently, two different in vitro studies observed that an insertion (ATTG2) of an ATTG sequence at position -94 of the promoter region of the *NFKB1* gene increases transcriptional activity compared to the allele with the deletion (ATTG1). A Chinese study suggested that -94 insertion/deletion ATTG polymorphism in NFKB1 is associated with congenital heart disease (Zhang et al., 2013). In three independent studies, totaling 1008, 428, and 439 cases, respectively, NFKB1 promoter variant was associated with a higher risk of CHD (Vogel et al., 2011). ATTG1/ATTG1 genotype may modulate risk of HF by increasing ventricular remodeling and worsening LV function (Mishra et al., 2013).

A study from our group reported that NFKB1 ATTG1/ATTG1 genotype was significantly associated with LVD (Fisher's method p-value = 0.007, Mantel–Haenszel OR = 2.34), LV end diastole (p-value = 0.013), end systole (p-value = 0.011) dimensions,L V mass (p-value = 0.024), mean LVEF (p-value = 0.001), and MI (p-value = 0.043). Our data suggests that NFKB1-94 ATTG ins/del polymorphism plays a significant role in conferring susceptibility of LVD.

14.3 Sarcomeric Proteins

A sarcomere is the fundamental unit of striated and cardiac muscle tissue. Muscle fibers are composed of tubular myofibrils. The myofibrils comprise sarcomeres, which appear as dark and light bands under the microscope. In one sarcomere unit, C-terminus of titin attaches to M-line and N-terminus of titin anchors to Z-disk, which spans a half sarcomere from the Z-disk to the center of the sarcomere. Titin anchor to Z-line by attaching both actin and myosin proteins. Myosin is in the center of the sarcomere while actin is cross-linked in the Z-lines and overlaps with myosin (Gregorio et al., 1998; Guo et al., 2010). During muscle contraction, calcium ions bind to TnC to generate a conformational change, finally allowing myosin binding on actin, leading to cross-bridge formation with the help of energy provided from adenosine triphosphate (ATP) hydrolysis (Hamdani et al., 2008; Gordon, Homsher & Regnier, 2000).

All muscle proteins show slow turnover and require replacement by new synthesis. Any deficiency of these proteins will result in the dysfunction of muscle contraction, which may result in HF.

14.3.1 Sarcomeric Cytoskeletal Proteins

14.3.1.1 Titin

Titin, also known as connectin, is a huge muscle protein expressed in vertebrate muscle. It is the largest protein and third most abundant sarcomeric protein with an average about 10% of myofibril mass (Wang, McClure & Tu, 1979; Maruyama, 1976). Titin spans the entire half of the sarcomere from Z-line to M-line, and two titin molecules form a continuous filament along the whole length of the sarcomere by overlapping at the M-line (Gregorio et al., 1998; Guo et al., 2010). The three elements of titin in the extensible I-band region are the key determinants of myocardial passive tension and play a major role in elastic recoil of the cardiac myocytes. These also contribute to diastolic function during LV filling phase (LeWinter and Granzier, 2014). These three elements are 1) tandem Ig segments consisting of serially linked immunoglobulin (Ig)-like domains, 2) the spring-like PEVK segment (with high percentages of proline, glutamic acid, valine, and lysine), and 3) the N2B element with its extensible unique sequence (N2B-Us) (Guo et al., 2010; LeWinter and Granzier, 2014; Bang et al., 2001).

Titin is coded by a single gene but distinct isoform classes result from alternate splicing of titin mRNAs (Bang et al., 2001). There are three major isoform classes in mammalian cardiac muscle (LeWinter and Granzier, 2014). The titin isoforms show development and function-specific expression. Alteration in the cardiac titin isoform expression ratios has been linked to cardiac disease. In animal models, a canine tachycardia-induced model of dilated cardiomyopathy (DCM) indicates increased N2B titin after two to four weeks of pacing (Wu et al., 2002). A spontaneously hypertensive rat model also showed a reduced ratio of N2BA/N2B titin in response to pressure overload (Warren et al., 2003). In humans, left ventricle biopsies from patients with diastolic HF had a reduced N2BA/N2B titin (van Heerebeek et al., 2006). Chronically ischemic LVs of CAD patients with congestive HF had nearly 50% N2BA titin (compared to total titin (N2BA+N2B) while approximately 30% N2BA was found in the LVs of control donor patients (Neagoe et al., 2002). Analysis of explanted nonischaemic human DCM hearts again demonstrated increased proportions of N2BA/N2B (Makarenko et al., 2004; Nagueh et al., 2004). Higher expression of compliant isoforms has also been found in patients with HF with preserved ejection fraction (HFpEF), a group accounting for about half of all HF cases and characterized by increased diastolic stiffness (Borbely et al., 2009; Borbely et al., 2005). Recently, a muscle-specific splicing factor, RNA binding motif 20 (Rbm20), was reported to regulate titin alternative splicing (Guo et al., 2012). The Rbm20-deficient rats express largest titin isoform (~3.83Mda) and develop DCM (Guo et al., 2013; Guo et al., 2012; Li et al., 2013), which was confirmed by studies on Rbm20 knockout mice (Methawasin et al., 2014). RBM20 mutations in patients with severe DCM also lead to the expression of the larger, compliant fetal cardiac titin isoform (Guo et al., 2012).

14.3.1.2 *Myosin Binding Protein-C*

Myosin binding protein-C (MyBP-C) is a thick filament-associated protein localized to the cross-bridge containing C zones of striated (and cardiac) muscle sarcomeres, where it binds to myosin and titin. Titin act as a molecular ruler of the sarcomeric proteins (Whiting, Wardale & Trinick 1989), and MyBP-C as a spatially defined regulatory protein (Craig and Offer, 1976; Gautel et al., 1995; Hartzell and Glass, 1984; Schlender and Bean, 1991). Myosin, MyBP-C, and titin form a stable ternary complex (Okagaki et al., 1993). There are multiple genes of MYBP-C. In adult striated muscle, there are three isoforms of MyBP-C. The fsMyBP-C is the fast skeletal isoform encoded by gene MYBPC2 in human. The ssMyBP-C is the slow form in skeletal muscle encoded by MYBPC1 (Weber et al., 1993). Human cardiac MyBP-C (cMyBP-C) is encoded by gene MYBPC3 (Gautel et al., 1995). The fast and slow skeletal muscle isoforms can be co-expressed in the same sarcomeres (Dhoot et al., 1985). However, the cardiac isoform is expressed only in cardiac muscle throughout development, and the cardiac isoform of MyBP-C cannot be trans-complemented by skeletal MyBP-Cs (Gautel et al., 1998). The mutation-caused truncated cardiac MyBP-C isoforms have been a cause of hypertrophic cardiomyopathy (Ackermann and Kontrogianni-Konstantopoulos, 2011; Flashman et al., 2004; James and Robbins, 2011; Oakley et al., 2004; Sadayappan and de Tombe, 2014). Since MyBP-C undergoes reversible phosphorylation by cyclic AMP-dependent protein kinase and calcium/calmodulin-dependent protein kinase II, its role in the adrenergic regulation of cardiac contraction has also been suggested (McClellan, Kulikovskaya & Winegrad, 2001; Sadayappan et al., 2006).

14.3.2 Genetic Polymorphisms in Sarcomeric Genes and LVD

Due to the importance of sarcomere genes in heart function, Kumar et al. (2016) selected four important genetic variants from four different sarcomeric genes (Table 14.1) to explore the role of three common variants of sarcomeric genes, namely MYBPC3 25 bp deletion, TTN 18 bp I/D, TNNT2 5bp I/D, and Myosprn K2906N gene in the development of LVD in CAD patients.

MYBPC3: A common polymorphic intronic deletion of 25-base-pair in *MYBPC3* at the 3′ region of the gene has been reported to be associated with DCM and HCM in populations of Southeast Asia (Dhandapany et al., 2009). The deletion located in intron 32 causes skipping of the downstream exon 33 and results in incorporation of missense amino acids at C-terminal region of cardiac MYBPC3 (Dhandapany et al., 2009). The deletion is present in 2–6% of individuals in Indian populations with high incidence of cardiac diseases in India. In case control association studies, we observed significant association of MYBPC3 25 bp gene deletion with CAD. MYBPC3 25 bp deletion is significantly associated with high risk of LVD (non-LVD vs. LVD: OR=1.62, p-value=0.033; and controls vs. LVD: OR=3.83, p-value < 0.001) (Kumar et al., 2016; Table 14.2).

On further analysis, a significant association of this deletion polymorphism was seen with severity of LVD as significantly higher percentage of deletion genotype was found in the patients in groups LVEF = 31-40% and below 31%. Moreover, in-depth analysis of different clinical characteristics showed that this deletion polymorphism is not only associated with EF but also with other echocardiographic parameters such as LV end diastole dimension (LVEDD) and LV end systolic dimension (LVESD). All these results strongly support the hypothesis that MYBPC3 25 bp deletion allele is associated with LVD. Multivariate analysis results confirm that MYBPC3 25 bp deletion allele may be alone or in combination with other factors such as hypertension be responsible for development of LVD in CAD patients, and ruled out any possibilities of involvement of confounding factors such as smoking, diabetes, hypertension, and STEMI (ST-elevation MI). On evaluating other factors of LV remodeling, patients with MYBPC3 25 bp deletion genotype had significantly higher LV end systolic and diastolic dimensions, which shows that the patients with DW genotype were at higher risk of developing LV remodeling (Tables 14.3-14.5).

Previous studies also established that cardiac MyBP-C plays an important role in the genesis of cardiac muscle disorders (Dhandapany et al., 2009). The 25-bp intronic deletion results in skipping of exon 33 and incorporation of missense of amino acids at the C-terminal (Dhandapany et al., 2009; Waldmuller et al., 2003). The mutated protein may cause breakdown of sarcomere byintegration in the myofibrils (Dhandapany et al., 2009). Moreover, on interpreting the protein model, we found that the 25-bp gene deletion disturbs the alpha helical section in the cMyBP-C and further there is integration of an additional alpha helix as well as extra β-pleated sheets in the mutated protein. Since cardiac MyBP-C C8, C9, and C10 domains are known to directly bind to a subset of Ig domains of titin/connectin and also to myosin any conformational changes in the mutated protein may result in change of direction or conformation of the C10 domain, which is very important for myosin filament binding. Lack of myosin binding may

TABLE 14.1

Candidate Genes and Genetic Variants Related to Genes Encoding Sarcomeric Proteins

Gene	Position	Polymorphism	Functional Role
MYBPC3	11p11.2	25bp Ins/del	MYBPC3 mutationsare associated with heritable cardiomyopathies
Myospryn	5q14.1	K2906N	Myospryn K2906N(rs6859595) polymorphism is shown to associate with left ventricular hypertrophy, cardiac adaptation in response to pressure overload, and left ventricular diastolic dysfunction in hypertensive patients
TTN	2q31	18bp Ins/del	18-bp deletion within the PEVK region that regulates extensibility of titin
TNNT2	1q32	5bp Ins/del	5bp (CTTCT) polypyrimidine tract deletion in intron 3 of the TNNT2 affect the branch site selection and splicing.

TABLE 14.2

Sarcomeric Gene Polymorphisms Analysis in Healthy Controls, CAD And LVD Patients

Genotypes	Controls (300)	CAD (988)	Non-LVD (LVEF ≥ 45%)	LVD (LVEF < 45%)	OR (95% CI) p-value[a]	OR (95% CI) p-value[b]	OR (95% CI) p-value[c]	OR (95% CI) p-value[d]
***MYBPC3* 25 bp deletion**								
WW	287 (95.7)	898 (90.9)	676 (92.0)	222 (87.7)	-	-	-	-
DW+DD	13 (4.3)	90 (9.1)	59 (8.0)	31 (12.3)	**2.29 (1.21-4.33) 0.011**	1.87 (0.96-3.64) 0.065	**3.83 (1.83-8.12) < 0.001**	**1.62 (1.04-2.62) 0.033**
***TTN*18 bp I/D Polymorphism**								
II	287 (95.7)	951 (96.3)	707 (96.2)	244 (96.4)	-	-	-	-
ID+DD	13 (4.3)	37 (3.7)	28 (3.8)	9 (3.6)	1.00 (0.51-1.98) 0.994	0.99 (0.49-2.02) 0.998	0.91 (0.36-2.29) 0.847	0.97 (0.45-2.11) 0.949
***TNNT2* 5bp I/D Polymorphism**								
II	57 (19.0)	223 (22.6)	172 (23.4)	51 (20.2)	-	-	-	-
ID	153 (51.0)	454 (45.9)	339 (46.1)	115 (45.5)	1.19 (0.82-1.75) 0.362	0.82 (0.56-1.20) 0.310	0.93 (0.57-1.53) 0.780	0.85 (0.58-1.24) 0.396
DD	90 (30.0)	311 (31.5)	224 (30.5)	87 (34.4)	1.34 (0.90-2.00) 0.147	0.82 (0.54-1.24)0.347	0.99 (0.58-1.67) 0.967	0.87 (0.58-1.31) 0.510
***Myospryn* K2906N polymorphism**								
AA	245 (81.7)	810 (82.0)	606 (82.4)	204 (80.6)	-	-	-	-
AC+CC	55 (18.3)	178 (18.0)	129 (17.6)	49 (19.4)	0.94 (0.65-1.34) 0.715	0.93 (0.65-1.34) 0.715	1.03 (0.65-1.64) 0.911	1.18 (0.82-1.71) 0.368

Significant values are shown in bold

p-value [a] = p-value between healthy controls and CAD

p-value [b] = p-value between healthy controls and Non-LVD

p-value [c] = p-value between healthy controls and LVD

p-value [d] = p-value between Non-LVD and LVD

TABLE 14.3

Left Ventricular Ejection Fraction (LVEF) Subgroup-Based Analysis of MYBPC3 25 bp Deletion Polymorphism

Genotype ↓	> 55% N(%)	51–55%, N(%)	46–50%, N(%)	41–45%, N(%)	31–40%, N(%)	< 31% N (%)	p-value
WW	224 (24.8%)	152 (16.8%)	229 (25.6%)	87 (9.7%)	141 (15.6%)	65 (7.3%)	-
DW+DD	12 (13.3%)	14 (15.5%)	28 (31.1%)	5 (5.5%)	21 (23.3%)	10 (11.1%)	**0.035**

LVEF subgroups →

Significant value is shown in bold

TABLE 14.4

Comparative Analysis of *MYBPC3* 25 bp Deletion in CAD Patients with Clinical Attributes

Clinical Characteristics	WW N (%)	DW+DD N (%)	p-value
Patients	898(90.89)	90(0.09)	-
*Age (in years) at CAD diagnosis	56.14 ± 9.10	56.70 ± 9.52	0.58
Male	793 (88.3)	74(82.2)	0.12
Risk Factors			
Hypertensive	395 (44.3)	42 (46.6)	0.65
Diabetes	301 (33.5)	33 (36.7)	0.56
Smoking	228 (25.4)	30 (33.3)	0.10
*BMI, kg/m^2	24.27±3.12	24.78±2.75	0.45
Myocardial Infarction (MI)	501(55.8)	42 (46.7)	0.11
Angiographic Profiles			
Single vessel disease	500 (55.7)	43 (47.8)	-
Double vessel disease	177 (19.7)	23 (25.6)	-
Triple vessel disease	221 (24.6)	24 (26.7)	0.29
*Echocardiographic traits			
LV end diastole dimension (mm)	44.66±6.91	46.46±5.82	**0.03**
LV end systolic dimension (mm)	32.74±5.64	34.90±6.12	**0.03**
LV posterior wall thickness (mm)	9.56±1.41	9.61±1.22	0.79
LV intraventricular septum (mm)	9.87±1.63	9.82±1.35	0.84
LV mass (gm)	152.41±47.59	168.20±47.03	0.10
LV ejection fraction	49.24±10.10	46.40±10.18	**0.01**
Reduced LVEF (< 45%)	222(24.7)	31(34.4)	**0.03**

Significant values are shown in bold

LVD – Left Ventricular Dysfunction, MI – Myocardial Infarction, STEMI – ST elevation MI,*
Values are mean ± SD

cause severe effects on sarcomere incompetence suggesting its involvement in the morphological and functional changes of cardiac muscle.

Several other mechanisms have also been suggested to describe pathogenesis of cardiac muscle due to truncated and missense MyBP-C such as haplo-insufficiency and poison peptides. The mutant MYBPC3 mRNA may go through nonsense-mediated mRNA decay. It has been suggested that these missense

TABLE 14.5

Multivariate Analysis of LVD and Non-LVD Patients

Genotypes	Non-LVD	LVD	OR (95%CI)	p-value	FDR p_{corr}
Nonsmoker CAD patients					
WW	522 (92.9)	148 (88.1)	Reference	-	-
DW+DD	40 (7.1)	20 (11.9)	1.83 (1.04-3.25)	**0.038**	**0.044**
Nondiabetic CAD patients					
WW	460 (92.7)	137 (86.7)	Reference	-	-
DW+DD	36 (7.3)	21 (13.3)	2.06 (1.16-3.67)	**0.014**	**0.040**
Normotensive CAD patients					
WW	372 (92.1)	131 (89.1)	Reference	-	-
DW+DD	32 (7.9)	16 (10.9)	1.51 (0.79-2.87)	0.207	-
Non-STEMI CAD patients					
WW	455 (91.2)	91 (84.3)	Reference	-	-
DW+DD	44 (8.8)	17 (15.7)	2.06 (1.12-3.79)	**0.020**	**0.040**
Nondiabetic and non-STEMI CAD patients					
WW	296 (91.9)	50 (84.7)	Reference	-	-
DW+DD	26 (8.1)	9 (15.3)	2.22 (0.96-5.06)	0.052	0.052
Nonsmoker and non-STEMI CAD patients					
WW	352 (92.1)	57 (82.6)	Reference	-	-
DW+DD	30 (7.9)	12 (17.4)	2.70 (1.29-5.66)	**0.008**	**0.040**
Nondiabetic and nonsmoker CAD patients					
WW	348 (94.1)	88 (88.0)	Reference	-	-
DW+DD	22 (5.9)	12 (12.0)	2.31 (1.09-4.90)	**0.029**	**0.040**
CAD patients without STEMI, Diabetes, and Smoking					
WW	224 (93.7)	32 (84.2)	Reference	-	-
DW+DD	15 (6.3)	6 (15.8)	3.26 (1.15-9.23)	**0.026**	**0.040**
CAD patients without STEMI, Diabetes, Smoking, and Hypertensive					
WW	135 (93.8)	22 (84.6)	Reference	-	-
DW+DD	9 (6.2)	4 (15.4)	3.34 (0.91-12.22)	0.069	-

Significant values are shown in bold, OR – odds ratio, CI – confidence interval

MYBPC3 mutations uses an ubiquitin-proteasome system (UPS) to destabilize its proteins, which may contribute to cardiac dysfunction (Sarikas et al., 2005). Also, taking into consideration the decline in function of the UPS with age and oxidative stress (Bulteau, Szweda & Friguet, 2002; Okada K, 1999) the mutated protein may simply accumulate, disrupt the cellular homeostasis, and initiate LVD.

It is quite interesting that the MYBPC3 25-bp deletion is relatively common in South Asia and its frequency varies across this limited region. The time to the most recent common ancestor (TMRCA) estimate, based on previous haplotype analysis, is ~33,000 (−/+23,000) years (Dhandapany et al., 2009), suggesting that the deletion might have arisen in India and was possibly not present in the initial inhabitants that arrived in this region from Africa some 50,000 to 20,000 years ago (Simonson et al., 2010). It is somewhat surprising that a deleterious mutation would be found at such a high frequency. The carrier frequency of 2–8% gradation from North to South India suggests that this variation may contribute significantly to the burden of cardiac diseases in the subcontinent.

Some single nucleotide polymorphisms in TNNT2 and TTN genes have been studied with different cardiac remodelling phenotypes. A 5bp I/D polymorphism in intron 3 of TNNT2 gene has been clinically assessed in relation to cardiac hypertrophy (Komamura et al., 2004). The authors reported that the DD genotype of above was associated with a larger LV mass and wall thickness in the hypertrophy population.

The deletion allele frequency was considerably higher in the hypertrophy population as compared with the healthy controls. However, in contrast, there was no significant association reported in cardiac hypertrophy (Farza et al., 1998). Rani et al. (2012) reported that 5 bp deletion polymorphism was found to be significantly higher in HCM patients, which results in skipping of exon 4 during splicing. A study by Nakagami et al. (2007) reported the possible association between myospryn polymorphisms and cardiac hypertrophy. The authors established that AA genotype in K2906N was a risk allele in left ventricle diastolic dysfunction in hypertensive patients (Nakagami et al., 2007).

In order to explore the association of titin, troponin T2, and myosporin gene deletion polymorphisms, we carried out a case control association study involving 988 consecutive patients with angiographically confirmed CAD and 300 healthy controls. Among the 988 CAD patients, 253 with reduced left ventricle ejection fraction (LVEF $\leq$4 5%) were categorized as LVD. We selected titin (TTN) 18 bp I/D, troponin T type 2 (TNNT2) 5 bp I/D, and myospryn K2906N polymorphisms for our study. Our results suggested that TTN 18 bp I/D, TNNT2 5 bp I/D, and myospryn K2906N polymorphisms do not show any significant association with LVD. Thus, among sarcomeric gene polymorphisms, MYBPC3 25-bp deletion polymorphism is significantly associated with LVD, while TTN, TNNT2, and myosporin genetic variants do not seem to play a significant role in conferring LVD as well as CAD risk in north Indian population.

14.4 Signalling Pathway

14.4.1 Renin-Angiotensin-Aldosterone System

The renin-angiotensin-aldosterone system (RAAS) plays a vital role in regulating the physiological processes of the cardiovascular system (van Berlo and Pinto, 2003). It does not only function as an endocrine system, but in tissues and organs, it also serves local paracrine and autocrine functions. Angiotensin II (ANG II), which is the primary effector molecule of this system, has emerged as a critical hormone that affects the functions of almost all organs, and it has both positive and pathological effects. ANG II regulates salt/water homeostasis and vasoconstriction, modulating blood pressure with acute stimulation, though with chronic stimulus, it promotes hyperplasia and hypertrophy of vascular smooth muscle cells (Geisterfer, Peach & Owens, 1988; Xi et al., 1999). In addition, long-term exposure to ANG II influences cardiac hypertrophy and remodeling. RAAS is a candidate for modifying expression of left ventricular hypertrophy (LVH) because it has a regulatory role in cardiac function, blood pressure, and electrolyte homeostasis and hence maintains vascular tone and cardiovascular remodeling (Griendling, Murphy & Alexander, 1993; Johnston, 1992). This system is one of the major neuroendocrine axes involved in the development of cardiac failure. Thus, inhibition of this RAAS system has important therapeutic effects. Angiotensin converting enzyme inhibitors have a dual mechanism. Primarily, they inhibit the conversion of ANG I to ANG II and hence reduce vasoconstriction and cell proliferation. Furthermore, they inhibit the metabolism of bradykinin and thus increase the production of prostaglandins and nitric oxide.

14.4.1.1 Components of RAAS

The RAAS is composed of a cascade of hormones initially triggered by the release of renin from the kidney (Figure 14.2) (Perazella and Setaro, 2003). Renin is a proteolytic enzyme that has a local action in the kidney as well as the substrate angiotensinogen, which is a protein precursor that is produced in and secreted by the liver. Angiotensinogen is cleaved by renin to form the biologically inactive peptide angiotensin I (AngI). This circulating decapeptide is then efficiently converted to the active octapeptide angiotensin II (AngII) by angiotensin-converting enzyme (ACE). ACE is a tissue-based zinc metalloprotease. AngII is produced in a number of organs, largely from locally generated AngI. Two well-characterized subtypes of AngII receptors mediate the major physiologic actions of AngII in humans: these have been termed angiotensin type 1 (AT1) and angiotensin type 2 (AT2) receptors. Both receptors are G-coupled polypeptides. In the human body, the AT1 receptors are more widely distributed and thus more important than the AT2 receptors. Stimulation of either the AT1 or the AT2 receptor results in activation of

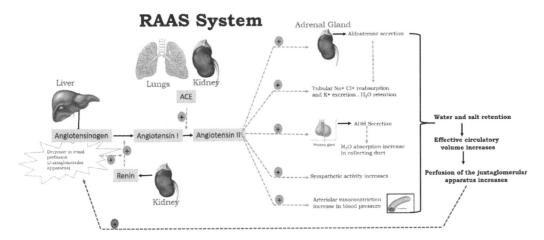

FIGURE 14.2   Renin-angiotensin-aldosterone system (RAAS): Renin, normally secreted in response to underperfusion of the kidneys, cleaves the decapeptide Angiotensin I from angiotensinogen, and Angiotensin I is converted to Angiotensin II by ACE. The red dashed line indicates feedback inhibition of renin secretion. ACE=Angiotensin converting enzyme.

different signal transduction pathways, which results in antagonizing effects. For example, AngII, stimulating the AT1 receptor, is a potent vasoconstrictor, whereas AT2 receptor stimulation by AngII results in vasodilatation. In addition to its vasoconstriction and other effects, AngIIcan activate AT1 receptors in the adrenal gland, which results in synthesis of the steroid hormone aldosterone (Atlas, 2007). It is generally accepted that excessive stimulation of the AT1 receptor by AngII results in unfavorable effects, whereas stimulation of the AT2 receptor is beneficial. The overall effect of activation of the RAAS is an increase in effective circulating volume, resulting in an increase in perfusion of the juxtaglomerular apparatus. Through this phenomenon, the release of renin by the kidney is inhibited by feedback mechanism.

In the adrenal cortex, aldosterone is synthesized from deoxy-corticosterone by a mitochondrial cytochrome P450 enzyme, aldosterone synthase (CYP11B2) (Curnow et al., 1991). Aldosterone helps to regulate blood pressure by controlling sodium balance and intravascular volume (White, 1994). Mutations in CYP11B2 gene can cause aldosterone deficiency (Pascoe, Curnow, Slutsker, Rosler, et al., 1992). Therefore, any genetic variation in the aldosterone synthesis pathway might impact on the structure and function of the left ventricle. Conversely, an inherited form of hypertension, glucocorticoid-suppressible hyperaldosteronism, is caused by genetic recombination between CYP11B1 and CYP11B2, which increases expression of CYP11B2 and leads to inappropriate secretion of aldosterone (Lifton, Dluhy, Powers, Rich, Gutkin, et al., 1992; Pascoe, Curnow, Slutsker, Connell, et al., 1992; Lifton, Dluhy, Powers, Rich, Cook, et al., 1992). Therefore, it is plausible that polymorphisms in CYP11B2 might affect aldosterone biosynthesis and thus perhaps influence LV mass or size. On the basis of this information, some researchers have analyzed the aldosterone synthase gene for more frequent genetic polymorphisms in LVD (Kupari et al., 1998).

14.4.1.2 RAAS Gene Polymorphisms

ACE I/Dgene Polymorphisms
The ACE gene is located on chromosome 17q23. The intron 16 of the ACE gene shows I/D polymorphism, which contains an insertion (I) and deletion (D) (i.e., the presence or absence of 287 bpAlu repeat). Serum ACE levels have been found to be higher in homozygotes for the deletion allele (DD) in comparison to those homozygous for the insertion allele (II); however, intermediate levels have been found in heterozygotes (ID). Subjects with the DD genotype have higher cardiac ACE activity (Danser et al., 1995, Tiret et al., 1992, Rigat et al., 1990). After MI, if early treatment of ACE inhibitor is given, it decreases the chance of adverse remodeling of the left ventricle, the incidence of HF, and mortality (Borghi, Cicero & Ambrosioni 2008; Kober et al., 1995; Pfeffer et al., 1992; Ertl et al., 1982).

14.4.1.3 ACE I/D Polymorphism and LV Remodeling after MI

Ischemic heart disease is one of the most frequent causes of dilated cardiomyopathy. When the ACE gene was cloned and the association between the polymorphism of this gene and the levels of angiotensin II was recognized, any possible association of this genetic variant with CVD was tested. In a French multicenter study designed to identify variants of candidate genes predisposing to MI, the association of the ACE polymorphism with ischemic heart disease was documented for the first time (Cambien et al., 1992). Cambien et al. (1992) reported that the DD genotype was significantly more frequent in patients with MI than in controls, especially among subjects with low body mass index and low levels of Apo lipoprotein (Cambien et al., 1992). Several smaller studies found an increased risk of LV enlargement or remodeling among individuals with the ID/DD genotype after MI (Ulgen et al., 2007; Palmer et al., 2003; Nagashima et al., 1999; Ohmichi et al., 1996;, Pinto et al., 1995); others were negative, but in the presence of ACEI therapy (Zee et al., 2002). Several studies of CVD phenotypes have suggested that the D allele from the insertion/deletion (I/D) polymorphism within the ACE gene confers increased risk for CVD including LVH (Montgomery, 1997; Perticone et al., 1997; Iwai et al., 1994, Soubrier, Nadaud & Williams, 1994; Schunkert et al., 1994; Evans et al., 1994) while various contrasting studies showed no association with D allele (Lindpaintner et al., 1996). One study also reported that the *ACE* I/D polymorphism was associated with the development of Lvdys function in the acute phase after STEMI (Parenica et al., 2010).

14.4.1.4 ACE I/D Polymorphism and HF Severity and Progression

To assess whether the ACE *DD* genotype is a risk factor for the development of end-stage HF due to cardiomyopathy, a study found the ACE genotype in 214 patients with end-stage failure caused by ischemic (n=102) and oridiopathic (n=112) DCM and compared these genotypes of 79 organ donors with normally functioning hearts. The results suggested that an ACE gene variant may contribute to the pathogenesis of both types of cardiomyopathy (Raynolds et al., 1993). Other studies did not confirm these results (Vancura et al., 1999; Montgomery et al., 1995). Notwithstanding a limited sample size, Candy et al. (1999) documented inpatients with idiopathic DCM, an effect of the ACEgene *ID* variants, on LV systolic performance and dimensions in 171 consecutive patients in NYHA functional class II or III. The results of this study indicate that the DD genotype of the ACE gene is independently associated with both a reduced LV systolic performance and an increased LV cavity size in patients with idiopathic DCM (Candy et al., 1999). Probably the higher circulating angiotensin II concentrations associated with the ACEgene deletion polymorphism may influence LV remodeling through either direct myocardial or load-induced effects (Ueda et al., 1995). Possible reasons include a role for the insertion sequence as a silencer motif, which could invalidate the action of a possible other polymorphism (Hunley et al., 1996), or that the absence of this sequence is in linkage disequilibrium with an as yet unidentified polymorphism of the ACE or another gene that controls ACE expression (Montgomery et al., 1995).

14.4.1.5 AT1 A1166C Gene Polymorphism

AT1 A1166C gene polymorphism is located in the 3' untranslated region (3' UTR) of the angiotensin II receptor type 1 gene *AT1*, which is also known as *AGTR1*, AT2R1, or AT1R. It is among the most studied of over 50 SNPs in *AT1* gene.

    AT1 A1166C has been characterized and investigated in relation to arterial hypertension (Kikuya et al., 2003; Ono et al., 2003), hypertension-induced hypertrophy (Takami et al., 1998), aortic stiffness (Benetos et al., 1996), MI (Tiret et al., 1994; Nakauchi et al., 1996), and carotid intimal-medial thickening (Chapman et al., 2001). Since the +1166 A/C polymorphism does not appear to be functional, it is postulated to be a genetic marker or in linkage disequilibrium with an unidentified functional locus, which would affect the regulation of the gene in response to Ang II. Moreover, various studies have also focused on other locus of *AT1* gene (Lajemi et al., 2001; Takahashi et al., 2000; Erdmann et al., 1999; Zhang et al., 2000; Poirier et al., 1998). The *AT1*1166C allele is associated with increased risk for essential hypertension in Caucasian populations (Wang, Zee & Morris, 1997; Bonnardeaux et al., 1994). There are likely to be ethnic differences in risk; while the *AT1*1166C allele was associated with hypertension in a Chinese population (Jiang et al., 2001), it was not observed as a risk in a Japanese population (Ono et al., 2003). Age and gender may also influence risk, as discussed in a review of *AT1* single nucleotide polymorphisms (SNPs) and their role in hypertension and related disorders (Baudin, 2005).

Pregnant women who are A1166C rs5186(C) allele carriers are more likely to develop pregnancy-induced hypertension (Nalogowska-Glosnicka et al., 2000). However, *AT1* A1166C does not appear to modify risk for developing coronary heart disease (CHD). A literature-based meta-analysis of over 20,000 CHD cases concluded that there were no significant associations of AT1 A1166C gene polymorphism in CHD (Xu et al., 2010).

14.4.1.6 *CYP11B2 T-344C Gene Polymorphisms*

CYP11B2 T-344C gene polymorphism is located in the promoter region of the Aldosterone synthase gene, CYP11B2. Takai et al. (2002) showed that CYP11B2 T-344C gene polymorphism is significantly associated with LV volume in patients with DCM (Takai et al., 2002), while Tiret and colleagues reported that T-344C polymorphism was not associated with severity of DCM (Tiret et al., 2000). This discrepancy may be due to either the difference of methods used for the evaluation of the disease severity, or ethnic differences. A Finnish population sample of 84 persons (44 women) aged 36 to 37 years was studied by M-mode and Doppler echocardiography to assess LV size, mass, and function. In another study, CYP11B2 promoter polymorphism reported statistically significant variations in LV end-diastolic diameter, end-systolic diameter, and LV mass. All these effects were independent of potentially confounding factors, like-physical activity, smoking, ethanol consumption, sex, body size, and blood pressure. Genotype groups also differed in a measure of LV diastolic function, the heart rate-adjusted atrial filling fraction (Kupari et al., 1998). However, in another study no association was found between a polymorphism of the aldosterone synthase gene and LV structure (Schunkert et al., 1999).

14.4.1.7 *Genetic Polymorphisms in RAAS and LVD*

Since the range of physiologic effects of ACE, AT1 and CYP11B2, genetic variations that affect baseline RAAS activity, are candidates for increasing risk of and adverse outcomes in heart disease and could probably affect a wide variety of clinical phenotypes. Therefore, we carried out a study to assess the association of ACE insertion/deletion (ACE I/D rs4340), AT1 (A1166C rs5186), and CYP11B2 (T-344C rs1799998) polymorphisms with LVD in CAD patients (Mishra et al., 2012b). Our results showed that ACE I/D was significantly associated with CAD but not with the LVD subgroup. The AT1 1166C variant was significantly associated with LVD (LVEF 45) (p value = 0.013; OR = 3.69). However, CYP11B2 (rs1799998) was not associated with either CAD or LVD (Mishra et al., 2012b).

Earlier it was reported that A1166C polymorphism is located within the target sites of miRNA binding (Sethupathy et al., 2007). With the help of reporter silencing assays, it was reported that miR155 downregulates the expression of AT1 gene only with the 1166A allele, and not with the 1166C allele. With 1166C allele, AT1 expression increases, resulting in arteriolar vasoconstriction and increased blood pressure, which finally results in reduced cardiac output. It has also been reported that AT1 receptor density increases in MI (Maczewski, Maczewska & Duda, 2008). The higher expression of AT1 receptors with 1166C allele may lead to higher susceptibility for MI, which may later progress to LVD.

14.4.2 β-Adrenergic Signalling Pathway

Sympathetic activation plays a vital role in cardiovascular homeostasis. In disease conditions such as hypertension, ischemic heart disease, and congestive HF, catecholamine stimulation of β-adrenoceptors has numerous adverse effects. β-blockers have been used as an effective therapy for hypertension, ischemic heart disease, and congestive HF (Bristow, 2000).

Adrenergic receptors are divided into α- and β-adrenergic receptors. adrenergic receptors are mediators of cardiomyocyte hypertrophy, whereas α2-adrenergic receptors are presynaptic inhibitors of norepinephrine release (Port and Bristow, 2001). β1- and β2-adrenergic receptors increase cardiac inotropy and chronotropy, and the β1-receptor are the dominant subtype (Liggett, 2000c). In HF, chronic sympathetic activation leads to selective downregulation of β1-adrenergic receptors and uncoupling of β1- and β2-adrenergic receptors, markedly blunting both signaling pathways (Port and Bristow, 2001). Therefore, it can be hypothesized that genetic variants of adrenergic receptors may also play a role in HF. In addition, β-adrenergic receptor blockers have been found to improve symptoms and mortality in HF, albeit with substantial inter-individual variation (Liggett, 2000c).

14.4.2.1 β1-Adrenoceptor

Due to their predominance in the normal and failing myocardium, recent work has focused on the genetic diversity of β1-ARs. The two most common polymorphisms are Ser49> Gly and Arg389> Gly (Maqbool et al., 1999). The relative allele frequency for the Arg389> Gly variant is approximately 0.70/0.30 and for the Ser49> Gly polymorphism 0.85/0.15. As well as the two most common variants, multiple amino acid polymorphisms have been documented for the β1-receptor including Ala59> Ser, Arg399> Cys, His402> Arg, Thr404> Ala, and Pro418> Ala. The codon 49 polymorphism is located in the extracellular domain of the receptor, and no reports have addressed its potential functional significance. In contrast, amino acid 389 is located near the carboxyl-terminus cytoplasmic tail, and in vitro studies demonstrate a higher basal adenylcyclase activity with the Arg389 receptor. With agonist stimulation this distinction was greatly magnified, suggesting that the Arg389 variant results in a gain of function in terms of G-protein coupling (Mason et al., 1999).

14.4.2.2 β2-Adrenoceptor

Recent investigations have focused on the β2-AR, because of its importance in the pharmacologic treatment of asthma (Hall, 1996; Liggett, 2000b). Sequencing of the β2-AR in populations revealed four polymorphisms that result in amino acid substitution: Arg16> Gly, Glu27> Gln,Val34> Met, and Thr164> Ile. The Met34 variant is extremely rare and found in less than 1% in populations. In vitro studies of the three more common polymorphisms demonstrate significant functional consequences in terms of receptor function or regulation (Liggett, 1998).

The Ile164 receptor has a significantly lower binding affinity for epinephrine, norepinephrine, and isoproterenol (Green et al., 1993). The change of Ile for Thr occurs with a minor allele frequency of approximately 3 to 5% of the general population. Agonist stimulation studies also suggest a much lower level of adenylcyclase activity with the Ile164 variant. The data from murine models appear consistent with in vitro studies, as transgenic mice that overexpress the Ile164 receptor in the heart have a decrease in resting and agonist-stimulated contractile function in vivo when compared with transgenic controls overexpressing the wild-type Thr164 receptor (Turki et al., 1996).

The most common polymorphisms are at position 16 (Arg16> Gly, allele frequency approximately 0.40/0.60) and position 27 (Gln27> Glu, allele frequency approximately 0.55/0.45). Neither polymorphism appears to influence agonist binding affinity nor coupling to Gs protein; however, both appear to affect receptor downregulation. Agonist stimulation of β-receptors generally results in downregulation or a reduction in the number of available receptors. Studies of agonist stimulation of cultured cells reveal that Gly16 receptors have a greater reduction in receptor number or enhanced downregulation when compared with Arg16. In contrast, the Glu27 receptor appears to be resistant to downregulation when compared with the Gln27variant (Green et al., 1995).

14.4.2.3 Adnergic Receptors and Congestive HF

β-adrenergic signaling plays an important role in the development of the HF syndrome, and use of adrenoceptor blockade improves survival. These facts led researchers to take much interest in the effects of β-AR variants in HF progression. In a study of 259 patients with class II to class IV HF, it was found that the presence of the Ile164 receptor polymorphism markedly decreased transplant-free survival, with a relative risk of death or transplant of 4.8 as compared to those homozygous for Thr164 (Liggett et al., 1998). The polymorphisms at amino acid positions 16 and 27 had no effect on HF survival. The data from the same population revealed a marked reduction in functional capacity, as measured by metabolic stress

TABLE 14.6

Frequency and Function of β1- and β2-Adrenoceptor Polymorphisms

(A)

Codon	Region	Polymorphism	Minor Allele frequency (Humma et al., 2001, Liggett 2000a)	Function in vitro	Ref.
Β1-adrenoceptor					
389	Cytoplasmic	Arg/Gly	0.30	Gly389 = gain of function (↑cAMP)	(Mason et al., 1999)
49	Extracellular	Ser/Gly	0.15	No data	
β2-adrenoceptor					
16	Extracellular	Arg/Gly	0.60	Gly16 = enhanced downregulation	(Green et al., 1995)
27	Extracellular	Gln/Glu	0.45	Glu27 = resistance to downregulation	(Green et al., 1995)
164	Transmembrane domain	Thr/Ile	0.05	Ile164 = loss of function (↓ agonist binding, ↓ cAMP)	(Green et al., 1993)

testing, among patients with the Ile164 and a more modest reduction for patients with Gly16 (Badenhorst et al., 2007). A study of normal Thr164/Ile heterozygotes demonstrated blunted agonist responsiveness compared with individuals homozygous for Thr164 (Brodde et al., 2001; Feldman, 2001), which may underlie the negative impact of the Ile164 variant on HF survival. Recently, the effects of the Ile164 variant on transplant-free survival were re-evaluated in 458 patients at the University of Pittsburgh, and this analysis confirmed the negative impact initially reported; it appears this may be reduced by β-blocker therapy (McNamara, MacGowan & London, 2002).

14.4.2.4 β1-Adrenoceptor Variants and LVD

Functional Variation
We conducted a hospital-based case-control study (600 CAD patients and 200 controls) to investigate the role of adrenergic receptor (ADR) gene variants in susceptibility of LVD risk in CAD patients in North Indian population. The studied ADR gene polymorphisms with their locations, rs numbers, and functional roles are given in Table 14.7.

On comparing the genotype frequency distribution in CAD patients with that of controls, no significant difference was observed in the distribution of ADRA2A C-1291G and ADRB1 C1165G polymorphisms both at the genotypic and allelic level. However, on comparing the frequency distribution of ADRB3 T190C in CAD patients and healthy controls, significant association was observed with CC genotype of ADRB3 T190C polymorphism (p-value=0.040, OR=1.5; Table 14.8) Also, at allelic level C allele of ADRB3 T190C conferred risk for CAD (p-value=0.005, OR=1.7; Table 14.8).

Further, a case study was performed to estimate the correlation between the genotypes of ADRB3 T190C, ADRA2AC-1291G, and ADRB1 C1165G and the established risk factors (i.e., diabetes mellitus, hypertension, and smoking status, and lipid levels) for CAD. The subjects were compared for the distribution of ADRB3 T190C, ADRA2AC-1291G, and ADRB1 C1165G genotypes with risk factors. However, the three selected genetic variants in adrenergic receptors were not found to modulate the CAD risk by diabetes, hypertension, smoking, and lipid levels (Table 14.9).

CAD is an established risk factor for LVD so we segregated CAD patients on the basis of reduced (≤ 45%) and preserved (> 45%) LVEF and compared their status with ADRB3 T190C, ADRA2AC-1291G, and ADRB1 C1165G polymorphisms. There were no significant differences in the distributions of ADRB3 T190C, ADRA2AC-1291G, and ADRB1 C1165G polymorphisms in both reduced and preserved left

TABLE 14.7

Candidate Genes and Polymorphisms Selected

Genes	Type of Polymorphism	rs no.	Functional Role
ADRB1	Arg389Gly (C1165G)	rs1801253	These adrenergic receptors polymorphisms increase cardiac inotropy and chronotropy.
ADRA2A	C-1291G (promoterregion)	rs1800544	Causing vasoconstriction and vasodilation
ADRB3	C190T (Arg64Try)	rs 4994	

TABLE 14.8

Adrenergic Receptor Gene Polymorphisms Analysis of CAD Patients and Controls

Genotypes/Alleles	Controls n (%)	Cases n (%)	p-value	OR (95% CI)
ADRB3 190 T> C				
TT	158 (79.0)	422 (70.3)	-	1 (reference)
TC	42 (21.0)	162 (27.3)	**0.040**	**1.5 (1.0-2.2)**
CC	0	16 (2.7)	-	-
TC+CC	42 (21.0)	178 (29.7)	**0.012**	**1.6 (1.1-2.4)**
T	358 (89.5)	1006 (83.8)	-	1 (reference)
C	42 (11.5)	194(16.2)	**0.005**	**1.7 (1.1-2.4)**
ADRA2A -1291 C> G				
CC	46 (23.0)	137 (22.8)	-	1 (reference)
CG	100 (50.0)	325 (54.2)	0.494	1.1 (0.7-1.7)
GG	54 (27.0)	138 (23.0)	0.718	0.9 (0.6-1.5)
CG+GG	154 (77.0)	463 (77.2)	0.728	1.0 (0.7-1.6)
C	192 (48.0)	599 (49.9)	-	1 (reference)
G	208 (52.0)	601 (50.1)	0.316	0.9 (0.7-1.1)
ADRB1 1165C> G				
CC	109 (54.5)	292 (48.7)	-	1 (reference)
CG	85 (42.5)	278 (46.3)	0.298	1.2 (0.9-1.6)
GG	6 (3.0)	30 (5.0)	0.202	1.8 (0.7-4.5)
CG+GG	91 (45.5)	308 (51.3)	0.207	1.2 (0.9-1.7)
C	303 (75.7)	862(71.8)	-	1 (reference)
G	97 (24.3)	338(28.2)	0.112	1.3 (0.9-1.7)

Significant values sown in Bold

OR odds ratio, CI confidence interval

ventricle ejection fraction (p-value=0.093, p-value=0.856, p-value=0.595). Thus, the adrenergic receptor sequence variants conferred no risk of LVD in CAD patients (Table 14.10).

14.4.3 JAK-STAT Signaling Pathway

The Janus kinase/signal transducers and activators of transcription (JAK/STAT) pathway is a pleiotropic cascade that plays a very important role in development and homeostasis in animals. Cytokines and growth factors are mainly regulated by the JAK/STAT pathway in mammals. JAK activation stimulates cell proliferation, differentiation, cell migration, and apoptosis. These processes are affected by mutations that reduce JAK/STAT pathway activity.

TABLE 14.9

Adrenergic Receptor Genetic Polymorphism Influence on CAD Risk Due to Established Risk Factors

ADRB3 **T190C**

Clinical Characteristics	TT (N%)	TC (N%)	CC (N%)	p-value
Hypertensive	193(71.2)	68(25.1)	10(3.7)	0.264
Diabetic	116(65.9)	54(30.7)	6(3.4)	0.293
Smoker	106(71.1)	40(26.8)	3(2.0)	0.845
*TC	138.9±37.3	131.8±43.3	131.5±26.7	0.466
*TG	147.6±63.9	142.0±57.2	111.0±36.6	0.179
*LDL	75.1±27.7	72.3±28.8	76.9±24.8	0.787
*HDL	33.5±7.8	33.4±9.2	31.1±6.0	0.671
*BMI	24.5±3.1	23.8±2.9	24.3±3.0	0.271

ADRA2A **C-1291G**

Clinical Characteristics	CC	CG	GG	p-value
Hypertensive	66(24.4)	147(54.2)	58(21.4)	0.592
Diabetic	40(22.7)	95(54.0)	41(23.3)	0.994
Smoker	30(20.1)	88(59.1)	31(20.8)	0.382
*TC	140.7±47.1	135.9±35.1	135.6±37.5	0.736
*TG	144.5±58.7	145.9±65.2	141.8±56.3	0.923
*LDL	76.5±31.0	74.1±26.1	73.8±28.9	0.854
*HDL	33.0±7.4	33.4±8.2	33.4±8.4	0.951
*BMI	24.0±3.2	24.5±3.0	24.1±3.0	0.523

ADRB1 **C1165G**

Clinical Characteristics	CC	CG	GG	p-value
Hypertensive	66(24.4)	147(54.2)	58(21.4)	0.960
Diabetic	40(22.7)	95(54.0)	41(23.3)	0.893
Smoker	30(20.1)	88(59.1)	31(20.8)	0.380
*TC	137.5±40.4	136.2±37.6	137.0±21.9	0.970
*TG	144.9±59.1	142.9±64.0	159.1±71.4	0.733
*LDL	73.5±28.5	76.2±28.2	71.1±8.3	0.720
*HDL	32.3±7.3	34.4±8.7	34.5±8.3	0.167
*BMI	24.6±2.9	24.0±3.2	23.0±3.0	0.156

* Values are mean ± SD

RAAS plays a vital role in regulating cardiovascular functions, such as in hypertension (Mascareno et al., 2001), LV hypertrophy (Lavie, Ventura & Messerli, 1991), ischemic DCM, and HF (Raynolds et al., 1993). The JAK/STAT signaling pathway among other second-messenger systems at the cellular level (Raynolds et al., 1993; Sadoshima and Izumo, 1993; Sadoshima et al., 1993; Booz and Baker, 1995) is associated with activation of the autocrine loop of the heart tissue–localized RAAS (Mascareno, Dhar & Siddiqui 1998; Hirota et al., 1995; Pennica et al., 1995). It is a major signal transduction pathway of the cytokine superfamily (Ihle, 1995), activated by several hypertrophicagonists (Kodama et al., 1997; Pennica, Wood & Chien, 1996) including Angiotensin II (Hirsch et al., 1999). It has been shown that activation and translocation of three specific members of the STAT family, STAT 3, 5A, and STAT 6, are facilitated by Angiotensin II, which results in activation of the autocrine RAAS loop via transcriptional activation of the ANG gene promoter in the hypertrophied myocardium (Mascareno et al., 2001).

TABLE 14.10

Adrenergic Receptor Gene Polymorphism Analysis of Patients with Preserved (LVEF > 45%) and Reduced (LVEF ≤45%) Left Ventricular Ejection Fraction

Genotypes	LVEF> 45% N (%)	LVEF≤45% N (%)	p–value[a] OR (95% CI)
ADRB3 190 T> C			
TT	281 (68.4)	141 (74.6)	1(reference)
TC+CC	130 (31.6)	48 (25.4)	0.093
			0.7 (0.5 – 1.0)
ADRA2A -1291 C> G			
CC	90 (21.9)	47 (24.9)	1 (reference)
CG	228 (55.5)	97 (51.3)	0.435
			0.8 (0.5-1.3)
GG	93 (22.6)	45 (23.8)	0.856
			1.0 (0.6-1.5)
ADRB11165C> G			
CC	210 (51.1)	82(43.4)	1 (reference)
CG	181 (44.0)	97 (51.3)	0.095
			1.3 (0.9-1.9)
GG	20 (4.9)	10 (5.3)	0.595
			1.2 (0.6-2.7)

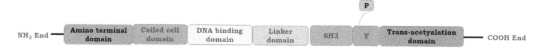

FIGURE 14.3 Schematic illustrations of STATs domains and structural features. N-terminal domain; coiled–coil domain (CCD); DNA binding domain (DBD); Linker domain; Src homology domain 2 (SH2) and the tyrosine residue (Y) phosphorylation sites.

14.4.3.1 STATs

In mammals, seven STATs (STATs 1, 2, 3, 4, 5A, 5B, and 6) have been identified ranging from 750 to 900 amino acids (Kisseleva et al., 2002). These proteins share a common feature. The structural and functional analysis of these proteins suggest that they have six conserved domains (Figure 14.3). This includes the N-terminal domain (NH2), the coiled-coiled domain (CCD), the DNA binding domain (DBD), the tyrosine activation domain (SH2), and the linker domain. In contrast, the carboxyl-terminal transcriptional activation domain (TAD) is very divergent and controls STAT specificity (Figure 14.3). The N-terminal half of the STAT consists of two relatively poorly characterized domains. This domain is well conserved between these families of protein and is reported to promote cooperativity in DNA binding and to regulate nuclear translocation. It represents an independently folded and stable moiety, which can be cleaved from the full-length molecule by limited proteolysis (Vinkemeier et al., 1996).

14.4.3.2 STAT Signaling in Cardiovascular Diseases

It has been reported that all seven members of the STAT family are expressed in the heart and/or cultured cardiac myocytes, fibroblasts, and endothelial cells (Xuan et al., 2001; Boengler et al., 2008).

Most of the available information about cardiovascular involvement relates to STAT1 and three family members. Various stimuli that activate hypertrophic growth of cardiac myocytes and/or provide cardioprotection have been demonstrated to activate JAK-STAT signaling in the heart. Studies have established that these stimuli also enhance cardiac STAT functional activity, as assessed by electrophoretic mobility shift assays of DNA binding activity, or promoter-reporter assays of transcriptional activity (Booz, Day & Baker, 2002).

14.5 Myocardial Remodeling

14.5.1 Matrixmetalloproteinases

The founding member of the matrix metalloproteinase (MMP) family, collagenase, was identified in 1962 by Gross and Lapiere, who found that tadpole tails during metamorphosis contained an enzyme that could degrade fibrillar collagen (Gross and Lapiere, 1962). Subsequently, an interstitial collagenase, collagenase-1 or MMP1, was found in diseased skin and synovium (Birkedal-Hansen et al., 1993). In vitro, MMP1 initiates degradation of native fibrillar collagens, crucial components of vertebrate extracellular matrix (ECM), by cleaving the peptide bond between Gly775–Ile776 or Gly775–Lys776 in native type I, II, or III collagen molecules (Welgus, Kobayashi & Jeffrey, 1983). Further research led to the discovery of a family of structurally related proteinases (23 in human, 24 in mice), now referred to as the MMP family. Interest in MMPs increased in the late 1960s and early 1970s following observations that MMPs are upregulated in diverse human diseases including cardiovascular, rheumatoid arthritis, and cancer.

MMPs are members of the met-zinc group of proteases, which are named after the zinc ionand the conserved Met residue at the active site (Stocker et al., 1995). Mammalian MMPs share a conserved domain structurethat consists of a catalytic domain and an auto inhibitory pro-domain. The pro-domain contains a conserved Cys residue that coordinates the active-site zinc to inhibit catalysis. When the pro-domain is destabilized or removed, the active site becomes available to cleave substrates. Most MMP-family members also contain a hemopexindomain, attached at their C-termini by a flexible hinge. The hemopexin domain encodes a four-bladed β-propeller structure that mediates protein–protein interactions. This domain also contributes to proper substraterecognition, activation of the enzyme, protease localization, internalization, and degradation (Overall, 2002). The structures of the catalytic and hemopexin domains of several MMPs, including MMP1, MMP2, MMP3, and MMP14 (also known as membrane type 1 MMP (MT1-MMP), have been solved (Maskos, 2005). MMP2 and MMP9 also have fibronectin type II repeats, which mediate binding to collagens, inserted into the catalytic domain. Most MMPs are secreted proteins; however, six MT-MMPs, MMP14, MMP15, MMP16, and MMP24, have transmembrane domains and short cytoplasmic tails, and MMP17 and MMP25 have glycosylphosphatidyl inositol (GPI) linkages. The activity of MMPs is controlled at many levels and the regulation of MMP activity remains a topic of intense research (Page-McCaw, Ewald & Werb, 2007).

14.5.1.1 Matrix MMPs and HF Process

The MMPs are zinc-dependent endopeptidases with varying substrate specificity and the capacity to degrade many components of the ECM. The cardiac ECM, the connective tissue scaffold on which cellular elements are arranged, plays a vital role in the maintenance of myocardial structure and function, particularly that of the left ventricle (LV). The physiological integrity of the ECM structure is largely under the control of the matrix MMP family of endopeptidases, the activity of which maintains a balance between connective tissue synthesis and degradation. Altered MMP expression and activity under pathological conditions may lead to a situation favoring proteolysis. The result is adverse ventricular remodelling, leading to LV dilatation, loss of contractile function, and progressive clinical HF. The severity of this process of LV remodelling is linked intimately to adverse prognosis (Lindsey et al., 2002; Rohde et al., 1999). The balance between ECM synthesis and degradation has been considered to play a key role in maintaining LV geometry and function. The ECM provides structural support for myocyte alignment and blood vessels. It also coordinates the conversion of myocyte contraction into myocardial force. Furthermore, it can affect myocardial stiffness and diastolic function (Romanic et al., 2001; Ducharme et al., 2000). Several studies have demonstrated that MMPs are involved not only in LV remodeling and failures (Newby, 2005; Henney et al., 1991; Woessner 1991) but also in cardiac rupture (Heymans et al., 1999). The MMPs have been identified in normal and failing myocardium (Spinale, 2002; Creemers et al., 2001; Spinale et al., 2000). An important structural milestone in patients with progressive HF is myocardial remodelling, although the inciting stimuli can be diverse. Pharmacological interventions targeted at altering this adverse LV myocardial remodelling process hold therapeutic promise.

In patients with end-stage cardiomyopathic disease, changes in a number of MMP subtypes have been documented (Spinale, 2002; Spinale et al., 2000). Specifically, increased myocardial levels ofMMP-3, MMP-2, and MMP-9 have been identified in patients with cardiomyopathic disease due to both ischaemic and non-ischaemica etiologies. In addition, circulating plasma levels of MMP-2 and MMP-9 have been reported in patients with cardiomyopathy and related to the severity of the disease process (Wilson et al., 2002). In animal models of HF, a cause–effect relationship has been demonstrated through the use of MMP transgenic constructs as well as pharmacological MMP inhibition (Spinale, 2002; Creemers et al., 2001). Based on these studies and clinical observational reports, a consensus is building that the induction and activation of myocardial MMPs contribute to adverse LV remodelling and thereby contribute to the progression of the HF process.

14.5.1.2 MMP Gene Polymorphisms

Interestingly, in the promoters of MMP-1, -3, -7, -9, and -1 polymorphisms have been identified, which appear to influence MMP gene expression (Ye, 2000; Horne et al., 2007; Jormsjo et al., 2001). These observations also indicate that variations in the levels of MMP transcription inpatients suffering from MI might contribute to differences in infarct healing, LV remodeling, and the transition to end-stage HF or cardiac rupture. Further research is needed to identify a possible correlation between these events after MI and MMP polymorphisms.

14.5.1.3 Matrix Metalloproteinases-2 (MMP2)

MMP2 gene is located on long arm of chromosome 16q13-q21. MMP-2 (72-kD gelatinase or gelatinase A) is ubiquitously distributed in cardiac myocytes and fibroblasts and it has been shown to be persistently upregulated after MI (Carlyle et al., 1997; Podesser et al., 2001; Dixon et al., 1996). Therefore, MMP-2 may play an important role in early myocardial healing and the late post-infarct remodelling process. However, no studies have yet determined the pathophysiological significance of MMP-2 in post-MI hearts. Only a few genetic studies on MMP-2 showing the role it plays in atheroschlerosis or atherothrombosis, despite the fact that MMP-9 and MMP-2 generally act upon the same substrates (Newby, 2005; Galis and Khatri, 2002; Nagase and Woessner, 1999). A cardiac rupture usually occurs unexpectedly, and it is often fatal. Several studies in mice with the deletion of MMP-2 may provide some insight regarding the pathophysiological role of MMP-2 activation in cardiac rupture and thus help to establish an effective therapeutic strategy (Hayashidani et al., 2003; Mukherjee et al., 2003; Rohde et al., 1999). In addition, myocardial MMP-2 activation after MI is also involved in the process of LV structural remodeling, which is a central feature of HF progression (Lee and Libby, 2000).

To date several association studies on CVD phenotype and promoter region polymorphisms of *MMP2* gene have been explored but with conflicting results. *MMP2* rs17859821 A allele has been associated with better prognosis of systolic HF in the northern Han Chinese population (Alp et al., 2011). *MMP2* rs243866 A allele has been associated with lower risk of systolic HF in Han Chinese (Hua et al., 2009). Two *MMP2* promoter polymorphisms (−790T/G and −735C/T) have been associated with chronic HF (Vasku et al., 2003). A haplo type comprised of four *MMP2* promoter polymorphisms (−1575G/A, −1306C/T, −790T/G, and −735C/T) have been associated with coronary triple-vessel disease (Vasku et al., 2004). *MMP2* C-735T polymorphism has been associated with CAD and MI (Alp et al., 2011).

14.5.1.4 Matrix Metalloproteinases-7 (MMP7)

MMP 7 gene, located on the long arm of chromosome 11q21-q22.MMP-7 (also known as matrilysin or PUMP-1), is a protease with broad substrate specificity; it can degrade fibronectin, proteoglycans, elastin, and type IVcollagen. It is among the smallest members of the MMP family (Quantin, Murphy & Breathnach, 1989). MMP-7 was found to be overexpressed in colorectal cancer and it was first characterized from a humanrectal carcinoma cell line (Miyazaki et al., 1990). In CAD, it has been suggested that increased activity ofMMP-7 can play an important role in development of CAD. The increased proteolytic activities within the coronary arterial wall that are linked with CHD suggest that functional polymorphisms in genes involved in matrix remodeling may account for part of thegenetic predisposition to atherosclerosis and its clinical indicators (Thompson and Parks, 1996).

14.5.1.5 Matrix Metalloproteinases-9 (MMP9)

MMP9 gene is located on the long arm of chromosome 20q11.2-q13.1. Gelatinase B (also known as 92-kDa type IV collagenase and MMP9) is one of the MMPs found to be highly expressed in the disruption-prone regions of atherosclerotic plaques (Zaltsman and Newby, 1997; Brown et al., 1995; Galis et al., 1994). It has a broad substrate specificity, being particularly active against gelatines (denatured collagens that have lost the typical triple helix) and type IV collagen (a major component of the basement membrane underlining the endothelium and surrounding each vascular smooth muscle cell). It also possesses proteolytic activity against proteoglycan core protein and elastin, which are resistant to degradation by some other MMPs (Birkedal-Hansen et al., 1993). Expression of gelatinase B is regulated primarily at the level of transcription, where the promoter of the gene responds to different regulators such as interleukin-1, platelet-derived growth factor, tumor necrosis factor-a, and epidermal growth factor (Fabunmi et al., 1996; Birkedal-Hansen et al., 1993; Huhtala et al., 1991). The hypothesis of a causal role of MMP-9 in CVDs is supported by genetic studies showing that functional promoter variations of the *MMP9* gene were related to presence and severity of CVDs (Pollanen et al., 2001; Peters et al., 1999). On the other hand, little is known about the clinical significance of circulating MMP-9 in CVDs. Elevated levels of MMP-9 have been reported in patients with unstable angina (Kai et al., 1998). However, prospective data on the impact of MMP-9 plasma levels on future CV prognosis are lacking. Several other studies demonstrated a prominent role of MMP-9 in myocardial ECM remodeling in cardiac rupture (Heymans et al., 1999) and LV remodeling (Kelly et al., 2007; Ducharme et al., 2000; Heymans et al., 1999).

The *MMP9*R279Q (or G836A), *MMP9* P574R (or C1721G,) and *MMP9* R668Q (or G2003A) polymorphisms are located on exon 6, exon 10, and exon 12 of *MMP9* gene, respectively. *MMP9*R279Q (or G836A) polymorphism has been associated with increased risk for MI, but not with CAD (Horne et al., 2007). We explored the association of MMP2 (C-735T, rs2285053), MMP7 (A-181G, rs11568818), and MMP9 (R279Q, rs17576), (P574R, rs2250889), (R668Q, rs17577) genetic polymorphisms with LVD in CAD (Mishra et al., 2012a). We found that among them, only MMP9 R668Q was significantly associated with LVD (LVEF ≤ 45) (p value=0.009; OR=3.82). To validate our results, we performed a replication study in additional cases and results again confirmed consistent findings (p value=0.033; OR=3.59). Also the frequency of haplotype R, P, Q comprising R668Q variation in MMP 9 was significantly higher in reduced LVEF subjects (p value=0.008; OR=1.83) (Mishra et al., 2012a).

14.6 Multigenetic and Multianalytical Approach in LVD

From the ongoing discussion, it appears that LVD is a very complex condition that is caused by multiple factors like mechanical, neurohormonal, and genetic factors. We have already discussed the association of inflammatory, matrix MMPs, and RAAS pathway genes with LVD. In complex multifactorial diseases, most genetic variants are known to exert small but significant effect on disease phenotype. Therefore, a statistical methodology should be applied to identify the combination of genetic variants and their possible interactions contributing towards genetic susceptibility to LVD in the background of CAD. We used our genotyping data for 11 SNPs in 9 genes belonging to the above three pathway genes (i.e., RAAS, MMPs, and inflammatory pathways). We then calculated G score and gene-gene interactions using multifactor dimensionality reduction (MDR) and classification and regression tree (CART) for LVD susceptibility.

On assessing the mean G-score in individual SNP between non-LVD and LVD groups, we found a significant difference in mean G-scores of AT1 A1166C, MMP9 R668Q, and NFKB1-94 ATTG ins/del

TABLE 14.11

Studied SNPs Mean G Scores with Their Corresponding P-Values

Polymorphisms	Non-LVD	LVD	p-value
ACEI/D	1.86±0.73	1.86±0.75	0.922
AT1 A1166C	1.22±0.48	1.44±0.66	**< 0.001**
*CYP11B2*T-344C	1.76±0.68	1.73±0.64	0.639
*MMP2*C-735T	1.22±0.47	1.28±0.52	0.177
MMP7 A-181G	1.79±0.68	1.91±0.70	0.066
MMP9 R279Q	2.07±0.70	2.02±0.72	0.405
MMP9 P574R	1.36±0.53	1.33±0.53	0.650
MMP9 R668Q	1.64±0.56	1.81±0.62	**0.002**
NFKB1-94 ATTG ins/del	1.46±0.64	1.60±0.70	**0.023**
IL6 G-174C	1.32±0.51	1.33±0.53	0.961
TNFα G-308A	1.18±0.0.38	1.11±0.31	0.054
Collective G-Scores of associated SNPs	4.31±0.92	4.85±1.09	**< 0.001**
Collective G-Scores of non-associated SNPs	12.58±1.80	12.58±1.95	0.999

Significant values are shown in bold

TABLE 14.12

Multifactor Dimensionality Reduction (MDR) Analysis to Find Association of High-Order Gene-Gene Interactions with LVD Risk

Interaction best Models	Testing Accuracy	#CVC score	χ^2 (p-value)	(95% CI) OR
[a]*AT1* A1166C	0.568	10/10	15.42 (< 0.0001)	(1.5-3.5) 2.30
ACE I/D, *AT1*A1166C	0.526	4/10	18.13 (< 0.0001)	(1.6-3.3) 2.28
*AT1*A1166C, *MMP7 A-181G*, *MMP* R668Q	0.549	5/10	35.12 (< 0.0001)	(2.2-4.8) 3.24
[b]*AT1* A1166C, *MMP7* A-181G, *MMP* R668Q, *NFKB1*ATTGI/D	0.568	9/10	59.71 (< 0.0001)	(3.1-6.8) 4.57

CVC: Cross-Validation Consistency

a *AT1* A1166 Cmodel, with the maximum testing accuracy and maximum CVC was considered as the best interection model.

b In addition to this, the four-factor model including *AT1* A1166C, *MMP7* A-181G, *MMP* R668Q, *NFKB1*ATTGI/D polymorphisms with high testing accuracy and CVC was considered as the best interaction model.

polymorphisms. The combined mean G-scores of risk-associated SNPs (from single locus analysis) were highly significant and conferred increased risk for LVD (4.85 ± 1.09 vs. 4.31 ± 0.92; p < 0.001) while combined G-scores of non-associated SNPs were not found to be significant between LVD and non-LVD patients (12.58 ± 1.95 vs. 12.58 ± 1.80; p = 0.999) (Table 14.11) (Mishra et al., 2014).

For CART analysis, we generated a tree structure for all studied genetic variations of three pathways named RAAS, MMPs, and inflammatory. All SNPs of these three pathway genes resulted in ten terminal nodes in the final tree. The first splitting node contains a single AT1 A1166C genotype, separating individuals with the wild-type genotypes (low risk) from subjects with the homozygous variant genotype (high risk), which suggests that this SNP is the strongest risk factor for LVD among the all polymorphisms examined. However, individuals carrying AT1 1166 AA, NFKB1 ID+DD, MMP2 279RQ+QQ, and TNFα-308GA+AA genotypes had the lowest case rate and considered as reference (Mishra et al., 2014).

In MDR, a one-factor model for predicting LVD risk was AT1 A1166C SNP (testing accuracy = 0.568, CVC = 10/10, permutation p < 0.001, Table 14.12). The two-factor model of ACE I/D and AT1A1166C

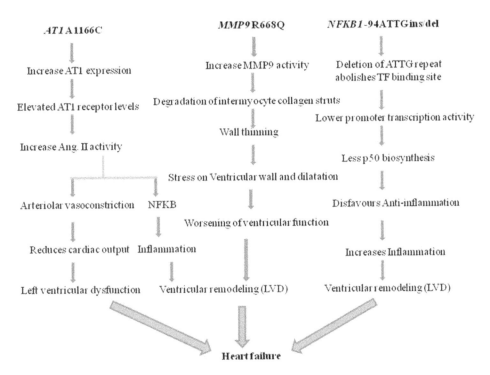

FIGURE 14.4 Proposed heart failure model:Angiotensin II activity can be enhanced by AT1 A1166C polymorphism through increasing AT1 expression. MMP9 activity can be increased by MMP9 R668Q and Angiotensin II polymorphisms. An increased or dysregulated activity of MMP9 contributes to pathological remodeling states linked with heart failure. Inflammation also increased by the increased angiotensin II activity and MMP9 expression in myocardium. NFKB1-94 ATTG ins/del, AT1 A1166C, and MMP9R668Q polymorphisms collectively increase inflammation in myocardium, which leads to development and progression of ventricular remodeling and hence LVD.

had testing accuracy of 0.526 but with CVC = 4/10 (permutation p < 0.001, Table 14.12). The three-factor model including AT1A1166C, MMP7 A-181G, and MMP R668Q SNPs yielded testing accuracy of 0.549 and the CVC of 05/10 (permutation p = < 0.001, Table 14.12). Furthermore, the four-factor interaction model consisted of AT1 A1166C, MMP7 A-181G, MMP9 R668Q, and NFKB1 ATTG ins/del polymorphisms with an improved testing accuracy of 0.568 and CVC = 9/10 with permutation p < 0.001 (Mishra et al., 2014).

We have have proposed a model for ventricular remodeling following LVD and/or HF based on the above findings (Figure 14.4). Increased AT1, MMP9, and NFkB1 p50 subunit expression favors inflammation that aids in the development and progression of ventricular remodeling and LVD (Mishra et al., 2014).

At present, there is no clinical test for identification of CAD patients who have high risk of developing severe cardiac disorder in later stages. The late onset symptoms and influence of secondary risk factors may cause a lasting threat for HF. However, these gene-based insights may make it possible to develop tests that can be useful in diagnosis of disease before clinical manifestations. Furthermore, genetic tests may be useful for identification of persons at risk of severe LVD and HF.

Acknowledgements

Financial support for the research work was provided by Department of Biotechnology (DBT) Government of India. BM and RM were Emeritus Medical Scientists of ICMR, New Delhi.

REFERENCES

Ackermann, M. A., and A. Kontrogianni-Konstantopoulos. 2011. "Myosin binding protein-C: a regulator of actomyosin interaction in striated muscle." *J Biomed Biotechnol* 2011:636403. doi: 10.1155/2011/636403.

Alp, E., S. Menevse, M. Tulmac, A. Yilmaz, R. Yalcin, and A. Cengel. 2011. "The role of matrix metalloproteinase-2 promoter polymorphisms in coronary artery disease and myocardial infarction." *Genet Test Mol Biomarkers* 15 (4):193–202. doi: 10.1089/gtmb.2010.0113.

Atlas, S. A. 2007. "The renin-angiotensin aldosterone system: pathophysiological role and pharmacologic inhibition." *J Manag Care Pharm* 13 (8 Suppl B):9–20. doi: 10.18553/jmcp.2007.13.s8-b.9.

Badenhorst, D., G. R. Norton, K. Sliwa, R. Brooksbank, R. Essop, P. Sareli, and A. J. Woodiwiss. 2007. "Impact of beta2-adrenoreceptor gene variants on cardiac cavity size and systolic function in idiopathic dilated cardiomyopathy." *Pharmacogenomics J* 7 (5):339–45. doi: 10.1038/sj.tpj.6500426.

Bang, M. L., T. Centner, F. Fornoff, A. J. Geach, M. Gotthardt, M. McNabb, C. C. Witt, D. Labeit, C. C. Gregorio, H. Granzier, and S. Labeit. 2001. "The complete gene sequence of titin, expression of an unusual approximately 700-kDa titin isoform, and its interaction with obscurin identify a novel Z-line to I-band linking system." *Circ Res* 89 (11):1065–72.

Bastard, J. P., M. Maachi, C. Lagathu, M. J. Kim, M. Caron, H. Vidal, J. Capeau, and B. Feve. 2006. "Recent advances in the relationship between obesity, inflammation, and insulin resistance." *Eur Cytokine Netw* 17 (1):4–12.

Baudin, B. 2005. "Polymorphism in angiotensin II receptor genes and hypertension." *Exp Physiol* 90 (3):277–82. doi: 10.1113/expphysiol.2004.028456.

Benetos, A., S. Gautier, S. Ricard, J. Topouchian, R. Asmar, O. Poirier, E. Larosa, L. Guize, M. Safar, F. Soubrier, and F. Cambien. 1996. "Influence of angiotensin-converting enzyme and angiotensin II type 1 receptor gene polymorphisms on aortic stiffness in normotensive and hypertensive patients." *Circulation* 94 (4):698–703.

Birkedal-Hansen, H., W. G. Moore, M. K. Bodden, L. J. Windsor, B. Birkedal-Hansen, A. DeCarlo, and J. A. Engler. 1993. "Matrix metalloproteinases: a review." *Crit Rev Oral Biol Med* 4 (2):197–250.

Boengler, K., D. Hilfiker-Kleiner, H. Drexler, G. Heusch, and R. Schulz. 2008. "The myocardial JAK/STAT pathway: from protection to failure." *Pharmacol Ther* 120 (2):172–85. doi: 10.1016/j.pharmthera.2008.08.002.

Bonnardeaux, A., E. Davies, X. Jeunemaitre, I. Fery, A. Charru, E. Clauser, L. Tiret, F. Cambien, P. Corvol, and F. Soubrier. 1994. "Angiotensin II type 1 receptor gene polymorphisms in human essential hypertension." *Hypertension* 24 (1):63–9.

Booz, G. W., and K. M. Baker. 1995. "Molecular signalling mechanisms controlling growth and function of cardiac fibroblasts." *Cardiovasc Res* 30 (4):537–43.

Booz, G. W., J. N. Day, and K. M. Baker. 2002. "Interplay between the cardiac renin angiotensin system and JAK-STAT signaling: role in cardiac hypertrophy, ischemia/reperfusion dysfunction, and heart failure." *J Mol Cell Cardiol* 34 (11):1443–53.

Borbély, A., I. Falcao-Pires, L. van Heerebeek, N. Hamdani, I. Édes, C. Gavina, A. F. Leite-Moreira, J. G. Bronzwaer, Z. Papp, J. van der Velden, G. J. Stienen, and W. J. Paulus. 2009. "Hypophosphorylation of the Stiff N2B titin isoform raises cardiomyocyte resting tension in failing human myocardium." *Circ Res* 104 (6):780–6. doi: 10.1161/CIRCRESAHA.108.193326.

Borbély, A., J. van der Velden, Z. Papp, J. G. Bronzwaer, I. Edes, G. J. Stienen, and W. J. Paulus. 2005. "Cardiomyocyte stiffness in diastolic heart failure." *Circulation* 111 (6):774–81. doi: 10.1161/01.CIR.0000155257.33485.6D.

Borghi, C., A. F. Cicero, and E. Ambrosioni. 2008. "Effects of early treatment with zofenopril in patients with myocardial infarction and metabolic syndrome: the SMILE Study." *Vasc Health Risk Manag* 4 (3):665–71.

Bristow, M. R. 2000. "beta-adrenergic receptor blockade in chronic heart failure." *Circulation* 101 (5):558–69.

Brodde, O. E., R. Buscher, R. Tellkamp, J. Radke, S. Dhein, and P. A. Insel. 2001. "Blunted cardiac responses to receptor activation in subjects with Thr164Ile beta(2)-adrenoceptors." *Circulation* 103 (8):1048–50.

Brown, D. L., M. S. Hibbs, M. Kearney, C. Loushin, and J. M. Isner. 1995. "Identification of 92-kD gelatinase in human coronary atherosclerotic lesions. Association of active enzyme synthesis with unstable angina." *Circulation* 91 (8):2125–31.

Bulteau, A. L., L. I. Szweda, and B. Friguet. 2002. "Age-dependent declines in proteasome activity in the heart." *Arch Biochem Biophys* 397 (2):298–304. doi: 10.1006/abbi.2001.2663.

Cambien, F., O. Poirier, L. Lecerf, A. Evans, J. P. Cambou, D. Arveiler, G. Luc, J. M. Bard, L. Bara, S. Ricard, and et al., 1992. "Deletion polymorphism in the gene for angiotensin-converting enzyme is a potent risk factor for myocardial infarction." *Nature* 359 (6396):641–4. doi: 10.1038/359641a0.

Candy, G. P., D. Skudicky, U. K. Mueller, A. J. Woodiwiss, K. Sliwa, F. Luker, J. Esser, P. Sareli, and G. R. Norton. 1999. "Association of left ventricular systolic performance and cavity size with angiotensin-converting enzyme genotype in idiopathic dilated cardiomyopathy." *Am J Cardiol* 83 (5):740–4. doi: 10.1016/s0002-9149(98)00981-3.

Cao, D., H. Li, J. Yi, J. Zhang, H. Che, J. Cao, L. Yang, C. Zhu, and W. Jiang. 2011. "Antioxidant properties of the mung bean flavonoids on alleviating heat stress." *PLoS One* 6 (6):e21071. doi: 10.1371/journal.pone.0021071.

Carlyle, W. C., A. W. Jacobson, D. L. Judd, B. Tian, C. Chu, K. M. Hauer, M. M. Hartman, and K. M. McDonald. 1997. "Delayed reperfusion alters matrix metalloproteinase activity and fibronectin mRNA expression in the infarct zone of the ligated rat heart." *J Mol Cell Cardiol* 29 (9):2451–63. doi: 10.1006/jmcc.1997.0482.

Chapman, C. M., L. J. Palmer, B. M. McQuillan, J. Hung, J. Burley, C. Hunt, P. L. Thompson, and J. P. Beilby. 2001. "Polymorphisms in the angiotensinogen gene are associated with carotid intimal-medial thickening in females from a community-based population." *Atherosclerosis* 159 (1):209–17. doi: 10.1016/s0021-9150(01)00499-3.

Chrysohoou, C., C. Pitsavos, J. Barbetseas, I. Kotroyiannis, S. Brili, K. Vasiliadou, L. Papadimitriou, and C. Stefanadis. 2009. "Chronic systemic inflammation accompanies impaired ventricular diastolic function, detected by Doppler imaging, in patients with newly diagnosed systolic heart failure (Hellenic Heart Failure Study)." *Heart Vessels* 24 (1):22–6. doi: 10.1007/s00380-008-1080-7.

Craig, R., and G. Offer. 1976. "The location of C-protein in rabbit skeletal muscle." *Proc R Soc Lond B Biol Sci* 192 (1109):451–61.

Creemers, E. E., J. P. Cleutjens, J. F. Smits, and M. J. Daemen. 2001. "Matrix metalloproteinase inhibition after myocardial infarction: a new approach to prevent heart failure?" *Circ Res* 89 (3):201–10.

Curnow, K. M., M. T. Tusie-Luna, L. Pascoe, R. Natarajan, J. L. Gu, J. L. Nadler, and P. C. White. 1991. "The product of the CYP11B2 gene is required for aldosterone biosynthesis in the human adrenal cortex." *Mol Endocrinol* 5 (10):1513–22.

Danser, A. H., M. A. Schalekamp, W. A. Bax, A. M. van den Brink, P. R. Saxena, G. A. Riegger, and H. Schunkert. 1995. "Angiotensin-converting enzyme in the human heart. Effect of the deletion/insertion polymorphism." *Circulation* 92 (6):1387–8.

Dhandapany, P. S., S. Sadayappan, Y. Xue, G. T. Powell, D. S. Rani, P. Nallari, T. S. Rai, M. Khullar, P. Soares, A. Bahl, J. M. Tharkan, P. Vaideeswar, A. Rathinavel, C. Narasimhan, D. R. Ayapati, Q. Ayub, S. Q. Mehdi, S. Oppenheimer, M. B. Richards, A. L. Price, N. Patterson, D. Reich, L. Singh, C. Tyler-Smith, and K. Thangaraj. 2009. "A common MYBPC3 (cardiac myosin binding protein C) variant associated with cardiomyopathies in South Asia." *Nat Genet* 41 (2):187–91. doi: 10.1038/ng.309.

Dhoot, G. K., M. C. Hales, B. M. Grail, and S. V. Perry. 1985. "The isoforms of C protein and their distribution in mammalian skeletal muscle." *J Muscle Res Cell Motil* 6 (4):487–505.

Diwan, A., Z. Dibbs, S. Nemoto, G. DeFreitas, B. A. Carabello, N. Sivasubramanian, E. M. Wilson, F. G. Spinale, and D. L. Mann. 2004. "Targeted overexpression of noncleavable and secreted forms of tumor necrosis factor provokes disparate cardiac phenotypes." *Circulation* 109 (2):262–8. doi: 10.1161/01.CIR.0000109642.27985.FA.

Dixon, I. M., H. Ju, D. S. Jassal, and D. J. Peterson. 1996. "Effect of ramipril and losartan on collagen expression in right and left heart after myocardial infarction." *Mol Cell Biochem* 165 (1):31–45.

Ducharme, A., S. Frantz, M. Aikawa, E. Rabkin, M. Lindsey, L. E. Rohde, F. J. Schoen, R. A. Kelly, Z. Werb, P. Libby, and R. T. Lee. 2000. "Targeted deletion of matrix metalloproteinase-9 attenuates left ventricular enlargement and collagen accumulation after experimental myocardial infarction." *J Clin Invest* 106 (1):55–62. doi: 10.1172/JCI8768.

Elster, S. K., E. Braunwald, and H. F. Wood. 1956. "A study of C-reactive protein in the serum of patients with congestive heart failure." *Am Heart J* 51 (4):533–41. doi: 10.1016/0002-8703(56)90099-0.

Erdmann, J., K. Riedel, K. Rohde, I. Folgmann, T. Wienker, E. Fleck, and V. Regitz-Zagrosek. 1999. "Characterization of polymorphisms in the promoter of the human angiotensin II subtype 1 (AT1) receptor gene." *Ann Hum Genet* 63 (Pt 4):369–74.

Ertl, G., R. A. Kloner, R. W. Alexander, and E. Braunwald. 1982. "Limitation of experimental infarct size by an angiotensin-converting enzyme inhibitor." *Circulation* 65 (1):40–8.

Evans, A. E., O. Poirier, F. Kee, L. Lecerf, E. McCrum, T. Falconer, J. Crane, D. F. O'Rourke, and F. Cambien. 1994. "Polymorphisms of the angiotensin-converting-enzyme gene in subjects who die from coronary heart disease." *Q J Med* 87 (4):211–4.

Fabunmi, R. P., A. H. Baker, E. J. Murray, R. F. Booth, and A. C. Newby. 1996. "Divergent regulation by growth factors and cytokines of 95 kDa and 72 kDa gelatinases and tissue inhibitors or metalloproteinases-1, -2, and -3 in rabbit aortic smooth muscle cells." *Biochem J* 315 (Pt 1):335–42.

Farza, H., P. J. Townsend, L. Carrier, P. J. Barton, L. Mesnard, E. Bahrend, J. F. Forissier, M. Fiszman, M. H. Yacoub, and K. Schwartz. 1998. "Genomic organisation, alternative splicing and polymorphisms of the human cardiac troponin T gene." *J Mol Cell Cardiol* 30 (6):1247–53. doi: 10.1006/jmcc.1998.0698.

Feldman, R. D. 2001. "Adrenergic receptor polymorphisms and cardiac function (and dysfunction): a failure to communicate?" *Circulation* 103 (8):1042–3.

Ferrucci, L., R. D. Semba, J. M. Guralnik, W. B. Ershler, S. Bandinelli, K. V. Patel, K. Sun, R. C. Woodman, N. C. Andrews, R. J. Cotter, T. Ganz, E. Nemeth, and D. L. Longo. 2010. "Proinflammatory state, hepcidin, and anemia in older persons." *Blood* 115 (18):3810–6. doi: 10.1182/blood-2009-02-201087.

Flashman, E., C. Redwood, J. Moolman-Smook, and H. Watkins. 2004. "Cardiac myosin binding protein C: its role in physiology and disease." *Circ Res* 94 (10):1279–89. doi: 10.1161/01.RES.0000127175.21818.C2.

Frantz, S., A. Ducharme, D. Sawyer, L. E. Rohde, L. Kobzik, R. Fukazawa, D. Tracey, H. Allen, R. T. Lee, and R. A. Kelly. 2003. "Targeted deletion of caspase-1 reduces early mortality and left ventricular dilatation following myocardial infarction." *J Mol Cell Cardiol* 35 (6):685–94. doi: 10.1016/S0022-2828(03)00113-5.

Frantz, S., K. Hu, B. Bayer, S. Gerondakis, J. Strotmann, A. Adamek, G. Ertl, and J. Bauersachs. 2006. "Absence of NF-kappaB subunit p50 improves heart failure after myocardial infarction." *FASEB J* 20 (11):1918–20. doi: 10.1096/fj.05-5133fje.

Galis, Z. S., and J. J. Khatri. 2002. "Matrix metalloproteinases in vascular remodeling and atherogenesis: the good, the bad, and the ugly." *Circ Res* 90 (3):251–62.

Galis, Z. S., G. K. Sukhova, M. W. Lark, and P. Libby. 1994. "Increased expression of matrix metalloproteinases and matrix degrading activity in vulnerable regions of human atherosclerotic plaques." *J Clin Invest* 94 (6):2493–503. doi: 10.1172/JCI117619.

Gautel, M., D. O. Furst, A. Cocco, and S. Schiaffino. 1998. "Isoform transitions of the myosin binding protein C family in developing human and mouse muscles: lack of isoform transcomplementation in cardiac muscle." *Circ Res* 82 (1):124–9.

Gautel, M., O. Zuffardi, A. Freiburg, and S. Labeit. 1995. "Phosphorylation switches specific for the cardiac isoform of myosin binding protein-C: a modulator of cardiac contraction?" *EMBO J* 14 (9):1952–60.

Geisterfer, A. A., M. J. Peach, and G. K. Owens. 1988. "Angiotensin II induces hypertrophy, not hyperplasia, of cultured rat aortic smooth muscle cells." *Circ Res* 62 (4):749–56.

Glorieux, G., G. Cohen, J. Jankowski, and R. Vanholder. 2009. "Platelet/Leukocyte activation, inflammation, and uremia." *Semin Dial* 22 (4):423–7. doi: 10.1111/j.1525-139X.2009.00593.x.

Gordon, A. M., E. Homsher, and M. Regnier. 2000. "Regulation of contraction in striated muscle." *Physiol Rev* 80 (2):853–924.

Green, S. A., G. Cole, M. Jacinto, M. Innis, and S. B. Liggett. 1993. "A polymorphism of the human beta 2-adrenergic receptor within the fourth transmembrane domain alters ligand binding and functional properties of the receptor." *J Biol Chem* 268 (31):23116–21.

Green, S. A., J. Turki, P. Bejarano, I. P. Hall, and S. B. Liggett. 1995. "Influence of beta 2-adrenergic receptor genotypes on signal transduction in human airway smooth muscle cells." *Am J Respir Cell Mol Biol* 13 (1):25–33. doi: 10.1165/ajrcmb.13.1.7598936.

Gregorio, C. C., K. Trombitas, T. Centner, B. Kolmerer, G. Stier, K. Kunke, K. Suzuki, F. Obermayr, B. Herrmann, H. Granzier, H. Sorimachi, and S. Labeit. 1998. "The NH2 terminus of titin spans the Z-disc: its interaction with a novel 19-kD ligand (T-cap) is required for sarcomeric integrity." *J Cell Biol* 143 (4):1013–27.

Griendling, K. K., T. J. Murphy, and R. W. Alexander. 1993. "Molecular biology of the renin-angiotensin system." *Circulation* 87 (6):1816–28.

Gross, J., and C. M. Lapiere. 1962. "Collagenolytic activity in amphibian tissues: a tissue culture assay." *Proc Natl Acad Sci U S A* 48:1014–22.

Guo, W., S. J. Bharmal, K. Esbona, and M. L. Greaser. 2010. "Titin diversity—alternative splicing gone wild." *J Biomed Biotechnol* 2010:753675. doi: 10.1155/2010/753675.

Guo, W., J. M. Pleitner, K. W. Saupe, and M. L. Greaser. 2013. "Pathophysiological defects and transcriptional profiling in the RBM20-/-rat model." *PLoS One* 8 (12):e84281. doi: 10.1371/journal.pone.0084281.

Guo, W., S. Schafer, M. L. Greaser, M. H. Radke, M. Liss, T. Govindarajan, H. Maatz, H. Schulz, S. Li, A. M. Parrish, V. Dauksaite, P. Vakeel, S. Klaassen, B. Gerull, L. Thierfelder, V. Regitz-Zagrosek, T. A. Hacker, K. W. Saupe, G. W. Dec, P. T. Ellinor, C. A. MacRae, B. Spallek, R. Fischer, A. Perrot, C. Ozcelik, K. Saar, N. Hubner, and M. Gotthardt. 2012. "RBM20, a gene for hereditary cardiomyopathy, regulates titin splicing." *Nat Med* 18 (5):766–73. doi: 10.1038/nm.2693.

Hall, I. P. 1996. "Beta 2 adrenoceptor polymorphisms: are they clinically important?" *Thorax* 51 (4):351–3.

Hamdani, N., V. Kooij, S. van Dijk, D. Merkus, W. J. Paulus, C. D. Remedios, D. J. Duncker, G. J. Stienen, and J. van der Velden. 2008. "Sarcomeric dysfunction in heart failure." *Cardiovasc Res* 77 (4):649–58. doi: 10.1093/cvr/cvm079.

Hartzell, H. C., and D. B. Glass. 1984. "Phosphorylation of purified cardiac muscle C-protein by purified cAMP-dependent and endogenous Ca2+-calmodulin-dependent protein kinases." *J Biol Chem* 259 (24):15587–96.

Hayashidani, S., H. Tsutsui, M. Ikeuchi, T. Shiomi, H. Matsusaka, T. Kubota, K. Imanaka-Yoshida, T. Itoh, and A. Takeshita. 2003. "Targeted deletion of MMP-2 attenuates early LV rupture and late remodeling after experimental myocardial infarction." *Am J Physiol Heart Circ Physiol* 285 (3):H1229–35. doi: 10.1152/ajpheart.00207.2003.

Henney, A. M., P. R. Wakeley, M. J. Davies, K. Foster, R. Hembry, G. Murphy, and S. Humphries. 1991. "Localization of stromelysin gene expression in atherosclerotic plaques by in situ hybridization." *Proc Natl Acad Sci U S A* 88 (18):8154–8.

Heymans, S., A. Luttun, D. Nuyens, G. Theilmeier, E. Creemers, L. Moons, G. D. Dyspersin, J. P. Cleutjens, M. Shipley, A. Angellilo, M. Levi, O. Nube, A. Baker, E. Keshet, F. Lupu, J. M. Herbert, J. F. Smits, S. D. Shapiro, M. Baes, M. Borgers, D. Collen, M. J. Daemen, and P. Carmeliet. 1999. "Inhibition of plasminogen activators or matrix metalloproteinases prevents cardiac rupture but impairs therapeutic angiogenesis and causes cardiac failure." *Nat Med* 5 (10):1135–42. doi: 10.1038/13459.

Hirota, H., K. Yoshida, T. Kishimoto, and T. Taga. 1995. "Continuous activation of gp130, a signal-transducing receptor component for interleukin 6-related cytokines, causes myocardial hypertrophy in mice." *Proc Natl Acad Sci U S A* 92 (11):4862–6.

Hirsch, A. T., J. A. Opsahl, M. M. Lunzer, and S. A. Katz. 1999. "Active renin and angiotensinogen in cardiac interstitial fluid after myocardial infarction." *Am J Physiol* 276 (6 Pt 2):H1818–26.

Horne, B. D., N. J. Camp, J. F. Carlquist, J. B. Muhlestein, M. J. Kolek, Z. P. Nicholas, and J. L. Anderson. 2007. "Multiple-polymorphism associations of 7 matrix metalloproteinase and tissue inhibitor metalloproteinase genes with myocardial infarction and angiographic coronary artery disease." *Am Heart J* 154 (4):751–8. doi: 10.1016/j.ahj.2007.06.030.

Hua, Y., L. Song, N. Wu, X. Lu, X. Meng, D. Gu, and Y. Yang. 2009. "Polymorphisms of MMP-2 gene are associated with systolic heart failure risk in Han Chinese." *Am J Med Sci* 337 (5):344–8. doi: 10.1097/MAJ.0b013e31818eb2a2.

Huhtala, P., A. Tuuttila, L. T. Chow, J. Lohi, J. Keski-Oja, and K. Tryggvason. 1991. "Complete structure of the human gene for 92-kDa type IV collagenase. Divergent regulation of expression for the 92-and 72-kilodalton enzyme genes in HT-1080 cells." *J Biol Chem* 266 (25):16485–90.

Humma, L. M., B. J. Puckett, H. E. Richardson, S. G. Terra, T. E. Andrisin, B. L. Lejeune, M. R. Wallace, J. F. Lewis, D. M. McNamara, L. Picoult-Newberg, C. J. Pepine, and J. A. Johnson. 2001. "Effects of beta1-adrenoceptor genetic polymorphisms on resting hemodynamics in patients undergoing diagnostic testing for ischemia." *Am J Cardiol* 88 (9):1034–7.

Hunley, T. E., B. A. Julian, J. A. Phillips, 3rd, M. L. Summar, H. Yoshida, R. G. Horn, N. J. Brown, A. Fogo, I. Ichikawa, and V. Kon. 1996. "Angiotensin converting enzyme gene polymorphism: potential silencer motif and impact on progression in IgA nephropathy." *Kidney Int* 49 (2):571–7.

Ihle, J. N. 1995. "Cytokine receptor signalling." *Nature* 377 (6550):591–4. doi: 10.1038/377591a0.

Ito, M., H. Takahashi, K. Fuse, S. Hirono, T. Washizuka, K. Kato, F. Yamazaki, K. Inano, T. Furukawa, M. Komada, and Y. Aizawa. 2000. "Polymorphisms of tumor necrosis factor-alpha and interleukin-10 genes in Japanese patients with idiopathic dilated cardiomyopathy." *Jpn Heart J* 41 (2):183–91.

Iwai, N., N. Ohmichi, Y. Nakamura, and M. Kinoshita. 1994. "DD genotype of the angiotensin-converting enzyme gene is a risk factor for left ventricular hypertrophy." *Circulation* 90 (6):2622–8.

James, J., and J. Robbins. 2011. "Signaling and myosin-binding protein C." *J Biol Chem* 286 (12):9913–9. doi: 10.1074/jbc.R110.171801.

Jha, R. K., Q. Ma, H. Sha, and M. Palikhe. 2009. "Acute pancreatitis: a literature review." *Med Sci Monit* 15 (7):RA147–56.

Jiang, Z., W. Zhao, F. Yu, and G. Xu. 2001. "Association of angiotensin II type 1 receptor gene polymorphism with essential hypertension." *Chin Med J (Engl)* 114 (12):1249–51.

Johnston, C. I. 1992. "Franz Volhard Lecture. Renin-angiotensin system: a dual tissue and hormonal system for cardiovascular control." *J Hypertens Suppl* 10 (7):S13–26.

Jormsjo, S., C. Whatling, D. H. Walter, A. M. Zeiher, A. Hamsten, and P. Eriksson. 2001. "Allele-specific regulation of matrix metalloproteinase-7 promoter activity is associated with coronary artery luminal dimensions among hypercholesterolemic patients." *Arterioscler Thromb Vasc Biol* 21 (11):1834–9.

Kai, H., H. Ikeda, H. Yasukawa, M. Kai, Y. Seki, F. Kuwahara, T. Ueno, K. Sugi, and T. Imaizumi. 1998. "Peripheral blood levels of matrix metalloproteases-2 and -9 are elevated in patients with acute coronary syndromes." *J Am Coll Cardiol* 32 (2):368–72. doi: 10.1016/s0735-1097(98)00250-2.

Karin, M., T. Lawrence, and V. Nizet. 2006. "Innate immunity gone awry: linking microbial infections to chronic inflammation and cancer." *Cell* 124 (4):823–35. doi: 10.1016/j.cell.2006.02.016.

Kawano, S., T. Kubota, Y. Monden, T. Tsutsumi, T. Inoue, N. Kawamura, H. Tsutsui, and K. Sunagawa. 2006. "Blockade of NF-kappaB improves cardiac function and survival after myocardial infarction." *Am J Physiol Heart Circ Physiol* 291 (3):H1337–44. doi: 10.1152/ajpheart.01175.2005.

Kelly, D., G. Cockerill, L. L. Ng, M. Thompson, S. Khan, N. J. Samani, and I. B. Squire. 2007. "Plasma matrix metalloproteinase-9 and left ventricular remodelling after acute myocardial infarction in man: a prospective cohort study." *Eur Heart J* 28 (6):711–8. doi: 10.1093/eurheartj/ehm003.

Kikuya, M., K. Sugimoto, T. Katsuya, M. Suzuki, T. Sato, J. Funahashi, R. Katoh, I. Kazama, M. Michimata, T. Araki, A. Hozawa, I. Tsuji, T. Ogihara, T. Yanagisawa, Y. Imai, and M. Matsubara. 2003. "A/C1166 gene polymorphism of the angiotensin II type 1 receptor (AT1) and ambulatory blood pressure: the Ohasama Study." *Hypertens Res* 26 (2):141–5.

Kiowski, W., G. Sutsch, P. Hunziker, P. Muller, J. Kim, E. Oechslin, R. Schmitt, R. Jones, and O. Bertel. 1995. "Evidence for endothelin-1-mediated vasoconstriction in severe chronic heart failure." *Lancet* 346 (8977):732–6. doi: 10.1016/s0140-6736(95)91504-4.

Kisseleva, T., S. Bhattacharya, J. Braunstein, and C. W. Schindler. 2002. "Signaling through the JAK/STAT pathway, recent advances and future challenges." *Gene* 285 (1-2):1–24.

Kober, L., C. Torp-Pedersen, J. E. Carlsen, H. Bagger, P. Eliasen, K. Lyngborg, J. Videbaek, D. S. Cole, L. Auclert, and N. C. Pauly. 1995. "A clinical trial of the angiotensin-converting-enzyme inhibitor trandolapril in patients with left ventricular dysfunction after myocardial infarction. Trandolapril Cardiac Evaluation (TRACE) Study Group." *N Engl J Med* 333 (25):1670–6. doi: 10.1056/NEJM199512213332503.

Kodama, H., K. Fukuda, J. Pan, S. Makino, A. Baba, S. Hori, and S. Ogawa. 1997. "Leukemia inhibitory factor, a potent cardiac hypertrophic cytokine, activates the JAK/STAT pathway in rat cardiomyocytes." *Circ Res* 81 (5):656–63.

Komamura, K., N. Iwai, K. Kokame, Y. Yasumura, J. Kim, M. Yamagishi, T. Morisaki, A. Kimura, H. Tomoike, M. Kitakaze, and K. Miyatake. 2004. "The role of a common TNNT2 polymorphism in cardiac hypertrophy." *J Hum Genet* 49 (3):129–33. doi: 10.1007/s10038-003-0121-4.

Krishnamurthy, P., J. Rajasingh, E. Lambers, G. Qin, D. W. Losordo, and R. Kishore. 2009. "IL-10 inhibits inflammation and attenuates left ventricular remodeling after myocardial infarction via activation of STAT3 and suppression of HuR." *Circ Res* 104 (2):e9–18. doi: 10.1161/CIRCRESAHA.108.188243.

Kubota, T., D. M. McNamara, J. J. Wang, M. Trost, C. F. McTiernan, D. L. Mann, and A. M. Feldman. 1998. "Effects of tumor necrosis factor gene polymorphisms on patients with congestive heart failure. VEST Investigators for TNF Genotype Analysis. Vesnarinone Survival Trial." *Circulation* 97 (25):2499–501.

Kumar, S., A. Mishra, A. Srivastava, M. Bhatt, N. Garg, S. K. Agarwal, S. Pande, and B. Mittal. 2016. "Role of common sarcomeric gene polymorphisms in genetic susceptibility to left ventricular dysfunction." *J Genet* 95 (2):263–72.

Kundu, J. K., and Y. J. Surh. 2008. "Inflammation: gearing the journey to cancer." *Mutat Res* 659 (1-2):15–30. doi: 10.1016/j.mrrev.2008.03.002.

Kupari, M., A. Hautanen, L. Lankinen, P. Koskinen, J. Virolainen, H. Nikkila, and P. C. White. 1998. "Associations between human aldosterone synthase (CYP11B2) gene polymorphisms and left ventricular size, mass, and function." *Circulation* 97 (6):569–75.

Lajemi, M., C. Labat, S. Gautier, P. Lacolley, M. Safar, R. Asmar, F. Cambien, and A. Benetos. 2001. "Angiotensin II type 1 receptor-153A/G and 1166A/C gene polymorphisms and increase in aortic stiffness with age in hypertensive subjects." *J Hypertens* 19 (3):407–13.

Lavie, C. J., H. O. Ventura, and F. H. Messerli. 1991. "Regression of increased left ventricular mass by antihypertensives." *Drugs* 42 (6):945–61.

Lee, R. T., and P. Libby. 2000. "Matrix metalloproteinases: not-so-innocent bystanders in heart failure." *J Clin Invest* 106 (7):827–8. doi: 10.1172/JCI11263.

Lerman, A., F. L. Hildebrand, Jr., L. L. Aarhus, and J. C. Burnett, Jr. 1991. "Endothelin has biological actions at pathophysiological concentrations." *Circulation* 83 (5):1808–14.

Levine, B., J. Kalman, L. Mayer, H. M. Fillit, and M. Packer. 1990. "Elevated circulating levels of tumor necrosis factor in severe chronic heart failure." *N Engl J Med* 323 (4):236–41. doi: 10.1056/NEJM199007263230405.

LeWinter, M. M., and H. L. Granzier. 2014. "Cardiac titin and heart disease." *J Cardiovasc Pharmacol* 63 (3):207–12. doi: 10.1097/FJC.0000000000000007.

Li, S., W. Guo, C. N. Dewey, and M. L. Greaser. 2013. "Rbm20 regulates titin alternative splicing as a splicing repressor." *Nucleic Acids Res* 41 (4):2659–72. doi: 10.1093/nar/gks1362.

Lifton, R. P., R. G. Dluhy, M. Powers, G. M. Rich, S. Cook, S. Ulick, and J. M. Lalouel. 1992. "A chimaeric 11 beta-hydroxylase/aldosterone synthase gene causes glucocorticoid-remediable aldosteronism and human hypertension." *Nature* 355 (6357):262–5. doi: 10.1038/355262a0.

Lifton, R. P., R. G. Dluhy, M. Powers, G. M. Rich, M. Gutkin, F. Fallo, J. R. Gill, Jr., L. Feld, A. Ganguly, J. C. Laidlaw, and et al., 1992. "Hereditary hypertension caused by chimaeric gene duplications and ectopic expression of aldosterone synthase." *Nat Genet* 2 (1):66–74. doi: 10.1038/ng0992-66.

Liggett, S. B. 1998. "Pharmacogenetics of relevant targets in asthma." *Clin Exp Allergy* 28 Suppl 1:77–9; discussion 80–1.

Liggett, S. B. 2000a. "Beta(2)-adrenergic receptor pharmacogenetics." *Am J Respir Crit Care Med* 161 (3 Pt 2):S197–201. doi: 10.1164/ajrccm.161.supplement_2.a1q4-10.

Liggett, S. B. 2000b. "The pharmacogenetics of beta2-adrenergic receptors: relevance to asthma." *J Allergy Clin Immunol* 105 (2 Pt 2):S487–92.

Liggett, S. B. 2000c. "Pharmacogenetics of beta-1-and beta-2-adrenergic receptors." *Pharmacology* 61 (3):167–73. doi: 10.1159/000028397.

Liggett, S. B., L. E. Wagoner, L. L. Craft, R. W. Hornung, B. D. Hoit, T. C. McIntosh, and R. A. Walsh. 1998. "The Ile164 beta2-adrenergic receptor polymorphism adversely affects the outcome of congestive heart failure." *J Clin Invest* 102 (8):1534–9. doi: 10.1172/JCI4059.

Lindpaintner, K., M. Lee, M. G. Larson, V. S. Rao, M. A. Pfeffer, J. M. Ordovas, E. J. Schaefer, A. F. Wilson, P. W. Wilson, R. S. Vasan, R. H. Myers, and D. Levy. 1996. "Absence of association or genetic linkage between the angiotensin-converting-enzyme gene and left ventricular mass." *N Engl J Med* 334 (16):1023–8. doi: 10.1056/NEJM199604183341604.

Lindsey, M. L., J. Gannon, M. Aikawa, F. J. Schoen, E. Rabkin, L. Lopresti-Morrow, J. Crawford, S. Black, P. Libby, P. G. Mitchell, and R. T. Lee. 2002. "Selective matrix metalloproteinase inhibition reduces left ventricular remodeling but does not inhibit angiogenesis after myocardial infarction." *Circulation* 105 (6):753–8.

Lusis, A. J. 2003. "Genetic factors in cardiovascular disease. 10 questions." *Trends Cardiovasc Med* 13 (8):309–16. doi: 10.1016/j.tcm.2003.08.001.

Maczewski, M., J. Maczewska, and M. Duda. 2008. "Hypercholesterolaemia exacerbates ventricular remodelling after myocardial infarction in the rat: role of angiotensin II type 1 receptors." *Br J Pharmacol* 154 (8):1640–8. doi: 10.1038/bjp.2008.218.

Makarenko, I., C. A. Opitz, M. C. Leake, C. Neagoe, M. Kulke, J. K. Gwathmey, F. del Monte, R. J. Hajjar, and W. A. Linke. 2004. "Passive stiffness changes caused by upregulation of compliant titin isoforms in human dilated cardiomyopathy hearts." *Circ Res* 95 (7):708–16. doi: 10.1161/01.RES.0000143901.37063.2f.

Maqbool, A., A. S. Hall, S. G. Ball, and A. J. Balmforth. 1999. "Common polymorphisms of beta1-adrenoceptor: identification and rapid screening assay." *Lancet* 353 (9156):897. doi: 10.1016/s0140-6736(99)00549-8.

Maruyama, K. 1976. "Connectin, an elastic protein from myofibrils." *J Biochem* 80 (2):405–7.

Mascareno, E., M. Dhar, and M. A. Siddiqui. 1998. "Signal transduction and activator of transcription (STAT) protein-dependent activation of angiotensinogen promoter: a cellular signal for hypertrophy in cardiac muscle." *Proc Natl Acad Sci U S A* 95 (10):5590–4.

Mascareno, E., M. El-Shafei, N. Maulik, M. Sato, Y. Guo, D. K. Das, and M. A. Siddiqui. 2001. "JAK/STAT signaling is associated with cardiac dysfunction during ischemia and reperfusion." *Circulation* 104 (3):325–9.

Maskos, K. 2005. "Crystal structures of MMPs in complex with physiological and pharmacological inhibitors." *Biochimie* 87 (3-4):249–63. doi: 10.1016/j.biochi.2004.11.019.

Mason, D. A., J. D. Moore, S. A. Green, and S. B. Liggett. 1999. "A gain-of-function polymorphism in a G-protein coupling domain of the human beta1-adrenergic receptor." *J Biol Chem* 274 (18):12670–4.

McClellan, G., I. Kulikovskaya, and S. Winegrad. 2001. "Changes in cardiac contractility related to calcium-mediated changes in phosphorylation of myosin-binding protein C." *Biophys J* 81 (2):1083–92. doi: 10.1016/S0006-3495(01)75765-7.

McNamara, D. M., G. A. MacGowan, and B. London. 2002. "Clinical importance of beta-adrenoceptor polymorphisms in cardiovascular disease." *Am J Pharmacogenomics* 2 (2):73–8.

Methawasin, M., K. R. Hutchinson, E. J. Lee, J. E. Smith, 3rd, C. Saripalli, C. G. Hidalgo, C. A. Ottenheijm, and H. Granzier. 2014. "Experimentally increasing titin compliance in a novel mouse model attenuates the Frank-Starling mechanism but has a beneficial effect on diastole." *Circulation* 129 (19):1924–36. doi: 10.1161/CIRCULATIONAHA.113.005610.

Mishra, A., A. Srivastava, T. Mittal, N. Garg, and B. Mittal. 2012a. "Association of matrix metalloproteinases (MMP2, MMP7 and MMP9) genetic variants with left ventricular dysfunction in coronary artery disease patients." *Clin Chim Acta* 413 (19-20):1668–74. doi: 10.1016/j.cca.2012.05.012.

Mishra, A., A. Srivastava, T. Mittal, N. Garg, and B. Mittal. 2012b. "Impact of renin-angiotensin-aldosterone system gene polymorphisms on left ventricular dysfunction in coronary artery disease patients." *Dis Markers* 32 (1):33–41. doi: 10.3233/DMA-2012-0858.

Mishra, A., A. Srivastava, T. Mittal, N. Garg, and B. Mittal. 2013. "Role of inflammatory gene polymorphisms in left ventricular dysfunction (LVD) susceptibility in coronary artery disease (CAD) patients." *Cytokine* 61 (3):856–61. doi: 10.1016/j.cyto.2012.12.020.

Mishra, A., A. Srivastava, T. Mittal, N. Garg, and B. Mittal. 2014. "Genetic predisposition to left ventricular dysfunction: a multigenic and multi-analytical approach." *Gene* 546 (2):309–17. doi: 10.1016/j.gene.2014.05.060.

Miyazaki, K., Y. Hattori, F. Umenishi, H. Yasumitsu, and M. Umeda. 1990. "Purification and characterization of extracellular matrix-degrading metalloproteinase, matrin (pump-1), secreted from human rectal carcinoma cell line." *Cancer Res* 50 (24):7758–64.

Montgomery, H. 1997. "Should the contribution of ACE gene polymorphism to left ventricular hypertrophy be reconsidered?" *Heart* 77 (6):489–90.

Montgomery, H. E., P. J. Keeling, J. H. Goldman, S. E. Humphries, P. J. Talmud, and W. J. McKenna. 1995. "Lack of association between the insertion/deletion polymorphism of the angiotensin-converting enzyme gene and idiopathic dilated cardiomyopathy." *J Am Coll Cardiol* 25 (7):1627–31. doi: 10.1016/0735-1097(95)00109-h.

Mukherjee, R., T. A. Brinsa, K. B. Dowdy, A. A. Scott, J. M. Baskin, A. M. Deschamps, A. S. Lowry, G. P. Escobar, D. G. Lucas, W. M. Yarbrough, M. R. Zile, and F. G. Spinale. 2003. "Myocardial infarct expansion and matrix metalloproteinase inhibition." *Circulation* 107 (4):618–25.

Nagase, H., and J. F. Woessner, Jr. 1999. "Matrix metalloproteinases." *J Biol Chem* 274 (31):21491–4.

Nagashima, J., H. Musha, T. So, T. Kunishima, S. Nobuoka, and M. Murayama. 1999. "Effect of angiotensin-converting enzyme gene polymorphism on left ventricular remodeling after anteroseptal infarction." *Clin Cardiol* 22 (9):587–90.

Nagueh, S. F., G. Shah, Y. Wu, G. Torre-Amione, N. M. King, S. Lahmers, C. C. Witt, K. Becker, S. Labeit, and H. L. Granzier. 2004. "Altered titin expression, myocardial stiffness, and left ventricular function in patients with dilated cardiomyopathy." *Circulation* 110 (2):155–62. doi: 10.1161/01.CIR.0000135591.37759.AF.

Nakagami, H., Y. Kikuchi, T. Katsuya, R. Morishita, H. Akasaka, S. Saitoh, H. Rakugi, Y. Kaneda, K. Shimamoto, and T. Ogihara. 2007. "Gene polymorphism of myospryn (cardiomyopathy-associated 5) is associated with left ventricular wall thickness in patients with hypertension." *Hypertens Res* 30 (12):1239–46. doi: 10.1291/hypres.30.1239.

Nakauchi, Y., T. Suehiro, M. Yamamoto, N. Yasuoka, K. Arii, Y. Kumon, N. Hamashige, and K. Hashimoto. 1996. "Significance of angiotensin I-converting enzyme and angiotensin II type 1 receptor gene polymorphisms as risk factors for coronary heart disease." *Atherosclerosis* 125 (2):161–9. doi: 10.1016/0021-9150(96)05866-2.

Nalogowska-Glosnicka, K., B. I. Lacka, M. J. Zychma, W. Grzeszczak, E. Zukowska-Szczechowska, R. Poreba, B. Michalski, B. Kniazewski, and J. Rzempoluch. 2000. "Angiotensin II type 1 receptor gene A1166C polymorphism is associated with the increased risk of pregnancy-induced hypertension." *Med Sci Monit* 6 (3):523–9.

Neagoe, C., M. Kulke, F. del Monte, J. K. Gwathmey, P. P. de Tombe, R. J. Hajjar, and W. A. Linke. 2002. "Titin isoform switch in ischemic human heart disease." *Circulation* 106 (11):1333–41.

Newby, A. C. 2005. "Dual role of matrix metalloproteinases (matrixins) in intimal thickening and atherosclerotic plaque rupture." *Physiol Rev* 85 (1):1–31. doi: 10.1152/physrev.00048.2003.

Niebauer, J., H. D. Volk, M. Kemp, M. Dominguez, R. R. Schumann, M. Rauchhaus, P. A. Poole-Wilson, A. J. Coats, and S. D. Anker. 1999. "Endotoxin and immune activation in chronic heart failure: a prospective cohort study." *Lancet* 353 (9167):1838–42. doi: 10.1016/S0140-6736(98)09286-1.

Oakley, C. E., B. D. Hambly, P. M. Curmi, and L. J. Brown. 2004. "Myosin binding protein C: structural abnormalities in familial hypertrophic cardiomyopathy." *Cell Res* 14 (2):95–110. doi: 10.1038/sj.cr.7290208.

Ohmichi, N., N. Iwai, K. Maeda, H. Shimoike, Y. Nakamura, M. Izumi, Y. Sugimoto, and M. Kinoshita. 1996. "Genetic basis of left ventricular remodeling after myocardial infarction." *Int J Cardiol* 53 (3):265–72. doi: 10.1016/0167-5273(96)02562-4.

Okada K, Wangpoengtrakul C, Osawa T, Toyokuni S, Tanaka K, Uchida K. 1999. "4-Hydroxy-2-nonenal-mediated impairment of intracellular proteolysis during oxidative stress. Identification of proteasomes as target molecules." *J. Biol.Chem.* 274:23787–23793.

Okagaki, T., F. E. Weber, D. A. Fischman, K. T. Vaughan, T. Mikawa, and F. C. Reinach. 1993. "The major myosin-binding domain of skeletal muscle MyBP-C (C protein) resides in the COOH-terminal, immunoglobulin C2 motif." *J Cell Biol* 123 (3):619–26.

Ono, K., T. Mannami, S. Baba, N. Yasui, T. Ogihara, and N. Iwai. 2003. "Lack of association between angiotensin II type 1 receptor gene polymorphism and hypertension in Japanese." *Hypertens Res* 26 (2):131–4.

Overall, C. M. 2002. "Molecular determinants of metalloproteinase substrate specificity: matrix metalloproteinase substrate binding domains, modules, and exosites." *Mol Biotechnol* 22 (1):51–86. doi: 10.1385/MB:22:1:051.

Page-McCaw, A., A. J. Ewald, and Z. Werb. 2007. "Matrix metalloproteinases and the regulation of tissue remodelling." *Nat Rev Mol Cell Biol* 8 (3):221–33. doi: 10.1038/nrm2125.

Pahl, H. L. 1999. "Activators and target genes of Rel/NF-kappaB transcription factors." *Oncogene* 18 (49):6853–66. doi: 10.1038/sj.onc.1203239.

Palmer, B. R., A. P. Pilbrow, T. G. Yandle, C. M. Frampton, A. M. Richards, M. G. Nicholls, and V. A. Cameron. 2003. "Angiotensin-converting enzyme gene polymorphism interacts with left ventricular ejection fraction and brain natriuretic peptide levels to predict mortality after myocardial infarction." *J Am Coll Cardiol* 41 (5):729–36. doi: 10.1016/s0735-1097(02)02927-3.

Parenica, J., M. P. Goldbergova, P. Kala, J. Jarkovsky, M. Poloczek, J. Manousek, K. Prymusova, L. Kubkova, D. Tomcikova, O. Toman, M. Tesak, J. Tomandl, A. Vasku, and J. Spinar. 2010. "ACE gene insertion/deletion polymorphism has a mild influence on the acute development of left ventricular dysfunction in patients with ST elevation myocardial infarction treated with primary PCI." *BMC Cardiovasc Disord* 10:60. doi: 10.1186/1471-2261-10-60.

Pascoe, L., K. M. Curnow, L. Slutsker, J. M. Connell, P. W. Speiser, M. I. New, and P. C. White. 1992. "Glucocorticoid-suppressible hyperaldosteronism results from hybrid genes created by unequal crossovers between CYP11B1 and CYP11B2." *Proc Natl Acad Sci U S A* 89 (17):8327–31.

Pascoe, L., K. M. Curnow, L. Slutsker, A. Rosler, and P. C. White. 1992. "Mutations in the human CYP11B2 (aldosterone synthase) gene causing corticosterone methyloxidase II deficiency." *Proc Natl Acad Sci U S A* 89 (11):4996–5000.

Pennica, D., K. L. King, K. J. Shaw, E. Luis, J. Rullamas, S. M. Luoh, W. C. Darbonne, D. S. Knutzon, R. Yen, K. R. Chien, and et al., 1995. "Expression cloning of cardiotrophin 1, a cytokine that induces cardiac myocyte hypertrophy." *Proc Natl Acad Sci U S A* 92 (4):1142–6.

Pennica, D., W. I. Wood, and K. R. Chien. 1996. "Cardiotrophin-1: a multifunctional cytokine that signals via LIF receptor-gp 130 dependent pathways." *Cytokine Growth Factor Rev* 7 (1):81–91.

Perazella, M. A., and J. F. Setaro. 2003. "Renin-angiotensin-aldosterone system: fundamental aspects and clinical implications in renal and cardiovascular disorders." *J Nucl Cardiol* 10 (2):184–96. doi: 10.1067/mnc.2003.392.

Perticone, F., R. Ceravolo, C. Cosco, M. Trapasso, A. Zingone, P. Malatesta, N. Perrotti, D. Tramontano, and P. L. Mattioli. 1997. "Deletion polymorphism of angiotensin-converting enzyme gene and left ventricular hypertrophy in southern Italian patients." *J Am Coll Cardiol* 29 (2):365–9. doi: 10.1016/s0735-1097(96)00485-8.

Peters, D. G., A. Kassam, P. L. St Jean, H. Yonas, and R. E. Ferrell. 1999. "Functional polymorphism in the matrix metalloproteinase-9 promoter as a potential risk factor for intracranial aneurysm." *Stroke* 30 (12):2612–6.

Pfeffer, M. A., E. Braunwald, L. A. Moye, L. Basta, E. J. Brown, Jr., T. E. Cuddy, B. R. Davis, E. M. Geltman, S. Goldman, G. C. Flaker, and et al., 1992. "Effect of captopril on mortality and morbidity in patients with left ventricular dysfunction after myocardial infarction. Results of the survival and ventricular enlargement trial. The SAVE Investigators." *N Engl J Med* 327 (10):669–77. doi: 10.1056/NEJM199209033271001.

Pinto, Y. M., W. H. van Gilst, J. H. Kingma, and H. Schunkert. 1995. "Deletion-type allele of the angiotensin-converting enzyme gene is associated with progressive ventricular dilation after anterior myocardial infarction. Captopril and Thrombolysis Study Investigators." *J Am Coll Cardiol* 25 (7):1622–6. doi: 10.1016/0735-1097(95)00090-q.

Podesser, B. K., D. A. Siwik, F. R. Eberli, F. Sam, S. Ngoy, J. Lambert, K. Ngo, C. S. Apstein, and W. S. Colucci. 2001. "ET(A)-receptor blockade prevents matrix metalloproteinase activation late postmyocardial infarction in the rat." *Am J Physiol Heart Circ Physiol* 280 (3):H984–91.

Poirier, O., J. L. Georges, S. Ricard, D. Arveiler, J. B. Ruidavets, G. Luc, A. Evans, F. Cambien, and L. Tiret. 1998. "New polymorphisms of the angiotensin II type 1 receptor gene and their associations with myocardial infarction and blood pressure: the ECTIM study. Etude Cas-Temoin de l'Infarctus du Myocarde." *J Hypertens* 16 (10):1443–7.

Pollanen, P. J., P. J. Karhunen, J. Mikkelsson, P. Laippala, M. Perola, A. Penttila, K. M. Mattila, T. Koivula, and T. Lehtimaki. 2001. "Coronary artery complicated lesion area is related to functional polymorphism of matrix metalloproteinase 9 gene: an autopsy study." *Arterioscler Thromb Vasc Biol* 21 (9):1446–50.

Port, J. D., and M. R. Bristow. 2001. "Altered beta-adrenergic receptor gene regulation and signaling in chronic heart failure." *J Mol Cell Cardiol* 33 (5):887–905. doi: 10.1006/jmcc.2001.1358.

Quantin, B., G. Murphy, and R. Breathnach. 1989. "Pump-1 cDNA codes for a protein with characteristics similar to those of classical collagenase family members." *Biochemistry* 28 (13):5327–34.

Rani, D. S., P. Nallari, P. S. Dhandapany, S. Tamilarasi, A. Shah, V. Archana, M. AshokKumar, C. Narasimhan, L. Singh, and K. Thangaraj. 2012. "Cardiac Troponin T (TNNT2) mutations are less prevalent in Indian hypertrophic cardiomyopathy patients." *DNA Cell Biol* 31 (4):616–24. doi: 10.1089/dna.2011.1366.

Raynolds, M. V., M. R. Bristow, E. W. Bush, W. T. Abraham, B. D. Lowes, L. S. Zisman, C. S. Taft, and M. B. Perryman. 1993. "Angiotensin-converting enzyme DD genotype in patients with ischaemic or idiopathic dilated cardiomyopathy." *Lancet* 342 (8879):1073–5. doi: 10.1016/0140-6736(93)92061-w.

Rigat, B., C. Hubert, F. Alhenc-Gelas, F. Cambien, P. Corvol, and F. Soubrier. 1990. "An insertion/deletion polymorphism in the angiotensin I-converting enzyme gene accounting for half the variance of serum enzyme levels." *J Clin Invest* 86 (4):1343–6. doi: 10.1172/JCI114844.

Rohde, L. E., A. Ducharme, L. H. Arroyo, M. Aikawa, G. H. Sukhova, A. Lopez-Anaya, K. F. McClure, P. G. Mitchell, P. Libby, and R. T. Lee. 1999. "Matrix metalloproteinase inhibition attenuates early left ventricular enlargement after experimental myocardial infarction in mice." *Circulation* 99 (23):3063–70.

Romanic, A. M., C. L. Burns-Kurtis, B. Gout, I. Berrebi-Bertrand, and E. H. Ohlstein. 2001. "Matrix metalloproteinase expression in cardiac myocytes following myocardial infarction in the rabbit." *Life Sci* 68 (7):799–814. doi: 10.1016/s0024-3205(00)00982-6.

Ross, R. 1993. "The pathogenesis of atherosclerosis: a perspective for the 1990s." *Nature* 362 (6423):801–9. doi: 10.1038/362801a0.

Sadayappan, S., and P. P. de Tombe. 2014. "Cardiac myosin binding protein-C as a central target of cardiac sarcomere signaling: a special mini review series." *Pflugers Arch* 466 (2):195–200. doi: 10.1007/s00424-013-1396-8.

Sadayappan, S., H. Osinska, R. Klevitsky, J. N. Lorenz, M. Sargent, J. D. Molkentin, C. E. Seidman, J. G. Seidman, and J. Robbins. 2006. "Cardiac myosin binding protein C phosphorylation is cardioprotective." *Proc Natl Acad Sci U S A* 103 (45):16918–23. doi: 10.1073/pnas.0607069103.

Sadoshima, J., and S. Izumo. 1993. "Molecular characterization of angiotensin II--induced hypertrophy of cardiac myocytes and hyperplasia of cardiac fibroblasts. Critical role of the AT1 receptor subtype." *Circ Res* 73 (3):413–23.

Sadoshima, J., Y. Xu, H. S. Slayter, and S. Izumo. 1993. "Autocrine release of angiotensin II mediates stretch-induced hypertrophy of cardiac myocytes in vitro." *Cell* 75 (5):977–84.

Sakai, S., T. Miyauchi, M. Kobayashi, I. Yamaguchi, K. Goto, and Y. Sugishita. 1996. "Inhibition of myocardial endothelin pathway improves long-term survival in heart failure." *Nature* 384 (6607):353–5. doi: 10.1038/384353a0.

Sarikas, A., L. Carrier, C. Schenke, D. Doll, J. Flavigny, K. S. Lindenberg, T. Eschenhagen, and O. Zolk. 2005. "Impairment of the ubiquitin-proteasome system by truncated cardiac myosin binding protein C mutants." *Cardiovasc Res* 66 (1):33–44. doi: 10.1016/j.cardiores.2005.01.004.

Schlender, K. K., and L. J. Bean. 1991. "Phosphorylation of chicken cardiac C-protein by calcium/calmodulin-dependent protein kinase II." *J Biol Chem* 266 (5):2811–7.

Schunkert, H., C. Hengstenberg, S. R. Holmer, U. Broeckel, A. Luchner, M. W. Muscholl, S. Kurzinger, A. Doring, H. W. Hense, and G. A. Riegger. 1999. "Lack of association between a polymorphism of the aldosterone synthase gene and left ventricular structure." *Circulation* 99 (17):2255–60.

Schunkert, H., H. W. Hense, S. R. Holmer, M. Stender, S. Perz, U. Keil, B. H. Lorell, and G. A. Riegger. 1994. "Association between a deletion polymorphism of the angiotensin-converting-enzyme gene and left ventricular hypertrophy." *N Engl J Med* 330 (23):1634–8. doi: 10.1056/NEJM199406093302302.

Seta, Y., K. Shan, B. Bozkurt, H. Oral, and D. L. Mann. 1996. "Basic mechanisms in heart failure: the cytokine hypothesis." *J Card Fail* 2 (3):243–9.

Sethupathy, P., C. Borel, M. Gagnebin, G. R. Grant, S. Deutsch, T. S. Elton, A. G. Hatzigeorgiou, and S. E. Antonarakis. 2007. "Human microRNA-155 on chromosome 21 differentially interacts with its polymorphic target in the AGTR1 3' untranslated region: a mechanism for functional single-nucleotide polymorphisms related to phenotypes." *Am J Hum Genet* 81 (2):405–13. doi: 10.1086/519979.

Simonson, T. S., Y. Zhang, C. D. Huff, J. Xing, W. S. Watkins, D. J. Witherspoon, S. R. Woodward, and L. B. Jorde. 2010. "Limited distribution of a cardiomyopathy-associated variant in India." *Ann Hum Genet* 74 (2):184–8. doi: 10.1111/j.1469-1809.2010.00561.x.

Singh, T., and A. B. Newman. 2011. "Inflammatory markers in population studies of aging." *Ageing Res Rev* 10 (3):319–29. doi: 10.1016/j.arr.2010.11.002.

Soubrier, F., S. Nadaud, and T. A. Williams. 1994. "Angiotensin I converting enzyme gene: regulation, polymorphism and implications in cardiovascular diseases." *Eur Heart J* 15 Suppl D:24–9.

Spinale, F. G. 2002. "Matrix metalloproteinases: regulation and dysregulation in the failing heart." *Circ Res* 90 (5):520–30.

Spinale, F. G., M. L. Coker, L. J. Heung, B. R. Bond, H. R. Gunasinghe, T. Etoh, A. T. Goldberg, J. L. Zellner, and A. J. Crumbley. 2000. "A matrix metalloproteinase induction/activation system exists in the human left ventricular myocardium and is upregulated in heart failure." *Circulation* 102 (16):1944–9.

Stocker, W., F. Grams, U. Baumann, P. Reinemer, F. X. Gomis-Ruth, D. B. McKay, and W. Bode. 1995. "The metzincins--topological and sequential relations between the astacins, adamalysins, serralysins, and matrixins (collagenases) define a superfamily of zinc-peptidases." *Protein Sci* 4 (5):823–40. doi: 10.1002/pro.5560040502.

Takahashi, N., H. Murakami, K. Kodama, F. Kasagi, M. Yamada, T. Nishishita, and T. Inagami. 2000. "Association of a polymorphism at the 5'-region of the angiotensin II type 1 receptor with hypertension." *Ann Hum Genet* 64 (Pt 3):197–205. doi: 10.1017/S0003480000008083.

Takai, E., H. Akita, K. Kanazawa, N. Shiga, M. Terashima, Y. Matsuda, C. Iwai, Y. Miyamoto, H. Kawai, A. Takarada, and M. Yokoyama. 2002. "Association between aldosterone synthase (CYP11B2) gene polymorphism and left ventricular volume in patients with dilated cardiomyopathy." *Heart* 88 (6):649–50.

Takami, S., T. Katsuya, H. Rakugi, N. Sato, Y. Nakata, A. Kamitani, T. Miki, J. Higaki, and T. Ogihara. 1998. "Angiotensin II type 1 receptor gene polymorphism is associated with increase of left ventricular mass but not with hypertension." *Am J Hypertens* 11 (3 Pt 1):316–21. doi: 10.1016/s0895-7061(97)00457-3.

Thompson, R. W., and W. C. Parks. 1996. "Role of matrix metalloproteinases in abdominal aortic aneurysms." *Ann N Y Acad Sci* 800:157–74.

Tiret, L., A. Bonnardeaux, O. Poirier, S. Ricard, P. Marques-Vidal, A. Evans, D. Arveiler, G. Luc, F. Kee, P. Ducimetiere, and et al., 1994. "Synergistic effects of angiotensin-converting enzyme and angiotensin-II type 1 receptor gene polymorphisms on risk of myocardial infarction." *Lancet* 344 (8927):910–3.

Tiret, L., C. Mallet, O. Poirier, V. Nicaud, A. Millaire, J. B. Bouhour, G. Roizes, M. Desnos, R. Dorent, K. Schwartz, F. Cambien, and M. Komajda. 2000. "Lack of association between polymorphisms of eight candidate genes and idiopathic dilated cardiomyopathy: the CARDIGENE study." *J Am Coll Cardiol* 35 (1):29–35. doi: 10.1016/S0735-1097(99)00522-7.

Tiret, L., B. Rigat, S. Visvikis, C. Breda, P. Corvol, F. Cambien, and F. Soubrier. 1992. "Evidence, from combined segregation and linkage analysis, that a variant of the angiotensin I-converting enzyme (ACE) gene controls plasma ACE levels." *Am J Hum Genet* 51 (1):197–205.

Towbin, J. A., and N. E. Bowles. 2001. "Molecular genetics of left ventricular dysfunction." *Curr Mol Med* 1 (1):81–90.

Turki, J., J. N. Lorenz, S. A. Green, E. T. Donnelly, M. Jacinto, and S. B. Liggett. 1996. "Myocardial signaling defects and impaired cardiac function of a human beta 2-adrenergic receptor polymorphism expressed in transgenic mice." *Proc Natl Acad Sci U S A* 93 (19):10483–8.

Ueda, S., H. L. Elliott, J. J. Morton, and J. M. Connell. 1995. "Enhanced pressor response to angiotensin I in normotensive men with the deletion genotype (DD) for angiotensin-converting enzyme." *Hypertension* 25 (6):1266–9.

Ulgen, M. S., O. Ozturk, S. Alan, M. Kayrak, Y. Turan, S. Tekes, and N. Toprak. 2007. "The relationship between angiotensin-converting enzyme (insertion/deletion) gene polymorphism and left ventricular remodeling in acute myocardial infarction." *Coron Artery Dis* 18 (3):153–7. doi: 10.1097/mca.0b013e328010a4c4.

Valen, G., Z. Q. Yan, and G. K. Hansson. 2001. "Nuclear factor kappa-B and the heart." *J Am Coll Cardiol* 38 (2):307–14. doi: 10.1016/s0735-1097(01)01377-8.

Valgimigli, M., C. Ceconi, P. Malagutti, E. Merli, O. Soukhomovskaia, G. Francolini, G. Cicchitelli, A. Olivares, G. Parrinello, G. Percoco, G. Guardigli, D. Mele, R. Pirani, and R. Ferrari. 2005. "Tumor necrosis factor-alpha receptor 1 is a major predictor of mortality and new-onset heart failure in patients with acute myocardial infarction: the Cytokine-Activation and Long-Term Prognosis in Myocardial Infarction (C-ALPHA) study." *Circulation* 111 (7):863–70. doi: 10.1161/01.CIR.0000155614.35441.69.

van Berlo, J. H., and Y. M. Pinto. 2003. "Polymorphisms in the RAS and cardiac function." *Int J Biochem Cell Biol* 35 (6):932–43. doi: 10.1016/S1357-2725(02)00369-2.

van Heerebeek, L., A. Borbély, H. W. Niessen, J. G. Bronzwaer, J. van der Velden, G. J. Stienen, W. A. Linke, G. J. Laarman, and W. J. Paulus. 2006. "Myocardial structure and function differ in systolic and diastolic heart failure." *Circulation* 113 (16):1966–73. doi: 10.1161/CIRCULATIONAHA.105.587519.

Vančura, V., J. Hubáček, I. Málek, M. Gebauerová, J. Pit'ha, Z. Dorazilová, M. Langová, M. Želízko, and R. Poledne. 1999. "Does angiotensin-converting enzyme polymorphism influence the clinical manifestation and progression of heart failure in patients with dilated cardiomyopathy?" *Am J Cardiol* 83 (3):461–2, A10. doi: 10.1016/s0002-9149(98)00889-3.

Vasků, A., M. Goldbergova, L. I. Holla, L. Spinarova, J. Spinar, J. Vitovec, and J. Vacha. 2003. "Two MMP-2 promoter polymorphisms (-790T/G and -735C/T) in chronic heart failure." *Clin Chem Lab Med* 41 (10):1299–303. doi: 10.1515/CCLM.2003.197.

Vasku, A., M. Goldbergová, L. Izakovicová Hollá, L. Sisková, L. Groch, M. Beránek, S. Tschöplová, V. Znojil, and J. Vácha. 2004. "A haplotype constituted of four MMP-2 promoter polymorphisms (-1575G/A, -1306C/T, -790T/G and -735C/T) is associated with coronary triple-vessel disease." *Matrix Biol* 22 (7):585–91. doi: 10.1016/j.matbio.2003.10.004.

Vinkemeier, U., S. L. Cohen, I. Moarefi, B. T. Chait, J. Kuriyan, and J. E. Darnell, Jr. 1996. "DNA binding of in vitro activated Stat1 alpha, Stat1 beta and truncated Stat1: interaction between NH2-terminal domains stabilizes binding of two dimers to tandem DNA sites." *EMBO J* 15 (20):5616–26.

Vogel, U., M. K. Jensen, K. M. Due, E. B. Rimm, H. Wallin, M. R. Nielsen, A. P. Pedersen, A. Tjønneland, and K. Overvad. 2011. "The NFKB1 ATTG ins/del polymorphism and risk of coronary heart disease in three independent populations." *Atherosclerosis* 219 (1):200–4. doi: 10.1016/j.atherosclerosis.2011.06.018.

Waldmüller, S., S. Sakthivel, A. V. Saadi, C. Selignow, P. G. Rakesh, M. Golubenko, P. K. Joseph, R. Padmakumar, P. Richard, K. Schwartz, J. M. Tharakan, C. Rajamanickam, and H. P. Vosberg. 2003. "Novel deletions in MYH7 and MYBPC3 identified in Indian families with familial hypertrophic cardio-myopathy." *J Mol Cell Cardiol* 35 (6):623–36. doi: 10.1016/s0022-2828(03)00050-6.

Wang, K., J. McClure, and A. Tu. 1979. "Titin: major myofibrillar components of striated muscle." *Proc Natl Acad Sci U S A* 76 (8):3698–702.

Wang, W. Y., R. Y. Zee, and B. J. Morris. 1997. "Association of angiotensin II type 1 receptor gene poly-morphism with essential hypertension." *Clin Genet* 51 (1):31–4.

Warren, C. M., M. C. Jordan, K. P. Roos, P. R. Krzesinski, and M. L. Greaser. 2003. "Titin isoform expression in normal and hypertensive myocardium." *Cardiovasc Res* 59 (1):86–94. doi: 10.1016/s0008-6363(03)00328-6.

Weber, F. E., K. T. Vaughan, F. C. Reinach, and D. A. Fischman. 1993. "Complete sequence of human fast-type and slow-type muscle myosin-binding-protein C (MyBP-C). Differential expression, conserved domain structure and chromosome assignment." *Eur J Biochem* 216 (2):661–9.

Wei, C. M., A. Lerman, R. J. Rodeheffer, C. G. McGregor, R. R. Brandt, S. Wright, D. M. Heublein, P. C. Kao, W. D. Edwards, and J. C. Burnett, Jr. 1994. "Endothelin in human congestive heart failure." *Circulation* 89 (4):1580–6.

Welgus, H. G., D. K. Kobayashi, and J. J. Jeffrey. 1983. "The collagen substrate specificity of rat uterus collagenase." *J Biol Chem* 258 (23):14162–5.

White, P. C. 1994. "Disorders of aldosterone biosynthesis and action." *N Engl J Med* 331 (4):250–8. doi: 10.1056/NEJM199407283310408.

Whiting, A., J. Wardale, and J. Trinick. 1989. "Does titin regulate the length of muscle thick filaments?" *J Mol Biol* 205 (1):263–8. doi: 10.1016/0022-2836(89)90381-1.

Wilson, A. G., F. S. di Giovine, A. I. Blakemore, and G. W. Duff. 1992. "Single base polymorphism in the human tumour necrosis factor alpha (TNF alpha) gene detectable by NcoI restriction of PCR product." *Hum Mol Genet* 1 (5):353.

Wilson, A. G., J. A. Symons, T. L. McDowell, H. O. McDevitt, and G. W. Duff. 1997. "Effects of a polymorphism in the human tumor necrosis factor alpha promoter on transcriptional activation." *Proc Natl Acad Sci U S A* 94 (7):3195–9.

Wilson, E. M., H. R. Gunasinghe, M. L. Coker, P. Sprunger, D. Lee-Jackson, B. Bozkurt, A. Deswal, D. L. Mann, and F. G. Spinale. 2002. "Plasma matrix metalloproteinase and inhibitor profiles in patients with heart failure." *J Card Fail* 8 (6):390–8. doi: 10.1054/jcaf.2002.129659.

Woessner, J. F., Jr. 1991. "Matrix metalloproteinases and their inhibitors in connective tissue remodeling." *FASEB J* 5 (8):2145–54.

Wu, Y., S. P. Bell, K. Trombitas, C. C. Witt, S. Labeit, M. M. LeWinter, and H. Granzier. 2002. "Changes in titin isoform expression in pacing-induced cardiac failure give rise to increased passive muscle stiffness." *Circulation* 106 (11):1384–9.

Xi, X. P., K. Graf, S. Goetze, E. Fleck, W. A. Hsueh, and R. E. Law. 1999. "Central role of the MAPK pathway in ang II-mediated DNA synthesis and migration in rat vascular smooth muscle cells." *Arterioscler Thromb Vasc Biol* 19 (1):73–82.

Xu, M., P. Sham, Z. Ye, K. Lindpaintner, and L. He. 2010. "A1166C genetic variation of the angiotensin II type I receptor gene and susceptibility to coronary heart disease: collaborative of 53 studies with 20,435 cases and 23,674 controls." *Atherosclerosis* 213 (1):191–9. doi: 10.1016/j.atherosclerosis.2010.07.046.

Xuan, Y. T., Y. Guo, H. Han, Y. Zhu, and R. Bolli. 2001. "An essential role of the JAK-STAT pathway in ischemic preconditioning." *Proc Natl Acad Sci U S A* 98 (16):9050–5. doi: 10.1073/pnas.161283798.

Ye, S. 2000. "Polymorphism in matrix metalloproteinase gene promoters: implication in regulation of gene expression and susceptibility of various diseases." *Matrix Biol* 19 (7):623–9. doi: 10.1016/s0945-053x(00)00102-5.

Zaltsman, A. B., and A. C. Newby. 1997. "Increased secretion of gelatinases A and B from the aortas of cholesterol fed rabbits: relationship to lesion severity." *Atherosclerosis* 130 (1-2):61–70. doi: 10.1016/s0021-9150(96)06046-7.

Zee, R. Y., S. D. Solomon, U. A. Ajani, M. A. Pfeffer, and K. Lindpaintner. 2002. "A prospective evaluation of the angiotensin-converting enzyme D/I polymorphism and left ventricular remodeling in the 'Healing and Early Afterload Reducing Therapy' study." *Clin Genet* 61 (1):21–5. doi: 10.1034/j.1399-0004.2002.610104.x.

Zhang, D., L. Li, Y. Zhu, L. Zhao, L. Wan, J. Lv, X. Li, P. Huang, L. Wei, and M. Ma. 2013. "The NFKB1-94 ATTG insertion/deletion polymorphism (rs28362491) contributes to the susceptibility of congenital heart disease in a Chinese population." *Gene* 516 (2):307–10. doi: 10.1016/j.gene.2012.12.078.

Zhang, X., J. Erdmann, V. Regitz-Zagrosek, S. Kurzinger, H. W. Hense, and H. Schunkert. 2000. "Evaluation of three polymorphisms in the promoter region of the angiotensin II type I receptor gene." *J Hypertens* 18 (3):267–72.

15

Genetics of Diabetic Nephropathy: A Review

Gurvinder Singh
Department of Human Genetics, Guru Nanak Dev University, Amritsar, India

Priyanka Raina
Integrative Genomics of Ageing Group, Institute of Ageing and Chronic Disease, University of Liverpool, Liverpool, UK,

A.J.S. Bhanwer
Department of Genetics, Sri Guru Ram Das University of Health Sciences, Amritsar, India

15.1 Introduction

Diabetic nephropathy (DN)/diabetic kidney disease (DKD) is the foremost or the root cause for the development of end-stage renal disease (ESRD) in the Western world as well as in other parts of the world (Sagoo and Gnudi, 2020). It is a chronic, morbid, and a dreadful complication of diabetes. This microvascular complication has affected approximately 45% of type 1 diabetes (T1D) and type 2 diabetes (T2D) patients (Hovind et al., 2001). A recent study found that at the time of diagnosis, approximately one third of newly diagnosed T2D patients have already progressed towards secondary complications (i.e., either micro- or macrovascular complications) (Gedebjerg et al., 2018). Diabetic nephropathy (DN) is also the primary cause for patients who undergo renal replacement therapy worldwide (Gnudi et al., 2016). Reduction in the number of podocytes and their loss has been considered as the earliest sign of DN in diabetic patients (Pagtalunan et al., 1997). It has also been demonstrated that glomerular podocytes are essential in the development of DN (Wolf et al., 2005). According to previous and recent reports in both developed or developing nations, diabetes is the most common cause of chronic kidney disease (CKD), and cases are also increasing. The current situation may also have arisen due to any of the following (ADA, 2018; Vujičić et al., 2012; Hemanth et al., 2011):

a) The prevalence of diabetes, particularly T2D is increasing.
b) The prolonged life expectancy of diabetic patients due to newly developed therapies/technologies.
c) Diabetic ESRD patients are now allowed to recruit for treatment in ESRD programs where they were not allowed to register before.

The inheritability of DN has been observed in families supporting the fact of a genetic background of the disease. International collaborations are important milestones towards unravelling the genetic basis of DN, which has led to the discovery of specific genes involved in the development of nephropathy condition in diabetic patients (McKnight et al., 2015). Even after the discovery of a few genes, collaborative efforts, and the advancements of techniques, new treatments for DN are limited. The increases in the prevalence of diabetes and its complications like DN (Hill et al., 2014) are encouraging researchers to explore the genome to diagnose the disease at its early stages. Knowledge of the genetic markers responsible for DN progression can also led to the development of personalized medication.

DOI: 10.1201/9781003220404-17

15.2 Epidemiology of Diabetic Nephropathy

The prevalence of DN is increasing in parallel with the increase in T2D prevalence (Ritz and Zeng, 2011). About 40% of patients with T2D have been reported to develop CKD. T2D has also become the leading cause of ESRD worldwide and accounts for approximately 40% of the patients receiving renal replacement therapy each year. ESRD and dialysis treatment incur substantial cost in health, social, and financial terms (Luk and Chan, 2008; IDF, 2017; Scirica, 2017). In a recent study it was observed that adults with T2D have hyper-renal filtration and early progression to DN, thus indicating an increased impact of diabetes on adults with T2D (Bjornstad and Cherney, 2018). The number of DN patients undergoing kidney replacement therapy increased two folds in the United States in the period 1991–2001. The European Diabetes (EURODIAB) Prospective Complications Study Group and an 18-year Danish study showed that the overall prevalence of microalbuminuria in T1D and T2D patients was 12.6% and 33%, respectively. According to the United Kingdom Prospective Diabetes Study (UKPDS) in Great Britain the annual incidence of microalbuminuria in patients with T2D is 2% and its prevalence is 25% after ten years of diagnosis (Vujičić et al., 2012; Zoungas et al., 2017). At present, diabetes is the primary root cause of ESRD in the Western world and the principal cause for patients requiring renal replacement therapy worldwide. However, due to the strong association between DN and cardiovascular disease, a majority of patients with DN will die even before progression to ESRD, as a result of cardiovascular-related events (Gnudi et al., 2016).

Various countries such as Hong Kong, Finland, and the United Kingdom have adopted renal registries, which show that diabetic renal disease remains the single most common cause of renal failure, amounting to 24.8% of all the different causes. Epidemiology studies of T2D patients has shown that DN prevalence ranges from 7.6% to 55% globally, while in different international registries, it varies between 11.5% in the United Kingdom to 42.9% in Thailand (Al-Rubeaan et al., 2014; Shen et al., 2009; Parving et al., 2006). In India, DN is expected to develop in 6.6 million of the 30 million patients suffering from T2D (Baig et al., 2011). In a recent study, prevalence of CKD in Asian Indians is 39.8%, whereas in elderly people, DN accounts for more than 46% of CKD. In the Chennai Urban Rural Epidemiology Study (CURES), the prevalence of overt nephropathy and microalbuminuria was 2.2% and 26.9%, respectively, in urban residents with T2D (Ritz and Zeng, 2011; Luk et al., 2016).

15.3 Diagnosis of Diabetic Nephropathy

The clinical diagnosis for DN is based on the presence of albuminuria and/or reduced estimated glomerular filtration rate (eGFR), when there are no visible signs or symptoms of any other root causes for damage of renal cells. There are some known specific markers for the diagnosis of DN, including long-standing duration of diabetes (T2D), albuminuria without haematuria, evidence of retinopathy, and gradually progressive kidney disease (Table 15.1). However, the symptoms of DN may be present at the diagnosis, which could be either with or without the presence of retinopathy in T2D, but the most remarkable emblem is reduced eGFR without albuminuria, which has been frequently reported in both T1D and

TABLE 15.1

Different Markers for Detecting the Development of DN (ADA, 2018)

a. Albuminuria (AER $\geq$ 30mg/24 hours; ACR $\geq$ 30mg/g)	Markers of renal damage
b. Urine sediment abnormalities	
c. Electrolyte and other abnormalities due to tubular disorders	
d. Abnormalities detected by histology	
e. Structural abnormalities detected by imaging	
f. History of renal transplantation	
g. GFR < 60ml/min/1.73m^2	

T2D and is becoming a more common factor over the time as the prevalence of diabetes increases in United States and other parts of the world (Afkarian et al., 2016; de Boer et al., 2011; Kramer et al., 2003; Molitch et al., 2010). The nomenclature for "nephropathy" was replaced by "Diabetic Kidney Disease (DKD)" to emphasize that, while nephropathy may stem from a different range of causes, thus attention is placed on kidney disease, which is directly related to diabetes. There are several minor edits to this section by ADA (2016); the significant ones, based on evidence, are as follows (ADA, 2016):

- Guidance to the patients, when to refer to physicians experienced in the care of diabetic kidney disease
- When to refer for dialysis or kidney replacement treatment

Urinary sediment with red or white blood cells or cellular casts, swiftly increasing albuminuria or nephrotic syndrome, fast declining eGFR, or the absence of retinopathy (in T1D) may suggest alternative or additional causes for kidney disease. Patients with these conditions should be referred to a nephrologist and renal biopsy should be considered as an important factor for further diagnosis. It is rare for patients with T1D to develop renal complication without retinopathy, whereas in T2D patients, retinopathy is moderately sensitive and specific for nephropathy caused by diabetes (DN), as confirmed by kidney biopsies (He et al., 2013).

15.4 Classification of Diabetic Nephropathy

The natural history of DN in T2D is very similar to that in T1D with the exception that a small amount of albumin is already excreted in urine (microalbuminuria stage) at the time of diagnosis in T2D. This reflects the certainty that most T2D patients have had the hyperglycaemia for longer before its diagnosis (Parchwani and Upadhyah, 2012). The revised classification takes into account the findings on the prognosis of T2D patients from a "historical cohort study" from Japan. Patients with microalbuminuria are diagnosed as having incipient nephropathy and all patients with GFR of < 30 mL/min/1.73 m^2 are classified as kidney failures, regardless of their urinary albumin/protein values (Haneda et al., 2015). Pooled data from 54 countries show that at least 80% cases of ESRD are caused by diabetes, hypertension, or a combination of both (USRDS, 2014). DN has been categorized into five stages as described in Table 15.2 (Gupalli, 2015; Vujičić et al., 2012).

15.5 Pathophysiology of Diabetic Nephropathy

Multiple factors are involved in the pathophysiological mechanisms for the development of DN. It has been apparent for more than a decade that DN and its outcomes involve several mechanisms and

TABLE 15.2

Different Stages of DN

	Designation	Characteristics	GFR (ml/min/1.73m²)	Albumin Excretion	Chronology
Stage 1	Hyperfunction and hypertrophy	Glomerular Hyperfiltration	> 90	May be increased	Present at the time of diagnosis
Stage 2	Silent stage	Thickened GBM Expanded mesangium	60-90	< 200 mg/dl	First five years
Stage 3	Incipient stage	Microalbuminuria	30-59	30-300 mg/dl	6-15 years
Stage 4	Overt diabetic nephropathy	Macroalbuminuria	15-29	> 380 mg/dl	15-25 years
Stage 5	Uremic	ESRD	< 15	Decreasing	25-30 years

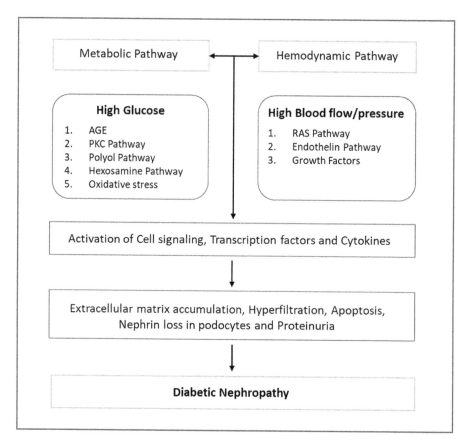

FIGURE 15.1   Metabolic pathways involved in diabetic nephropathy.

distinctive levels of development (Dronavalli et al., 2008). Hyperglycaemia is the initiating event that causes structural and functional changes, followed by the development of glomerular basement membrane (GBM) thickening, accumulation of mesangial matrix, overt proteinuria, and finally glomerulosclerosis and ESRD (Vinod, 2012). The pathophysiological mechanisms occurring in DN are further divided into hemodynamic and metabolic factors as shown in Figure 15.1.

15.5.1 Metabolic Factors

Prolonged hyperglycaemia in diabetic patients is the root cause of all microvascular complications, which develop at the later stage of the disease (Campos, 2012). Optimized glucose control can reduce the risk or slow the progression of diabetic kidney disease (ADA, 2016). However, achieving and maintaining normal blood glucose levels in diabetic patients remains a challenge. High glucose-induced upregulation of angiotensin II and several other growth factors such as transforming growth factor beta (TGF-β), vascular endothelial growth factor (VEGF) in mesangial cells, and in proximal tubular cells has been confirmed in in vitro studies (Hsieh et al., 2002). In addition, high glucose is also believed to induce the production of superoxide by the mitochondrial electron transport chain, which further activates transcription factor nuclear factor-kappa B (NF-κB) through the stimulation of protein kinase C (PKC) activity. All these events eventually contribute to the progression and development of DN (Nishikawa et al., 2000).

15.5.2 Hemodynamic Factors

Hemodynamic changes associated with T2D are responsible for increased glomerular pressure and hyperfiltration resulting in stress-related glomerular damage, loss of podocytes, hypertrophy, and glomerular changes in diabetic kidneys (Hostetter, 2003; Kanwar et al., 2011). Altered hemodynamic factors act independently and in concert with metabolic pathways, to activate intracellular second messengers and various growth factors. These molecular mechanisms ultimately lead to increased renal albumin permeability and extracellular matrix (ECM) accumulation (Luis-Rodríguez et al., 2012; Lenoir et al., 2014).

15.6 Genetics of Diabetic Nephropathy

There are multiple disparities in the process of progression of nephropathy in diabetic patients. Studies have shown that some patients feel a rapid decline in kidney function while others do not suffer and instead experience suboptimal glycaemic control. It has also been observed that DN aggregates in families, thus signalling the contribution of genetics in its development and progression (van Zuydam et al., 2018). In the United Kingdom, diabetes now accounts for 10% of the budget, with 80% of patient spending on controlling the secondary complications of diabetes like DN (dialysis), blindness (retinopathy), amputation (neuropathy), heart problems, and stroke (McKnight et al., 2015). In 2013, 25% of ESRD patients had suffered renal complications because of diabetes, whereas in the United States 40% of individuals were following the dialysis treatment because of DN, and this percentage had further raised to 50% in countries like South Korea, Malaysia, and Mexico (USRDS, 2014; Gilg et al., 2015). However, there is no such data available in India even with the improving healthcare system, which points towards the need to perform a collaborative study in India as well.

Epidemiological studies have revealed that genetic predisposition is an important factor in the development of DN in patients with both T1D and T2D (Breyer, 2007; Noura Al-Jameel, 2014). In a few studies of parent-offspring pairs, sibling-pairs, or studies of extended families, increased aggregation of DN was seen. The chance of developing DN increases 2–3 times if the sibling of a T2D patient has developed nephropathy (Vujičić et al., 2012; Zelmanovitz et al., 2009; Ayodele et al., 2004). The exact genetic mechanisms involved in the pathogenesis of DN development are unknown, but some studies have reported that few genes might interact with environmental factors and lead to the progression of DN. These genes may take part in the development of proteinuria, a few are related to decrease in eGFR, and some genes are known to cause both situations. Understanding the function of these genes can be helpful to recognize individuals susceptible to DN, therefore the preventive interventions can be given to prolong the onset of DN and increase life expectancy (Zelmanovitz et al., 2009). In a recent study it was observed that even low-frequency and rare variants located at coding regions provide essential information in understanding the genetic architecture of complex diseases such as DN (Guan et al., 2018).

During the last decade innovation and advancement in genetic approaches have led researchers to explore and identify T2D and its complications in detail. Previously different techniques like TaqMan, Sequenom MassARRAY iPLEX, and Sanger sequencing (McKnight et al., 2009a; McKnight et al., 2009b) were used to identify the single nucleotide polymorphisms (SNPs), but today's higher throughput techniques like high-density arrays and next-generation sequencing (NGS) help us in studying the genetics behind the complex disorders like diabetes and its complications with more precision and accuracy. The collaboration between the different scientists is also an emerging factor to uncover the risk factors replicated across different populations (Chan et al., 2014; Germain et al., 2015; Sandholm et al., 2014; Sandholm et al., 2017; van Zuydam et al., 2018). The role of genetics is poorly understood, but it is very important to understand the underlying molecular mechanism leading to DN. Different factors such as hemodynamic changes and metabolic pathways are known to be involved in the pathogenesis of DN. Excessive glucose influx activates cellular signaling pathways, including advanced glycation endproducts (AGE), protein kinase C (PKC) pathway, oxidative stress, polyol pathway, hexosamine pathway, renin angiotensin system, and endothelin pathway (Kawanami et al., 2016). The susceptibility genes involved in the development of DN are related to following pathways.

15.6.1 Advanced Glycation End Products

Sustained hyperglycaemia also leads to non-enzymatic glycation resulting in Amadori's products known as advanced glycation end products (AGEs) (Tan et al., 2007). AGEs can modulate cellular functions by interacting with their cognate receptor, RAGE (receptor for AGE) (Kanwar et al., 2011). AGEs are known to be one of the major contributors in the progression of DN and other complications associated with diabetes (Gugliucci and Bendayan, 1995). AGEs are produced in small amount under normal physiological conditions, but their levels markedly increase in a chronic hyperglycemic environment (Jakus and Rietbrock, 2004). Almost all renal structures are susceptible to accumulate AGEs including basement membranes, mesangial and endothelial cells, podocytes, and renal tubules (Busch et al., 2010). Several studies have suggested that inhibition of AGE formation prevents the development and progression of DN among animal models (Fukami et al., 2007). AGEs have been reported to induce apoptotic cell death, quenching of nitric oxide (NO), activation of TGF-β-Smad signaling pathways, and monocyte chemoattractant protein-1 (MCP-1) production in mesangial cells (Yamagishi et al., 2002). AGEs are also involved in inducing chronic immune imbalance in diabetic patients, by attracting immune cells into diffused glycated tissue (Hu et al., 2015).

15.6.2 Oxidative Stress

Growing evidence indicates that metabolic abnormalities in diabetes lead to increase in oxidative stress and the overproduction of reactive oxygen species (ROS) (Giacco and Brownlee, 2010). This ROS production results in the activation of harmful biochemical pathways, including increased AGE formation, activation of PKC, increased flux through the polyol pathway, and overactivity of the hexosamine pathway, which initiates cellular ROS generation (Vasavada and Agarwal, 2005; Forbes et al., 2008). Oxidative stress may activate the transcription factor NF-κB, which is involved in the induction of MCP-1 in both T cells and monocytes (Li and Karin, 1999; Aukrust et al., 2001). Oxidative stress also mediates fibrogenesis by increasing TGF-β expression as well as its activation from the latent complex (Liu and Gaston Pravia, 2010). Mitochondria are found in abundance in renal proximal tubules as there is always a higher demand of energy in the process of reabsorption. They are also known to produce large amount of oxygen radicals (Gyuraszova et al., 2020). Thus, during hyper-filtration in diabetic condition more oxygen radicals are produced and the kidneys are under more oxidative stress. These radicals may cause acute or chronic injury to renal cells, which can further lead to the condition of nephropathy (DN) under diabetic stress (Gyuraszova et al., 2020).

15.6.3 Hexosamine Pathway

The hexosamine biosynthetic pathway has been hypothesized to be involved in the development of insulin resistance and diabetic vascular complications (Schleicher and Weigert, 2000). The hexosinase converts fructose-6-phosphate into glucosamine-6-phosphate. Glutamine-fructose-6-phosphateamidotransferase (GFAT) is the rate-limiting enzyme of this pathway (Singh et al., 2008). Current data indicates that the flux through the hexosamine pathway, regulated by GFAT, may be causally involved in the development of diabetic vascular disease, particularly DN (Zheng et al., 2008, Bran et al., 2010). Both high glucose and angiotensin II activate the GFAT enzyme in mesangial cells leading to overexpression of GFAT in kidney glomeruli (Hao et al., 2012).

15.6.4 Aldose Reductase (Polyol) pathway

When intracellular glucose levels increase, the polyol pathway of glucose metabolism becomes active (Luis-Rodríguez et al., 2012). The first and rate-limiting enzyme in this pathway is aldose reductase (AR), which reduces glucose to sorbitol using nicotinamide adenine dinucleotide phosphate (NADPH) as a cofactor; sorbitol is then metabolized to fructose by sorbitol dehydrogenase that uses nicotinamide adenine dinucleotide (NAD+) as a cofactor (Ramana et al., 2005). The polyol pathway is activated under hyperglycemic conditions and is considered to play an important role in the development of DN (Iso et al., 2001). Intracellular sorbitol accumulation and decline in NADPH contents caused by increased AR flux has been postulated to induce osmotic damage and oxidative stress, respectively (Chung et al., 2003). Activation of AR itself is able to cause damage by activating mechanisms such as activation of PKC and protein glycosylation (Haneda et al., 2003). Some studies have shown that the inhibition of AR may have a beneficial effect on proteinuria and GFR (Chung et al., 2003).

15.6.5 Renin Angiotensin System

The intrarenal renin angiotensin system (RAS) is an important regulator of renal function and structure (Fukami et al., 2007). Angiotensin II exerts growth stimulatory and profibrogenic effects, most likely via upregulation of growth factors such as TGF-β, platelet-derived growth factor (PDGF), CTGF, and VEGF and can also act as a pro-inflammatory factor (Ruiz-Ortega et al., 1998). A close relationship between the RAS and AGE systems in DN has been described. Treatment with valsartan, an angiotensin II type 1 receptor (AT1R) antagonist, ameliorated the accumulation of AGEs in kidney glomeruli and tubules (Thomas et al., 2005; Chawla et al., 2010). Moreover, angiotensin II infusion has been shown to accelerate the accumulation of AGEs in glomeruli and tubules as well (Gurley and Coffman, 2007).

15.6.6 Endothelin Pathway

DN is associated with enhanced renal synthesis of endothelin (ET), one of the most potent endogenous vasoconstrictors (Benz and Amann, 2011). In addition to its direct vasoconstrictor effects, enhanced levels of ET-1 may also contribute to endothelial dysfunction through inhibitory effects on NO production (Mildenberger et al., 2003). In the kidney, ET-1 exerts a number of physiological functions including control of water and sodium (Na+) homeostasis. Very similar to the RAS, the ET system is complex, comprising a converting enzyme and two functionally active receptors (i.e., the ETA receptor (ETA-R) and the ETB (ETB-R) (Lenoir et al., 2014). These receptors are equally important from a kidney perspective since both are present in the kidney with different localization and function. The ETA-R is localized to renal vessels whereas the ETB-R is present mainly in the medulla, but also expressed in mesangial cells, endothelial cells, and podocytes of glomeruli (Rebibou et al., 1992; Uchida et al., 1997).

15.7 Strategies to Identify Genes Associated with Diabetic Nephropathy

With the passage of time different techniques like sequencing of the human genome, the annotation and detection of commonly observed SNPs, haplotype blocks, and development of innovative techniques have facilitated the detailed study of complex diseases to an unimaginable level (Wang and Furey, 2009). As just described DN is a complex disorder involving multiple genes, and different combinations of gene defects exist among diabetic patients (Dronavalli et al., 2008). Numerous studies performed in the last decade have provided different evidence of genetic architecture underlying T2D (Parchwani et al., 2013). Human genetic research is confronting with multiple challenges to track down the fundamental cause of T2D, but one of the foremost challenges is to explicate the influence of specific underlying genetic variations in complex disorders like T2D (Conway and Maxwell, 2009). Different approaches and advanced methodologies are being utilised or applied to uncover genetic risk factors involved in the development of this epidemic. Some of these are described below.

15.7.1 Linkage Analysis

Genetic linkage is a potent contrivance exploited by different researchers and scientists to find out the location of the suspected (diseased) gene on a chromosome. The basis of this technique is to observe the genes being collectively passed on to the next generation as their physical location on the chromosome is close to each other, thus remaining linked during meiosis (Pulst, 1999). Observations from different genetic studies steadily indicate that DN is familial in nature. In the initial stages of the gene hunt for diabetes, researchers applied linkage analysis approach to track down potential risk genes showing association with diabetes (Grant et al., 2009). Genetic linkage analysis is best suited for uncovering genes in small studies like family-based studies, which involve genotyping of the members affected in a family for a selected set of markers to locate the regions, which inherit together frequently in a family, consequently pointing towards a potential genomic region having the susceptibility locus (Parchwani et al., 2013). Two different studies have identified and linked chromosome 10 and 18 with DN susceptibility (Iyengar et al., 2003; McDonough et al., 2009).

15.7.2 Association Studies

These type of studies are used to track down different candidate genes or genomic regions that might play a potential role in developing a specific disease and is confirmed by unearthing the correlation between status of the disease and genetic variations (Lewis and Knight, 2012). Association studies are classified into two different types: the Genome Wide Association Study (GWAS) and candidate gene studies. The GWAS follows a wide and thorough pursuit of the genome for genes and its variants that are specifically related to the disease (Ardlie et al., 2002). The candidate gene study, involving the rigorous and collected genetic analysis, which is confined or restricted to single or multiple candidate genes at a time is done; however, these genes are typically selected on the basis of their known or presumed functions and the biologic characteristics of the disease in query (McCarthy, 2010).

15.7.2.1 Genome Wide Association Studies

The Genome Wide Association Study (GWAS) is a hypothesis-free approach as the putative genes are not selected on the basis of their physiology (Malecki, 2005; Gulati and Yeo, 2013). In this approach millions of variants or polymorphisms are tested collectively to find the association with a specific disease in hundreds or thousands of patients at a time (Hardy and Singleton, 2009). It has revolutionized research and predicted the influence of genetics on complex traits such as T2D with high impact (Manolio, 2010). Complex disorders are usually considered as a geneticist's nightmare, because in contrast to single-gene disorders, complex diseases are caused by multiple genes along with environmental factors, each having a relatively small effect (Manolio, 2010). GWAS has screened more than 120 susceptibility loci for T2D (van Zuydam et al., 2018).

15.7.2.2 Candidate Gene Studies

Candidate gene studies have an imperative role to play in uncovering genetic associations. These are the potential surveys that can identify and uncover the risk-associated variants with a particular disease (Patnala et al., 2013). These kinds of studies are performed swiftly and are cost effective as they target those genes that are already known to be linked to the disease previously, and thus are applied only when prior knowledge about the functions of the gene is known (Kwon and Goate, 2000). In this approach a gene is selected on the basis of its association or relevance in the mechanism of the disease to be examined (Kwon and Goate, 2000). After the selection of a gene, specific polymorphisms are selected (usually tag SNPs) on the basis of their functional relevance (i.e., either affecting gene regulation or its protein product) (Collins et al., 1997). Finally, the selected genetic polymorphisms or variants are validated for the disease association by comparing their frequency in cases and the random control subjects.

15.7.3 Next-Generation Sequencing

In the past few years, next-generation sequencing (NGS) has appeared as a swift, germane, and apropos tool for the elucidation of genetic defects underlying both rare and common human diseases. Easy availability and declined costs of NGS have enabled researchers to exploit this approach for screening large cohorts or populations for the genetic determinants of T2D (de Bruin and Dauber, 2015). NGS is further classified into whole exome sequencing (WES) and RNA-sequencing (RNA-Seq).

15.7.3.1 Exome Sequencing

Exons are the coding regions, thus the mutations or variants in these regions are more important and actionable as compared to the variants found in the non-coding regions. This technique covers the selective regions responsible for coding proteins as compared to the whole genome sequencing in which all coding and non-coding regions are sequenced collectively. Since only 3–5% of the human genome is coding, this approach is cost effective and provides better per base coverage (Choi et al., 2009). In the recent past, studies have discovered a large number of coding variants associated with T2D and DN risk using this approach (Bailey et al., 2014).

15.7.3.2 RNA Sequencing

RNA-Seq affords broader insights about gene expression regulatory networks in DN. To better explore the molecular basis of DN RNA-Seq is a high-throughput alternative to the traditional RNA/cDNA cloning and sequencing strategies. Furthermore, RNA-Seq also provides information on the expression levels of the transcripts and the alternate splice variants. RNA-Seq also allows robust comparison between diseased and normal tissues, as well as the subclassification of disease states (Wang et al., 2009).

15.8 Differentially Expressed Genes in Diabetic Nephropathy

In a recent study, it was observed that 566 genes were expressed in glomerulus and 581 genes were expressed in tubulointerstitium regions in kidney. Out of these 566 glomerular genes 453 genes are upregulated and 105 genes are downregulated while in the case of tubulointerstitial region genes 287 genes were upregulated and 290 were downregulated (Cai et al., 2020). Pathway enrichment analysis has revealed that 13 (54.2%) of 24 enrichment pathways and 8 of 16 in tubulointerstitium were involved in immune system regulation including chemokine signalling pathway, complement, and coagulation cascades, cell-mediated cytotoxicity, NOD-like receptor signaling pathway, and platelet activation, whereas the downregulated genes were involved in amino acid and carbohydrate metabolism (Cai et al., 2020).

In the early stages of the studies, most of the groups focused on candidate genes, which have a biologically plausible role in the pathogenesis of the DN (McKnight et al., 2015). Candidate gene studies have a significant impact as these studies and help in the validation of results obtained from the advanced techniques and thus are being performed often and being published frequently. Meta-analysis is another technique used to track down the genes involved in different studies, but it is usually with the hurdles of different statistical tests performed by different studies (McKnight et al., 2015). Candidate gene studies were followed by linkage studies involving genome-wide approaches. These studies were conducted using multigenerational families and then tracked down the genetic risk loci for DN in a specific chromosome (McKnight et al., 2015). The linkage studies were then followed by GWAS, whole genome sequencing, whole exome sequencing, and NGS. In these techniques millions of single-nucleotide polymorphisms are targeted and checked for the association with a specific disease. NGS is a comprehensive technique with increasing sample size to hunt down the rare variants that may have higher impact in the development of DN (McKnight et al., 2015). The candidate genes that are involved in pathogenesis of DN are given in Table 15.3. These genes need more replication and functional-based studies to validate their function.

15.9 Genes Involved in Diabetic Nephropathy

Genes involved in the development of nephropathy related to T2D are lipid metabolism genes (*ACACB* and *ADIPOQ*), glucose metabolism genes (*GCKR* and *TCF7L2*), angiogenesis-related genes (*EPO* and *VEGFA*), renal structure and functional genes (*SHROOM*, *FERM* and *FRMD3*), inflammation and oxidative stress genes (*ELMO1* and *TGF-β1*), and other susceptible genes (*SLC12A3*, *KCNJ11,* and *CTSC*) (Wei et al., 2018). The roles of some of the important genes involved in the development of DN are explained below.

15.9.1 *ADIPOQ*

ADIPOQ codes for adiponectin and has been as a known susceptible gene for T2D, insulin resistance, and obesity (Fisman and Tenenbaum, 2014). Adiponectin is a vital modular in insulin resistance and is mainly secreted by podocytes. It is also believed that it aids in β-oxidation and has both anti-inflammatory and

TABLE 15.3

Key Candidate Genes Involved in Renal Function and Development

Genes	Effects
C3, CCR2, CCL5, CXCL1, CCL19, and *CCL21*	Inflammation
COL1A1, COL1A2, COL3A1, and *COL15A1*	Fibrosis
EHHADH, HAO2 and *PECR*	Cellular lipid metabolic process
ACOX2, EHHADH and *SLC27A2*	Fatty acid beta-oxidation
DHRS4, DAO, PECR, and *PIPOX*	Oxidation reduction
CXCL1, CCL5 and *CCL21*	Kidney function and mRNA expression of cytokines
COL1A1, COL1A2, and *COL3A1*	Collagens
ACOX2, EHHADH and *HAO2*	mRNA expression in metabolic process
DAO, PECR and *PIPOX*	mRNA expression in oxidative-reduction
Genes identified through GWAS and Meta-analysis	
AFF3, COX6A1, ELMO1, EPO, ERBB4, GLRA3, and *SORBS1*	Fibrosis, Oxidative stress, cellular motility, erythropoiesis and angiogenesis, tubulogenesis, glucagon secretion, insulin secretion, and resistance
TGF-β, MCP-1 and *eNOS*	Inflammation
ELMO1, CD2AP, NPHS1, TCF7L2, HLA-G, and *VEGF-A*	Inflammation and signalling

This list is based on data generated by (McKnight et al., 2015; Cai et al., 2020; Raina et al., 2015b; Raina et al., 2015a; Raina, 2015; Singh, 2019)

anti-atherogenic effects. In an experiment in *ADIPOQ* knockdown mice showed increased albuminurea and oxidative stress (Liu and Liu, 2014; Wei et al., 2018). Also, increased glucose induction in Ankita/ APN$^{-/-}$mice led to the inhibition of TGF-β/Smad2 adiponectin pathway and activated the NF-κB in mesangial cells (Fang et al., 2015).

15.9.2 *TGF-β1*

TGF-β1 is one of the isoforms of the TGF-β family. It is a cytokine with multiple functions that plays an imperative role in different cellular processes involving cell proliferation, differentiation, immune processes, ECM formation, angiogenesis, and apoptosis (Zhou et al., 2014). Its mode of action is through different signaling pathways like MAPK and Smad pathways (Barnette et al., 2013). In the case of renal malfunctioning, higher expression of *TGF-β1* can trigger renal hypertrophy and aid in the sedimentation of ECM proteins causing renal fibrosis (Mou et al., 2016). More specifically in DN patients this process occurs in mesangial cells of glomeruli (El-Sherbini et al., 2013). Thus, these changes may lead to the development and progression of nephropathy in diabetic patients (Wei et al., 2018).

15.9.3 *TCF7L2*

TCF7L2 is positioned on the 10th chromosome (10q25.2) in the human genome. *TCF7L2*, also known as *TCF4* (T-cell transcription factor 4) gene, is a nuclear receptor gene, and has a pivotal role in Wnt/ β-catenin signalling pathway. Along with glucose homoeostasis, *TCF7L2* is also involved in insulin secretion, islet β-cell proliferation, and differentiation (Wei et al., 2018). A study of a Taiwanese population observed that both *TCF7L2* and *ADIPOQ* may interact collectively in the development of nephropathy in diabetic patients (Fu et al., 2012). Another study observed that the effect of *TCF7L2* on DN is via ALK1/Smad1 pathway. *TCF7L2* expression has also been enhanced by AGEs through *TGF-β1*, which lead to the transfer of *TCF7L2* from cytoplasm to nucleus. Consequently, the expression of *TCF7L2* enhances after its interaction with *ALK1* promoter. This enhanced effect of *TGF-β1* by *ALK1* promoted the phosphorylation of cellular Smad1, which ultimately causes glomerular sclerosis (Araoka et al., 2010).

15.9.4 *VEGFA*

The *VEGFA* gene is positioned on chromosome number 6 (6p21.3). Cytokines play an important role in the pathophysiology of an organism and *VEGFA* being a cytokine plays a pivotal role in microvascular diseases like the proliferation of endothelial cells in glomeruli, migration, and modulation of the permeability of different tissues in the body. Its expression has also been observed in the renal cells and is mainly involved in the podocytes and vascular endothelial cells. Thus, *VEGFA* may have an association with DN in T2D patients (Wei et al., 2018).

15.9.5 *ELMO1*

ELMO1 is an essential factor aiding in the pathogenesis of DN in diabetic patients. First of all, it was identified by Shimazaki et al. (2005) in a Japanese population, which was then confirmed by Leak et al. (2009) in an African American population, and in American Indian population by Hanson et al. (2010). *ELMO1* can help in the pathogenesis of DN by two different ways: either by oxidative stress or by renal fibrosis. In the first case, it can activate Rac pathway and enhance the expression of NAD(P)H oxidase, which can increase the oxidative stress in the kidney, thus leading to damage to the renal cells. Whereas, in the second case *ELMO1* increases the expression of fibrogenic genes (e.g., TGF-B1) and suppresses the expression of anti-fibrotic genes (e.g., MMP), which can lead to the accumulation of ECM proteins followed by the thickening of the glomerular basement membrane, ultimately causing diabetic glomerulosclerosis (Shimazaki et al., 2005). However, recently, one study showed that *ELMO1* shows a protective effect in both zebrafish and human samples for glomerular cells. According to this study, *ELMO1* gene helped the renal cells to survive in diabetic condition by reducing the rate of apoptosis (Sharma et al., 2016). The contradictory results favor the fact that the genetics of DN still need to be explored at higher level with more sample size considering functional aspects and collaboration of different laboratories to cover multiple ethnicities and get a clear picture of the role of genetics in DN.

15.10 Epigenetics and DN

Most of the protein coding genes in human genome are regulated by micro-RNAs (miRNAs) (Landgraf et al., 2007). At present the diagnosis of DN is performed by detecting micro-albuminurea, but not all patients develop micro-albuminurea, so the technique must be modified to trace the symptoms of developing DN (Parving et al., 2015). Detection of circulating miRNAs in the body has been described (Arroyo et al., 2011) and it was shown in another study that urinary miRNAs is a promising and novel source of biomarkers that were stabilised with argonaute 2 protein and rapidly detectable by RT-qPCR (reverse-transcription quantitative polymerase-chain reaction) (Beltrami et al., 2015). Recently a protocol was developed by Newbury et al. (2020) to detect the candidate DN biomarkers from the patient's urine samples, which is very accurate and a rapid test to diagnose the DN in diabetic patients. It has also been previously discovered that miR-192, miR-194, miR-215, miR-216, miR-146a, miR-204, and miR-886 were elevated in the kidney of patients suffering from diabetes (Landgraf et al., 2007). miR-192 was also observed in diminished amount in the biopsies of patients with diabetic kidney disease (Krupa et al., 2010). This emphasizes that miRNAs are potential biomarkers to detect renal damage in earlier stages in the case of diabetes and as well as other renal disorders (Newbury et al., 2020).

15.11 Concluding Remarks

The human genome is an ocean of genes in which locating the genes to a specific disorder is a cumbersome process. According to the currently available data there are about 600 genes related to DN. The available resources also provide significant opportunities for researchers to explore and discover new methods to delay or hinder the progression of the disease affecting kidneys frequently. DN pathophysiology involves complex interaction of both environmental as well as genetic factors. In addition, different polymorphisms show different results in different populations, thus making it more difficult to understand its mode of action. This chapter has made an effort to shed light on the different susceptible genes known to be associated with DN to distinguish their functions and make this process simpler as well as comprehensible. Still there are numerous challenges to address to uncover the role of genetic factors in the progression of the disease in different ethnicities. Thus, a wide range of studies involving multiple gene variants in different ethnicities with functional analyses is the need of the hour to decipher the role of genetics in DN. More studies in the future with emerging and advanced technologies will also help in locating further novel regions associated with the disease and aid in finding a cure to this renal disorder.

REFERENCES

ADA. 2016. Standards of Medical Care in Diabetes. *Diabetes Care,* 39, 1–119.

ADA. 2018. Standards of Medical Care in Diabetes. *Diabetes Care,* 41, 1–172.

Afkarian, M., Zelnick, L. R., Hall, Y. N. et al. 2016. Clinical Manifestations of Kidney Disease Among US Adults With Diabetes, 1988-2014. *Jama,* 316, 602–610.

Al-Rubeaan, K., Youssef, A. M., Subhani, S. N. et al. 2014. Diabetic nephropathy and its risk factors in a society with a type 2 diabetes epidemic: Saudi National Diabetes Registry-based study. *PLoS One,* 9, e88956.

Araoka, T., Abe, H., Tominaga, T. et al. 2010. Transcription factor 7-like 2 (TCF7L2) regulates activin receptor-like kinase 1 (ALK1)/Smad1 pathway for development of diabetic nephropathy. *Molecules and Cells,* 30, 209–218.

Ardlie, K. G., Kruglyak, L. & Seielstad, M. 2002. Patterns of linkage disequilibrium in the human genome. *Nat Rev Genet,* 3, 299–309.

Arroyo, J. D., Chevillet, J. R., Kroh, E. M. et al. 2011. Argonaute2 complexes carry a population of circulating microRNAs independent of vesicles in human plasma. *Proc Natl Acad Sci USA,* 108, 5003–5008.

Aukrust, P., Berge, R. K., Ueland, T. et al. 2001. Interaction between chemokines and oxidative stress: possible pathogenic role in acute coronary syndromes. *J Am Coll Cardiol,* 37, 485–491.

Ayodele, O. E., Alebiosu, C. O. & Salako, B. L. 2004. Diabetic nephropathy - a review of the natural history, burden, risk factors and treatment. *J Natl Med Assoc,* 96, 1445–1454.

Baig, M. R., Gillani S. W., Sulaiman S. A. S., Krishna, D. R. & K, N. 2011. Epidemiology of diabetic nephropathy in the poor patients from rural south-east india. *International Journal of Food, Nutrition and Public Health,* 4, 9.

Bailey, J. N. C., Palmer, N. D., Ng, M. C. Y. et al. 2014. Analysis of coding variants identified from exome sequencing resources for association with diabetic and non-diabetic nephropathy in African Americans. *Hum Genet,* 133, 769–779.

Barnette, D. N., Hulin, A., Ahmed, A. S. et al. 2013. Tgfβ-Smad and MAPK signaling mediate scleraxis and proteoglycan expression in heart valves. *J Mol Cell Cardiol,* 65, 137–146.

Beltrami, C., Clayton, A., Newbury, L. J. et al. 2015. Stabilization of urinary micrornas by association with exosomes and argonaute 2 protein. *Noncoding RNA,* 1, 151–166.

Benz, K. & Amann, K. 2011. Endothelin in diabetic renal disease. *Contrib Nephrol,* 172, 139–148.

Bjornstad, P. & Cherney, D. Z. 2018. Renal hyperfiltration in adolescents with type 2 diabetes: physiology, sex differences, and implications for diabetic kidney disease. *Curr Diab Rep,* 18, 22.

Bran, G. M., Goessler, U. R., Schardt, C. et al. 2010. Effect of the abrogation of TGF-beta1 by antisense oligonucleotides on the expression of TGF-beta-isoforms and their receptors I and II in isolated fibroblasts from keloid scars. *Int J Mol Med,* 25, 915–921.

Breyer, M. D. 2007. Diabetic nephropathy: introduction. *Semin Nephrol,* 27, 129.

Busch, M., Franke, S., Rüster, C. & Wolf, G. 2010. Advanced glycation end-products and the kidney. *Eur J Clin Invest,* 40, 742–755.

Cai, F., Zhou, X., Jia, Y. et al. 2020. Identification of key genes of human advanced diabetic nephropathy independent of proteinuria by transcriptome analysis. *BioMed Research International,* 2020, 7283581.

Campos, C. 2012. Chronic hyperglycemia and glucose toxicity: pathology and clinical sequelae. *Postgrad Med,* 124, 90–97.

Chan, Y., Lim, E. T., Sandholm, N. et al. 2014. An excess of risk-increasing low-frequency variants can be a signal of polygenic inheritance in complex diseases. *Am J Hum Genet,* 94, 437–452.

Chawla, T., Sharma, D. & Singh, A. 2010. Role of the renin angiotensin system in diabetic nephropathy. *World J Diabetes,* 1, 141–145.

Choi, M., Scholl, U. I., Ji, W. et al. 2009. Genetic diagnosis by whole exome capture and massively parallel DNA sequencing. *Proc Natl Acad Sci U S A,* 106, 19096–19101.

Chung, S. S., Ho, E. C., Lam, K. S. & Chung, S. K. 2003. Contribution of polyol pathway to diabetes-induced oxidative stress. *J Am Soc Nephrol,* 14, S233–236.

Collins, F. S., Guyer, M. S. & Charkravarti, A. 1997. Variations on a theme: cataloging human DNA sequence variation. *Science,* 278, 1580–1581.

Conway, B. R. & Maxwell, A. P. 2009. Genetics of diabetic nephropathy: are there clues to the understanding of common kidney diseases? *Nephron Clin Pract,* 112, c213–221.

De Boer, I. H., Rue, T. C., Hall, Y. N. et al. 2011. Temporal trends in the prevalence of diabetic kidney disease in the United States. *Jama,* 305, 2532–2539.

De Bruin, C. & Dauber, A. 2015. Insights from exome sequencing for endocrine disorders. *Nat Rev Endocrinol,* 11, 455–464.

Dronavalli, S., Duka, I. & Bakris, G. L. 2008. The pathogenesis of diabetic nephropathy. *Nat Clin Pract Endocrinol Metab,* 4, 444–452.

El-Sherbini, S. M., Shahen, S. M., Mosaad, Y. M., Abdelgawad, M. S. & Talaat, R. M. 2013. Gene polymorphism of transforming growth factor-beta1 in Egyptian patients with type 2 diabetes and diabetic nephropathy. *Acta Biochim Biophys Sin (Shanghai),* 45, 330–338.

Fang, F., Bae, E. H., Hu, A. et al. 2015. Deletion of the gene for adiponectin accelerates diabetic nephropathy in the Ins2 (+/C96Y) mouse. *Diabetologia,* 58, 1668–1678.

Fisman, E. Z. & Tenenbaum, A. 2014. Adiponectin: a manifold therapeutic target for metabolic syndrome, diabetes, and coronary disease? *Cardiovasc Diabetol,* 13, 103.

Forbes, J. M., Coughlan, M. T. & Cooper, M. E. 2008. Oxidative stress as a major culprit in kidney disease in diabetes. *Diabetes,* 57, 1446–1454.

Fu, L. L., Lin, Y., Yang, Z. L. & Yin, Y. B. 2012. Association analysis of genetic polymorphisms of TCF7L2, CDKAL1, SLC30A8, HHEX genes and microvascular complications of type 2 diabetes mellitus. *Zhonghua Yi Xue Yi Chuan Xue Za Zhi,* 29, 194–199.

Fukami, K., Yamagishi, S., Ueda, S. & Okuda, S. 2007. Novel therapeutic targets for diabetic nephropathy. *Endocr Metab Immune Disord Drug Targets,* 7, 83–92.

Gedebjerg, A., Almdal, T. P., Berencsi, K. et al., 2018. Prevalence of micro-and macrovascular diabetes complications at time of type 2 diabetes diagnosis and associated clinical characteristics: A cross-sectional baseline study of 6958 patients in the Danish DD2 cohort. *J Diabetes Complications,* 32, 34–40.

Germain, M., Pezzolesi, M. G., Sandholm, N. et al. 2015. SORBS1 gene, a new candidate for diabetic nephropathy: results from a multi-stage genome-wide association study in patients with type 1 diabetes. *Diabetologia,* 58, 543–548.

Giacco, F. & Brownlee, M. 2010. Oxidative stress and diabetic complications. *Circ Res,* 107, 1058–1070.

Gilg, J., Pruthi, R. & Fogarty, D. 2015. UK Renal Registry 17th annual report: chapter 1 UK renal replacement therapy incidence in 2013: national and centre-specific analyses. *Nephron,* 129 Suppl 1, 1–29.

Gnudi, L., Gentile, G. & Ruggenenti, P. 2016. *The Patient with Diabetes Mellitus,* Oxford, Oxford University Press.

Grant, R. W., Moore, A. F. & Florez, J. C. 2009. Genetic architecture of type 2 diabetes: recent progress and clinical implications. *Diabetes Care,* 32, 1107–1114.

Guan, M., Keaton, J. M., Dimitrov, L. et al. 2018. An exome-wide association study for type 2 diabetes-attributed end-stage kidney disease in African Americans. *Kidney Int Rep,* 3, 867–878.

Gugliucci, A. & Bendayan, M. 1995. Reaction of advanced glycation endproducts with renal tissue from normal and streptozotocin-induced diabetic rats: an ultrastructural study using colloidal gold cytochemistry. *J Histochem Cytochem,* 43, 591–600.

Gulati, P. & Yeo, G. S. 2013. The biology of FTO: from nucleic acid demethylase to amino acid sensor. *Diabetologia,* 56, 2113–2121.

Gupalli, L. N. 2015. Prospective and retrospective study of diabetes and its complications. *World Journal of Pharmaceutical Research,* 4, 2010–2028.

Gurley, S. B. & Coffman, T. M. 2007. The renin-angiotensin system and diabetic nephropathy. *Semin Nephrol,* 27, 144–152.

Gyuraszova, M., Gurecka, R., Babickova, J. & Tothova, L. 2020. Oxidative stress in the pathophysiology of kidney disease: implications for noninvasive monitoring and identification of biomarkers. *Oxid Med Cell Longev*, 2020, 5478708.

Haneda, M., Koya, D., Isono, M. & Kikkawa, R. 2003. Overview of glucose signaling in mesangial cells in diabetic nephropathy. *J Am Soc Nephrol*, 14, 1374–1382.

Haneda, M., Utsunomiya, K., Koya, D. et al. 2015. A new classification of diabetic nephropathy 2014: a report from Joint Committee on Diabetic Nephropathy. *J Diabetes Investig*, 6, 242–246.

Hanson, R. L., Millis, M. P., Young, N. J. et al. 2010. ELMO1 variants and susceptibility to diabetic nephropathy in American Indians. *Mol Genet Metab*, 101, 383–390.

Hao, H. H., Shao, Z. M., Tang, D. Q. et al. 2012. Preventive effects of rutin on the development of experimental diabetic nephropathy in rats. *Life Sci*, 91, 959–967.

Hardy, J. & Singleton, A. 2009. Genomewide association studies and human disease. *N Engl J Med*, 360, 1759–1768.

He, F., Xia, X., Wu, X. F., Yu, X. Q. & Huang, F. X. 2013. Diabetic retinopathy in predicting diabetic nephropathy in patients with type 2 diabetes and renal disease: a meta-analysis. *Diabetologia*, 56, 457–466.

Hemanth, K. N., Prashanth, S. & Vidya Sagar, J. 2011. Diabetic nepropathy-pathogenesis and newer targets in treatment. *Diabetic Nephropathy-Pathogenesis and Newer Targets in Treatment*, 6, 15.

Hill, C. J., Cardwell, C. R., Patterson, C. C. et al. 2014. Chronic kidney disease and diabetes in the national health service: a cross-sectional survey of the U.K. national diabetes audit. *Diabet Med*, 31, 448–454.

Hostetter, T. H. 2003. Hyperfiltration and glomerulosclerosis. *Semin Nephrol*, 23, 194–199.

Hovind, P., Rossing, P., Tarnow, L., Smidt, U. M. & Parving, H. H. 2001. Progression of diabetic nephropathy. *Kidney Int*, 59, 702–709.

Hsieh, T. J., Zhang, S. L., Filep, J. G. et al. 2002. High glucose stimulates angiotensinogen gene expression via reactive oxygen species generation in rat kidney proximal tubular cells. *Endocrinology*, 143, 2975–2985.

Hu, H., Jiang, H., Ren, H. et al. 2015. AGEs and chronic subclinical inflammation in diabetes: disorders of immune system. *Diabetes Metab Res Rev*, 31, 127–137.

IDF. 2017. International Diabetes Federation (IDF) Diabetes Atlas. *Diabetes Res Clin Pract*, 8, 1–150.

Iso, K., Tada, H., Kuboki, K. & Inokuchi, T. 2001. Long-term effect of epalrestat, an aldose reductase inhibitor, on the development of incipient diabetic nephropathy in type 2 diabetic patients. *J Diabetes Complications*, 15, 241–244.

Iyengar, S. K., Fox, K. A., Schachere, M. et al. 2003. Linkage analysis of candidate loci for end-stage renal disease due to diabetic nephropathy. *J Am Soc Nephrol*, 14, S195–201.

Jakus, V. & Rietbrock, N. 2004. Advanced glycation end-products and the progress of diabetic vascular complications. *Physiol Res*, 53, 131–142.

Kanwar, Y. S., Sun, L., Xie, P., Liu, F. Y. & Chen, S. 2011. A glimpse of various pathogenetic mechanisms of diabetic nephropathy. *Annu Rev Pathol*, 6, 395–423.

Kawanami, D., Matoba, K. & Utsunomiya, K. 2016. Signaling pathways in diabetic nephropathy. *Histol Histopathol*, 31, 1059–1067.

Kramer, H. J., Nguyen, Q. D., Curhan, G. & Hsu, C. Y. 2003. Renal insufficiency in the absence of albuminuria and retinopathy among adults with type 2 diabetes mellitus. *Jama*, 289, 3273–3277.

Krupa, A., Jenkins, R., Luo, D. D. et al. 2010. Loss of MicroRNA-192 promotes fibrogenesis in diabetic nephropathy. *J Am Soc Nephrol*, 21, 438–447.

Kwon, J. M. & Goate, A. M. 2000. The candidate gene approach. *Alcohol Res Health*, 24, 164–168.

Landgraf, P., Rusu, M., Sheridan, R. et al. 2007. A mammalian microRNA expression atlas based on small RNA library sequencing. *Cell*, 129, 1401–1414.

Leak, T. S., Perlegas, P. S., Smith, S. G. et al. 2009. Variants in intron 13 of the ELMO1 gene are associated with diabetic nephropathy in African Americans. *Ann Hum Genet*, 73, 152–159.

Lenoir, O., Milon, M., Virsolvy, A. et al. 2014. Direct action of endothelin-1 on podocytes promotes diabetic glomerulosclerosis. *J Am Soc Nephrol*, 25, 1050–1062.

Lewis, C. M. & Knight, J. 2012. Introduction to genetic association studies. *Cold Spring Harb Protoc*, 2012, 297–306.

Li, N. & Karin, M. 1999. Is NF-kappaB the sensor of oxidative stress? *Faseb Jj*, 13, 1137–1143.

Liu, M. & Liu, F. 2014. Regulation of adiponectin multimerization, signaling and function. *Best Pract Res Clin Endocrinol Metab*, 28, 25–31.

Liu, R. M. & Gaston Pravia, K. A. 2010. Oxidative stress and glutathione in TGF-beta-mediated fibrogenesis. *Free Radic Biol Med*, 48, 1–15.

Luis-Rodríguez, D., Martínez-Castelao, A., Górriz, J. L., De-Álvaro, F. & Navarro-González, J. F. 2012. Pathophysiological role and therapeutic implications of inflammation in diabetic nephropathy. *World J Diabetes*, 3, 7–18.

Luk, A. & Chan, J. C. 2008. Diabetic nephropathy--what are the unmet needs? *Diabetes Res Clin Pract*, 82 Suppl 1, S15–20.

Luk, A. O., Li, X., Zhang, Y. et al. 2016. Quality of care in patients with diabetic kidney disease in Asia: The Joint Asia Diabetes Evaluation (JADE) Registry. *Diabet Med*, 33, 1230–1239.

Malecki, M. T. 2005. Genetics of type 2 diabetes mellitus. *Diabetes Res Clin Pract*, 68 Suppl1, S10–21.

Manolio, T. A. 2010. Genomewide association studies and assessment of the risk of disease. *N Engl J Med*, 363, 166–176.

McCarthy, M. I. 2010. Genomics, type 2 diabetes, and obesity. *N Engl J Med*, 363, 2339–2350.

Mcdonough, C. W., Bostrom, M. A., Lu, L. et al. 2009. Genetic analysis of diabetic nephropathy on chromosome 18 in African Americans: linkage analysis and dense SNP mapping. *Hum Genet*, 126, 805–817.

Mcknight, A. J., Currie, D., Patterson, C. C. et al. 2009a. Targeted genome-wide investigation identifies novel SNPs associated with diabetic nephropathy. *The HUGO Journal*, 3, 77–82.

Mcknight, A. J., Duffy, S. & Maxwell, A. P. 2015. Genetics of diabetic nephropathy: a long road of discovery. *Curr Diab Rep*, 15, 41.

Mcknight, A. J., Woodman, A. M., Parkkonen, M. et al. 2009b. Investigation of DNA polymorphisms in SMAD genes for genetic predisposition to diabetic nephropathy in patients with type 1 diabetes mellitus. *Diabetologia*, 52, 844–849.

Mildenberger, E., Biesel, B., Siegel, G. & Versmold, H. T. 2003. Nitric oxide and endothelin in oxygen-dependent regulation of vascular tone of human umbilical vein. *Am J Physiol Heart Circ Physiol*, 285, H1730–1737.

Molitch, M. E., Steffes, M., Sun, W. et al. 2010. Development and progression of renal insufficiency with and without albuminuria in adults with type 1 diabetes in the diabetes control and complications trial and the epidemiology of diabetes interventions and complications study. *Diabetes Care*, 33, 1536–1543.

Mou, X., Liu, Y., Zhou, D. et al. 2016. Different risk indictors of diabetic nephropathy in transforming growth factor-beta1 T869C CC/CT genotype and TT genotype. *Iran J Public Health*, 45, 761–767.

Newbury, L. J., Wonnacott, A., Simpson, K., Bowen, T. & Fraser, D. 2020. Assessment of urinary microRNAs by quantitative polymerase chain reaction in diabetic nephropathy patients. *Methods Mol Biol*, 2067, 277–285.

Nishikawa, T., Edelstein, D., Du, X. L. et al. 2000. Normalizing mitochondrial superoxide production blocks three pathways of hyperglycaemic damage. *Nature*, 404, 787–790.

Noura Al-Jameil, F. A. K., Arjumand, S., Khan, M. F., Tabassum, H. 2014. Dyslipidemia and its correlation with type 2 diabetic patients at different stages of proteinuria. *Biomedical Research*, 25, 227–231.

Pagtalunan, M. E., Miller, P. L., Jumping-Eagle, S. et al. 1997. Podocyte loss and progressive glomerular injury in type II diabetes. *The Journal of Clinical Investigation*, 99, 342–348.

Parchwani, D., Murthy, S., Upadhyah, A. & Patel, D. 2013. Genetic factors in the etiology of type 2 diabetes: linkage analyses, candidate gene association, and genome-wide association – still a long way to go! *National Journal of Physiology, Pharmacy and Pharmacology*, 3.

Parchwani, D. N. & Upadhyah, A. A. 2012. Diabetic nephropathy: progression and pathophysiology. *International Journal of Medical Science and Public Health*, 1, 59–70.

Parving, H. H., Lewis, J. B., Ravid, M., Remuzzi, G. & Hunsicker, L. G. 2006. Prevalence and risk factors for microalbuminuria in a referred cohort of type II diabetic patients: a global perspective. *Kidney Int*, 69, 2057–2063.

Parving, H. H., Persson, F. & Rossing, P. 2015. Microalbuminuria: a parameter that has changed diabetes care. *Diabetes Res Clin Pract*, 107, 1–8.

Patnala, R., Clements, J. & Batra, J. 2013. Candidate gene association studies: a comprehensive guide to useful in silico tools. *BMC Genet*, 14, 39.

Pulst, S. M. 1999. Genetic linkage analysis. *Arch Neurol*, 56, 667–672.

Raina, P. 2015. *TGF MCP 1 eNOS Polymorphisms and Conventional Risk Factors in T2D and ESRD*. Ph.D., Guru Nanak Dev University.

Raina, P., Matharoo, K. & Bhanwer, A. J. 2015a. Monocyte chemoattractant protein-1 (MCP-1) g.-2518A> G polymorphism and susceptibility to type 2 diabetes (T2D) and end stage renal disease (ESRD) in the North-West Indian population of Punjab. *Ann Hum Biol,* 42, 276–282.

Raina, P., Sikka, R., Kaur, R. et al. 2015b. Association of transforming growth factor beta-1 (TGF-beta1) genetic variation with type 2 diabetes and end stage renal disease in two large population samples from North India. *Omics: A Journal of Integrative Biology,* 19, 306–317.

Ramana, K. V., Friedrich, B., Tammali, R. et al. 2005. Requirement of aldose reductase for the hyperglycemic activation of protein kinase C and formation of diacylglycerol in vascular smooth muscle cells. *Diabetes,* 54, 818–829.

Rebibou, J. M., He, C. J., Delarue, F. et al. 1992. Functional endothelin 1 receptors on human glomerular podocytes and mesangial cells. *Nephrol Dial Transplant,* 7, 288–292.

Ritz, E. & Zeng, X. 2011. Diabetic nephropathy – Epidemiology in Asia and the current state of treatment. *Indian J Nephrol,* 21, 75–84.

Ruiz-Ortega, M., Bustos, C., Hernández-Presa, M. A. et al. 1998. Angiotensin II participates in mononuclear cell recruitment in experimental immune complex nephritis through nuclear factor-kappa B activation and monocyte chemoattractant protein-1 synthesis. *J Immunol,* 161, 430–439.

Sagoo, M. K. & Gnudi, L. 2020. Diabetic nephropathy: an overview. *Methods Mol Biol,* 2067, 3–7.

Sandholm, N., Forsblom, C., Mäkinen, V. P. et al. 2014. Genome-wide association study of urinary albumin excretion rate in patients with type 1 diabetes. *Diabetologia,* 57, 1143–1153.

Sandholm, N., Van Zuydam, N., Ahlqvist, E. et al. 2017. The genetic landscape of renal complications in type 1 diabetes. *J Am Soc Nephrol,* 28, 557–574.

Schleicher, E. D. & Weigert, C. 2000. Role of the hexosamine biosynthetic pathway in diabetic nephropathy. *Kidney Int Suppl,* 77, S13–18.

Scirica, B. M. 2017. Use of biomarkers in predicting the onset, monitoring the progression, and risk stratification for patients with type 2 diabetes mellitus. *Clin Chem,* 63, 186–195.

Sharma, K. R., Heckler, K., Stoll, S. J. et al, 2016. ELMO1 protects renal structure and ultrafiltration in kidney development and under diabetic conditions. *Sci Rep,* 6, 37172.

Shen, F-C., Chen, C-Y., Su, S-C. & Liu, R. T. 2009. The prevalence and risk factors of DN in Taiwanese T2D-a hospital based study. *Acta Nephrologica,* 23, 90–95.

Shimazaki, A., Kawamura, Y., Kanazawa, A. et al. 2005. Genetic variations in the gene encoding ELMO1 are associated with susceptibility to diabetic nephropathy. *Diabetes,* 54, 1171–1178.

Singh, G. 2019. *Association Analysis of Genetic Variants of Various Candidate Genes in Diabetic Nephropathy Patients from North India.* PhD, Guru Nanak Dev University.

Singh, V. P., Baker, K. M. & Kumar, R. 2008. Activation of the intracellular renin-angiotensin system in cardiac fibroblasts by high glucose: role in extracellular matrix production. *Am J Physiol Heart Circ Physiol,* 294, H1675–1684.

Tan, A. L., Forbes, J. M. & Cooper, M. E. 2007. AGE, RAGE, and ROS in diabetic nephropathy. *Semin Nephrol,* 27, 130–143.

Thomas, M. C., Tikellis, C., Burns, W. M. et al. 2005. Interactions between renin angiotensin system and advanced glycation in the kidney. *J Am Soc Nephrol,* 16, 2976–2984.

Uchida, K., Uchida, S., Nitta, K., Yumura, W. & Nihei, H. 1997. Regulated expression of endothelin converting enzymes in glomerular endothelial cells. *J Am Soc Nephrol,* 8, 580–585.

USRDS. 2014. International comparisons in United States renal data system. 2014 USRDS annual data report: epidemiology of kidney disease in the United States. Bethesda (MD). *National Institutes of Health, National Institute of Diabetes and Digestive and Kidney Diseases,* 188–210.

Van Zuydam, N. R., Ahlqvist, E., Sandholm, N. et al. 2018. A Genome-Wide Association Study of Diabetic Kidney Disease in Subjects with Type 2 Diabetes. 67, 1414–1427.

Vasavada, N. & Agarwal, R. 2005. Role of oxidative stress in diabetic nephropathy. *Adv Chronic Kidney Dis,* 12, 146–154.

Vinod, P. B. 2012. Pathophysiology of diabetic nephropathy. *Clinical Queries: Nephrology* 102, 121–126.

Vujičić, B., Turk, T., Crnčević-Orlić, Z., Đorđević, G. & Rački, S. 2012. Diabetic nephropathy, pathophysiology and complications of diabetes mellitus. *Intech Open* 27.

Wang, T. & Furey, T. S. 2009. Analysis of complex disease association and linkage studies using the University of California Santa Cruz Genome Browser. *Circ Cardiovasc Genet,* 2, 199–204.

Wang, Z., Gerstein, M. & Snyder, M. 2009. RNA-Seq: a revolutionary tool for transcriptomics. *Nat Rev Genet,* 10, 57–63.

Wei, L., Xiao, Y., Li, L.et al., 2018. The susceptibility genes in diabetic nephropathy. *Kidney Dis (Basel),* 4, 226–237.

Wolf, G., Chen, S. & Ziyadeh, F. N. 2005. From the periphery of the glomerular capillary wall toward the center of disease: podocyte injury comes of age in diabetic nephropathy. *Diabetes,* 54, 1626–1634.

Yamagishi, S., Inagaki, Y., Okamoto, T.et al. 2002. Advanced glycation end product-induced apoptosis and overexpression of vascular endothelial growth factor and monocyte chemoattractant protein-1 in human-cultured mesangial cells. *J Biol Chem,* 277, 20309–20315.

Zelmanovitz, T., Gerchman, F., Balthazar, A. P. et al. 2009. Diabetic nephropathy. *Diabetol Metab Syndr,* 1, 10.

Zheng, J. M., Zhu, J. M., Li, L. S. & Liu, Z. H. 2008. Rhein reverses the diabetic phenotype of mesangial cells over-expressing the glucose transporter (GLUT1) by inhibiting the hexosamine pathway. *Br J Pharmacol,* 153, 1456–1464.

Zhou, T. B., Jiang, Z. P., Qin, Y. H. & Drummen, G. P. 2014. Association of transforming growth factor-β1 T869C gene polymorphism with diabetic nephropathy risk. *Nephrology (Carlton),* 19, 107–115.

Zoungas, S., Gerstein, H. C., Holman, R. R. et al. 2017. Microvascular outcomes in type 2 diabetes – Authors' reply. *Lancet Diabetes Endocrinol,* 5, 580.

16

Human Y Chromosome: Genetic Markers, Implications, and Pathologies

Yogesh Thapen and Vijay Kumar
Department of Zoology, Panjab University, Chandigarh, India

Swarkar Sharma and Ekta Rai
School of Biotechnology, Shri Mata Vaishno Devi University, Katra, Ondoa

16.1 Introduction

Variations in DNA of individuals can be used to understand the genetic diversity of a population and to reconstruct its history and evolution (Crawford and Beaty, 2013). Understanding genetic diversity is most important in studies of human ancestry, migrations, and evolutionary studies (Romero et al., 2009). Knowing the genetic structure and diversity in humans is not only of evolutionary importance but is also of medical relevance as some disease susceptibility alleles occur at a greater frequency in some populations of specific geographical regions (Wilson et al., 2001; Tishkoff and Verrelli, 2003). The difference in allelic frequencies between subpopulations in a population are mainly due to different ancestry results into population stratification. Various association studies have shown the impact of population stratification on different disease susceptibilities (Cardon and Bell, 2001; Thomas and Witte, 2002; Bittles, 2005; Ghosh, 2007; Price et al., 2010; Sharma et al., 2013; Kaul et al., 2015; Sokhi et al., 2016; Hu et al., 2017; Erzurumluoglu et al., 2018).

In order to analyze genetic diversity, autosomes and allosomes both play a very important role but for evolutionary or phylogenetic studies, Y chromosome and mitochondrial DNA (mtDNA) play a pivotal role. The Y chromosome mainly represents the patrilineal lineage as its major part does not show any recombination. This part is known as the non-recombining portion of Y chromosome (NRY) or male-*specific region* of the Y chromosome (MSY) and passes through generations from father to son. Mitochondrial DNA is mainly helpful in understanding the matrilineal lineage and it also remains uninterrupted by recombination process and passes from the mother to its progenies carrying the variations from one generation to another. The Y chromosome is the most informative loci for investigating genetic diversity and population substructure. The DNA variations found within the NRY reflects a simple paternal history revealed by the pattern of alleles at informative loci (i.e., markers, comprising the haplotype) (Underhill et al., 2000).

Ninety-eight percent of the human genome is diploid, with the chromosomes coming in coordinating sets, and these sets take part in recombination, the reshuffling of portions when eggs and sperms are made. The Y chromosome is unique: particular for male sex-assurance, it stands unapproachable and haploid, and, for a large portion of its length, demandingly keeps away from the chaotic business of recombination. This is the reason the Y chromosome is so generally utilized in human populace considers. As it goes from father to child down fatherly heredities, the main changes happening are because of transformation and the molecular record of the past due to which it is moderately simple to decipher contrasted with the recombining X chromosome and autosomes. The human Y chromosome decides maleness by causing the advancement of the testis and is male-explicit, haploid, and avoids recombination. These exceptional properties of the Y have significant ramifications for its genes, mutations, and its populace hereditary genes.

Markers basically utilized in evaluating the paternal history are short tandem repeat (STR) and single-nucleotide polymorphisms (SNP). A STR is an example of at least two nucleotides that are repeated straightforwardly adjacent to one another and repeats can go long from two to six base sets. A STR polymorphism happens when homologous STR loci vary in the quantity of repeats between people. By recognizing repeats of a particular arrangement at specific areas in the genome, it is conceivable to make a hereditary profile of a person. SNP is a DNA sequence variation happening at a locus when a solitary nucleotide in the genome contrasts between individuals from an animal types or matched chromosomes in a person. Hereditary variations in this uniparentally acquired Y chromosome can be utilized to characterize gatherings of Y-DNA haplotypes (fundamentally known as haplogroups), which share a typical progenitor (Sachidanandam et al., 2001; Suh and Vig, 2005). Uniform analysis of a vast number of randomly selected Y-chromosome SNPs on various populations of the world has provided better insights on genetic affinities, disease diagnosis, forensic analysis, and population genetic studies (Mills et al., 2006b; 1000 Genomes Project Consortium, 2012; Ferragut et al., 2016).

16.2 Evolution of Y Chromosome

The mammalian X and Y chromosomes are thought to have developed from a conventional pair of autosomes (Graves and Schmidt, 1992). It is thought that X-Y separation would have started simply after X-Y crossing over stopped, which may have happened around 240 to 320 million years ago. All NRY X-degenerate genes and pseudogenes appear to be results of suppression of crossing over in genealogical autosomes, with ensuing separation of the Y from the X chromosome (Lahn and Page, 1999).

16.3 Structure of Y Chromosome

The human Y chromosome comprises a short (Yp) and a long (Yq) arm (Figure 16.1). This chromosome consists of some distinctive regions like pseudoautosomal region (PAR1 and PAR2), euchromatic and heterochromatic regions. The two pseudoautosomal regions (PAR1 and PAR2) are situated on both telomeric ends spread on around 5% of the chromosome. They are indistinguishable with the telomeric portions of the X chromosome and the genes restricted in PARs shows an autosomal example of inheritance (Seda et al., 2005). Euchromatic portion comprise of Yp and the proximal piece of Yq corresponding to Yq11, while the distal piece of the long-arm Yq12 is made of a hereditarily dormant area called heterochromatin. Yq12 may vary in size in various male individuals of different populations (Bachtrog and Charlesworth, 2001). Important genes required for male sex assurance and spermatogenesis are present in a particular portion of Y chromosome called the male-specific region (MSY) (previously called the non-combining region of Y (NRY)) spans both Yp and Yq arms as depicted in Figure 16.1 (Seda et al., 2005; Repping et al., 2002).

The heterochromatic part of the Y chromosome comprises of three regions: centromere, DYZ19 in Yq, and major portion of distal Yq. Each region contains a number of tandem repeats of DNA sequences. The distal Yp heterochromatin has high variation in its length and can be used in identification of males and their profiling (Rahman et al., 2004). Similarly length of centromeric heterochromatin has also been shown to vary among different male genealogies. Moreover, these Y-chromosome regions contain many hereditary markers normally utilized in evolutionary studies (Santos et al., 1995). The euchromatic region of MSY includes 23 Mb and is comprised of three major groups of genes (Skaletsky et al., 2003). The first group is made out of X-transposed genes having two coding units with around 99% character to the relating X chromosome. The second group comprises 16 coding genes. These genes are likely relics of the primitive autosome pair from which X and Y advanced. However, the vast majority of them have X-chromosome similarity. The third group of genes is a multicopy class that covers roughly 10.2 Mb of Yp and Yq. In this region duplicated genes show ~99.9% similarity. There are eight palindromic portions, six of which have genes that are expressed distinctly in testis. The second and third groups of genes have

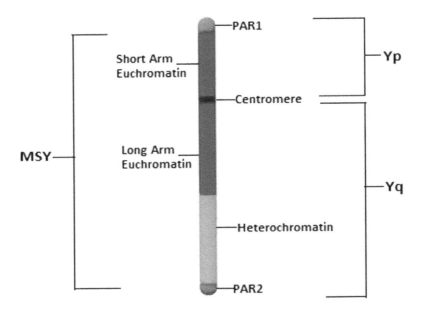

FIGURE 16.1 Structure of Y chromosome displaying pseudo-autosomal regions (PARs), male specific region (MSY or NRY) and the heterochromatin.

(Adapted from Seda et al 2005)

diverse expression pattern: the second group is engaged with cell housekeeping exercises and the third group is solely made out of genes identified with male-specific functions, predominantly spermatogenesis (Skaletsky et al., 2003).

16.4 Y Chromosome: Functions and Associated Pathologies

Y chromosome has its role explicitly in defining male phenotype. This chromosome has its implications in male sex assurance and in male germ cell formation and maintenance.

16.4.1 Testis Development and *SRY* Gene

The gene *SRY* (sex-determining region on the Y chromosome) is responsible for testis development. It is situated on the short arm of the Y chromosome near the pseudoautosomal region. This gene contains single exon encoding a 204 amino acid long polypeptide, which consists of a DNA binding domain suggesting that this protein manages gene expression of other genes. This gene has been shown to be pivotal for differentiation of gonad and starting testis development (Sinclair et al., 1990).

16.4.2 Hostile to Turner Syndrome Impact

The individual with Turner syndrome is a female with 45, X karyotype, also known as monosomy of X chromosome. The key appearances of this disorder are development disorders including sterility. In humans, although every female cell has two X chromosomes, only one of them undergoes inactivation resulting in expression of genes of only one X chromosome in all the cells. However, this condition does not really mean that only one X chromosome is enough for normal development of females. It is now known with certainty that alleles of both the X genes are required for normal development in females. This happens in such a way that either X chromosome out of two can be inactivated and thus a tissue has gene expression on both the chromosomes. Keeping in view this condition, the males that have only one X chromosome may have some Turner syndrome-like impact. In reality that does not happen because males who have 46, XY karyotype, the genes responsible for Turner syndrome impact, are present on the Y chromosome. Despite the fact that there is no clear identification of genes engaged with the Turner condition, there is an impression of various loci on the X and Y chromosome related with Turner syndrome (e.g., *SHOX/PHOG* (Rao et al., 1997; Ellison et al., 1996), *ZFX/ZFY* (Page, 1988) *GCY,* and *TCY)* (Barbaux et al., 1995).

16.4.3 Oncogenic Effects of Y Chromosome

The role of the Y chromosome in malignant growth is still speculative. However, Y-chromosome loss and rearrangements have been related with various kinds of malignancies, such as bladder cancer (Sauter et al., 1995), male sex cord stroma tumors (de Graaff et al., 1999), lung malignancy (Center et al., 1993), and esophageal carcinoma (Hunter et al., 1993). In spite of the fact that these adjustments of this chromosome are moderately present in various sorts of malignancy, there is no immediate proof for the role of Y in tumor development since any proto-oncogenes and tumor suppresser genes have not been localized to the Y chromosome.

16.4.4 Other Pathological Conditions

Various genes on the Y chromosome have associated pathologies such as SHOX (short stature homebox-containing) associated with short stature, Lerf-Weill syndrome, SRY (sex reversal Y) related to sex reversal, RPS4Y (ribosomal protein S4, Y), ZFY (zinc-finger Y) and BPY1 (basic protein, Y1) associated with Turner syndrome, TSPY (testis-specific protein, Y) associated with gonadoblastoma, USP9Y (or DFFRY) {ubiquitin-specific protease (or drosophila fat-facets related, Y)} related to azoospermia, PRY (putative tyrosine phosphatase protein-related Y), DBY (DEAD box, Y), UTY (ubitiquitous TRY motif, Y), CDY (chromodomain, Y), EIF1AY (translation initiation factor 1A, Y), VCY2 (variably charged protein, Y2), RBM (RNA-binding motif, Y), and XKRY (XK-related, Y) are mainly associated with infertility in males (Rao et al., 1997; Sinclair et al., 1990; Fisher et al., 1990; Page et al., 1987; Arnemann et al., 1987; Reijo et al., 1995; Lahn and Page, 1997; Ma et al., 1993).

16.5 Y-Chromosome Markers

Evolutionary or population genetics studies centered explicitly on males clearly require hereditary markers from the Y chromosome. Human genome projects have progressed delivering a great deal of Y-chromosome sequences (International Human Genome Sequencing Consortium, 2002; Skaletsky et al., 2003; Mouse Genome Sequencing Consortium et al., 2002). Without genome sequence data, elective methodologies are required to study Y-chromosome markers. Two of them are random amplified polymorphic DNA (RAPD) and amplified fragment length polymorphism (AFLP). RAPD is a quick technique with minimal efforts but results are sometime difficult to reproduce. AFLP is exceptionally steady yet tedious and more costly than RAPD. The two strategies can be utilized with a practically boundless arrangement of groundwork that will deliver limitless source of conceivable outcomes to create Y markers (Hadrys et al., 1992; Mueller and Wolfenbarger, 1999).

16.5.1 Types of Y-Chromosome Markers

The genetic polymorphism of the Y chromosome is generally grouped into biallelic markers and polymorphisms of tandem repeats or multi-allelic markers (Jobling and Tyler-Smith, 2000). Biallelic markers include SNPs and insertions and deletions (indels). SNPs are the most well-known kind of polymorphisms, consisting of about 90% of all polymorphisms of DNA (Collins et al., 1997). SNPs have low rate of change and are thus very suitable for studying early evolutionary history of mankind. The change rate for SNP markers is about 2×10^{-8} for every base for each generation (Nachman and Crowell, 2000).

Indels in Y chromosome are also of great significance. Mostly deletions in areas of Y-explicit genes (*AZFa, AZFb, AZFc*) have been known as reasons for diseases like male infertility, spermatogenic failure, oligospermia, and azoospermia. All of these diseases seriously disable male reproductive wellness (Fernandes et al., 2002; 2004; Repping et al., 2003). Not all indels influence male fertility; they continue over ages and are adequately considered as polymorphisms. One such indel is a 2kb deletion in 12f2 marker (Casanova et al., 1985), utilized for characterizing haplogroup J as indicated by the current classification (YCC, 2002). Some indels have emerged autonomously more than once in mankind's history. For instance, the deletion or duplication of the 50f2/C (DYS7C) area out of sight of various haplogroups is believed to emerged inany event 7–8 times (Jobling et al., 1996). Another example is the deletion of the *DAZ3/DAZ4* loci that has been shown in people with haplogroup N (Fernandes et al., 2004), generally present in northern Eurasia.

Another genetic polymorphism in humans is present in the form of repeated DNA sequences. The repetitive sequences are either tandem or are interspersed. Long interspersed nucleotide elements (LINEs) and short interspersed nucleotide elements (SINEs) are the most abundant repetitive sequences. The best instances of the LINEs and SINEs are L1 and Alu components. Around 55,000 Alu and 12,000 L1 insertions are explicit to humans and are not found in chimpanzees (Mills, et al., 2006a; Treangen and Salzberg, 2011).

The tandemly repeated classes of polymorphism incorporate minisatellites and microsatellites that possess a moderately lesser portion of the genome. Since these repeats are spread all through the genome; they are broadly utilized in human genetic diversity studies. As per their length, these repeats are classified as satellite-DNA (repeat lengths of one to a few thousand base pairs), minisatellites or a variable number of tandem repeats running from 10 to 100 bp, and microsatellites or STRs, under 10 bp, for the most part 2 to 6 bp long (Chambers and MacAvoy, 2000). In Y-chromosomal examinations microsatellites are generally utilized, while minisatellites have been utilized distinctly in certain examinations (Jin et al., 2003).

Microsatellites are multi-allelic markers with various allele numbers run from 3 to 49 in the locus. Their change rate is a lot higher than that for biallelic markers and, in this way, are generally utilized in phylogenetic examinations to research events that have happened in a recent time in evolutionary history (de Knijff et al., 1997; Litt and Luty, 1989).

In evolutionary studies, STRs are significant in combination with haplogroup information (de Knijff, 2000), as they empower to consider diversity within haplogroup. STRs are especially investigated in criminological work (Jobling et al., 1997). So far the quantity of broadly utilized Y-chromosomal STRs has been very low (around 30) yet in a study by Kayser et al. (2004), 166 conceivably helpful STRs were depicted. Various investigations have indicated that the normal change rate for autosomal tetranucleotide repeats is about 2.0×10^{-3} for every generation (Weber and Wong, 1993). Comparable outcomes (2.0×10^{-3} for every age) were obtained for Y-chromosomal tetranucleotide repeats in pedigree family studies that were in concordance with one of the study for autosomal microsatellites (Heyer et al., 1997; Weber and Wong, 1993). However, the change rate was assessed, utilizing information on microsatellite variations in Y-chromosome haplogroups characterized by SNPs in populations with recorded histories (the African Bantu extension, the dissimilarity of Polynesian population, and the inception of Gypsy peoples from Bulgaria), just as utilizing similar information on overall SNP variety, both at autosomal and Y-chromosome loci. The assessed transformation rate for a normal Y-chromosome STR locus was seen as 6.9×10^{-4} for every generation (Zhivotovsky et al., 2004).

16.6 Y Chromosome as Population Marker

The Y-linked loci in the MSY area are haploid and without recombination with the X chromosome. In view of these specific attributes, there is accumulation of changes along the ages called paternal or male heredities. Population geneticists have widely contemplated human male genealogies to follow relocations and recreate mankind's history (Jobling and Tyler-Smith, 2003). Numerous Y-chromosome polymorphisms, additionally called unique event polymorphisms, are biallelic markers and can be consolidated in haplogroups that characterize Y genealogies with explicit geographic dispersions around the globe (Y Chromosome Consortium – YCC 2002). The haplogroup conveyances reflect past segment occasions and human relocation courses. The overall example of dispersion of the haplogroups recommends an ongoing inception (somewhere in the range of 60,000 and 150,000 years prior) in Africa for all present-day human Y chromosomes (Underhill et al., 2000; Wilder et al., 2004).

The overall distribution of Y-chromosome-based heredities is believed to be an outcome of irregular transformative powers, such as genetic drift, population extension, and migration. In any case, one can not excuse natural selection so effectively in light of the fact that the Y chromosome conveys significant genes associated with spermatogenesis, which can be an objective for adaptive processes. Two potential selection components could possibly have strongly affected the population hereditary variety of Y chromosomes: hitchhiking and background selection. The hitchhiking impact happens when allele increments in its frequency occurs since it is connected to a valuable allele at a neighboring locus exposed to positive selection, regardless of whether it assumes itself any immediate role in wellness (Otto, 2000). The background selection process is the inverse; in this procedure, an allele is more averse to persevere in a population and might be dispensed with on the grounds that it is linked to deleterious alleles. The result of these two procedures would thus be able to be the spread and inevitable obsession, or the reduction and possible elimination of a specific Y haplogroup or ancestry.

16.7 Y-Chromosome Haplogrouping

Steady revelation of new markers in the human Y chromosome prompted the development of a few irrelevant and nonsystematic terminologies for Y-chromosomal haplogroups (Jobling and Tyler, 2000; Semino et al., 2000; Underhill et al., 2000; Hammer et al., 2001). To resolve the issue, the Y Chromosome Consortium (YCC) made a single most Y-chromosomal phylogenetic tree of binary haplogroups (YCC 2002), joining essentially all past nomenclatures. The ancestral conditions of Y-chromosomal binary markers were dictated by correlation of homologous areas of the NRY in firmly related species like chimpanzees, gorillas, and orangutans (Underhill et al., 2000; Hammer et al., 2001). A various leveled classification framework and a basic arrangement of rules were developed to unambiguously mark the various clades settled inside this tree (YCC, 2002). Now a reexamined variant of the Y-chromosome haplogroup tree containing 311 particular haplogroups joining around 600 binary markers has been distributed in which new markers and haplogroups were presented and past haplogroups essentially adjusted observing the principles introduced in YCC 2002 (Karafet et al., 2008).

16.8 Conclusion

The Y chromosome has driven the route in human molecular evolution and its genetic markers are important for measuring admixture among populations. There is lot of information with respect to the geographical origins of Y-SNPs and investigations of human populations dependent on these SNPs. Due to the high specificity, Y SNPs can be utilized to measure admixture among different population groups without depending on more complicated models of admixture. Specifically data on the Y chromosome may reveal more about the path followed by modern humans after they left Africa and settled in different mainlands. Notwithstanding, the next coherent advance would be to recognize genetic variants associated with complex multigenic illnesses and even those caused by microbes like malaria, viral hepatitis, HIV, tuberculosis, etc.

REFERENCES

1000 Genomes Project Consortium. 2012. An integrated map of genetic variation from 1,092 human genomes. *Nature* 491: 56–65.

Arnemann, A. J., Epplen. J., Cooke, H. et al. 1987. A human Y chromosomal DNA sequence expressed in testicular tissue. *Nucl Acids Res* 15:8713–8724.

Bachtrog, D., and Charlesworth, B. 2001. Towards a complete sequence of the human Y chromosome. *Genome Biology* 2(5):1016.1–1016.5.

Barbaux, S., Vilain, E., Raoul, O. et al. 1995. Proximal deletions on the long arm of the Y chromosome suggest a critical region associated with a specific subset of characteristic Turner stigmata. *Hum Mol Genet* 4:1565–1568.

Bittles, A. H. 2005. Population stratification and genetic association studies in South Asia. *J Mol Genet Med* 1:43–48.

Cardon, L. R. and Bell, J. I. 2000. Association study designs for complex diseases. *Nature Reviews Genetics* 2:91–99.

Casanova, M., Leroy, P., Boucekkine, C. et al. 1985. A human Y -linked DNA polymorphism and its potential tor estimating genetic and evolutionary distance. *Science* 230:1403–1406.

Center, R., Lukeis, R., Vrazas, V. et al. 1993. Y chromosome loss and rearrangement in non-small lung cancer. *Int J Cancer* 55:390–393.

Chambers, G. K., and MacAvoy, E. S. 2000 Microsatellites: consensus and controversy. *Comp Biochem Physiol B Biochem Mol Bio* 126:455–476.

Collins, F. S., Guyer, M. S., Charkravarti, A. 1997. Variations on a theme: cataloging human DNA sequence variation. *Science* 278:1580–1581.

Crawford, M. H., Beaty, K. G. 2013. DNA fingerprinting in anthropological genetics: past, present, future. *Investigative Genetics* 4:1–10.

de G raaff, W. E., van E chten, J., van der V een, A. Y. et al. 1999. Loss of the Y-chromosome in the primary metastasis of a male sex cord stromal tumor: pathogenetic implications. *Cancer Genet Cytogenet* 112:21–25.

deKnijff, P. 2000. Messages through bottlenecks: on the combined use of slow and fast evolving polymorphic markers on the human Y chromosome. *Ann J Hum Gen* 67:1055–1061

deKnijff, P., Kayser, M., Caglia, A. et al. 1997. Chromosome Y microsatellites: population genetics and evolutionary aspects. *Int J Legal Med* 110:134–149

Ellison, J., Li, X., Francke, U. et al. 1996. Rapid evolution of pseudoautosomal genes and their mouse homologs. *Mammal Genome* 7:25–30.

Erzurumluoglu, A., Baird, D., Richardson, T. et al. 2018. Using Y-chromosomal haplogroups in genetic association studies and suggested implications. *Genes* 9:45.

Fernandes, S., Huellen, K., Goncalves, J. et al. 2002. High frequency of DAZ1/DAZ2 gene deletions in patients with severe oligozoospermia. *Mol Hum Reprod* 8:286–298.

Fernandes, S., Paracchini, S., Meyer, L. H. et al. 2004. A large AZFc deletion removes DAZ3/DAZ4 and nearby genes from men in Y haplogroup N. *Ann J Hum Genet* 74:180–187.

Ferragut, J. F., Pereira, R., Castro, J. A. et al. 2016. Genetic diversity of 38 insertion-deletion polymorphisms in Jewish populations. *Forensic Sci Int Genet* 21:1–4.

Fisher, E. M. C., Beer-Romero, P., Brown, L. G. et al. 1990. Homologous ribosomal protein genes on the human X and Y chromosome: escape from X inactivation and possible implication for Turner Syndrome. *Cell* 63:1205–1218.

Ghosh, S. 2007. Interpreting a genetic case-control finding: What can be said, what cannot be said and implications in Indian populations. *Ind J Hum Genet* 13:1–4.

Graves, J. A., Schmidt, M. M. 1992. Mammalian sex chromosomes: design or accident? *Genet Dev* 2:890–901.

Hadrys, H., Balick, M., Schierwater, B. 1992. Applications of random amplified polymorphic DNA (RAPD) in molecular ecology. *Mol Ecol* 1:55–63

Hammer, M. F., Karafet T. M., Redd, A. J. et al. 2001. Hierarchical patterns of global human Y-chromosome diversity. *Mol Biol Evol* 18:1189–1203.

Heyer, E., Puymirat, J., Dieltes, P. et al. 1997. Estimating Y chromosome specific microsatellite mutation frequencies using deep rooting pedigrees. *Hum Mol Genet* 6:799–803.

Hu, W., Chen, M., Ji, J. et al. 2017. Interaction between Y chromosome haplogroup O3* and 4-n-octylphenol exposure reduces the susceptibility to spermatogenic impairment in Han Chinese. *Ecotoxicol Environ Saf* 144:450–455.

Hunter, S., Gramlich, T., Abbott, K. et al. 1993. Y chromosome loss in oesophageal carcinoma: an in situ hybridization study. *Genes Chromosomes Cancer* 8:172–177.

International Human Genome Sequencing Consortium. 2002. Initial sequencing and comparative analysis of the mouse genome. *Nature* 420:520–562.

Jin, Z. B., Huang, X. L., Nakajima, Y. et al. 2003. Haploid allele mapping of Y-chromosome minisatellite, MSY1 (DYF155S1), to a Japanese population. *Leg Med (Tokyo)* 5:87–92.

Jobling, M. A., and Tyler-Smith, C. 2003. The human Y chromosome: an evolutionary marker comes of age. *Nat Rev Genet* 4:598–612.

Jobling, M. A., Samara, V., Pandya, A. et al. 1996. Recurrent duplication and deletion polymorphisrns on the long ann of the Y chromosome in normal males. *Hum Mol Genet* 5:1767–1775.

Jobling, M. A., and Tyler-Smith, C. 2000. New uses for new haplotypes the human Y chromosome, disease and selection. *Trends Genet* 16:356–362.

Jobling, M. A., Pandya, A., Tyler-Smith, C. 1997. The Y chromosome in forensic analysis and paternity testing. *Int J Legal Med* 110:118–124.

Karafet, T. M., Mendez, F. L., Meilerman, M. B. et al. 2008. New binary polymorphisms reshape and increase resolution of the human Y chromosomal haplogroup tree. *Genome Res* 18:830–838.

Kaul, N., Singh, Y. P., Bhanwer, A. J. S. (2015) The influence of ethnicity in the association of WC, WHR, hypertension and PGC-1α (Gly482Ser), UCP2 -866 G/A and SIRT1 -1400 T/C polymorphisms with T2D in the population of Punjab. *Gene* 563:150–154.

Kayser, M., Kittler, R., Erler, A. et al. 2004. A comprehensive survey of human Y -chromosomal microsatellites. *Ann J Hum Genet* 74:1183–1197.

Lahn, B. T., and Page, D. C. 1999. Four evolutionary strata on the human X chromosome. *Science* 286:964–967.

Lahn, B. T., and Page, D. 1997. Functional coherence of the human Y chromosome. *Science* 278:675–680.

Litt, M., and Luty, J. A. 1989. A hypervariable microsatellite revealed by in vitro amplification of a dinucleotide repeat within the cardiac muscle actin gene. *Am J Hum Genet* 44:397–401.

Ma, K., Inglis, J. D., Sharkey, A. et al. 1993. A Y chromosome gene family with RNA-binding protein homology: candidates for the azoospermia factor AZF controlling spermatogenesis. *Cell* 75:1287–1295.

Mills, R. E., Bennett, E. A., Iskow R. C. et al. 2006a. Recently mobilized transposons in the human and chimpanzee genomes. *Ann J Hum Genet* 78:671–679.

Mills, R. E., Luttig, C. T., Larkins, C. E. et al. 2006b. An initial map of insertion and deletion (INDEL) variation in the human genome. *Genome Research* 16:1182–1190.

Mouse Genome Sequencing Consortium, Waterston, R. H., Lindblad-Toh, K. et al. 2002. Initial sequencing and comparative analysis of the mouse genome. *Nature* 420:520–562

Mueller, U. G. and Wolfenbarger, L. L. 1999. AFLP genotyping and fingerprinting. *Trends Ecol Evol* 14:389–394.

Nachman, M. W., and Crowell, S. L. 2000. Estimate of the mutation rate per nucleotide in humans. *Genetics* 156:297–304.

Otto, P. S. 2000. Detecting the form of selection from DNA sequence data. *Trends Genet* 16: 526–529.

Page, D. C. 1988. Is ZFY the sex-detennining gene on the human Y chromosome? *Philos Trans R Soc Land B Biol Sci* 322:155–157.

Page, D. C., Mosher, R., Simpson, et al. 1987. The sex-determining region of the human Y chromosome encodes a finger protein. *Cell* 51:1091–1104.

Price, A. L., Zaitlen, N. A., Reich, D. et al. 2010 New approaches to population stratification in genome-wide association studies. *Nat Rev Genet* 11:459–463.

Rahman, M. M., Bashamboo, A., Prasad, A. et al. 2004. Organizational variation of DYZ1 repeat sequences on the human Y chromosome and its diagnostic potentials. *DNA Cell Biol* 23:561–571.

Rao, E., Weiss, B., Fukami, M. et al. 1997. Pseudoautosomal deletions encompasing a novel gene cause growth failure in idiopatic short stature and Turner syndrome. *Nat Genet* 16:54–63.

Reijo, R., Lee, T. Y., Salo, P. et al. 1995. Diverse spermatogenic defects in humans caused by Y chromosome deletions encompassing a novel RNA-binding protein gene. *Nat Genet* 10:383–395.

Repping, S., Skaletsky, H., Brown, L. et al. 2003. Polymorphism for a 1.6-Mb deletion o f the human Y chromosome persists through balance between recurrent mutation and haploid selection. *Nat Genet* 35:247–251.

Repping, S., Skaletsky, H., Lange, J. et al. 2002. Recombination between palindromes P5 and P1 on the human Y chromosome causes massive deletions and spermatogenic failure. *Am J Hum Genet* 71: 906–922.

Romero, I. G., Manica, A., Goudet, J. et al. 2009. How accurate is the current picture of human genetic variation and quest. *Heredity* 102:120–126.

Sachidanandam, R., Weissman, D., Schmidt, S. C. et al. 2001. A map of human genome sequence variation containing 1.42 million single nucleotide polymorphisms. *Nature* 409: 928–933.

Santos, F. R., Pena, S. D. and Tyler-Smith, C. 1995. PCR haplotypes for the human Y chromosome based on alphoid satellite DNA variants and heteroduplex analysis. *Gene* 165:191–198.

Sauter, G., Moch, H., Wagner, U. et al. 1995. Y chromosome loss detected by FISH in bladder cancer. *Cancer Genet Cytogenet* 82:163–169.

Seda, O., Liska, F. and Sedova, L. 2005. Sex Determination. Multimedia E-textbook of Medical Biology, Genetics and Genomics. Czech Republic: Institute of Biology and Medical Genetics of the First Faculty of Medicine of Charles University and the General Teaching Hospital.

Semino, O., Passarino, G., Oefner, P. J. et al. 2000. The genetic legacy of Paleolithic Homo sapiens sapiens in extant Europeans: a Y chromosome perspective. *Science* 290:1155–1159.

Sharma, R., Matharoo, K., Kapoor, R. et al. 2013. Ethnic differences in CAPN10 SNP-19 in type 2 diabetes: a North-West Indian case control study and evidence from meta-analysis. *Genetics Research* 95:146–155.

Sinclair, A. H., Berta, P., Palmer, M. S. et al. 1990. A gene from the human sex-determining region encodes a protein with homology to a conserved DNA-binding motif. *Nature* 346:240–244.

Skaletsky, H., Kuroda-Kawaguchi, T., Minx, P. J. et al. 2003. The male-specific region of the human Y chromosome is a mosaic of discrete sequence classes. *Nature* 423:825–837.

Sokhi, J., Sikka, R., Raina, P. et al. 2016. Association of genetic variants in INS (rs689), INSR (rs1799816) and PP1G. G (rs1799999) with type 2 diabetes (T2D): a case-control study in three ethnic groups from North-West India. *Mol Genet Genomics* 291:205–216.

Suh, Y. and Vijg, J. 2005. SNP discovery in associating genetic variation with human disease phenotypes. *Mutat Res* 573:41–53.

The Y Chromosome Consortium. 2002. A nomenclature for the tree of human Y-chromosomal binary haplogroups. *Genome Res* 12:339–348.

Thomas, D. C. and Witte, J. S. 2002. Point: population stratification: a problem for case-control studies of candidate-gene associations? *Cancer Epidemiol Biomarkers Prev* 11:505–512.

Tishkoff, S. A. and Verrelli, B. C. 2003. Patterns of human genetic diversity: implications for human evolutionary history and disease. *Annu Rev Genomics Hum Genet* 4:293–340

Treangen, T. J. and Salzberg, S. L. 2011. Repetitive DNA and next-generation sequencing: computational challenges and solutions. *Nat Rev Genet* 13:36–46.

Underhill, P. A., Shen, P., Lin, A. A. et al. 2000. Y chromosome sequence variation and the history of human populations. *Nat Genet* 26:358–361.

Weber, J. L. and Wong, C. 1993. Mutation of human short tandem repeats. *Hum Mol Genet* 2:1123–1128.

Wilder, J. A., Mobasher, Z. and Hammer, M. F. 2004. Genetic evidence for unequal effective population sizes of human females and males. *Mol Biol Evol* 21:2047–2057.

Wilson, J. F., Weale, M. E., Smith, A. C. et al. (2001) Population genetic structure of variable drug response. *Nat Genet* 29:265–269.

Zhivotovsky, L. A., Underhill, P. A., Cinnioğlu, C. et al. 2004. The effective mutation rate at y chromosome short tandem repeats, with application to human population-divergence time. *Am J Hum Genet* 74:50–61.

17

Role of Repair Gene Polymorphism and Hypermethylation of GSTP Gene in the Risk of Prostate Cancer

Sukhjeet Sidhu and Jagdeep S. Deep
Indian Institute of Science Education and Research, Mohali, Chandigarh, India

R.C. Sobti
Department of Biotechnology, Panjab University, Chandigarh, India

17.1 Introduction

Prostate cancer is one of the most prevalent and least understood of all malignancies in men. Prostatic tumors are androgen-dependent, resulting in the death of the patient. Since the late 1940s, there has been a dramatic increase in the identification of prostatic cancer cases. The reasons are many, like increased elderly population, cancer registration and improved methods of prognosis of the disease, use of new diagnostic technologies including transrectal ultrasound guided needle biopsy, computer tomography, greater frequency of operations for benign disease, and serum testing of prostate-specific antigen (PSA) (Jemal et al., 2004).

17.2 Historical Background

The prevalence of histological prostate cancer is remarkably similar in the whole world, but clinical incidence widely varies. This indicates that although the initiation rate of prostate cancer is the same, that of progression of clinically evident disease varies. This suggests that prostate cancer is an interplay of genetic and epigenetic events both of which may be affected by environmental risk factors that act as promoters or activators. It is a multistep process involving three stages (i.e., initiation, promotion, and progression), mediated through various cellular, biochemical, and molecular changes. It involves activation of oncogenes, loss of function of tumour suppressor gene, modulations in genes related to growth regulation, cell cycle, apoptosis, metastases, and angiogenesis as well as alteration of modifier genes (i.e., metabolic, hormonal, DNA repair genes, methylation, and genomic stability). Epigenetics refers to altered levels of a gene's transcriptional activity without directly affecting its primary DNA nucleotide sequence. Individuals with defects in mutation repair pathways are often susceptible to spontaneous or induced cancer. The molecular machinery of the repair pathways has slowly been unraveled over the past few decades. Understanding these molecular pathways improves the prognosis of the disease and may help in finding genes involved in initiation and progression.

A malignant tumour results after a series of DNA alterations in a single cell, or clones of that cell, which lead to loss of normal function, aberrant or uncontrolled cell growth, and often metastases. Several of the genes, which are frequently lost or mutated, have been identified including those whose function is to induce cell proliferation under specific circumstances (e.g., *ras* and *myc* proto-oncogenes) and genes that are programmed to halt proliferation in damaged cells (e.g., *p53* and *APC* tumour suppressor genes). In addition, mutations in genes involved in DNA repair, cell-cycle control, angiogenesis, and

DOI: 10.1201/9781003220404-19

telomerase production also play an important role in cancer genesis. With the exception of rare familial cancers, which are primarily caused by a germline inheritance of a specific mutation, a sporadic cancer may acquire mutations as a result of genotoxic exposure to external or internal agents (e.g., tobacco, chemicals, dietary factors, pollutants, and sex hormones) resulting in DNA aberrations. The likelihood of a mutation(s) occurring and persisting in subsequent clones may be heavily dependent on the efficiency with which potentially toxic exposures are metabolized and excreted, and also the efficiency with which small mistakes in DNA replication are rectified. This progress of carcinogenesis is likely to vary strongly between individuals because of the population variability in polymorphic genes that regulate these processes. Changes in the patterns of methylationhave been associated with the altered expression of a number of genes involved in cell cycle control and apoptosis, including *p16, GSTP1, INK4a, RASSFIA, RAR-β, FHIT, APC, MGMT,* and H- and E-cadherins among many others in various carcinomas (Esteller et al., 2001). Silencing of tumour suppressor and tumour-related genes by hypermethylation at promoter CpG islands is one of the major events in human tumourigenesis.

The present chapter is an effort to analyze polymorphisms in *XPC* and *XPD* repair genes, *GSTP1* exon 5 and exon 6 metabolic genes, and their association with the etiology of prostate cancer and correlation of the same. The methylation pattern of *GSTP1* and *MGMT* gene has also been studied in prostate cancer, BPH patients, and healthy controls to correlate it with the incidence and progression of this cancer.

17.2.1 What is a Prostate?

A prostate is a firm grey to reddish, partly glandular, partly fibro-muscular body surrounding the beginning of the male urethra. It lies at a low level in the inferior border of the symphysis pubis and pubic arch and rectal ampulla through which it may be palpated. The gland is somewhat conical, the base measuring 4 cm transversely. It has 2 cm anterio-posterior and 3 cm vertical diameters and weighs about 8 gm. It is enveloped in a thin, but strong fibrous capsule. The capsule is firmly adherent to the gland and continuous with a median septum in the urethral crest. It is also continuous with numerous fibromuscular septa enmeshing the glandular tissue.

The prostate is traversed by the urethra and ejaculatory ducts and contains the prostatic utricle. The urethra usually passes between its anterior and middle thirds. The ejaculatory ducts pass antero-inferiorly through its posterior region to open into the prostatic urethra. Histological sections show two concentric zones of glandular tissue (Franks, 1954; Fergusson and Gibson, 1956). The larger peripheral zone has long, branched glands whose ducts curve posterior to open mainly into the prostatic sinuses. The internal zone consists of submucosal glands. Peripheral and internal zones are said to be separated by an ill-defined capsule. Carcinoma affects almost exclusively the peripheral zone, the internal being prone to benign hypertrophy.

At birth the prostate has a system of ducts embedded in a stroma that forms a large part of the gland. At puberty, the prostate gland enters a maturation phase and in approximately 12 months during this time it more than doubles in size, due almost entirely to follicular development. During the third decade, the glandular epithelium grows by irregular multiplication of the endothelial infoldings into the lumen of the follicles. The size remains unaltered until 45–50 years, when the epithelial folding tends to disappear, follicular outlines become more regular, and amyloidal bodies increase in number, all signs being of prostatic involution. After 45–50 years, the prostate may undergo benign hypertrophy, increasing in size until death, or alternatively it may undergo progressive atrophy. After middle age, the prostate often enlarges projecting into the bladder to impede urination by distorting the prostatic urethra. The median lobe may enlarge the most, with even a small enlargement obstructing the internal urethral orifice, the more the patient strains the more the prostatic mass, acting like a valve, blocks the opening. The hypertrophied part may be removed surgically (prostatectomy).

There are valve-less venous communications between the prostatic and extra dural venous plexuses, which are probably an important factor in the metastasis of prostatic neoplasms to the vertebral bodies (Batson, 1940; Franks, 1953).

Prostate carcinoma is a major health problem in western industrialized countries, where around 10% of men are diagnosed with this cancer usually in their old age out of which 10% die from the disease. The introduction of good serum-marker, prostate-specific antigen (PSA) has allowed detection of many cancers, while they are still locally confined and can be cured by surgery or radiotherapy. Those cancers that have spread too extensively locally or have developed distant metastases cannot be cured by current procedures. A third and apparently large graph of prostate cancer takes a very slow course and will not lead to clinical symptoms during the life term of an elderly man and need to be actively monitored. Molecular research on prostate cancer therefore faces three major tasks:

1. Detecting the cancer
2. Distinguishing both locally confined and indolent, locally confined, but likely to progress, or has progressed beyond reach of current treatment
3. Developing effective treatment for metastasis and locally progressive cases

17.2.2 Benign Prostatic Hyperplasia

Benign prostatic hyperplasia (BPH) and prostate cancer are common diseases of aged men. Both diseases appear to be androgen-dependent for growth, but BPH commonly arises in the central and transitional zone of the prostate while cancer is most often found in the peripheral zone of the gland.

It has been reported that more than half of the population aged 75 years has histologic evidence of BPH, while prostate cancer is amongst the most common male cancers. Both share important anatomic, pathologic, and genetic links. Prostate is now the most common site of cancer in men (excluding melanoma skin cancers), while BPH affects as many as 62% of men aged 75 year (European National registry data). Studies have identified prolonged history of BPH as a risk factor for prostate cancer (Armenian et al., 1974).

17.2.3 Tumor-specific Antigens and Antibodies

17.2.3.1 Prostate-Specific Antigens

PSA is a serum protease that is secreted from prostate epithelial cells (Cohen et al., 1992). PSA levels have prognostic value for men with prostate cancer. Approximately 30 years ago, it was first proposed as serum marker for early detection of prostate cancer. The medial levels are approximately 0.7 ng/ml in men aged 60 yr and modest elevation of blood level of PSA to 4.0ng/ml is strongly associated with an increased risk of cancer (Meitz et al., 2002). PSA is an important marker for diagnosis and follow-up of prostate cancer patients (Ware, 1994). Specific germ line genetic polymorphisms in the promoter region of the PSA gene have been reported to be associated with higher serum PSA levels. The same may be used for screening of prostate cancer. However, the specificity of total serum PSA is limited particularly in rising incidence of clinically relevant prostate cancer in patients with low PSA serum levels (less than 4.0 ng/ml). The specificity of PSA determination is essentially required in cancer patients for which there is a dire need for new tools.

17.2.3.2 Tumor-Specific Antibodies

Proteomic serum profiling as a diagnostic tool and platform for biomarker discovery in prostate cancer is an emerging research area (Banez et al., 2005). Changes in serum protein composition reflecting the pathological state of organs/tissues will facilitate the discovery and quantification of protein biomarkers for differentiation between malignant and normal cells (Petricoin et al., 2002). Tumours are known to induce release of many proteins into the blood and due to various modifications, they appear as foreign molecules and thus lead to the activation of immune system. The presence of auto-antibodies in the sera of high-risk individuals foretells the onset of cancer development and marks their significance as molecular signatures for useful clinical diagnostic and prognostic information. Multiple prostate cancer-specific antigens were identified via the detection of auto-antibodies in the serum of patients with prostate cancer via high throughput phage peptide microarray analysis. The measurement of serum auto-antibodies against a panel of 22 tumor-associated peptides detected prostate cancer with 88.2% specificity and 81.6% sensitivity in a case-control study (Leushner, 2001). Compared to PSA, this auto-antibody signature had significantly better performance suggesting its use against peptides derived from prostate cancer tissue as better tool for screening of prostate cancer.

The regulation of gene expression by aberrant methylation has been well established in tumour biology. The epigenetic phenomenon of hypermethylation in tumor-related genes has been implicated in cancer development and progression (Nelson et al., 1997; Lou et al., 1999; Sasaki et al., 2002) and is therefore one of the most promising means of identifying marker candidates for the early detection of cancer. The diagnostic potential of cancer-specific methylated markers for prostate and bladder cancers have been evaluated in urine and serum samples (Nelson et al., 1997).

Prostate growth depends on synergistic interactions between estrogen and androgens. The ratio of estrogen to androgens in the prostate increases by 40% in ageing men, and this may influence the natural history of both BPH and prostate cancer. Asian men who follow a traditional diet (which provides a rich supply of phytoestrogens) have a lower prevalence of BPH and prostate cancer than men following a modern western diet (Sim and Cheng, 2005) and that is why prostate cancer incidence among Asian immigrants to the United States is higher than in their respective native population (Cook et al., 1999). Inflammation contributes to the development of BPH. In one study, it was suggested that inflammation plays a role in the pathogenesis of prostate cancer. Needle biopsy specimens from men with clinical signs to suggest malignancy revealed a significant link between inflammation and serum PSA (Maclennan et al., 2006).

Mapping the whole genome made it possible to identify genes related to specific disease states and using biomarker technology based on molecular signatures of gene expression feasibility for discovering and predicting cancer classes has been demonstrated (Golub et al., 1999). Genetic alterations damage the structure of DNA and thereby induce mutations that manifest in abnormally functioning proteins that, thereby, precipitate diseased conditions. Malignancy is characterized by genomic alterations that allow proliferation. A number of such alterations have been identified in prostate cancer. Genes that encode enzymes involved in steroid hormone synthesis or function such as cytochrome P-45017 alpha (CYP17), steroid 5-X reductase type II (SRD5A2), and PSA have attracted attention as potential markers of prostate cancer and BPH (Habuchi et al., 2000; Salam et al., 2005). Gene rearrangements have also been implicated in a number of cancers and have recently been uncovered in patients with prostate cancer; however, similar incidences have been rarely reported in BPH (Laxman et al., 2006; Perner et al., 2007). Epigenetic processes such as DNA methylation represent another mechanism of gene regulation. A number of genes are commonly hypermethylated and therefore inactivated during prostate cancer progression (Doboxy et al., 2007). Some of these are tumour suppressor genes (adenomatous polyposis coli, *APC* and Ras-association domain family 1A gene, *RASSF1A*), while others have a role in cell cycle regulation (14-3-3σ) or heavy metal binding (MTG) or encode for proteins such as ATP-binding cassette (ABC) transporters (MDR 1) glutathione-S-transferase (GSTP), and glutathione peroxidases (GPX3). Some genes like endothelin receptor type B (*EDNRB*), cell adhesion molecules (*cadherin-4; CDH4*), and estrogen receptor (*ER*) are selectively methylated in many prostate cancers in their 5' promoter regions. Epigenetic technologies in cancer studies are helping to increase the number of cancer candidate genes and allow to examine changes in 5-methyl cytosine DNA and histone modifications at a genome-wide level.

17.3 Epidemiology of Prostate Cancer

Aging populations as well as introduction of more sensitive diagnostic procedures and cancer registration have resulted in an increase in incidence of prostate cancer at a higher pace (Vercelli et al., 2000). Worldwide, a remarkable increase in the identification of prostate cancer cases has been reported. The use of new diagnostic techniques including serum PSA, transrectal ultrasound guided needle biopsy, computer tomography, and greater frequency of operation for benign diseases may be the major reasons of this increase. This has led to a substantial increase in number of cancer cases observed as compared to earlier time (Hankey et al., 1990). Also the mortality rate has declined mainly due to incidental discovery and timely detection (Miller et al., 1993). Moreover, increasing incidence rate and reaterg public awareness of prostate cancer has created an explosion of prostate cancer screening in western countries. It has certainly affected several epidemiologic features of the disease like its incidence, tumour staging, patient characteristics as well as care and outcome (Mettlin, 2000).

17.3.1 International Statistics

Prostate cancer is the second most common cancer in Europe and the United States. Its incidence and mortality rates vary worldwide. It accounts for 33% of all recently diagnosed malignancies among men in United States. It is considered as the most common malignancy in men followed by lung and colorectal cancer in European Union (Ferlay et al., 2007). More than 30,000 men are diagnosed with prostate cancer every year in the UK (http://info.cancerresearchuk.org.pdf). A 15% higher incidence rate and 38% higher death rate are reported in African American men than in white men. As compared to whites, the death rate from prostate, stomach, and cervical cancers is more than double in black Americans. Factors known to contribute to racial disparities in mortality vary by cancer site (Jemal et al., 2007). According to the World Health Organization, death from cancer is expected to increase manifold worldwide by the year 2020. People living in developing countries (i.e., Latin America, the Caribbean, Asia, the Middle East, and Africa) are predicted to be at higher risk than those in developed countries. Although actual cancer incidence rates are still lower in developing countries than in North America and Europe, the rise in cancer-related deaths will represent a significant burden to the already overwhelmed health systems in developing countries (Rastogi et al., 2004). Thus, prostate cancer is going to be an actual health burden worldwide.

17.3.2 Asian Statistics

Although Asian people have the lowest incidence and mortality rates of prostate cancer in the world, these rates have rapidly risen in the past two decades in most Asian countries. Prostate cancer has become one of the leading male cancers in some Asian countries. In 2000, the age-adjusted incidence was over 10 per 100000 men in Japan, Taiwan, Singapore, Malaysia, the Philippines, and Israel (Pu et al., 2004). According to a recent study, the incidence of prostate cancer in Asian countries is still increasing rapidly due to a more lifestyle. Prostate cancer mortality is expected to continue to increase in Asian countries as the percentage of advanced-stage prostate cancers remains high (Namiki et al., 2010). There has been a significant increase in the incidence of prostate cancer in Korea (Jung et al., 2010). High incidence rate of prostate cancer has also been reported in Turkey (Ceber et al., 2008). The increase in the incidence and mortality rates in Asian countries from 1973–1997 was estimated to be 4.8–9.8 (Singapore), 4.9–9.0 (Miyagi, Japan), 5.1–7.9 (Hong Kong), 1.6–2.3 (Shanghai, China), and 6.8–7.9 (Bombay, India) per 100,000 men. In Japan, Taiwan, Singapore, Malaysia, Philippines, and Israel, the age-adjusted incidence of prostatic cancer was over 10 per 100,000 men in 2002. In Taiwan and Singapore, prostate cancer is the sixth leading male cancer, population of both the places being 23 and 4.6 millions, respectively (as per the 2003 data), with Chinese people being the largest proportion of this population (Pu et al., 2004).

17.3.3 Indian Statistics

In the year 2000, nearly 550,000 deaths due to cancer occurred in Indian population. While in 2001, 6,605 cases of prostate cancer and a total of 565,682 cases of all types of cancer were predicted in India. In developing countries like India, 80% of victims when detected are already at an incurable stage (Pal and Mittal, 2004).

The epidemiology of prostate cancer is poorly understood in India and very few reports are available on the survival data inspite of being the largest country in south-central Asia (population 1.05 billion in 2003). This may be because of poor patient follow-up and inadequate reporting system of cancer incidence rate among all male cancers in India. The survival of prostate cancer patients is relatively poor in India, being 40% for localized disease, 24% for direct extension and regional node involvement, and 13% for metastasis diseases (Sunny et al., 2004).

A Delhi urban resident population-based cancer registry reveals an ASR of 9.0 per 100,000 men in prostate cancer and the incidence of prostate cancer in males was the highest among the Indian registries (Manoharan et al., 2009).

17.4 Risk Factors Involved in Prostate Cancer

Inthe past several decades, the epidemiology and screening studies have shown concern about the pathogenesis of prostate cancer, but no definitive cause has been established. The clinical effect of prostate cancer is increasing. Growing public awareness has raised questions concerning the cause of prostate cancer as well as ways to screen for and prevent this disease. The ultimate goal of epidemiologic studies is to identify risk factors to guide disease prevention strategies. The prevailing risk factors that may be important in the development of prostate cancer supported by scientific literature are being cited as follows.

17.4.1 Age and Ethnicity

Diagnosis and mortality rate of prostate cancer is very rare in men below 50 years of age, which after this age shows an exponential increase (Haas & Sakr, 1997). The probability of developing prostate cancer increases with age. Studies have revealed that the probability increases from 0.005% among individuals who are less than 39 years of age to 2.2% for those aged 40–59 years and 13.7% for those aged 60–79 years. Twenty percent of men in the age of 50–60 years and 50% of those in the age of 70–80 years showed histological evidence of malignancy (Carter et al., 1990). In United States, more than 70% of all cases of prostate cancer are diagnosed in men above 65 years of age.

As far as ethnicity is concerned, the highest rates of prostate cancer in the world have been found in African Americans (275.3 per 100,000 men). This incidence is 60% higher than among whites, which in turn is higher than the rates in Hispanics and Asian/Pacific Islanders (Table 17.1).

Scandinavian countries show the highest rate of prostate cancer, while Asian countries show the lowest (American Cancer Society, 2003; Crawford, 2003). Prostate cancer is ranked as second leading cause of deaths in Spain (11%) and fourth in Italy (8%). It is the most common cancer among males in France (19%) (Reddy et al., 2003). Age-adjusted incidence rates as well as death rates from clinical prostate cancer vary dramatically from country to country, considering the difference in and availability of screening programmes (Haas and Sakr, 1997). Waterhouse (1982) and Muir et al. (1991) found a 25-fold difference between incidence rates in American black men living in San Francisco and in Japanese men. In 1988, the age-adjusted death rate per 100,000 population was 15.7 for men in the United States and 3.5 for those in Japan. This interpretation is further supported by the observation that immigrants moving from low-risk areas to the United States gradually assume higher risk of the US population (Haenszel and Kirihoro, 1968; Dunn, 1975; Flanders, 1984; Miekle and Smith, 1990; Muir et al., 1991; Yu et al., 1991; Shimizu et al., 1991). Thus, despite the presence of histologic cancer appearing to be related to age, other risk factors that increase the development of prostate cancer probably affect the 'Promotion' steps of the transformation pathway.

17.4.2 Family History

The incidence of prostate cancer in male relatives of patients with prostate cancer is increased. Higher incidence of prostate cancer was found among male relatives of patients with breast cancer (Woolf, 1960;

TABLE 17.1

Rate of Incidence of Prostate Cancer Amongst Different Ethnic Groups

Ethnic Group	Incidence (per 1,00,000)
White	172.9
African American	275.3
Asians/Pacific Islander	107.2
American Indian/Alaskan Native	60.7
Hispanics	127.6

Krain, 1974; Theisseu, 1974; Schuman et al., 1977; Canon et al., 1982; Miekle and Stanish, 1982; Miekle et al., 1985; Steinberg et al., 1990; Carter et al., 1990, 1992; Spitz et al., 1991).

Familial clustering of prostate cancer was also reported by Canon et al. (1982) in Utah Mormons. Men with a father or brother with prostate cancer have double the risk of developing prostate cancer as men without affected relatives and the risk increases with increasing number of affected relatives (Carter et al., 1990; Steinberg et al., 1990; Carter et al., 1992). Studies in Japan reported that the age at diagnosis of prostate cancer was significantly lower in patients with a positive family history than those without it (69.4+7.5 vs. 74.2+8.2 years; p 0.001) (Smith et al., 1996; Xu et al., 1998). Segregation and linkage analysis have shown that early onset of prostate cancer may be inherited in an autosomal-dominant fashion of a rare high-risk allele suggesting that the autosomal-dominant form of prostate cancer accounts for a significant number of early-onset cases (Steinberg et al., 1990), though these cases represent only a small proportion of prostate cancer (Carter et al., 1993). To date, two familial susceptibility loci have been mapped to the X chromosome and to a region of chromosome 1q. About 0.6% of white men inherit a mutated allele of one or more predisposing genes (Gronberg et al., 1996; Ghadirian et al., 1997).

17.4.3 Socio-Economic Conditions

Baquet et al. (1991) at the National Cancer Institute while investigating the incidence of prostate cancer and correlating it with population density, education, and income level in African Americans and whites found it to be higher in former than in the latter group. No statistically significant association was found between socio-economic status and prostate cancer incidence (Baquet et al., 1991). Ernster et al. (1978) using data from Third National Cancer Survey (1969–1971 in Alameda County) also found no association of prostate cancer incidence and socio-economic status in African American and white men. Similar studies by McWhorter et al. (1989) and many others with positive and negative results (Clemmesen & Nielsen, 1951; Buell et al., 1960; Richardson, 1965; Seidman, 1970; Ernster et al., 1977) in general support the view that socio-economic status is not an important risk factor for the development of prostate cancer. No doubt, factors like poverty, lack of education, and health insurance are important causative factors of cancer because they activate risk and affect the prognosis and diagnosis as well as palliative care. Mortality rate has also been found to be higher in developing countries than in developed ones (Ward et al., 2004).

17.4.4 Occupation

One consistent data set from a large body of literature shows that farmers and other agricultural workers have a 7–12% increased risk of cancer (Steinberg et al., 1990; Carter et al., 1990). This may be due to lifestyle factors such as increased intake of meat and fats. It can also be attributed to exposure to chemicals. Though the epidemiologic evidence linking specific pesticide or herbicide exposure to prostate cancer is weak, organochlorines present in these can affect circulating hormone levels. Workers in heavy industry, rubber manufacturing, and newspaper printing may also have higher risk of prostate cancer (Steinberg et al., 1990).

17.4.5 Physical Activity

Overweight and obesity due to lack of physical activity increases the risk of certain cancers. Physical activity and sports play an important role in preventing genitourinary tumors (Sommer et al., 2004). This may be attributed to the fact that physical activity decreases levels of total and free testosterone, reduces obesity, and enhances immune protection (Canon et al., 1982). Physical activity reduces physical role limitation, decreases falls, elevates mood, reduces fatigue, and attenuates losses in bone density promoting weight loss for cancer risk.

17.4.6 Diet

Research in epidemiology and studies on migrants have revealed the influence of diet on prostate cancer risk. Japanese men, who in their native country manifested low incidence of prostate cancer, and had migrated to the United States at younger age started reflecting the prevailing local incidence and mortality rates (Shimizu et al., 1991; Whittemore et al., 1995; Cook et al., 1999). This may have been attributed to higher intake of fat, meat, and dairy products. Studies on whites, African Americans, and Asian Americans have shown association of prostate cancer risk with total fat intake (Giovannucci et al., 1993). A red meat-rich diet has been linked with prostate cancer risk (Veierod et al., 1997). A nonvegetarian diet has been associated with an increased risk of prostate cancer (Sobti et al., 2009).

Dairy products and beef are major sources of dietary branched fatty acids. An enzyme, α-methyl-coenzyme-M-reductase, which plays a key role in the peroxisomal oxidation of these fatty acids, has been found to be up regulated in prostate cancer, but not in normal prostate. Hydrogen peroxide, generated by oxidation process, may be a source of oxidative damage to the prostate genome (Gronberg, 2003). A low-fat, high-fibre diet has been shown to affect male sex hormone metabolism by decreasing circulating testosterone. Altered hormone metabolism plays a role in the progression of prostate cancer from histo-logic to clinically significant forms and it has been observed that the incidence of prostate cancer is very low in eunuchs and castrated men as the growth and differentiation of prostate is under androgenic control (Hill et al.,1979; Wynder et al., 1984).

Soybean products are found to be rich in isoflavones such as genistin and daidzin. It has been suggested that isoflavones inhibit protein tyrosine kinase, which are important for cell proliferation and transform-ation and also for angiogenesis, thus limiting the development and metastasis of prostate tumours (Shirai et al., 2002). This factor may be one of the major reasons for lower incidence of prostate cancer in Japan than in the United States as Japanese people consume a soybean-rich diet. In general, a high-fibre and low-fat diet may protect men against the development of prostate cancer. High calcium intake has also been related to an increased risk of prostate cancer (Rodriguez et al., 2003).

Armstrong and Doll (1975) found that prostate cancer deaths from 32 countries were highly correlated with total fat consumption. Rose et al. (1986) determined this correlation to animal fat and not vegetable fat. Consumption of beans, lentils, pear, tomatoes, raisins, dates, and dried fruits have been reported to decrease risk for prostate cancer significantly (Mills et al., 1989). Increased vitamin A intake has been reported with an increased risk for prostate cancer (Armenian et al., 1974; Graham et al., 1983; Heshmet et al., 1985; Kolonel et al., 1988; Ohno et al., 1988; Mills et al., 1989). Some studies have contradicted these results (Hirayama., 1979; Ohno et al., 1988). Vitamin A found in plants (beta carotene) has been observed to be pro-tective, whereas its intake from animal sources increases the risk (Shekelle et al., 1981; Mettlin et al., 1989).

Slightly reduced risk with regular supplements of vitamin E has also been reported (Heinonen et al., 1998). Polyphenols in green tea act as powerful antioxidants, reducing the risk of prostate cancer. The increased frequency, duration, and quantity of green tea decline prostate cancer risk (Gupta et al., 1999). It has been suggested that a high body mass index (BMI) and bone mass may be associated with prostate cancer. Men with BMI of 35.0 to 39.9 had a 34% greater risk of dying of prostate cancer than those with a normal BMI (Calle et al., 2003). Selenium, an essential trace element found largely in grains, fish, and meat, is protective against prostate cancer (Leitzmann et al., 2003; Klein, 2004). Interestingly, men with diabetes mellitus have been observed to have a lower risk of developing prostate cancer. In a hospital-based case-control study on whites and Hispanics, diabetes was associated with a 40% lower risk of prostate cancer and a 53% lower risk of regional or advanced prostate cancer (Rosenberg et al., 2002a).

17.4.7 Smoking

A number of studies have reported that cigarette smoking may be a risk factor for the development of prostate cancer (Shaarawy and Mahmoud., 1982; Dai et al., 1988; Honda et al., 1988; Fincham et al., 1990; Hsing et al., 1990). Relative risks of 1.8 and 2.1 for cigarette smoking and tobacco chewing, respectively, have been reported by Hsing et al. (1990). Significantly higher risk in prostate cancer cases and in BPH cases has been reported in previous studies (Sobti et al., 2009, 2010; Thakur et al., 2011).

A study has also proposed a higher risk in smokers with an increased exposure to cadmium (Honda et al., 1988). Cadmium is a trace element found in cigarette smoke and alkaline batteries. People working in the welding and electroplating occupations are exposed to high levels of cadmium. However, a case-control study by Fincham et al. (1990) found no link between smoking and prostate cancer. It has also been proposed that cigarette smoking may alter circulating levels of steroid hormones. It is associated with enhanced levels of bio-available testosterone and also lowers estradiol in men. Significant positive association between cigarettes smoked per day and total serum and rostenedione and total and free testosterone in men has been reported (Dai et al., 1988). The overall data for cigarette smoking risk are complicated by conflicting reports on the effect of cigarette smoking on serum sex hormone (Shaarawy et al., 1982; Dai et al., 1988).

17.4.8 Vasectomy

Vasectomized men have higher levels of circulating testosterone, which may have an increased risk for prostate cancer. A large cohort study on 5332 men, each matched with three non-vasectomized comparison controls, showed no increased risk either for prostate cancer or benign prostatic hypertrophy (Giovannucci et al., 1992).

Mettlin et al. (1990) reported a relative risk of 1.7 for reporting a vasectomy at any age and a relative risk of 2.2 for men reporting vasectomy 13 to 18 years before being diagnosed with cancer. Honda et al. (1988) have also reported the same association. Two other larger studies have confirmed this positive trend between the number of years since vasectomy and prostate cancer risk (Giovannucci et al., 1992). Thus, vasectomy appears to confer an increased risk for the development of prostate cancer.

17.4.9 Benign Prostatic Hyperplasia

It is difficult to determine the role of BPH in the risk of prostate cancer. A history of BPH has been reported to carry a relative risk of 13.5% by Mischina et al. (1985) and a relative risk of 5.1 for prostate cancer by Armenian et al. (1974). Not knowing the reasons, the authors of these retrospective and prospective studies have found a higher death rate from prostate cancer in men with a history of benign prostatic hyperplasia (Armenian et al., 1974). However, Greenwald et al. (1974) found no association between BPH and prostate cancer.

17.4.10 Alcohol Consumption

Alcohol affects hormone metabolism disturbing the balance between androgen and estrogen. Repeated high dose of alcohol in non-alcoholic men suppresses testicular production and increases clearance of testosterone. It also increases circulating estrogen levels leading to development of feminine characters (Purohit, 2000).

Alcohol may influence risk of prostate cancer by enhancing the solubility and absorption of mutagens and inhibiting cytochrome P-450 detoxification enzymes. Acetaldehyde, the product of ethanol metabolism, also inhibits enzymes in the DNA methylation pathway.

Dennis (2000) found no association between prostate cancer risk and alcohol consumption. Certain cohort studies have reported a moderately increased risk for prostate and bladder cancers from specific types of alcohol (Sommer et al., 2004).

Antioxidant and anticarcinogenic properties of red wine due to high concentration of polyphenols have been observed to decrease tumor formation. Prostate cancer risk is reduced by 6% by consuming a glass of red wine each week. Schuurman et al. (1999) observed an increased risk with white and fortified, but no association with red wine. A statistically significant rise in relative risk was observed in men consuming 22 or more drinks per week (Hayes, 2000). Direct association was suggested in some studies (Knowles et al., 2000), while inverse association by others (Albertsen and Gronbeck, 2002). Men having 5–6 drinks of alcohol per week showed a moderately higher risk of prostate cancer than those who were non-alcoholics or who drank less than 1 day per week (Sesso et al., 2001).

17.5 Polymorphisms of DNA Repair Genes

Repair mechanisms protect the genome from DNA damage caused by endogenous and environment agents. Polymorphisms and defects in many genes affect the efficiency and accuracy of DNA repair.

Genetic polymorphisms of DNA repair genes have been reported to lead to amino acid substitution in various cancers. The discovery of an increasing number of single nucleotide polymorphisms (SNPs) in perhaps all the genes of an organism highlights the bewildering diversity between individuals and the potential differences in molecular responses of humans to DNA lesions.

Estimates of daily number of DNA lesions in a human cell ranges from 100-500 spontaneous deaminations to 20,000 to 40,000 single-strand breaks (Mullaart et al., 1990). The repair of damage to DNA is essential for the survival of the cell and the health of the organism and over evolutionary periods, the cell has developed a diverse set of defense mechanisms to deal with a wide range of DNA lesions and adducts. Individuals with defects in a mutation repair pathway are often susceptible to spontaneous or induced cancers. The molecular machinery of the repair pathways has slowly been unraveled over the past few decades.

A number of DNA repair pathways are involved in the maintenance of genetic stability. Nucleotide excision repair pathway is the most versatile and important (Sarasin, 2003), especially for DNA damage induced by cigarette smoking. Many diseases are associated with dysfunction of this pathway suggesting it to also be important in the general population. The base excision pathway involves removal of modified bases such as single-strand breaks, non-bulky adducts, oxidative damage, alkylation, or methylation. The oxoguanine glycosidase 1 (*hOGG1*) gene encodes a DNA glycosylase/AP lyase. It suppresses the mutagenic effects of 8-hydroxyguanine by catalyzing its removal from reactive oxygen species. In this regard, Xu et al. (2002) found two sequence variants of this gene and showed an association between these polymorphisms and risk of prostate cancer. Mismatch repair pathway removes unrepaired bases and partially recognizes bulky adducts. Finally recombination pathways are able to remove or bypass bulky lesions allowing the cells to tolerate them (Hoeijmakers, 2001). Abnormal recombination may produce mutations or genetic instability leading eventually to cancer. Susceptibility to cancer is determined by two types of genes: low penetrance and high penetrance genes. Alterations in high penetrance DNA repair genes generally result in inherited disorders such as xeroderma pigmentosum and hereditary non-polyposis colorectal cancer. Genetic polymorphisms are generally found in low-penetrance genes in which the sensitivity is more subtly affected (Shields and Harris, 2000).

17.5.1 Role of Xeroderma Pigmentosum Group D (*XPD*) Gene

The nucleotide excision repair (NER) pathway repairs bulky DNA adducts and includes xeroderma pigmentosum group D (*XPD*) and xeroderma pigmentosum group C (*XPC*) repair genes. NER is especially important as it plays a critical role in repairing DNA damage induced by several suspected human prostate carcinogens, including tobacco-related polycyclic aromatic hydrocarbons (PAHs) and heterocyclic aromatic amines (HAAs) from well done meats and pesticides. Prostate cells can activate PAHs and HAAs.

Khan et al. (2000) and Van Hoffen et al. (2003) explained the basic mechanism of NER in which recognition of DNA lesion is the first step followed by single-strand incision at both sides of the lesion. The lesion containing the single-stranded DNA fragment undergoes excision and the excised nucleotides are replaced by the DNA repair synthesis and ligation of the remaining single-stranded nick. The two NER subpathways, global genome repair (GGR) pathway (which repairs DNA lesions across the genome) and transcription coupled repair (TCR) pathway (which repairs DNA lesions that are specific to the transcribed strand of active genes), differ in damage recognition step. The XPD protein is absolutely necessary in nucleotide excision repair. Once the DNA lesion has been recognized by specific proteins, the helicase activity of XPD, in concerted action with the xeroderma pigmentosum group B helicase, allows the opening of double helix so that the damaged strand can be cut and removed. XPD activity is essential for life; total absence of the *XPD* gene results in embryonic lethality (Friedberg, 2003).

Point mutations in the human XPD protein play a causative role in DNA repair-deficiency diseases (i.e., xeroderma pigmentosum, trichothiodystrophy, and Cockayne syndrome), which are characterized by high ultraviolet-light hypersensitivity, a high mutation frequency, and cancer-proneness, as well as some mental and growth retardation and probably aging (Stary et al., 2002). Most of these mutations are located in the C-terminal part of the protein, which is the domain of interaction, inside the transcription factor IIH complex, with the p44 protein being necessary for activating the helicase activity (Tirode et al., 1999). The very high cancer-proneness of xeroderma pigmentosum patients shows clearly the relevant association between DNA repair efficiency and cancer risk. Because the XPD protein is absolutely necessary for efficient nucleotide excision repair, DNA repair-deficient cells arising from a mutation in the *XPD* gene exhibit low unscheduled DNA synthesis and low survival following ultraviolet irradiation.

Moreover, point mutations that cause diseases and are found in the homozygous state in patients or on only one *XPD* allele in asymptomatic parents, seven polymorphisms in exons 6, 8, 10, 17, 22, and 23 of the *XPD* gene, have been identified by sequencing the DNA of individuals (Broughton et al., 1996; Shen et al., 1998; Mohrenweiser et al., 2002). Three of these polymorphisms are silent, and the remaining four result in amino acid changes. Whereas the codons 199, 201, and 575 polymorphisms are rare (allele frequency ~1%), those in codons 156, 312, 711, and 751 are common (allele frequencies > 25%) (Shen et al., 1998; Mohrenweiser et al., 2002). Following the study by Shen et al. (1998), three *XPD* polymorphisms, *arg*156*arg*, *asp*312*asn*, and *lys*751*gln*, were mainly investigated in genetic epidemiologic studies because of their high frequencies and amino acid substitution variants.

With regard to the *XPDlys*751*gln* polymorphism, the *gln* allele is common in Europe and North America; approximately 50% of the subjects carrying the heterozygous *lys/gln* genotype and 10–15% carrying homozygous *gln/gln* genotype. The *gln* allele was less frequently reported in African Americans, with 5.6% *gln/gln* homozygosity (David-Beabes et al., 2001). This allele is uncommon in China (Liang et al., 2003), South Korea (Park et al., 2002), and Japan (Hamajima et al., 2002) with nearly 90% of the subjects carrying the *lys/lys* genotype, while the *gln/gln* genotype was rarely observed. However, this pattern of genotype frequencies was very different in another Chinese population (Chen et al., 2002), with approximately 18% of subjects carrying the homozygous *gln/gln* genotype. The discrepancy in results may be due to technical errors or ethnic differences in the pattern of mutations.

A large number of SNPs in different DNA repair genes have been identified and some of them have been studied for human cancer susceptibility (Mohrenweiser et al., 2002). However, only a few of them have been evaluated in prostate cancer risk. SNPs in a base excision repair (BER) gene, oxoguanine glycosidase 1 (*hOGG1*), were associated with prostate cancer in both sporadic and familial cases (Sanyal et al., 2004). A genetic variant in another *BER* gene, X-ray cross-complementation group 1 (*XRCC1*) R399G, was associated with elevated prostate cancer risk in individuals with lower vitamin E and lycopene intake (Hu et al., 2005).

To date more than 40 genes and 200 SNPs have been identified in the NER pathway (Rybicki et al., 2004). Rybicki et al. (2004) while evaluating a NER polymorphism and prostate cancer risk demonstrated that combined variant genotypes of *ERCC2/XPD* D312N in NER and *XRCC1* R399G in BER greatly increased the risk of prostate cancer.

17.5.2 Role of Xeroderma Pigmentosum Group C (*XPC*) Gene

The XPC protein, involved in the NER pathway, binds to HR23B to form the XPC-HR23B complex and is thought to be an early damage detector and initiator of NER (Melton et al., 1998). The *XPC* codon 939 polymorphism (*A-C* transition, exon 15) results in a Lys to Gln alteration, which has been found to be associated with an increased risk of bladder and lung (Sanyal et al., 2004; Hu et al., 2005) cancer.

The *XPC* gene product contributes to the global genome repair pathway (GGR). It is a member of the NER pathway and is tightly associated with one of the two human homologues of *Saccharomycescerevisiae* RAD23 protein (HR23B) (Melton et al., 1998). The XPC-HR23B complex has a structure-specific affinity for certain defined lesions, including UV-induced photoproducts, the acetyl amino fluorescence adduct, and artificial cholesterol moieties. There are six core NER factors (XPC HR23B, TF11H, XPA, RPA, XPG, and ERCC 1-XPF). Among these factors, only the XPC-HR23B complex can bind damaged DNA, changing the DNA conformation around the lesion (Melton et al., 1998; Sanyal et al., 2004). Studies have shown that in global genome repair (GGR), damage is initially recognized by the XPC-hHR23B complex in association with the XPA-RPA complex as well as XPE protein (Chavanne et al., 2000; Khan et al., 2000; Gozukara et al., 2001). XPA-RPA may aid in positioning other repair factors and guiding the nucleases to proper incision sites between single-stranded and duplex DNA (Goode et al., 2002). Lesions on the transcribed strand of DNA result in the stalling of RNA polymerase II. Thus XPC-HR23B complex is the DNA damage detector and initiator of the GGR reaction (Melton et al., 1998; Sanyal et al., 2004).

Amongst all identified SNPs of *XPC*, two are commonly studied: *Lys* 939 *Gln* (A33512C, rs2228001) and *Ala* 499 *Val* (c21151T, rs2228000). *XPC-PAT*, a novel variant in intron 9 first reported by Khan et al. (2004), was found to be in linkage disequilibrium with an A to C substitution in exon 15 that gives risk to a Lys to Gln substitution at position 939 and this variant was later investigated for its functional relevance and its association in DNA repair capacity.

The knowledge of mutated *XP660C* gene suggested that normal *XPC* gene is critical for the cells to complete excision repair of bulky DNA lesions (Berneberg and Lehmann, 2001). Several epidemiological studies have been conducted to explore the associations of *XPC* polymorphisms with cancer risk, but results are contradictory (e.g., Vogel et al. (2005) found an increased risk of lung cancer associated with the 939 *Gln* allele in a Danish population).

Sanyal et al. (2004) reported that carriers with C allele had an increased risk of bladder cancer in a Swedish population and Shen et al. (2005) found *XPC* variant 939Gl4 genotype to be associated with a borderline significant risk of lung cancer in a Chinese population. Many mutations in the *XPC* gene were reported by Chavanne et al. (2000). A R579 top variant was found in the *XPC* gene in a xeroderma pigmentosum family in Turkey and Italy (Gozukara et al., 2001). Studies have reported that extracts from XP patients showed delayed repair with a particularly strong decrease in the activity of XPC extracts for all lesions tested.

Hirata et al. (2007) reported an association between the polymorphism of *XRCC1Arg* 399 *Gln* and risk of renal cell carcinoma. Van Gils et al. (2002) found no discernible difference between prostate cancer cases and controls for the *XRCC1* codon 399 variants. However, they found a remarkable risk for the combination of low dietary intake of vitamin E and the *XRCC1* codon 399 *Gln/Gln* genotypes (Van Gils et al., 2002). Rybicki et al. (2004) and Ritchey et al. (2005) also investigated the *XRCC1* codon 399 polymorphism in prostate cancer. Wang et al. (2004) found the *XRCC7* gene polymorphism to be associated with glioma. Hirata et al. (2007) hypothesized that the polymorphisms of DNA repair genes could be risk factors for prostate cancer.

The combined analysis of XPC Lys939Gln and XPC-PAT variants showed that patients who inherited (Lys/Gln + PAT D/D) genotypes were protected against prostate cancer development compared to controls. On the other hand, no significant association has been found between XPC polymorphisms and clinical parameters or between XPC polymorphisms and lifestyle factors (Said et al., 2019).

17.6 Polymorphisms of Metabolic Genes

The GST pi class, most relevant in human cancers, is encoded by a single gene, mapped to chromosome 11q13 (Board et al., 1989; Islam et al., 1989). The GSTP1 protein catalyzes the glutathione conjugation of several anti-cancer agents (Ishikawa et al., 1993; Ishimoto et al., 2002). A random population analysis demonstrated *GSTP1* to be polymorphic at amino acid 105. Polymorphism in *GSTP1* is associated with drug resistance, failures of therapy, and poor patient survival (Oguchi et al., 1994; Yasuno et al., 1999). Because of the functional importance and widespread nature of *GSTP1*, a number of studies have been carried out to investigate the role of polymorphisms in disease susceptibility, particularly in cancer. In gliomas, the nuclear localization of *GSTP1* showing its high expression is considered as a determinant of poor survival (Ali-Osman et al., 1997).

It has been found that mothers with Ala 113 polymorphism of *GSTP1A* had an increased risk of having children born with autistic disorder, suggesting its potential role in neurodevelopment (Williams et al., 2007). A highly significant increase in frequency of *GSTP1b/GSTP1b* genotype was observed in a cohort of bladder cancer patients. An increase in the proportion of individuals homozygous for the low activity of *GSTP1b* allele was observed in a COPD population (Palmer et al., 2006). A highly significant increase in the proportion of individuals homozygous for *GSTP1b* allele was found in teratoma and seminoma cancer samples. The study showed no significant increase in susceptibility associated with *GSTP1b* allele compared to controls in breast and colon cancers. The same study showed marked reduction in frequency of *GSTP1b* homozygotes, and a highly significant reduction in homozygotes for the *GSTP1a* alleles in prostate cancer. The observations indicate that polymorphism at the *GSTP1* locus may be an important factor in susceptibility to different types of cancer.

A meta-analysis on 17 studies with 5281 cases and 7176 controls of colorectal cancer demonstrated that the *GSTP1* polymorphism is unlikely to be a major risk for susceptibility to colorectal cancer (Gao et al., 2009) consistent with a previous meta-analysis of 2005 on four comparisons (Chan et al., 2005). Four allelic variants have been described for the *GSTP1-1* gene (*A, B, C, D*) leading to different amino acid substitutions in position 105 and 114 of the protein sequence. The proteins encoded by different alleles show different abilities to metabolize carcinogens and anticancer agents, suggesting an association between *GSTP1* polymorphism and the risk for a variety of cancers as well as between said polymorphism and varying responses to cancer treatments.

The *ile*105*val* allele has been shown to influence the risk of Barret's oesophagus and oesophageal carcinoma (Van Licshout et al., 1999). The polymorphisms have also been shown to modulate the response to chemotherapy in patients with metastatic colorectal cancer (Stoehlmacher et al., 2002) and multiple myeloma (Dasgupta et al., 2003). The ile105val allele modulates the risk of chemotherapy-related acute myeloid leukemia in patients treated for breast cancer and other cancers (Allan et al., 2001). Latest meta analysis on 30 published case control studies including 15,901 cases and 18,757 controls performed in 2010 suggests that *GSTP1ile/val* polymorphism may increase susceptibility to breast cancer in Asian population (Lu et al., 2011).

Several studies have shown that these *GSTP1* polymorphisms may be linked to susceptibility to inflammatory diseases such as asthma (Palmer et al., 2006), allergies (Gilliland et al., 2004), and systemic sclerosis (Palmer et al., 2003). Variations in GSTs (glutathione S-transferases) have also been associated with liver diseases. Homozygosity for the *GSTP1 Ile*105*val* allele is increased in cystic fibrosis patients with significant liver disease (Henrion-Caude et al., 2002). GST expression is also altered in the liver of patients with alcohol liver disease (ALD) (Harrison et al., 1990). This disease has a degree of inter-individual variation of reactive oxygen species (ROS) and their toxic metabolites due to raised oxidative stress.

Not much work has been done on the association of exon 6 in prostate cancer, however, a few studies in other cancers have been done. Transition of cytosine to thymidine in exon 6 changes *ala*114 to *val* at the protein level. Wang et al. (2003) performed a study of 582 Caucasian lung cancer cases and reported that *GSTP1* exon 6 polymorphism was associated with lung cancer. A study on COPD in Japanese population did not report 114 *val* allele in either group of subjects showing that the allele was not a significant contributor to the development of COPD in the population (Ishii et al., 1999). One of the studies has also reported significantly better survival in patients who had exon 6 variant genotype (*ala/val* or *val/val*) as compared to patients who had the wild-type genotype (*ala/ala*; p=0.037), thus concluding that *GSTP1* exon 6 variant genotypes may be associated with improved survival among patients with stage III and IV non-small cell lung carcinoma, the protective association being found in younger patients (< 62 years) and in males (Lu et al., 2006).

A regression analysis on the number of risk-associated alleles per individual (*GSTM1*active*, *GSTT1*null*, *GSTP1*Val rs1695*, and *GSTP1*Val rs1138272*) showed a significant increase in the risk of developing PC, from 3.65-fold in carriers of two risk alleles (95% CI = 1.55-8.61, $p = 0.003$) to an approximately 12-fold increase in carriers of all four risk alleles (95% CI = 3.05-44.93, $p < 0.001$) (Santric et al., 2020).

17.7 Methylation

Cancer arises through a series of not only genetic, but also epigenetic alterations. Hypermethylation of DNA plays a key role in gene silencing. DNA hypermethylation patterns are frequently altered in human cancers. Changes in methylation pattern have a central role in tumorigenesis, particularly the methylation of CpG islands has been shown to be important in transcriptional repression of numerous genes that function to prevent tumor growth or development. The first tumor suppressor gene found to be silenced through promoter hypermethylation was *Rb1* (Sakai et al., 1991). Almost half of the tumor suppressor genes implicated in familial cancer are known to be inactivated by DNA hypermethylation and it seems that this is as frequent an event as mutations occurring within the coding region of genes. These methylation changes include genome wide-hypomethylation as well as regional hypermethylation (Ehrlich, 2002). Aberrant hypermethylation in cancer cells occurs at CpG islands that are generally protected from methylation in normal tissues. Each tumor has its own characteristic set of genes with an increased propensity to become methylated. Moreover, an individual tumor within a single patient has a unique epigenetic fingerprint that reflects/visualizes the gradual formation (evolution) of tumor as compared to the tumor of the same type in a different patient population. Development of cancer is closely related to DNA methylation and its presence or absence affects its prognosis. Studies have shown several methylated genes to be closely related to the prognosis of cancer. As per one study, p16 promotor methylation was detected in 42% of tumors (Yi et al., 2001). Hence, due to the abovementioned characteristics, CpG methylation provides important information to study changes and can also be an invaluable tool in cancer diagnosis and prognosis.

Mutations in individual genes have outlined critical aspects of tumourigenesis. Global genome screens have provided important information about molecular events occurring in tumourigenesis, but do not provide any universal markers. On the other hand, a single type of DNA alteration (i.e., aberrant methylation of gene promoter) can point to the pathway disrupted in every type of cancer and can provide marker for sensitive detection.

Multiple key cancer genes have been studied to obtain a map of this alteration in malignant transformation. Clusters of CpG sites found dispersed in the genome are called CpG islands, DNA stretches ranging from 0.5 to 5 kb with GC content of at least 50% (Cross and Bird, 1995). Most of these CpG islands are unmethylated in the promoter region as compared to those present in introns and repetitive sequences where they are heavily methylated and inactivated. As methylation occurs early and can be detected in body fluids, it may be of potential use in early detection of tumours and for determining the prognosis. Because DNA methylation is reversible, drugs like 5' azacitidine (Jackson et al., 1997; Villar-Garea et al., 2003), decitabine, and histone deacetylase inhibitors are being used to treat a variety of tumors. Novel demethylating agents such as antisense DNA methyltransferases and small interference RNAs are being developed, making the field of DNA methylation wider and more exciting. Analysis of candidate gene can be seen as only a partial picture of the methylation changes in cancer. Completion of human genomes sequencing and discovery of new techniques to study new genes like methylation-sensitive arbitrarily primed PCR, methylated-CpG island amplification, restriction landmark genomic scanning, and differential methylation hybridization will be extremely useful.

In cancer, CpG island cytosine hypermethylation has been observed in more than 60 genes, including known tumor suppressor genes. The factors underlying CpG island hypermethylation are not known, however, evidence has suggested the existence of a CpG island methylator phenotype (CIMP) involving the silencing and inactivating of multiple genes by promoter hypermethyltion (Shen et al., 2002), possibly through upregulation of DNMTI (Kanai et al., 2001), which is a maintenance methyltransferase (Mtase) and exhibits its effects on hemi-methylated DNA. Colorectal carcinogenesis is frequently characterized by CIMP positivity. Even premalignant adenomas (Rashid et al., 2001) and serrated adenomas (Chan et al., 2002) exhibit CIMP positivity, suggesting this phenotype to be an early event in colon carcinogenesis (Toyota et al., 1999).

Hypermethylation at CpG sites can also predispose to mutations because 5-methyl cytosine (5-MeC) can spontaneously undergo hydrolytic deamination, causing C to T transitions. Increased mutation rates such as those observed at CpG sites in the *p53* gene (Robertson et al., 1997) have been associated with endogenous and exogenous exposures to mutagen. Methylation of *CDH13* by itself or in combination with *ASC* is related to recurrence in patients who have undergone radical prostatectomy. Methylation in CpG dinucleotides in the promoter region of human *RTVP-1* is largely responsible for the downregulation of human RTVP-1 (Ren et al., 2004). In fact, methylation resistance is inversely correlated to the expression of Msh2, the initial mismatch repair factor. O^6-methylguanine-DNA methyltransferase (MGMT) plays a crucial role in the defense against alkylating agents that generate O^6-alkylguanine in DNA, a major trigger of genotoxicity and apoptosis. Therefore, screening the individuals' *MGMT* expression levels in tumors and normal tissue should predict efficacy of methylation-based cancer therapies.

17.7.1 Methylation in GSTP1 Gene

Serum PSA level, digital rectal examination (DRE), and transrectal ultrasonography in combination have increased the ability to detect prostate cancer in its initial stage (Brawer et al., 2000). Thus it accounts for the decreased mortality rate related to prostate cancer (Jemal et al., 2004). However, the limitations of PSA level as a screening tool has limited diagnostic value as its sensitivity and specificity is at the most 75% (Neal and Donovan, 2000). The test is unable to distinguish between malignant and benign lesions accounting for unnecessary biopsies (Catalona et al., 2000).

Similarly the value of DRE and imaging techniques are also limited in early disease detection. Thus none of the procedures above or in conjunction have been able to diagnose prostate cancer. To establish a small set of reliable diagnostic investigation in prostate cancer, effort has been made to quantitatively assess the methylation status of CpG islands in regulating region of *GSTP1* gene.CpG island methylation of *GSTP1* has been detected in several cancer types, including breast and hepatocellular, but only in prostate cancer has this abnormality been constantly detected with a prevalence of more than 90% as quoted in some reviews. This is the most frequent epigenetic alteration reported in prostate cancer and also in high-grade prostate intraepithelial neoplasia (HGPIN), a prostate cancer precursor lesion (Jeronimo et al., 2001; Virmani et al., 2002; Lin et al., 2001a,b; Jeronimo et al., 2002; Brooks et al., 1998). Since induced *GSTP1* expression in prostate cancer cell lines did not suppress cell growth, *GSTP1* is not recognized as a tumor suppressor gene (TSG), it instead was proposed to act as a "caretaker gene" (Nelson et al., 2001). This suggests that prostate cells devoid of *GSTP1* expression are more susceptible to endure DNA damage induced by oxidants and electrophiles whether originated endogenously or from dietary intake (Nelson et al., 2001). CpG island methylation of *GSTP1* is an attractive biomarker for prostate cancer screening for several reasons. First, that *GSTP1* promoter methylation is rarely found in non-cancerous prostatic tissue, potentially giving the test a high specificity. Secondly, *GSTP1* hypermethylation is considerably less frequent in other genitourinary malignancies as bladder and renal cancer (Esteller et al., 1998; Maruyama et al.,2001; Chan et al., 2002), although it has been identified in many breast and liver carcinomas (Tchou et al., 2000; Estellar et al., 2001).

Goessl et al. (2000) using a non-quantitative fluorogenic MSP assay detected *GSTP1* hypermethylation in 72% of plasma samples, 50% of ejaculates, and 36% of voided urine samples from prostate cancer patients with BPH. Not only limited to body fluids, the role of *GSTP1* hypermethylation is now firmly established for tissue samples also. The alteration has subsequently been reported in non-cancerous prostate tissue (Brooks et al., 1998). A study on frozen tissue samples of 69 patients with clinically localized prostate cancer, 28 with paired HGPIN lesions, and 31 patients with BPH screened for *GSTP1* methylation using quantitative assay revealed methylation in 29% of BPH tissue samples and 91.3% of prostate cancer tissue samples (Jeronimo et al., 2001). Maruyama and coworkers (2002) reported *GSTP1* methylation frequency of 36% in prostate carcinoma, whereas Yamanaka et al. (2003) reported a methylation frequency of 88% for the same gene. The latter value being in range with the reports by previous researchers (Lee et al., 1994; Brooks et al., 1998; Jeronimo et al., 2001; Lin et al., 2001; Jeronimo et al., 2002; Harden et al., 2003; Woodson et al., 2003). The discrepant results may be attributed to different methodologies and also to population differences.

All studies reported a consistent link between *GSTP1* methylation and prostate cancer. Detection of this methylation marker in urine or serum samples can be a valuable screening tool and its analysis might increase the accuracy of diagnosis of the malignancy in prostate biopsies. It can also help stratify patients with initial morphologically negative biopsies into high- and low-risk groups, thus improving patient care and reducing follow-up cost. Although the strength of the association has varied in tissues samples, it has been detected in 70 to 90% with sample numbers varying from 8 to 105 patients.

17.8 Conclusions

In the past several decades, epidemiological and screening studies have shown concerns about the pathogenesis of prostate cancer, but definitive causes have not been established. A number of genetic and environmental factors is known to influence individual susceptibility towards the formation of prostatic tumors. Unlike genetics, epigenetic mechanisms such as DNA methylation confer different functional status to the same genes under different environmental conditions. Knowledge of such gene-environment interaction may lead to established biomarkers that will perform better than the standards of PSA, Gleason score, and TNM (tumour, node, metastasis) staging. The present chapter was an endeavor to unravel the polymorphic genes implicated in the etiology of prostate cancer and the prevalence of aberrant promoter methylation in GSTP gene along with their environment interactions.

REFERENCES

Albertsen K, Grønbaek M (2002). Does amount or type of alcohol influence the risk of prostate cancer? *Prostate* 52:297–304.

Ali-Osman F, Brunner JM, Kutluk TM, Hess K (1997). Prognostic significance of glutathione-S-transferase pi expression and subcellular localization in human gliomas. *Clin Cancer Res* 3:2253–2261.

Allan JM et al. (2001). Polymorphism in glutathione-S-transferase Pi is associated with susceptibility to chemotherapy induced leukemia. *Proc Natl Sci USA* 98:11592–11597.

American Cancer Society (2003). *Cancer Facts and Figures*. Atlanta G.A.: American Cancer Society.

Armenian HK, Lilienfeid AM, Diamond EL, Bross ID (1974). Relation between benign prostatic hyperplasia and cancer of prostate. *Lancet* 115:7.

Armstrong B, Doll R (1975). Environment factors and cancer incidence and mortality in different countries with special reference to dietary practices. *Int J Cancer* 15:617–631.

Banez LL, Srivastava S, Moul JW (2005). Proteomics in prostate cancer. *CurrOpinUrol* 15:151.

Baquet CR, Horm JW, Gibbe T, Greenwald P (1991). Socioeconomic factors and cancer incidence among blacks and whites. *J Natl Cancer Inst* 83:551–557.

Batson OV (1940). The function of the vertebral veins and their role in the spread of metastases. *Ann Surg* 112:138–149.

Berneberg M, Lehmann AR (2001). Xeroderma pigmentosum and related disorders: Defects in DNA repair and transcription. *Adv Genet* 43:71–102.

Board PG, Webb GC, Coggan M (1989). Isolation of a DNA clone and localization of the human glutathione-S-transferase 3 genes to chromosome bonds 11q13 and 12q13-14. *Ann Hum Genet* 53:205–213.

Brawer MK (2000). Screening for prostate cancer. *Semin Surg Oncol* 18:29–36.

Brooks JD, Weinstein M, Lin X, Su Y, Pin SS, Bova GS (1998). CG island methylation changes near the GSTP1 gene in prostatic intraepithelial neoplasia. *Cancer Epidemiol Biomarkers Prev* 7:531–536.

Broughton BC, Steingrimsdottir H, Lehmann AR (1996). Five polymorphisms in the coding sequence of the xeroderma pigmentosum group D gene. *Mutat Res* 362:209–211.

Buell P, Dunn JE, Breslow L (1960). The occupational-social class risks of cancer mortality in men. *J Choronic Dis* 12:600–621.

Calle EE, Rodriguez C, Walker-Thurmond K, Thun MJ (2003). Overweight, obesity, and mortality from cancer in a prospectively studied cohort of U.S. adults. *N Engl J Med* 348:1625–1638.

Canon I, Bishop DT, Skolnick M, Hunt S, Lyon JL, Smart CR (1982). Genetic epidemiology of prostate cancer in the Utah mormon genealogy. *Cancer Surv* 1:47–69.

Carter BS, Beaty TH, Steinberg GD, Childs B, Walsh PC (1992). Mendelian inheritance of familial prostate cancer. *Proc Natl Acad Sci USA* 89:3367–3371.

Carter BS, Bova GS, Beaty TH, Steinberg GD, Childs B, Isaacs WB, Walsh PC (1993). Hereditary prostate cancer: epidemiologic and clinical features. *J Urol* 150:797–802.

Carter BS, Carter HB, Isaacs JT (1990). Epidemiologic evidence regarding predisposing factor to prostate cancer. *Prostate* 16:187–197.

Catalona WJ, Southwick PC, Slawin KM, Partin AW Brawer MK, Flanigan RC (2000). Comparison of percent free PSM, PSA density and age-specific PSA cutoffs for prostate cancer detection and staging. *Urology* 56:255–260.

Ceber E, Cakir D, Ogce F, Simsir A, Cal C, Ozentürk G (2008). Why do men refuse prostate cancer screening? Demographic analysis in Turkey. *Asian Pac J Cancer Prev* 9:387–390.

Chan K, Jiang ZT, He HQ (2005). Relationship between metabolic enzyme polymorphism and colorectal cancer. *World J Gastroenterol* 11:331–335.

Chan MW, Chan LW, Tang NL, Tong JH, Lo KW, Lee TL (2002). Hypermethylation of multiple genes in tumor tissue and voided urine in urinary bladder cancer patients. *Clin Cancer Res* 8:464–470.

Chavanne F, Broughton BC, Pietra D, Narde T, Browitt A, Lehmann A, Stefanini M (2000). Mutation in the XPC gene in families with xeroderma pigmentosum and consequences at the cell, protein and transcript levels. *Cancer Res* 60:1974–1982.

Chen S, Tang D, Xue K, Xu L, Ma G, Hsu Y, Cho SS (2002). DNA repair gene XRCC1 and XPD polymorphisms and risk of lung cancer in a Chinese population. *Carcinogenesis* 23:1321–1325.

Clemmesen J, Neilsen A (1951). The social distribution of cancer in Copenhagen, 1943-1947. *Br J Cancer* 5:159–171.

Cohen P, Graves H, Peehl D, Kamarei M, Guidice L, Rosenfeld R (1992). Prostate specific antigen (PSA) is an insulin like growth factor binding protein-3-protease found in seminal plasma. *J Clin Endo Met* 75:1046–1053.

Cook LS, Goldoft M, Schwartz SM, Weiss NS (1999). Incidence of adenocarcinoma of the prostate in Asian immigrants to the United States and their descendants. *J Urol* 161:152–155.

Crawford, ED (2003). Epidemiology of prostate cancer. Urology 62(6 suppl 1):3–12.

Cross SH, Bird AP (1995). CpG islands and genes. *CurrOpin Genet Dev* 5:309–314.

Dai WS, Gutai JP, Kuller LH, Cauley JA (1988). Cigarette smoking and serum sex-hormones in men. *Am J Epidemiol* 128:796–805.

Dasgupta RK et al. (2003). Polymorphic variations in GSTP1 modulates outcome following therapy of multiple myeloma. *Blood* 102:2345–2350.

David-Beabes GL, Lunn RM, London SJ (2001). No association between the XPD (Lys751Gln) polymorphism or the XRCC3 (Thr241Met) polymorphism and lung cancer risk. *Cancer Epidemiol Biomarkers Prev* 10:911–912.

Dennis LK (2000). Meta-analysis for combining relative risks of alcohol consumption and prostate cancer. *Prostate* 42:56–66.

Doboxy JR, Roberts JL, Fuvx W, Jarrard DF (2007). The expanding role of epigenetic in the development diagnosis and treatment of prostate cancer and benign prostatic hyperplasia. *J Urol* 177:822–831.

Dunn JE (1975). Cancer Epidemiology in populations of the United States. *Cancer Res* 35:3240–3245.

Ehrlich M (2002). DNA methylation in cancer: too much, but also too little. *Oncogene* 21:5400–5413.

Ernster VL, Selvin S, Sacks ST, Austin DF, Brown SM, Winkelstein W Jr (1978). Prostatic cancer: Mortality and incidence rates by race and social class. *Am J Epidemiol* 107:311–320.

Ernster VL, Winkelstein W Jr, Selvia S, Brown SM, Sacks ST, Austin DF (1977). Race, socioeconomic status and prostate cancer. *Cancer Treat Rep* 61:187–191.

Esteller M, Corn PG, Baylin SB, Herman JG (2001). A gene hypermethylation profile of human cancer. *Cancer Res* 61:3225–3229.

Esteller M, Corn PG, Urena JM, Gabrielson E, Baylin SB, Herman JG (1998). Inactivation of glutathione S-transferase P1 gene by promoter hypermethylation in human neoplasia. *Cancer Res* 58:4515–4518.

Fergusson JD, Gibson EC (1956). Prostatic smear diagnosis. *Br Med J* 1:822–825.

Ferlay J, Autier P, Boniol M, Heanue M, Colombet M, Boyle P (2007). Estimates of the cancer incidence and mortality in Europe in 2006. *Ann Oncol* 18:581–592.

Fincham SM, Hill GB, Hanson J, Wijayasinghe C (1990). Epidemiology of prostate cancer: A case control study. *Prostate* 17:189–206.

Flanders WD (1984). Review Prostate Cancer Epidemiology. *Prostate* 5:621–629.

Franks LM (1954). Atrophy and hyperplasia in the prostate proper. *J PatholBacteriol* 68:617–621.

Franks LM (1953). The spread of prostatic carcinoma to the bones. *J PatholBacteriol* 66:91–93.

Friedberg EC (2003). DNA damage and repair. *Nature* 421:436–440.

Gao Y, Pan X, Su T, Mo Z, Cao Y, Gao F (2009). Glutathione-S-transferase P1 Ile105Val polymorphisms and colorectal cancer risk: A meta analysis and HuGE review. *Europeon J Cancer* 45:3303–3314.

Ghadirian P, Howe GR, Hislop TG, Maisonneuve P (1997). Family history of prostate cancer: A multi-center case-control study in Canada. *Int J Cancer* 70:679–681.

Gilliland FD, Li YF, Saxon A, Diaz-Sanchez D (2004). Effect of glutathione-S-transferase M1 and P1 genotypes on xenobiotics enhancement of allergic responses: Randomized, placebo-controlled crossover study. *Lancet* 363:119–125.

Giovannucci E, Ascherio A, Rimm EB, Colditz GA, Stamfer MJ, Willet WC (1992). A prospective cohort study of vasectomy and prostate cancer in US men. *JAMA* 269:873–877.

Giovannucci E, Rimm EB, Colditz GA (1993). A prospective study of dietary fat and risk of prostate cancer. *J Natl Cancer Inst* 85:1571–1579.

Goessl C, Krause H, Muller M, Heicappell R, Schrader M, Sachsinger J (2000). Flourescent methylation specific polymerase chain reaction for DNA based detection of prostate cancer in body fluids. *Cancer Res* 60:5941–5945.

Golub TR et al. (1999). Molecular classification of cancer: Class discovery and class prediction by gene expression monitoring. *Science* 286:531–537.

Goode EL, Ulrich CM, Potter JD (2002). Polymorphisms in DNA repair genes and associations with cancer risk. *Cancer Epidemiol Biomarkers Prev* 11:1513–1530.

Gozukara EM et al. (2001). A stop codon in xeroderma pigmentosum group C families in Turkey and Italy: Molecular genetic evidence for a common ancestor. *J Invest Dermatol* 117:197–204.

Graham S, Haughey B, Marshall J, Priore R, Byers T, Rzepka T, Mettlin C, Pontes JE (1983). Diet in the epidemiology of carcinoma of the prostate gland. *J Natl Cancer Inst* 70:687–692.

Greenwald P, Kirmiss V, Polan AK, Diek VS (1974). Cancer of the prostate among men with benign prostate hyperplasia. *J Natl Cancer Inst* 53:335–340.

Grönberg H, Damber L, Damber JE (1996). Familial prostate cancer in Sweden. A nationwide register cohort study. *Cancer* 77:138–143.

Grönberg H (2003). Prostate cancer epidemiology. *Lancet* 361:859–864.

Gupta S, Ahmad N, Mukhtar H (1999). Prostate cancer chemoprevention by green tea. *Semin Urol Oncol* 17:70–76.

Haas GP, Sakr WA (1997). Epidemiology of prostate cancer. *CA Cancer J Clin* 47:273–278.

Habuchi T, Liging Z, Suzuki T (2000). Increased risk of prostate cancer and benign prostatic hyperplasia associated with a CYP17 gene polymorphism with a gene dosage effect. *Cancer Res* 60:5710–5713.

Haenszel W, Kirihoro M (1968). Studies of Japanese migrants *J Natl Cancer Inst* 40:43–68.

Hamajima N, Saito T, Matsuo K, Suzuki T, Nakamura T, Matsuura A, Okuma K, Tajima K (2002). Genotype frequencies of 50 polymorphisms for 241 Japanese non-cancer patients. *J Epidemiol* 12:229–236.

Hankey BA, Miller B, Clegg L, Edwards BK (1990). SEER cancer statistics review-PC: Family history and the risk of prostate cancer. *Prostate* 17:337–347.

Harden SV, Sanderson H, Goodman SN, Partin AA, Walsh PC, Epstein JL (2003). Quantitative GSTP1 methylation and the detection of prostate adenocarcinoma in sextant biopsies. *J Natl Cancer Inst* 95:1634–1637.

Harrison DJ, May L, Hayer C, Haque MM, Heyes JD (1990). Glutathione-S-transferase in alcoholic liver disease. *Grid* 31:909–912.

Hayes JD, Strange RC (2000). Glutathione-S-transferase polymorphisms and their biological consequences. *Pharmacology* 61:154–166.

Heinonen OP et al. (1998). Prostate cancer and supplementation with alpha-tocopherol and beta-carotene: incidence and mortality in a controlled trial. *J Natl Cancer Inst* 90:440–446.

Henrion-Caude A, Flamant C, Roussey M, Housset C, Flahault A, Fryer AA, Chadelat K, Strange RC, Clement A (2002). Liver disease in pediatric patients with cystic fibrosis is associated with glutathione S-transferase P1 polymorphism. *Hepatology* 36:913–917.

Heshmat MY, Kaul L, Kavi J, Jackson MP, Jackson AG, Jones GW (1985). Nutrition and prostate cancer: A case control study. *Prostate* 6:7–17.

Hill P, Wynder EL, Garbaczewski L, Garnes H, Walker ARP (1979). Diet and urinary steroids in black and white North American men and black South African men. *Cancer Res* 39:5101–5105.

Hirata H et al. (2007). Polymorphisms of DNA repair genes are risk factors for prostate cancer. *Eur J Cancer* 43:231–237.

Hirayama T (1979). Epidemiology of prostate cancer with special reference to the role of diet. *Natl Cancer Inst Monogr* 53:149–155.

Hoeijmakers JH (2001). Genome maintenance mechanisms for preventing cancer. *Nature* 411:366–374.

Honda GD, Bernstein L, Ross RK, Greenland S, Gerkins V, Henderson BE (1988). Vasectomy, cigarette smoking, and age at first sexual intercourse as risk factors for prostate cancer in middle aged men. *Br J Cancer* 57:326–331.

Hsing AW, McLaughlin JK, Schuman LM, Bjelke E, Gridley G, Wacholder S (1990). Diet, tobacco use and fatal prostate cancer: Results from the Lutheran brotherhood cohort study. *Cancer Res* 50:6836–6840.

Hu X, Chen X, Ping H, Chen Z, Zeng F, Lu G (2005). Immunohistochemical analysis of Omi/HtrA2 expression in prostate cancer and benign prostatic hyperplasia. *J Huazhong Univ Sci Tech Med Sci* 25:671–673.

Ishii T, Matsuse T, Teramoto S, Matsui H, Miyao M, Hosoi T, Takahashi H, Fukuchi Y, Ouchi Y (1999). Glutathione-S-transferase P1 (GSTP1) polymorphism in patients with chronic obstructive pulmonary disease. *Thorax* 54:693–696.

Ishikawa T, Ali-Osman F (1993). Glutathione associated cis-diaminedichloroblatinum II metabolism and ATP-dependent efflux from leukemia cells. Molecular characterization of glutathione-platinum complex and its biological significance. *J Biol Chem* 268:20116–20125.

Ishimoto TM, Ali-Osman F (2002). Allelic variants of human glutathione-S-transferase Pi gene confer differential cytoprotection against anticancer agents in *Escherichia coli. Pharmacogenetics* 12:543–553.

Islam MQ, Platz A, Szpirer J, Szpirer C, Levan G, Mannervik B (1989). Chromosomal localization of human Glutathione transferase genes of classes alpha, mu and pi. *Hum Genet* 82:338–342.

Jackson-Grusby L, Laird PW, Magge SN, Moeller BJ, Jaenisch R (1997). Multigenecity of 5-aza-2'-deoxycitidine is mediated by the mammalian DNA methyltransferase. *Proc NatlAcadSci USA* 94:4681–4685.

Jemal A, Siegel R, Ward E, Murray T, Xu J, Thun MJ (2007). Cancer statistics, 2007. CA *Cancer J Clin* 57:43–66.

Jemal A, Tiwani RC, Murray T, Ghafoor A, Samuels A, Ward E (2004). Cancer Statistics, 2004. CA. *Cancer J Clin* 54:8–29.

Jerónimo C, Usadel H, Henrique R, Oliveira J, Lopes C, Nelson WG, Sidransky D (2001). Quantitation of GSTP1 methylation in non-neoplastic prostatic tissue and organ-confined prostate adenocarcinoma. *J Natl Cancer Inst* 93:1747–1752.

Jerónimo C, Usadel H, Henrique R, Silva C, Oliveira J, Lopes C, Sidransky D (2002). Quantitative GSTP1 hypermethylation in bodily fluids of patients with prostate cancer. *Urology* 60:1131–1135.

Jung KW, Park S, Kong HJ, Won YJ, Boo YK, Shin HR, Park EC, Lee JS (2010). Cancer statistics inKorea: incidence, mortality and survival in 2006-2007. *J Korean Med Sci* 25:1113–1121.

Kanai Y, Ushijima S, Kondo Y, Nakanishi Y, Hirohashi S (2001). DNA methyltransferase expression and DNA methylation of CPG islands and peri-centromeric satellite regions in human colorectal and stomach cancers. *Int J Cancer* 91:205–212.

Khan SG, Metter EJ, Tarone RE, Bohr VA, Grossman L, Hedayati M, Bale SJ, Emmert S, Kraemer KH (2000). A new xeroderma pigmentosum group C poly (AT) insertion/deletion polymorphism. *Carcinogenesis* 21:1821–1825.

Klein EA (2004). Selenium: Epidemiology and basic science. *J Urol* 171:s50–s53, discussion s53.

Knowles LM, Zigrossi DA, Tauber RA, Hightower C, Milner JA (2000). Flavonoids suppress androgen-independent human prostate tumor proliferation. *Nutr Cancer* 38:116–122.

Kolonel LN, Yoshizama CN, Hankin JH (1988). Diet and prostatic cancer: A case control study in Hawai. *Am J Epidemiol* 127:999.

Krain LS (1974). Some epidemiologic variables in prostatic carcinoma in California. *Prev Med* 3:154–159.

Laxman B et al. (2006).Noninvasive detection of TMPRSS2:ERG fusion transcripts in the urine of men with prostate cancer. *Neoplasia* 8:885–888.

Lee WH, Marton RA, Epstein JI, Brooks JD, Campbell PA, Bova GS (1994). Cytidine methylation of regulatory sequences near the pi-class glutathione-S-transferase gene accompanies human prostatic carcinogenesis. *Proc Natl Acad Sci USA* 91:11733–11737.

Leitzmann ME, Stampfer MJ, Wu K, Coliditz GA, Willett WC, Giovannucci EL (2003). Zinc supplement use and risk of prostate cancer. *J Natl Cancer Inst* 95:1004–1007.

Leushner J (2001). MALDI TOF mass spectrometry: an emerging platform for genomics and diagnostics. *Expert Rev Mol Diagn* 1:11.

Liang G, Xing D, Niao X, Tan W, Yu C, Lu W, Lin D (2003). Sequence variations in the DNA repair gene XPD and risk of lung cancer in a Chinese population. *Int J Cancer* 105:669–673.

Lin X et al. (2001a). Reversal of GSTP1 CpG island hypermethylation and reactivation of pi-class glutathione-S-transferase (GSTP1) expression in human prostate cancer cells by treatment with procainamide. *Cancer Res* 61:8611–8616.

Lin X, Tascilar M, Lee WH, Vles WJ, Lee BH, Veeraswamy R (2001b). GSTP1 CpG island hypermethylation is responsible for the absence of GSTPI expression in human prostate cancer cells. *Am J Pathol* 159:1815–1826.

Lou W, Krill D, Dhir R, Becich MJ, Dong JT, Frierson HF Jr, Isaacs WB, Isaacs JT, Gao AC (1999). Methylation of the CD44 metastasis suppressor gene in human prostate cancer. *Cancer Res* 59:2329–2331.

Lu C, Spitz MR, Zhao H, Dong Q, Truong M, Chang JY, Blumenschein GR Jr, Hong WK, Wu X (2006). Association between glutathione S-transferase pi polymorphisms and survival in patients with advanced nonsmall cell lung carcinoma. *Cancer* 106:441–447.

Lu S, Wang Z, Cui D, Liu H, Hao X (2011). Glutathione S-transferase P1 Ile105Val polymorphism and breast cancer risk: a meta-analysis involving 34,658 subjects. *Breast Cancer Res Treat* 125:253–259.

Maclennan GT et al. (2006). The influence of chronic inflammation in prostatic carcinogenesis: A 5 year follow up study. *I Uro* 176:1012–1016.

Manoharan N, Tyagi BB, Raina V (2009). Cancer incidences in urban Delhi – 2001-05. *Asian Pac J Cancer Prev* 10:799–806.

Maruyama R et al. (2001). Aberrant promoter methylation profile of bladder cancer and its relationship to clinicopathological features. *Cancer Res* 61:8659–8663.

Maruyama R et al. (2002). Aberrant promoter methylation profile of prostate cancers and its relationship to clinicopathological features. *Clin Cancer Res* 8:514–519.

Mcwhorter WP, Schatzkin AG, Horn JW, Brown CC (1989). Contribution of socioeconomic status to black/white difference in cancer incidence. *Cancer* 63:982–987.

Meikle AW, Smith JA Jr (1990). Epidemiology of prostate cancer. *Urol Clin North Am* 17:709–718.

Meikle AW, Stanish WM (1982). Familial prostatic cancer risk and low testosterone. *J Clin EndocrinMetab* 54: 1104–1108.

Meitz JC et al. (2002). Cancer Research UK/BPG UK Familial Prostate Cancer Study Collaborators. HPC2/ELAC2 polymorphisms and prostate cancer risk: Analysis by age of onset of disease. *Br J Cancer* 87:905–908.

Melton DW, Ketchen AM, Núñez F, Bonatti-Abbondandolo S, Abbondandolo A, Squires S, Johnson RT (1998). Cells from ERCC1-deficient mice show increased genome instability and a reduced frequency of S-phase-dependent illegitimate chromosome exchange but a normal frequency of homologous recombination. *J Cell Sci* 111:395–404.

Mettlin C, Selenskas S, Natarajan N, Hubeu R (1989). Beta carotene and animal fats and their relationship to prostate cancer risk: A case-control study. *Cancer* 64:605–612.

Mettlin C, Natarajan N, Huben R (1990). Vasectomy and prostate cancer risk. *Am. J. Epidemiol.* 132:1056–1061

Mettlin C (2000). Impact of screening on prostate cancer rates and trends. *Microsc Res Tech* 51:415–418.

Miller EB, Ladaga LE, el-Mahdi AM, Schellhammer PF (1993). Reevaluation of prostatic biopsy after definitive radiation therapy. *Urology* 41:311–316.

Mills PK, Beeson WL, Phillips RL, Fraser GE (1989). Cohort study of diet, lifestyle, and prostate cancer in Adventist men. *Cancer* 64:598–604.

Mischina T, Watanabe H, Araki H, Nakao M (1985). Epidemiological study of Prostate cancer by matched pair analysis. *Prostate* 6:423–446.

Mohrenweiser HW, Xi T, Vázquez-Matías J, Jones IM (2002). Identification of 127 amino acid substitution variants in screening 37 DNA repair genes in humans. *Cancer Epidemiol Biomarkers Prev* 11:1054–1064.

Muir CS, Nectous J, Staszewski J (1991). The epidemiology of prostate cancer. Geographical distribution and time trends. *Acta Oncol* 30:133–140.

Mullaart E, Lohman PH, Berends F, Vijg J (1990). DNA damage metabolism and ageing. *Mutat Res* 237:189–210.

Namiki M et al. (2010). Prostate Cancer Working Group report. *Jpn J Clin Oncol* 40:i70–75.

Neal DE, Donovan JL (2000). Prostate cancer: To screen or not to screen? *Lancet Oncol* 1:17–24.

Nelson CP, Kidd LC, Sauvageot J, Isaacs WB, De Marzo AM, Groopman JD, Nelson WG, Kensler TW (2001). Protection against 2-hydroxyamino-1-methyl-6-phenylimidazo (4,5-b) pyridine cytotoxicity and DNA adduct formation in human prostate by glutathione s-transferase P1. *Cancer Res* 61:103–109.

Nelson JB, Lee WH, Nguyen SH, Jarrard DF, Brooks JD, Magnuson SR, Opgenorth TJ, Nelson WG, Bova GS (1997). Methylation of the 5' CpG island of the endothelin B receptor gene is common in human prostate cancer. *Cancer Res* 57:35–37.

Oguchi H. Kikkawa F, Kajima M., Maeda O, Mizuno K, Suganuma N, Kawai M, Tomoda Y (1994). Glutathione related enzymes in cis-diamminedichloroplatinum(II) sensitive and resistant human ovarian carcinoma cells. *Anticancer Res* 14:193–200.

Ohno Y, Yashida O, Oishi K, Okada K, Yamabe H, Schroeder FH (1988). Dietary beta carotene and cancer of the prostate: A case control study in Kyoto, Japan. *Cancer Res* 48:1331–1336.

Pal SK, Mittal B (2004). Fight against cancer in countries with limited resources: the post-genomic era scenario. *Asian Pac J Cancer Prev* 5:328–333.

Palmer CN, Doney AS, Lee SP, Murrie I, Ismail T, Macgregor DF, Mukhopadhyay S (2006). Glutathione-S-transferase M1 and P1 genotype, passive smoking, and peak expiratory flow in asthma. *Pediatrics* 118:710–716.

Palmer CN, Young V, Ho M, Doney A, Belch JJ (2003). Association of common variations in glutathione s-transferase genes with premature development of cardiovascular disease in patients with systemic sclerosis. *Arthritis Rheum* 48:854–855.

Park JY et al. (2002). Lys 751 Gln polymorphism in the DNA repair gene XPD and risk of primary lung cancer. *Lung Cancer* 36:15–16.

Perner S et al. (2007). TMPRSS2-ERG fusion prostate cancer: an early molecular event associated with invasion. *Am J SurgPathol* 31:882–888.

Petricoin EF 3rd et al. (2002). Serum proteomic patterns for detection of prostate cancer. *J Natl Cancer Inst* 94:1576–1578.

Pu YS, Chiang HS, Lin CC, Huang CY, Huang KH, Chen J (2004). Changing trends of prostate cancer in Asia. *Aging Male* 7:120–132.

Purohit V (2000). Can alcohol promote aromatization of androgens to estrogens? A review. *Alcohol* 22:123–127.

Rashid A, Shen L, Morris JS, Issa JP, Hamilton SR (2001). CpG island methylation in colorectal adenomas. *Am J Pathol* 159:1129–1135.

Rastogi T, Hildesheim A, Sinha R (2004). Opportunities for cancer epidemiology in developing countries. *Nat Rev Cancer* 4:909–917.

Reddy S, Shapiro M, Morton R Jr, Brawley OW (2003). Prostate cancer in black and white Americans. *Cancer Metastasis Rev* 22:83–86.

Ren C et al. (2004). RTVP-1, a Tumor Suppressor Inactivated by Methylation in Prostate Cancer. *Cancer Research* 64:969–976.

Richardson IM (1965). Prostatic cancer and social class. *Br J Prev Soc Med* 19:140–142.

Ritchey JD, Huang WY, Chokkalingam AP, Gao YT, Deng J, Levine P, Stanczyk FZ, Hsing AW (2005). Genetic variants of DNA repair genes and prostate cancer: a population-based study. *Cancer Epidemiol Biomarkers Prev* 14:1703–1709.

Robertson KD, Jones PA (1997). Dynamic interrelationships between DNA replication, methylation, and repair.*Am J Hum Genet* 61:1220–1224.

Rodriguez C, McCullough ML, Mondul AM, Jacobs EJ, Fakhrabadi-Shokoohi D, Giovannucci EL, Thun MJ, Calle EE (2003). Calcium, dairy products and risk of prostate cancer in a prospective cohort of United States men. *Cancer Epidemiol Biomarkers Prev* 12:597–603.

Rose DP, Boyar AP, Wynder EL (1986). International comparisons of mortality rates for cancer of the breast, ovary, prostate and colon, and per capita food consumption. *Cancer* 58:2363–2371.

Rosenberg DJ, Neugut AI, Ahsan H, Shea S (2002a). Diabetes mellitus and the risk of prostate cancer. *Cancer Invest* 20:157–165.

Rybicki BA, Conti DV, Moreira A, Cicek M, Casey G, Witte JS (2004). DNA repair gene XRCC1 and XPD polymorphisms and risk of prostate cancer. *Cancer Epidemiol Biomarkers Prev* 13:23–29.

Said R, Bougatef K, SettiBoubaker N, Jenni R, Derouiche A, Chebil M, Ouerhani S (2019). Polymorphisms in XPC gene and risk for prostate cancer. *Mol Biol Rep* 46:1117–1125.

Sakai T, Toguchida J, Ohtani N, Yandell DW, Rapaport JM, Dryja TP (1991). Allele-specific hypermethylation of the retinoblastoma tumor-suppressor gene. *Am J Hum Genet* 48:880–888.

Salam MT, Ursin G, Skinner EC, Dessiss T, Rcichard JK (2005). Associations between polymorphisms in the steroid 5-X reductase type 11 (SRD5A2) gene and benign prostaic hyperplasia and prostate cancer. *Urol Oncol* 23:246–253.

Santric V et al. (2020). *GSTP1* rs1138272 Polymorphism Affects Prostate Cancer Risk. *Medicina* 56:128.

Sanyal S et al. (2004). Polymorphisms in DNA repair and metabolic genes in bladder cancer. *Carcinogenesis* 25:729–734.

Sarasin A (2003). An overview of the mechanisms of mutagenesis and carcinogenesis. *Mutat Res* 544:99–106.

Sasaki M, Tanaka Y, Perinchery G, Dharia A, Kotcherguina I, Fujimoto S, Dahiya R (2002). Methylation and inactivation of estrogen, progesterone, and androgen receptors in prostate cancer. *J Natl Cancer Inst* 94:384–390.

Schumann L, Mandel M, Blackard C, Bauer H, Scarlett J, Mchugh R (1977). Epidemiologic study of Prostate Cancer: A preliminary report. *Cancer Treat Rep* 61:181–186.

Schuurman AG, Goldbohm RA, Van den Brandt PA (1999). A prospective cohort study on consumption of alcoholic beverages in relation to prostate cancer incidence (The Netherlands). *Cancer Causes Control* 10:597–605.

Seidman H (1970). Cancer death rates by site and sex for religious and socioeconomic groups in New York City. *Environ Res* 3:234–250.

Sesso HD, Paffenbarger RS Jr, Lee IM (2001). Alcohol consumption and risk of prostate cancer: The Harvard Alumni Health Study. *Int J Epidemiol* 30:749–755.

Shaarawy M, Mahmoud KZ (1982). Endocrine profile and semen characteristics in male smokers. *FertilSteril*38:255–257.

Shekelle RB, Lepper M, Lin S, Maliza C, Raynor WJ Jr, Rossof AH (1981). Dietary vitamin A and risk of cancer in the western electric study. *Lancet* 2:1185–11900

Shen M et al. (2005). Polymorphisms in the DNA nucleotide excision repair genes and lung cancer risk in Xuan Wei, China. *Int J Cancer* 116:768–773.

Shen MR, Jones IM, Mohrenweiser H (1998). Nonconservative amino acid substitution variants exist at polymorphic frequency in DNA repair genes in healthy humans. *Cancer Res* 58:604–608.

Shen W, Waldschmidt M, Zhao X, Ratliff T, Krieg AM (2002). Antitumor mechanisms of oligodeoxynucleotides with CpG and polyG motifs in murine prostate cancer cells: decrease of NF-kappaB and AP-1 binding activities and induction of apoptosis. *Antisense Nucleic Acid Drug Dev* 12:155–164.

Shields PG, Harris CC (2000). Cancer risk and low-penetrance susceptibility genes in gene-environment interactions. *J Clin Oncol* 18:2309–2315.

Shimizu H, Ross RK, Bernstein L, Yatani R, Henderson BE, Mack TM (1991). Cancers of the prostate and breast among Japanese and White Immigrants in Los Angeles County. *Br J Cancer* 63:963–966.

Shirai T, Asamoto M, Takahashi S, Imaida K (2002). Diet and prostate cancer. *Toxicology* 181–182:89–94.

Sim HG, Cheng CW (2005). Changing demography of prostate cancer in Asia. *Eur J Cancer* 41:834–845.

Smith JR et al. (1996). Major susceptibility locus for prostate cancer on chromosome 1 suggested by a genome-wide search. *Science* 274:1371–1374.

Sobti RC, Gupta L, Thakur H, Seth A, Singh SK, Kaur P (2009). CYP17 gene polymorphism and its association in north Indian prostate cancer patients. *Anticancer Res* 29:1659–1663.

Sobti RC, Thakur H, Gupta L, Janmeja AK, Seth A, Singh SK (2010). Polymorphisms in the HPC/ELAC-2 and alpha 1-antitrypsin genes that correlate with human diseases in a North Indian population. *Mol Biol Rep.* Feb 2 (Epub ahead of print)

Sommer F, Klotz T, Schmitz-Drager BJ (2004). Lifestyle issues and genitourinary tumors. *World J Urol* 21:402–413.

Spitz MR, Currier RD, Fueger JJ, Babaian RJ, Newell GR (1991). Familial pattern of prostate cancer: A case control of analysis. *J Urol* 146:1305–1307.

Stary A, Sarasin A (2002). The genetics of the hereditary xeroderma pigmentosum syndrome. *Biochemie* 84:49–60.

Steinberg GD, Carter BS, Beaty TH, Chids B, Walsh PC (1990). Family history and the risk of prostate cancer. *Prostate* 17:337.

Stoehlmacher J, Park DJ, Zhang W, Groshen S, Trao-wes DD, Yu MC, Lenz HJ (2002). Association between glutathione-S-transferase Pi, Ti and Mi genetic polymorphism and survival of patients with metastatic colorectal cancer. *J Natl Cancer Inst* 94:936–942.

Sunny L, Yeole BB, Kurkure AP, Hakama M, Shiri R, Mathew SS, Shastri NG, Advani SH (2004). Cummulative risk and trends in prostate cancer incidence in Mumbai, India. *Asian PacJ Cancer Prev* 5:401–405.

Tchou JC et al. (2000). GSTP1 CpG island DNA hypermethylation in hepatocellular carcinoma. *Int J Oncol* 16:663–676.

Thakur H, Gupta L, Sobti RC, Janmeja AK, Seth A, Singh SK (2011). Association of GSTM1T1 genes with COPD and prostate cancer in north Indian population. *Mol Biol Rep* 38:1733–1739.

Theisseu E (1974). Concerning a familial association between breast cancer and both prostatic and uterine malignancies. *Cancer* 34:1102–1107.

Tirode F, Busso D, Coin F, Egly JM (1999). Reconstitution of the transcription factor TFIIH: assignment of functions for the three enzymatic subunits, XPB, XPD, and cdk7. *Mol Cell* 3:87–95.

Toyota M, Ahuja N, Ohe-Toyota M, Herman JG, Baylin SB, Issa JP (1999). CpG island methylator phenotype in colorectal cancer. *Proc Natl Acad Sci USA* 96:8681–8686.

Van Gils CH, Bostick RM, Stern MC, Taylor JA (2002). Differences in base excision repair capacity may modulate the effect of dietary antioxidant intake on prostate cancer risk: an example of polymorphisms in the XRCC1 gene. *Cancer Epidemiol Biomarkers Prev* 11:1279–1284.

Van Hoffen A, Balajee AS, van Zeeland AA, Mullenders LH (2003). Nucleotide excision repair and its interplay with transcription. *Toxicology* 193:79–90.

Van Licshout EM, Roelofs HM, Dekkar S, Mulder CJ, Wobbes T, Jansen JB, Peters WH (1999). Polymorphic expression of the glutathione s-transferase Pi gene and its susceptibility to Barret's oesophagus and oesophageal Carcinoma. *Cancer Res* 59:586–589.

Veierød MB, Laake P, Thelle DS (1997). Dietary fat intake and risk of prostate cancer: A prospective study of 25,708 Norwegian men. *Int J Cancer* 73:634–638.

Vercelli M, quaglia A, Marani E, Parodi S (2000). Prostate cancer incidence and mortality trends among elderly and adult Europeans. *Crit. Rev. Oncol Hematol* 35:133–144.

Villar-Garea A, Fraga MF, Espada J, Esteller M (2003). Procaine is a DNA-demethylating agent with growth-inhibitory effects in human cancer cells. *Cancer Res* 63:4984–4989.

Virmani AK, Tsou JA, Siegmund KD, Shen LY, Long TI, Laird PW, Gazdar AF, Laird-Offringa IA (2002). Hierarchical clustering of lung cancer cell lines using DNA methylation markers. Cancer Epidemiol. *Biomarkers Prev* 11:291–297.

Vogel U, Overvad K, Wallin H, Tjønneland A, Nexø BA, Raaschou-Nielsen O (2005). Combinations of polymorphisms in XPD, XPC and XPA in relation to risk of lung cancer. *Cancer Lett* 222:67–74.

Wang LE et al. (2004). Polymorphisms of DNA repair genes and risk of glioma. *Cancer Res* 64:5560–5563.

Wang Y, Spitz MR, Schabath MB, Ali-Osman F, Mata H, Wu X (2003). Association between glutathione-S-transferase Pi polymorphisms and lung cancer risk in Caucasians: a case-control study. *Lung Cancer* 40:25–32.

Ward E, Jemal A, Cokkinides V, Singh GK, Cardinez C, Ghafoor A, Thun M (2004). Cancer disparities by race/ethnicity and socioeconomic status. *CA Cancer J Clin* 54:78–93.

Ware JL (1994). Prostate cancer progression. Implications of histopathology. *Am J Pathol* 145:983–993.

Waterhouse J, Muir C, Shanmugaratnam K (1982). Cancer incidence in five continents. In: Cancer Incidence. Lyon, France: International Agency for Research in Cancer 6.

Whittemore AS et al. (1995). Prostate cancer in relation to diet, physical activity, and body size in blacks, whites, and Asians in the United States and Canada. *J Natl Cancer Inst* 87:652–661.

Williams TA, Mars AE, Buysike SG, Stenroos ES, Wang R, Factura-Santiago MF, Lambert GH, Johnson WG (2007). Risk of autistic disorder in affected offspring of mothers with a glutathione-S-transferase Pi haplotype. *Arch PaditrAddescMed* 161:356–361.

Woodson K. Hayes R, Wideroff L, Villaruz L, Tangrea J (2003). Hypermethylation of GSTPI, CDUU, and E-cadherin genes in prostate cancer among US Black and Whites. *Prostate* 55:199–205.

Woolf CM (1960). An investigation of the familial aspects of carcinoma of the prostate. *Cancer* 13:739–744.

Wynder EL, Laakso K, Sotarauta M, Rose DP (1984). Metabolic epidemiology of prostatic cancer. *Prostate* 5:47–53.

Xu J et al. (1998). Evidence for a prostate cancer susceptibility locus on the X Chromosome. *Nat Genet* 20:175–179.

Xu J et al. (2002). Associations between hOGG1 sequence variants and Prostate Cancer susceptibility. *Cancer Res* 62:2253–2257.

Yamanaka M et al. (2003). Altered methylation of multiple genes in carcinogenesis of the prostate. *Int J Cancer* 106:382–387.

Yasuno T, Mobsumura T, Mabsumura T, Shikata T, Inazawa J, Sakabi T, Truchida S, Takahata A (1999). Cisplatin resistant human neuroblastoma cell line. *Anticancer Res* 19:4049–4057.

Yi J, Wang ZW, Cang H, Chen YY, Zhao R, Yu BM, Tang XM (2001). p16 gene methylation in colorectal cancers associated with Duke's staging. *World J Gastroenterol* 7:722–725.

Yu H, Harris RE, Gaoy, Gao R, Wynder EL (1991). Comparative epidemiology of Cancer of the Colon, Rectum, prostate and breast in Shanghai, China versus the United States. *Inst J Epidemiol* 20:76–81.

18

Lymphatic Filariasis-Visceral Leishmaniasis Coinfection

Vikas Kushwaha
Department of Biotechnology, Panjab University, Chandigarh, India.

18.1 Introduction

Both lymphatic filariasis (LF) and visceral leishmaniasis (VL) are vector-borne neglected tropical diseases. In various regions of the world, coinfection of these diseases is emerging and affecting public health. These two diseases share a common mode of transmission (i.e., transmission through different species of mosquitoes or sandflies). Therefore, the distribution of LF and VL in the world occurs in almost the same geographical locations. The filarial parasite belongs to the family Filariidae (phylum Nematoda) and causing agents are *Brugia malayi, B. timori,* and *Wuchereria bancrofti.* The disease is transmitted by different mosquito species of *Culex, Aedes, Mansonia,* and *Anopheles* (Murthy, 2019). Lymphatic filariasis affects people in 72 countries throughout the tropics and sub-tropics of Asia, Africa, the Western Pacific, and parts of the Caribbean and South America. The lifecycles of the LF parasite is complicated. Adult worms lodge in the host's lymphatic system where fecund females release larvae (first-stage larvae: microfilaria; mf), which periodically circulate in the blood system of the host. Mosquitoes pick up circulating mf in the blood during blood feeding, where they metamorphose to form infectious larvae (third-stage larvae: L3). Infective larvae (L3) are then transmitted by the mosquitoes to new hosts during feeding (WHO, 2016).

The WHO proposed mass drug administration (MDA) to combat disease development, involving the treatment of people in endemic areas with the following combinations of anthelmintic medicines: Albendazole: 400 mg + Diethylcarbamazine citrate: 6 mg/kg; Albendazole: 400 mg+ Ivermectin: 150–200 µg/kg; or Albendazole: 400 mg, preferably twice a year (WHO, 2006).

Leishmania is a protozoan parasite that belongs to the family *Trypanosomatidae.* They are unicellular eukaryotes having a well-defined nucleus and other cell organelles including kinetoplasts and flagella. They are spread to their host (mainly vertebrates) by female phlebotomine sandflies of the genus *Phlebotomus* (Rostamian et al., 2018). Visceral leishmaniasis is also known as kala-azar, which is caused by the *Leishmania donovani* in the Indian subcontinent and Africa and *L. infantum* in the Mediterranean basin, Central and South America. The majority (about 90%) of cases reported from five countries: Sudan, Nepal, India, Brazil, and Ethiopia (Keerti et al., 2018). The free-swimming procyclic promastigote type undergoes differentiation into an infective metacyclic stage during the parasite's digenetic life cycle, and eventually, after infection during blood feeding, differentiates into the disease-causing rounded amastigote forms that reside within the macrophages. In the macrophages, amastigotes split, release after rupturing from the cell, and macrophages are further engulfed. During feeding, sandflies ingest the amastigote from the infected host and transmit the disease. For the treatment of VL, various medicines such as pentavalent antimonials (sodium stibogluconate and meglumine antimoniate), Liposomal amphotericin B, Miltefosine, Paromomycin, and Sitamaquine are used, but current drugs have notable safety, resistance, stability, and cost disadvantages. They are poorly tolerated, have a long period of treatment, and are difficult to administer (Alves et al., 2018).

DOI: 10.1201/9781003220404-20

Leishmania/filarial coinfection cases are reported in certain parts of the world. People living in endemic areas are more vulnerable to helminth infections while *Leishmania* infection occurs due to their genetic susceptibility. The diagnosis of lymphatic filariasis is distinct from visceral leishmaniasis due to different clinical presentations. Thus, the patients suspected with visceral leishmaniasis and/or filarial infection should be tested for both the disease especially in the endemic areas. The diagnosis of filariasis includes the presence of the microfilariae to be checked in a blood smear of the individual. When parasites are not found in the blood, the adult worms may occasionally be found in a lymph node sample from an infected individual. Somewhat easier diagnostic tests like antibody test, antigen test, and radiology (lymphoscintigraphy) were recently developed to diagnose the presence of filarial infection. Visceral leishmaniasis diagnosis involves antibody detection using the rK39 rapid diagnostic test (RDT) and the alternative direct agglutination test (DAT) to confirm infection. People with VL symptoms but negative diagnostic findings are referred to hospitals for microscopic examination of the tissue aspirate from spleen, bone marrow, or lymph node.

18.2 Clinical Manifestations

The majority of people infected with lymphatic filariasis do not have flu, fever, or vomiting as clinical symptoms or signs. In fact, the majority of LF patients are totally unaware that they have the disease. Affected people can experience high temperatures, trembling chills, body aches, and swollen lymph nodes, as well as episodes of acute lymphatic vessel inflammation (lymphangitis). Excess fluid may accumulate (edema) in the affected areas (i.e., arms and/or legs), but this usually goes away after the other symptoms have subsided. During acute episodes of symptoms, some people with filariasis have abnormally elevated levels of some white blood cells (eosinophilia). Even if there are no other signs, filariasis may cause chronic lymph node swelling (lymphadenopathy). Long-term lymphatic vessel obstruction can lead to a number of other problems. Males can experience inflammation, pain, and swelling of the testes (orchitis), sperm track (funiculitis), and/or sperm ducts as a result of attacks (epididymitis). It is likely that the scrotum will swell abnormally and become painful. Hydrocele, the presence of lymphatic fluid in the urine (chyluria), and/or abnormally swollen lymphatic vessels are examples of these (varices). Progressive edema (elephantiasis) of the female external genitalia (vulva), breasts, and/or arms and legs are also potential symptoms (WHO, 2016). These signs have been linked to a longer duration of exposure and the accumulation of worms, according to experts.

There are three categories of filarial symptoms:

a. **Asymptomatic microfilaremic (Mf carriers):** People who live in endemic areas have mf in their peripheral blood and remain asymptomatic microfilaremic (mf carriers) throughout their lives. They are vulnerable to lymphatic pathology such as dilation, kinking, collateral formation, and so on. They play a part in disease transmission.

b. **Chronic symptomatic:** Symptoms of amicrofilaremia are typical in these people. Lymphangitis (inflammation of the infected area), generalized malaise, and fever characterize this acute stage. Hydrocoele, chyluria, lymphoedema, and elephantiasis are the main chronic symptoms that occur later. Blockage of the abdominal or thoracic lymph vessels, which leads to chyluria or hematochyluria and is typically incurable, is a more severe condition.

c. **Endemic normal (EN):** People of endemic areas are free from both disease symptoms and microfilariae (mf).

The majority of people who are infected with the parasite never show any symptoms. As a consequence, the term leishmaniasis refers to being ill as a result of a *Leishmania* infection rather than actually becoming infected with the parasite. There are three main types of disease patterns of leishmaniasis:

a. **Visceral leishmaniasis** (VL; kala azar/Black fever/Dum Dum fever) is lethal if not treated properly in over 95% of cases. Common symptoms are irregular bouts of fever, pyrexia, anemia, emaciation, heavy skin pigmentation, and enlargement of the spleen and liver.

b. **Cutaneous leishmaniasis** (CL; Jericho boil/Baghdad button/Delhi sore/Oriental sore) is a common form with some symptoms like lesions on skin, ulcers on exposed parts of the body, lifelong scars, and serious infirmity.

c. **Mucocutaneous leishmaniasis** (MCL; Espunidia) causes total or partial devastation of mucous membranes of the mouth, nose, and throat.

Signs of visceral leishmaniasis develop steadily over a period of weeks or even months: persistent fever, hepatosplenomegaly (enlarged liver spleen), severe weight loss, pancytopenia, progressive anaemia (low red blood cell count), leukopenia (low white blood cell count), thrombocytopenia (low platelet count), hypergammaglobulinemia (high protein), and lymphadenopathy. Some patients develop post-kala-azar dermal leishmaniasis (PKDL), a condition characterized by skin lesions (such as erythematous or hypo pigmented macules, papules, nodules, and patches) that occur at varying intervals after (or during) treatment for visceral leishmaniasis. People with PKDL that have been diagnosed for a long time may be valuable tools (www.who.int/csr/resources/publications/CSR_ISR_2000_1leish/en/).

18.3 Lymphatic Filariasis and Visceral Leishmaniasis Coinfection in Rodents

Coinfection of LF and VL is caused by two different organisms. Both LF and VL, parasites infective stages replicate in the mosquito or sandfly and can deliver concomitantly infectious particles in a single bite via saliva.

Coinfection of these two diseases has been studied in vivo in mice using *Brugia malayi* and *Leishmania donovani* as a LF and VL agent, respectively. Mice were infected with the rodent filarial nematode *Litomosoides sigmodontis* followed by footpad infection with the protozoan parasite *Leishmania major* to see if coinfection had an effect on disease progression. This research shows that *L. sigmodontis* affects the development of *L. major* (Lamb et al., 2005). In BALB/c mice, a pork worm, *Trichinella spiralis*, inhibits VL progression, implying that filarial infections have a direct impact on *Leishmania* parasite growth (Rousseau et al., 1997). In another study, L3 stage of filarial parasite *B. malayi* was found to inhibit the progression of *L. donovani* amastigote in mice (Porthouse et al., 2006). In addition, filarial adult parasite has been assumed to modulate the immune response and encourage the development of amastigote *L. donovani* in the mouse (Verma et al., 2015). It was subsequently studied to find out whether BmAFII (adult parasite extract fraction) and F6 (54.2–67.8 kDa) of *B. malayi* BmAFII fraction inhibits the progression of amastigotes in mice (Murthy et al., 2008; Verma et al., 2015). Researchers recently found that cross-reactive fraction Ld1 of *L. donovani* (52.9–93.6 kDa) and *B. malayi* facilitate filarial infection (Verma et al., 2018). A comprehensive picture of the interaction of these two pathogens in the progression or inhibition of the disease is necessary for further elaborate investigations.

18.4 Lymphatic Filariasis and Visceral Leishmaniasis Coinfection in Human

Lymphatic filariasis infection is usually non-fatal, whereas visceral leishmaniasis can cause serious complications, including death. As a consequence, coinfection with these two diseases may result in a disease with similar symptoms. Hence, diagnosis and treatment of such patients becomes complicated. As a result, clinical manifestations in cases of coinfection with these infections must be properly treated. Early identification of these coinfections is important for better patient care. The role of coinfection in the clinical presentation of the disease has only been studied in a few studies. In the splenic aspirate of one of 28 patients from 29 sites, both *L. donovani* bodies and microfilariae (mf) coexisted (Jain et al., 2001). In cases of pyrexia of unknown origin (PUO), both parasites were reported singly, particularly in patients from endemic areas; mixed infection by both parasites was rare (Ahmed et al., 2014). According to recent investigations, patients having lymphatic filariasis and leishmaniasis coinfection present severe disease condition with higher mortality rate than single infection. The prevalence of filariasis and leishmaniasis coinfection has recently been reported from Mali, Sudan. Individuals with overlapping infections (microfilariae; mf+/leishmanin skin test; LST +) had an average incidence of 1.51%, 6.24% mf/LST+, and

13.76% mf+/LST. Men (8/6 ratio) were more affected by coinfection than women (Sangare et al., 2018). To fully comprehend the pathogenesis and severity of the dual viral infections, more thorough research involving a larger patient population is needed.

18.5 Immune Response Against Lymphatic Filariasis and Visceral Leishmaniasis

Lymphedema, hydrocele, and elephantiasis are the most common symptoms of LF infection. T cells are the major players of the filarial infection immune system. IL-4, IL-4R, or Stat 6 mice are more susceptible to brugian infection, which indicates that Th2 immune response types are essential for filarial infection eradication (Spencer et al., 2001; Babu and Nutman, 2014). Filarial parasites invade and destroy host tissue during the immune response to LF, resulting in the release of cytokines such as thymic stromal lymphopoietin (TSLP), which activates innate lymphoid cells (ILCs) and other cell populations to secrete IL-4, IL-5, IL-9, IL-10, and IL-13, the development of IgE and IgG1 or IgG4 (Grencis, 2015; Kalyanasundaram et al., 2020). IFN-γ and NO, interestingly, tend to play a crucial defensive role in filarial infection in mice (Dixit et al., 2006; Sahoo et al., 2009). As a result, for defense against filarial infection, both Th1 and Th2 responses must be in sync (Kwarteng et al., 2017). The clearance of filarial parasites in all types of filarial patients is aided by the antibody-dependent cell-mediated cytotoxicity (ADCC) action of IgG antibody (Kalyanasundaram et al., 2020). IgE specific to filarial parasites plays a critical and defensive function in helminths that facilitate parasite killing and IgA also protects host from against filariasis Gurish et al., 2004; Sahu et al., 2008). To summarize, immunity to lymphatic filariasis necessitates a Th2 response from immune system cells.

Leishmania infection is dependent on the cooperation of different cells in the immune system (neutrophils, lymphocytes, macrophages, and so on). Th1 responses are primarily responsible for protective immunity against *Leishmania* infection in humans and mice (Garg et al., 2005). When natural killer (NK) and T cells interact with IL-12, Th1 responses are activated, lymphocyte proliferation, cytotoxic responses, and IFN-γ production are restored (Bacellar et al., 1996; Ghalib et al., 1995; De Almeida et al., 2003). IFN-γ released from Th1 cells causes macrophages to produce H2O2 and nitric oxide (NO), which promotes disease resolution through NO-mediated parasite killing, while TNF-α with IFN-γ induces macrophages to produce NO and iNOS (Murray and Nathan, 1999). Several studies have shown that producing IFN-γ, TNF-α, and IL-12 increased the expression of nitric oxide synthase, which is essential for parasite clearance and the development of parasite resistance/protection (Wilhelm et al., 2019). CD4+ Th17 cells, on the other hand, have been linked to host resistance and susceptibility to leishmaniasis (Pitta et al., 2009). High levels of IL-4, IL-5, IL-13, and anti-inflammatory cytokines are linked to chronic infection and VL pathogenesis, respectively (Kumar et al., 2017). IL-13 enhances host defense in VL, according to studies with IL-13 knockout mice infected with *L. donovani* infection (Dayakar et al., 2019). In conclusion, *Leishmania* infection affects the immune system by eliciting strong Th1 and Th17 responses.

18.6 Immune Responses in *Leishmania*–Filaria Coinfection

The immunological impact of filarial and leishmanial coinfection on immune responses has been demonstrated in a mouse model. Various studies from various research labs have shown that the existence of filarial infection has a substantial impact on the efficiency of the immune response elicited by the *Leishmania* parasite. In mice, the L3 stage of the filarial parasite induces proinflammatory cytokine (IFN-γ, TNF-α, IL-1, IL-8) release, while BmAFII (adult parasite extract fraction) activates proinflammatory mediators (IL-1β, IL-8, IFN-γ, TNF-α), NO release, and cellular proliferative responses, inhibiting the amastigote progression of *L. donovani* (Porthouse et al., 2006; Murthy et al., 2008). Due to upregulated Th1 cytokines (IFN-γ, TNF-α, IL-12), lymphocyte proliferation, NO development, high IgG, IgG2/3 levels, and downregulated Th2 cytokine expression (TGF-β), F6 (54.2–67.8 kDa) of *B. malayi* BmAFII fraction inhibit *L. donovani* infection (Verma et al., 2015).

In mice, filarial adult parasites facilitate the progression and development of *L. donovani* amastigote by producing TGF-β and IL-10 (Verma et al., 2015). Apart from the filarial parasite's microfilariae stage, which has no effect on immune modulation in mice. Filarial cross-reactive fraction Ld1 (52.9–93.6 kDa) of *L. donovani* facilitates filarial infection progression by downregulating IL-5, IL-13, IFN-γ, TNF-α, and IL-2 cytokine levels, and upregulating IL-4 and TGF-β (Verma et al., 2018).

18.7 Conclusion

By measuring and diagnosing each infecting agent, the significance of the LF and VL coinfection can be determined. Furthermore, larger patient groups and more elaborate clinical trials are required to determine the impact of disease severity in the case of coinfection. In endemic areas, clinically suspicious cases should also be screened for both pathogens. This knowledge is critical for diagnosing the infecting pathogen early and accurately, as well as correlating clinical symptoms with coinfection for proper patient management. Furthermore, the initiation, progression, and development of host immune responses to filarial and leishmanial coinfection indicate that filarial parasites induce Th1 and Th2 responses in coinfection, which influence the host immune system's ability to fight *Leishmania* infection. This knowledge will also aid in the implementation of effective controls to prevent outbreaks caused by this emerging coinfection.

REFERENCES

Ahmed, N. H., Shwetha, J., Samantaray, J. C., Jana, K., 2014. A case of mixed infection with filariasis and visceral leishmaniasis. Trop. Parasitol. 4 (1), 62–64. http://doi.org/10.4103/2229-5070.129191.

Alves, F., Bilbe, G., Blesson, S., Goyal, V., Monnerat, S., Mowbray, C., Muthoni Ouattara, G., et al., 2018. Recent development of visceral leishmaniasis treatments: successes, pitfalls, and perspectives. Clin Microbiol Rev. 31(4):e00048–18. doi: 10.1128/CMR.00048-18

Babu, S., Nutman, T. B., 2014. Immunology of lymphatic filariasis. Parasite Immunol. 36 (8), 338–346. http://doi.org/10.1111/pim.12081.

Bacellar, O., Brodskyn, C., Guerreiro, J., Barral-Netto, M., Costa, C. H., Coffman, R., et al., 1996. Interleukin-12 restores interferon-gamma production and cytotoxic responses in visceral leishmaniasis. J. Infect. Dis. 173 (6), 1515–1518.

Dayakar, A., Chandrasekaran, S., Kuchipudi, S. V., Kalangi, S. K., 2019. Cytokines: key determinants of resistance or disease progression in visceral leishmaniasis: opportunities for novel diagnostics and immunotherapy. Frontiers in Immunology 10, 670. https://doi.org/10.3389/fimmu.2019.00670

De Almeida, M. C., Cardoso, S. A., Barral-Netto, M., 2003. Leishmania (Leishmania) chagasi infection alters the expression of cell adhesion and costimulatory molecules on human monocyte and macrophage. Int. J. Parasitol. 33 (2), 153–162. http://doi.org/10.1016/S0020-7519(02)00266-7.

Dixit, S., Gaur, R. L., Sahoo, M. K., Joseph, S. K., Murthy, P. S., Murthy, P. K., 2006. Protection against L3 induced *Brugia malayi* infection in *Mastomys coucha* pre-immunized with BmAFII fraction of the filarial adult worm. Vaccine 24 (31-32), 5824–5831. http://doi.org/10.1016/j.vaccine.2006.05.003.

Garg, R., Gupta, S. K., Tripathi, P., Naik, S., Sundar, S., Dube, A., 2005. Immunostimulatory cellular responses of cured Leishmania-infected patients and hamsters against the integral membrane proteins and non-membranous soluble proteins of a recent clinical isolate of Leishmania donovani. Clin. Exp. Immunol. 140 (1), 149–156. http://doi.org/10.1111/j.1365-2249.2005.02745.x.

Ghalib, H. W., Whittle, J. A., Kubin, M., Hashim, F. A., el-Hassan, A. M., Grabstein, K. H., et al., 1995. IL-12 enhances Th1-type responses in human Leishmania donovani infections. J. Immunol. 154 (9), 4623–4629.

Grencis, R. K., 2015. Immunity to helminths: resistance, regulation, and susceptibility to gastrointestinal nematodes. Annu. Rev. Immunol. 33, 201–225. http://doi.org/10.1146/annurev-immunol-032713-120218.

Gurish, M. F., Bryce, P. J., Tao, H., Kisselgof, A. B., Thornton, E. M., Miller, H. R., et al., 2004. IgE enhances parasite clearance and regulates mast cell responses in mice infected with Trichinella spiralis. J. Immunol. 172 (2), 1139–1145. http://doi.org/10.4049/jimmunol.172.2.1139.

Jain, S., Sodhani, P., Gupta, S., Sakhuja, P., Kumar, N., 2001. Cytomorphology of filariasis revisited. Expansion of the morphologic spectrum and coexistence with other lesions. Acta Cytol. 45 (2), 186–191. http://doi.org/10.1159/000327275.

Kalyanasundaram, R., Khatri, V., Chauhan, N., 2020. Advances in Vaccine Development for human lymphatic filariasis. Trends in Parasitology 36 (2), 195–205. https://doi.org/10.1016/j.pt.2019.11.005

Keerti, Yadav, N. K., Joshi, S., Ratnapriya, S., Sahasrabuddhe, A. A., Dube, A., 2018. Immunotherapeutic potential of leishmania (leishmania) donovani Th1 stimulatory proteins against experimental visceral leishmaniasis. Vaccine 36 (17), 2293–2299. http://doi.org/10.1016/j.vaccine.2018.03.027.

Kumar, R., Bhatia, M., Pai, K., 2017. Role of cytokines in the pathogenesis of visceral leishmaniasis. Clin. Lab. 63 (10), 1549–1559. http://doi.org/10.7754/Clin.Lab.2017.170404.

Kwarteng, A., Ahuno, S.T., 2017. Immunity in filarial infections: lessons from animal models and human studies. Scand J Immunol 85, 251–257. https://doi.org/10.1111/sji.12533

Lamb, T. J., Graham, A. L., Le Goff, L., Allen, J. E., 2005. Co-infected C57BL/6 mice mount appropriately polarized and compartmentalized cytokine responses to Litomosoides sigmodontis and Leishmania major but disease progression is altered. Parasite. Immunol. 27 (9), 317–324. http://doi.org/10.1111/j.1365-3024.2005.00779.x.

Murray, H. W., Nathan, C. F., 1999. Macrophage microbicidal mechanisms in vivo: reactive nitrogen versus oxygen intermediates in the killing of intracellular visceral Leishmania donovani. J. Exp. Med. 189 (4), 741–746. http://doi.org/10.1084/jem.189.4.741.

Murthy, P. K., 2019. Strategies to control human lymphatic filarial infection: tweaking host's immune system. Curr. Top. Med. Chem. 19 (14), 1226–1240. http://doi.org/10.2174/1568026619666190618110613.

Murthy, P. K., Dixit, S., Gaur, R. L., Kumar, R., Sahoo, M. K., Shakya, N., et al., 2008. Influence of *Brugia malayi* life stages and BmAFII fraction on experimental *Leishmania donovani* infection in hamsters. Acta Trop. 106 (2), 81–89. http://doi.org/10.1016/j.actatropica.2008.01.007.

Pitta, M. G., Romano, A., Cabantous, S., Henri, S., Hammad, A., Kouriba, B., Argiro, L., el Kheir, M., Bucheton, B., Mary, C., Hassan El-Safi, S., Dessein, A., 2009. IL-17 and IL-22 are associated with protection against human kala azar caused by Leishmania donovani. J. Clin. Invest. 119 (8), 2379–2387. http://doi.org/10.1172/JCI38813.

Porthouse, K. H., Chirgwin, S. R., Coleman, S. U., Taylor, H. W., Klei, T. R., 2006. Inflammatory responses to migrating Brugia pahangi third-stage larvae. Infect. Immun. 74 (4), 2366–2372. http://doi.org/10.1128/IAI.74.4.2366-2372.2006.

Rostamian, M., Bahrami, F., Niknam, H. M., 2018. Vaccination with whole-cell killed or recombinant leishmanial protein and toll-like receptor agonists against Leishmania tropica in BALB/c mice. PLoS One 13 (9), e0204491. http://doi.org/10.1371/journal.pone.0204491.

Rousseau, D., Le Fichoux, Y., Stien, X., Suffia, I., Ferrua, B., Kubar, J., 1997. Progression of visceral leishmaniasis due to Leishmania infantum in BALB/c mice is markedly slowed by prior infection with Trichinella spiralis. Infect. Immun. 65 (12), 4978–4983. http://doi.org/10.1016/S1383-5769(98)80724-1.

Sahoo, M. K., Sisodia, B. S., Dixit, S., Joseph, S. K., Gaur, R. L., Verma, S. K., et al., 2009. Immunization with inflammatory proteome of Brugia malayi adult worm induces a Th1/Th2-immune response and confers protection against the filarial infection. Vaccine 27 (32), 4263–4271. http://doi.org/10.1016/j.vaccine.2009.05.015.

Sahu, B. R., Mohanty, M. C., Sahoo, P. K., Satapathy, A. K., Ravindran, B., 2008. Protective immunity in human filariasis: a role for parasite-specific IgA responses. J. Infect. Dis. 198 (3), 434–443. http://doi.org/10.1086/589881.

Sangare, M. B., Coulibaly, Y. I., Coulibaly, S. Y., Coulibaly, M. E., Traore, B., Dicko, I., et al., 2018. A cross-sectional study of the filarial and Leishmania co-endemicity in two ecologically distinct settings in Mali. Parasit. Vectors 11 (1), 18. http://doi.org/10.1186/s13071-017-2531-8.

Spencer, L., Shultz, L., Rajan, T. V., 2001. Interleukin-4 receptor-Stat6 signaling in murine infections with a tissue-dwelling nematode parasite. Infect. Immun. 69 (12), 7743–7752. http://doi.org/10.1128/IAI.69.12.7743-7752.2001.

Verma, R., Joseph, S. K., Kushwaha, V., Kumar, V., Siddiqi, M. I., Vishwakarma, P., et al., 2015. Cross reactive molecules of human lymphatic filaria Brugia malayi inhibit Leishmania donovani infection in hamsters. Acta Trop. 152, 103–111. http://doi.org/10.1016/j.actatropica.2015.08.018.

Verma, R., Kushwaha, V., Pandey, S., Thota, J. R., Vishwakarma, P., Parmar, N., et al., 2018. Leishmania donovani molecules recognized by sera of filaria infected host facilitate filarial infection. Parasitol. Res. 117 (9), 2901–2912. http://doi.org/10.1007/s00436-018-5981-9.

WHO 2006. Preventive chemotherapy in human helminthiasis. (Geneva).

WHO 2016. Global programme to eliminate lymphatic filariasis: progress report. Geneva: World Health Organization. www.who.int/csr/resources/publications/CSR_ISR_2000_1leish/en/

Wilhelm, P., Ritter, U., Labbow, S., Donhauser, N., Rollinghoff, M., Bogdan, C., 2001. Rapidly fatal leishmaniasis in resistant C57BL/6 mice lacking TNF. J Immunol. 166, 4012–4019. http://doi.org/10.4049/jimmunol.166.6.4012

19

Metabolic Dysregulation, Oncogenes, and Tumor Suppressors: A Highly Orchestrated Performance to Induce Carcinogenesis

Mani Chopra, Era Seth, and Sanchita Khurana
Department of Zoology, Panjab University, Chandigarh, India

R.C. Sobti
Department of Biotechnology, Panjab University, Chandigarh, India

Abbreviations

6PGDH	6-phosphogluconate dehydrogenase
ATP	Adenosine tri-phosphate
DNA	Deoxyribose nucleic acid
E-4-P	Erythrose-4-phosphate
F-2, 6-BP	Fructose 2, 6 bisphosphate
F-6-P	Fructose-6-phosphate
FAD	Flavin Adenine dinucleotide
FH	Fumarate hydratase
GAPDH	Glyceraldehyde-3-phosphate dehydrogenase
GAPDH	Glyceraldehyde-3-phosphate dehydrogenase
GLUT	Glucose transporters
HIF	Hypoxia Inducible Factor
HK	Hexokinase
IDH	Isocitrate dehydrogenase
IMM	Inner mitochondrial membrane
LDH	Lactate dehydrogenase
MCT	Monocarboxylate transporter
NAD$^+$	Nicotinamide adenine dinucleotide
NADPH	Nicotinamide adenine dinucleotide phosphate
OMM	Outer mitochondrial membrane
NRF-2	Nuclear factor erythroid factor-2
PDH	Pyruvate dehydrogenase complex
PDK	Pyruvate dehydrogenase complex kinase
PFK	Phosphofructo kinase
PGK	Phosphoglycerate kinase
PGK	Phosphoglycerate kinase
PGM	Phosphoglycerate mutase
PHDGH	Phosphoglycerate dehydrogenase
PI	Phosphohexose isomerase
PK	Pyruvate kinase
PPP	Pentose phosphate pathway

DOI: 10.1201/9781003220404-21

RuPE	Ribulose-5-phosphate epimerase
RuPI	Ribulose-5-phosphate isomerise
S-7-P	Seduheptulose-7-phosphate
SDH	Succinate dehydrogenase
SIRT3	Sirturin 3
TALDO	Transaldolase
TCA	Tricarboxylic acid cycle
TIGAR	T*P53*-induced glycolysis and apoptosis regulator
TKT	Transketolase
TPI	Triose phosphate isomerase
VEGF	Vascular endothelial growth factor
VHL	Von Hippel Lindau tumor suppressor gene
Xu-5-P	Xylulose-5-phosphate

19.1 Introduction

Metabolism is the set of chemical transformations within the cells that are indispensable for life of all organisms. Every cell engages itself in metabolism and they constantly recycle biomolecules such as lipids and proteins and damaged organelles and synthesize new molecules as per its requirements. Alteration in metabolism is an attribute of cancer cells (Nagarajan et al., 2016). Otto Warburg, a German physiologist in the early nineteenth century, first devised the correspondence between transformed cellular metabolism and cancer (Warburg, 1927). He reasoned that the impelling cause for this transformation was the irreversible damage to respiration (Warburg, 1956). Mitochondria are utmost source of energy resources in all cells, function in cell signalling, redox regulation, apoptosis, and origination of various metabolites crucial for the production of macromolecules that sustain survival of normal cells. Alterations in the functioning of mitochondria contributes significantly to the remodelling of cellular metabolic machinery from oxidative phosphorylation to aerobic glycolysis, thus commencing carcinogenesis. Aerobic glycolysis assisted by proliferative metabolic mediators not only fulfils the energy requirements of cancer cells but also generates intermediates for biosynthesis of metabolites required for maintaining the highly proliferative state of cancer cells due to their integral role in forming components of various organelles. Hence, the transformed metabolism is a characteristic feature of all cancer cells and a stepwise study of these pathways can be fruitful in the treatment of this disease.

19.2 Glucose Metabolism in Cancer Cells

Warburg discovered that cancer cells exhibit a specific metabolic pattern characterised by a shift from respiration to fermentation even in the ample supply of oxygen (Warburg, 1956). Cancer cells utilise glucose in a different manner as compared to normal cells utilising 85% of glucose for aerobic glycolysis, 10% for oxidative phosphorylation, and 5% for biosynthetic pathways (Hu et al., 2017). This increased dependence on aerobic glycolysis and reduced dependence on oxidative phosphorylation is termed "The Warburg Effect" (Racker, 1972). Initially, it seems to be controversial as oxidative phosphorylation produces 36 molecules of ATP from one glucose molecule whereas the Warburg phenotype produces two molecules of ATP per glucose molecule. In spite of this, cancer cells utilize aerobic glycolysis as it benefits them in bioenergetics by compensating for the ATP deficit and in biosynthesis by facilitating the simultaneous production of intermediates required for biosynthesis of lipids, amino acids, and nucleotides (Warburg, 1956). It promotes tumor initiation, invasion, and progression. It also aids in resisting apoptosis by impeding pro-apoptotic factors and enhancing expression of anti-apoptotic genes.

The Warburg Effect or aerobic glycolysis is of great significance due to its ability to function even under hypoxic conditions. Hypoxia-inducible factor-1 (HIF-1) is a heterodimeric protein that contributes to the creation of hypoxic conditions in cells even though an ample supply of oxygen is available. It consists of two subunits: HIF-1α and HIF-1β.

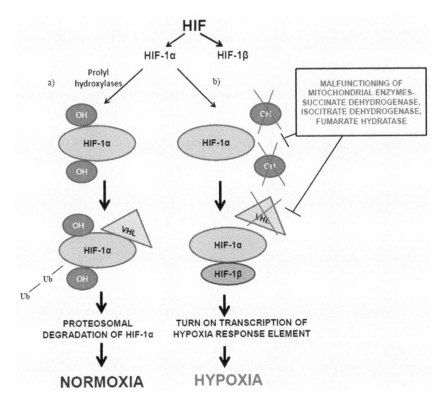

FIGURE 19.1 a) Degradation of HIF under normal conditions. b) Stabilisation of HIF induced by dysfunctioning of mitochondrial enzymes leading to hypoxia.

Under normal conditions or normoxia, the HIF-1α subunit is degraded continuously in a way that it is first produced, then hydroxylated by prolyl hydroxylases, and finally it is rapidly degraded by a mechanism that involves ubiquitylation via the product of tumor suppressor gene, Von Hippel-Lindau (VHL) (Strowitzki et al., 2019). Due to loss of activity of mitochondrial enzymes that drive Kreb's cycle and oxidative phosphorylation, HIF-1α is not hydroxylated and instead of being degraded, it binds to HIF-1β. The HIF-1α-HIF-1β heterodimer complex turns on the transcription of hypoxia response element a total of 800 genes, thus creating hypoxic conditions that drive cancer cell proliferation (Mucaj et al., 2012; Huang and Zhou, 2020). Hypoxic conditions possess the ability to increase the rate of glycolysis manifolds by upregulating glycolytic transporters and enzymes (Tameemi et al., 2019) (Figure 19.1). The corresponding mechanisms are discussed in the later part of this review.

19.3 Aerobic Glycolysis Pathway

As proliferating cells have an increased demand for glucose, a large number of glucose molecules derived from glycogenolysis, fatty acid metabolism, and gluconeogenesis are diverted towards the glycolytic pathway wherein it enters the cells via glucose transporters (GLUT) to initiate glycolysis. Out of the 12 isoforms of GLUT, GLUT 1 is overexpressed in most cancers like breast, lung, and prostate cancer (Haber et al., 1998; Jun et al., 2011). Hexokinase II (HKII), the predominant isoform of hexokinase, catalyses the first committed step in glycolysis by converting glucose to glucose-6-phosphate (Rempel et al., 1996; DeWaal et al., 2018). Upregulated hexokinase in cancer cells also drives more glucose molecules towards this glycolytic pathway (Marbaniang and Kma, 2018). Glucose-6-phosphate after being isomerised to fructose-6-phoshate (F-6-P) by phosphohexose isomerase serves as a substrate for phosphofructokinase (PFK). PFK-1, also called the pacemaker of glycolysis, catalyses the rate-limiting step by converting fructose-6-phosphate to fructose-1,6-bisphosphate by utilising ATP (Zancan et al., 2008). PFK-1 is allosterically upregulated by F-2,6-BP whereas it is downregulated by ATP and F-6-P. Another enzyme that plays a critical role in amplifying glycolysis is phosphofructo kinase 2 (PFK-2) that converts F-6-P to F2,6-BP, which is the most potent activator of PFK-1. Enhanced levels of F-2,6-BP in cancer cells eradicates the feedback inhibition on PFK-1 by ATP and F-6-P, thus causing glycolysis to move forward in an unhindered manner (Ghanbari-Movahed et al., 2019). Fructose 1,6 bisphosphate is broken down into dihydroxyacetone phosphate and glyceraldehyde-3-phosphate by aldolase. Dihydroxyacetone phosphate is further converted to glyceraldehyde-3-phosphate to carry forward glycolysis. Glyceraldehye-3-phosphate is the substrate for glyceraldehyde-3-phosphate dehydrogenase (GADPH). GADPH is a

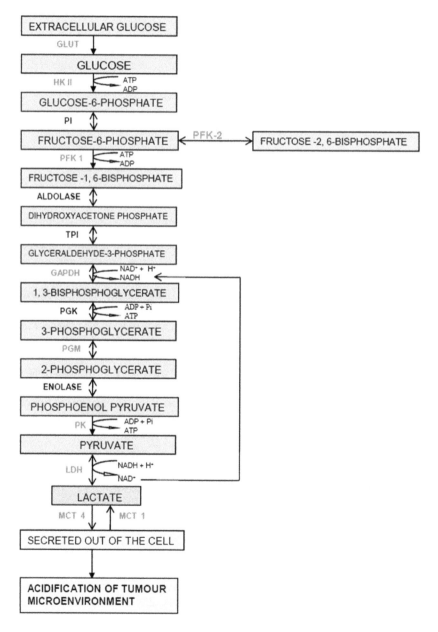

FIGURE 19.2 Deregulated aerobic glycolysis in cancer cells. The enzymes highlighted in red are upregulated to drive carcinogenesis.

housekeeping enzyme in the glycolytic pathway and is elevated in cancer cells. It mediates the conversion of glyceraldehdye-3-phosphate to 1,3 bisphosphoglycerate (Tarrado-Castellarnau et al., 2017). NADH is generated at this step and participates in a variety of biosynthetic reactions required to sustain the rapid rate of cancer cell proliferation (Schek et al., 1988; Yaku et al., 2018). Phoshoglycerate mutase (PGM) is involved in the conversion of 3-phosphoglycerate to 2-phosphoglycerate and is also elevated in cancer cells. Intensified levels of pyruvate kinase (most commonly its M2 isoform-PKM2) catalyse the irreversible conversion of phosphoenol pyruvate to pyruvate. This reaction is accompanied by a simultaneous generation of ATP. This rapid rate of ATP generation compensates for the high energetic demands of cancer cells (Lu et al., 2016). Pyruvate also functions in maintaining the glycolytic flux by preventing the degradation of HIF-1α and maintain hypoxic conditions (Singh et al., 2017). Elevated levels of pyruvate, also the end products of glycolysis, are now deflected from TCA cycle towards lactate generation in a reaction catalysed by lactate dehydrogenase (LDH) enzyme (Le et al., 2010). This step is accompanied by replenishment of NAD^+ by oxidation of NADH to NAD^+. NAD^+ serves as fuel that drives the conversion of glyceraldehyde-3-phosphate (G-3-P) to 1,3-bisphosphoglycerate via positive feedback loop to enhance glycolysis (Heiden et al., 2009).

The amplified rate of glycolysis increases lactate production up to 40 fold as compared to normal cells (Brizel et al., 2001; Tanner et al., 2018). Lactate produced in the cells as a consequence of aerobic glycolysis or Warburg phenotype is transported inside and outside of the cells by monocarboxylate transporters (MCT) 1 and 4. MCT 1 is responsible for uptake of lactate into the cells whereas MCT 4 the extrusion of lactate from the cell (Halestrap, 2012). Lactate itself is also responsible for increasing the expression of MCTs (Bonen, 2001) (Figure 19.2). The release of lactate from the cells also leads to acidification of tumor microenvironment. The highly acidic environment eases the path for cell migration, invasion, and tumor growth, thus enhancing the metastatic potential of cancer cells (San-Millán and Brooks, 2017). Intensified lactate levels have the ability to escape immune responses of the body by inhibiting T-cells (Morrot et al., 2018), natural killer cells (la Cruz-López et al., 2019), differentiation of leukocytes, and release of cytokines (Santos et al., 2019). Cancer cells possess a unique property of displaying angiogenesis (i.e., the formation of new blood vessels). Lactate contributes significantly to angiogenesis by upregulation of vascular endothelial growth factor (VEGF) (Kumar et al., 2007; Dhup et al., 2012).

19.4 Kreb's Cycle

As stated by Warburg, the root cause of cancer was dysfunctioning in respiration. Mitochondria are responsible for executing the respiratory mechanisms in the cell to generating ATP. The tricarboxylic acid cycle (TCA) or the Kreb's cycle occurs in the mitochondria normally to generate metabolic intermediates including NADPH, NADH, and precursors for synthesis of amino acids. Alterations in the functioning of enzymes in the TCA cycle lead to accumulation of metabolites that have high potential to trigger carcinogenesis. This is implicated in a variety of cancers including prostate, renal, and thyroid cancers. Succinate dehydrogenase (SDH), also called respiratory complex II, is localised in the inner mitochondrial membrane (Moosavi et al., 2019) and catalyses reactions in TCA cycle as well as in the electron transport chain. In the TCA cycle, it converts succinate to fumarate with a simultaneous reduction of FAD to $FADH_2$. Dysfunctioning of SDH results in accumulation of succinate. Further another enzyme, dysfunctioning of fumarate hydratase, a mitochondrial enzyme that is responsible for converting fumarate to malate, leads to accumulation of fumarate. Accumulated succinate (Selak et al., 2005) and fumarate (Isaacs et al., 2005) inhibit the activity of prolyl hydroxylases responsible for creation of hypoxic conditions in cells via stabilisation of HIF-1α. Also, the loss of fumarate hydratase activity leads to low mitochondrial oxidative phosphorylation, increased glucose consumption, and lactate production by the cell in cancers cells like kidney cancer cells.

Isocitrate dehydrogenase (predominantly IDH-1) located in the mitochondrial matrix carries out the decarboxylation of isocitrate to generate α-ketoglutarate and is mutated in cancer cells (Tommasini-Ghelfi et al., 2019). Mutations in the activity of this enzyme result in the formation of an enantiomer of α-ketoglutarate, 2-hydroxyglutarate (Ward et al., 2010; Xu et al., 2011) Accumulation of 2-hydroxyglutarate

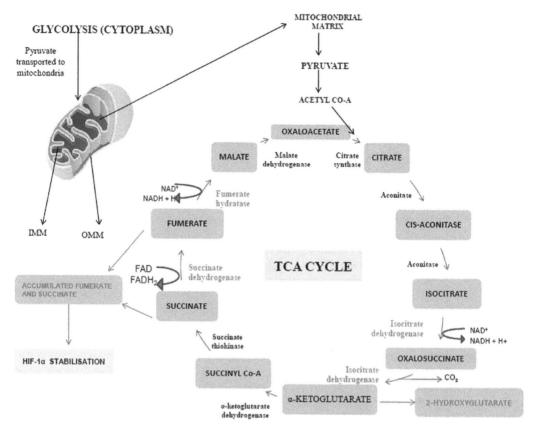

FIGURE 19.3   Figure depicts the altered enzymes in the TCA cycle in cancer cells. The enzymes highlighted in red are mutated and are responsible for driving carcinogenesis by reducing the utilisation capacity of the cell and creating hypoxic conditions.

inhibits the activity of all other enzymes in the TCA cycle (Ugele et al., 2019). It inhibits the enzymatic activity of cytochrome c oxidase complex (complex IV) and ATP synthase (complex V) in the process of oxidative phosphorylation (Fu et al., 2015). This further reduces the dependence on oxidative phosphorylation and causes the cell to switch over to aerobic glycolysis to promote the Warburg Effect (Figure 19.3).

19.4 Role of Oncogenes and Tumor Suppressor Genes in Aerobic Glycolysis

19.4.1 Hypoxia Inducible Factor

HIF as mentioned earlier drives cancer cell proliferation by creating hypoxic conditions in the cell and also by regulating glycolytic transporters and enzymes. HIF upregulates GLUT to maintain a continuous influx of glucose into the cell (Ren et al., 2008; Chen et al., 2012) to be utilised for hexokinase II. HIF-1 elevates the levels of hexokinase for the rapid conversion of glucose to glucose-6-phosphate for maintaining the high rate of glycolysis. HIF-1 in the glycolytic pathway induces the transcription of pyruvate dehydrogenase kinase 1(PDK-1) that phosphorylates pyruvate dehydrogenase complex (PDH). Phosphorylated PDH is unable to convert pyruvate to acetyl Co-A, thus inhibiting Kreb's cycle and subsequent oxidative phosphorylation (Eyassu and Angione, 2017). Instead, pyruvate is converted to lactate under the influence of elevated levels of lactate dehydrogenase to drive the Warburg Effect. HIF also upregulates the expression of MCTs for transporting lactate (Miranda-Gonçalves et al., 2016). As discussed earlier, lactate participates in angiogenesis via upregulation of VEGF where HIF-1α plays a

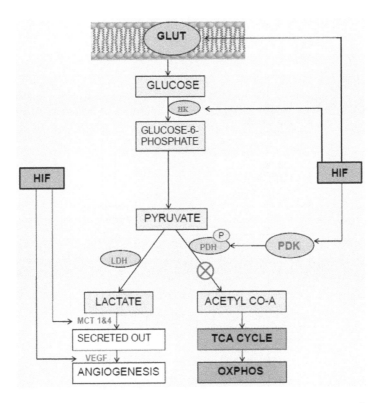

FIGURE 19.4 Role of HIF-1 in cancer cell metabolism. HIF-1 regulates expression of GLUT, hexokinase (HK), pyruvate dehydrogenase kinase (PDK), MCTs, and VEGF.

cardinal role in increasing the transcription of VEGF (Francesco et al., 2017). Thus, stabilised HIF-1 is a major contributing factor in operating the metabolic pathways of cancer (Figure 19.4).

19.4.2 Protein Kinase B

AKT/Protein kinase B play a crucial role in cancer cell metabolism that influence its survival. Hyperactivated AKT in cancer cells facilitates elevation of ATP to meet their high energy demands. AKT influences aerobic glycolysis and enhances hexokinase expressions of GLUT diverting more glucose towards glycolysis and enhances hexokinase expressions. It indirectly stimulates PFK-1 by increase in F-2, 6-BP activity by phosphorylation of PFK-2 (Deprez et al., 1997; Bartrons et al., 2018). mTOR is a downstream target of AKT. AKT via mTOR activation increases HIF-1 levels and its associated pathways that promote growth under hypoxic conditions (Zhang et al., 2018). Another oncogene, *c-Myc*, is also a downstream target of AKT which functions in the upregulation of glycolytic enzymes to increase the ability of cells to enhance glycolytic rate. *c-Myc* upregulates HK II and PDK-1 by working in synergism with HIF for conversion of glucose to G-6-P and to halt the conversion of pyruvate to acetyl Co-A, respectively (Huang, 2008). *c-Myc* is also involved in the upregulation of LDH to stimulate growth under hypoxic conditions by strengthening the conversion of pyruvate to lactate swiftly (Semenza et al., 1996; Valvona et al., 2015).

19.4.3 Tumor Protein p53

p53 is a tumor suppressor gene that encodes transcription factors that regulate metabolic pathways by influencing the key enzymes involved in oxidative phosphorylation and glycolysis. Hence, a loss in the function of *p53* contributes significantly to alterations in the metabolic pathways that function normally

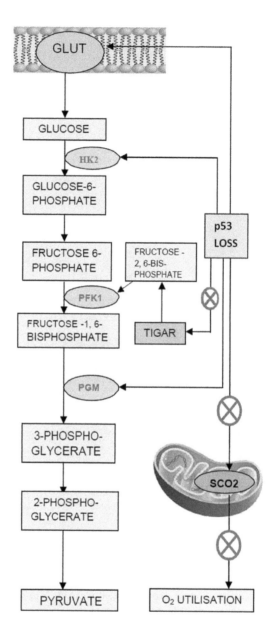

FIGURE 19.5 Role of p53 in cancer cell metabolism. Loss of p53 disrupts the functional ability of SCO2 protein and increases the expression of GLUT, phosphofructokinase 1 (PFK), and phosphoglycerate mutase (PGM).

in all cells. A decline in the levels of *p53* is a major contributor to the switch over from mitochondrial oxidative phosphorylation to aerobic glycolysis in a way that it reduces the oxygen consumption capacity of the cells.

Loss of *p53* reduces the ability of cytochrome c oxidase assembly 2 protein (SCO2) in the cytochrome c oxidase complex of mitochondria to utilise oxygen for cellular metabolism, thus initiating carcinogenesis by increasing the dependence of cells on aerobic glycolysis (Simabuco et al., 2018).

Down-regulation of *p53* influences glucose metabolism such that it upregulates enzymes in the aerobic glycolytic pathway and inhibits the metabolites from entering into Kreb's cycle. It increases the expression of GLUT by allowing more glucose molecules to enter the cell to be utilised by hexokinase for rapid conversion to glucose-6-phosphate (Ohnishi et al., 2020). Declined levels of *p53* inhibit T*P53*-induced glycolysis and apoptosis regulator (TIGAR) gene and hence contribute to upregulation of fructose-2, 6-bisphosphate to enhance the levels of PFK-1 for conversion of F-6-P to F-1, 6-BP (Ros and Schulze, 2013). Loss of *p53* also increases the expression of phosphoglycerate mutase and facilitates glycolysis to proceed unobstructed (Itahana and Itahana, 2018). Depletion of *p53* enhances rate cell invasion and metastasis by altering activity of integrins and also assisting in immune escape. *p53* loss is also associated with increased angiogenesis by elevation of VEGF (Farhang Ghahremani et al., 2013).

19.5 Pentose Phosphate Pathway

Highly proliferating cancer cells require a continuous supply of glucose to fulfil their energy demands and for biosynthesis of macromolecules to sustain new cells (Warburg, 1956). Hence, cancer cells channelise some of the glucose towards the pentose phosphate pathway/hexose monophosphate shunt to yield precursors for nucleotides and NADPH. The pentose phosphate pathway (PPP) branches from the first committed step of glycolysis in a reaction catalysed by hexokinase II that converts glucose to glucose-6-phosphate. PPP consists of two phases: oxidative phase and nonoxidative phase. The irreversible oxidative branch generates NADPH and ribose-5-phosphate; a precursor for synthesis of DNA and RNA (Kruger and von Schaewen, 2003; Patra and Hay, 2014). The reversible non-oxidative branch generates F-6-P and G-3-P that can either reform pentose phosphates or are diverted towards glycolysis (Riganti et al., 2012). The PPP enzymes are significantly elevated in cancers such that they continuously assist in the generation of these intermediates.

During the oxidative phase, glucose-6-phosphate dehydrogenase (G6PD) catalyses the rate-limiting step in PPP by converting G-6-P into 6-phosphoglucanolactone with a simultaneous generation of NADPH at this step (Cohen and Rosemeyer, 1969; Jin and Jin, 2019). G6PD is upregulated in many cancers owing to the high demands of NADPH by cancer cells (Ayala et al., 1991; Yang et al., 2019). NADPH is required in cancer cells for DNA and fatty acid synthesis and also aids in protecting them from oxidative stress by detoxification of ROS (Schafer et al., 2009). 6-phosphogluconate dehydrogenase (6PGDH) converts 6-phosphogluconate to ribulose-5-phosphate accompanied with a reduction of NADP to NADPH (Patra and Hay, 2014). 6PGDH is upregulated in cancers (Lucarelli et al., 2015). Ribulose-5-phosphate (Ru-5-P) is then isomerised to ribose-5-phosphate (R-5-P) and xylulose-5-phosphate (Xu-5-P) in a reaction catalysed ribulose-5-phosphate isomerase and ribulose-5-phosphate epimerase, respectively (Figure 19.6).

The expressions of these enzymes are elevated in cancer cells such that their reaction products: -R-5-P serve as a precursor for generation of nucleotides, which is utilised by cancer cells for DNA synthesis and Xu-5-P is implicated in the amplification of PFK-2 in glycolysis by activating its phosphatase activity (now called F-2, 6BPase). PFK-2 through its phosphatase activity upregulates F-2,6-BP leading to enhancement in the levels of PFK-1 for rapid conversion of F-6-P to F-1, 6-bisphosphate in order to amplify the rate of glycolysis (Nishimura and Uyeda, 1995; Marbaniang and Kma, 2018).

The non-oxidative phase consists of reversible reactions in which R-5-P and Xu-5-P are converted to G-3-P and seduheptulose-7-phosphate (S-7-P) by transketolase and is elevated in cancer cells. Transaldolase facilitates the conversion of G-3-P and S-7-P to erythrose-4-phosphate (E-4-P) and F-6-P. These can be used later on for synthesis of pentoses by reversing the abovementioned reactions when the requirements in cancer cells for nucleotides are high (Bouzier-Sore and Bolaños, 2015). Cancer cells derive 80% of the ribonucleotides from this non-oxidative pathway. Another transketolase mediates the reactions between Xu-5-P and E-4-P to form G-3-P and F-6-P (Riganti et al., 2012). When the cancer cells require more NADPH and ATP instead of nucleotides, G-3-P is diverted towards the glycolytic pathway, thus intensifying the Warburg Effect whereas F-6-P is converted back to G-6-P to carry forward PPP and generate more NADPH (Bouzier-Sore and Bolaños, 2015). Thus, transketolase and transaldolase concerned with the non-oxidative phase play an important role in the manipulation of cancer cell metabolic

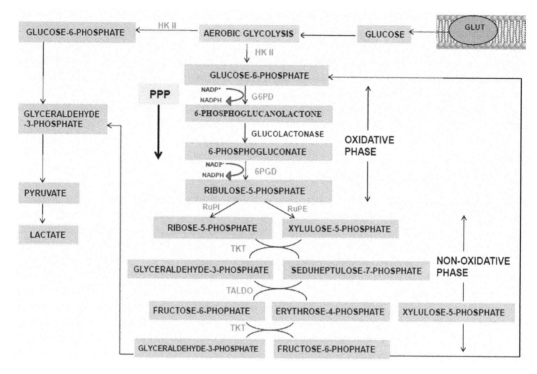

FIGURE 19.6 Deregulated pentose phosphate pathway in cancer cells. The enzymes depicted in red, HKII, G6PD, RuPI, RuPE, TKT, and TALDO, are upregulated in cancer cells.

machinery depending on its needs. Therefore, the pentose phosphate pathway is crucial for cancer cells by synthesising key intermediates required to sustain cell proliferation (Figure 19.6).

19.6 Role of Oncogenes and Tumor Suppressor Genes in Pentose Phosphate Pathway

19.6.1 Ras

Ras mutations are involved in a variety of cancers including lung and colon cancer. Oncogenic *Ras* drives more glucose molecules into the cell via GLUT. It also modulates the expressions of HK to generate more G-6-P to be diverted towards PPP (Patra et al., 2013). *Ras* mutations upregulate ribulose-5-phosphate isomerase and ribulose-5-phosphate epimerase in the non-oxidative phase increase the output of PPP (Ying et al., 2012) (Figure 19.7).

19.6.2 Nuclear Factor Erythroid 2-related Factor-2

Nrf-2 is a transcription factor that operates under conditions of oxidative stress. It normally remains associated with kelch-like erythroid cell-derived protein (Keap 1) wherein Keap 1 degrades Nrf-2 by ubiquitination. Under conditions of oxidative stress Nrf-2 dissociates from Keap-1 and translocates to the nucleus to turn on the transcription of antioxidant response element to activate antioxidant defences (Tu et al., 2019; Wei et al., 2019). It is activated by *Ras*, *c-Myc,* and AKT. Nrf-2 is also implicated in the elevation of PPP enzymes in both oxidative (G6PDH and 6PGDH) and non-oxidative pathways (TKT and TALDO) for rapid synthesis of ribose-5-phosphate and NADPH (DeNicola et al., 2011; Mitsuishi et al., 2012; Jin and Jin, 2019) (Figure 19.7).

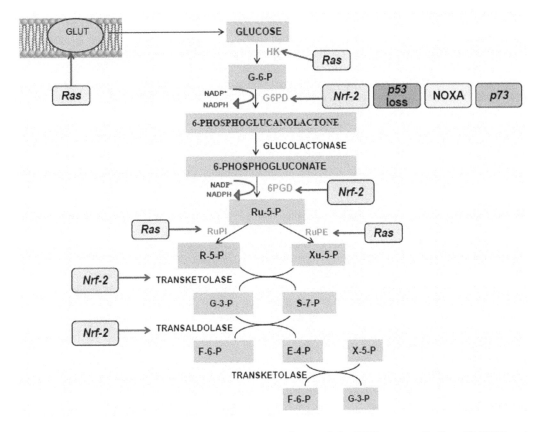

FIGURE 19.7 Role of oncogenes and loss of tumor suppressors in upregulating PPP in cancer cells. *Ras, p73*, NOXA, and Nrf-2 influence various enzymes in PPP to generate pentose phosphates and NADPH.

19.6.3 Tumor Protein *p53*

As mentioned earlier, *p53* is involved in the suppression of cancer cell proliferation. *p53* interacts with PPP enzyme glucose-6-phosphate dehydrogenase (G6PD) to reduce the output of NADPH and pentose phosphates (Yang et al., 2019). Hence, loss of *p53* evades the inhibitory effect on G6PD and causes G-6-P to enter PPP for biosynthesis of NADPH and R-5-P. Other *p53* targets, NOXA (Lowman et al., 2010) and *p73*, a *p53*-related protein (Du et al., 2013), are also implicated in the upregulation of PPP in cancer cells. NOXA normally functions as a pro-apoptotic factor, but when an abundant supply of glucose is available as in cancer cells, it supports cell survival. Both NOXA and *p73* induce the first step in PPP by converting glucose-6-phosphate to 6-phosphogluconolactone. Hence, *p53* and its related targets function in a coordinated manner to regulate the flux through PPP in cancer cells (Figure 19.7).

The altered glucose metabolism plays a crucial role in driving the carcinogenesis by fulfilling its requirements to maintain a highly proliferative state. Activated oncogenes and loss of tumor suppressors in cancer cells work in an orchestrated manner to stimulate reprogramming of the cellular metabolism in such a way that reduces the cell's dependence on oxidative phosphorylation. Instead, aerobic glycolysis is their preferred pathway over normoxic conditions that leads to excessive lactate production and accumulation and thus contribute to the Warburg Effect. Lactate favours cell migration, metastasis, immune escape, and angiogenesis to potentially trigger carcinogenesis. This transformed glycolytic/neoplastic phenotype also diverts some of the molecules towards biosynthetic pathways including PPP to yield precursors for important biomolecules and can withstand its rapid multiplication rate. Thus, this symphony of dysregulated metabolism, tumor suppressors, and oncogenes works in synergism to induce neoplastic transformations.

REFERENCES

Ayala, Antonio, Isabel Fabregat, and Alberto Machado. 1991. "The Role of NADPH in the Regulation of Glucose-6-Phosphate and 6-Phosphogluconate Dehydrogenases in Rat Adipose Tissue." *Molecular and Cellular Biochemistry*. Springer. 105(1):1–5. doi:10.1007/BF00230368. PMID:1922005.

Bartrons, Ramon, Helga Simon-Molas, Ana Rodríguez-García, Esther Castaño, Àurea Navarro-Sabaté, et al. 2018. "Fructose 2,6-Bisphosphate in Cancer Cell Metabolism." *Frontiers in Oncology*. Frontiers Media S.A. doi:10.3389/fonc.2018.00331.

Bonen, Arend. 2001. "The Expression of Lactate Transporters (MCT1 and MCT4) in Heart and Muscle." *European Journal of Applied Physiology* 86 (1). Springer Verlag: 6–11. doi:10.1007/s004210100516.

Bouzier-Sore, Anne Karine, and Juan P. Bolaños. 2015. "Uncertainties in Pentose-Phosphate Pathway Flux Assessment Underestimate Its Contribution to Neuronal Glucose Consumption: Relevance for Neurodegeneration and Aging." *Frontiers in Aging Neuroscience*. Frontiers Media S.A. doi:10.3389/fnagi.2015.00089.

Brizel, David M., Thies Schroeder, Richard L. Scher, Stefan Walenta, Robert W. Clough, Mark W. Dewhirst, and Wolfgang Mueller-Klieser. 2001. "Elevated Tumor Lactate Concentrations Predict for an Increased Risk of Metastases in Head-and-Neck Cancer." *International Journal of Radiation Oncology Biology Physics* 51 (2). Elsevier: 349–353. doi:10.1016/S0360-3016(01)01630-3.

Chen, Jin Qiang, and Jose Russo. 2012. "Dysregulation of Glucose Transport, Glycolysis, TCA Cycle and Glutaminolysis by Oncogenes and Tumor Suppressors in Cancer Cells." *Biochimica et Biophysica Acta – Reviews on Cancer*. Elsevier. doi:10.1016/j.bbcan.2012.06.004.

Cohen, P., and M. A. Rosemeyer. 1969. "Subunit Interactions of Glucose-6-Phosphate Dehydrogenase from Human Erythrocytes." *European Journal of Biochemistry* 8 (1): 8–15. John Wiley & Sons, Ltd. doi:10.1111/j.1432-1033.1969.tb00488.x.

la Cruz-López, Karen G. de, Leonardo Josué Castro-Muñoz, Diego O. Reyes-Hernández, Alejandro García-Carrancá, and Joaquín Manzo-Merino. 2019. "Lactate in the Regulation of Tumor Microenvironment and Therapeutic Approaches." *Frontiers in Oncology*. Frontiers Media S.A. doi:10.3389/fonc.2019.01143.

DeNicola, Gina M., Florian A. Karreth, Timothy J. Humpton, Aarthi Gopinathan, Cong Wei, Kristopher Frese, Dipti Mangal, et al., 2011. "Oncogene-Induced Nrf2 Transcription Promotes ROS Detoxification and Tumorigenesis." doi:10.1038/nature10189.

Deprez, Johan, Didier Vertommen, Dario R. Alessi, Louis Hue, and Mark H. Rider. 1997. "Phosphorylation and Activation of Heart 6-Phosphofructo-2-Kinase by Protein Kinase B and Other Protein Kinases of the Insulin Signaling Cascades." *Journal of Biological Chemistry* 272 (28). J Biol Chem: 17269–17275. doi:10.1074/jbc.272.28.17269.

DeWaal, Dannielle, Veronique Nogueira, Alexander R. Terry, Krushna C. Patra, Sang Min Jeon, Grace Guzman, et al. 2018. "Hexokinase-2 Depletion Inhibits Glycolysis and Induces Oxidative Phosphorylation in Hepatocellular Carcinoma and Sensitizes to Metformin." *Nature Communications* 9 (1). Nature Publishing Group: 1–14. doi:10.1038/s41467-017-02733-4.

Dhup, Suveera, Rajesh Kumar Dadhich, Paolo Ettore Porporato, and Pierre Sonveaux. 2012. "Multiple Biological Activities of Lactic Acid in Cancer: Influences on Tumor Growth,Angiogenesis and Metastasis." *Current Pharmaceutical Design* 18 (10). Bentham Science Publishers Ltd.: 1319–1330. doi:10.2174/138161212799504902.

Du, Wenjing, Peng Jiang, Anthony Mancuso, Aaron Stonestrom, Michael D. Brewer, Andy J. Minn, et al. 2013. "TAp73 Enhances the Pentose Phosphate Pathway and Supports Cell Proliferation." *Nature Cell Biology* 15 (8). Nature Publishing Group: 991–1000. doi:10.1038/ncb2789.

Eyassu, Filmon, and Claudio Angione. 2017. "Modelling Pyruvate Dehydrogenase under Hypoxia and Its Role in Cancer Metabolism." *Royal Society Open Science* 4 (10). Royal Society Publishing. doi:10.1098/rsos.170360.

Fu, Xudong, Randall M. Chin, Laurent Vergnes, Heejun Hwang, Gang Deng, Yanpeng Xing, et al., 2015. "2-Hydroxyglutarate Inhibits ATP Synthase and MTOR Signaling." *Cell Metabolism* 22 (3). Cell Press: 508–515. doi:10.1016/j.cmet.2015.06.009.

Farhang Ghahremani, M., S. Goossens, D. Nittner, X. Bisteau, S. Bartunkova, A. Zwolinska, et al., 2013. "P53 Promotes VEGF Expression and Angiogenesis in the Absence of an Intact P21-Rb Pathway." *Cell Death and Differentiation* 20 (7). Nature Publishing Group: 888–897. doi:10.1038/cdd.2013.12.

Francesco, Ernestina M. De, Andrew H. Sims, Marcello Maggiolini, Federica Sotgia, Michael P. Lisanti, and Robert B. Clarke. 2017. "GPER Mediates the Angiocrine Actions Induced by IGF1 through the HIF-1α/VEGF Pathway in the Breast Tumor Microenvironment." *Breast Cancer Research: BCR* 19 (1). BioMed Central: 129. doi:10.1186/s13058-017-0923-5.

Haber, R. S., A. Rathan, K. R. Weiser, A. Pritsker, et al. 1998. "GLUT1 Glucose Transporter Expression in Colorectal Carcinoma: A Marker for Poor Prognosis." *Wiley Online Library*. Accessed May 31. https://acsjournals.onlinelibrary.wiley.com/doi/abs/10.1002/(SICI)1097-0142(19980701)83:1%3C34::AID-CNCR5%3E3.0.CO;2-E.

Halestrap, Andrew P. 2012. "The Monocarboxylate Transporter Family-Structure and Functional Characterization." *IUBMB Life*. John Wiley & Sons, Ltd. doi:10.1002/iub.573.

Heiden, Matthew G. Vander, Lewis C. Cantley, and Craig B. Thompson. 2009. "Understanding the Warburg Effect: The Metabolic Requirements of Cell Proliferation." *Science*. Science. doi:10.1126/science.1160809.

Hu, Xun, Ming Chao, and Hao Wu. 2017. "Central Role of Lactate and Proton in Cancer Cell Resistance to Glucose Deprivation and Its Clinical Translation." *Signal Transduction and Targeted Therapy* 2 (1). Springer Nature: 1–8. doi:10.1038/sigtrans.2016.47.

Huang, L. E. 2008. "Carrot and Stick: HIF-α Engages c-Myc in Hypoxic Adaptation." *Cell Death and Differentiation* 15, 672–677 doi:10.1038/sj.cdd.4402302.

Huang, Ruixue, and Ping-Kun Zhou. 2020. "HIF-1 Signaling: A Key Orchestrator of Cancer Radioresistance." *Radiation Medicine and Protection* 1 (1). Elsevier BV: 7–14. doi:10.1016/j.radmp.2020.01.006.

Isaacs, Jennifer S., Jin Jung Yun, David R. Mole, Sunmin Lee, Carlos Torres-Cabala, Yuen Li Chung, et al., 2005. "HIF Overexpression Correlates with Biallelic Loss of Fumarate Hydratase in Renal Cancer: Novel Role of Fumarate in Regulation of HIF Stability." *Cancer Cell* 8 (2). Cell Press: 143–153. doi:10.1016/j.ccr.2005.06.017.

Itahana, Yoko, and Koji Itahana. 2018. "Emerging Roles of P53 Family Members in Glucose Metabolism." *International Journal of Molecular Sciences*. MDPI AG. doi:10.3390/ijms19030776.

Jin, Lin, and Yanhong Zhou. 2019. "Crucial Role of the Pentose Phosphate Pathway in Malignant Tumors (Review)." *Oncology Letters* 17 (5). Spandidos Publications: 4213–4221. doi:10.3892/ol.2019.10112.

Jun, Young Jin, Se Min Jang, Hu Lin Han, Kang Hong Lee, Ki Seok Jang, and Seung Sam Paik. 2011. "Clinicopathologic Significance of GULT1 Expression and Its Correlation with Apaf-1 in Colorectal Adenocarcinomas." *World Journal of Gastroenterology* 17 (14). Baishideng Publishing Group Co: 1866–1873. doi:10.3748/wjg.v17.i14.1866.

Kruger, Nicholas J. and Antje Von Schaewen. 2003. "The Oxidative Pentose Phosphate Pathway: Structure and Organisation." *Current Opinion in Plant Biology*. Elsevier Ltd. doi:10.1016/S1369-5266(03)00039-6.

Kumar, V. B. Sameer, R. I. Viji, M. S. Kiran, and P. R. Sudhakaran. 2007. "Endothelial Cell Response to Lactate: Implication of PAR Modification of VEGF." *Journal of Cellular Physiology* 211 (2). John Wiley & Sons, Ltd: 477–485. doi:10.1002/jcp.20955.

Le, Anne, Charles R. Cooper, Arvin M. Gouw, Ramani Dinavahi, Anirban Maitra, Lorraine M. Deck, et al., 2010. "Inhibition of Lactate Dehydrogenase A Induces Oxidative Stress and Inhibits Tumor Progression." *Proceedings of the National Academy of Sciences of the United States of America* 107 (5). National Academy of Sciences: 2037–2042. doi:10.1073/pnas.0914433107.

Lowman, Xazmin H., Maureen A. McDonnell, Ashley Kosloske, Oludare A. Odumade, Christopher Jenness, Christine B. Karim, et al., 2010. "The Proapoptotic Function of Noxa in Human Leukemia Cells Is Regulated by the Kinase Cdk5 and by Glucose." *Molecular Cell* 40 (5). Cell Press: 823–833. doi:10.1016/j.molcel.2010.11.035.

Lu, Wei, Yang Cao, Yijian Zhang, Sheng Li, Jian Gao, Xu An Wang, et al., 2016. "Up-Regulation of PKM2 Promote Malignancy and Related to Adverse Prognostic Risk Factor in Human Gallbladder Cancer." *Scientific Reports* 6 (June). Nature Publishing Group. doi:10.1038/srep26351.

Lucarelli, Giuseppe, Vanessa Galleggiante, Monica Rutigliano, Francesca Sanguedolce, Simona Cagiano, Pantaleo Bufo, et al., 2015. "Metabolomic Profile of Glycolysis and the Pentose Phosphate Pathway Identifies the Central Role of Glucose-6-Phosphate Dehydrogenase in Clear Cell-Renal Cell Carcinoma." *Oncotarget* 6 (15). Impact Journals LLC: 13371–86. doi:10.18632/oncotarget.3823.

Lu, Wei, Yang Cao, Yijian Zhang, Sheng Li, Jian Gao, Xu An Wang, et al., 2016. "Up-Regulation of PKM2 Promote Malignancy and Related to Adverse Prognostic Risk Factor in Human Gallbladder Cancer." *Scientific Reports* 6 (June). Nature Publishing Group. doi:10.1038/srep26351.

Marbaniang, Casterland and Lakhan Kma. 2018. "Dysregulation of Glucose Metabolism by Oncogenes and Tumor Suppressors in Cancer Cells." *Asian Pacific Journal of Cancer Prevention*. Asian Pacific Organization for Cancer Prevention. doi:10.22034/APJCP.2018.19.9.2377.

Miranda-Gonçalves, Vera, Sara Granja, Olga Martinho, Mrinalini Honavar, Marta Pojo, Bruno M. Costa, et al., 2016. "Hypoxia-Mediated Upregulation of MCT1 Expression Supports the Glycolytic Phenotype of Glioblastomas." *Oncotarget* 7 (29). Impact Journals LLC: 46335–46353. doi:10.18632/oncotarget.10114.

Mitsuishi, Yoichiro, Keiko Taguchi, Yukie Kawatani, Tatsuhiro Shibata, Toshihiro Nukiwa, Hiroyuki Aburatani, et al., 2012. "Nrf2 Redirects Glucose and Glutamine into Anabolic Pathways in Metabolic Reprogramming." *Cancer Cell* 22 (1). Cancer Cell: 66–79. doi:10.1016/j.ccr.2012.05.016.

Movahed, Zahra Ghanbari, Mohsen Rastegari-Pouyani, Mohammad Hossein Mohammadi, and Kamran Mansouri. 2019. "Cancer Cells Change Their Glucose Metabolism to Overcome Increased ROS: One Step from Cancer Cell to Cancer Stem Cell?" *Biomedicine and Pharmacotherapy*. Elsevier Masson SAS. doi:10.1016/j.biopha.2019.108690.

Moosavi, Behrooz, Edward A. Berry, Xiao Lei Zhu, Wen Chao Yang, and Guang Fu Yang. 2019. "The Assembly of Succinate Dehydrogenase: A Key Enzyme in Bioenergetics." *Cellular and Molecular Life Sciences*. Birkhauser Verlag AG. doi:10.1007/s00018-019-03200-7.

Morrot, Alexandre, Leonardo Marques da Fonseca, Eduardo J. Salustiano, Luciana Boffoni Gentile, Luciana Conde, Alessandra Almeida Filardy, et al. 2018. "Metabolic Symbiosis and Immunomodulation: How Tumor Cell-Derived Lactate May Disturb Innate and Adaptive Immune Responses." *Frontiers in Oncology*. Frontiers Media S.A. doi:10.3389/fonc.2018.00081.

Mucaj, Vera, Jessica E.S. Shay, and M. Celeste Simon. 2012. "Effects of Hypoxia and HIFs on Cancer Metabolism." *International Journal of Hematology* 95 (5): 464–70. doi:10.1007/s12185-012-1070-5.

Nagarajan, Arvindhan, Parmanand Malvi, and Narendra Wajapeyee. 2016. "Oncogene-Directed Alterations in Cancer Cell Metabolism." *Trends in Cancer*. Cell Press. doi:10.1016/j.trecan.2016.06.002.

Nishimura, Motonobu, and Kosaku Uyeda. 1995. "Purification and Characterization of a Novel Xylulose 5-Phosphate-Activated Protein Phosphatase Catalyzing Dephosphorylation of Fructose-6-Phosphate,2-Kinase:Fructose-2,6-Bisphosphatase." *Journal of Biological Chemistry* 270 (44). American Society for Biochemistry and Molecular Biology Inc.: 26341–46. doi:10.1074/jbc.270.44.26341.

Ohnishi, Tomokazu, Joji Kusuyama, Kenjiro Bandow, and Tetsuya Matsuguchi. 2020. "Glut1 Expression Is Increased by P53 Reduction to Switch Metabolism to Glycolysis during Osteoblast Differentiation." *Biochemical Journal* 477 (10). Portland Press Ltd: 1795–1811. doi:10.1042/BCJ20190888.

Patra, Krushna C., and Nissim Hay. 2014. "The Pentose Phosphate Pathway and Cancer." *Trends in Biochemical Sciences*. Elsevier Ltd. doi:10.1016/j.tibs.2014.06.005.

Patra, Krushna C., Qi Wang, Prashanth T. Bhaskar, Luke Miller, Zebin Wang, Will Wheaton, et al., 2013. "Hexokinase 2 Is Required for Tumor Initiation and Maintenance and Its Systemic Deletion Is Therapeutic in Mouse Models of Cancer." *Cancer Cell* 24 (2). Cancer Cell: 213–28. doi:10.1016/j.ccr.2013.06.014.

Racker, E. 1972. "Bioenergetics and the Problem of Tumor Growth: An Understanding of the Mechanism of the Generation and Control of Biological Energy May Shed Light on the Problem of Tumor Growth." *American Scientist* 60(1) 56–63. Sigma Xi. https://pubmed.ncbi.nlm.nih.gov/4332766/.

Rempel, Annette, Saroj P. Mathupala, Constance A. Griffin, Anita L. Hawkins, and Peter L. Pedersen. 1996. "Glucose Catabolism in Cancer Cells: Amplification of the Gene Encoding Type II Hexokinase." *Cancer Research* 56 (11).

Ren, Bu Fang, Lian Fu Deng, Jun Wang, Ya Ping Zhu, Li Wei, and Qi Zhou. 2008. "Hypoxia Regulation of Facilitated Glucose Transporter-1 and Glucose Transporter-3 in Mouse Chondrocytes Mediated by HIF-1α." *Joint Bone Spine* 75 (2). Joint Bone Spine: 176–181. doi:10.1016/j.jbspin.2007.05.012.

Riganti, Chiara, Elena Gazzano, Manuela Polimeni, Elisabetta Aldieri, and Dario Ghigo. 2012. "The Pentose Phosphate Pathway: An Antioxidant Defense and a Crossroad in Tumor Cell Fate." *Free Radical Biology and Medicine*. Pergamon. doi:10.1016/j.freeradbiomed.2012.05.006.

Ros, Susana, and Almut Schulze. 2013. "Balancing Glycolytic Flux: The Role of 6-Phosphofructo-2-Kinase/Fructose 2,6-Bisphosphatases in Cancer Metabolism." *Cancer & Metabolism* 1 (1). Springer Science and Business Media LLC. doi:10.1186/2049-3002-1-8.

San-Millán, Iñigo, and George A. Brooks. 2017. "Reexamining Cancer Metabolism: Lactate Production for Carcinogenesis Could Be the Purpose and Explanation of the Warburg Effect." *Carcinogenesis*. Oxford University Press. doi:10.1093/carcin/bgw127.

Santos, N., Pereira-Nunes, A., Baltazar, F. and Granja, S. 2019. "Lactate As A Regulator of Cancer Inflammation and Immunity." Immunometabolism, 1(2).

Schafer, Zachary T., Alexandra R. Grassian, Loling Song, Zhenyang Jiang, Zachary Gerhart-Hines, Hanna Y. Irie, et al. 2009. "Antioxidant and Oncogene Rescue of Metabolic Defects Caused by Loss of Matrix Attachment." *Nature* 461 (7260). Nature Publishing Group: 109–13. doi:10.1038/nature08268.

Schek, Nancy, Bruce Lee Hall, and Olivera J. Finn. 1988. "Increased Glyceraldehyde-3-Phosphate Dehydrogenase Gene Expression in Human Pancreatic Adenocarcinoma." *Cancer Research* 48 (22).

Selak, Mary A., Sean M. Armour, Elaine D. MacKenzie, Houda Boulahbel, David G. Watson, Kyle D. Mansfield, et al. 2005. "Succinate Links TCA Cycle Dysfunction to Oncogenesis by Inhibiting HIF-α Prolyl Hydroxylase." *Cancer Cell* 7 (1). Cell Press: 77–85. doi:10.1016/j.ccr.2004.11.022.

Semenza, Gregg L., Bing Hua Jiang, Sandra W. Leung, Rosa Passantino, Jean Paul Concordat, Pascal Maire, and Agata Giallongo. 1996. "Hypoxia Response Elements in the Aldolase A, Enolase 1, and Lactate Dehydrogenase a Gene Promoters Contain Essential Binding Sites for Hypoxia-Inducible Factor 1." *Journal of Biological Chemistry* 271 (51). American Society for Biochemistry and Molecular Biology Inc.: 32529–37. doi:10.1074/jbc.271.51.32529.

Simabuco, Fernando M., Mirian G. Morale, Isadora C. B. Pavan, Ana P. Morelli, Fernando R. Silva, and Rodrigo E. Tamura. 2018. "P53 and Metabolism: From Mechanism to Therapeutics." *Oncotarget*. Impact Journals LLC. doi:10.18632/oncotarget.25267.

Singh, Davinder, Rohit Arora, Pardeep Kaur, Balbir Singh, Rahul Mannan, and Saroj Arora. 2017. "Overexpression of Hypoxia-Inducible Factor and Metabolic Pathways: Possible Targets of Cancer." *Cell and Bioscience*. BioMed Central Ltd. doi:10.1186/s13578-017-0190-2.

Strowitzki, Moritz, Eoin Cummins, and Cormac Taylor. 2019. "Protein Hydroxylation by Hypoxia-Inducible Factor (HIF) Hydroxylases: Unique or Ubiquitous?" *Cells* 8 (5). MDPI AG: 384. doi:10.3390/cells8050384.

Tameemi, Wafaa Al, Tina P. Dale, Rakad M. Kh Al-Jumaily, and Nicholas R. Forsyth. 2019. "Hypoxia-Modified Cancer Cell Metabolism." *Frontiers in Cell and Developmental Biology* 7 (January). Frontiers Media SA: 4. doi:10.3389/fcell.2019.00004.

Tanner, Lukas Bahati, Alexander G. Goglia, Monica H. Wei, Talen Sehgal, Lance R. Parsons, Junyoung O. Park, et al. 2018. "Four Key Steps Control Glycolytic Flux in Mammalian Cells." *Cell Systems* 7 (1). Cell Press: 49–62.e8. doi:10.1016/j.cels.2018.06.003.

Tarrado-Castellarnau, Míriam, Santiago Diaz-Moralli, Ibrahim H. Polat, Rebeca Sanz-Pamplona, Cristina Alenda, Víctor Moreno, et al. 2017. "Glyceraldehyde-3-Phosphate Dehydrogenase Is Overexpressed in Colorectal Cancer Onset." *Translational Medicine Communications* 2 (1). Springer Science and Business Media LLC. doi:10.1186/s41231-017-0015-7.

Tommasini-Ghelfi, Serena, Kevin Murnan, Fotini M. Kouri, Akanksha S. Mahajan, Jasmine L. May, and Alexander H. Stegh. 2019. "Cancer-Associated Mutation and beyond: The Emerging Biology of Isocitrate Dehydrogenases in Human Disease." *Science Advances* 5 (5). American Association for the Advancement of Science: eaaw4543. doi:10.1126/sciadv.aaw4543.

Tu, Wenjun, Hong Wang, Song Li, Qiang Liu, and Hong Sha. 2019. "The Anti-Inflammatory and Anti-Oxidant Mechanisms of the Keap1/Nrf2/ARE Signaling Pathway in Chronic Diseases." *Aging and Disease*. International Society on Aging and Disease. doi:10.14336/AD.2018.0513.

Ugele, Ines, Zugey Elizabeth Cárdenas Conejo, Kathrin Hammon, Monika Wehrstein, Christina Bruss, et al., 2019. "D-2-Hydroxyglutarate and L-2-Hydroxyglutarate Inhibit IL-12 Secretion by Human Monocyte-Derived Dendritic Cells." *International Journal of Molecular Sciences* 20 (3). MDPI AG. doi:10.3390/ijms20030742.

Valvona, Cara J., Helen L. Fillmore, Peter B. Nunn, and Geoffrey J. Pilkington. 2016. "The Regulation and Function of Lactate Dehydrogenase A: Therapeutic Potential in Brain Tumor." *Brain Pathology*. Blackwell Publishing Ltd. doi:10.1111/bpa.12299.

Warburg, O. 1956. "On respiratory impairment in cancer cells." *Science*, 124.

Warburg, Otto, Franz Wind, and Erwin Negelein. 1927. "The Metabolism of Tumors in the Body." *Journal of General Physiology* 8 (6). The Rockefeller University Press: 519–30. doi:10.1085/jgp.8.6.519.

Ward, Patrick S., Jay Patel, David R. Wise, Omar Abdel-Wahab, Bryson D. Bennett, Hilary A. Coller, et al., 2010. "The Common Feature of Leukemia-Associated IDH1 and IDH2 Mutations Is a Neomorphic Enzyme Activity Converting α-Ketoglutarate to 2-Hydroxyglutarate." *Cancer Cell* 17 (3). Cell Press: 225–34. doi:10.1016/j.ccr.2010.01.020.

Wei, Ran, Mayu Enaka, and Yasuteru Muragaki. 2019. "Activation of KEAP1/NRF2/P62 Signaling Alleviates High Phosphate-Induced Calcification of Vascular Smooth Muscle Cells by Suppressing Reactive Oxygen Species Production." *Scientific Reports* 9 (1). Nature Publishing Group: 1–13. doi:10.1038/s41598-019-46824-2.

Xu, Wei, Hui Yang, Ying Liu, Ying Yang, Ping Wang, Se Hee Kim, et al., 2011. "Oncometabolite 2-Hydroxyglutarate Is a Competitive Inhibitor of α-Ketoglutarate-Dependent Dioxygenases." *Cancer Cell* 19 (1). Cancer Cell: 17–30. doi:10.1016/j.ccr.2010.12.014.

Yaku, Keisuke, Keisuke Okabe, Keisuke Hikosaka, and Takashi Nakagawa. 2018. "NAD Metabolism in Cancer Therapeutics." *Frontiers in Oncology*. Frontiers Media S.A. doi:10.3389/fonc.2018.00622.

Yang, Hung-Chi, Yi-Hsuan Wu, Wei-Chen Yen, Hui-Ya Liu, Tsong-Long Hwang, Arnold Stern, et al. 2019. "Cells The Redox Role of G6PD in Cell Growth, Cell Death, and Cancer." *Cells* 8. doi:10.3390/cells8091055.

Ying, Haoqiang, Alec C. Kimmelman, Costas A. Lyssiotis, Sujun Hua, Gerald C. Chu, Eliot Fletcher-Sananikone, et al. 2012. "Oncogenic Kras Maintains Pancreatic Tumors through Regulation of Anabolic Glucose Metabolism." *Cell* 149 (3). Elsevier B.V.: 656–70. doi:10.1016/j.cell.2012.01.058.

Zancan, Patricia, Monica M. Marinho-Carvalho, Joana Faber-Barata, João M.M. Dellias, and Mauro Sola-Penna. 2008. "ATP and Fructose-2,6-Bisphosphate Regulate Skeletal Muscle 6-Phosphofructo-1-Kinase by Altering Its Quaternary Structure." *IUBMB Life* 60 (8). IUBMB Life: 526–33. doi:10.1002/iub.58.

Zhang, Zhen, Li Yao, Jinhua Yang, Zhenkang Wang, and Gang Du. 2018. "PI3K/Akt and HIF-1 Signaling Pathway in Hypoxia-Ischemia (Review)." *Molecular Medicine Reports*. Spandidos Publications. doi:10.3892/mmr.2018.9375.

20

Transthyretin Cardiac Amyloidosis: Recent Advances in Diagnosis and Treatment

Shreya Ghosh and Ashwani Kumar Thakur
Department of Biological Sciences and Bioengineering, Mehta Family Center for Engineering in Medicine, Indian Institute of Technology, Kanpur, India

Dibbendhu Khanra
Heart and Lung Centre, New Cross Hospital, Royal Wolverhampton NHS Trust, UK

Abbreviations

ATTR-CM	transthyretin amyloid cardiomyopathy
TTR	transthyretin
BNP	brain natriuretic peptide
NT-BNP	N-terminal brain natriuretic peptide
ISA	international society for amyloidosis
M	million
ATTR	amyloidogenic transthyretin
ATTRwt	wild-type transthyretin
ATTRmt	mutant transthyretin
US	United States
kDa	kilo dalton
EFSR	ejection fraction strain rate
NMR	nuclear magnetic resonance
β	beta
Tc	technetium
PYP	pyrophosphate
DPD	3,3-diphosphono-1,2-propanodicarboxylic acid
HMDP	hydroxymethylene diphosphonate
OLT	orthotopic liver transplantation
TUDCA	tauro-ursodeoxycholic acid
EGCG	epigallocatechin-3-gallate.

20.1 Introduction

Proteins undergo folding to attain functionally active native conformation. Various factors like stress, aging, mutations, and defects in molecular chaperones often perturb the protein folding process and thus function. Subsequently, some proteins get misfolded and tend to deposit as amyloid fibrils in various tissues and organs. About 42 proteins in humans are known to be involved in amyloid formation (Buxbaum, Dispenzieri et al., 2020). Amyloid fibrillar deposits can damage several organs especially kidney, nervous system, and heart in the majority of cases. Most amyloid patients eventually suffer from cardiac distress as the amyloid disease progresses. Clinicians often prefer assessment of cardiac

DOI: 10.1201/9781003220404-22

biomarkers to know the degree of heart involvement. But these biomarkers are commonly altered in any heart failure conditions like cardiovascular diseases, ischemic heart diseases, and many others (Ghantous, Kamareddine et al., 2020). Hence, the majority of cases are often misdiagnosed as age-related problems.

According to guidelines laid down by the International Society for Amyloidosis (ISA), cardiac amyloidosis can be classified either as systemic or localised. Systemic amyloidosis is characterised by the involvement of several organs, as represented in Table 20.1. In localised form, amyloid deposition is mainly restricted to the organ producing the amyloid precursor protein, as represented in Table 20.2. Monoclonal immunoglobulin light chain (primarily kappa and lambda) and transthyretin protein mainly drives the systemic form, whereas medin, atrial natriuretic peptide, and lactadherin drives the localised form (Guan, Mishra et al., 2012). Among these, transthyretin-associated cardiac amyloidosis is generally an unexplored cause of heart failure in aged individuals. Various known point mutations trigger the dissociation of monomers from the biologically active tetramer of transthyretin, thereby initiating systemic amyloid formation through a complex aggregation pathway. Wild-type form of the protein also undergoes slow aggregation and causes the onset of symptoms in aged individuals, especially octagenerians (Ritts, Cornell et al., 2017; Bhogal, Ladia et al., 2018). Various TTR variants are associated with cardiac dysfunction as shown in Table 20.3 (Connors, Lim et al., 2003). However, Val30Met, Val122Ile, and Thr60Ala are the most predominant transthyretin variants associated with cardiac phenotype (Kittleson, Maurer et al., 2020). Prevalence rate of ATTR amyloidosis in the recent years is reported to increase across the world. Val122Ile is the most prevalent transthyretin mutation associated with cardiac phenotype among

TABLE 20.1

List of Systemic Amyloid Disease and its Associated Amyloid Precursor Proteins (Benson, Buxbaum et al., 2020)

Disease	Precursor Proteins	Target organs
Primary amyloidosis	Immunoglobulin light and heavy chain	All organs except CNS
Secondary amyloidosis	Serum amyloid A	All organs except CNS
Familial and Senile systemic amyloidosis	Transthyretin (variant and wild type)	Peripheral nervous system, ANS, heart,eye, leptomen, kidney, heart, ligaments, and tenosynovium
Haemodialysis-related amyloidosis	β_2 microglobulin (variant and wild type)	Musculoskeleton system and ANS
Apo-lipoprotein associated amyloidosis	Plasma apo-lipoproteins (Apo AI [variants], Apo AII [variants] and Apo AIV [wild-type])	Heart, liver, kidney, PNS, testis, larynx, skin, and kidney medulla
Gelsolin-derived hereditary amyloidosis (Finnish amyloidosis)	Gelsolin (variants)	Kidney, PNS, and cornea
Hereditary apolipoprotein CII amyloidosis	Apolipoprotein CII (variants)	Kidney
Hereditary apolipoprotein CIII amyloidosis	Apolipoprotein CIII (variants)	Kidney
Hereditary fibrinogen Aα-chain amyloidosis	Fibrinogen Aα-chain variants	Kidney primarily
Leukocyte chemotactic factor 2 amyloidosis	Leukocyte chemotactic factor-2	Kidney primarily
Cerebral amyloid angiopathy	Cystasin C (variants)	CNS, PNS, and Skin
Familial British Dementia	BriPP (variants)	CNS
Prions disease	Prion protein (variants)	PNS

TABLE 20.2

List of Localised Amyloid Disease and its Associated Amyloid Precursor Proteins (Benson, Buxbaum et al., 2020)

Disease	Precursor Proteins	Target organs
Familial Danish dementia	Danish amyloid precursor protein/DanPP (variants)	CNS
Alzheimer's disease	Amyloid β precursor protein (variants and wild type)	CNS
Parkinson's disease	α-Synuclein	CNS
Alzheimer's disease	Tau protein	CNS
Prion's disease	Prion proteins (wild type and variants)	CNS
Hungtington's disease	Hungtingtin protein	CNS
Medullary thyroid carcinoma (MTC)	Calcitonin	Thyroid
Type 2 diabetes mellitus	Islet amyloid polypeptide (IAPP)	Islet of langerhans, Insulinomas
Isolated atrial amyloidosis (IAA)	Atrial natriuretic peptide	Cardiac atria
Prolactinomas	Prolactin	Pitutitary prolactinomas, aging pituitary
Insulin-derived amyloidosis associated with diabetes mellitus	Insulin	Pancreas, subcutaneous skin tumours, amyloidomas near injection site (insulin ball)
Chronic lung disease	Lung surfactant protein	Lung
Hypotrichosis simplex of the scalp (HSS)	Corneodesmosin (CDSN)	Cornified epithelia, hair follicles
Aortic medial amyloidosis (AMA)	Lactadherin (specifically medin)	Senile aortic media
Lattice corneal dystrophy	Keratoepithelin	Cornea
Familial subepithelial corneal amyloidosis	Lactoferrin	Cornea
Calcifying epithelial Odontogenic or Pindborg tumour (CEOT)	Odontogenic ameloblast-associated protein (OAAP)	Odontogenic tumours
Senile vesicle seminalis amyloidosis	Semenogelin I (sgI)	Seminal vesicles
Enfurvitide-associated amyloidosis	Enfurvitide	Site of Enfurvitide injection
Tumour-associated amyloidosis	Cathepsin K	Associated with local tumour
Age-related venous amyloidosis	EGF-containing fibulin-like extracellular matrix protein 1 (EFEMP1)	Aging-associated portal veins

African Americans with an allele frequency of 0.0173 (Jacobson, Alexander et al., 2015). A nine-year retrospective study carried out in Japan reported 70.3 to 86.1 ATTRwt cases and 50 to 61 ATTRmt cases per million of adult heart failure patients, respectively (Winburn, Ishii et al., 2019). In a US population-based study, the prevalence of ATTRwt was estimated as 1014 per 1 million general population. Similarly, ATTRmt prevalence was estimated as 89/1M population in Portugal, 19/1M population in Cyprus, and 11/1M population in Sweden. Out of all the variants, the prevalence of Val122Ile mutation in aged individuals was highest in the United States (1293/1M) and West Africa (1059/1M) (Grogan, Siepen et al., 2017). Recent developments in both diagnostic techniques and therapeutic interventions for ATTR cardiac amyloidosis have instilled the need for understanding the pathophysiology of this disease. Keeping this notion in mind, researchers in collaboration with clinicians across the world have already started taking initiatives to untangle the knots of this disease pathology.

TABLE 20.3

List of TTR Variants Associated with Cardiac Phenotype (Connors, Lim et al., 2003)

Mutant variants	Phenotype	Geographic focus
Cys10Arg	Autonomic neuropathy, eye, heart, polyneuropathy	USA
Asp18Asn	Heart	USA
Val120Ile	Carpal tunnel syndrome, heart	Germany, USA
Ser23Asn	Eye, heart, polyneuropathy	USA
Pro24Ser	Carpal tunnel syndrome, heart, polyneuropathy	USA
Ala25Ser	Heart, polyneuropathy	USA
Val30Ala	Autonomic neuropathy, heart	USA
Val30Leu	Autonomic neuropathy, heart, kidney, polyneuropathy	Japan, USA
Phe33Cys	Carpal tunnel syndrome, eye, kidney, heart	USA
Arg34Thr	Heart, polyneuropathy	Italy
Lys35Asn	Autonomic neuropathy, heart, polyneuropathy	France
Glu42Asp	Heart	France
Ala45Asp	Heart, polyneuropathy	Ireland, Italy, USA
Ala45Ser	Heart	Sweden
Ala45Thr	Heart	Ireland, Italy, USA
Gly47Ala	Autonomic neuropathy, heart, polyneuropathy	Germany, Italy, France
Gly47Glu	Heart, kidney, polyneuropathy	Germany, Italy
Thr49Ile	Heart, polyneuropathy	Japan
Thr49Pro	Heart	USA
Ser50Arg	Autonomic neuropathy, heart, polyneuropathy	France, Italy, Japan
Ser50Ile	Autonomic neuropathy, heart, polyneuropathy	Japan
Glu51Gly	Heart	USA
Ser52Pro	Autonomic neuropathy, heart, kidney, polyneuropathy	England
Glu54Lys	Autonomic neuropathy, heart, polyneuropathy	Japan
His56Arg	Heart	USA
Leu58His	Carpal tunnel syndrome, heart	Germany, USA
Thr59Lys	Autonomic neuropathy, heart, polyneuropathy	Italy, USA
Thr60Ala	Carpal tunnel syndrome, heart, polyneuropathy	Australia, Germany, Ireland, UK, USA, Japan
Phe64Leu	Carpal tunnel syndrome, heart, polyneuropathy	Italy, USA
Ile68Leu	Heart	Germany, USA
Tyr69Ile	Carpal tunnel syndrome, heart	Japan
Ser77Tyr	Heart, kidney, polyneuropathy	France, Germany, USA
Ala81Thr	Heart	USA
Ile84Thr	Autonomic neuropathy, heart, polyneuropathy	Germany, UK
Gln92Lys	Heart	Japan
Ala97Gly	Heart, polyneuropathy	Japan
Ala97Ser	Heart, polyneuropathy	China, France, Taiwan
Arg103Ser	Heart	USA
Ile107Met	Heart, polyneuropathy	Germany
Ile107Val	Carpal tunnel syndrome, heart, polyneuropathy	Germany, USA, Japan
Leu111Met	Carpal tunnel syndrome, heart	Denmark
Ser112Ile	Heart, polyneuropathy	Italy
Ala120Ser	Autonomic neuropathy, heart, polyneuropathy	Caribbean
Val122Ile	Heart	Africa, Portugal, USA

20.2 Molecular Mechanism Driving Transthyretin Amyloidogenesis

Human transthyretin is a 55 kDa protein, primarily responsible for the systemic transport of retinol binding protein and thyroxin hormone (Buxbaum, Reixach et al., 2009). Both the variant and wild-type form of this protein can drive the aggregation resulting in subsequent amyloid deposition and organ dysfunction. More than 130 mutations triggering amyloid formation have been identified in transthyretin protein to date (http://amyloidosismutations.com). The amyloidogenic precursor states of both the wild-type and mutant TTR adopts a native folded structure but differ in stability. Mutant precursor state is less stable than wild-type transthyretin (Lim et al., 2017). The monomeric form of transthyretin comprises two β-sheets and each β-sheet comprises four strands, namely D/A/G/H and C/B/E/F, respectively. Both these intra and inter β-strands interact with each other via loops (Jiang, Smith et al., 2001). The presence of mutations have been reported to perturb the conformational stability of the CD loops in the monomer, triggering amyloid formation of the protein (Yee, Aldeghi et al., 2019). Monomeric intermediates generated from the dissociation of tetrameric wild-type protein rapidly aggregates under mild acidic conditions at physiological temperature (Sun, Dyson et al., 2018). Various structural changes occur during amyloid formation and are often characterised by various biophysical techniques. NMR studies have revealed that the two β-sheet (CBEF and DAGH) structures initially present in the tertiary structure of transthyretin protein remains intact even after the amyloid formation (Lim et al., 2016b). But the loop regions and the helical structures are disrupted in the final aggregate state (Dasari, Hung et al., 2020). Moreover, the interaction of AB loop region with strand A often lead to its conformational change and destabilisation of the main DAGH β sheet (Lim et al., 2016a). Moreover, a mechanism-based study on TTR aggregation depicted that the F and H strands on transthyretin monomers are the drivers of amyloid formation (Saelices, Johnson et al., 2015). The proposed mechanism for transthyretin amyloidogenesis generally involves the formation of dimers, followed by hexamers and thereby self-assembled toxic oligomers. These oligomers consist of 6 to 10 monomers and initiate formation of fibrillar-enriched species (Faria, Almeida et al., 2015; Dasari, Hughes et al., 2019).

Researchers have started connecting the in vitro mechanism of transthyretin aggregation with cellular perspective. In a recent study, it was depicted that the fibrils derived from a C-terminal fragment of transthyretin protein was also identified in affected tissues (Ueda, Okada et al., 2019). Moreover, other studies have also depicted that the fibrils extracted from the human cardiac tissue exhibited identical structural features and stability like the fibrils formed under in vitro conditions (Dasari, Hung et. al. 2020; Raimondi, Mangione et al., 2020). More studies are required to understand the in vivo mechanism of aggregation underlying pathogenesis of transthyretin amyloid cardiomyopathy. The perturbations of the structural integrity of transthyretin protein often lead to amyloid formation (Figure 20.1) and the early onset of this disease.

20.3 Diagnostic Approaches for Transthyretin Cardiac Amyloidosis

Early and accurate diagnosis of transthyretin amyloid cardiomyopathy (ATTR-CM) could be the key factor in estimating its actual prevalence rate. Heart failure symptoms are commonly found in ATTR-CA patients. Apart from cardiac symptoms, neurological, gastro-intestinal, and ophthalmological manifestations are also common in ATTR-CM cases (Witteles, Bokhari et al., 2019; Hafeez and Bavry, 2020). ATTR-CM is a multi-systemic disorder and also involves infiltration of amyloid fibrils in soft tissues, thereby causing nerve entrapment. Hence, both ATTRwt and ATTRmt patients often show extra-cardiac symptoms like carpal tunnel syndrome, lumbar spinal stenosis, and biceps tendon rupture (Westermark, Westermark et al., 2014; Geller, Singh et al., 2017; Sperry, Reyes et al., 2018). Cardiac biomarkers like N-terminal proBNP, BNP, and troponins are often measured in patient blood to support diagnosis (Kumar, Dispenzieri et al., 2012; Kristen, Maurer et al., 2017; Ritts, Cornell et al., 2017). Moreover, the cut-off level of NT-proBNP and troponin T have been utilised by the clinicians for staging the disease (González-López et al., 2017b; Gillmore, Damy et al., 2018). Absence of M spike, an indicator of monoclonal gammopathy in the serum free light-chain assay profile, confirms the non-involvement of

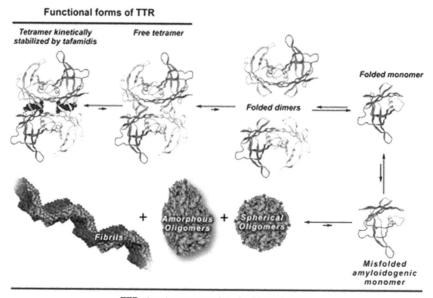

FIGURE 20.1   Mechanism for aggregation and amyloid formation of transthyretin protein (Bulawa, Connelly et al., 2012). (Reprint permission license number: permission granted.)

immunoglobin light chain and involvement of transthyretin in the majority of cases (Witteles, Bokhari et al., 2019). But monoclonal gammopathy of unknown significance has also been reported in ATTR-CM patients (Phull, Sanchorawala et al., 2018). Hence, it depicts the importance of systematic evaluation of blood parameters in these patients. Clinicians also depend on certain electrocardiographic and echo-cardiographic findings for preliminary screening of amyloid presence in heart failure patients (Macedo, Schwartzmann et al., 2020). The presence of left ventricular hypertrophy (both symmetric and asymmetric) in echocardiogram and pseudo-infarct pattern along with sinus rhythm in the electrocardiogram are the most common features found in ATTR-CM patients (Damy, Maurer et al., 2016; González-López, et al., 2017a). Ventricular granular speckling pattern in echocardiography shows 87% sensitivity and 81% specificity in defining amyloid presence in heart. Similarly, reduced global longitudinal strain along with apical sparing value can differentially diagnose cardiac amyloidosis from other causes of left ventricular hypertrophy and heart failure with 87% sensitivity and 72% specificity, respectively (Tsang and Lang 2010; Pagourelias, Mirea et al., 2017). Moreover, the presence of a "cherry on top" pattern in the bull's eye plot in two-dimensional speckle tracking echocardiographic findings also provides significant cues for ATTR-CM (Ruberg, Grogan et al., 2019). Nevertheless, ejection fraction to strain rate (EFSR) is 90% sensitive and 92% specific in distinguishing cardiac amyloidosis from other causes of heart failure (Pagourelias, Mirea et al., 2017). Increased interventricular septal wall thickness is also considered as a strong indicator for transthyretin involvement, despite the absence of low voltage in electrocardiogram in the majority of cases (Damy, Maurer et al., 2016; González-López, et al., 2017a; Ruberg, Grogan et al., 2019). Heterogeneous late gadolinium enhancement pattern is often observed in cardiac magnetic resonance (CMR) imaging of cardiac amyloidosis patients. However, there is no clinical validity for differentiation of ATTR from AL type on the basis of LGE pattern (Saelices, Nguyen et al., 2019). Hence, the correlation between the amount of amyloid load and marked extracellular volume expansion and abnormal nulling time for the myocardium is significantly evaluated in CMR imaging of ATTR-CM patients (Witteles, Bokhari et al., 2019).

In recent years, advanced radionuclide (technetium labelled) imaging scans using bone tracers like 3,3-diphosphono-1,2-propanodicarboxylic acid (DPD), pyrophosphate (PYP), and hydroxymethylene diphosphonate (HMDP) are often employed to differentiate transthyretin-related cardiac amyloidosis from immunoglobulin light-chain cardiac amyloidosis (Singh, Falk et al., 2019). Grade 2 to 3 cardiac uptake of ^{99m}Tc-PYP or a heart/contralateral chest ratio of greater than 1.5 in bone scintigraphy scan is a strong indicator for ATTR-CM (Castano, Haq et al., 2016). However, these diagnostic imaging techniques solely cannot confirm ATTR-CM (Wisniowski and Wechalekar, 2020). Therefore, the clinicians mostly rely on immune-histochemical staining and mass spectrometry-based analysis on biopsy specimen, preferably endomyocardial biopsy (Gilbertson, Theis et al., 2015). Mass spectrometry helps in identification of the proteins involved in driving the amyloid formation. Moreover, genetic analysis is often carried out to detect mutations, if involved. In some cases, genetic profiles of the asymptomatic carriers are also screened to predict the onset of disease symptoms. Thus, the combination of tissue biopsy-based invasive and non-invasive imaging methods can successfully identify ATTR-CM patients as shown in Figure 20.2.

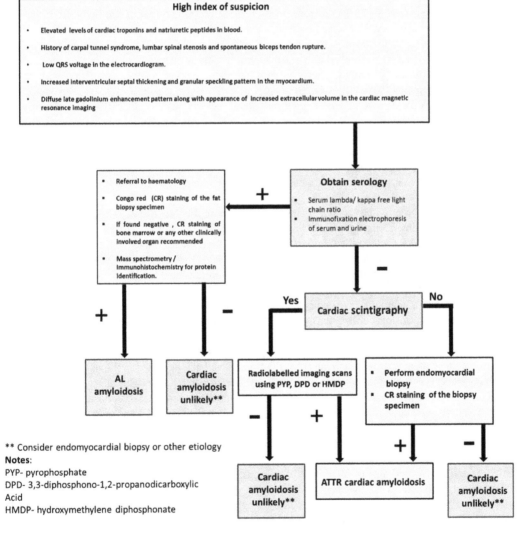

FIGURE 20.2 Outline of systematic diagnostic approaches for ATTR-CM (Hafeez and Bavry, 2020). (Reprint permission license number: No need. Open access.)

20.4 Therapeutic Strategies Undertaken for Transthyretin Cardiac Amyloidosis

Researchers across the globe are actively taking initiatives in development of therapeutic strategies to tackle the disease pathology and symptoms. Symptom management is the primary care undertaken for ATTR patients in terms of tackling fluid balance and impairment of diastolic filling (period in which the ventricle fills with blood from the left atrium). Moreover, cardiac arrhythmias are tackled in ATTR-CM patients by the use of catheter ablation and amiodarone therapy (Ruberg and Berk 2012; Mints, Doros et al., 2018). However, the systolic hypertension cannot be controlled in ATTR-CM patients by administration of diuretics as they are highly sensitive to diuretics like calcium channel blockers, beta blockers, and angiotensin converting enzyme inhibitors. Moreover, they often suffer from severe hypotension and fatigue upon taking these medications (Siddiqi and Ruberg, 2018). Orthotopic liver transplantation (OLT) is the first disease-modifying treatment used for ATTR amyloidosis since 1990s. But it can only tackle the mutant form and not the wild-type form of the protein (Ando, Coelho et al., 2013). This is because wild-type protein will be naturally produced even after transplantation, as liver is the only source of circulating TTR. Moreover, in some cases, the progression of wild-type transthyretin-associated cardiomyopathy was observed even after liver transplantation (Yazaki, Mitsuhashi et al., 2007; Kay, Menachem et al., 2018). Hence, for patients with hereditary ATTR-CM, combination of heart and liver transplantation can be considered as a feasible option. This combined transplantation approach not only stops the production of amyloidogenic protein but also the complications associated with downstream organ dysfunction (heart) (Strouse, Briasoulis et al., 2019). However, for the wild-type cases this approach is rare as the disease occurs in aged individuals (Davis, Kale et al., 2015). Yet, the survival rate after liver transplantation varies among hereditary ATTR patients. For some mutant variants like Leu111Met, Ala25Ser, and Phe33Cys transplantation improved the survival rate of patients. But for some other mutations like Thr60Ala, Val30Met, Ser50Arg, and Ser77Tyr no improvement in survival of ATTR patients occurred even after transplantation (Suhr et al., 2016). Hence, researchers have embarked on the journey of discovering therapeutic strategies to enhance stabilisation of structurally altered mutant transthyretin protein.

Recently, a lot of progress has been achieved in transthyretin drug development programs. Drugs like Tafamidis and RNA-interfering agents like Patisiran are effective in treating transthyretin-related cardiac amyloidosis. Tafamidis binds to the thyroxin binding site of tetrameric transthyretin thereby stabilising it and inhibiting its dissociation into amyloidogenic monomers (Kim, Choi et al., 2021). Similarly, Patisiran is a small interfering RNA, directed against the 3′-untranslated region of mutant and wild-type transthyretin coding RNA thereby reducing the level of circulating transthyretin in blood (Hoy, 2018). The clinical trials for Tafamidis have depicted it as an effective therapy for treating transthyretin amyloid cardiomyopathy in terms of reducing the overall rate of mortality and cardiovascular-related hospitalisation in these patients (Park et al., 2020). Similarly, the APOLLO-B clinical trial for Patisiran revealed its high efficiency in treating transthyretin amyloidosis patients with cardiomyopathy (Holis et al., 2020). Recently, both of them received approval from FDA and have been launched in the market (Hoy, 2018; Urquhart, 2019). TTR amyloid disruptors like doxycycline in combination with tauro-ursodeoxycholic acid (TUDCA) can synergistically reduce the load of fibrillar aggregates (Cardoso, Martins et al., 2010). Similarly, natural compounds like epigallocatechin-3-gallate (EGCG) and curcumin are efficient disruptors of transthyretin-derived mature amyloid fibrils in vitro (Pullakhandam, Srinivas et al., 2009; Ferreira, Saraiva et al., 2011). Currently these natural molecules are under clinical trials for evaluation of their efficacy (Ciccone, Tonali et al., 2020; Bezerra, Saraiva et al., 2020). Conformation-specific novel anti-TTR antibody raised against its amyloid-driving segments along with transthyretin stabiliser molecule termed AG10 are in development and will soon undergo preclinical and clinical trials (Ruberg, Grogan et al., 2019). However, these therapeutic strategies are unable to prevent amyloid formation via seeding mechanism. To tackle this problem researchers have recently designed an inhibitor peptide, TabFH2. It is a mixture of two peptides, TabF2 and TabH2, directed against the amyloid driving F and H β-strands of transthyretin and inhibits self-association under in vitro conditions in a tissue-independent

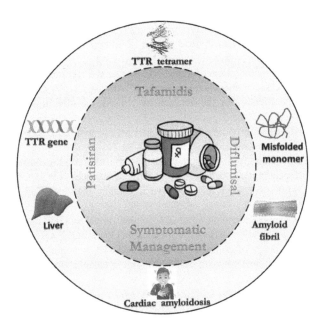

FIGURE 20.3 Illustration of specific treatment options available for ATTR-CM.

manner (Saelices, Nguyen et al., 2019). It may soon undergo preclinical study for treatment of ATTR-CM. Currently clinicians are advised to follow a treatment algorithm for ATTR-CM patients comprising specific treatment options as highlighted in Figure 20.3.

20.5 Conclusion

ATTR-CM is a fatal cardiac disorder, characterised by the deposition of transthyretin-derived amyloid fibrils. The diagnosis begins with the assessment of cardiac biomarkers followed by electrocardiographic, echocardiographic, and radiolabelled imaging. Finally, amyloid typing is done on the endomyocardial or adipose tissue biopsy of the suspected patients. Combination of various non-invasive radiolabelled imaging methods and tissue-based mass spectroscopy are required for the identification of precursor proteins and accurate diagnosis at various stages of this disease. Moreover, current progress in drug development programs for transthyretin cardiac amyloidosis has offered new hope of targeted therapy in ATTR-CM patients. This also strengthens the urgent need for early and correct diagnosis of this disease to prevent disease progression. Clinicians should follow the systematic diagnostic approach to avoid misdiagnosis of ATTR-CM (Hafeez and Bavry, 2020). Further, the population must be sensitised about the disease pathology and the severe outcomes of disease progression along with median survival rate. Genetic screening studies should be undertaken in patients suffering from cardiac problems to identify asymptomatic carriers of mutation, if any. Moreover, population-based genetic screening should also be undertaken. This might help the patients to approach the clinicians for diagnosis and treatment to establish the accurate statistics on the current and future epidemiology of this disease. Moreover, age is another important factor to be considered by the clinicians at the time of diagnosis. Although wild-type transthyretin-associated cardiac amyloidosis is reported in octagenerians, some research studies have started highlighting the early age of onset for wild-type-associated ATTR-CM (Ghosh, Khanra et al., 2021; Grogan, Scott et al., 2016). Hence, early diagnosis followed by targeted therapy might enable the clinicians to treat higher numbers of such patients in the future. This is only possible if researchers join hands with clinicians across the world and actively participate in the global amyloid diagnosis program (Thakur, Ghosh et al., 2019; Thakur, Ghosh et al., 2021).

REFERENCES

Ando, Y. et al. (2013). "Guideline of transthyretin-related hereditary amyloidosis for clinicians." Orphanet Journal of Rare Diseases 8(1): 1–18.

Benson, M. D. et al. (2020). "Amyloid nomenclature 2020: update and recommendations by the International Society of Amyloidosis (ISA) nomenclature committee." Amyloid 27(4): 217–222.

Bezarra, F. et al. (2020). "Modulation of the mechanisms driving transthyretin amyloidosis." Frontiers in Molecular Neuroscience 13(234).

Bhogal, S. et al. (2018). "Cardiac amyloidosis: an updated review with emphasis on diagnosis and future directions." Current Problems in Cardiology 43(1): 10–34.

Bulawa, C. E. et al. (2012). "Tafamidis, a potent and selective transthyretin kinetic stabilizer that inhibits the amyloid cascade." Proceedings of the National Academy of Sciences 109(24): 9629–9634

Buxbaum, J. N. et al. (2009). "Transthyretin: the servant of many masters." Cellular and Molecular Life Sciences 66(19): 3095–3101.

Buxbaum J. N. et al. (2022) "Amyloid nomenclature 2022: update, novel proteins, and recommendations by the International Society of Amyloidosis (ISA) Nomenclature Committee." *Amyloid*. 1–7.

Cardoso, I. et al. (2010). "Synergy of combined doxycycline/TUDCA treatment in lowering Transthyretin deposition and associated biomarkers: studies in FAP mouse models." Journal of Translational Medicine 8(1): 74.

Castano, A. et al. (2016). "Multicenter study of planar technetium 99m pyrophosphate cardiac imaging: predicting survival for patients with ATTR cardiac amyloidosis." JAMA Cardiology 1(8): 880–889.

Ciccone, L. et al. (2020). "Natural compounds as inhibitors of transthyretin amyloidosis and neuroprotective agents: analysis of structural data for future drug design." Journal of Enzyme Inhibition and Medicinal Chemistry **35**(1): 1145–1162.

Connors, L. H. et al. (2003). "Tabulation of human transthyretin (TTR) variants, 2003." Amyloid 10(3): 160–184.

Damy, T. et al. (2016). "Clinical, ECG and echocardiographic clues to the diagnosis of TTR-related cardiomyopathy." Open Heart 3(1).

Dasari, A. K. et al. (2019). "Transthyretin aggregation pathway toward the formation of distinct cytotoxic oligomers." Scientific Reports 9(1): 1–10.

Dasari, A. K. R. et al. (2020). "Structural characterization of cardiac ex vivo transthyretin amyloid: insight into the transthyretin misfolding pathway in vivo." Biochemistry 59(19): 1800–1803.

Davis, M. K. et al. (2015). "Outcomes after heart transplantation for amyloid cardiomyopathy in the modern era." Am J Transplant 15(3): 650–658.

Faria, T. Q. et al. (2015). "A look into amyloid formation by transthyretin: aggregation pathway and a novel kinetic model." Physical Chemistry Chemical Physics 17(11): 7255–7263.

Ferreira, N. et al. (2011). "Natural polyphenols inhibit different steps of the process of transthyretin (TTR) amyloid fibril formation." FEBS letters 585(15): 2424–2430.

Geller, H. I. et al. (2017). "Association between ruptured distal biceps tendon and wild-type transthyretin cardiac amyloidosis." Jama 318(10): 962–963.

Ghantous, C. M. et al. (2020). "Advances in cardiovascular biomarker discovery." Biomedicines 8(12): 552.

Ghosh, S. et al. (2021) "Wild type transthyretin cardiac amyloidosis in a young individual: A case report." Medicine 100(17).

Gilbertson, J. et al. (2015). "A comparison of immunohistochemistry and mass spectrometry for determining the amyloid fibril protein from formalin-fixed biopsy tissue." Journal of Clinical Pathology 68(4): 314–317.

Gillmore, J. D. et al. (2018). "A new staging system for cardiac transthyretin amyloidosis." European Heart Journal 39(30): 2799–2806.

González-López, E. et al. (2017a). "Clinical characteristics of wild-type transthyretin cardiac amyloidosis: disproving myths." European Heart Journal 38(24): 1895–1904.

González-López, E. et al. (2017b). "Diagnosis and treatment of transthyretin cardiac amyloidosis. Progress and hope." Revista Española de Cardiología (English Edition) 70(11): 991–1004.

Grogan, M. et al. (2016). "Natural history of wild-type transthyretin cardiac amyloidosis and risk stratification using a novel staging system." Journal of the American College of Cardiology 68(10): 1014–1020.

Grogan, M. et al. (2017). "Estimating population-level prevalence of wild-type and variant transthyretin amyloid cardiomyopathy." Journal of Cardiac Failure 23(8): S73.

Guan, J. et al. (2012). "Current perspectives on cardiac amyloidosis." American Journal of Physiology. Heart and Circulatory Physiology 302(3): H544–H552.

Hafeez, A. S. and A. A. Bavry (2020). "Diagnosis of transthyretin amyloid cardiomyopathy." Cardiology and Therapy 9(1): 85–95.

Holis, L. et al. (2020). "Experience of patisiran with transthyretin stabilizers in patients with hereditary transthyretin-mediated amyloidosis." Neurodegenerative Disease Management 10(5): 289–300

Hoy, S. M. (2018). "Patisiran: first global approval." Drugs 78(15): 1625–1631.

Jacobson, D. R. et al. (2015). "Prevalence of the amyloidogenic transthyretin (TTR) V122I allele in 14 333 African–Americans." Amyloid 22(3): 171–174.

Jiang, X. et al. (2001). "An engineered transthyretin monomer that is nonamyloidogenic, unless it is partially denatured." Biochemistry 40(38): 11442–11452.

Kay, J. et al. (2018). "Progressive cardiomyopathy in ttr amyloidosis after liver transplant." Journal of Cardiac Failure 24(8): S81.

Kim, D. et al. (2021). "Tafamidis for cardiac transthyretin amyloidosis." Cardiovascular Prevention and Pharmacotherapy 3(1): 1–9.

Kittleson, M. M. et al. (2020). "Cardiac amyloidosis: evolving diagnosis and management: a scientific statement from the American Heart Association." Circulation 142(1): e7-e22.

Kristen, A. V. et al. (2017). "Impact of genotype and phenotype on cardiac biomarkers in patients with transthyretin amyloidosis – Report from the Transthyretin Amyloidosis Outcome Survey (THAOS)." PLOS ONE 12(4): e0173086.

Kumar, S. et al. (2012). "Revised prognostic staging system for light chain amyloidosis incorporating cardiac biomarkers and serum free light chain measurements." Journal of Clinical Oncology: Official Journal of the American Society of Clinical Oncology 30(9): 989–995.

Lim, K. H. et al. (2016a). "Structural changes associated with transthyretin misfolding and amyloid formation revealed by solution and solid-state NMR." Biochemistry 55(13): 1941–1944.

Lim, K. H. et al. (2016b). "Solid-state NMR studies reveal native-like β-sheet structures in transthyretin amyloid." Biochemistry 55(37): 5272–5278.

Lim, K. H. et al. (2017). "Pathogenic mutations induce partial structural changes in the native β-sheet structure of transthyretin and accelerate aggregation." Biochemistry 56(36): 4808–4818.

Macedo, A. V. S. et al. (2020). "Advances in the treatment of cardiac amyloidosis." Current Treatment Options in Oncology 21(5): 1–18.

Mints, Y. Y. et al. (2018). "Features of atrial fibrillation in wild-type transthyretin cardiac amyloidosis: a systematic review and clinical experience." ESC Heart Failure 5(5): 772–779.

Pagourelias, E. D. et al. (2017). "Echo parameters for differential diagnosis in cardiac amyloidosis: a head-to-head comparison of deformation and nondeformation parameters." Circulation: Cardiovascular Imaging 10(3): e005588.

Park J. et al. (2020). "Tafamidis: a first-in-class transthyretin stabilizer for transthyretin amyloid cardiomyopathy." Annals of Pharmacotherapy 54(5): 470–477.

Phull, P. et al. (2018). "Monoclonal gammopathy of undetermined significance in systemic transthyretin amyloidosis (ATTR)." Amyloid 25: 1–6.

Pullakhandam, R. et al. (2009). "Binding and stabilization of transthyretin by curcumin." Archives of Biochemistry and Biophysics 485(2): 115–119.

Raimondi, S. et al. (2020). "Comparative study of the stabilities of synthetic in vitro and natural ex vivo transthyretin amyloid fibrils." Journal of the Biological Chemistry 295(33): 11379–11387

Ritts, A. J. et al. (2017). "Current concepts of cardiac amyloidosis: diagnosis, clinical management, and the need for collaboration." Heart Failure Clinics 13(2): 409–416.

Ruberg, F. L. and J. L. Berk (2012). "Transthyretin (TTR) cardiac amyloidosis." Circulation 126(10): 1286–1300.

Ruberg, F. L. et al. (2019). "Transthyretin amyloid cardiomyopathy: JACC state-of-the-art review." Journal of the American College of Cardiology 73(22): 2872–2891.

Saelices, L. et al. (2015). "Uncovering the mechanism of aggregation of human transthyretin." Journal of Biological Chemistry 290(48): 28932–28943.

Saelices, L. et al. (2019). "A pair of peptides inhibits seeding of the hormone transporter transthyretin into amyloid fibrils." Journal of Biological Chemistry 294(15): 6130–6141.

Siddiqi, O. K. and F. L. Ruberg (2018). "Cardiac amyloidosis: an update on pathophysiology, diagnosis, and treatment." Trends in Cardiovascular Medicine 28(1): 10–21.

Singh, V. et al. (2019). "State-of-the-art radionuclide imaging in cardiac transthyretin amyloidosis." Journal of Nuclear Cardiology 26(1): 158–173.

Sperry, B. W. et al. (2018). "Tenosynovial and cardiac amyloidosis in patients undergoing carpal tunnel release." Journal of the American College of Cardiology 72(17): 2040–2050.

Strouse, C. et al. (2019). "Approach to a patient with cardiac amyloidosis." Journal of Geriatric Cardiology: JGC 16(7): 567–574.

Suhr, O. B. et al. (2016). "Survival after transplantation in patients with mutations other than Val30Met: extracts from the FAP World Transplant Registry." Transplantation 100(2): 373.

Sun, X. et al. (2018). "Kinetic analysis of the multistep aggregation pathway of human transthyretin." Proceedings of the National Academy of Sciences 115(27): E6201-E6208.

Thakur, A. K. et al. (2019). "Amyloidosis: a strong need for clinical diagnosis in India." Amyloid 26(3): 175–176.

Thakur, A. K. et al. (2021). "TTR cardiac amyloidosis: A right time to start clinical diagnosis globally." Current Science (Manuscript accepted).

Tsang, W. and R. M. Lang (2010). "Echocardiographic evaluation of cardiac amyloid." Current Cardiology Reports 12(3): 272–276.

Ueda, M. et al. (2019). "A cell-based high-throughput screening method to directly examine transthyretin amyloid fibril formation at neutral pH." Journal of Biological Chemistry 294(29): 11259–11275.

Urquhart, L. (2019). "FDA new drug approvals in Q2 2019." Nature Reviews Drug Discovery 18(8): 575.

Westermark, P. et al. (2014). "Transthyretin-derived amyloidosis: probably a common cause of lumbar spinal stenosis." Upsala Journal of Medical Sciences 119(3): 223–228.

Winburn, I. et al. (2019). "Estimating the prevalence of transthyretin amyloid cardiomyopathy in a large in-hospital database in Japan." Cardiology and Therapy 8(2): 297–316.

Wisniowski, B. and A. J. A. H. Wechalekar (2020). "Confirming the diagnosis of amyloidosis." Acta Haematologica 143(4): 312–321.

Witteles, R. M. et al. (2019). "Screening for transthyretin amyloid cardiomyopathy in everyday practice." JACC: Heart Failure 7(8): 709–716.

Yazaki, M. et al. (2007). "Progressive wild-type transthyretin deposition after liver transplantation preferentially occurs onto myocardium in FAP patients." American Journal of Transplantation 7(1): 235–242.

Yee, A. W. et al. (2019). "A molecular mechanism for transthyretin amyloidogenesis." Nature Communications 10(1): 1–10.

21

Pathophysiology of Diabetes-Induced Foot Ulcers and Therapy Options

Reena Badhwar
Delhi Pharmaceutical Science and Research University, New Delhi, India
Shree Guru Gobind Singh Tricentenary University, Gurugram, India

Harvinder Popli
Delhi Pharmaceutical Science and Research University, New Delhi, India

Harpal S. Buttar and Istvan G. Telessy
Department of Pathology and Laboratory Medicine, University of Ottawa, Ottawa, Canada

Vijay Bhalla
Shree Guru Gobind Singh Tricentenary University, Gurugram, India

21.1 Introduction

Diabetes is a metabolic disorder characterized by hyperglycemia, insulin resistance, or unregulated system of insulin and hyperlipidemia. This disease is growing rapidly, which may responsible for 2.70% of compromised lifestyle and 2.45% of deaths worldwide in 2017 (IHME, 2017). Prevalence rates are higher in developing countries than developed countries as in the case of India, around 61.2 million of the population are diabetic and this number is likely to increase to 101.2 million by 2030 (Frykberg RG et al., 2007). This disturbed metabolism is also responsible for many other macrovascular diseases, including retinopathy, cardiovascular, and nephropathy, and microvascular diseases, such as nephropathy and neuropathy. Among these complications a major and very distressing problem is foot infection (Singh S et al., 2013), which further develops into diabetic foot ulcer (DFU) and affects 15% of patients with diabetes and if not treated in a timely manner becomes a major cause of partial or complete limb amputation resulting in poor quality of life and premature mortality (Pendsey SP, 2010). According to the United State survey, approximately 38% of amputations are linked to diabetic ulcers. This disease has been a severe problem because this disease accounts for ~25% of hospitalizations and has become a major cause of increased healthcare costs (Raghav A et al., 2018).

21.2 Classification of Diabetic Foot Ulcers

It is necessary to understand the characteristics of a wound such as type, location, appearance, size, and depth before starting treatment. This evaluation is helpful to understand the ulcer etiology and whether the lesions are ischemic, neuropathic, or neuro-ischemic (Margolis DJ et al., 1999). There are numerous classification systems such as Wagner–Meggit, Brodsky, University of Texas, and International Working Group Classification to classify and understand the severity of the diabetic wound (Brodsky JW, 2007; Kaufman J et al., 1987). The Wagner's classification is the most commonly used system to describe ulcer depth, tissue necrosis level, extent of ulcer, and the occurrence of gangrene (Cuzzell J, 2003) as shown

DOI: 10.1201/9781003220404-23

TABLE 21.1

Wagner–Meggit Classification System of Diabetic Foot Lesions

Grades	Foot lesions
0	No open lesions or cellulitis
1	Ulcer on foot local surface with full thickness but not in tissues
2	Wound up to muscles, joints tissues, tendon and ligaments but absence of abscess development and bone penetration
3	Severe ulcers with abscess, joint sepsis, cellulitis formation, and sometimes osteomyelitis can be noticed
4	Gangrene appearance on surface of heel or forefoot
5	Complete foot gangrene

TABLE 21.2

University of Texas Classification System of Diabetic Ischemia and Wound Infection

	Grades			
Stages	**0**	**1**	**2**	**3**
A	Cured pre- or post-ulcerative lesion entirely epithelialized	Local, non-infectious, superficial, and non-ischemic	Wound penetration up to tendon and capsule	Wound penetrating to bone or joint
B	Infection occurrence (α)	(α)	(α)	(α)
C	Presence of ischemia (β)	(β)	(β)	(β)
D	Presence of both infection and ischemia (γ)	(γ)	(γ)	(γ)

α = infection occurrence; β = ischemia presence; γ = presence of both infection and ischemia.

in Table 21.1, but cant not explain the infection and level of ischemia. Thus, these days the University of Texas Antonio classification system (UTSA) or Texas classification are preferable to Wagner because they provide full information such as depth and ischemic and infection stages of ulcers associated with DFUs, which is helpful to better understand ulcer lesion and developing successful strategies for ulcer treatment (Frykberg RG, 2002). But the Texas system, is not able to find the selection of necessary antibiotics totreat the infection (Shaw JE et al., 1997). The Texas system is classified into stages and grades (A to D) and (0 to 3), respectively. When a wound comes into higher stages of a grading system, it is not able to heal without risk of amputation and vascular repair (Armstrong DG et al., 1998) (Table 21.2).

21.3 Microbial Loading in Diabetic Foot Ulcer

The microbial load refers to the occurrence of 10^5 or more than the organism per gram of tissue (Bendy RH et al., 1964). There is not a single organism responsible for diabetic foot infection; it is a cluster of gram-positive, gram-negative bacteria and fungi including *Pseudomonas aeruginosa, S. aureus, Klebsiella pneumoniae, Proteobacteria, beta-hemolytic streptococci, Staphylococcus, E. coli*, and *coli form bacteria*. It is reported that the most frequently obtained bacteria in diabetic ulcer are *S. aureus and Staphylococcus*. It is necessary to identify the specific organism present in the wound before starting the treatment so that appropriate antimicrobial therapy and management of the ulcer can be started. Different studies have different views. For example, Citron et al. reported that chronic and unhealed ulcers have monomicrobial burden and chronic infections are monomicrobial such as *S. aureus* (Citron DM et al., 2007). Whereas Hunt JA suggested that severe or chronic wounds are polymicrobial including anaerobic such as gram-negative rods and enterococci and mild wounds have monomicrobial load (Hunt JA, 1992).

Some studies also reported that polymicrobial loading on ulcer is further becoming a leading cause of the virulence factor generation such as proteases, hemolysins, and collagenases resulting in enhanced inflammation and delayed healing (Wall IB et al., 2002). Some western countries suggest that DFU is

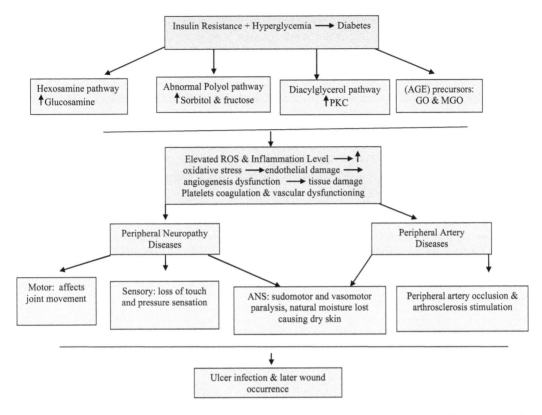

FIGURE 21.1 Diagrammatic Representation of Diabetic Foot Ulcer Pathophysiology. Decrease =; Result →; Increase = ↑; PKC = roteinkinase C; AGE = advanced glycation end product; GO = glyoxal; MGO= methyl glyoxal; ROS = reactive oxygen species; ANS = autonomic nervous system.

a cluster of gram-positive aerobic organism whereas some eastern countries state it is a hub of gram-negative aerobes microorganism. Thus, a study conducted based on duration of ulcer, Wagner system, and diabetic wound healing time found that amount of aerobic organism and anaerobic pathogens was 66.8% and 33.2%, respectively. The total number of diverse pathogens was 728 in 654 diabetes patients (Viswanathan V et al., 2002).

21.4 Pathophysiology of the Diabetic Foot Ulcer

DFU is a multifactorial pathophysiological state characterized by infection, deep tissue damage, and ulcer. These complications are not noticeable by patients at initial stage of ulcer due to occurrence of peripheral neuropathy disease (PND) and ischemia induced from peripheral arterial disease (PAD) or lower limb deformities or both (Pedrosa HC, 2010). In these situations, mild ischemia can be a major cause of ulcer and impaired wound healing. Several degenerative factors like insulin resistance, immune suppression, and hyperglycemia (Apelqvist J et al., 1994), and many pathways including polyol pathway, hexosamine pathways, inflammatory cytokines (IL-6, IL-10 & TNF-α), and glycoxation may hasten vascular changes and peripheral neuropathy by bacterial infection stimulation (Eslami MH et al., 2007). Nitric oxide is a wound healing booster but hyperglycemia disturbs the endothelial reaction resulting in decreased nitric oxide level causing soft tissue damage of bone and impaired wound healing (Ollendrof DA et al., 1998).

21.4.1 Peripheral Neuropathy

Peripheral neuropathy is a nerve impairment disorder affecting movement (especially toe movement), sensations, and temperature of body. There are numbers of related factors that cause foot problems but among them peripheral neuropathy is a major precursor for DFU (Honing ML et al., 1998). There is no specific cause of neuropathy, but it is a result of many body disorders like hyperglycemia, insulin resistancy, reactive oxygen species, and many activation pathways and inhibition (Cameron NE et al., 1997). The conversion of glucose to sorbitol and fructose happens in the presence of aldose reductase (ALR2). Hence, ALR2 is an important factor to initiate the polyol pathway (Kumar, H et al., 2012). In diabetic patients neuropathy is manifested into three components of the nervous system: motor, sensory, and autonomic (Canal N et al., 1997).

In the case of **motor** neuropathy small muscles of the foot are affected causing claw's toe, hammer toe, loss of ankle reflexes, and Charcot's foot problems (Steed DL, 2001). Body balance is also altered due to a which patient's gait is affected. There is imbalance between flexion and leg extension due to damaged foot muscles causing anatomic foot deformities, which leads skin cracking and further becomes a cause reason of DFU (Watson JC et al., 2015).

Sensory: Sensory neuropathy is loss of protective, vibration, touch, and pressure sensations due to damage of sensory nerve present in extremities. Sometimes high sensation of pain takes place at night called "burning feet syndrome," but in the case of chronic sensory neuropathy pain feeling is diminished showing high risk of trauma (Gardner SE et al., 2008). This insensitivity of ulcer makes doctor and patient unaware for a longer time and chronic ulceration can occur suddenly. In sensory neuropathy, skin breakdown occurs due to which microbial growth takes place resulting in reoccurrence and lack of wound healing (Alavi A et al., 2014).

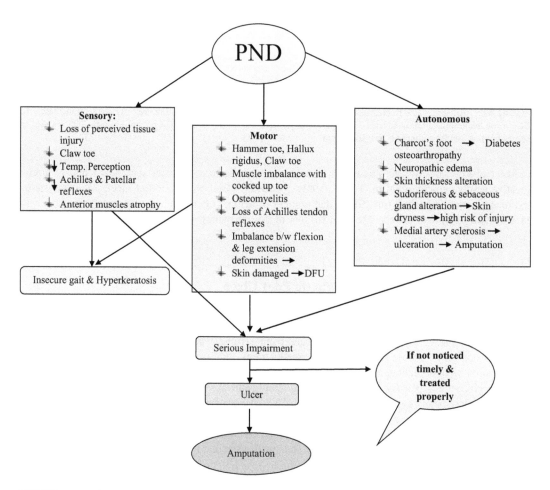

FIGURE 21.2 Diagrammatic representation of pathophysiology of peripheral neuropathic diseases. Decreased =; ↓ Result = →; Diabetic Foot Ulcer = DFU.

TABLE 21.3

Different Strategies and Treatments for Diabetic Foot Ulcer (Perez-Favila A et al., 2019)

Therapy	Method	Advantage	Disadvantage	References
Neuropathic Ulcer	Alpha lipoic acid	Delay or chances of peripheral nerves damaged	Absence of data evaluating long-term treatment	(Bartkoski S et al., 2016)
	(IL-6)	Peripheral nerve fibers regeneration	Inflammation at (high doses)	(Cox AA et al., 2017)
	Antidepressants: Amitriptyline, Venlafaxin, Duloxetine, and Nortriptyline	Effective against neuropathic pain. Similar effects to pregabalin and gabapentin	Muscarinic effect, sleep disturbance, and depression	(Javed S et al., 2015)
	Mesenchymal stem cells	Neuroprotective, can be isolated from adipose tissue and has cell plasticity	Less cost effective, the number of transplanted cells that are integrated and reachable into the organ functioning are low	(Oses C et al., 2017)
	Anticonvulsants: Pregabalin, Gabapentin	Reduction of neuropathic pain	Effective after the second week, drowsiness, dyspnea, and fatigue	(Dworkin RH. et al., 2007). (Raskin P et al., 2016)
	Analgesics: Tramadol, Oxycodone, Tapentadol, and Acetaminophen	Diabetic poly neuropathic tenderness reduction	Sedation, confusion, and opioids misuse is possible	(Tang HY et al., 2019)

ANP: In this case, neuropraxia stimulation causing sensation and strength of muscles defects as well as sudomotor and vasomotor paralysis occurs at the affected nerve site. Autonomic neuropathy is a major cause of sweat and sebaceous gland imbalance causing loss of natural moisture of feet due to which skin breakdown and fissure predisposition takes place (Clayton W et al., 2009). Further, this imbalance is responsible for ulcer infection, tissue necrosis, lesser humidification, and inflammation resulting in DFU development. In this neuropathy, medial artery sclerosis occurs, which is a serious cause of severe ulceration and amputation (Lavery LA et al., 2007).

21.4.1.1 Treatment of Peripheral Neuropathic Disease

Peripheral neuropathy including sensory, motor, and autonomic is a symbolic cause of DFU. This condition is responsible for loss of temperature and sensation in lower limbs of patients due and patients are often unaware of infection and DFU develops (Boulton AJ et al., 1998). The first step for PND management is to control glucose level. Pharmacologically, there are only three FDA-approved treatments available, namely, Pregabalin, Duloxetine and Tapentadol (Games G et al., 2013). Some analgesics (Tramadol, Acetaminophen), antidepressants (Amitriptyline, Venlafaxinand, Nortriptyline), and opioids (Oxycodone) are also included with these therapies to avoid body and neuron pain (Attal N et al., 2010; Javed S et al., 2015).

21.5 Peripheral Arterial Disease

PAD is a vascular and lower extremity disease found in 25–30% of DFU patients (Javed S et al., 2015). In peripheral arteries, endothelial and smooth cell dysfunction occurs due to dyslipidemia and hyperglycemia, which is a leading cause of DFU and its complications. It is also responsible for plasma

TABLE 21.4

Treatment Strategies for Diabetic Foot Ulcers (Adapted from Perez-Favila A et al., 2019)

Therapy	Method	Advantage	Disadvantage	Reference
	Percutaneous transluminal angioplasty	Increases the limb recovery rate and beneficiary for aged patients	Not appropriate for young patients, limited scientific facts, Requirement of adjuvant treatment to avoid restenosis with platelet inhibitors or vitamin antagonist K	(Iida O et al., 2012). (Lee V et al., 2014)
Ischemic Ulcer: (a). Endovascular therapy	Angioplasty	Increases the vessel primary permeability, target lesion revascularization	Cost effectiveness is less, rate of amputation is not decreased, and restenosis rate is high	(Kayssi A et al., 2016)
	Angiosoma	Helpful in ischemic ulcer, increases arterial flow to the ischemic limb, improves mobility, and minimize pain at rest and amputation rate is also decreased.	Very long arterial segments, difficulties in identifying affected angiosoma, diffuse, calcified, and multiple lesions, small arterial caliber, and slow distal beds flow.	(Fernández-Samos Gutiérrez R, 2012). (Iida O et al., 2012)
	Bypass:autologous human umbilical vein and synthetic materials with or without heparin	Helpful in primary permeability improvement and foot preservation.	No scientific data available	(Ambler GK et al 2018). (Albers M et al., 2005)
	Vitamin E	Increases blood flow and body's capacity to renovate, cost effective without any side effects	Authentic scientific data is not available	(Kleijnen J et al., 2000)
Anticoagulant Therapy	Beta-blockers	Does not affect, blood flow, walking distance, leg vascular resistance and temperature of the skin.	Not satisfactory scientific data available	(Paravastu SC et al., 2013)
	Cilostazol	Vasodilator, antiproliferative activity; it prevents arterial leg ulcers and restenosis, improves claudication and long-term patency after infra-inguinal endovascular interventions	Expensive and contraindicated with congestive heart failure patients	(Bedenis R et al., 2014). (De Franciscis S et al., 2013). (Soga Y et al., 2012)

TABLE 21.4 (Continued)

Treatment Strategies for Diabetic Foot Ulcers (Adapted from Perez-Favila A et al., 2019)

Therapy	Method	Advantage	Disadvantage	Reference
	Levocarnitine	Improves walking distance, claudication	Dose and duration of treatment is not decided	(Robertson L et al., 2012). (Alonso-Coello P et al., 2012)
	Hyperbaric oxygen therapy (HOT)	Helpful in ulcer healing and minimizes patient time in hospital	Adjuvant therapy with antibiotics, small amount of studies evidence and high risk of bias	(Park SJ et al., 2010). (Matas M et al., 2013)
Drug Therapy for Symptomatic Relief:				
Naftidrofuryl oxalate	(selective serotonin (5-hydrroxytryptamine 2[5-HT2]) receptor antagonist)	Aerobic metabolism efficiency increased and minimizes erythrocyte rigidity, and improves the transcutaneous oxygen pressure in areas of ischemia	Diarrhoea, nausea, and vomiting and skin rash	(Barradell LB et al., 1996)
Pentoxifylline	Affects the blood cell rheology and decreases the blood thickness	Walking distance improvement	Cost effectiveness and clinical benefit are limited	(Stevens JW et al., 2012). (Salhiyyah K et al., 2012)
Analgesics	Transdermal patches (Buprenorphine), neuromodulation using spinal cord activators	Relief in pain and help in limb salvage	Expensive	(Ubbink DT et al., 2013)
Prostaglandin and prostacyclin (e.g., iloprost & beraprost)	Antiplatelets, antiproliferative, and vasodilator	improve the rest pain, rate of ulcer healing ultimately less chance of amputation	Not appropriate for endovascular or surgical revascularization	(Téllez GA and Castaño JC, 2010)

coagulation due to the increased vasoconstrictor thromboxane A2 and also affects the leukocyte and macrophage mechanism (IDF, 7th ed., 2015). The abnormalities in endothelial function and extended inflammatory response can affect microcirculation, may increase basement membrane thickness or capillary thickness, increase blood coagulation, cause improper blood flow, and diminish levels of nitric oxide. Nitric oxide regulates vasodilation and keeps blood vessels safe from endogenous injury. Thus, in the case of nitric oxide shortage vasoconstriction and arthrosclerosis are caused resulting in ischemia (Singh S et al., 2013). It has been added that ischemia is a major cause of amputation in 80–90% of diabetes patients. PAD is not only a responsible factor for DFU it is a combination of many other abnormalities including DNP, reactive oxygen species, trauma, uncontrolled infection, and severe inflammation (Eskelinen E et al., 2004). PAD is a severe disorder causing lower limb artery damage and poor blood flow in arteries and veins, which ultimately leads to lower limb loss. The therapeutic approaches are based on location and types of ischemia as well as treatment-associated risks and results (Armstrong DG et al., 2017). There is no single treatment for these disorders; these days multidisciplinary treatment therapies including bypass surgery, open surgery, or revascularization, arterial repair, endovascular treatment such as catheter-directed thrombolytic (CDT), percutaneous mechanical thrombectomy (PMT), and percutaneous thromboaspiration (PAT) are in practice for ischemia. These efforts are to improve survival prognosis, to save the lower limb, to prevent ischemia occurrence, and to enhance blood flow (Ouriel K et al., 1998).

21.6 Role of Reactive Oxygen Species in Diabetic Foot Ulcer

Various studies have documented that elevated levels of reactive oxygen species (ROS) including singlet oxygen, hydrogen peroxide (H_2O_2), and superoxide anions disturb the endothelial function and prevent angiogenesis, which leads to delayed wound healing (Grether-Beck S et al., 1996). Wlaschek and Scharffetter-Kochanek (2005) hypothesized that elevation in macrophages and neutrophils in chronic wounds could cause accumulation in ROS. The imbalance between pro-oxidants and antioxidants is also a cause of oxidative stress and superoxide production. Oxidative stress and superoxides are more prevalent in chronic wounds than in acute wounds (Wlaschek M et al., 2005). This increased level of ROS leads to tissue damage following proteolytic pathway activation (James TJ et al., 2003). To detoxify ROS there is a need for natural antioxidant molecules including vitamins A and E (Rojas AI et al., 1999) and glutathione (Mudge BP et al., 2002), but these are deficient in chronic wounds, resulting in high accumulation of ROS, which causes tissue degeneration. Keratinocyte migration and re-epithelialization is also affected due to increased ROS level in chronic wounds (O'Toole EA et al., 1996).

21.6.1 Treatment of Reactive Oxygen Species

Tur E et al. (1995) performed in vitro studies and suggested that topical application of H_2O_2, benzyl peroxide, and tetra chlorodecaoxides is helpful in wound healing. Kwakman PH et al. (2012) impregnated the glucose oxidase into a wound dressing, tested it on an excision model diabetic rat wound, and reported that glucose oxidase also has the capacity for ROS generation. Another study (Arul V et al., 2012) also concluded that glucose oxidase is also helpful in nitric oxide stimulation, which plays a major role in wound fibroblast and keratin formation.

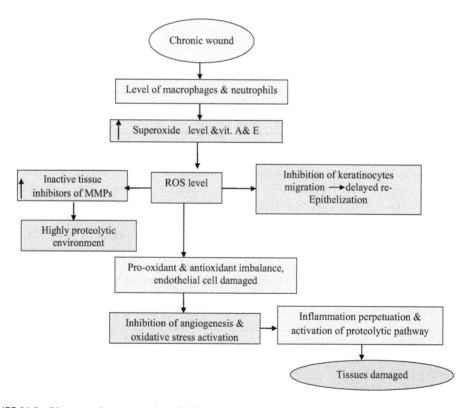

FIGURE 21.3 Diagrammatic representation of ROS pathophysiology. Decrease = ↓; MMPs = Matrix metalloproteinases; Result =;→ Increased = ↑.

TABLE 21.5

Therapeutic Strategies Based on ROS Function Modulation from Dunnill C. et al., 2017

ROS-modulating therapeutic approach	Positive physiological (ROS) effects on ulcer	References
Topical H_2O_2	Anti-bacterial increases angiogenesis, O_2 level enhancement, keratinocyte proliferation, and migration numerousimmunocyte recruitment.	(Klyubin IV et al., 1996). (Tur E et al., 1995)
Honey	Anti-bacterial and H_2O_2-related effect and immunocyte recruitment.	(Kwakman PH et al., 2012)
Hyperbaric O_2 therapy	Wound hypoxia reduction causing enhanced anabolism, H_2O_2-related effects efficient, and phagocytic respiratory bursts.	(Berner J et al., 2014)
Recombinant PDGF	Improved perfusion through nitric oxide, angiogenesis, macrophages, fibroblast, neutrophils endothelial cell migration resulting in wound healing.	(Kaltalioglu K et al., 2013)
Recombinant glucose oxidase	H_2O_2-related effects, enhanced perfusion through nitric oxide, better keratinocytes differentiation, and collagen arrangement resulting ulcer healing at early stage.	(Jull AB et al., 2015)

(NADPH)Nicotinamide adenine dinucleotide phosphate; (ROS) reactive oxygen species. (PDGF) platelet-derived growth factor.

21.7 Charcot Foot Pathophysiology

Neuropathic osteoarthropathy is also called Charcot neuropathy (CN) or Charcot foot. It is a continuous degenerative condition in which joints, soft tissues, and bone are affected at the initial stage and further cause deformity, dislocation, and deep ulcer of the foot and ankle joints (Rogers CL et al., 2011). Current studies suggest that proprioception loss is not the only cause of Charcot arthropathy, but there are numerous leading factors including peripheral neuropathy, vascular neuropathy, neuropeptides, hyperglycemia, genetics and microvascular structure, bone turnover, and abnormal bone metabolism, which further cause severe inflammation and its amplification leading to osteolysis. Some studies report that imbalance between pro-and anti-inflammatory cytokines are responsible for bone damage (Chantelau E et al., 2006).

The increased level of proinflammatory tumor necrosis factor-a (TNF-α), interleukin-6 (IL-6), and interleukin-1 β (IL-1β), mainly the receptor activator of the nuclear factor kappa B (NF-kB), receptor activator of nuclear factor kappa ligand L (RANKL) and decreased level of anti-inflammatory (IL-4 & IL-10) cytokines are the leading cause of osteoclast (Mabilleau G et al., 2008; Baumhauer JF et al., 2006). The elevated amount of (TNF-α) stimulates the (NF-kB), (RANK) ligand (RANKL), which further activates the osteoclast precursor cells leading to matured osteoclast cell division resulting in osteolysis, osteoporosis, imbalanced bone turnover, and rheumatoid arthritis.

A depletion of capcaisin-induced neuropeptides like substance P (SP) and calcitonin gene-related peptide (CGRP) in unmyelinated sensory neurons also leads to large bone loss and fragility (Offley SC et al., 2005). It is also suspected that neuropeptides are linked with bone metabolism process. The increased level of nitric oxide (NO) plays an important role in osteoblasts but decreases are also responsible for osteocytes to apoptosis causing increased osteoclast formation and bone resorption (Nilforoushan D et al., 2009). The major consequences of diabetes mellitus, i.e., hyperglycemia (where sugar is accumulated in large amounts, stimulating hyperlipidemia) and free radical formation (such as ROS and AGEs), trigger the RANK/RANKL cytokine system (Jeffcoate W et al., 2005). The activation and stimulation of these factors further cause neuropathy, vasculopathy, and finally lower limb ulcer and bone damage.

21.7.1 The microvascular structure and bone turnover

Charcot also mentioned that elevations in bone perfusion as well as sympathetic denervation also play an important role in bone resorption (Charcot JM et al., 1868). This sympathetic denervation unregulates the arterial-venous shunt flow due to which fluid starts to ooze out from leaked capillary because of increased venous pressure by disturbed shunt (Rajbhandari SM et al., 2002). This process leads to severe tissue edema and improper microcirculation causing tissue ischemia (Schaper NC et al., 2008). In Charcot foot the increased alkaline phosphate level and deficiency of vitamin D cause osteopenia by activation of para-thyroid hormone, which is responsible for calcium loss (Rangel ÉB et al., 2012).

21.7.2 Charcot Treatment

Before starting the treatment and therapies it is necessary to diagnose Charcot foot properly as inflam-mation is the primary sign of joint and bone injury, which may resemble cellulitis, gout, and vein throm-bosis, which may result in wrong diagnosis (Eichenholtz SN, 1966; Charcot J-M et al., 1883; Cofield RH et al., 1983; Johnson JT et al., 1967; Armstrong DG et al., 1997; Henderson VE et al., 1905). The Charcot diagnosis is based on clinical images, which were scanned using techniques like radiographic imaging, magnetic resonance imaging (MRI), and positron emission tomography scanning. Offloading is also a good therapy to manage deformity progression. In Charcot foot, it is necessary to avoid weight or plantar pressure and mobilization of the foot (Caputo GM et al., 1998; Jeffcoate W, 2008). Thus, there are some options like half-shoes, orthoses, and wheelchairs prescribed but they are not very efficient. The one and only gold standard and efficient technique of offloading is a removable total contact cast (TCC) (Fejfarová V et al., 2019). This cast should be used continuously until edema, skin temperature, and erythema (Frykberg RG et al., 2010) are under control and replaced every three days to avoid pistoning (Armstrong DG et al., 1997). These days instant TCC (iTCC) or removable walking casts are also in use, which are easy to remove (Armstrong DG et al., 2005).

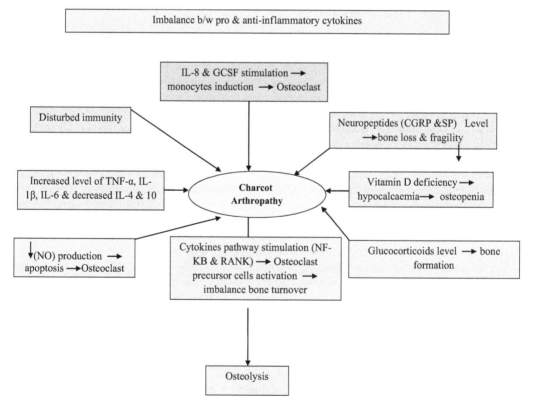

FIGURE 21.4 Diagrammatical representation of Charcot foot pathophysiology. Granulocyte colony-stimulating factor = GCSF; tumor necrosis factor-a = TNF-α; interleukin-1 β = (IL-1β); interleukin-6 = (IL-6); interleukin – 4 & 10 = (IL-4 & 10); nitric oxide =NO; calcitonin gene-related peptide = CGRP; nuclear factor kappa B = NF-KB), receptor activator for nuclear factor κ B ligand = RANKL.

TABLE 21.6

Primary Diagnosis Techniques and Pharmacological Treatments of Bone Healing

Techniques	Advantages	
Positron emission tomography scanning (X-rays)	Easily affordable and available, information regarding bone structure, mineralization, and bone alignment can be obtained.	(Morrison WB et al., 2002)
Magnetic resonance imaging (MRI)	More efficient than X-ray detection, provides detailed information and images of protons in fat and water, and can portray anatomy and pathology of bone and soft tissues as well. Osteomyelitis sensitivity and specificity is intense.	(Morrison WB et al., 2001)
Positron emission tomography scanning	Helpful to differentiate charcot foot and osteomyelitis	(Keidar Z et al., 2005). (Höpfner S et al., 2004)
Total contact casting (TCC)	Plantar pressure redistribution diminishes mechanical forces, local inflammation and edema, decreased osteoclast, and progression of deformity regulation	(Jude E et al., 2001). (Pakarinen TK et al., 2011). (Pitocco D et al., 2005). (Bem R et al., 2006)
Bisphosphonates (pamidronate, alendronate, and zolendronate) and calcitonin	Reduction of bone turnover and temperature	(Petrova NL, et al., 2012)

21.8 Role of Flavonoids in the Treatment of Diabetic Foot Ulcers

Flavonoids are natural polyphenolic antioxidant and anti-inflammation substances present in a large number of plants. Over 7000 to 8000 different flavonoid compounds have been isolated and identified. On the basis of chromane ring (i.e., ring C and hydroxylation structure) they are divided into different subgroups like isoflavones, anthocyanins, flavan-3-ol, chalcones, flavonols, flavanones, flavanonols, and flavones (Khoo HE et al., 2017). Several bioactive flavonoids have shown antidiabetic, wound healing (Chirumbolo S, 2012), antioxidant (Procházková D et al., 2011), anti-inflammatory (Kim HP et al., 2004), and antimicrobial activities (Cushnie TPT et al., 2005). Many flavonoids have been used for a long time in traditional medicine. The presence of these properties has generated interest in using flavonoids to treat different ailments including DFU. Flavonoids have also secured their place in the phytotherapeutic market in the form of tablets, granules, capsules, topical gels, and solutions (e.g., Hesperidin, Hidrosmin for edema and venous insufficiency) (Caro-Ordieres et al., 2020).

The various flavonoids tested for treating diabetic foot complications are listed in Table 21.4. Their effects consist of diabetic peripheral neuropathy, which is a leading cause of ischemia, ulcer, gangrene, and amputation. Diabetic peripheral neuropathy is a symptom of nerve damage causing insensitivity to pain, temperature, and numbness, which leads to severe ulcer formation because patients remain unaware of ulcer at initial stages (Tesfaye S et al., 2013). There are some leading causes of PAD generation such as hyperglycemia, insulin resistance, endothelial and protein kinase dysfunction, and polyol pathway activation, which further generate oxidative stress, ROS, and inflammatory cytokine activation. These pathway activations and their disturbance further cause NO accumulation and NF κB activation (Du X et al., 2003; Obrosova IG et al., 2005). Thus, flavonoids play major roles between enzymes and genes to regulate various pathways. Some flavonoids and their subgroups like anthocyanins and quercetin are helpful to regulate the inflammatory mediators (TNF-α and IL-6) (Brown TJ et al., 2019) whose downregulation may be responsible for diabetic foot complications like PAD and PND. The increased level of oxidative stress and ROS also leads to DFU and related ailments so flavonoids such as naringenin (Al-Rajaie SS et al., 2015), fisetin, hesperidin (Zhao X et al., 2015), catechin (Addepalli V and Suryavanshi SV,

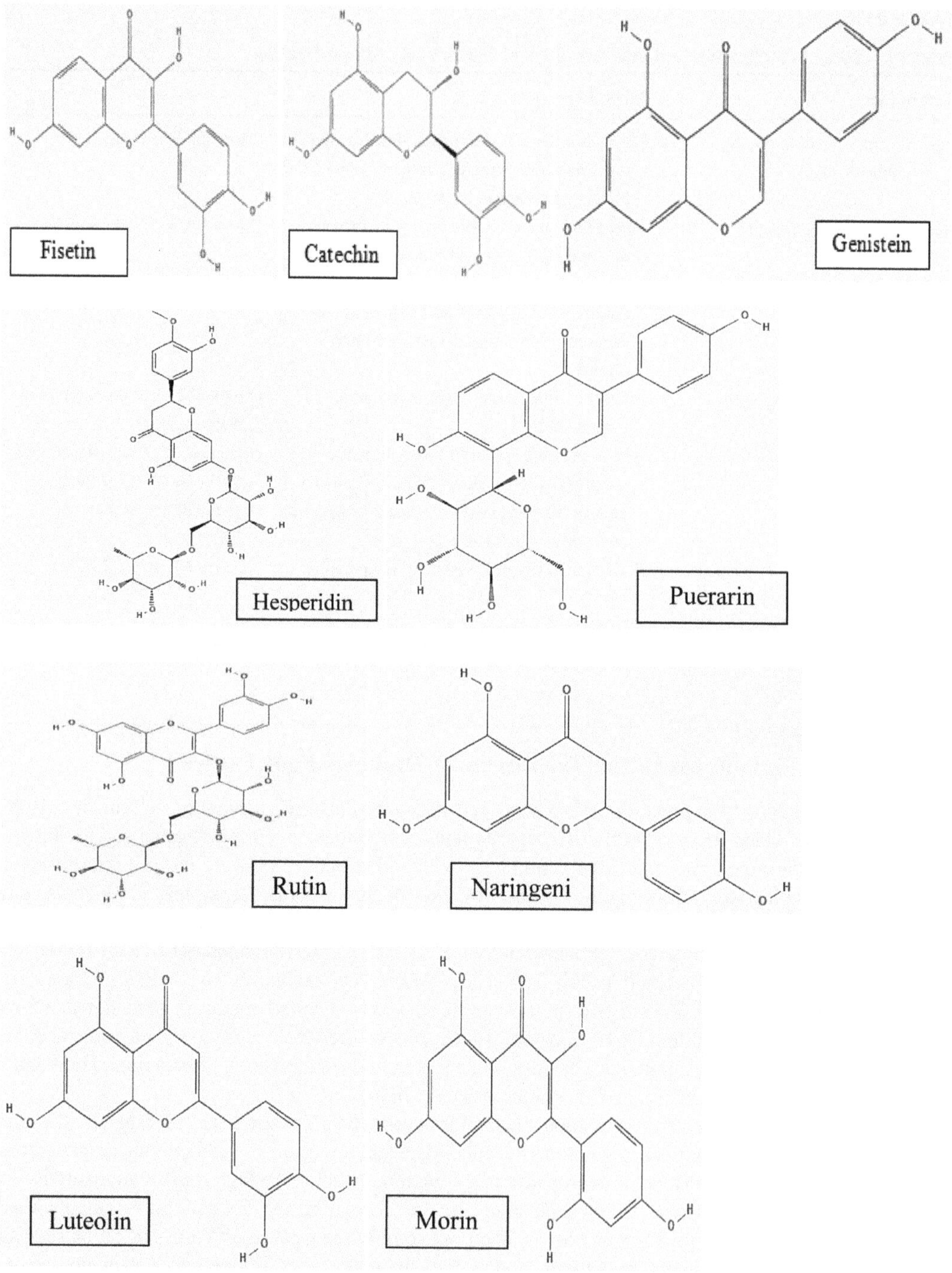

FIGURE 21.5 Chemical structure of different flavonoids.

2018), genistein (Valsecchi AE et al., 2011), morin (Bachewal P et al., 2018), rutin (Tian R et al., 2016), kaempferol (Kishore L et al., 2018), and luteolin (Li M et al., 2015) works as cell apoptosis inhibitors resulting in ROS and inflammatory cytokine reduction by inhibiting extrinsic (death receptor-mediated) as well as intrinsic (mitochondria-mediated) pathways (Maestri A et al., 2005). These flavonoids also stimulate antioxidant enzymes such as CAT and SOD, which are helpful in ROS and oxidative stress

TABLE 21.7

List of Flavonoids and Their Effects on Diabetic Peripheral Neuropathy (Basu P and Basu A, 2020)

Flavonoids	Flavonoids (Dose mg/kg and Route of administration in rats & mice models)	Histopathological/Biochemical/Molecular Parameters	Reference
Catechin	25 mg/kg and 50 mg/kg Oral	Improved left (ventricular systolic pressure and hemodynamic parameters mean arterial pressure and heart rate), oxidative stress parameters (MDA, GSH, CAT, SOD), reversed diabetes-induced neuronal damage and reduced MMP-9 level	(Addepalli V and Suryavanshi SV, 2018)
Morin	50 and 100 mg/kg Oral gavage	↑Mitochondrial-specific superoxide dismutase 2 ↓ (SOD2) expression in high glucose-treated N2A cells ↓Glucose-induced ROS by improving Nrf2 expression and its downstream HO-1expressor in N2A cells IKK (ser176/180) phosphorylation, TNF-α and IL-6 level, X translocation and expression of NF-κB in N2A cells resulting in decreased IL-6 and TNF-α levels	(Bachewal P et al., 2018)
Naringenin	20 and 50 and 100 mg/kg/day Oral gavage	↑Level of, IL-1β and IL-6, TNF-α, and NO GSH, SOD, CAT, GPx, and GR levels in sciatic nerves Enhancement in diminished sciatic expressions of insulin, Growth factor and NGF levels	(Al-Rejaie SS et al., 2015)
Rutin	5, 25, and 50 mg/kg Oral	↓NF-κB, Iκ-Bα, p -, Iκ-Bα, IL-6, and TNF-α in DRG neurons of ↓ diabetic rats, Na+, K+-ATPase activities in sciatic nerves↓ Caspase-3 expression in DRG neurons ↓MDA and ↓ ROS levels, partially increased antioxidant enzymes SOD, GPx, glutathione-S-transferase (GST), and CAT in sciatic nerves ↑ H₂S, Nrf2, and HO-1 in DRG neurons	(Tian R et al., 2016)
Luteolin	50 mg/kg, 100 mg/kg, and 200 mg/kg (*i.p*)	↓ ROS and MDA levels,↑ Antioxidant enzymes SOD, ↓GST, GPx, and CAT along with Nrf2 and HO-1 in nerve tissues in diabetic rats	(Li M et al., 2015)
Fisetin	10 mg/kg Oral	Exacerbated oxidative stress by reducing lipid peroxide, ROS production, co-administration of ROS scavenger, ↓phenyl-N-tert-butylnitrone potentiated antinociceptive activity, CAT activity in spinal cord, DRG, and sciatic nerve	(Zhao X et al., 2015)
Hesperidin	25, 50, and 100 mg/kg (*p.o*)	↓ Serum glucosuria, cholesterol, and triglyceride levels, mRNA expressions of TNF-α and IL-6, ↓Elevated glycated hemoglobin and aldose reductase levels, hemodynamic parameters (SBP, DBP, and MABP, neural lipid peroxidase, NO, and total calcium levels) Serum insulin, neural SOD, glutathione, and Na+K+ATPase levels	(Visnagri A et al., 2014)
Puerarin	4, 20, and 100 nM intrathecal	↓ NF-κB, IL-6, IL-1B, and TNF-α in spinal cord, ↓Diabetes-induced elevation of TNF-α, IL-1B, and IL-6 and NF-κB DNA-binding activities, X overexpression of NF-κB p65 and p65 nucleus translocation	(Liu M et al., 2014)

(continued)

TABLE 21.7 (Continued)

List of Flavonoids and Their effects on Diabetic Peripheral Neuropathy (Basu P and Basu A, 2020)

Flavonoids	Flavonoids (Dose mg/kg and Route of administration in rats & mice models)	Histopathological/Biochemical/Molecular Parameters	Reference
Genistein	3 and 6 mg/kg subcutaneous	↓ Pro-inflammatory cytokines TNF-α, IL-1,and IL-6, ROS levels in sciatic nerves; MDA and ROS levels in brain and liver; iNOS in thoracic aorta NGF, eNOS, and SOD, did not modify decreased cerebral activities of CAT and GPx, restored hepatic GPx activity but it did not modify CAT activity decrease, restored the GSH content and the GSH and GSSG ratio in liver but did not modify total glutathione content	(Valsecchi AE et al., 2011)
Naringin	40 and 80 mg/kg (*i.p*)	↓ SOD level, TNF-α, ↑ lipid peroxide, elevated neural nitrite, Na-K-ATPase levels along with percentage of apoptosis	(Kandhare AD et al., 2012)

X = inhibited/prevented. (decreased = ↓); MMPs = Matrix metalloproteinases; (result = →); (increased =↑); ROS = Reactive oxygen species; TBARS = thiobarbituric acid reactive substances; SOD = superoxide dismutase 2; MDA = malondialdehyde; GSH = glutathione; CAT = catalase;NFR2 = Nuclear factor-related factor 2; GPx = glutathione peroxidase; TNF-α = tumor necrosis factor-α; IL-1β = interleukin-1 β; IL-6 = interleukin-6; IL-4 & IL-10 = interleukin – 4 & 10; NO = nitric oxide; NF-KB = nuclear factor kappa B; SBP= systolic blood pressure; DBP = diastolic blood pressure; MA = mean artery pressure.

reduction. Cardozo, L.F. et al. (2013) conducted a study using a diabetic animal model. The results of this study concluded that (Nrf2) -/HO-1 play a defensive role against neuroinflammation and oxidative stress.

Flavonoids like rutin, luteolin, and morin are able to lessen oxidative stress. The decreased level of anti-inflammatory (IL-4 and IL-10) cytokines and increased level of transforming growth factor β (TGF-β), NO, TNF-α, (IL-6), and (IL-1β) stimulate NF-kB and RANK, which are further responsible for oxidative stress and ROS generation resulting in bone injury and osteoclast. Thus, in these cases different flavonoids have a specific role to regulate these species. Kaempferol regulates NO level and rutin, morin, and puerarin are helpful in NF-κB level reduction (Agca CA et al., 2014).

21.8.1 Catechin

Source: Green tea

Mechanism of Action: Catechin is a polyphenolic component of green tea. It is a good antioxidant with various pharmacological and biological activities. Catechin is helpful in antioxidant enzyme stimulation and is actively reduces oxidative stress and ROS level resulting in less neuronal degradation. The stimulation of ROS, inflammatory cytokines (TNF-α, NF-κβ), and leukocytes (IL-1, IL-β and IL-6) is a major cause of neuropathic damage or pain. The antioxidant capability of this component can control the apoptosis process as well as the plasma glucose level by glucose transporter modulation (Bernatoniene J and Kopustinskiene DM, 2018). Some studies have explained that antioxidative effect of catechins (obtained from green tea) has the capacity to alter subcellular ROS production, cytochrome (P450, 2E1) activity, and glutathione metabolism. This process further inhibits the protein degradation process, which is also a leading cause of PND. Li et al. (2015) agreed that catechin from green tea is helpful in ameliorating insulin resistance by acting as peroxisome proliferator-activated receptor ligands (PPAR-L) with a dual alpha/gamma agonistic effect.

Preclinical Study: A preclinical study was performed in which diabetes was induced in male rats using streptozotocin. After diabetes confirmation, the catechin dose (25 and 50 mg/kg) was given to the animal for 28 days. The catechin (50 mg/kg) enhanced hemodynamic parameters such as mean arterial blood pressure, heart rate, and left ventricular systolic pressure. Additionally this dose was successful in oxidative stress and plasma glucose levels (p < 0.01) reduction. It was noticed that this dose (50mg/kg) of catechin was able to decrease the circulatory MMP-9 level in experimental animals. Further, the result of histopathology showed that ingestion of catechin up to 28 days can prevent neuronal damage. Finally, from the study result, it was concluded that catechin has the ability to manage diabetic neuropathic diseases in experimental rats (Addepalli V and Suryavansh, SV., 2018).

21.8.2 Morin

Source: Seaweeds, guavava (indian), onion, almond, red wine, and osage orange

Mechanism of Action: Morin is a bioflavonoid compound and contains numerous pharmacological activities such as antioxidant, anticancer, anti-inflammatory, and chemoprotective. Komirishetty et al. (2016) reported that morin exhibited anti-inflammatory and antioxidant action against chronic constriction injury (CCI)-induced peripheral neuropathy by regulating ROS. Morin has anti-inflammatory and detoxifying effects against ROS antioxidant effect by regulation of NF-j B and Nrf2 pathways.

Preclinical Study: Bachewal et al. (2017) evaluated the pharmacological action of morin on metabolic mitochondrial ROS production on NF-j B, Nrf2 pathways in diabetic rats (Streptozotocin-induced) and in high glucose-insulted mouse neuroblastoma cell line Neuro 2A (N2A). There was increased in hypersensitivity as well as impairment in sensory nerve conduction velocities (SNCV), motor nerve conduction velocities (MNCV), and normalized blood flow (NBF). The morin oral dose (50 and 100 mg/kg) reduced the sensory motor alteration and an improvement was seen in SNCV, MNCV, and NBF in experimental diabetic animals. In another mouse model it was reported that morin has antioxidant and anti-inflammatory action by changing the mitochondrial function via regulation and NF-j B and Nrf2 pathways. Moreover, it was concluded that morin has a neuroprotective effect in experimental DN.

21.8.3 Hesperidin (hesperetin-7-rhamnoglucoside)

Source: Citrus species with *C. sinensis, C. unshiu, and citrus aurantium L.*

Mechanism of Action: Hesperidin is a flavonoid component found in numerous citrus plants. The deficiency of hesperidin can cause capillary leakiness and extremity pain, which further becomes a main cause of weakness, ache, and night leg cramps.

Hesperidin has biological and pharmacological activities including anti-cancer, hepatoprotective, antifungal, antihyperlipidemic, anti-inflammatory, antimicrobial, antioxidant, analgesic, antiulcer, and antidiabetic (Visnagri A et al., 2014). The efficacy of hesperidin has been proved against diabetes-induced complications such as PAD, PND, encephalopathy, and cardiomyopathy. It can regulate the TGF-β, Smad-2/3 mRNA and VEGF-c, and Ang-1/Tie-2 expression resulting in vasculogenesis and angiogenesis of skin, which is a sign of ulcer healing.

Preclinical Studies: Kandhare et al. (2018) examined the hesperidin wound healing potential in DFU. For this study diabetes was induced in rat using STZ, 55 mg/kg, i.p. After confirmation of diabetes into experimental animals the ulcer was created in each animal. Further, hesperidin dose (25, 50, and 100 mg/kg, p.o.) was given for 21 days. The resulted showed that hesperidin has vasculogenesis and angiogenesis activities leading to early wound healing. It is also helpful in management of neuropathic and ischemic ailment via NO and SOD regulation.

21.8.4 Genistein

Source: Legumes species

Mechanism of Action: Genistein is an isoflavone obtained from soybean. It is known for tyrosine kinase inhibitory and estrogen-like effect. Additionally, it also has antioxidative potential via antioxidant enzymes activities including (GPx), (HO-1), and SOD regulation. A study reported that genistein in the form of dietary supplement enhanced the wound healing rate by regulating pro-inflammatory cytokines (TNF-α, IL-1α, IL-1β-, IL-6, and IL-10) and antioxidant protection mechanism (Mezei et al., 2003). In diabetic wound, disturbance in antioxidant defense system such as GPx and SOD leads to ROS stimulation, which further help in wound impairment. The Nrf2 is a key regulator of oxidative stress and also helpful in management of antioxidant defense system. Thus, it is regarded as a targeted factor in wound treatment in diabetic ailments. The targeted factor in diabetic condition is NFκB, which is responsible for inflammatory cytokine (NO and COX2) stimulation. It also plays an important role in regulation of NOD-like receptor protein-3 (NLRP3), cryopyrin, and CIAS1, which are helpful in ulcer healing and are known for native immunity. However, these are important parameters of diabetic wound healing and should be regulated properly so that complete and early wound healing takes place (Park et al., 2011).

Preclinical Studies: Hyeyoon E et al. (2016) conducted genistein effect on rate-limiting stage or (inflammatory phase) of diabetic wound. It was reported that dietary intake of genistein accelerated the delayed ulcer healing in diabetic animals via regulation of Nrf2-associated antioxidant defense system and NFκB-related inflammatory response. Thus, it was suggested that genistein may be helpful in wound management due to its improving action of protein stage of anti-inflammatory cytokines and antioxidant activities, which are the main cause of any ulcer unhealing (Hyeyoon et al., 2016).

21.8.5 Rutin: (3, 30, 40, 5, 7-pentahydroxyflavone-3-rhamnoglucoside)

Source: Apples, red wine, onion, and tea

Mechanism of Action: Rutin or Vitamin P is a common flavonoid glycoside that is readily available in the human diet. It also contains disaccharides rutinose and quercetin flavonols called quercetin -3-rutinosid. Rutin contains numerous pharmacological and biological activities such as anticarcinogenic, antibacterial, antidiabetic, antioxidant anti-inflammatory, and antiviral. Additionally, it has blood pressure-lowering and capillary reinforcement effect as well as can decrease lycogenolytic and gluconeogenic enzyme activity (Schwingel TE et al., 2014). By protecting pancreatic β cells and improving insulin resistance system rutin acts as an antihyperglycemic agent. It can suppress adipocyte differentiation via inhibition of membrane lipid peroxidation and scavenging oxidative stress. In addition, rutin can prevent DN via regulation of TGF-β1/CTGF/ECM and TGF-β1/Smad/ECM signaling pathways and oxidative stress. Vitamin P can also minimize ischemic neural apoptosis via increasing antioxidant enzymes action as well as decreasing p53 expression (Kamalakkannan N et al., 2006).

Preclinical Studies: Al-Enazi MM et al. (2013) evaluated rutin effect as an antiinflammatory and anti-oxidant agent by inducing DN in male Wistar rats. After completion of study, it was reported that rutin has antioxidant activities and ameliorated hyperglycemia-stimulated thermal hyperalgesia and improved diabetic neuropathic pain. Finally, a study suggested that rutin may be beneficial in DN management and treatment. Tian et al. (2016) evaluated the effect of rutin in DN-induced experimental rats. The rutin dose (5 mg/kg, 25 mg/kg, and 50 mg/kg) was introduced in the animals for 2 weeks. After completion of the study it was concluded that rutin can significantly reduced the plasma glucose and oxidative stress level, and can inhibit neuroinflammation via Nrf2 and hydrogen sulphide stimulation. Niture et al. (2014) observed the rutin potential on diabetic neuropathic rats. The STZ (55 mg/kg i.p.) was administered for four weeks to induce diabetes in rats. Then, for three weeks, sertraline (30 mg/kg, p.o.), metformin (200 mg/kg, p.o.), and rutin (50 and 100 mg/kg, p.o.) were injected into experimental animals. The glycosylated hemoglobin, serum glucose, and serum triglyceride levels were checked to determine the rutin antidiabetic action. Further, some parameters such as walking function test, TNF-α level, cold allodynia, thermal hyperalgesia, antioxidant enzymes including MDA, SOD, GSH, and NO level, and sciatic nerve axonal degeneration were followed. The conclusion of this study was that rutin regulated TNF-α as well as antioxidant enzyme level in diabetic experimental animals. Overall, these three studies showed that rutin is significantly effective against DN.

21.8.6 Naringenin: (NA), (4′, 5, 7-trihydroxy flavanones 7-rhamnoglucoside)

Source: Oranges, tomatoes, and grapefruits

Mechanism of Action: Naringenin is an important flavanone obtained from citrus fruits. It is also popular for its beneficial biological properties like antidiabetic, antiulcer, anti-inflammatory, antioxidant or free radical absorber, and immunity modulator (Grayer RJ et al., 2005). It can also activate peroxisome proliferator-activator receptors (PPARs) and carbohydrate metabolism. Naringenin is helpful in DN reduction by regulating the antioxidant enzyme SOD, catalase (CAT), paraoxonase (PON), and GPx activities (Al-Rejaie SS et al., 2015).

Preclinical Studies: In DN, allodynia and hyperalgesia are the main ailments. Hasanein P and Fazeli F (2014) observed the potential of NA to treat hyperalgesia and allodynia on STZ-induced diabetes animals. The NA doses (20, 50, and 100 mg/kg. p.o.) were given to rats (O.D.) for 8 weeks. After dose completion the superoxide dismutase and plasma glucose level were measured and complete allodynia and hyperalgesia was noticed in animals.

Finally, this study reported that NA (50–100 mg/kg) ameliorated DN via regulation of NO and glucose level as well as antioxidant enzyme stimulation.

21.8.7 Puerarin

Source: *Radix Puerariae lobata*

Mechanism of action: puerarin is a flavonoid obtained from Gegen (Radix Puerariae lobata) extraction and is known for its numerous pharmacological activities such as antioxidant, anti-inflammatory, antipyretic, and vasodilator and anticancer. Additionally, it has bone formation capacity and antidiabetic effect via improving insulin sensitive receptor activity. Some studies reported that puerarin can lessen blood viscosity and platelet aggregation as well as enhance microcirculation and decrease blood sugar level and enlarge coronary artery. It is also effective against proinflammatory cytokine production, which ultimately leads to diabetic neuropathic condition (Zhou YX ey al., 2014).

Preclinical Studies: Liu M et al. (2014) evaluated the potential of puerarin on diabetic neuropathic pain and chronic constriction injury (CCI) on animals. The intrathecal dose (4–100 nM) of puerarin was administered into experimental animals for one week. After completion of this study, it was reported that puerarin can inhibit proinflammatory cytokine (TNF-α, IL-1α, IL-1β, and IL-6) response as well as (NF-κB) upregulation. However, puerarin can be effective in DN pain via anti-inflammatory cytokine and NF-κB inhibition. Turer A and Onger ME (2018) conducted a study to examine the puerarin effect by oral ingestion on diabetic rat wound healing. For this study diabetes was induced using STZ dose (200 mg/kg). After confirmation of diabetes a full thickness wound was created in paravertebral area of experimental rats and sterile plaster was used to cover the wound. The diabetic rats were given Puerarin dose (200 mg/kg) via oral gavage for one week. After euthanization animal's stereological analysis was measured. Finally, it was concluded that puerarin is beneficial in new vessel formation and diabetic wound treatment in experimental rats.

21.8.8 Luteolin

Source: From *Martyniaccae* family plant

Mechanism of Action: Luteolin is a flavonoid extracted from the *Martynia annua (M. annua) Linn.* plant. It is known for its free radical scavenging, antioxidant, and neuroprotective properties via upregulation of (Nrf2) protein level. The antioxidant properties of luteolin are associated with (Nrf2) activation. Thus, some studies suggest that (Nrf2) is a targeted agent for the treatment of DN (Cardozo LF et al., 2013).

Preclinical Studies: Li et al. (2015) conducted a study to determine the effect of luteolin on DN. For this observation STZ was used to induce diabetes in experimental rats. The luteolin doses (50 mg/kg, 100 mg/kg, and 200 mg/kg) were injected (i.p) in animals for three weeks. Further, to examine the luteolin effect on DN, electrophysiological, biochemical, and behavioral parameters were tested. The data obtained from biochemical testing proved that luteolin has antioxidant action and can reduce the malondialdehyde and ROS stimulation. Moreover, luteolin can upregulate the protein level of (Nrf2) and (HO-1) in diabetic animals. Hence, it can reduce DN as well as encephalopathy.

21.8.9 Fisetin: (3, 39, 49, 7-tetrahydroxyflavone)

Source: Strawberries, onion

Mechanism of Action: Fisetin is a natural flavonoid found in the human diet including vegetables and fruits. Fisetin has many pharmacological activities such as anti-inflammatory, antiallergic, anticancer, antioxidant, and neuroprotective. Fisetin was able to reduce diabetes complications via lowering the methylglyoxal-dependant protein glycation, and in vitro it can downregulate gluconeogenesis and glycogenolysis (Khan N et al., 2013).

Preclinical Studies: Zhao et al. (2015) performed a study to observe the fisetin potential on DN and to investigate its mechanism. Diabetes was generated using a single dose of STZ (200 mg/kg i.p.) and to explore mechanical thermal hyperalgesia or allodynia Hargreaves test or von Frey test were performed. It was noticed that low dose of fisetin ameliorated neuropathic pain as well as reduced mechanical allodynia and thermal hyperalgesia symptoms in diabetic animals. Further, at higher doses fisetin showed antioxidant effect on rat tissue such as sciatic verve and dorsal root ganglion (DRG) but was not effective against hyperglycemia. Finally, it was reported that at higher dose, fisetin can manage or treat DN, allodynia, and hyperalgesia in diabetic type 1 mice via regulating antioxidant enzymes and spinal (GABA) receptors, which may be targets in DN.

21.8.10 Naringin: Naringin: (4′, 5, 7-trihydroxy flavanones 7-rhamno glycoside)

Source: Citrus species

Mechanism of Action: Naringin is an essential flavanone extracted from citrus fruits like grape and it contains pharmacological properties such as antioxidant, neuroprotective, anti-inflammatory, antiatherogenic, cholesterol lowering, antiulcer, antimicrobial, antimutagenic, anticancer, and cardioprotective properties [195]. It is also known as a free radical scavenger and metal chelating agent. Alam et al. (2014) suggested that naringin can ameliorate (TNF-a) level and transform growth factor-b (TGF-b) level, which is a major pathogenesis factor for numerous interstitial diseases. Naringin can reduce neuronal apoptosis and DNA damage via Bax-Bcl-2 pathway modulation. It is estimated that antioxidant and free radical absorbance action help naringin in wound healing.

Kandhare et al. (2015) conducted a study to investigate the naringin ointment (NO) potential in wound healing. For this study, a cream was formulated containing soft paraffin as a base and naringin concentration was 1, 2, to 4% w/w. The NO efficacy was assessed by topical application on incision and excision wound for twenty days. After completion of the study, some parameters were followed including histological, biochemical, and molecular. At the end of the experiment it was reported that naringin (2 & 4%) is helpful in re-epithelization and wound contraction resulting in effective wound healing. Additionally, NO has oxido-nitrosative stress (SOD, MPO, GSH, NOs, and MDA)-restoring ability. The Bax mRNA expression and proinflammatory cytokine level was also downregulated by NO treatment. The upregulation of VEGF and TGF-b, polymerase gamma (pol-g), collagen-1 mRNA, and Smad-3 level was also noticed using naringin application on wound. However, NO can be a good wound healing agent.

Conflict of Interest: All authors declare no conflict of interest.

REFERENCES

Addepalli V, Suryavanshi SV (2018) Catechin attenuates diabetic autonomic neuropathy in streptozotocin induced diabetic rats. Biomed Pharma cother. (108):1517–1523. https://doi: 10.1016/j.biopha.2018.09.179. Epub 2018 Oct 9. PMID: 30372853.

Agca CA, Tuzcu M, Hayirli A, Sahin K (2014) Taurine ameliorates neuropathy via regulating NF-κB and Nrf2/HO-1 signaling cascades in diabetic rats. Food and Chemical Toxicology. International Journal Published for the British Industrial Biological Research Association. (71):116–121. https://doi: 10.1016/j.fct.2014.05.023.

Alam MA, Subhan N, Rahman MM, Uddin SJ, Reza HM, Sarker SD (2014) Effect of citrus flavonoids, naringin and naringenin, on metabolic syndrome and their mechanisms of action. Adv Nutr.5 (4):404–417. doi: 10.3945/an.113.005603. PMID: 25022990

Alavi A, Sibbald RG, Mayer D, Goodman L, Botros M, Armstrong DG, et al. (2014) Diabetic foot ulcers: Part I. Pathophysiology and prevention. J Am Acad Dermatol. 70 (1):11–18. https://doi: 10.1016/j.jaad.2013.06.055. PMID: 24355275.

Al-Enazi MM (2014) Protective effects of combined therapy of rutin with silymarin on experimentallyinduced diabetic neuropathy in rats. Pharmacology & Pharmacy. (5): 876–889. doi: 10.4236/pp.2014.59098

Albers M, Romiti M, Brochado-Neto FC, Pereira, CAB (2005) Meta-analysis of alternate autologous vein bypass grafts to infrapopliteal arteries. J. Vasc. Surg. (42): 449–455. https://doi.org/10.1016/j.jvs.2005.05.031. [CrossRef].

Alonso-Coello P, Bellmunt S, McGorrian C, Anand SS, Guzman R, Criqui MH, et al. (2012) Antithrombotic therapy in peripheral artery disease: Antithrombotic Therapy and Prevention of Thrombosis. American College of Chest Physicians Evidence-Based Clinical Practice Guidelines. 141 (2 Suppl): 669S–690S. doi: 10.1378/chest.11-2307. PMID: 22315275; PMCID: PMC3278062.

Al-Rejaie SS, Aleisa AM, Abuohashish HM, Parmar MY, Ola MS, Al-Hosaini AA, Ahmed MM (2015) Naringenin neutralises oxidative stress and nerve growth factor discrepancy in experimental diabetic neuropathy. Neurol Res. 37 (10):924–933. https://doi: 10.1179/1743132815Y.0000000079. Epub 2015 Jul 17. PMID: 26187552.

Ambler GK, Twine CP (2018) Graft type for femoro-popliteal bypass surgery. Cochrane Database Syst Rev. 2 (2):CD001487. doi: 10.1002/14651858.CD001487.pub3. PMID: 29429146; PMCID: PMC6491197.

Apelqvist J, Ragnarson-Tennvall G, Persson U, Larsson J (1994) Diabetic foot ulcers in a multidisciplinary setting. An economic analysis of primary healing and healing with amputation. J Intern Med. 235 (5):463–471. doi: 10.1111/j.1365-2796.1994.tb01104.x. PMID: 8182403.

Armstrong DG, Boulton AJM, Bus SA (2017) Diabetic foot ulcers and their recurrence. N Engl J Med. 376 (24):2367–2375. doi: 10.1056/NEJMra1615439. PMID: 28614678.

Armstrong DG, Lavery LA (1997). Monitoring healing of acute Charcot's arthropathy with infrared dermal thermometry. J Rehabil Res Dev. 34 (3):317–321. PMID: 9239625.

Armstrong DG, Lavery LA, Harkless LB (1998) Validation of a diabetic wound classification system. The contribution of depth, infection, and ischemia to risk of amputation. Diabetes Care. (5):855–859. doi: 10.2337/diacare.21.5.855. PMID: 9589255.

Armstrong DG, Lavery LA, Wu S, Boulton AJ (2005) Evaluation of removable and irremovable cast walkers in the healing of diabetic foot wounds: a randomized controlled trial. Diabetes Care. 28 (3):551–554. doi: 10.2337/diacare.28.3.551. PMID: 15735186.

Armstrong DG, Todd WF, Lavery LA, Harkless LB, Bushman TR (1997) The natural history of acute Charcot's arthropathy in a diabetic foot specialty clinic. Diabet Med. (5):357–363. doi: 10.1002/(SICI)1096-9136 (199705)14:5 < 357::AID-DIA341> 3.0.CO;2-8. PMID: 9171250.

Arul V, Masilamoni JG, Jesudason EP, Jaji PJ, Inayathullah M, Dicky John DG, et al. (2012) Glucose oxidase incorporated collagen matrices for dermal wound repair in diabetic rat models: a biochemical study. J Biomater Appl. (8):917–938. doi: 10.1177/0885328210390402. Epub 2011 Mar 1. PMID: 21363874.

Attal N, Cruccu G, Baron R, Haanpää M, Hansson P, Jensen TS, Nurmikko T (2010) European Federation of Neurological Societies. EFNS guidelines on the pharmacological treatment of neuropathic pain: 2010 revision. Eur J Neurol. (9):1113-e88. doi: 10.1111/j.1468-1331.2010.02999.x. Epub 2010 Apr 9. PMID: 20402746.

Atturu G, Homer-Vanniasinkam S, Russell DA (2014) Pharmacology in peripheral arterial disease: what the interventional radiologist needs to know. Semin Intervent Radiol. (4):330–337. doi: 10.1055/s-0034-1393969. PMID: 25435658; PMCID: PMC4232431.

Bachewal P, Gundu C, Yerra VG, Kalvala AK, Areti A, Kumar A (2018) Morin exerts neuroprotection via attenuation of ROS induced oxidative damage and neuroinflammation in experimental diabetic neuropathy. Biofactors. 44 (2):109–122. doi: 10.1002/biof.1397. Epub 2017 Nov 28. PMID: 29193444.

Barradell LB, Brogden RN (1996) Oral naftidrofuryl. A review of its pharmacology and therapeutic use in the management of peripheral occlusive arterial disease. Drugs Aging. 8 (4):299–322. doi: 10.2165/00002512-199608040-00005. PMID: 8920176.

Bartkoski S, Day M (2016) Alpha-lipoic acid for treatment of diabetic peripheral neuropathy. Am. Fam. Physician; 2016; 93: 786.

Basu P, Basu A (2020) In vitro and in vivo effects of flavonoids on peripheral neuropathic pain. Molecules. 25 (5):1171. https://doi.org/10.3390/molecules25051171

Baumhauer JF, O'Keefe RJ, Schon LC, Pinzur MS (2006) Cytokine-induced osteoclastic bone resorption in charcot arthropathy: an immunohistochemical study. Foot Ankle Int. 27 (10):797–800. doi: 10.1177/107110070602701007. PMID: 17054880.

Bedenis R, Stewart M, Cleanthis M, Robless P, Mikhailidis DP, Stansby G (2014) Cilostazol for intermittent claudication. Cochrane Database Syst Rev. (10):CD003748. doi: 10.1002/14651858.CD003748.pub4. PMID: 25358850; PMCID: PMC7173701.

Bem R, Jirkovska A, Fejfarova V, Skibova J, Jude EB (2006) Intranasal Calcitonin in the treatment of acute Charcot neuro osteoarthropathy. Diabetes Care. (29): 1392–1394. https://doi.org/10.2337/dc06-0376

Bendy RH Jr, Nuccio PA, Wolfe E, Collins B, Tamburro C, Glass W, Martin CM. Relationship of quantitative wound bacterial counts to healing of decubiti: effect of topical gentamicin. Antimicrob Agents Chemother (Bethesda). (10):147–55. PMID: 14287920.

Bernatoniene J, Kopustinskiene DM (2018) the role of catechins in cellular responses to oxidative stress. Molecules.23 (4):965. doi: 10.3390/molecules23040965. PMID: 29677167; PMCID: PMC6017297.

Berner JE, Vidal P, Will P, Castillo P (2014) Uso de oxígenohiperbárico para el manejo de heridas: bases físicas, biológicas y evidencia disponible [Use of hyperbaric oxygenation for wound management]. Rev Med Chil. 142 (12):1575–83. Spanish. doi: 10.4067/S0034-98872014001200011. PMID: 25693440.

Boulton AJ, Gries FA, Jervell JA (1998) Guidelines for the diagnosis and outpatient management of diabetic peripheral neuropathy. Diabet Med. 15 (6):508–14. doi: 10.1002/(SICI)1096-9136 (199806)15:6 < 508::AID-DIA613> 3.0.CO;2-L. PMID: 9632127.

Brodsky JW (2007) Classification of foot lesions in diabetic patients. The Diabetic Foot. Philadelphia: Mosby Elsevier; 227–39. doi: 10.1016/B978-0-323-04145-4.50016-8

Brown TJ, Sedhom R, Gupta A (2019) Chemotherapy-induced peripheral neuropathy. JAMA Oncol. 5 (5):750. doi: 10.1001/jamaoncol.2018.6771. PMID: 30816956.

Cameron NE, Cotter MA, Basso M, Hohman TC (1997) Comparison of the effects of inhibitors of aldose reductase and sorbitol dehydrogenase on neurovascular function, nerve conduction and tissue polyol pathway metabolites in streptozotocin-diabetic rats. Diabetologia. 40 (3):271–81. doi: 10.1007/s001250050674. PMID: 9084964.

Canal N, Nemni R (1997) Autoimmunity and diabetic neuropathy. Clin Neurosci. (4):371–3.

Caputo GM, Ulbrecht J, Cavanagh PR, Juliano P (1998) The Charcot foot in diabetes: six key points. American Family Physician. 57 (11):2705–2710.

Cardozo LF, Pedruzzi LM, Stenvinkel P, Stockler-Pinto MB, Daleprane JB, Leite M Jr, Mafra D (2013) Nutritional strategies to modulate inflammation and oxidative stress pathways via activation of the master antioxidant switch Nrf2. Biochimie. 95 (8):1525–33. doi: 10.1016/j.biochi.2013.04.012. Epub 2013 May 1. PMID: 23643732.

Caro-Ordieres T, Marín-Royo G, Opazo-Ríos L, Jiménez-Castilla L, Moreno JA, Gómez-Guerrero C, Egido J (2020) The coming age of flavonoids in the treatment of diabetic complications. J Clin Med. 27;9 (2):346. doi: 10.3390/jcm9020346. PMID: 32012726; PMCID: PMC7074336.

Chantelau E, Onvlee GJ (2006) Charcot foot in diabetes: farewell to the neurotrophic theory. Horm Metab Res. 38 (6):361–7. doi: 10.1055/s-2006-944525. PMID: 16823717.

Charcot J-M (1868) Sur quelques arthropathies qui paraissent dépendre d'une lésion du cerveau ou de la moelle épinière. [On some arthropathies apparently related to a lesion of the brain or spinal cord]. Arch Physiol Norm Pathol 1868; 1: 161–178.

Charcot J-M, Fere C (1883) Affectionsosse use set articulaires du pied chez les tabétiques (Pied tabétique). Archives de Neurologie 1883; 6:305–319.

Chirumbolo S (2012) Flavonoids in propolis acting on mast cell-mediated wound healing. Inflammopharmacology. 20 (2):99–101. doi: 10.1007/s10787-012-0125-9. Epub 2012 Feb 17. PMID: 22349997.

CIMA (2019) Available online: https://cima.aemps.es (accessed on 24 May 2019).

Citron DM, Goldstein EJ, Merriam CV, Lipsky BA, Abramson MA (2007) Bacteriology of moderate-to-severe diabetic foot infections and in vitro activity of antimicrobial agents. J Clin Microbiol. 45 (9):2819–2828. doi: 10.1128/JCM.00551-07. Epub 2007 Jul 3. PMID: 17609322; PMCID: PMC2045270.

Clayton W, Elasy TA (2009) A review of pathophysiology, classification and treatment of foot ulcers in diabetic patients. Clin Diabetes. (27):52–58

Cofield RH, Morrison MJ, Beabout JW (1983) Diabetic neuroarthropathy in the foot: patient characteristics and patterns of radiographic change. Foot Ankle. 4 (1):15–22. doi: 10.1177/107110078300400104. PMID: 6618351.

Comerota AJ, Froehlich J, Turpie AGG, and White JV (1994) Results of a prospective randomized trial evaluating surgery versus thrombolysi for ischemia of the lower extremity. The STILE Trial. Ann. Surg. (220): 251–268. https://doi: 10.1097/00000658-199409000-00003

Cox AA, Sagot Y, Hedou G, Grek C, Wilkes T, Vinik AI, Ghatnekar G (2017) Low-dose pulsatile interleukin-6 as a treatment option for diabetic peripheral neuropathy. Front Endocrinol (Lausanne). (2): 8:89. doi: 10.3389/fendo.2017.00089. PMID: 28512447; PMCID: PMC5411416.

Cushnie TP, Lamb AJ (2005) Antimicrobial activity of flavonoids. Int J Antimicrob Agents. 26 (5):343–356. Erratum in: Int J Antimicrob Agents. doi: 10.1016/j.ijantimicag.2005.09.002. 2006 Feb;27 (2):181. PMID: 16323269; PMCID: PMC7127073.

Cuzzell J (2003) Wound assessment and evaluation: diabetic ulcer protocol. Dermatol Nurs. 15 (2):153. PMID: 12751351.

de Franciscis S, Gallelli L, Battaglia L, Molinari V, Montemurro R, Stillitano DM, et al. (2015) Cilostazol prevents foot ulcers in diabetic patients with peripheral vascular disease. Int Wound J. 12 (3):250–253. doi: 10.1111/iwj.12085. Epub 2013 May 15. PMID: 23672237.

Drel V, Szabo C, Stevens, M, Obrosova I. (2005) Low-dose poly (ADP-Ribose) polymerase inhibitor-containing combination therapies reverse early peripheral diabetic neuropathy. Diabetes. (54): 1514–1522. https://doi:10.2337/diabetes.54.5.1514.

Du X, Matsumura T, Edelstein D, Rossetti L, Zsengellér Z, Szabó C, Brownlee M (2003) Inhibition of GAPDH activity by poly (ADP-ribose) polymerase activates three major pathways of hyperglycemic damage in endothelial cells. J Clin Invest. 112 (7):1049–57. doi: 10.1172/JCI18127. PMID: 14523042; PMCID: PMC198524.

Dunnill C, Patton T, Brennan J, Barrett J, Dryden M, Cooke J, et al. (2017) Reactive oxygen species (ROS) and wound healing: the functional role of ROS and emerging ROS-modulating technologies for augmentation of the healing process. Int Wound J. 14 (1):89–96. doi: 10.1111/iwj.12557. Epub 2015 Dec 21. PMID: 26688157.

Dworkin RH, O'Connor AB, Backonja M, Farrar JT, Finnerup NB, Jensen TS, et al. (2007) Pharmacologic management of neuropathic pain: evidence-based recommendations. Pain. 132 (3):237–251. doi: 10.1016/j.pain.2007.08.033. Epub 2007 Oct 24. PMID: 17920770.

Eichenholtz SN (1966) Charcot Joints. Springfield, IL, Charles C. Thomas.

Eskelinen E, Lepäntalo M, Hietala EM, Sell H, Kauppila L, Mäenpää I, et al. (2004) Lower limb amputations in southern Finland in 2000 and trends up to 2001. Eur J Vasc Endovasc Surg. 27 (2):193–200. doi: 10.1016/j.ejvs.2003.10.011. PMID: 14718903.

Eslami MH, Zayaruzny M, Fitzgerald GA (2007) The adverse effects of race, insurance status, and low income on the rate of amputation in patients presenting with lower extremity ischemia. J Vasc Surg. 45 (1):55–9. doi: 10.1016/j.jvs.2006.09.044. PMID: 17210382.

Fejfarová V, Pavlů., Bém R, Wosková V, Dubský M, Němcová A, et al. (2019) The superiority of removable contact splints in the healing of diabetic foot during postoperative care. Journal of Diabetes Research; 2019: 10. https://doi.org/10.1111/j.1742-481X.2012.01022.x

Fernández-Samos Gutiérrez R (2012) The angiosome model in the revascularization strategy of critical limb ischemia. Angiología. 64: 173–182. http://dx.doi.org/10.1016/j.angio.2012.03.003

Frykberg RG (2002) Diabetic foot ulcers: pathogenesis and management. Am Fam Physician. 66 (9):1655–62. doi: 10.1016/j.cpm.2002.04.001 PMID: 12449264.

Frykberg RG, Eneroth M (2010) Principles of conservative management. In The Diabetic Charcot Foot: Principles and Management. Frykberg RG, Ed. Brooklandville, MD, Data Trace Publishing Company. pp. 93–116

Frykberg RG, Wittmayer B, Zgonis T (2007) Surgical management of diabetic foot infections and osteomyelitis. Clin Podiatr Med Surg. 24 (3):469–82, viii-ix. doi: 10.1016/j.cpm.2007.04.001. PMID: 17613386.

Games G, Hutchison A (2013) Tapentadol-ER for the treatment of diabetic peripheral neuropathy. Consult Pharm. 28 (10):672–5. doi: 10.4140/TCP.n.2013.672. PMID: 24129223.

Gardner SE, Frantz RA (2008) Wound bioburden and infection-related complications in diabetic foot ulcers. Biol Res Nurs. 10 (1):44–53. doi: 10.1177/1099800408319056. PMID: 18647759; PMCID: PMC3777233.

Grayer RJ, Veitch NC (2008) Flavanones and dihydroflavonols. In Flavonoids; CRC Press: Boca Raton, FL, USA. pp. 924–1009. DOI: 10.1039/b718040n PMID: 18497898

Grether-Beck S, Olaizola-Horn S, Schmitt H, Grewe M, Jahnke A, Johnson JP, et al. (1996) Activation of transcription factor AP-2 mediates UVA radiation-and singlet oxygen-induced expression of the human intercellular adhesion molecule 1 gene. Proc Natl Acad Sci USA. 93 (25):14586–14591. doi: 10.1073/pnas.93.25.14586. PMID: 8962096; PMCID: PMC26177.

Hasanein P, Fazeli F (2014) Role of naringenin in protection against diabetic hyperalgesia and tactile allodynia in male Wistar rats. J Physiol Biochem. (70):997–1006. doi: 10.1007/s13105-014-0369-5. Epub 2014 Nov 19.

Henderson VE (1905) Joint affections in tabes dorsalis. J Pathol. (10):211–264. https://doi.org/10.1002/path.1700100302

Honing ML, Morrison PJ, Banga JD, Stroes ES, Rabelink TJ (1998) Nitric oxide availability in diabetes mellitus. Diabetes Metab Rev.14 (3):241–9. doi: 10.1002/(sici)1099-0895 (1998090)14:3 < 241::aid-dmr216> 3.0.co;2-r. PMID: 9816472.

Höpfner S, Krolak C, Kessler S, Tiling R (2004) Präoperative Bildgebung bei diabetisch-neuropathischer Osteoarthropathie: Ist der zusätzliche Einsatz von (18)F-FDGPET sinnvoll? [Preoperative imaging of Charcot neuroarthropathy: Does the additional application of (18)F-FDG-PET make sense?] Nuklearmedizin. 45 (1):15–20. German. doi: 10.1267/nukl06010015. PMID: 16493510.

Hunt JA (1992) Foot infections in diabetes are rarely due to a single microorganism. Diabet Med. 9 (8):749–752. doi: 10.1111/j.1464-5491.1992.tb01885.x. PMID: 1395469.

Hyeyoon E, Lee HJ, Lim Y (2016) Ameliorative effect of dietary genistein on diabetes induced hyper-inflammation and oxidative stress during early stage of wound healing in alloxan induced diabetic mice. Biochem Biophys Res Commun. 478 (3):1021–1027. doi: 10.1016/j.bbrc.2016.07.039. Epub 2016 Jul 16. PMID: 27431618.

IDF (2015) International Diabetes Federation 7th edition. 2015. ISBN: 978–2-930229-81-2

Iida O, Soga Y, Hirano K, Kawasaki D, Suzuki K, Miyashita Y, et al. (2012) Long-term results of direct and indirect endovascular revascularization based on the angiosome concept in patients with critical limb ischemia presenting with isolated below-the-knee lesions. J Vasc Surg. 55 (2):363–370.e5. doi: 10.1016/j.jvs.2011.08.014. Epub 2011 Nov 1. PMID: 22051875.

Institute for Health Metrics and Evaluation (IHME) (2017) GBD Compare Data Visualization.

James TJ, Hughes MA, Cherry GW, Taylor RP (2003) Evidence of oxidative stress in chronic venous ulcers. Wound Repair Regen.11 (3):172–6. doi: 10.1046/j.1524-475x.2003.11304.x. PMID: 12753597.

Javed S, Alam U, Malik RA (2015) Burning through the pain: treatments for diabetic neuropathy. Diabetes ObesMetab.17 (12):1115–25. doi: 10.1111/dom.12535. Epub 2015 Sep 10. PMID: 26179288.

Jeffcoate W (2008) The causes of the Charcot syndrome. Clin Podiatr Med Surg.25 (1):29–42, vi. doi: 10.1016/j.cpm.2007.10.003. PMID: 18165109.

Jeffcoate W, Game F, Cavanagh PR (2005) The role of proinflammatory cytokines in the cause of neuropathic osteoarthropathy (acute Charcot foot) in diabetes. Lancet. 366 (9502):2058–61. doi: 10.1016/S0140-6736 (05)67029-8. Epub 2005 Aug 10. PMID: 16338454.

Johnson JT (1967) Neuropathic fractures and joint injuries. Pathogenesis and rationale of prevention and treatment. J Bone Joint Surg Am. 49 (1):1–30. PMID: 4163089.

Jude EB, Selby PL, Burgess J, Lilleystone P, Mawer EB, Page SR, et al. (2001) Bisphosphonates in the treatment of Charcot neuroarthropathy: a double-blind randomised controlled trial. Diabetologia.44 (11):2032–7. doi: 10.1007/s001250100008. PMID: 11719835.

Jull AB, Cullum N, Dumville JC, Westby MJ, Deshpande S, Walker N (2015) Honey as a topical treatment for wounds. Cochrane Database Syst Rev. 6; (3):CD005083. doi: 10.1002/14651858.CD005083.pub4. PMID: 25742878.

Kaltalioglu K, Coskun-Cevher S, Tugcu-Demiröz F, Celebi N (2013) PDGF supplementation alters oxidative events in wound healing process: A time course study. Archives of dermatological research. 305. https://doi10.1007/s00403-013-1326-9.

Kamalakkannan N, Prince PS (2006) Antihyperglycaemic and antioxidant effect of rutin, a polyphenolic flavonoid, in streptozotocin-induced diabetic wistar rats. Basic Clin PharmacolToxicol.98 (1):97–103. doi: 10.1111/j.1742-7843.2006.pto_241.x. PMID: 16433898.

Kandhare AD, Raygude KS, Ghosh P, Ghule AE, Bodhankar SL (2012) Neuroprotective effect of naringin by modulation of endogenous biomarkers in streptozotocin induced painful diabetic neuropathy. Fitoterapia.83 (4):650–659. doi: 10.1016/j.fitote.2012.01.010. Epub 2012 Feb 9. PMID: 22343014.

Kaufman J, Breeding L, Rosenberg N (1987) Anatomical location of acute diabetic foot infection: its influence on the outcome of treatment. Am J Surg. (53): 109–112. doi: 10.11648/j.ajim.20150302.11

Kayssi A, Al-Atassi T, Oreopoulos G, Roche-Nagle G, Tan KT, Rajan DK (2016) Drug-eluting balloon angioplasty versus uncoated balloon angioplasty for peripheral arterial disease of the lower limbs. Cochrane Database Syst Rev.4; (8):CD011319. doi: 10.1002/14651858.CD011319.pub2. PMID: 27490003.

Keidar Z, Militianu D, Melamed E, Bar-Shalom R, Israel O (2005) The diabetic foot: initial experience with 18F FDG PET/CT. J Nucl. Med. (46):444–449.

Khoo HE, Azlan A, Tang ST, Lim SM (2017) Anthocyanidins and anthocyanins: colored pigments as food, pharmaceutical ingredients, and the potential health benefits. Food Nutr Res. 61 (1):1361779. doi: 10.1080/16546628.2017.1361779. PMID: 28970777; PMCID: PMC5613902.

Kim HP, Son KH, Chang HW, Kang SS (2004) Anti-inflammatory plant flavonoids and cellular action mechanisms. J Pharmacol Sci. 96 (3):229–245. doi: 10.1254/jphs.crj04003x. Epub 2004 Nov 12. PMID: 15539763.

Kishore L, Kaur N, Singh R (2018) Effect of Kaempferol isolated from seeds of Eruca sativa on changes of pain sensitivity in Streptozotocin-induced diabetic neuropathy. Inflammopharmacology. 26 (4):993–1003. doi: 10.1007/s10787-017-0416-2. Epub 2017 Nov 20. PMID: 29159712.

Kleijnen J, Mackerras D (2000) Vitamin E for intermittent claudication. Cochrane Database Syst Rev. (2):CD000987. doi: 10.1002/14651858.CD000987. PMID: 10796571.

Klyubin IV, Kirpichnikova KM, Gamaley IA (1996) Hydrogen peroxide-induced chemotaxis of mouse peritoneal neutrophils. Eur J Cell Biol. 70 (4):347–351. PMID: 8864663.

Komirishetty P, Areti A, Sistla R, Kumar A (2016) Morin mitigates chronic constriction injury (CCI)-induced peripheral neuropathy by inhibiting oxidative stress induced parp over-activation and neuroinflammation. Neurochem Res. 41 (8):2029–2042. doi: 10.1007/s11064-016-1914-0. Epub 2016 Apr 15. PMID: 27084773.

Khan N, Syed DN, Ahmad N, Mukhtar H (2013) Fisetin: a dietary antioxidant for health promotion. Antioxid Redox Signal.19 (2):151–162. doi: 10.1089/ars.2012.4901. Epub 2012 Dec 18. PMID: 23121441; PMCID: PMC3689181.

Kumar, H, Anup S, Sobhia, ME (2012) Novel insights into the structural requirements for the design of selective and specific aldose reductase inhibitors. Journal of Molecular Modeling. 18. 1791–9. 10.1007/s00894-011-1195-0.

Kwakman PH, Zaat SA (2012) Antibacterial components of honey. IUBMB Life. (64):48–55. https://doi.org/10.1002/iub.578

Lavery LA, Higgins KR, Lanctot DR, Constantinides GP, Zamorano RG, Athanasiou KA, et al. (2007) Preventing diabetic foot ulcer recurrence in high-risk patients: use of temperature monitoring as a self-assessment tool. Diabetes Care. 30 (1):14–20. doi: 10.2337/dc06-1600. PMID: 17192326.

Lee V, Singh G, Trasatti JP, Bjornsson C, Xu X, Tran TN, et al. (2014) Design and fabrication of human skin by three-dimensional bioprinting. Tissue Eng Part C Methods. 20 (6):473–484. doi: 10.1089/ten. TEC.2013.0335. Epub 2013 Dec 31. PMID: 24188635; PMCID: PMC4024844.

Li M, Li Q, Zhao Q, Zhang J, Lin J (2015) Luteolin improves the impaired nerve functions in diabetic neuropathy: behavioral and biochemical evidence. Int J Clin Exp Pathol. 8 (9):10112–10120. PMID: 26617718; PMCID: PMC4637533.

Liu M, Liao K, Yu C, Li X, Liu S, Yang S (2014) Puerarin alleviates neuropathic pain by inhibiting neuroinflammation in spinal cord. Mediators of Inflammation. https://doi.org/10.1155/2014/485927

Mabilleau G, Petrova NL, Edmonds ME, Sabokbar A (2008) Increased osteoclastic activity in acute Charcot's osteoarthropathy: the role of receptor activator of nuclear factor-kappaB ligand. Diabetologia.51 (6):1035–1040. doi: 10.1007/s00125-008-0992-1. Epub 2008 Apr 4. PMID: 18389210; PMCID: PMC2362134.

Maestri A, De Pasquale Ceratti A, Cundari S, Zanna C, Cortesi E, Crinò L (2005) A pilot study on the effect of acetyl-L-carnitine in paclitaxel-and cisplatin-induced peripheral neuropathy. Tumori. 91 (2):135–8. PMID: 15948540.

Margolis DJ, Kantor J, Berlin JA (1999) Healing of diabetic neuropathic foot ulcers receiving standard treatment. A meta-analysis. Diabetes Care.22 (5):692–5. doi: 10.2337/diacare.22.5.692. PMID: 10332667.

Matas M, Domínguez González JM, Montull E (2013) Antiplatelet therapy in endovascular surgery: the Rendovasc study. Ann Vasc Surg 2013; 27 (2):168–177. doi: 10.1016/j.avsg.2011.11.045.

Matsuo H, Shigematsu H (2010) Patient-based outcomes using the Walking Impairment Questionnaire for patients with peripheral arterial occlusive disease treated with Lipo-PGE1. Circ J. 74 (2):365–70. doi: 10.1253/circj.cj-09-0376. Epub 2009 Dec 26. PMID: 20037256.

Mezei O, Banz WJ, Steger RW, Peluso MR, Winters TA, Shay N (2003) Soy isoflavones exert antidiabetic and hypolipidemic effects through the PPAR pathways in obese Zucker rats and murine RAW 264.7 cells. J Nutr. 133 (5):1238–1243. doi: 10.1093/jn/133.5.1238. PMID: 12730403.

Morrison WB, Ledermann HP (2002) Work-up of the diabetic foot. Radiol Clin North Am 2002; 40:1171–1192

Morrison WB, Ledermann HP, Schweitzer ME (2001) MR imaging of the diabetic foot. MagnReson Imaging Clin N Am. 9 (3):603–613, xi. PMID: 11694429.

Mudge BP, Harris C, Gilmont RR, Adamson BS, Rees RS (2002) Role of glutathione redox dysfunction in diabetic wounds. Wound Repair Regen. (10): 52–58. doi: 10.1046/j.1524-475x.2002.10803.x

Niture NT, Ansari AA, Naik SR (2014) Anti-hyperglycemic activity of rutin in streptozotocin-induced diabetic rats: an effect mediated through cytokines, antioxidants and lipid biomarkers. Indian J Exp Biol. 52 (7):720–727. PMID: 25059040.

Nilforoushan D, Gramoun A, Glogauer M, Manolson MF (2009) Nitric oxide enhances osteoclastogenesis possibly by mediating cell fusion. Nitric Oxide.21 (1):27–36. doi: 10.1016/j.niox.2009.04.002. Epub 2009 Apr 21. PMID: 19389479.

Obrosova IG, Julius UA (2005) Role for poly (ADP-ribose) polymerase activation in diabetic nephropathy, neuropathy and retinopathy. Curr VascPharmacol.3 (3):267–83. doi: 10.2174/1570161054368634. PMID: 16026323.

Offley SC, Guo TZ, Wei T, Clark JD, Vogel H, Lindsey DP, et al. (2005) Capsaicin-sensitive sensory neurons contribute to the maintenance of trabecular bone integrity. J Bone Miner Res. 20 (2):257–267. doi: 10.1359/JBMR.041108. Epub 2004 Nov 16. PMID: 15647820.

Ollendorf DA, Kotsanos JG, Wishner WJ, Friedman M, Cooper T, Bittoni M, Oster G (1998) Potential economic benefits of lower-extremity amputation prevention strategies in diabetes. Diabetes Care. 21 (8):1240–1245. doi: 10.2337/diacare.21.8.1240. PMID: 9702427.

Oses C, Olivares B, Ezquer M, Acosta C, Bosch P, Donoso M, et al. (2017) Preconditioning of adipose tissue-derived mesenchymal stem cells with deferoxamine increases the production of pro-angiogenic, neuroprotective and anti-inflammatory factors: Potential application in the treatment of diabetic neuropathy. PLoS One. 12 (5):e0178011. doi: 10.1371/journal.pone.0178011. PMID: 28542352;

O'Toole EA, Goel M, Woodley DT (1996) Hydrogen peroxide inhibits human keratinocyte migration. Dermatol Surg.22 (6):525–9. doi: 10.1111/j.1524-4725.1996.tb00368.x. PMID: 8646466.

Ouriel K, Veith FJ, Sasahara AA (1998) A comparison of recombinant urokinase with vascular surgery as initial treatment for acute arterial occlusion of the legs. Thrombolysis or Peripheral Arterial Surgery (TOPAS) Investigators. N Engl J Med. 338 (16):1105–1011. doi: 10.1056/NEJM199804163381603. PMID: 9545358.

Pakarinen TK, Laine HJ, Mäenpää H, Mattila P, Lahtela J (2011) The effect of zoledronic acid on the clinical resolution of Charcot neuroarthropathy: a pilot randomized controlled trial. Diabetes Care.34 (7):1514–1516. doi: 10.2337/dc11-0396. Epub 2011 May 18. PMID: 21593295; PMCID: PMC3120211.

Paravastu SC, Mendonca DA, Da Silva A (2013) Beta blockers for peripheral arterial disease. Cochrane Database Syst Rev. (9):CD005508. doi: 10.1002/14651858.CD005508.pub3. PMID: 24027118; PMCID: PMC7271644.

Park E, Lee SM, Jung IK, Lim Y, Kim JH (2011) Effects of genistein on early-stage cutaneous wound healing. BiochemBiophys Res Commun.410 (3):514–519. doi: 10.1016/j.bbrc.2011.06.013. Epub 2011 Jun 7. PMID: 21679688.

Park SJ, Park DW, Kim YH, Kang SJ, Lee SW, Lee CW, et al. (2010) Duration of dual antiplatelet therapy after implantation of drug-eluting stents. N Engl J Med.362 (15):1374–1382. doi: 10.1056/NEJMoa1001266. Epub 2010 Mar 15. PMID: 20231231.

Pedrosa HC (2010) Diabetic polyneuropathy: new strategies for early diagnosis and therapeutic intervention – guidelines Neur-ALAD (in Portuguese) in The Latin America Congress on Controversies to Consensus in Diabetes, Obesity and Hypertension (CODHy), Buenos Aires, Argentina, pp. 2–8.

Perez-Favila A, Martinez-Fierro ML, Rodriguez-Lazalde JG, Cid-Baez MA, Zamudio-Osuna MJ, Martinez-Blanco MAR, et al. (2019) Current Therapeutic Strategies in Diabetic Foot Ulcers. Medicina. (55):714. doi:10.3390/medicina55110714

Pendsey SP (2010) Understanding diabetic foot. Int J Diabetes Dev Ctries. 30 (2):75–79. doi: 10.4103/0973-3930.62596. PMID: 20535310; PMCID: PMC2878694.

Petrova NL, Edmonds ME (2013) Medical management of Charcot arthropathy. Diabetes Obes Metab.15 (3):193–197. doi: 10.1111/j.1463-1326.2012.01671.x. Epub 2012 Sep 20. PMID: 22862834.

Pitocco D, Ruotolo V, Caputo S (2005) Six-month treatment with alendronate in acute Charcot neuroarthropathy: a randomized controlled trial. Diabetes. (28): 1214–1215. doi: 10.2337/diacare.28.5.1214.

Procházková D, Boušová I, Wilhelmová N (2011) Antioxidant and prooxidant properties of flavonoids. Fitoterapia. 82 (4):513–523. doi: 10.1016/j.fitote.2011.01.018. Epub 2011 Jan 28. PMID: 21277359.

Raghav A, Khan ZA, Labala RK, Ahmad J, Noor S, Mishra BK (2018) Financial burden of diabetic foot ulcers to world: a progressive topic to discuss always. Ther Adv Endocrinol Metab.9 (1):29–31. doi: 10.1177/2042018817744513. Epub 2017 Dec 12. PMID: 29344337; PMCID: PMC5761954.

Rajbhandari SM, Jenkins RC, Davies C, Tesfaye S (2002) Charcot neuroarthropathy in diabetes mellitus. Diabetologia. 45 (8):1085–1096. doi: 10.1007/s00125-002-0885-7. Epub 2002 Jul 11. PMID: 12189438.

Rangel ÉB, Sá JR, Gomes SA, Carvalho AB, Melaragno CS, Gonzalez AM, Linhares MM, Medina-Pestana JO (2012) Charcot neuro-arthropathy after simultaneous pancreas kidney transplant. Transplantation 2012; 94: 642–645. doi: 10.1097/TP.0b013e31825cadbb.

Raskin P, Huffman C, Yurkewicz L, Pauer L, Scavone JM, Yang R, Parsons B (2016) Pregabalin in patients with painful diabetic peripheral neuropathy using an NSAID for other pain conditions: a double-blind crossover study. Clin J Pain.32 (3):203–210. doi: 10.1097/AJP.0000000000000254. PMID: 25968451.

Robertson L, Andras A (2013) Prostanoids for intermittent claudication. Cochrane Database Syst Rev. 30; (4):CD000986. doi: 10.1002/14651858.CD000986.pub3. PMID: 23633305.

Robertson L, Ghouri MA, Kovacs F (2012) Antiplatelet and anticoagulant drugs for prevention of restenosis/reocclusion following peripheral endovascular treatment. Cochrane Database Syst Rev.15 (8):CD002071. doi: 10.1002/14651858.CD002071.pub3. PMID: 22895926; PMCID: PMC7066628.

Rogers CL, Robert G, Frykberg GR, Armstrong GD, Boulton JM, Edmonds M, et al. (2011) The Charcot foot in diabetes. Diabetes Care. (34):2123–2129. doi: 10.2337/dc11-0844.

Rojas AI, Phillips TJ (1999) Patients with chronic leg ulcers show diminished levels of vitamins A and E, carotenes, and zinc. Dermatol Surg.25 (8):601–604. doi: 10.1046/j.1524-4725.1999.99074.x. PMID: 10491041.

Ruffolo AJ, Romano M, Ciapponi A (2010) Prostanoids for critical limb ischaemia. Cochrane Database Syst Rev. (1):CD006544. doi: 10.1002/14651858.CD006544.pub2. Update in: Cochrane Database Syst Rev. 2018 Jan 10;1:CD006544. PMID: 20091595.

Salhiyyah K, Senanayake E, Abdel-Hadi M, Booth A, Michaels JA (2012) Pentoxifylline for intermittent claudication. Cochrane Database Syst Rev.18;1:CD005262. doi: 10.1002/14651858.CD005262.pub2. Update in: Cochrane Database Syst Rev. 2015 Sep 29;9:CD005262. PMID: 22258961.

Schaper NC, Huijberts M, Pickwell K (2008) Neurovascular control and neurogenic inflammation in diabetes. Diabetes Metab Res Rev. 24 Suppl 1:S40–44. doi: 10.1002/dmrr.862. PMID: 18442183.

Shaw JE, Boulton AJ (1997) The pathogenesis of diabetic foot problems: an overview. Diabetes. 46 Suppl 2:S58–61. doi: 10.2337/diab.46.2.s58. PMID: 9285501.

Singh S, Pai DR, Yuhhui C (2013) Diabetic Foot Ulcer – Diagnosis and Management. Clin Res Foot Ankle 1:120. doi:10.4172/2329-910X.1000120

Soga Y, Iida O, Kawasaki D, Hirano K, Yamaoka T, Suzuki K. Impact of cilostazol on angiographic restenosis after balloon angioplasty for infrapopliteal artery disease in patients with critical limb ischemia. Eur J VascEndovasc Surg.44 (6):577–581. doi: 10.1016/j.ejvs.2012.09.020. Epub 2012 Oct 26. PMID: 23107298.

Steed DL (2001) Diabetic Wounds, Assessment, Classification, and Management. Chronic Wound Care: A Clinical Source Book for Healthcare Professionals. Wayne, PA: Health Management Publications; 575–581. doi: 10.1016/s0741-5214 (95)70245-8.

Stevens JW, Simpson E, Harnan S, Squires H, Meng Y, Thomas S, et al. (2012) Systematic review of the efficacy of cilostazol, naftidrofuryl oxalate and pentoxifylline for the treatment of intermittent claudication. Br J Surg. 99 (12):1630–1638. doi: 10.1002/bjs.8895. Epub 2012 Oct 3. PMID: 23034699.

Tang HY, Jiang AJ, Ma JL, Wang FJ, Shen GM (2019) Understanding the signaling pathways related to the mechanism and treatment of diabetic peripheral neuropathy. Endocrinology. (160): 2119–2127. doi: 10.1210/en.2019-00311. [CrossRef] [PubMed]

Téllez, GA and Castaño, JC (2010) Antimicrobial peptides. Infectio. 14 (1): 55–67. https://doi.org/10.1016/S0123-9392 (10)70093-X

Tesfaye S, Boulton AJ, Dickenson AH. Mechanisms and management of diabetic painful distal symmetrical polyneuropathy. Diabetes Care.36 (9):2456–2465. doi: 10.2337/dc12-1964. PMID: 23970715; PMCID: PMC3747929.

Tian R, Yang W, Xue Q, et al (2015) Rutin ameliorates diabetic neuropathy by lowering plasma glucose and decreasing oxidative stress via Nrf2 signaling pathway in rats. European Journal of Pharmacology. 771:84–92. doi: 10.1016/j.ejphar.2015.12.021.

Tur E, Bolton L, Constantine BE (1995) Topical hydrogen peroxide treatment of ischemic ulcers in the guinea pig: blood recruitment in multiple skin sites. J Am Acad Dermatol.33 (2 Pt 1):217–221. doi: 10.1016/0190-9622 (95)90238-4. PMID: 7622648.

Turer A and Onger ME (2018) The effect of oral puerarin administration on wound healing in diabetic rat model. Ann Med Res. 25 (4): 536–9. doi: 10.5455/annalsmedres.2018.05.074.

Ubbink DT, Vermeulen H (2013) Spinal cord stimulation for non-reconstructable chronic critical leg ischaemia. Cochrane Database Syst Rev.28;2013 (2):CD004001. doi: 10.1002/14651858.CD004001.pub3. PMID: 23450547; PMCID: PMC7163280.

Valsecchi AE, Franchi S, Panerai AE, Rossi A, Sacerdote P, Colleoni M (2011) The soy isoflavone genistein reverses oxidative and inflammatory state, neuropathic pain, neurotrophic and vasculature deficits in diabetes mouse model. Eur J Pharmacol. 15;650 (2-3):694–702. doi: 10.1016/j.ejphar.2010.10.060. Epub 2010 Nov 2. PMID: 21050844.

Visnagri A, Kandhare AD, Chakravarty S, Ghosh P, Bodhankar SL (2014) Hesperidin, a flavanoglycone attenuates experimental diabetic neuropathy via modulation of cellular and biochemical marker to improve nerve functions, Pharmaceutical Biology.52: (7):814–828, doi: 10.3109/13880209.2013.870584

Viswanathan V, Jasmine JJ, Snehalatha C, Ramachandran A (2002) Prevalence of pathogens in diabetic foot infection in South Indian type 2 diabetic patients. J Assoc Physicians India. (50):1013–1016. PMID: 12421021.

Wall IB, Davies CE, Hill KE, Wilson MJ, Stephens P, Harding KG, Thomas DW (2002) Potential role of anaerobic cocci in impaired human wound healing. Wound Repair Regen.10 (6):346–353. doi: 10.1046/j.1524-475x.2002.t01-1-10602.x. PMID: 12453137.

Watson JC, Dyck PJ (2015) Peripheral neuropathy: a practical approach to diagnosis and symptom management. Mayo Clin Proc. 90 (7):940–951. doi: 10.1016/j.mayocp.2015.05.004. PMID: 26141332.

Wlaschek M, Scharffetter-Kochanek K (2005) Oxidative stress in chronic venous leg ulcers. Wound Repair Regen. 13 (5):452–461. doi: 10.1111/j.1067-1927.2005.00065.x. PMID: 16176453.

Zhao X, Wang C, Cui WG, Ma Q, Zhou WH (2015) Fisetin exerts antihyperalgesic effect in a mouse model of neuropathic pain: engagement of spinal serotonergic system. Sci Rep. 5:9043. doi: 10.1038/srep09043. PMID: 25761874; PMCID: PMC4356956.

Zhou YX, Zhang H, Peng C (2014) Puerarin: a review of pharmacological effects. Phytother Res. Jul;28 (7):961–975. doi: 10.1002/ptr.5083. Epub 2013 Dec 13. PMID: 24339367.

22

Current Challenges in Immunobiology of Autoimmunity and Cancer

Kumari Anupam
Department of Biochemistry, AIIMS, Bilaspur, India,

Jyotsana Kaushal, Ankit Tandon, and Archana Bhatnagar
Department of Biochemistry, Panjab University, Chandigarh, India

22.1 Introduction

22.1.1 What is Autoimmunity?

Our body encounters many pathogenic and non-pathogenic micro-organisms daily, but we do not always catch a disease. This happens due to the very efficient immune system that works day and night to protect us from various infections. The immune system has a way of handling the mismanaged responses at a very early stage, but what happens if the system cannot combat these self-antigens? It is imperative to understand that the immune responses to self-antigens do not always result in autoimmune disorders. Only when the autoantibodies are generated due to the autoimmune response is a dysfunction in the body considered an autoimmune disorder. The failure of our immune system to recognize and tolerate the self-directed immune response is considered as autoimmunity (South, 2013; Smith, 2010).

The earliest realization that the effector mechanisms that occur during host defense against a particular antigen, if turned against the host, can have detrimental effects and cause severe tissue damage s was termed *horror autotoxicus* by Paul Ehrlich. The human body, when healthy, does not generate an adaptive immune response to the self-generated antigens and has a tolerance mechanism. When that tolerance is overpowered in some individuals, the body does generate a sustained immune response leading to extensive tissue damage (Silverstein, 2014). Autoimmunity has always been a mystery to researchers as it has a very subjective way of occurrence. Every individual with an autoimmune disorder is unique, as autoimmunity can be triggered via many different approaches in the body. Thus, the failure mechanism of the immune system for an individual is also unique. Immunologists worldwide have found a few explanations for those failures to explain the fundamental processes in autoimmunity as shown in Figure 22.1.

22.2 What are Self-Antigens?

A self-antigen is any molecule or chemical group of an organism that acts as an antigen in inducing antibody formation in another organism but to which the healthy immune system of the parent organism is tolerant. The alteration in the self-components can make them seem foreign to our system. The production of various immune cells (B and T cells) from the hematopoietic stem cell is a complex process and generates a diverse array of cells. During that process, several receptors are generated that recognize the body's own constituents as foreign. But the cells carrying such self-reactive receptors are eliminated by various mechanisms, so that the immune response in the form of autoantibodies can be prevented, leading to the protection of the individual from any dysfunction (South, 2013).

DOI: 10.1201/9781003220404-24

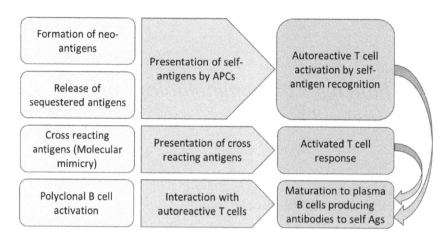

FIGURE 22.1   Major mechanisms of autoimmunity and disease.

22.3 Some of the Proposed Ways in which Self-Antigens Can Promote Autoimmunity

22.3.1 Alteration of Self-Antigens

Various mechanisms can alter self-components so that they seem foreign to the immune system. New antigenic determinants can be attached to self-proteins, or the shape of a self-antigen can shift for various reasons so that previously unresponsive helper T cells are stimulated and can cooperate with pre-existing B cells to secrete autoantibodies. Alteration of the shape of a self-protein has been shown to occur in experimental animals. It is the most probable explanation for producing the rheumatoid factors that are characteristic of rheumatoid arthritis. Infectious organisms also have the tendency to alter self-antigens, which may explain the development of autoantibodies against specialized cells and their hormonal products after viral infections; for example, the pancreatic cells that secrete insulin or those in the thyroid gland that make thyroid hormones.

22.3.2 Release of Sequestered Self-Antigens

Intracellular antigens and antigens found on tissues do not usually come in contact with the circulation and are segregated effectively from the immune system. Thus, they may be regarded as foreign if released into circulation due to tissue destruction caused by trauma or infection. For example, after sudden damage to the heart, antibodies against heart muscle membranes regularly appear in the blood.

22.3.3 Cross-Reaction with Foreign Antigens

When an infectious agent produces antigens similar to those on normal cells, the antibodies directed towards the foreign antigen also recognize the similar self-antigen; hence cross-reactivity leading to severe tissue damage. For example, the streptococci that cause rheumatic fever make antigens cross-reactive to those on heart muscle membranes, and antibodies that are supposed to be bound to the bacteria also bind to the heart muscle membrane and cause damage. Another instance of cross-reactivity is Chagas disease; the trypanosomes that cause the disease make cross-reactive antigens that produce autoantibodies against the surface of specialized nerve cells that help regulate orderly contraction of bowel muscles disrupting the normal bowel functioning. Some self-reactive TH cells (Helper T-cells) are generated during typical thymic selection; abnormalities in this process may generate even more self-reactive TH cells. The consecutive activation of the self-reactive T cells via different mechanisms and the polyclonal activation of B cells is thought to induce an autoimmune response, resulting in tissue damage (Küppers, 2010).

TABLE 22.1

Classification of Autoimmune Disorders Along with Their Target Self-Antigens and Affected Organs

Autoimmune disorders	Target self-antigens	Affected sites/organs
Organ-Specific Autoimmune Disorders		
Insulin-dependent Type 1 diabetes mellitus (T1DM)	Pancreatic β-cell antigens	Destruction of insulin producing cells in pancreas
Addison's disease	Cytoplasm adrenal cells 17a-/21 hydroxyase	Adrenal glands
Grave's disease	Thyroid stimulating hormone (TSH) receptor	Thyroid gland (hyperthyroidism)
Myasthenia gravis	Acetyl choline receptor	Neuromuscular paralysis affecting eyeand eyelid movements, facial expressions, and swallowing
Multiple sclerosis	Central nervous system antigens	Damaged myelin sheath, CNS inflammation
Pernicious anemia	Intrinsic factor	Vit B12 anemia (reduced RBCs)
Hashimoto's thyroiditis	Thyroglobulin, thyroid peroxidase	Thyroid gland (hypothyroidism)
Goodpasture's syndrome	Basement membrane antigens (Type IV collagen in GBM)	Kidneys, pulmonary implications
Systemic Autoimmune Disorders		
Systemic lupus erythematosus (SLE)	Nuclear antigens including DNA, RNA and proteins, RBCs and platelet membranes	Joints, kidneys, brain, and heart
Rheumatoid arthritis (RA)	Rheumatoid factor (RF) IgG immune complexes, citrullinated proteins, other joint antigens	Various joints of the body, eyes, lungs, and heart
Ankylosing spondylitis	CD41 cells, self-antigens (molecular mimicry, aberrant B27)	Spine and various joints
Sjögren's syndrome	SS-A (R0) SS-B (L0) (ducts, mitochondria, nuclei, and thyroid)	Eyes, mouth, and joints
Scleroderma (systemic sclerosis)	Nuclear IgG centromere, Scl70 (Topoisomerases, polymerases)	Skin fibrosis, arterial damage, vascular injury

22.4 Autoimmunity and Diseases

Autoimmune diseases can be classified according to several criteria; one of them is the location of the autoimmune attack. When the tolerance systems in an individual break down, an immune response against self-components is generated, which either targets one specific organ or generates a centralized response known as non-organ specific. Autoimmune diseases are distinguished into organ-specific and systemic (non-organ specific) as seen in Table 22.1. Recently these diseases have been more appropriately recharacterized into a spectrum of autoimmune diseases based on advances in their etiology and pathogenesis (Simmonds and Gough, 2004; Kono and Theofilopoulos, 2017; Actor, 2014).

22.5 The Fight Between Self and Non-Self

Immune tolerance is the in-built protection mechanism by which the unwanted immune responses to various self-antigens are contained. Various non-redundant checkpoints are engaged in this process to prevent the self-generated immune response and still maintain the efficiency to fight foreign pathogens. Even after the presence of such a system, autoimmune diseases contribute to a 3 to 9% of the health burden in the general population (Cooper et al., 2009; Kono and Theofilopoulos, 2017). A large section

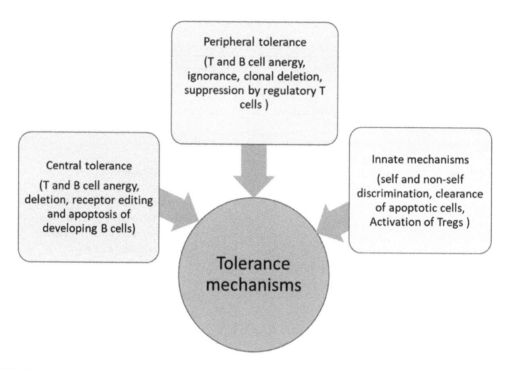

FIGURE 22.2 Mechanisms of tolerance: Tolerance can occur by various means including apoptosis of reactive cells, development of anergic response to antigen through loss of secondary signals, regulation of response as a result of antigen excess, and active suppression by regulatory T cells.

of the population is getting affected by autoimmunity, which makes it essential to decipher the pathways involved in immune tolerance to understand these diseases better and work towards the betterment of human society.

The concept of immunological tolerance has been around for more than 50 years, but its functionality and multifactorial basis is still being dissected. Most autoimmune disorders develop due to complex mechanisms guided by genetic, molecular, cellular, and environmental elements at varying stages of life, making it difficult for the tolerance mechanisms to protect, and thus its breakdown happens. Tolerance is generated at two different levels: the "upper level," being the central tolerance develops during the fetal life and eliminates potentially autoreactive lymphocytes that produce in the thymus to either clonal deletion (negative selection) or selection into the Treg lineage, and the second one is the "lower level" of peripheral tolerance that develops postnatally as a backup process, when some of the autoreactive lymphocytes (T cells) escape the upper level (Mackay, 2001).

The fault in the central tolerance sows the seed for the disease, but it is when the peripheral system also gives up, leading to the eruption of the autoimmune response. The peripheral tolerance also provides various checkpoints if the central tolerance becomes defective. This is achieved via T cell-intrinsic mechanisms of clonal deletion, anergy, immunological ignorance, or extrinsic mechanisms by a unique population of suppressor cells that regulate potentially response against the autoreactive T and B cells as described in Figure 22.2. Treg cells (CD4+CD25+Foxp3+) are amongst the first ones to play a role in the peripheral tolerance (Bluestone et al., 2015). The major cell killing is carried out by activated T and B cells that are inappropriately responding to self-antigens (Luo et al., 2019).

22.6 Etiology of Autoimmune Diseases

The studies have very evidently shown that the loss of tolerance and autoimmunity are closely intertwined, guided alongside by genetic predispositions. Another way of generating autoimmunity is a conventional

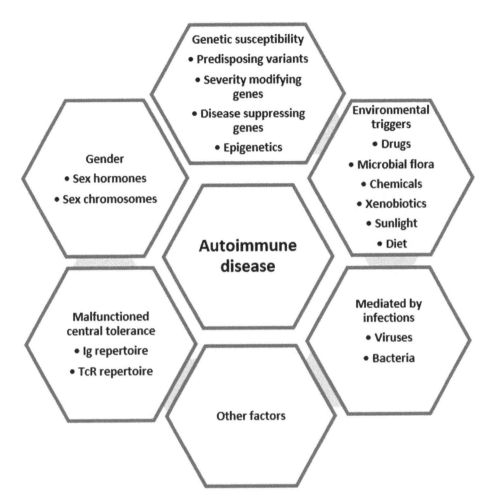

FIGURE 22.3 General etiology of autoimmune diseases. An autoimmune disease is usually the synergistic effect of multiple factors at one time making it difficult to understand a common basis of the pathogenesis of the disease.

one where the body produces an immune response to self-generated antigens for which the tolerance is not entirely established. Most of the systemic autoimmune diseases result from tolerance defects, while the organ-specific diseases can be mediated by either mechanism.

Most autoimmune disorders never occur by a single mechanism, and there is a multifold process and various checkpoints that have to be overcome to generate dysfunctionality. The incidence of an autoimmune disorder in an individual is driven by several factors, such as environmental, hormonal, and genetic factors, (as shown in Figure 22.3) leading to a breach in the self-tolerance mechanisms, resulting in autoimmunity.

22.6.1 Genetic Factors

Genetic susceptibility has been extensively studied in autoimmunity, and this was greatly facilitated by advancements in genomic studies during the last two decades. The best evidence for the genetic predisposition to autoimmune diseases in humans comes from family studies, especially monozygotic and dizygotic twins. For example, insulin-dependent diabetes mellitus (IDDM) has a prevalence of ~0.1% in the general population, whereas monozygotic twins are ~50% concordant, and human leukocyte antigen (HLA) identical siblings ~20% concordant for the disease. These numbers indicate that about half of the susceptibility factors are genetically determined and that almost half of the genetic predisposition is contributed by the major histocompatibility complex (MHC). Several autoimmune diseases have been studied in association with the HLA alleles, and the presentation of self-antigens by HLA gene products has been shown. Some examples include Grave's disease, Hashimoto disease, autoimmune gastritis (including pernicious anemia), type I (insulin-dependent) diabetes mellitus, and Addison disease. The presence of these diseases is more common in individuals that express MHC antigens on their cells. The concordance rate in rheumatoid arthritis (RA) is less than insulin-dependent diabetes mellitus-monozygotic twin concordance rate at ~20%, and the sibling occurrence risk at ~7%, at a population prevalence of ~1%, suggesting that the genetic susceptibility varies with a particular disease (Mackay, 2001; Pearce and Merriman, 2006; Holoshitz et al., 2013; Nagy, 2014; Cho and Feldman, 2015).

With the availability of genome sequences, a better understanding of genetic variations and haplotypes, along with high-throughput techniques, substantial insights into the genetic landscape of both humans and animals in autoimmune diseases have been observed. With the help of genome-wide association studies (GWAS), many cases can be studied at one time to observe genetic associations and capture common disease predisposing variants even with moderate effects. This has led to the identification of more than 100 candidate genes or loci in SLE and RA and other rheumatologic diseases such as systemic sclerosis, Kawasaki's disease, Behçet's disease, spondylitis, and antineutrophil cytoplasmic antibody (ANCA) associated vasculitis. Several general conclusions can be made about genetic susceptibility in the more common autoimmune diseases from GWAS and other studies, including those in animal models. First, autoimmune diseases are associated with a large number of susceptibility genes that have been shown to have an impact on a wide range of immunologic, cellular, and end-organ functions in ways that enhance, modify, or even suppress relevant pathophysiologic processes (Kochi, 2016; Gutierrez-Arcelus et al., 2016; Kono and Theofilopoulos, 2017).

As evidence suggests most autoimmune disorders are multifactorial, with complex etiology and pathogenesis consisting of an amalgamation of hereditary and environmental factors; identification and analysis of each element is still an ongoing process and comes with a unique set of challenges. For example, type I diabetes is believed to result from at least 14 genes. And even with the presence of several factors that could result in the autoimmune disease, it is not certain that it will.

22.6.2 Environmental Factors

Environmental factors are not the primary cause for autoimmune disorders; instead, they work synergistically. The already susceptible individuals – the genetically predisposed – are more likely to be affected by changes around them (Mackay, 2001). But the role of these environmental elements in the etiology is apparent as the studies conducted in monozygotic twins suggest that more than 50 and sometimes 70 or 80% of monozygotic twins are discordant for major autoimmune diseases.

Another major factor is "infection." The role of infections is strongly linked to the disruption of peripheral tolerance via the exposure of self-components to the immune system through the breakdown of vascular and cellular barriers, necrosis, leading to cell death and releasing the components into the system, increase in the costimulatory signals by activation of macrophages and T cells, and superantigen effects of various bacterial products. For example, mice infected with coxsackievirus that has a tropism for pancreatic islet cells or heart develop an autoimmune response (despite the clearance of the virus) to the breakdown products of islet cells or myocardium, resulting in chronic autoimmune inflammation. Various mechanisms by which the infections can promote autoimmunity are antigen mimicry, polyclonal lymphocyte activation, and increased immunogenicity of organ autoantigens secondary to infection-mediated inflammation.

The cross-reactive autoimmune response can be generated by a process of molecular (antigenic) mimicry, where an antigen of a microorganism of a constituent of food that sufficiently resembles a self-molecule of the individual leads to an aggravated immune system, thus generating a robust immune response. Many bacterial, viral, and parasitic infections are known to induce and aggravate the autoimmune response, mainly by molecular mimicry (Bach, 2005; Molina and Shoenfeld, 2005). Some of the examples include Reiter's syndrome after certain enteric infections, chronic Lyme arthritis resulting from *Borrelia burgdorferi*, and the association of oral *Porphyromonas gingivalis* that expresses a peptidyl arginine deiminase that can citrullinate proteins with RA, association between SLE and EBV infection, paediatric autoimmune neuropsychiatric disorders associated with streptococcal infection, etc. (Kono and Theofilopoulos, 2017). Some evidence also suggests that the lower incidence of infections in Western countries may have been responsible for increased incidence of allergic diseases- referred to as the "hygiene hypothesis". This trend has been particularly consistent in several diseases such as type 1 diabetes, inflammatory bowel disease, and multiple sclerosis, as observed from the epidemiological evidence. Early age onset (less than 2 to 3 years old) of type 1 diabetes has been observed in recent times and has been quite worrying since this is not observed in less developed countries (Gale, 2002; Bach, 2005).

There exist many other environmental triggers that might break tolerance and function, like infections causing tissue damage, as in the case of systemic lupus erythematosus (SLE), where sunlight acts as a trigger or alteration of the host molecules to render them immunogenic via chemicals or drug-induced mechanisms. Apart from all the information and studies available, what remains unknown is the specific environmental conditions and the extent to which they contribute to the induction and exacerbation of the autoimmune response. This is where the major challenge for understanding the etiology and the multifactorial pathogenesis of many autoimmune disorders exists. The reasons for this void are manifold. Several factors decide when and how and if the autoimmune response will be triggered.

22.6.3 Hormonal Factors

While considering the external environment as a factor for autoimmunity, one must not forget the internal environment, which may not be directly linked to a disease condition, but it certainly plays a part. Hormones influence the female disposition to autoimmune responses. Many cases have been studied where the eruption of disease occurs in the postpartum period (development of autoimmune thyroid disease, type 1 diabetes mellitus, or the psychological stress that may act through neuroendocrine pathways after pregnancy). This gender bias in autoimmunity has been a focus of research for quite some time now and can direct some crucial clues to disease pathogenesis. But the strength of this prevalence is varied in different disorders such as the 80% to 95% range for thyroiditis, SLE, Sjögren's syndrome, and anti-phospholipid syndrome; in the 60% to 75% range for RA, scleroderma, myasthenia gravis, and MS; and close to 50% for T1DM and autoimmune myocarditis. This is still under scrutiny as to why human autoimmune diseases afflict far more women than men, and it still proves to be a challenge to researchers (Kono and Theofilopoulos, 2017).

22.6.4 Co-Occurrence of Autoimmune Diseases

Autoimmune disorders with their multifactorial etiology and pathogenesis already present a significant challenge to identify and treat various diseases, but they have another tendency known as a co-occurrence. Their treatment has to be distinctively categorized based on organ system involvement and treated by varied medical specialties. But when one autoimmune disorder leads to another in an individual, it poses more threat to the particular individual, and the treatment methodology also becomes complicated. This may lead to multiple complications for the patients. Despite the need for more extensive and large-scale population based epidemiological research in the world of autoimmune disorders, much more is still left to be explored and understood (Cooper et al., 2009).

22.7 Selective Immunotherapies for Autoimmune Diseases (Mackay, 2001)

22.7.1 Monoclonal Antibodies or Blocking Antagonists

- Against cytokines such as tumor necrosis factor (TNF) (used for rheumatoid arthritis)
- Against cytokine receptors as tumor necrosis factor (used for rheumatoid arthritis)
- Against T-cell synapse (used for multiple sclerosis)
- Against chemokine receptors CCR5 and CXCR3

22.7.2 CTLA-4

- Downregulates activated T cells (trial use for psoriasis)

22.7.3 Regulatory Cytokines

- Interferon beta (IFN-β) possibly inhibits interleukin 12 (IL-12) (used for multiple sclerosis)
- Interleukins, IL-10 and IL-4 divert TH1 response to TH2 response (used in animal models)

22.7.4 Restoration of Tolerance

- Gene therapy (under development)
- Antigen-specific desensitization (used for multiple sclerosis, type 1 diabetes)
- Stem cell replacement (used for various diseases)

22.8 Cancer

The immune system is equipped with two major arms of innate and adaptive immunity interlinked that have overlapping functions. The key players of the innate immune system arm (dendritic cells, natural killer cells (NK), macrophages, neutrophils, eosinophils, basophils, and mast cells) can function without any pre-activation via antigens, and hence are designated as the first line of defense against antigens. On the other hand, adaptive arms have vital players such as B and T lymphocytes (CD4+ Helper and CD8+ cytotoxic T lymphocytes), which are activated upon the antigen-presentation by antigen-presenting cells (APCs) (Abbas AK, Lichtman AH, 2017). Antigen presentation leads to activation of antigen-specific T-and B-cell lymphocytes.

Usually, each cell in the body has specific DNA repair mechanisms that resolve over 20,000 DNA-damaging events (Loeb, 2011), leaving no lasting effects (Lindahl and Wood, 1999). Whenever these DNA damage events are not resolved in a cell, it leads to the development of malicious changes that can multiplicate into potentially malevolent changes. Cells infected with such malignant changes are marked and cleared of the body by a tumor immunosurveillance system via cell-mediated pathways, which are capable of recognizing foreign antigens. A malignant cell is created whenever it has accumulated over 11,000 mutations, leading to the expression of various tumor-associated antigens (TAAs) (Lindahl and Wood, 1999).

TAAs include the products of abnormally expressed products of erratic genes (proto-oncogenes, tumor suppressor genes, genes derived from oncogenic viruses, oncofetal antigens, erratic biomolecules including glycolipids and glycoproteins, and cell-specific differentiation antigens) that are the result of unresolved mutations. Receptor CD28 on antigen-presenting cells (APCs) recognize TAA via MHC-complexes and bind to B7 ligand on lymphocytes. B7 and CD28 receptors bind between T cells and APCs, respectively, leading to the formation of a junction called an immunological synapse, leading to the generation of costimulatory stimulus to kindle the proliferation and activation of T cells. Sometimes these immunological synapses formed with tumor cells lead to inhibitory interactions such as PD-1/PD-L1 and CTLA-4/B7.

22.9 Cancer Immunotherapy

The fact that the incidence of cancer is connected to the immune system of an individual was not known until in 19th century when Wilhelm Busch and Friedrich Fehleisen reported this interrelationship. It was from this report that the idea of targeting the immune system for cancer treatment came into play. Wilhelm Busch and Friedrich Fehleisen found that there is simultaneous regression of tumors after the eventual episode of erysipelas, a superficial skin infection caused by bacteria. In 1868, Busch was the first to infect the cancer patient with erysipelas and observe the tumor size. Fehleisen carried out the same experiment and discovered the causative bacteria of erysipelas Streptococcus pyogenes (Oelschlaeger, 2010; Oiseth and Aziz, 2017).

In 1891, irrespective of previous studies, William Coley treated sarcoma patients with extracts of heat-inactivated S. pyogenes and Serratia marcescens to boost immunity. Over a long-term follow-up of the patients under the study, Coley observed that the sarcoma size reduced after an erysipelas infection. Later on, this concoction or extract of heat-killed inactivated bacteria was named "Coley's toxins" (Coley, 1991). After this remarkable finding William Coley was named the "Father of Cancer Immunotherapy" as he established the fact that erysipelas results in improved outcomes in sarcoma patients. "Coley's toxin"represents the first documented active cancer immunotherapy intervention (Waldman et al., 2020). This extract had fascinating immunostimulatory attributes and accomplished promising responses in various cancers (Decker and Safdar, 2009).

In the 20th century, the idea of cancer immunotherapy reemerged, leading to significant progress with the beginning of new technology. A pioneering cancer immuno-oncologist, Professor Lloyd J. Old, observed that cancer cells differ from normal cells, and this difference is identified by the immunosurveillance system. He rightly projected that immunotherapy would be a fourth kind of cancer therapy along with other treatment branches (i.e., surgery, chemotherapy, and radiotherapy) (Dobosz and Dzieciątkowski, 2019). In 1909, Paul Ehrlich hypothesized that the defense system of an individual might avert the development of tumors from neoplastic cells (Ribatti, 2017; Decker et al., 2017). Lewis Thomas proposed that newly developing tumor cells are identified by the immune system through the neo-antigens expressed on the tumor cells in order to eradicate them. Later, Sir Frank Mac Farlane Burnet theorized that neo-antigens of tumor cells mediate the immunological response to counter the cancer cells. Lewis Thomas and Sir Frank Macfarlane Burnet self-reliantly comprehended the "cancer immunosurveillance hypothesis," affirming that TAAs are identified by immune systems in order to avert cancer development just like the case with graft rejection (Oiseth and Aziz, 2017). This theory, later on, led to the immune surveillance theory: "It is by no means inconceivable that small accumulation of tumor cells may develop and because they possessed new antigenic potentialities provoke an effective immunological reaction with regression of the tumor and no clinical hint of its existence" (Burnet, 1970).

Immunotherapy is defined as a branch of immunology that targets the immune system by suppressing, stimulating, and inducing the immune response.

Cancer immunotherapy has transformed the arena of oncology by lengthening the persistence of patients with rapidly lethal cancers. The number of cancer patients qualified for immunotherapy treatments is continuously rising as these therapies act as the first line of defense for many cancers. Due to these reasons, cancer immunotherapy has evolved as the "fifth pillar" of cancer therapy, joining the other players of surgery, cytotoxic chemotherapy, radiation, and targeted therapy (Oiseth and Aziz, 2017). In 2018 the importance of immunotherapy was established and rewarded when the Nobel Prize for physiology or medicine was awarded to James P. Allison and Tasuku Honjo for the discovery of a protein that is responsible for the evasion of malignant cells from the immune system. James P. Alison discovered the cytotoxic T-lymphocyte-associated protein (CTLA-4) and Tasuku Honjo discovered another protein called dthe programmed cell death protein 1/programmed cell death protein ligand 1 (PD-1/PD-L1) (Altmann, 2018; Kruger et al., 2019).

The body's defense mechanism against cancer involves recognition, identification, and clearance of newly developing malignant cells that express neoantigens or TAAs. TAAs form complex with human leukocyte antigens on the surface of T lymphocytes. Dendritic cells present the TAAs via HLA class-1 molecules to cytotoxic T lymphocytes and via HLA class-II molecules to activate helper T cells (CD4+) (Alatrash et al., 2013). A complex scheme of interactions involving immune system cells (dendritic cells (DCs), macrophages, plasma cells, and helper T cells) and immunomodulatory proteins (cytokines, antibodies) function continuously to avert tumor formation and growth (Klener et al., 2015).

Immunotherapies fit into one or more of the following five classes: checkpoint inhibitors, lymphocyte-promoting cytokines, engineered T cells such as CAR T and T cell receptor (TCR) T cells, agonistic antibodies against co-stimulatory receptors, cancer vaccines, and immunoadjuvants as described in Table 22.2.

TABLE 22.2

Different Types of FDA-Approved Immunotherapies

Name of therapy	Details	Year	Cancer type
Check-point inhibitors			
Anti-CTLA-4			
Ipilimumab	A human cytotoxic T-lymphocyte antigen 4 (CTLA-4)-blocking antibody	2011	Unresectable, late-stage melanoma (McDermott et al., 2013)
Anti-PD-1			
Pembrolizumab (Keytruda)	A humanized IgG4 antibody against PD1	2014	Aetastatic melanoma patients who are refractory to CTLA-4 therapy and BRAF inhibitor if they have BRAF mutation (Robert et al., 2014)
Nivolumab (Opdivo)	The first human IgG4 monoclonal antibody against PD-1	2014	Advanced, unresectable/metastatic melanoma (Hodi et al., 2018)
Cemiplimab (Libtayo)	A human monoclonal antibody against programmed death-1 (PD-1)	2015	Locally advanced, metastatic cutaneous squamous cell carcinoma (Migden et al., 2018)
Anti-PD-L1			
Atezolizumab (Tecentriq)	A humanized anti-PD-L1 mAb	2016	Advanced or metastatic urothelial carcinoma (Necchi et al., 2017)
Durvalumab (Imfinzi)	An IgG1κ anti-PD-L1 mAb	2017	Locally advanced or metastatic urothelial carcinoma (Massard et al., 2016)
Avelumab (Bavencio)	A fully human IgG1 anti-PD-L1 mAb and first FDA-approved treatment for metastatic MCC	2017	Metastatic Merkel cell carcinoma (MCC), in which patients' response to the therapy was not dependent on PD-L1 positivity. (Kaufman et al., 2016)
Cell Basedtherapy			
Idecabtagene vicleucel (Abecma)	B-cell maturation antigen (BCMA)-directed genetically modified autologous chimeric antigen receptor (CAR) T-cell therapy	2021	First cell-based gene therapy, for adult multiple myeloma patients (FDA, 2021a)
Brexucabtagene autoleucel (Tecartus)	A CD19-directed genetically modified autologous T cell immunotherapy	2020	It was approved for patients with mantle cell lymphoma (U.S. Food and Drug Administration (FDA, 2020)
Dendritic cell vaccine			
Sipuleucel-T	Consists of autologous antigen-presenting cell (APC) activated ex vivo by a fusion protein consisting of the antigen prostatic acid phosphatase (PAP) and granulocyte-macrophage colony stimulating factor (GM-CSF)	2010	Advanced prostate cancer (Cheever and Higano, 2011)
Immunomodulatory (Berraondo et al., 2019; Luke, 2020)			
Aldesleukin (Proleukin®):	A cytokine that targets the IL-2/IL-2R pathway	1992	Kidney cancer and melanoma (Clement and McDermott, 2009)
Granulocyte-macrophage colony-stimulating factor (GM-CSF)	Immunomodulatory cytokine	1991	Neuroblastoma (O Dillman, 2020)
Interferon-2α	Targets the IFNAR1/2 pathway;		leukemia and sarcoma

TABLE 22.2 (Continued)

Different Types of FDA-Approved Immunotherapies

Name of therapy	Details	Year	Cancer type
Peginterferon α-2b (Sylatron®/PEG-Intron®)	Targets the IFNAR1 pathway	2011	Melanoma (Di Trolio et al.,2012)
Pexidartinib (Turalio™)	a small molecule inhibitor of the KIT, CSF1R, and FLT3 pathways	2019	Tenosynovial giant cell tumor (Monestime and Lazaridis, 2020)
Chimeric Antigen Receptor (*CAR*) *T*-cell therapy			
Tisagenlecleucel (Kymriah)	target a protein on cancer cells known as CD19	2017	B cell acute lymphoblastic leukemia (FDA, 2021b)
Axicabtagene ciloleucel (Yescarta)	CD19-directed genetically modified autologous T cell	2017	Relapsed or refractory large B-cell lymphoma (Zhang et al., 2020)
Brexucabtagene autoleucel (Tecartus)	CD19-directed genetically modified autologous T cell	2020	Relapsed or refractory mantle cell lymphoma (U. S. Food and Drug Administration (FDA) (2020)

22.10 Divisions of Cancer Immunotherapy

22.10.1 Checkpoint Inhibitors

As discussed above, various components of the immune system protect the host from tumor development in a process called cancer immune-editing. Communications between the immune system and tumor growth are managed by an intricate network of biological pathways. Normally the immune system must inevitably remove the tumor cells by recognizing them as "foreign," as they exhibit exceptional and wide-ranging mutational profiles, but sometimes the immune system surpasses the tumor cell recognition and develops tolerance for such cells. In such cases the tumor cells start to act as self-cells and develop into tumors. This tolerance is upheld by several mechanisms involving regulatory cells, cytokines, chemokines, and immune checkpoints that function as immunosuppressants.

Appropriate activation of the immune system requires two signals: the first signal is generated upon the binding of T cell receptor to the antigen presented through major histocompatibility complex present on antigen presenting cells. Since this event is insufficient for complete T cell activation and lysis of tumor cells, the secondary costimulatory signals are generated upon the binding of costimulatory receptors (CD28) on T cells with CD80/CD86 receptors on APCs. In order to ensure that T cell activation occurs only through eligible antigens there are co-inhibitory signals to control this process. It is the balance between the co-stimulatory and co-inhibitory signals that determines if the T cell activation is ensued or T cell would become anergic to a particular antigen presented through MHC molecules. These checkpoints of the immune system are responsible for maintaining the homeostasis and tolerance in normal tissue and shielding organs from unnecessary damage yet are capable of removing pathogens competently.

A complex network of co-stimulatory and co-inhibitory signals that results in the battle of immune regulation and dysregulation in tumor grants the therapeutic prospects directing these to augment antitumor immunity. This process is regulated by immune checkpoints, which are basically receptors on the surface of immune system cells that control the stimulation or inhibition of immune response. Activation of the immune system works to control tumor development, which may procced to autoimmunity. Although tumors develop various strategies to evade these checkpoints of the immune system to circumvent recognition and abolition by the host immune system.

The most widely investigated class of immunotherapy agents is checkpoint inhibitors (ICIs) as shown in Figure 22.4. The most common target of ICIs is CTLA-4 and its ligand 1 (PD-1/PD-L1) and it has been employed for cancer treatment in combination with the standard of care regimens for patients with various types of tumors (Murciano-Goroff et al., 2020). Upon activation, T cells begin to express PD-1

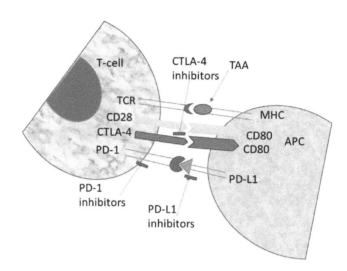

FIGURE 22.4 Targets of checkpoint inhibitors (ICIs).

in response to an event of inflammation, in order to identify atypical and malignant cells. As an evasion mechanism, the cancerous cells express PD-L1, the ligand for PD-1 on T cells, and render T cells inactive upon binding with PD-1. Hence obstructing this interaction with specific monoclonal antibodies (mAb) prohibits this evasion strategy of tumor cells and enable sthe T cells to intercede tumor cell death. On the other hand, CTLA-4 is a co-inhibitory receptor that controls the level of T cell activation upon binding with its counterparts CD80 and CD86 in T cells. This binding leads to the inhibition of T cells and hence blocks their protective function against malignant cells, promoting their survival and progression. Blocking the interaction of CTLA-4 with its ligand would restore the protective role of T cells from malignancies and enable T cells to identify and kill the malignant cells.

22.10.1.1 Key Challenges

Importantly, the exact cellular mechanisms responsible for CTLA4 blockade have yet to be investigated as different antibodies targeted for CTLA4 exhibit different attributes (Vargas et al., 2018). For example, some anti-CTLA4 antibodies may act two ways to deplete regulatory T cells and inhibit checkpoint functionality (Simpson et al., 2013).

Potent side effects in different organs is a major concern with the use of ICIs when administered in blood stream (Friedman et al., 2016). Many patients are non-responders to ICI treatment and patients who are responders have unpredictable potency of responses. Factors underlying responsiveness may include scarce T cell population infiltrating the tumor, derailed checkpoints in tumor cells as well as T cells and acquired resistance to ICI treatment (Restifo et al., 2016). Additionally, another challenge is that different tumors exhibit different microenvironments and hence possess distinctive pathways of immunosuppression. This calls for the need to develop new treatment strategies in order to achieve efficient and efficacious treatments (Joyce and Fearon, 2015).

As a matter of fact, the application of ICIs for broad range of cancers is yet an unachieved goal as a wide range of tumors are resistant to ICI-based immunotherapy. Therefore, the following areas need to be investigated: the diverse type of responses to ICIs among different cancer patients, most efficient combination of ICIs with other anticancer therapies, to expand the use of ICIs to include most of the cancer patients who have uncontrollable and not regressing tumors, and finally to find out the markers to predict the responsiveness of cancer patients towards the therapy.

22.10.2 Cytokines

Cytokines, the proteins with immunomodulatory properties, influence the immune system either by enhancing or inhibiting the effector cellular proteins mediators of immune system (Klener et al., 2015).

Cytokines are directly used in immunotherapy by injecting them into systemic circulation to elevate the immune response. As in 1986, the recombinant IFNα therapies received approval for clinical use, cytokines became the first immunotherapeutic agents ever to be employed in the clinic (Riley et al., 2019). Mainly three types of cytokines have been introduced and employed in immunotherapy: interferons (IFN-α), interleukins (IL-2), and granulocyte–macrophage colony-stimulating factor (GM-CSF) (Lee and Margolin, 2011).

GM-CSF improves the immune response by augmenting T cell homeostasis by improving the T cell survival, assisting in differentiation of dendritic cells so that these cells can present the TAAs efficiently. Both granulocyte colony-stimulating factor (G-CSF) and GM-CSF have been employed to potentiate and quicken the granulocyte replenishment postchemotherapy but GM-CSF may pose more potent pro-inflammatory effects as compared to G-CSF.

Today, IFN-α and IL-2 are employed in cancer treatment (Alatrash et al., 2013). To be more specific, IFN-α has immunostimulatory functions mediated via activation of DCs and enhancement of TAA presentation, hence augmenting helper T cell response, activity of cytotoxic lymphocytes, and natural killer cells (Alatrash et al., 2013). IFN-α is also employed with cancer vaccines to augment its therapeutic efficiency.

In a similar manner, IL-2 has been reported to boost the antitumor properties of the immune system by intensification of action of T cells, precisely those that work towards tumor infiltration and NK cell function. These two cytokines have been employed towards the augmentation of immune response, hence individual responses to this therapy depend on the strength of immune system of an individual. The recipient of the therapy should have a strong immune system for the therapy to be effective. Depending on the robustness of one's immune system the response rates to the therapy may vary. As such, cytokines are usually used in combination with other forms of immunotherapy (Klener et al., 2015).

Apart from these different cytokines agonists are being investigated by researchers that are capable of activating the immune cells through intracellular pathways. For example:

1. Inhibitors of TGFβ receptor type 1 (TGFβR1) that reestablish function of T cell and improves immune responses (e.g., SD-208).
2. Small-molecule agonists of TLR7/TLR8 that function by activating APCs.
3. Stimulator of interferon genes (STING) agonists has been employed to encourage the inflammatory cytokine production and type I interferon responses.

22.10.2.1 Key Challenges

A major drawback of using cytokines is their short half-life due to which very high doses are to be administered. Cytokine therapy usually comprises bolus injection with thigh dosage that results in vascular leakage and cytokine release syndrome (Rosenberg, 2014). Furthermore, cytokine therapy can ultimately invoke an autoimmune response against healthy tissues.

22.10.3 Cell-Based Immunotherapy

In cell-based immunotherapy natural or genetically modified T cells are expanded in ex vivo conditions in order to target TAAs (Karlitepe et al., 2015; Weiner, 2015). Ex vivo grown cells are injected into the patient and supplemented with external supply of cytokines (IL-2) to boost the effector function of these activated T cells (Klener et al., 2015). Chimeric antigen receptor T therapy (CAR-T) is among the most yielding cell-based immunotherapies. In CAR-T the T cells collected from patient blood are genetically engineered in ex vivo conditions, for improved specificity and action against the malignant cells. CAR-T cells re-infused into the patient to attack the malignant cells in a manner independent of HLA recognition. Now the reintroduced T cells are capable of recognizing the cancer cells and hence clearing them from the body. Hence, this type of therapy is able to deal with evasion strategies of cancer cells that lack HLA molecules. CAR-T is long-term therapy that is used once and lasts over a decade. Patients may have reemissions and prolonged survival, although the long-term consequences of this kind of therapy are yet under investigation. The primary target for CAR T cells was CD19, a B cell lineage marker, commonly expressed on B cell leukemias and lymphomas. A hostile consequence of anti-CD19 CAR T cells therapy is that it can lead to lead to B-cell aplasia by damaging the normal CD19 expressing B-lymphocytes. This can be lessened by antibody replacement therapy. At present, there are two FDA-approved CAR T cell therapies that target CD19: tisagenlecleucel for both diffuse large B cell lymphoma and acute lympho-blastic leukemia, and axicabtagene ciloleucel for diffuse large B cell lymphoma (Teijeira et al., 2012; Bartkowiak and Curran, 2015).

Furthermore, another type of cells for cell-based immunotherapy are TCR T cells that have entered clin-ical trials for both hematological and solid cancers. TCRs respond to intracellular TAAs when presented by MHCs (Cohen and Reiter, 2013). Unlike MHC-independent CAR T cells, TCR T cells require the MHC matched with the patient.

22.10.3.1 Key Challenges

A major challenge with this type of therapy is that the process of developing CAR T cells is extremely costly, complex, and time consuming. All these factors are actually inhibitory for the implementation of CAR T cell therapies for the benefit of more patients. Additionally, the injected cell does not survive for a longer time in the solid tumors that have unfavorable microenvironment. Due to the high affinity of TCR receptors of TCR T cells, there are off target bindings at non-specific ligands causing unpredictable toxicity (Linette et al., 2013).

Both types of cells pose two more major challenges: 1. CAR T and TCR T cells can evoke cytokine release syndrome and neurotoxicity (Van Den Berg et al., 2015; Fitzgerald et al., 2017). The second issue is inability of these engineered cells to have efficacy in solid tumors (Hege et al., 2017; O'Rourke et al., 2017; Migliorini et al., 2018). Until now only a few solid tumors have been successfully treated with CAR T cells, such as glioblastoma, which express higher levels of the target antigen EGFRvIII as compared with healthy cells. Translating adoptive T cell therapy into the treatment of solid tumors is going to be a futuristic goal of the utmost value.

However, immunotherapy has shown remarkable outcomes in a broad arena of cancer patients for targeting blood and skin cancers but applying the currently existing therapies to solid malignancies is yet to achieved with novel drug delivery innovations. More extensive knowledge of cell migration into solid tumors is of urgent need in order to apply T cell therapy in these malignancies. As an example, patients with certain diseases show increased permeability of CAR T cells through blood brain barrier, although the exact mechanism of this manifestation is still to be investigated. Novel approaches such as CRISPR–Cas for T cell engineering for expressing CARs can bring about a better basic understanding of delivery of these cells to targets.

22.10.4 Cancer Vaccines

Cancer vaccines comprise the fragments of tumor cells, dendritic cells, nucleic acid, or antigens to induce immune response against tumors. Just like therapies with monoclonal antibody, cancer vaccines are at present accessible as an immunotherapeutic treatment. Dendritic cell (DC) vaccines are the most com-monly investigated category of cell-based cancer vaccine. Dendritic cell vaccine is developed from the DCs collected from the patient; these cells are then genetically engineered to express TAAs so that they can directly activate T cell response against tumor cells.

Sipuleucel-T, the DC cancer vaccine for prostate cancer, showed longer survival of recipients. This vaccine was developed using extracted DCs from patient, activating them to prostate cancer antigen PA2024, then reintroducing them into the patient to target prostate cancer cells expressing the same antigen. This cancer vaccine constitutes prostatic acid phosphatase (PAP), which is expressed in 95% of this kind of tumor. The antigen is delivered along with GM-CSF so that DCs can present it to activate T cells to target PAP on the surface of tumor cells. A similar approach was employed for ovarian tumors expressing TAA CA-125 to activate DCs.

DNA- and RNA-based vaccines have emerged as a better option in comparison to conventional vaccines. The mechanism of action of DNA cancer vaccines involves uptake of DNA and mRNA by APCs, translation, and expressed as antigen. However, DNA vaccines also face challenges and are often unproductive due barriers to delivery of nucleic acids and immunogenicity. On the other hand, mRNAs possess advantages of being more self-molecule, non-infectious, and unable to integrate into the genome but also exhibit the limitations of shorter half-life and barrier to cellular internalization. Neoantigen vaccines are more specific to tumor cells and hence healthy cells are not attacked by the immune system. This type of vaccine is suitable for heterogenous tumors.

22.10.5 Immunoadjuvants

In order to alleviate the effects of targeted cancer therapies, immunomodulation is done using immunostimulatory molecules known as immunoadjuvants to invoke the immune response (Vermaelen, 2019). Immunoadjuvants recognize the TAAs on tumor cells to evoke the anti-tumor response (Hammerich et al., 2015). Immunoadjuvants are similar to pathogen-associated molecular patterns that are recognized by toll-like receptors (TLRs) on APCs. Generally, immunoadjuvants are processed through the lysosome and presented by MHC II to invoke humoral responses. However, TLR agonists, which act as immunoadjuvants, are processed through the endosomal pathway. Once these immunoadjuvants enter the DCs, they bypass the lysosomal degradation and are processed by cytoplasmic proteasomes (Song et al., 2020). Class I MHC molecules present the immunoadjuvant instigating dendritic cell maturation, a process called cross-presentation, which leads to the stimulation of cytotoxic T cells, hence invoking the adaptive immune response (Silva et al., 2019). Different types of immunoadjuvants are used for cancer immunotherapy: TLRs agonists, inorganic immunoadjuvants, plant-derived immunoadjuvants, exosomes, endogenous protein, and physical treatments.

22.10.5.1 Key Challenges

Alum-based immunoadjuvants are unable to produce anti-cancer effects as their cellular internalization is complex. Furthermore, allergic responses to Alum-based immunoadjuvants have been seen with elevated levels of IgE-mediated reactions. The use of TLR agonists is associated with a short half-life as these are rapidly degraded. The expression of TLRs on cancer cell surfaces causes tumor progression and metastasis (Wang et al., 2015).

It is now a well-established fact that the use of immunotherapies is restricted due to immune-related adverse events (irAEs). IrAEs are actually immunotherapy-induced activations of immune response and inflammation towards the healthy tissues of the recipient. It is a challenge to foresee, detect, and tackle the irAEs. In the scenario of metastatic melanoma, treatment with CTLA-4 antibody to block PD-1 undoubtedly results in a progressive upsurge in survival, but in turn, the incidence of irAEs doubles (Hodi et al., 2018). Several forecasters of irAEs have been anticipated, such as basal lymphopenia, eosinophilia, changes in B cell, T cell repertoire, systemic IL-17 level, and alterations in gut microbiota. However, all these factors have yet to be confirmed through future studies and clinical trials.

To combat the potent irAEs, there are guiding principles that endorse the use of corticosteroids for broad immunosuppression and, subsequently, TNF inhibitors or T cell suppressants. The checkpoint inhibitors (ipilimumab and nivolumab) routinely approved for melanoma are accompanied with toxicities of grade 3–4 (severe – life threatening) in less than 60% patients receiving the therapy (Wolchok et al., 2017). Furthermore, irAEs can be linked to mortality and noteworthy lifetime ailments, such as insulin-dependent diabetes, lasting pituitary malfunction, or inflamed joints. More studies and clinical trials are needed to develop prognosticators and innovative approaches to stop or decrease such toxic responses. Additionally, there is a need to develop innovative treatment options for patients who are non-responders and the ones who develop secondary resistance to immune checkpoint inhibitors. There are sparse treatment options apart from immune checkpoint inhibitors. Transfer of immune cells to the solid tumors by using cell-based therapies or cancer vaccines is still a struggle because the altered tumor microenvironment, which is immunosuppressive, exhibits high pressure of an interstitial fluid, which compresses its vascular setup and thick fibrotic tissue around the tumor that stop the T cell transport. Hence, the novel therapies with dual targets of the immune system and the tumor microenvironment could be more effective immunotherapies. Futuristically the basis of cancer immunotherapy would be the combination therapies involving checkpoint inhibitors and personalized cancer vaccines, and new therapies targeted would be developed towards the tumor microenvironment, tumor glycosylation, and the host microbiome.

22.11 Concluding Remarks

Cancer and autoimmunity are two manifestations of the failure of the immune response to the aberrant cells that escape the immunosurveillance system. Autoimmunity ensues due to multiple factors; hence understanding the etiology of these diseases is still under scrutiny. This is the reason that palliative therapies are the only option for disease management. However, cancer therapies are available but are harsh on patients leading to potentially adverse effects. Considerable efforts need to be made in the direction of making therapies more specific and targeted.

Acknowledgments

The authors would like to acknowledge Dr. Manish Kumar, Department of Biochemistry, All India Institute of Medical Sciences, Bilaspur, Himachal Pradesh for their help in grammatical corrections.

REFERENCES

Abbas A.K., Lichtman A.H., and Pillai S. (2017) Properties and overview of immune responses. *Cellular and Molecular Immunology*. pp. 1–11.

Actor, J.K. (2014) Autoimmunity: Regulation of response to self. In *Introd Immunol*. pp. 86–96.

Alatrash, G., Jakher, H., Stafford, P.D., and Mittendorf, E.A. (2013) Cancer immunotherapies, their safety and toxicity. *Expert Opin Drug Saf* 12: 631–645.

Altmann, D.M. (2018) A Nobel Prize-worthy pursuit: cancer immunology and harnessing immunity to tumour neoantigens. *Immunology* 155: 283–284.

Bach, J.F. (2005) Infections and autoimmune diseases. *J Autoimmun* 25: 74–80.

Bartkowiak, T. and Curran, M.A. (2015) 4-1BB agonists: Multi-potent potentiators of tumor immunity. *Front Oncol* 5: 1–16.

Berraondo, P., Sanmamed, M.F., Ochoa, M.C. Etxeberria, I., Aznar, M.A., Pérez-Gracia, J.L. et al. (2019) Cytokines in clinical cancer immunotherapy. *Br J Cancer* 120: 6–15 http://dx.doi.org/10.1038/s41 416-018-0328-y.

Bluestone, J.A., Bour-jordan, H., Cheng, M., and Anderson, M. (2015) Series Editor: Antonio La Cava. T cells in the control of organ-specific autoimmunity. *J Clin Invest* 125: 2250–2260.

Burnet, F.M. (1970) The concept of immunological surveillance. *Prog Exp Tumor Res* 13: 1–27.

Cho, J.H., and Feldman, M. (2015) Heterogeneity of autoimmune diseases: pathophysiologic insights from genetics and implications for new therapies. *Nat Med* 21: 730–738 www.ncbi.nlm.nih.gov/pmc/articles/PMC5716342/.

Cheever, M.A., and Higano, C.S. (2011) PROVENGE (sipuleucel-T) in prostate cancer: The first FDA-approved therapeutic cancer vaccine. *Clin Cancer Res* 17: 3520–3526.

Clement, J., and McDermott, D. (2009) The high-dose aldesleukin (IL-2) "select" Trial: A trial designed to prospectively validate predictive models of response to high-dose IL-2 treatment in patients with metastatic renal cell carcinoma. *Clin Genitourin Cancer* 7: E7–E9 http://dx.doi.org/10.3816/CGC.2009.n.014.

Cohen, M., and Reiter, Y. (2013) T-Cell Receptor-Like Antibodies: Targeting the Intracellular Proteome Therapeutic Potential and Clinical Applications. *Antibodies* 2: 517–534.

Coley, W.B. (1991) The treatment of malignant tumors by repeated inoculations of erysipelas: With a report of ten original cases. *Clin Orthop Relat Res* 3–11.

Cooper, G.S., Bynum, M.L.K., and Somers, E.C. (2009) Recent insights in the epidemiology of autoimmune diseases: Improved prevalence estimates and understanding of clustering of diseases. *J Autoimmun* 33: 197–207 http://dx.doi.org/10.1016/j.jaut.2009.09.008.

Da Silva, C.G., Camps, M.G.M., Li, T.M.W.Y., Zerrillo, L., Löwik, C.W., Ossendorp, F., and Cruz, L.J. (2019) Effective chemoimmunotherapy by co-delivery of doxorubicin and immune adjuvants in biodegradable nanoparticles. *Theranostics* 9: 6485–6500.

Decker, W.K. and Safdar, A. (2009) Bioimmunoadjuvants for the treatment of neoplastic and infectious disease: Coley's legacy revisited. *Cytokine Growth Factor Rev* 20: 271–281.

Di Trolio, R., Simeone, E., Di Lorenzo, G., Grimaldi, A.M., Romano, A., Ayala, F. et al. (2012) Update on PEG-interferon α-2b as adjuvant therapy in melanoma. *Anticancer Res* 32: 3901–3910.

Dobosz, P. and Dzieciątkowski, T. (2019) The intriguing history of cancer immunotherapy. *Front Immunol* 10.

FDA (2021a) ABECMA (idecabtagene vicleucel). US Food Drug Adm www.fda.gov/vaccines-blood-biolog ics/abecma-idecabtagene-vicleucel.

FDA (2021b) CAR T-Cell therapy approved by FDA for mantle cell lymphoma – National Cancer Institute. 1–7 www.cancer.gov/news-events/cancer-currents-blog/2020/fda-brexucabtagene-mantle-cell-lymphoma.

Fitzgerald, J.C., Weiss, S.L., Maude, S.L., Barrett, D.M., Lacey, S.F., Melenhorst, J.J. et al. (2017) Cytokine release syndrome after chimeric antigen receptor T cell therapy for acute lymphoblastic leukemia. *Crit Care Med* 45: e124–e131 http://journals.lww.com/00003246-201702000-00037.

Friedman, C.F., Proverbs-Singh, T.A., and Postow, M.A. (2016) Treatment of the immune-related adverse effects of immune checkpoint inhibitors: A review. *JAMA Oncol* 2: 1346–1353.

Gale, E.A.M. (2002) The rise of childhood type 1 diabetes in the 20th century. *Diabetes* 51: 3353–3361.

Gutierrez-Arcelus, M., Rich, S.S., and Raychaudhuri, S. (2016) Autoimmune diseases — connecting risk alleles with molecular traits of the immune system. *Nat Rev Genet* 17: 160–174 www.nature.com/artic les/nrg.2015.33.

Hammerich, L., Binder, A., and Brody, J.D. (2015) In situ vaccination: Cancer immunotherapy both personalized and off-the-shelf. *Mol Oncol* 9: 1966–1981.

Hege, K.M., Bergsland, E.K., Fisher, G.A., Nemunaitis, J.J., Warren, R.S., McArthur, J.G. et al. (2017) Safety, tumor trafficking and immunogenicity of chimeric antigen receptor (CAR)-T cells specific for TAG-72 in colorectal cancer. *J Immunother Cancer* 5: 1–14.

Hodi, F.S., Chiarion-Sileni, V., Gonzalez, R., Grob, J.J., Rutkowski, P., Cowey, C.L. et al. (2018) Nivolumab plus ipilimumab or nivolumab alone versus ipilimumab alone in advanced melanoma (CheckMate 067): 4-year outcomes of a multicentre, randomised, phase 3 trial. *Lancet Oncol* 19: 1480–1492.

Holoshitz, J., Liu, Y., Fu, J., Joseph, J., Ling, S., Colletta, A. et al. (2013) An HLA-DRB1-Coded signal trans-duction ligand facilitates inflammatory arthritis: A new mechanism of autoimmunity. *J Immunol* 190: 48–57 https://linkinghub.elsevier.com/retrieve/pii/S0022202X15370834.

Illman, R. O. (2020) An update on GM-CSF and its potential role in melanoma management. *Melanoma Manag* 7: MMT49.

Joyce, J.A., and Fearon, D.T. (2015) T cell exclusion, immune privilege, and the tumor microenvironment. *Science (80-)* 348: 74–80 www.cambridge.org/core/product/identifier/CBO9781107415324A009/type/ book_part.

Karlitepe, A., Ozalp, O., and Avci, C.B. (2015) New approaches for cancer immunotherapy. *Tumor Biol* 36: 4075–4078.

Kaufman, H.L., Russell, J., Hamid, O., Bhatia, S., Terheyden, P., D'Angelo, S.P. et al. (2016) Avelumab in patients with chemotherapy-refractory metastatic Merkel cell carcinoma: a multicentre, single-group, open-label, phase 2 trial. *Lancet Oncol* 17: 1374–1385 https://linkinghub.elsevier.com/retrieve/pii/ S1470204516303643.

Klener, P., Otahal, P., Lateckova, L., and Klener, P. (2015) Immunotherapy approaches in cancer treatment. *Curr Pharm Biotechnol* 16: 771–781 www.eurekaselect.com/openurl/content.php?genre=article&issn= 1389-2010&volume=16&issue=8&spage=738.

Kochi, Y. (2016) Genetics of autoimmune diseases: Perspectives from genome-wide association studies. *Int Immunol* 28: 155–161.

Kono, D.H., and Theofilopoulos, A.N. (2017) Chapter 19 – *Autoimmunity. Tenth Edit.*, Elsevier Inc. http:// dx.doi.org/10.1016/B978-0-323-31696-5.00019-X.

Kruger, S., Ilmer, M., Kobold, S., Cadilha, B.L., Endres, S., Ormanns, S. et al. (2019) Advances in cancer immunotherapy 2019 – Latest trends. *J Exp Clin Cancer Res* 38: 1–11.

Küppers, R. (2010) Overview of the immune system. *Lymphoid Neoplasms* 3ed 143–155.

Lee, S. and Margolin, K. (2011) Cytokines in cancer immunotherapy. *Cancers (Basel)* 3: 3856–3893.

Lindahl, T. and Wood, R.D. (1999) Quality control by DNA repair. *Science (80-)* 286: 1897–1905.

Linette, G.P., Stadtmauer, E.A., Maus, M. V., Rapoport, A.P., Levine, B.L., Emery, L. et al. (2013) Cardiovascular toxicity and titin cross-reactivity of affinity-enhanced T cells in myeloma and melanoma. *Blood* 122: 863–871.

Loeb, L.A. (2011) Human cancers express mutator phenotypes: origin, consequences and targeting. *Nat Rev Cancer* 11: 450–457 www.nature.com/articles/nrc3063.

Luke, J. (2020) Immunomodulators: checkpoint inhibitors, cytokines, agonists, and adjuvants. *Cancer Res Inst* 1–13 www.cancerresearch.org/immunotherapy/treatment-types/immunomodulators-checkpoint-inhibitors.

Luo, X., Miller, S.D., and Shea, L.D. (2019) Immune tolerance for autoimmune disease and cell transplantation. *Physiol Behav* 176: 139–148.

Mackay, I.R. (2001) Tolerance and autoimmunity. *West J Med* 174: 118–123 www.ncbi.nlm.nih.gov/pmc/articles/PMC1071274/.

Massard, C., Gordon, M.S., Sharma, S., Rafii, S., Wainberg, Z.A., Luke, J. et al. (2016) Safety and efficacy of durvalumab (MEDI4736), an anti-programmed cell death ligand-1 immune checkpoint inhibitor, in patients with advanced urothelial bladder cancer. *J Clin Oncol* 34: 3119–3125.

McDermott, D., Haanen, J., Chen, T.T., Lorigan, P., and O'Day, S. (2013) Efficacy and safety of ipilimumab in metastatic melanoma patients surviving more than 2 years following treatment in a phase III trial (MDX010-20). *Ann Oncol* 24: 2694–2698 https://doi.org/10.1093/annonc/mdt291.

Migden, M.R., Rischin, D., Schmults, C.D., Guminski, A., Hauschild, A., Lewis, K.D., et al. (2018) PD-1 blockade with cemiplimab in advanced cutaneous squamous-cell carcinoma. *N Engl J Med* 341–351.

Migliorini, D., Dietrich, P.Y., Stupp, R., Linette, G.P., Posey, A.D., and June, C.H. (2018) CAR T-cell therapies in glioblastoma: A first look. *Clin Cancer Res* 24: 535–540.

Molina, V., and Shoenfeld, Y. (2005) Infection, vaccines and other environmental triggers of autoimmunity. *Autoimmunity* 38: 235–245.

Monestime, S., and Lazaridis, D. (2020) Pexidartinib (TURALIO™): The first FDA-indicated systemic treatment for tenosynovial giant cell tumor. *Drugs R* D20: 189–195 https://doi.org/10.1007/s40268-020-00314-3.

Murciano-Goroff, Y.R., Warner, A.B., and Wolchok, J.D. (2020) The future of cancer immunotherapy: microenvironment-targeting combinations. *Cell Res* 30: 507–519.

Nagy, Z.A. Chapter 10 – Autoimmunity. In *A History of Modern Immunology*, Academic Press: 2014. pp. 281–325.

Necchi, A., Joseph, R.W., Loriot, Y., Hoffman-Censits, J., Perez-Gracia, J.L., Petrylak, D.P. et al. (2017) Atezolizumab in platinum-treated locally advanced or metastatic urothelial carcinoma: Post-progression outcomes from the phase II IMvigor210 study. *Ann Oncol* 28: 3044–3050.

O'Rourke, D.M., Nasrallah, M.P., Desai, A., Melenhorst, J.J., Mansfield, K., Morrissette, J.J.D. et al. (2017) A single dose of peripherally infused EGFRvIII-directed CAR T cells mediates antigen loss and induces adaptive resistance in patients with recurrent glioblastoma. *Sci Transl Med* 9: eaaa0984.

Oelschlaeger, T.A. (2010) Bacteria as tumor therapeutics? *Bioeng Bugs* 1: 146–147.

Oiseth, S.J., and Aziz, M.S. (2017) Cancer immunotherapy: a brief review of the history, possibilities, and challenges ahead. *J Cancer Metastasis Treat* 3: 250.

Pearce, S.H.S., and Merriman, T.R. (2006) Genetic progress towards the molecular basis of autoimmunity. *Trends Mol Med* 12: 90–98.

Restifo, N.P., Smyth, M.J., and Snyder, A. (2016) Acquired resistance to immunotherapy and future challenges. *Nat Rev Cancer* 16: 121–126.

Ribatti, D. (2017) The concept of immune surveillance against tumors. The first theories. *Oncotarget* 8: 7175–7180.

Riley, R.S., June, C.H., Langer, R., and Mitchell, M.J. (2019) Delivery technologies for cancer immunotherapy. *Nat Rev Drug Discov* 18: 175–196.

Robert, C., Ribas, A., Wolchok, J.D., Hodi, F.S., Hamid, O., Kefford, R. et al. (2014) Anti-programmed-death-receptor-1 treatment with pembrolizumab in ipilimumab-refractory advanced melanoma: A randomised dose-comparison cohort of a phase 1 trial. *Lancet* 384: 1109–1117.

Rosenberg, S.A. (2014) IL-2: The first effective immunotherapy for human cancer. *J Immunol* 192: 5451–5458.

Silverstein, A.M. (2014) *Autoimmunity: A History of the Early Struggle for Recognition*. Elsevier Inc., http://dx.doi.org/10.1016/B978-0-12-384929-8.00002-2.

Simmonds, M.J., and Gough, S.C.L. (2004) Genetic insights into disease mechanisms of autoimmunity. *Br Med Bull* 71: 93–113.

Simpson, T.R., Li, F., Montalvo-Ortiz, W., Sepulveda, M.A., Bergerhoff, K., Arce, F. et al. (2013) Fc-dependent depletion of tumor-infiltrating regulatory t cells co-defines the efficacy of anti-CTLA-4 therapy against melanoma. *J Exp Med* 210: 1695–1710.

Smith, K.A. (2010) Frontiers in immunology – grand challenges. *Front Immunol* 1: 1–2.

Song, C., Li, F., Wang, S., Wang, J., Wei, W., and Ma, G. (2020) Recent advances in particulate adjuvants for cancer vaccination. *Adv Ther* 3: 1900115.

South, M. (2013) Immune deficiencies. *Don't Forget The Bubbles* 1–17.

Teijeira, Á., Palazón, A., Garasa, S., Marré, D., Aubá, C., Rogel, A. et al. (2012) CD137 on inflamed lymphatic endothelial cells enhances CCL21-guided migration of dendritic cells. *FASEB J* 26: 3380–3392.

U.S. Food and Drug Administration (FDA) (2020) FDA approves brexucabtagene autoleucel for relapsed or refractory mantle cell lymphoma. *07/27/2020* 1–2 www.fda.gov/drugs/fda-approves-brexucabtagene-aut oleucel-relapsed-or-refractory-mantle-cell-lymphoma.

Van Den Berg, J.H., Gomez-Eerland, R., Van De Wiel, B., Hulshoff, L., Van Den Broek, D., Bins, A. et al. (2015) Case report of a fatal serious adverse event upon administration of T cells transduced with a MART-1-specific T-cell receptor. *Mol Ther* 23: 1541–1550.

Vargas, F.A., Furness, A.J.S., Litchfield, K., Joshi, K., Rosenthal, R., Ghorani, E. et al. (2018) Fc effector function contributes to the activity of human anti-CTLA-4 antibodies. *Cancer Cell* 33: 649–663.e4.

Vermaelen, K. (2019) Vaccine strategies to improve anticancer cellular immune responses. *Front Immunol* 10: 1–17.

Waldman, A.D., Fritz, J.M., and Lenardo, M.J. (2020) A guide to cancerimmunotherapy: from T cell basic science to clinical practice. *Nat Rev Immunol* 20: 651–668.

Wang, X.D., Gao, N.N., Diao, Y.W., Liu, Y., Gao, D., Li, W. et al. (2015) Conjugation of toll-like receptor-7 agonist to gastric cancer antigen MG7-Ag exerts antitumor effects. *World J Gastroenterol* 21: 8052–8060.

Weiner, L.M. (2015) Cancer immunology for the clinician. *Clin Adv Hematol Oncol* 13: 299–306.

Wolchok, J.D., Chiarion-Sileni, V., Gonzalez, R., Rutkowski, P., Grob, J.J., Cowey, C.L. et al. (2017) Overall survival with combined nivolumab and ipilimumab in advanced melanoma. *N Engl J Med* 377: 1345–1356.

Zhang, Q., Ping, J., Huang, Z., Zhang, X., Zhou, J., Wang, G. et al. (2020) CAR-T cell therapy in cancer: Tribulations and road ahead. *J Immunol Res* 2020: 1924379.

23

Human Papillomavirus (HPV): Molecular Epidemiology of Infection and its Associated Diseases

Abhishek Pandeya, Raj Kumar Khalko, Bharti Kotarya, Hema, Jitendra Kumar Yadav, and Sunil Babu Gosipatala
Department of Biotechnology, School of Life Sciences, Babasaheb Bhimrao Ambedkar University, Lucknow, India

Sudipta Saha
Department of Pharmaceutical Sciences, School of Pharmaceutical Sciences, Babasaheb Bhimrao Ambedkar University, Lucknow, India

R.C. Sobti
Department of Biotechnology, Panjab University, Chandigarh, India

23.1 Introduction

Papillomaviruses are a complex group of viruses that affects both humans and animals. Their origin seems to be related to changes in the epithelium of their ancestral host. The first reptiles appeared around 350 million years ago, and since then they have co-evolved with their respective hosts, with little Xeno transfer between species, which are now found in birds, reptiles, marsupials, and mammals. Thus, Human Papillomavirus (HPV) is an ancient DNA virus belonging to the *Papillomaviridae* family. The virions are small, non-enveloped, showing double-stranded DNA as the genome. They show circular DNA as the genome (approximately 8Kb), surrounded by an icosahedral capsid of 52–55 nm in diameter (Kirnbauer et al., 1992; Hagensee et al., 1993; Guan et al., 2017). These viruses are particularly tissue-specific and infect both the skin and the mucosal epithelium. More than 200 types of HPV strains/types have been characterized. The HPVs are classified into high-risk and low-risk types according to their propensity

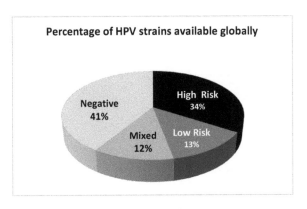

FIGURE 23.1 Distribution of different HPV strains based on their risk category globally.

DOI: 10.1201/9781003220404-25

forcausing cancers. The International Agency for Research on Cancer identifies 12 high-risk types of HPV associated with human cancer (types 16, 18, 31, 33, 35, 39, 45, 51, 52, 56, 58, 59), of which 70% are associated with cervical cancer and additional types for which there is insufficient evidence for carcinogenicity (i.e., types 68 and 73) (Doorbar et al., 2012). Low-risk HPV includes 26, 40, 42, 53, 54, 55, 61, 62, 64, 66, and 67, with HPV 6 and 11 being the most common, which are 90% associated with genital warts and later on rarely cause cancer. These HPVs are responsible for causing *Condylomata acuminata*, a type of genital wart (Celewicz et al., 2020). Both high-risk and low-risk strains are observed to be present in an individual. Different worldwide HPV strains and their percentages are shown in Figure 23.1 (Boda et al. 2016).

23.1.1 Historical Perspective and Evolution of Human Papillomaviruses

Papillomaviruses had millions of years ago and propagated in a range of different animal species, including humans. Over 200 papillomaviruses have been identified to date, including more than 150 distinct types and sub-types of HPVs. The expressions "serotype" and "strains" are not used to differentiate between papillomaviruses, and indeed, many papillomaviruses have not been distinguished beyond the level of their DNA sequence. Viruses that have co-evolved leisurely with their hosts commonly cause chronic infections, with virion production in the absence of apparent diseases. This can be seen in the cases for many β and γ HPV types. The α-papillomavirus types have developed immune evasion strategies that permit them to cause persistently visible papilloma. This virus results in the activation of the cell cycle, which leads to the differentiation of infected epithelial cells to create a replication-competent environment. Thus, it allows viral genome amplification and packaging into infectious particles.

HPV types (HPV 16 and 18) cause 97% of cancer in their infections, mostly cervical cancer. This is attributed to the studies of Harald Zur Hausen's group, for which he was awarded the Nobel Prize in 2008. Therefore, this finding paved the way for developing the cervical cancer vaccine, which was formerly the second most prevalent cancer in women (Zur Hausen, 1986 & 2006). Figure 23.2 indicates the discoveries and milestones achieved by researchers for HPV infections and their vaccine development.

23.1.2 Global Occurrence and Epidemiology of Human Papillomaviruses

HPVs are spreading across the world, and over 90% of the HPV infections may further lead to cancer. According to a CDC report (How Many Cancers Are Linked with HPV Each Year?, CDC, n.d.), out of all the specific cancer cases, 74% of cases were found due to HPV infections. Among which cervical cancer is the most prevalent type of cancer caused because of HPV infection. It was estimated that out of the total number of cervical cancer cases, 91% of cases are due to HPV infections (Basic Information about

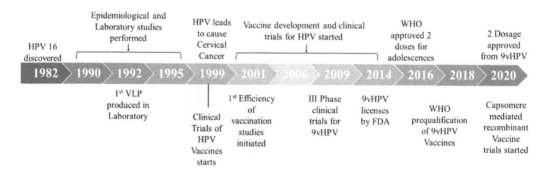

FIGURE 23.2 Timeline for HPV discovery, its associated studies, and vaccine developmental stages with reference to the time. (Source: Toh et al., 2019, Infection and Drug Resistance; Volume 12.)

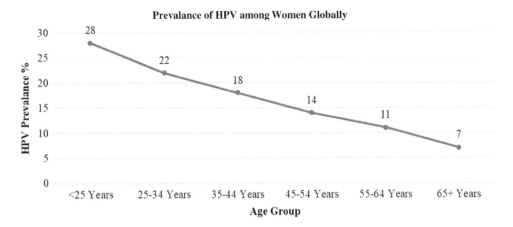

FIGURE 23.3 The graph indicates the prevalence of the HPV infection among the different age groups of women across the world.

HPV and Cancer, CDC, n.d.; Human Papillomavirus and Related Diseases, HPV Centre, n.d.). The age factor also plays a major role in HPV infection. The primary age group affected by the virus is less than 25 years. In Asia, young women are more susceptible than older women. Different studies have suggested that women of age group 55–64 show less infection than younger women (i.e., about 12–14% only). It was found that women less than 25 years of age show HPV prevalence of about 24% higher than older women across the globe as shown in the graph of Figure 23.3. Globally, HPV 16 is the most prevalent strain, which leads to cause cancer at its later infection stage (Serrano et al., 2018).

23.1.3 General Classification of HPV

HPV's classification is based on DNA sequence similarities, with individual types having a nucleotide sequence (sampled from L1 gene) that is at least 10% dissimilar from other papillomaviruses, including some biological and medical properties that served as the foundation for a formal nomenclature. They are classified on their oncogenic potential as high- and low-risk groups (Tommasino, 2014), further classified into α, β, γ, μ, and ν genera, which can be subdivided into various types depending on their infectivity (Bernard et al., 2010) as shown in Figure 23.4. In general, the cutaneous type infects the keratinizing epithelium, while mucosal types infect the non-keratinizing epithelium, primarily the ano-genital tract epithelium. They can also be found in the oral mucosa, conjunctiva, and respiratory tract (Bonnez and Reichman, 2000).

The immune system effectively counters HPVs infections. However, in some individuals, it causes benign genital warts, while in others affected by oncogenic types several types of cancers such as cervical, oropharyngeal, genital, head and neck may develop. HPV is associated with various clinical conditions that range from benign lesions to cancer (Bonnez and Reichman, 2000). Most HPV infections are benign, and infection of cutaneous epithelium can cause warts such as plantar warts, common warts, and flat warts. Among the 200 types of HPVs, more than 40 HPV types can be easily spread through direct sexual contact (i.e., from the skin and mucous membranes of infected people to the skin and mucous membranes of their partners). Other HPV types are responsible for non-genital warts, which are not sexually transmitted. They generally infect mucosal and cutaneous basal epithelial (skin or mucosal).

Sexually transmitted HPV types fall into two categories (as shown in Figure 23.5)

   (i) **Low-risk HPV,** which do not cause cancer but cause skin warts.
   (ii) **High-risk HPVs,** which can cause cancer.

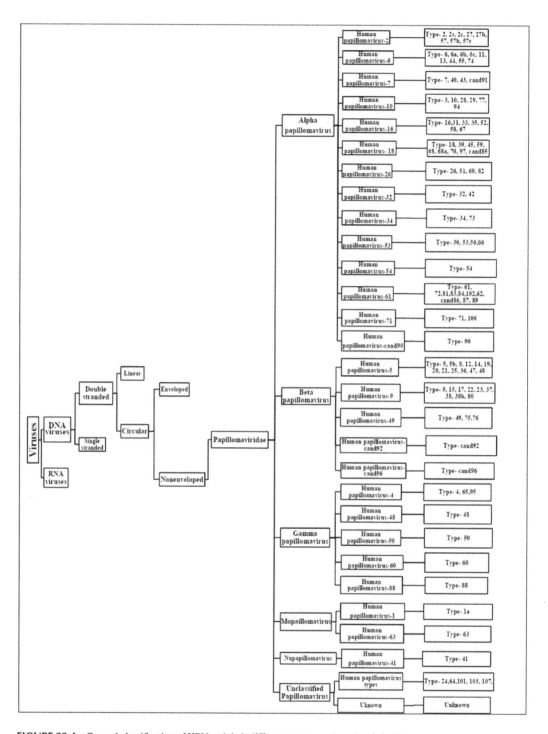

FIGURE 23.4 General classification of HPV and their different genotypes based on infectivity.

High-risk mucosal α-genus HPV types have been extensively studied and are the best-characterized group to date.

It has been estimated that up to 80% of sexually active individuals will get infected at some point in their lives, making HPV the most common sexually transmitted pathogen.

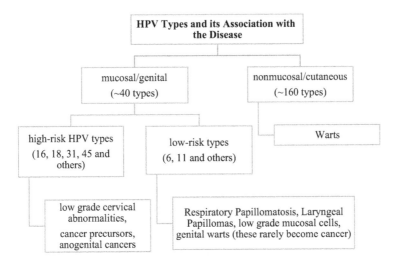

FIGURE 23.5 HPV types associated with different diseases/abnormalities.

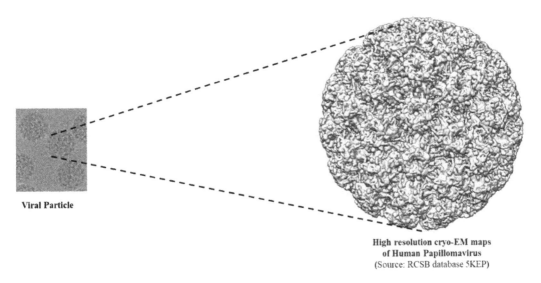

FIGURE 23.6 Electron microscopic view of the viral particle of HPV and its enlarged view through Cryo-EM imaging. (Source: Guan et al., 2017 and image taken from RCSB Database 5KEP.)

23.2 Structural Features

HPV shares a typical non-enveloped icosahedral structure 52–55 nm in diameter. Guan et al. (2017) identified the structure of HPV using advanced imaging technology, known as Cryo-EM (Cryo-Electron Microscopy), as depicted in Figure 23.6. Further, the arrangement of the different structural proteins is also known to produce viral particles as shown in Figure 23.7. The viral capsid of HPV contains two different proteins, L1 and L2. The structural protein L1 has 55 kDa size whereas L2 is 70 kDa (Kirnbauer et al., 1992; Hagensee et al., 1993). Each viral capsid has 360 L1 monomers, which combine to form 72 pentameric capsomeres, and each pentameric capsomere is coupled with a single L2 minor structural protein (72 pentameric capsomeres generated from 360 L1 protein and 72 minor L2 structural protein) to form a complete viral shell. Viral assembly occurs in the cell's nucleus; L1 protein self-assembles into virus-like particles, while L2 has a lesser-known role but may be involved with virion production

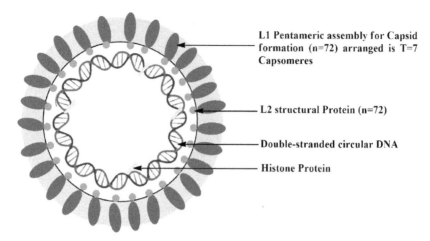

L1 Pentameric assembly for Capsid formation (n=72) arranged is T=7 Capsomeres

L2 structural Protein (n=72)

Double-stranded circular DNA

Histone Protein

Human Papillomavirus

FIGURE 23.7 Structure of HPV shows structural proteins major L1 and minor L2 proteins assembled in the pentameric form to produce capsomere. Whereas the minor L2 protein leads to the assembly with the L1 to provide the capsid stability of the virus. The virus contains double-stranded closed circular DNA having histones attached to it.

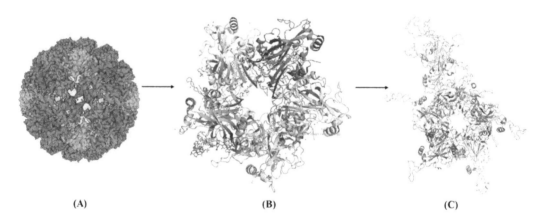

(A)   (B)   (C)

FIGURE 23.8 The capsid protein of the HPV 16 contains 360 molecules of L1 arranged in pentameric arrangement to produce capsomere of the virus particle. These L1 produces icosahedral lattices of L1. (A) Complete EM structure of capsomere of HPV. (B) L1 structural protein of HPV arranged in Pentameric form. (C) The monomeric L1 structure contains six different chains comprises A, B, C, D, E & F. (Source: Image taken from RCSB Databank (A) 35GR (B) 5W1O (C) 6I31.)

(Handler et al., 2015; Palefsky et al., 2016). These units are linked with each other via disulfide bonds (Chen et al., 2000 & 2001; Modis et al., 2002; Wolf et al., 2010). These 72 capsomeres are arranged as 12 capsomeres in 5 coordinated arrangements, while the other 60 capsomeres are arranged in 6 coordinated arragements and further arranged as a T=7d icosahedral surface lattice to produce complete viral capsid of the HPV as shown in Figure 23.8.

23.3 Genome Organization

The HPV genome is a double-stranded circular DNA molecule, and it is to be transcribed in the right direction (clockwise). It contains nine Open Reading Frames (**ORFs**) (Bernard et al., 2006) and encodes nine viral proteins, seven of which are early proteins (E1, E2, E4, E5A, E5B, E6, and E7) and two late

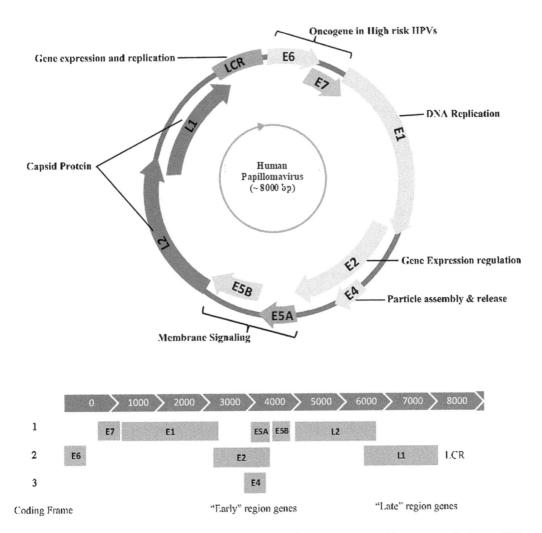

FIGURE 23.9 Genome organization of HPV and their Open Reading Frame (ORF) positions. (Source: Devi et al., 2019, Biomedical and Pharmacology Journal; 12(4).)

proteins (L1 & L2) as shown in Figure 23.9. Individual ORFs among the viral genome are designated as **early, late,** and **LCR** (Long Control Region) or **URR** (Upstream Regulatory Region). Despite some variations within the size and range of ORFs, all papillomaviruses contain well-conserved core genes. These genes are involved in replication (**E1 & E2**) and packaging (**L1 & L2**) with greater diversity in the remaining genes (**E6, E7, and E4**) that have roles in driving cell cycle entry, immune evasion, and virus release (Doorbar et al., 2012). The E1 cistron is highly preserved and encodes a protein that is a virus-specific DNA helicase. It is essential for viral genome replication and amplification. This gene additionally shows the helicase and DNA binding activity. The E2 cistron encodes a protein that binds to both the viral and cellular genome sites. It is conserved between HPV types in its N-terminal and C-terminal domains. It also functions in viral transcription, replication, and genome maintenance as well as partitioning. E6 & E7 interact with the different cellular proteins for their inhibition and act as a repressor. They help to reactivate the replication and inhibit cellular apoptosis for their non-recognition through the cellular genes for cleaning. The other two genes (L1 and L2) are the major structural proteins for the assembly and making of the capsid of the virus. The new HPV serological type is defined as having 90–98% homology to any existing types based on the E6, E7, and L1 regions. If between 2% and 10% DNA divergence is present, the two viruses are considered subtypes of the same HPV type. When they show less than 2% divergence, the viruses are considered variants (Galloway, 1999). Some variants have different biological and biochemical properties important in cervical cancer. There are 86 complete genomes of HPV characterized, and about 120 are partially characterized (de Villiers et al., 2004).

23.4 Pathophysiology: Mode of Infection and Transmission

The typical incubation period of HPV infection is around 8–12 months, while the immune response can vary from an infected person's immunological conditions and type of HPV infection. HPV is transmitted from skin-to-skin or mucosa to the mucosa and enters the body via cutaneous or mucosal trauma (Handler et al., 2015). It infects epithelial cells via interaction with cell surface receptors such as integrin-α 6, abundantly expressed in basal cells and epithelial cells. It is assumed that the HPV replication cycle commences with the virus's entry into the cell's epithelium. HPV entry into the epithelium requires mild abrasion or microtrauma of the epidermis. In the basal layer, viral replication is considered non-productive. The virus establishes itself as a low copy number episome by using the host DNA replication machinery to synthesize its DNA on average once per cycle (Flores et al., 1997). The virus converts to a rolling circle model of DNA replication in segregated keratinocytes of the suprabasal layer of the epithelium, amplifies its DNA to a large copy number, synthesizes capsid proteins, and releases virus assembly (Flores et al., 1999).

The antibodies are generated against the Major Capsid Protein L1 of the virus. Approximately 70–80% of women become seroconverted after natural infection. The antibody responses are typically slow to develop and of low titer and avidity. However, few men are seroconverted, and even after seroconversion, antibodies are not protective in humans, since they have no response to HPV infection. The available data denotes that whether natural infection with HPV induces protection against reinfection is equivocal. There appears to be a reduced risk of reinfection with the same HPV type, but infection does not seem to provide group-specific or general immune protection from reinfection with other HPV types. In most cases, those who develop lesions mount an effective cell-mediated immune (CMI) response, and the lesions regress.

23.4.1 Viral Entry into the Host Cell

HPV can interact with the extracellular matrix (ECM) through the laminin-332 molecule. Then the furin cleaved the L2 capsid protein of HPV from N-terminal to create its access to interact with the cell's receptors. Earlier studies found that the viral capsid undergoes conformational changes with HSPG binding (Giroglou et al., 2001; Selinka et al., 2003; Richards et al., 2006; Day et al., 2008; Horvath et al., 2010). One model shows that HSPG binding intends to cause conformational changes necessary for a secondary binding event, leading to infectious virus absorption via an unspecified receptor or receptor complex (Day et al., 2008; Kines et al., 2009; Richards et al., 2013). The furin cleaved on the N-terminal of the structural L2 protein at the furin convertase site. The RG-1 epitope (residues 17–36) on the L2 protein is exposed upon furin cleavage. In an in vitro study, using the furin pre-cleaved virus (FPC virus), it had been shown that FPC PsVs (pseudovirions) would bind and infect HSPG-null cells, suggesting that the primary role of HSPG (Heparin Sulphate Proteoglycans) binding is to enable cell surface furin cleavage (Day et al., 2008). On the other hand, within the in vivo murine cervicovaginal challenge model, FPC PsV infection was inhibited when HSPGs were cleaved with heparinase III treatment. Under heparinase III treatment, it was shown that FPC PsVs still bind to the cell surface but not to the basement membrane (BM) (Kines et al., 2009). These findings indicate that the BM-bound FPC PsVs is an active infection and not FPC cell-surface bound PsV.

The two well-studied endocytic pathways used by any non-enveloped virus are clathrin- and caveolin-mediated endocytic pathways, which make the virion enter inside the host cells. Dynamin pinches off the endocytic vesicles via clathrin or caveolin-mediated endocytosis from the plasma membrane.

Earlier studies by various research groups suggested that HPV type 16 used clathrin-mediated endocytosis to invade the host cells (Bousarghin et al., 2003; Smith et al., 2007; Day et al., 2003). After removing the HPV genome's capsid from the nucleus, only some L2 is required to transport the HPV genome to the host cell nucleus. The HPV genome is likely retained within the TGN (trans-Golgi-network) after uncoating. It waits for the host cell to decrease its protective mechanism following the onset of mitosis. Structural reorganization during cell division requires coordinated trafficking of vesicles from various compartments and enrichment of mitotic associated proteins along microtubules. HPV uses this time to traffick its genome to the nucleus. Two well-studied endocytic pathways are clathrin- and caveolin-mediated endocytosis used by non-enveloped viruses (Bousarghin et al., 2003).

Further, the L2 membrane destabilizes the peptides, and Syntex-18 egresses the L2 HPV genome complex. The Dynamin also supports the genome complex to enter inside the cell's nucleus for replication and making copies of the virion particle. After all the packaging and essential proteins are expressed, it is assembled, exocytosis happened, and the new copies of the infective virion come out in the body's circulatory system. Figure 23.10 demonstrates the complex pictorial representation of the infection cycle of HPV in the cells.

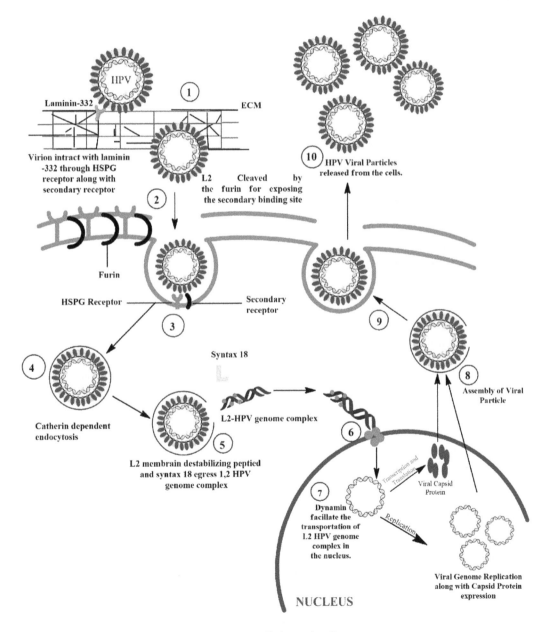

FIGURE 23.10 Pathway of HPV entry into the human cells for causing diseases.

23.4.2 Viral Genome Replication

The viral genome replication needs the helicase-ATPase activity of the viral initiator protein E1 and the multifunctional viral protein E2, which aids in the selective recruitment of E1 to the viral DNA. At the viral beginning of DNA replication, E1 oligomerizes and assembles as a double-hexamer, and it interacts with various host replication components, including polymerase-primase, replication protein A, topo-isomerase I, and cyclin E/Cdk2 (Hebner and Laimins, 2006). E2 is also a transcription factor that may transactivate and repress genes and also a regulator of genome segregation, which is necessary for viral survival (Bouvard et al., 1994; McBride et al., 2004). Late gene expression and viral genome replica-tion are induced when infected cells differentiate. Both E4 and E5 are necessary for viral amplification. The viral proteins E6 and E7 are expressed to keep the cellular replication machinery active, and they uncouple cell growth arrest and differentiation mainly by inactivating p53 and pRb. E7 inactivates pRb, forcing infected cells to stay proliferative and avoid cell cycle exit, whereas E6 abrogates p53, ensuring cell survival by avoiding apoptosis induced by this abnormal growth signal. After epithelial differen-tiation, the productive phase of the viral life cycle is increased even further, resulting in viral genome amplification to thousands of copies per cell in the suprabasal layers, along with stimulation of late gene regulation (Maglennon et al., 2011). The L1 and L2 proteins, which comprise the icosahedral capsid's components, subsequently wrap the amplified genomes into infectious virions. Furthermore, viral egress is most likely accomplished by spontaneous tissue shedding, which may be aided by E4's capacity to disrupt the keratin network (Doorbar et al., 2006). The control of the viral life cycle in this manner helps HPV to evade detection by the immune response because high levels of viral gene expression and virion generation are limited to the topmost layers of the epithelium, which are not really under immune surveil-lance (Stanley, 2010). HPV relies on the host DNA replication machinery to generate its DNA due to the viral genome's limited coding capacity. HPV uses a variety of techniques to disrupt important regulatory circuits that govern host cell replication, keeping developing cells active in the cell cycle. As a result, HPV can reactivate cellular proteins and signal transduction pathways required for late gene expression and viral DNA amplification.

23.5 HPV Diseases and Their Association with Cancer

23.5.1 Diseases Associated with HPV

HPV viruses propagate via contact with infected genital tissue, mucous membranes, or body fluids and can be transmitted sexually. The majority of HPV infections are asymptomatic and heal on their own within 1–2 years. If it is not diagnosed and treated properly, it can lead to chronic infection of high-risk types, which can develop into invasive carcinoma at the site of infection, most often in the genital tract. The chronic infection affects between 5–10% of all infected women. These infections will lead to premalignant glan-dular or squamous intraepithelial lesions within months or years, which are histopathologically classified as cervical intraepithelial neoplasia (CIN), and therefore to cancer. CIN is further graded as follows:

CIN 1: mild dysplasia;
CIN 2: moderate to marked dysplasia; and
CIN 3: severe dysplasia to carcinoma in situ.

Most CIN lesions on the cervix can slowly become cancerous.

The time duration between HPV and invasive carcinoma acquisition is generally 20 years or more. The basis for this progression is not well understood, but the predisposing conditions and risk factors include the following: HPV type; immune status (susceptibility is greater in persons who are immunocomprom-ised, HIV infected, or receiving immunosuppressive therapy); coinfection with other STI (herpes simplex, chlamydia, and gonococcal infections); parity and young age at first pregnancy; and tobacco smoking. HIV-infected women have a higher prevalence of persistent HPV infection, often with multiple HPV types, and are at increased risk of progression to high-grade CIN and cervical cancer compared to women without HIV infection (Denny et al., 2012). HPV infections are also implicated in other carcinomas such

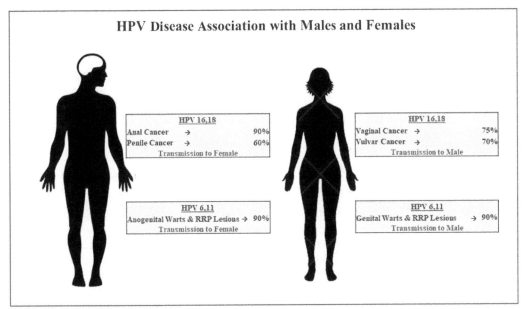

*RRP= Recurrent respiratory papillomatosis

FIGURE 23.11 The HPV and its associated diseases in males and females.

as anus carcinomas (90%), the vulva (70% depending on the age) and vagina (75%), the penis (60%), and the oropharynx (70% depending on the region). In the abovementioned cancers, HPV-16 is reported to be the predominant type to be found.

HPV infections with low-risk types cause anogenital warts in females and males. Over 90% of these are associated with HPV types 6 and 11. Anogenital warts can be difficult to treat and, in rare cases, can become malignant (Human Papillomavirus (HPV) Vaccination Coverage Among Adolescents, National Center for Immunization and Respiratory Diseases, 2017).

HPV6 and 11 can also cause a rare condition known as recurrent respiratory papillomatosis (RRP), in which warts form on the larynx or other parts of the respiratory tract with the risk of airway obstruction. RRP occurs in two forms: juvenile-onset RRP, which is caused by vertical transmission of HPV from other to a susceptible child prenatally and usually presents in childhood, and adult-onset RRP, which is probably transmitted horizontally through sexual activity with onsetin young adulthood, typically in the third decade of life (Larson and Derkay, 2010). RRP causes significant morbidity and may require multiple surgical interventions to maintain patient airway. It can be fatal, and lesions may undergo malignant changes, as shown in Figure 23.11.

23.5.2 HPV Cancer

HPV is the most prevalent viral infection of the reproductive system in both men and women, and it causes a variety of diseases. It includes precancerous lesions that may progress to cancer. Although most HPV infections do not cause symptoms and resolve spontaneously, persistent infection with HPV may result in disease. The association between HPV infection and the development of epithelial lesions or cancer is complex. Approximately 200 HPV types have been characterized, and particularly the alpha HPV types are classified into high-risk or low-risk types according to their association with anogenital malignancies. Also, an individual can be infected with multiple HPV types, which may also increase the risk of developing cervical cancer (Trottier et al., 2006).

Moreover, many HPVs have been identified from healthy individuals without any clinical systems. In women, persistent infection with specific HPV types (most frequently HPV-16 and HPV-18) may lead to precancerous lesions, and if it is untreated, may progress into cervical cancer. HPV infection is also associated with oropharyngeal and anogenital cancers and other conditions in men and women. Persistent infection with high-risk HPV genotypes is the cause of almost all cases of cervical cancer and is also associated with multiple other anogenital cancers (Bosch et al., 2013). Some individuals develop benign genital warts, while others are affected by specific oncogenic types and develop several types of cancers such as cervical, oropharyngeal, genital, head, and neck cancers. The HPVs belong to α genus reported to be oncogenic. Out of the 14 most common oncogenic HPV types, HPV16 is the most common and associated with the highest risk of progression to cancer (Palefsky et al., 2016). HPV infections were most of the time associated with the cancer.

23.5.3 Modulatory Role of HPV Proteins on Oncoproteins and Tumor Suppressor Genes in Cancer Progression

The early genes E6 and E7 play an important role in HPV-induced carcinogenesis by disrupting the two major tumor suppressor genes, p53, and pRb, which govern the normal cellular proliferation. The interaction of E7 with the pRb protein results in its destruction and the abnormal onset of S-phase, as well as the production of the E2F transcription factor, which induces the activation of cyclins and other S-phase regulators. The process of E6/E7-induced metamorphosis is not limited to the destruction of the critical cellular "guardians" pRb and p53. E7 also interacts with histone deacetylases, components of the AP1 transcription complex, and the cyclin-dependent kinase inhibitors p21 and p27, all of which are implicated in cell proliferation (Antinore et al., 1996; Funk et al., 1997). Simultaneously, the E6 protein recruits p53 for proteasomal degradation, hindering apoptosis and DNA repair, both of which are essential in the HPV life cycle. E6-mediated p53 degradation is significant because p53 is a transcription factor that governs the expression of genes encoding the cell cycle, DNA repair mechanism, metabolism, and apoptosis. This is crucial in the development of cervical malignancies because it reduces the efficiency of the cellular DNA damage response and permits secondary mutations to accumulate (Doorbar et al., 2006).

E6 and E7 viral oncoproteins have been found to cause DNA damage, centrosome abnormalities, and genomic segregation problems, resulting in chromosomal instability (Klingelhutz et al., 1996; Gewin et al., 2004). The catalytic component of telomerase [hTERT (human telomerase reverse transcriptase)], which inserts hexamer repeats into the telomeric ends of chromosomes, is activated by high-risk E6 (Shay et al., 2005). HPV16-E6 binds to E6AP, promoting the degradation of the transcriptional repressor NFX1-91 and, as a result, activating hTERT transcription; this repressor also plays a key role in HPV16-E6 stimulation of the carcinogenic transcription factor NF-kB (Unger et al., 2004). HPV-infected cells have a high amount of telomerase activity, which allows them to maintain telomere length and proliferate indefinitely (Wentzensen and von Knebel Doeberitz, 2007). Telomerase activity is generally limited to the proliferative fraction of the epithelium, and its stimulation is linked to cellular immortalization and carcinogenesis (Heselmeyer-Haddad et al., 2003). Numerous areas are lost in cervical carcinogenesis (2q, 3p, 4p, 5q, 6q, 11q, 13q, and 18q) while others are amplified (1q, 3q, 5p, and 8q) (Caraway et al., 2008). The 3q26 region contains sequences for the RNA component of the human telomerase gene, which acts as a template for the insertion of telomeres, which is the foundation for telomerase-based cell immortalization (Sharma et al., 2010). The degree of cervical neoplasia has been reported to enhance the frequency of 3q26 gain (Baylin and Jones, 2011). In addition to genetic changes, epigenetic mechanisms also have a significant impact on oncogenic processes. Epigenetic changes are frequently discovered early in carcinogenesis and are thought to represent essential starting events in certain malignancies (Jones and Baylin, 2002). Epigenetic processes contribute to tumor progression. A variety of epigenetic abnormalities have been reported in both the HPV and the cellular genome, such as DNA hypomethylation, hypermethylation of tumor suppressor genes, histone modifications, and changes in non-coding RNAs.

23.6 Diagnosis of Human Papilloma Viral Infections

Most HPV infections cause no symptoms and people are able to recover naturally. However, in some people, HPV infection persists and results in warts or precancerous lesions. The precancerous lesions increase the risk of cervix, vulva, vagina, penis, anus, mouth/oral, or throat cancer (HPV Information Centre Report, 2022; Ljubojevic and Skerlev, 2014). Nearly all cervical cancers are caused due to the two specific strains of HPV (i.e., HPV-16 and HPV-18), accounting for 70% of cases. There are over 181 different types of HPV strains having the capability to infect humans, out of which 15 have the capability to cause cancer and two strains cause common warts during their infection (Bernard et al., 2010). Therefore, diagnosing HPV infections is crucial in managing HPV-associated diseases and HPV-induced carcinogenesis.

In India, the diagnosis of HPV is mainly based on cytological methods (Sur and Chakravorty, 2015). However, other tests like visual inspection with Lugol's iodine (VILI) (Sankaranarayanan et al., 2004; Parashari et al., 2014) and Pap smear tests are routine. A study in the Chandigarh region showed that the HPV prevalence rates were more in the age group of 20–60 years (Sobti et al., 2001), with males comprising 65%. Further, it high expression of STAT3 levels in individuals infected with high-risk HPV types (i.e., HPV-16 &18) (Sobti et al., 2009) was also observed. The data from the All India Institute of Medical Sciences (AIIMS), New Delhi, indicate the wide spectrum of HPV infection throughout India. HR-HPV-16 & 18 genotypes are causing cervical cancer in India. All three variants of vaccines (i.e., bivalent, quadrivalent, and nonavalent vaccines) are available in India and are given in three doses over a six-month period (Golikeri, 2009). In 2016, the government of Punjab initiated the HPV vaccination campaign in the Bathinda (incidence 17.5 per 100,000 women) and Mansa (17.3 per 100,000 women) districts. In phase 1, nearly 10,000 girls studying in class 6 of government schools were covered. A total of 261 schools in Bathinda and 187 schools in Mansa were involved in the program. In total, 5,851 girls were vaccinated at Bathinda and 4,002 at Mansa, constituting 97.5% and 98.5% coverage, respectively. In the second phase, plans are afoot to include five more districts, which have the next highest incidence rates of the disease, thereby covering all districts that have a reported incidence of > 10 per 100,000 women (Prasad, 2017). The program will be gradually scaled up to include all girls in class 6 in both government and private schools across the state. The program is adopting both a facility-based and school-based approach to vaccination in the second phase (HPV Information Centre Report, 2022; Mehrotra et al., 2017). At the earlier stage of vaccination, the bivalent vaccine was given to people for curing cervical cancer by targeting the HR-HPV strains 16 and 18, and the quadrivalent vaccines are also administered nowadays. Figure 23.12 is a pictorial representation of the different diagnostic methods used for the identification of the HPV infection.

23.6.1 Presence of Warts in the Human Body Indicates HPV Infection

Both the low-risk and high-risk genotypes of HPV can induce different types of warts. Based on their infection sites, different types of warts are described. Common warts are usually found on the hands and feet but can also occur in other areas, such as the elbows or knees. They have a characteristic cauliflower-like

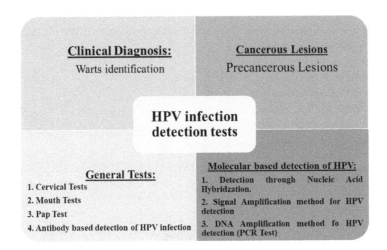

FIGURE 23.12 Different diagnostics methods for HPV infection.

surface and are typically slightly raised above the surrounding skin. Cutaneous HPV genotypes can cause genital warts; however, they are not associated with cancer development. Plantar warts are found on the soles of the feet, grow inward, causing pain while walking. Subungual or periungual warts form under the fingernail (subungual), around the fingernail, or on the cuticle (periungual). Plantar warts are caused due to low-risk HPV-type infections (de Koning et al., 2014). Flat warts are commonly found on the arms, face, or forehead. Similar to common warts, flat warts occur most frequently in children and teens. In people with normal immune function, flat warts are not associated with the development of cancer. However, during the infection of HPV, flat warts, later, lead to cancer (Lountzis and Rahman, 2008). Genital warts are quite contagious due to low-risk genital HPV and can be identified with a visual check. Five percent acetic acid (vinegar) is used to identify both warts, and squamous intraepithelial neoplasia (SIL) lesions with limited success by causing abnormal tissue to appear white. However, most doctors have found this technique helpful only in moist areas, such as the female genital tract.

Laryngeal papillomatosis is found in the larynx, caused by the infection of HPV 6 and 11 types, which leads to a rare condition known as recurrent laryngeal papillomatosis (Sinal and Woods, 2005) or other areas of the respiratory tract. These warts can recur frequently, may interfere with breathing, and in extremely rare cases, can progress to cancer. Surgical removal is highly preferable for these warts (Wu et al., 2003; Moore et al., 1999).

23.6.2 Clinical Laboratory Tests

   a. **Pap test:** Cervical test or Pap test is used to detect the HPV infection in the cervix, to identify HPV-16 and HPV-18 genotypes. In 2011, the FDA approved the Cobas HPV Test, which identifies many HPV genotypes such as HPV 16 & 18 and also detects the rest of the high-risk types (HPV 31, 33, 35, 39, 45, 51, 52, 56, 58, 59, 66, and 68). The above tests are DNA-based. RNA-based tests have also been developed. PreTect HPV-Proofer is for E6 and E7 mRNA detection. Recently p16 cell-cycle protein levels were also used to detect HPV infection, and these tests show high specificity and sensitivity in identifying the cells undergoing malignant transformation (Wentzensen and von Knebel Doeberitz, 2007; Molden et al., 2007).
   b. **Mouth test:** If the patient has lesions, the doctor can perform a biopsy to identify whether the lesions are cancerous or not. Further, they also test for HPV presence.
   c. **Antibody-based detection of HPV infection:** The IgG antibodies against the 16 L1 peptide in the sera from low-grade squamous intraepithelial lesion (LSIL) patients are used to diagnose high-risk HPV infections (Storey et al., 2013). The immune response to HPV's oncogene E7 found in NSCLC patients adds to the evidence linking HPV to NSCLC carcinogenesis.

23.6.3 Molecular Diagnosis

Molecular biology-based techniques have also been developed to detect HPV infections in the human body. There are the following methods:

   23.6.3.1 Methods based on nucleic acid hybridization
   23.6.3.2 Methods based on signal amplification
   23.6.3.3 Methods based on DNA amplification

23.6.3.1 Nucleic Acid Hybridization Method

HPV infections were first detected through Southern hybridization (Melchers et al., 1989) followed by in situ hybridization. HPV Card assay is based on in situ hybridization and exhibits high sensitivity (Villa et al., 2006).

23.6.3.2 Signal Amplification Detection Method

This method is based on the amplification of the signal produced by binding the probes with the sample DNA. Hybrid Capture II system (HCII, Digene, USA) is a non-radioactive signal amplification method based on the hybridization of the target HPV-DNA to labeled RNA probes in solution. The resulting RNA-DNA hybrids are captured onto microtiter wells and are detected by specific monoclonal antibodies and chemiluminescence substrate, providing a semi-quantitative measurement of HPV-DNA. Briefly in this test two different probe cocktails are used, one containing probes for low-risk genotype of HPV (i.e., HPV 6, 11, 42, 43, and 44) and the other containing probes for 13 high-risk genotypes: HPV 16, 18, 31, 33, 35, 39, 45, 51, 52, 56, 58, 59, and 68. This method has one limitation: though it detects high-risk and low-risk groups it does not permit the identification of specific HPV genotypes.

23.6.3.3 DNA Amplification Method

This method is based upon the amplification of L1gene fragment (MY09/MY11) and can detect a broad spectrum of the HPV strains with specific probes (Kleter et al., 1999; Gravitt et al., 2000). The INFORM HPV3 method used to detect the 13 different oncogenic HPVs is based on a PCR amplification system. The real-time-based methods increase the sensitivity and accuracy (Strauss et al., 2000; Cubie et al., 2001). The Real Time PCR assay was developed by Abbott to detect 14 high-risk HPV genotypes (16, 18, 31, 33, 25, 39, 45, 51, 52, 56, 58, 59, 66, 68) (Bihi et al., 2017).

23.7 HPV Vaccines

HPV vaccines were developed to protect individuals from the different HPV genotypes; depending on the groups of genotypes they protect against, the vaccines are called bivalent, quadrivalent or nonavalent. As per an HPV Information Centre report in 2022, the three prophylactic HPV vaccines that act against the high-risk HPV types are currently available and marketed in many countries around the globe and are used for the prevention of HPV-related disease: The first **quadrivalent vaccine** was approved in 2006 (McNeil, 2006), the **bivalent vaccine** in 2007, and the **nonavalent vaccine** in 2014. These vaccines are intended to be administered if possible before the onset of sexual activity (i.e., before first exposure to HPV infection). All vaccines available protect against HPV types 16 & 18, which can cause the greatest risk of cervical cancer. It has been estimated that these vaccines can prevent 70% of cervical cancer, 80% of anal cancer, 60% of vaginal cancer, 40% of vulvar cancer, and possibly some mouth cancer.

Using recombinant DNA technology, all three vaccines are prepared from the purified L1 structural protein that self-assemble to form HPV type-specific empty shells, termed virus-like particles (VLPs). None of the vaccines contains live biological products or viral DNA and are non-infectious; they do not contain antibiotics or preservative agents. The VLP-based vaccines are prepared from empty protein shells by recombinant technology (Zhou et al., 1991; Hagensee et al., 1993). These will be administered into the body along with the adjuvants. It will help to elicit the immune response in the host body. The process of VLP-based HPV vaccine against HPV 11 and the immunity developed through these vaccines are shown in Figure 23.13.

By 31st March 2017, globally, 71 countries (37%) had introduced the HPV vaccine in their national immunization programme for girls, and 11 countries (6%) also for boys, as described in Table 23.1.

All these HPV vaccines should be stored at 2–8°C, not frozen, and administered as soon as possible after being removed from the refrigerator. The stability of the HPV vaccines was observed to be different for a different type of vaccine. The shelf life for the bivalent vaccine has been demonstrated when stored outside the refrigerator for up to 3 days at temperatures between 8°C and 25°C, or up to 1 day at temperatures between 25°C and 37°C. For the quadrivalent vaccine, stability studies demonstrate that the vaccine is stable for 3 days when stored at temperatures from 8°C to 42°C. For the nonavalent vaccine, vaccine components are stable for up to 3 days when stored at temperatures from 8°C to 25°C. The WHO recognized the burden caused by cervical cancer and other HPV-related diseases, and reiterated the inclusion of HPV vaccines in national immunization programmes. Prevention of cervical cancer is best achieved through the immunization of girls, prior to sexual activity. All three HPV vaccines in use (bivalent, quadrivalent, and nonavalent) show excellent safety, efficacy, and effectiveness. Details of the different kinds of vaccines are given in Table 23.1.

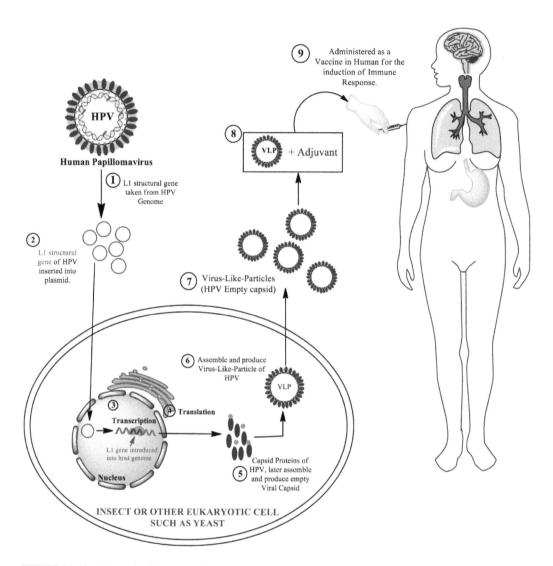

FIGURE 23.13 Schematic diagram showing the process of HPV L1 virus-like-particle (VLP) vaccine synthesis and immunity inside the host cell.

23.7.1 Bivalent Vaccine

This vaccine is administered for protection from cervical cancer. It is directed against high-risk HPV strains such as HPV-16 and HPV-18. The viral-like proteins are mixed with adjuvant aluminum hydroxide and 3-O desacyl-4' monophosphoryl lipid A. It is recommended for females of age 11–12 and females aged 13 through 26 who were not adequately vaccinated before. Bivalent vaccines are effective for about 10 years. It is important to get re-vaccinated every 7–7.5 years and screened again for HPV infection.

23.7.2 Quadrivalent Vaccine

This vaccine was first used for females in 2006, and from 2009 onwards, it was administered to males. It targets the four different high-risk strains of HPV (i.e., HPV-6, HPV-11, HPV-16, and HPV-18). The adjuvant used in this vaccine is amorphous aluminum hydroxyphosphate sulphate. It was assumed that

TABLE 23.1

Different Types of HPV Vaccines and Their Prevention of High-Risk HPVs

Type of Vaccine	Viral protein & expression system of Rec. protein	HPY Type (as per L1)	Route of administration	Age and Sex	Prevents
Bivalent vaccine (Cervarix)	L1 protein *Baculovirus* expression system in *Trichoplusiani* cells	HPV-16 &18	I.M.	Only Females from age 11 to 26 years	Premalignant lesions affecting the cervix
Quadrivalent (Gardasil 4)	L1 protein in the yeast expression system	HPV-6, 11, 16 & 18	I.M.	Both males & females	Cervical, vulvar, vaginal, and anal cancers by HPV-16 & 18
				Males (age): 13-22 years	Genital warts by HPV-6 & 11 Precancerous or dysplastic lesions by HPV-6,11,16 & 18
				Females (age): 9-45 years	CIN grade1; grade 2/3 and cervical adenocarcinoma in situ (AIS) (Vulvar intraepithelial neoplasia) VIN grade 2 & 3 Vaginal intraepithelial neoplasia (VaIN) grade 2 & 3 Anal intraepithelial neoplasia (AIN) grades 1, 2 & 3
Nona-valent Vaccine (Gardasil 9)	L1 protein In yeast expression systems	HPV-6, 11, 16, 18, 31, 33, 45, 52 & 58	I.M.		Anal cancer by HPV-16, 18, 31, 33, 45, 52 & 58 Genital warts (condyloma acuminate) by HPV-6&11 Premalignant lesions or dysplastic lesions by HPV-6, 11, 16, 18, 31, 33, 45, 52 & 58 AIN grades 1 ,2 & 3 CINgrade1, 2 & 3 VIN grades 2 & 3 VaIN grades 2 & 3

this vaccine protects against cervical, vulval, vaginal, and anal cancers. The recommended age for this vaccine is age 11–26 years females and 13–22 years in males.

23.7.3 Nonavalent Vaccine

This type of vaccine was introduced in 2014, directed against nine different strains of HPV (i.e., HPV-6, HPV-11, HPV-16, HPV-18, HPV-31, HPV-33, HPV-45, HPV-52, and HPV-58). The adjuvant used in this vaccine is amorphous aluminum hydroxyphosphate sulphate. It can be administered to both males and females (11–45 years for females; 13–22 years in males) (Joura et al., 2015; Serrano et al., 2018).

The nine-valent HPV vaccine was recently approved by the FDA and administration was recommended by the WHO. Following the administration of these 9vHPV vaccines, the titer peaked at roughly 7 months and subsequently declined over the next 90 months (Olsson et al., 2020). This study was performed on girls and boys at the age of 9 to 15 years. This shows the gradual increment of the immune capacity to overcome HPV infection in the host.

23.7.4 HPV Vaccine Dose Schedule

HPV vaccines should be administered to a person as per the dose recommended by the Advisory Committee on Immunization Practice (ACIP) (Markowitz et al., 2014). The dose for all types of vaccines is in a three-dose pack, and all three doses should be administered within 6 months. For the quadrivalent vaccine, the time interval between the first and second dose is about 2 months, and the final dose is administered after 4 months from the second dose of the vaccine. For the bivalent vaccine, the time interval between the first and second dose is about a 1 month, and the final dose is given 5 months after the second dose (Kreimer et al., 2015). For the nonavalent vaccine, the time interval between the first and second dose is about a 2-month gap and the final dose is given after 4 months from the second dose as shown in Table 23.1 (Petrosky et al., 2015).

Recently, the WHO issued a guideline for females about the dosage of the HPV vaccine. According to this guideline, the primary target group in most countries recommending HPV vaccination is young adolescent girls, aged 9–14. For all three vaccines, the vaccination schedule depends on the age of the vaccine recipient. For females, whose age is <15 years, a two-dose schedule (0, 6 months) is recommended. If the interval between doses is shorter than 5 months, then a third dose should be given at least 6 months after the first dose. For females whose age is ≥ 15 years at the time of the first dose, a three-dose schedule (0, 2, 6 months) is recommended. A three-dose schedule remains necessary for those known to be immunocompromised and/or HIV-infected.

23.8 HPV miRNAs

Like many double-strand DNA viruses, HPV is also reported to encode miRNAs. By using a bioinformatic approach, Gu et al.. (2011) predicted first time the presence of miRNAs inHPV. Later, Qian et al. (2013) reported 9-miRNAs in HPV based on a small RNA sequencing approach using libraries constructed from cultured cells and tissue samples as shown in Figure 23.14. Among them, five miRNAs were encoded by the HPV-16, one each by HPV-38, HPV-68, HPV-45, and HPV-6. HPV16-miR-H3 was encoded by the E6 region of HPV genome. HPV16-miR-H1, HPV16-miR-H5, and HPV6-miR-H1 were encoded from the E1 region of the HPV-16 and HPV-6; HPV16-miR-H2 was in a negative-strand corresponding to the LCR/URR at two different positions. The pre-miRNA sequence of HPV38-miR-H1 was encoded by the E7 region shared by the HPV-22, 23, 120, 104, and 115. The HPV45-miR-H1, HPV68-miR-H1, and HPV16-miR-H6 was encoded by L1 region. The miRNAs (i.e., HPV16-miR-H3, HPV16-miR-H5, HPV16-miR-H1, HPV68-miR-H1, and HPV45-miR-H1) were encoded by the plus (+) strand of the HPV genome while the rest four were encoded by the negative strand (-) (i.e., HPV38-miR-H1, HPV6-miR-H1, HPV16-miR-H6, and HPV16-miR-H2) as shown in Figure 23.14). The in silico studies of Tzong-Yi Lee and his research group (2018) revealed the functions of HPV-encoded miRNAs on various human pathways thereby helping the virus in its infection in humans. Further, it is speculated that they may play a crucial role in carcinogenesis. The hpv-miR-1 was reported to regulate various immunological processes of the host, whereas the hpv-miR-2 regulated the cellular metabolism, which further may lead to carcinogenic activity (Weng et al., 2018). The major role of hpv-miR-3 was to maintain the viral infection in the host by targeting the gene(s) responsible for cell death as shown in Table 23.2.

23.9 Conclusion

Human papillomaviruses (HPVs) have evolved with their human hosts and can cause latent/persistent infections. It is a common sexually transmitted infection around the globe that cause deleterious consequences among the human population. The implications of the HPV infection and its associated diseases are high in developing countries. Factors responsible for this high rate consist of germ-infested living conditions, co-infections with other pathogens, deprived healthcare facilities, and the high cost of vaccines. More than 200 genotypes of HPV have been identified to date, and most of the structural and genomic information were obtained from the alpha-HPV. HPVs exhibit tissue tropism and are divided into "mucous" and "cutaneous" type. Several studies have demonstrated that HPV type 16 and/or 18

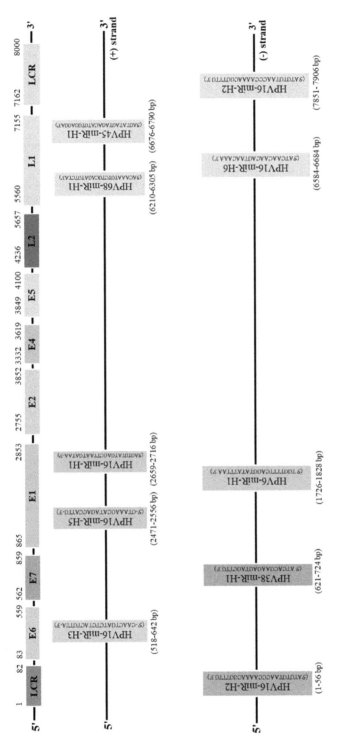

FIGURE 23.14 Schematic diagram showing the approximate genomic locations of the miRNAs encoded by the HPV. The HPV miRNAs position in the "+" strand and "−" strand shows separately. The squares represent the Pre-miRNAs names and their mature miRNAs sequences.

TABLE 23.2

HPV-Encoded miRNAs

HPV miRNAs	HPV strain/ Class of HPV	Position	Coding region	Sequence (5'→3')	Any other miRNAs ID
hpv-miR-1	HPV-16 *Alpha*-Papillomavirus	2659-2738 (+)	E1 Region	AGTGTATGAGCTTAATGATAA	hpv-miR-H1
hpv-miR-2	HPV-16 *Alpha*-papillomavirus	6694-6615 (-)	L1 Region	ATCAACAACAGTAACAAA	hpv-miR-H6
hpv-miR-3	HPV-16 *Alpha*- Papillomavirus	7903-7824 (-)	E6 Region	AUGUGUAACCCAAAAUC GGUUUG	hpv16-miR-H2

causes cancer, in which 97% of cases show cervical cancer is the most common type of cancer that prevails among the infected population. HPV may also lead to other types of cancers in which oropharyngeal and anogenital cancers are the most common. Recent reports also attribute the carcinogenicity to the HPV-58 subtype. The HPV infection rates were high in males, within the age group between 40–60 years. Several molecular, clinical diagnostic approaches are being used to detect HPV infections, and the frequent, accurate approach is a molecular-based approach.

Studies related to therapeutic interventions for HPV infections are ongoing for feasible and effective approaches to reduce the global burden of HPV infections, and minimize the prevalence cervical cancer. Though the currently available HPV vaccines have demonstrated satisfactory efficacy and safety, there is a need to develop broad-spectrum vaccines targeting other HPV variants and next-generation vaccines targeting other HPV proteins. RNAi based therapeutic approaches are also considered for HPV infections.

Acknowledgments

The authors would like to acknowledge the Indian Council of Medical Research, New Delhi for the Senior Research Fellowship Grant to Abhishek Pandeya IRIS No: 2017-2392; Award No.45/28/2018/IMM/BMS IRIS Cell No-2017-2392; Raj Kumar Khalko-National Fellowship for Scheduled Tribes (NFST), Ministry of Tribal Affairs, New Delhi (Award No: 201819-NFST-JHA-02141) & Babasaheb Bhimrao Ambedkar University, Lucknow for providing the necessary infrastructural and other essential facilities.

REFERENCES

Antinore M. J., Birrer M. J., Patel D., Nader L., McCance D. J. 1996. The human papillomavirus type 16 E7 gene product interacts with and trans-activates the AP1 family of transcription factors. *EMBO Journal* 15(8): 1950–1960. https://doi.org/10.1002/j.1460-2075.1996.tb00546.x

Basic Information about HPV and Cancer. n.d. CDC. Available from: www.cdc.gov/cancer/hpv/basic_info/ index.htm (Accessed September 8, 2022).

Baylin S. B., Jones P. A. 2011. A decade of exploring the cancer epigenome – biological and translational implications. *Nature Reviews Cancer* 11(10): 726–734. https://doi.org/10.1038/nrc3130

Bernard H-U., Calleja-Macias I. E., Dunn S. T. 2006. Genome variation of human papillomavirus types: phylogenetic and medical implications. *International Journal of Cancer* 118(5): 1071–1076. https://doi.org/ 10.1002/ijc.21655

Bernard H-U., Burk R. D., Chen Z., Van Doorslaer K., Zur Hausen H., de Villiers, E. M. 2010. Classification of papillomaviruses (PVs) based on 189 PV types and proposal of taxonomic amendments. *Virology* 401(1): 70–79. https://doi.org/10.1016/j.virol.2010.02.002

Bihi M. P., Tornillo L., Kind A. B., Obermann E., Noppen C., Chaffard R., Wynne P., et al. 2017. Human Papillomavirus (HPV) detection in cytologic specimens: similarities and differences of available methodology. *Applied Immunohistochemistry & Molecular Morphology* 25(3): 184–189. https://doi.org/ 10.1097/PAI.0000000000000290

Boda D., Neagu M., Constantin C., Nicolae Voinescu R., Caruntu C., Zurac S., et al. 2016. HPV strain distribution in patients with genital warts in a female population sample. *Oncology Letters* 12(3): 1779–1782. https://doi.org/10.3892/ol.2016.4903

Bonnez W., Reichman R. C. 2000. In Principles and practices of infectious diseases ed. G. L. Mandell, J. E. Bennet and R. Dolin. 2035–2049. Philadelphia: Churchill Livingstone.

Bosch F. X., Broker T. R., Forman D., Moscicki A-B., Gillison M. L., Doorbar J., Stern P. L. 2013. Comprehensive control of human papillomavirus infections and related diseases. *Vaccine* 31: H1–H31. https://doi.org/10.1016/j.vaccine.2013.10.003

Bousarghin L., Touzé A., Sizaret P-Y., Coursaget P. 2003. Human papillomavirus types 16, 31, and 58 use different endocytosis pathways to enter cells. *Journal of Virology* 77(6): 3846–3850. https://doi.org/10.1128/JVI.77.6.3846-3850.2003

Bouvard V., Storey A., Pim D., Banks L. 1994. Characterization of the human papillomavirus E2 protein: evidence of trans-activation and trans-repression in cervical keratinocytes. *EMBO Journal* 13(22): 5451–5459. https://doi.org/10.1002/j.1460-2075.1994.tb06880.x

Caraway N. P., Khanna A., Dawlett M., Guo M., Guo N., Lin E., Katz R. L. 2008. Gain of the 3q26 region in cervicovaginal liquid-based pap preparations is associated with squamous intraepithelial lesions and squamous cell carcinoma. *Gynecologic Oncology* 110, no. 1 (July): 37–42. https://doi.org/10.1016/j.ygyno.2008.01.040

Celewicz A., Celewicz, M., Michalczyk, M., Rzepka, R. 2020. Perspectives in HPV secondary screening and personalized therapy basing on our understanding of HPV-related carcinogenesis pathways. *Mediators of Inflammation* 2020: 2607594. https://doi.org/10.1155/2020/2607594

Chen X. S., Garcea R. L., Goldberg I., Casini G., Harrison, S. C. 2000. Structure of small virus-like particles assembled from the L1 protein of human papillomavirus 16. *Molecular Cell* 5(3): 557–567. https://doi.org/10.1016/S1097-2765(00)80449-9

Chen X. S., Casini G., Harrison S. C., Garcea, R. L. 2001. Papillomavirus capsid protein expression in Escherichia coli: purification and assembly of HPV11 and HPV16 L1. *Journal of Molecular Biology* 307(1): 173–182. https://doi.org/10.1006/jmbi.2000.4464

Cubie H. A., Seagar A. L., McGoogan E., Whitehead J., Brass A., Arends M. J., Whitley M. W. 2001. Rapid real time PCR to distinguish between high risk human papillomavirus types 16 and 18. *Molecular Pathology* 54(1): 24–29. https://doi.org/10.1136/mp.54.1.24

Day P. M., Lowy D. R., Schiller J. T. 2003. Papillomaviruses infect cells via a clathrin-dependent pathway. *Virology* 307(1): 1–11. https://doi.org/10.1016/S0042-6822(02)00143-5

Day P. M., Gambhira R., Roden R. B., Lowy D. R., Schiller J. T. 2008. Mechanisms of human papillomavirus type 16 neutralization by L2 cross-neutralizing and L1 type-specific antibodies. *J. Virol.* 82(9): 4638–4646.

de Koning M. N. C., Quint K. D., Bruggink S. C., Gussekloo J., Bouwes Bavinck J. N., Feltkamp M. C. W., et al. 2014. High prevalence of cutaneous warts in elementary school children and the ubiquitous presence of wart-associated human papillomavirus on clinically normal skin. *British Journal of Dermatology* 172(1): 196–201. https://doi.org/10.1111/bjd.13216

de Villiers E-M., Fauquet C., Broker T. R., Bernard H-U., Zur Hausen H. 2004. Classification of papillomaviruses. *Virology* 324(1): 17–27. https://doi.org/10.1016/j.virol.2004.03.033

Denny L. A., Franceschi S., de Sanjosé S., Heard I., Moscicki A. B., Palefsky J. 2012. Human papillomavirus, human immunodeficiency virus, and immunosuppression. *Vaccine* 30(Suppl 5): F168–F174. https://doi.org/10.1016/j.vaccine.2012.06.045

Devi, A., Bovilla V. R., Madhunapantula S. V. 2019. Current perspectives in human papilloma virus: where we are and what we need. *Biomed Pharmaco J* 12(4): 1683–1700. http://dx.doi.org/10.13005/bpj/1798

Doorbar J. 2006. Molecular biology of human papillomavirus infection and cervical cancer. *Clinical Science* 110(5): 525–541. https://doi.org/10.1042/CS20050369

Doorbar, J., Quint W., Banks L., Bravo I. G., Stoler M., Broker T. R., Stanley M. A. 2012. The biology and life-cycle of human papillomaviruses. *Vaccine* 30(Suppl 5): F55–F70. https://doi.org/10.1016/j.vaccine.2012.06.083

Flores E. R., Lambert P. F. 1997. Evidence for a switch in the mode of human papillomavirus type 16 DNA replication during the viral life cycle. *Journal of Virology* 71(10): 7167–7179. https://doi.org/10.1128/JVI.71.10.7167-7179.1997

Flores E. R., Allen-Hoffmann B. L., Lee D., Sattler C. A., Lambert P. F. 1999. Establishment of the human papillomavirus type 16 (HPV-16) life cycle in an immortalized human foreskin keratinocyte cell line. *Virology* 262(2): 344–354. https://doi.org/10.1006/viro.1999.9868

Funk J. O., Waga S., Harry J. B., Espling E., Stillman B., Galloway D. A. 1997. Inhibition of CDK activity and PCNA-dependent DNA replication by p21 is blocked by interaction with the HPV-16 E7 oncoprotein. *Genes & Development* 11(16): 2090–2100. https://doi.org/10.1101/gad.11.16.2090

Galloway D. A. 1999. Sexually Transmitted Diseases. Ed. K. K. Holmes, P. F. Sparling, P. A. Mardh, S. M. Lemon, W. E. Stamn, P. Piot, J. N. Wasserheit. New York: McGrawHill. 335–346.

Gewin L., Myers H., Kiyono T., Galloway D. A. 2004. Identification of a novel telomerase repressor that interacts with the human papillomavirus type-16 E6/E6-AP complex. *Genes & Development* 18(18): 2269–2282. https://doi.org/10.1101/gad.1214704

Giroglou T., Florin L., Schäfer F., Streeck R. E., Sapp, M. 2001. Human papillomavirus infection requires cell surface heparan sulfate. *Journal of Virology* 75(3): 1565–1570. https://doi.org/10.1128/JVI.75.3.1565-1570.2001

Golikeri P. 2009. A new vaccine for cervical Cancer and some good hope. http://cancersupport.aarogya.com/index.php?option=com_content&task=view&id=333&Itemid=361 (accessed May 5, 2021).

Gravitt P. E., Peyton C. L., Alessi T. Q., Wheeler C. M., Coutlee F., Hildesheim A., et al. 2000. Improved amplification of genital human papillomaviruses. *Journal of Clinical Microbiology* 38(1): 357–361. https://doi.org/10.1128/JCM.38.1.357-361.2000

Gu W., An J., Ye P., Zhao K-N., Antonsson A. 2011. Prediction of conserved microRNAs from the skin and mucosal human papillomaviruses. *Archives of Virology* 156(7): 1161–1171. https://doi.org/10.1007/s00705-011-0974-3

Guan J, Bywaters S. M., Brendle S. A., Ashley R. E., Makhov A. M., Conway J. F., et al. 2017. Cryoelectron microscopy maps of human papillomavirus 16 reveal L2 densities and heparin binding site. *Structure* 25(2): 253–263. https://doi.org/10.1016/j.str.2016.12.001

Hagensee M. E., Yaegashi N., Galloway D. A. 1993. Self-assembly of human papillomavirus type 1 capsids by expression of the L1 protein alone or by coexpression of the L1 and L2 capsid proteins. *Journal of Virology* 67(1): 315–322. https://doi.org/10.1128/JVI.67.1.315-322.1993

Handler M. Z., Handler N. S., Majewski S., Schwartz R. A. 2015. Human papillomavirus vaccine trials and tribulations: clinical perspectives. *Journal of the American Academy of Dermatology* 73(5): 743–756. https://doi.org/10.1016/j.jaad.2015.05.040

Hebner C. M., Laimins L. A. 2006. Human papillomaviruses: basic mechanisms of pathogenesis and oncogenicity. *Reviews in Medical Virology* 16(2): 83–97. https://doi.org/10.1002/rmv.488

Heselmeyer-Haddad K., Viktor Janz P. E., Castle N., Chaudhri N. W., Wilber K., Morrison L. E., et al. 2003. Detection of genomic amplification of the human telomerase gene (TERC) in cytologic specimens as a genetic test for the diagnosis of cervical dysplasia. *The American Journal of Pathology* 163(4): 1405–1416. https://doi.org/10.1016/S0002-9440(10)63498-0

Horvath C. A. J., Boulet G. A. V., Renoux V. M., Delvenne P. O., Bogers J-P. J. 2010. Mechanisms of cell entry by human papillomaviruses: an overview. *Virol J* 7, 11. https://doi.org/10.1186/1743-422X-7-1

How Many Cancers Are Linked with HPV Each Year? 2022. CDC. Available from: www.cdc.gov/cancer/hpv/statistics/cases.htm (Accessed September 8, 2022).

Human Papillomavirus and Related Diseases. 2022. HPV Information Centre, Spain. Available from: https://hpvcentre.net/statistics/reports/XWX.pdf (Accessed September 8, 2022).

Human Papillomavirus (HPV) Vaccination Coverage Among Adolescents 13-17 Years by State, HHS Region, and the United States, National Immunization Survey – Teen (NIS-Teen). 2017. National Center for Immunization and Respiratory Diseases. Available from: www.cdc.gov/vaccines/vpd/hpv/hcp/recommendations.html (Accessed April 18, 2021).

Jones P. A., Baylin S. B. 2002. The fundamental role of epigenetic events in cancer. *Nature Reviews Genetics* 3(6): 415–428. https://doi.org/10.1038/nrg816

Joura E. A., Giuliano A. R., Iversen O-E., Bouchard C., Mao C., Mehlsen J., et al., 2015. A 9-valent HPV vaccine against infection and intraepithelial neoplasia in women. *New England Journal of Medicine* 372(8): 711–723. https://doi.org/10.1056/NEJMoa1405044

Kines R. C., Thompson C. D., Lowy D. R., Schiller J. T., Day P M. 2009. The initial steps leading to papillomavirus infection occur on the basement membrane prior to cell surface binding. *Proceedings of the National Academy of Sciences of the United States of America* 106(48): 20458–20463. https://doi.org/10.1073/pnas.0908502106

Kirnbauer R., Booy F., Cheng N., Lowy D. R., Schiller J. T. 1992. Papillomavirus L1 major capsid protein self-assembles into virus-like particles that are highly immunogenic. *Proceedings of the National Academy of Sciences of the United States of America* 89(24): 12180–12184. https://doi.org/10.1073/pnas.89.24.12180

Kleter B., van Doorn L-J., Schrauwen L., Molijn A., Sastrowijoto S., ter Schegget J., et al. 1999. Development and clinical evaluation of a highly sensitive PCR-reverse hybridization line probe assay for detection and identification of anogenital human papillomavirus. *Journal of Clinical Microbiology* 37(8): 2508–2517. https://doi.org/10.1128/JCM.37.8.2508-2517.1999

Klingelhutz A. J., Foster S. A., McDougall J. K.1996. Telomerase activation by the E6 gene product of human papillomavirus type 16. *Nature* 380(6569): 79–82. https://doi.org/10.1038/380079a0

Kreimer A. R., Struyf F., Del Rosario-Raymundo M. R., Hildesheim A., Skinner S. R., Wacholder S., et al., 2015. Efficacy of fewer than three doses of an HPV-16/18 AS04-adjuvanted vaccine: combined analysis of data from the Costa Rica Vaccine and PATRICIA trials. *The Lancet Oncology* 16(7): 775–786. https://doi.org/10.1016/S1470-2045(15)00047-9

Larson D. A., Derkay C. S. 2010. Epidemiology of recurrent respiratory papillomatosis. *APMIS: acta pathologica, microbiologica, et immunologica Scandinavica* 118(6–7): 450–454. https://doi.org/10.1111/j.1600-0463.2010.02619.x

Ljubojevic S., Skerlev M. 2014. HPV-associated diseases. *Clinics in Dermatology* 32(2): 227–234. https://doi.org/10.1016/j.clindermatol.2013.08.007

Lountzis N. I., Rahman O. 2008. Images in clinical medicine: digital verrucae. *New England Journal of Medicine* 359(2): 177. https://doi.org/10.1056/NEJMicm071912

Maglennon G. A., McIntosh P, and Doorbar J. 2011. Persistence of viral DNA in the epithelial basal layer suggests a model for papillomavirus latency following immune regression. *Virology* 414(2): 153–163. https://doi.org/10.1016/j.virol.2011.03.019

Markowitz L. E., Dunne E. F., Saraiya M., Chesson H. W., Curtis C. R., Gee J., et al. 2014. Human papillomavirus vaccination: recommendations of the advisory committee on immunization practices (ACIP). *Morbidity and Mortality Weekly Report: Recommendations and Reports* 66(RR-05): 1–30.

McBride A. A., McPhillips M. G., Oliveira J. G. 2004. Brd4: tethering, segregation and beyond. *Trends in Microbiology* 12(12): 527–529. https://doi.org/10.1016/j.tim.2004.10.002

McNeil C. 2006. Who invented the VLP cervical cancer vaccines? *Journal of the National Cancer Institute* 98(7): 433. https://doi.org/10.1093/jnci/djj144

Mehrotra R., Hariprasad R., Rajaraman P., Mahajan V., Grover R., Kaur P., Swaminathan S. 2017. Stemming the wave of cervical cancer: human papillomavirus vaccine introduction in India. *Journal of Global Oncology* 4: 1–4. https://doi.org/10.1200/JGO.17.00030

Melchers W. J., Herbrink P., Walboomers J. M., Meijer C. J., vd Drift H., Lindeman J., Quint W. G. 1989. Optimization of human papillomavirus genotype detection in cervical scrapes by a modified filter in situ hybridization test. *Journal of Clinical Microbiology* 27(1): 106–110. https://doi.org/10.1128/JCM.27.1.106-110.1989

Modis Y., Trus B. L., Harrison S. C. 2002. Atomic model of the papillomavirus capsid. *The EMBO Journal* 21(18): 4754–4762. https://doi.org/10.1093/emboj/cdf494

Molden T., Kraus I., Skomedal H., Nordstrøm T., Karlsen F. 2007. PreTect™ HPV-Proofer: real-time detection and typing of E6/E7 mRNA from carcinogenic human papillomaviruses. *Journal of Virological Methods* 142(1–2): 204–212. https://doi.org/10.1016/j.jviromet.2007.01.036

Moore C. E., Wiatrak B. J., McClatchey K. D., Koopmann C. F., Thomas G. R., Bradford C. R., Carey T. E. 1999. High-risk human papillomavirus types and squamous cell carcinoma in patients with respiratory papillomas. *Otolaryngology — Head and Neck Surgery* 120(5): 698–705. https://doi.org/10.1053/hn.1999.v120.a91773

Olsson S-E., Restrepo J. A., Reina J. C., Pitisuttithum P., Ulied A., Varman M., Van Damme P., et al. 2020. Long-term immunogenicity, effectiveness, and safety of nine-valent human papillomavirus vaccine in girls and boys 9 to 15 years of age: interim analysis after 8 years of follow-up. *Papillomavirus Research* 10: 100203. https://doi.org/10.1016/j.pvr.2020.100203

Palefsky J. M., Hirsch M. S., Bloom A. 2016. Human Papillomavirus Infections: Epidemiology and Disease Associations. Waltham: UpToDate.

Parashari A., Singh V., Mittal T., Ahmed S., Grewal H., Gupta S., Sehgal A. 2014. Low cost technology for screening early cancerous lesions of oral cavity in rural settings. *Annals of Medical and Health Sciences Research* 4(1): 146–148. https://doi.org/10.4103/2141-9248.126628

Petrosky E., Bocchini J. A. Jr, Hariri S., Chesson H., Curtis C. R., Saraiya M., et al. 2015. Use of 9-valent human papillomavirus (HPV) vaccine: updated HPV vaccination recommendations of the advisory committee on immunization practices. MMWR. *Morbidity and Mortality Weekly Report* 64(11): 300–304.

Prasad R. 2017. A second chance for the HPV vaccine. www.thehindu.com/todays-paper/tp-opinion/a-second-chance-for-the-hpv-vaccine/article19821936 (accessed May 7, 2021).

Qian K., Pietilä T., Rönty M., Michon F., Frilander M. J., et al. 2013. Identification and validation of human papillomavirus encoded microRNAs. *PLOS One* 8(7): e70202. https://doi.org/10.1371/journal.pone.0070202

Richards K. F., Bienkowska-Haba M., Dasgupta J., Chen X. S., Sapp M. 2013. Multiple heparan sulfate binding site engagements are required for the infectious entry of human papillomavirus type 16. *Journal of Virology* 87(21): 11426–11437. https://doi.org/10.1128/JVI.01721-13

Richards R. M., Lowy D. R., Schiller J. T., Day P. M. 2006. Cleavage of the papillomavirus minor capsid protein, L2, at a furin consensus site is necessary for infection. *Proceedings of the National Academy of Sciences of the United States of America* 103(5): 1522–1527. https://doi.org/10.1073/pnas.0508815103

Sankaranarayanan R., Basu P., Wesley R. S., Mahe C., Keita N., Gombe Mbalawa C. C., et al. 2004. Accuracy of visual screening for cervical neoplasia: results from an IARC multicentre study in India and Africa. *International Journal of Cancer* 110(6): 907–913. https://doi.org/10.1002/ijc.20190

Selinka H-C., Giroglou T., Nowak T., Christensen N. D., Sapp M. 2003. Further evidence that papillomavirus capsids exist in two distinct conformations. *Journal of Virology* 77(24): 12961–12967. https://doi.org/10.1128/JVI.77.24.12961-12967.2003

Serrano B., Brotons M., Xavier Bosch F., Bruni L. 2018. Epidemiology and burden of HPV-related disease. *Best Practice & Research Clinical Obstetrics & Gynaecology* 47: 14–26. https://doi.org/10.1016/j.bpobgyn.2017.08.006

Sharma S., Kelly T. K., Jones P. A. 2010. Epigenetics in cancer. *Carcinogenesis* 31(1): 27–36. https://doi.org/10.1093/carcin/bgp220

Shay J. W., Wright W. E. 2005. Senescence and immortalization: role of telomeres and telomerase. *Carcinogenesis* 26(5): 867–874. https://doi.org/10.1093/carcin/bgh296

Sinal S. H., Woods C. R. 2005. Human papillomavirus infections of the genital and respiratory tracts in young children. *Seminars in Pediatric Infectious Diseases* 16(4): 306–316. https://doi.org/10.1053/j.spid.2005.06.010

Smith J. L., Campos S. K., Ozbun M. A. 2007. Human papillomavirus type 31 uses a caveolin 1-and dynamin 2-mediated entry pathway for infection of human keratinocytes. *Journal of Virology* 81(18): 9922–9931. https://doi.org/10.1128/JVI.00988-07

Sobti R. C., Kochar J., Singh K., Bhasin D., Capalash N. 2001. Telomerase activation and incidence of HPV in human gastrointestinal tumors in North Indian population. *Molecular and Cellular Biochemistry* 217(1–2): 51–56. https://doi.org/10.1023/a:1007224001047

Sobti R. C., Singh N., Hussain S., Suri V., Bharti A. C., Das B. C. 2009. Overexpression of STAT3 in HPV-mediated cervical cancer in a north Indian population. *Molecular And Cellular Biochemistry* 330(1–2): 193–199. https://doi.org/10.1007/s11010-009-0133-2

Stanley, M. 2010. HPV – immune response to infection and vaccination. *Infectious Agents and Cancer* 5: 19.

Storey R., Joh J., Kwon A., Jenson A. B., Ghim S., Kloecker G. H. 2013. Detection of immunoglobulin G against E7 of human papillomavirus in non-small-cell lung cancer. *Journal of Oncology* 2013: 240164. https://doi.org/10.1155/2013/240164

Strauss S., Desselberger U., Gray J. J. 2000. Detection of genital and cutaneous human papillomavirus types: differences in the sensitivity of generic PCRs, and consequences for clinical virological diagnosis. *British Journal of Biomedical Science* 57(3): 221–225.

Sur D., Chakravorty R. 2015. Present status of cervical neoplasia control and human papilloma virus epidemiology in India: The wind is blowing; unfolding the truth. *J Cancer Sci Ther* 8: 240–243. http://dx.doi.org/10.4172/1948-5956.1000375

Toh Z. Q., Kosasih J., Russell F. M., Garland S. M., Mulholland E. K., Licciardi P. V. 2019. Recombinant human papillomavirus nonavalent vaccine in the prevention of cancers caused by human papillomavirus. *Infection and Drug Resistance* 4;12: 1951–1967. http://doi.org/10.2147/IDR.S178381

Tommasino M. 2014. The human papillomavirus family and its role in carcinogenesis. *Seminars in Cancer Biology* 26: 13–21. https://doi.org/10.1016/j.semcancer.2013.11.002

Trottier H., Mahmud S., Costa M. C., Sobrinho J. P., Duarte-Franco E., Rohan T. E., et al. 2006. Human papillomavirus infections with multiple types and risk of cervical neoplasia. *Cancer Epidemiology and Prevention Biomarkers* 15(7): 1274–1280. https://doi.org/10.1158/1055-9965.EPI-06-0129

Unger E. R., Steinau M., Rajeevan M. S., Swan D., Lee D. R., Vernon S. D. 2004. Molecular markers for early detection of cervical neoplasia. *Disease Markers* 20(2): 103–116. https://doi.org/10.1155/2004/432684

Villa L. L., Denny L. 2006. Chapter 7: Methods for detection of HPV infection and its clinical utility. *International Journal of Gynecology & Obstetrics* 94 Suppl. 1: S71–S80. https://doi.org/10.1016/S0020-7292(07)60013-7

Weng S-L., Huang K-Y., Weng J. T-Y., Hung F-Y., Chang T-H., Lee T-Y. 2018. Genome-wide discovery of viral microRNAs based on phylogenetic analysis and structural evolution of various human papillomavirus subtypes. *Briefings in Bioinformatics* 19(6): 1102–1114.

Wentzensen N., von Knebel Doeberitz M. 2007. Biomarkers in cervical cancer screening. *Disease Markers* 23(4): 315–330. https://doi.org/10.1155/2007/678793

Wolf M., Garcea R. L., Grigorieff N., Harrison S. C. 2010. Subunit interactions in bovine papillomavirus. *Proceedings of the National Academy of Sciences* 107(14): 6298–6303. https://doi.org/10.1073/pnas.0914604107

Wu R., Sun S., Steinberg B. M. 2003. Requirement of STAT3 activation for differentiation of mucosal stratified squamous epithelium. *Molecular Medicine* 9 (3–4): 77–84. https://doi.org/10.2119/2003-00001.Wu

Zhou J., Sun X. Y., Stenzel D. J., Frazer I. H. 1991. Expression of vaccinia recombinant HPV 16 L1 and L2 ORF proteins in epithelial cells is sufficient for assembly of HPV virion-like particles. *Virology* 185(1): 251–257. https://doi.org/10.1016/0042-6822(91)90772-4

zur Hausen, H. 1986. Human papillomavirus infections and prospects for vaccination. In *Vaccine Intervention Against Virus-Induced Tumours*, ed. J. M. Goldman, and M. A. Epstein. London: Palgrave Macmillan, 63–80. https://doi.org/10.1007/978-1-349-08243-8_5

zur Hausen H. 2006. *Infections Causing Human Cancer*. Wiley-VCH: Weinheim. https://doi.org/10.1002/3527609318

24

Challenges of Multidrug-Resistant Microbes on Public Health

Ram Krishan Negi, Himani Khurana, Monika Sharma, Meghali Bharti, and Sonakshi Modeel
Fish Molecular Biology Laboratory, Department of Zoology, University of Delhi, Delhi, India

Tarana Negi
Department of Zoology, Government College, Bahadurgarh, India

24.1 Introduction

Penicillin was the first drug that was discovered in 1928 by Alexander Fleming (Fleming, 1929). Thereafter, a number of antibiotics have been commercialized to treat infection. Massive increase in the use of antibiotics as medicine has increased the occurrence and spread of multidrug-resistant bacteria. The ability of bacteria to protect and survive against an antibiotic is termed as antibiotic resistance and resistance to multiple antibiotics by a single bacterium is called multidrug resistance (MDR). Antibiotics that have been proved to be a miracle in the past by their virtue of saving millions of lives from an infectious disease are no longer the ultimate reason for their continuous use, leading to the development of antibiotic resistance to different kinds of drugs. Bacteria acquire this resistance either by random changes in the DNA (mutations) or by acquiring the resistance genes from the nearby bacteria through horizontal gene transfer (HGT) (Nikaido, 2009). To meet the increased food demand, the production is escalated ignoring the environmental and health hazards such as overuse of antimicrobials (Figure 24.1). Fish and seafood meet not only the protein need but also the need for animal-derived products among human beings, which is mostly sustained by the aquaculture sector, significantly contributing to the livelihood of many households. The aquaculture production is affected due to several bacterial diseases caused by both Gram-negative organisms such as *Aeromonas hydrophila*, *A. salmonicida*, *Vibrio harveyi*, *V. anguillarum*, *Edwardsiella tarda*, *Citrobacter freundii*, *Flavobacterium psychrophilum*, *Yersinia ruckeri*, *Pseudomonas fluorescens*, and Gram-positive bacteria belonging to genera *Streptococcus*, *Staphylococcus*, and *Mycobacterium*. The consumption of infected fish poses a serious threat to public health and to combat the stress of infections antibiotics are deployed in the aquaculture system (Preena et al., 2020). This leads to the emergence of antimicrobial-resistant pathogens. The aquaculture sector has been challenged by various kinds of infectious diseases that threaten the production and quality since to combat those there is expensive dependency on various kind of antibiotics (Aly & Albutti, 2014; Reverter et al., 2020). The combined use of antimicrobials and land-derived contamination in the aquatic system is significantly contributing to the selective selection of multidrug-resistant (MDR) bacteria, which further imposes an alarming threat to public health (Figure 24.2) (Miranda, Godoy, & Lee, 2018; Santos & Ramos, 2018). The common edible fish carp, salmon, tilapia, and catfish have been reported to possess antimicrobial-resistant pathogens (Čížek et al., 2010; Lozano, Díaz, Muñoz, & Riquelme, 2018; Monteiro et al., 2015). The possible threats of antimicrobial resistance (AMR) have also been observed in ornamental fish and possible zoonosis to fish handlers. The transfer of antimicrobial-resistant pathogens from aquatic environment to natural environment may lead to the development of AMR in wild fish and their related food products, which when consumed by humans will have serious health implications. Another major concern is its seriousness due to poor management practices (Preena et al., 2020). Use of antimicrobials and medicated food in aquaculture to increase animal weight and quality leads to the

DOI: 10.1201/9781003220404-26

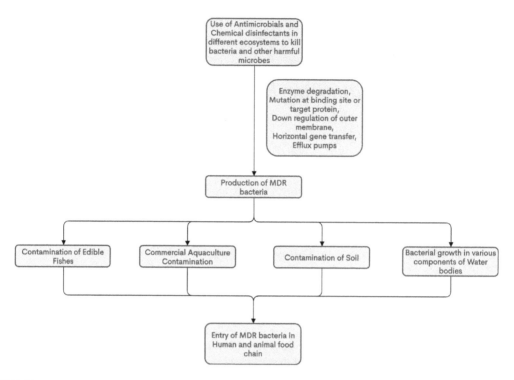

FIGURE 24.1   Representation of antimicrobial resistance in animal and human food chain through aquaculture.

emergence of reservoirs of antibiotic resistance in fish and other aquatic organisms and simultaneously in the surrounding aquatic environment (Thornber et al., 2020; Watts et al., 2017). Aquatic bacteria are able to transfer the antimicrobial resistance genes to other bacteria, and can ultimately be transferred to humans via the overlapping environment between human and aquaculture (Heuer et al., 2009). This problem needs

immediate attention as this might lead to the increased chances of infection to humans or increase the frequency of treatment failures and thus increased severity of infection (Laxminarayan et al., 2013). Several studies have reported multidrug resistance in common human pathogens isolated from aquaculture and their products. There is an urgent need to find alternative antimicrobials from potential sources including medicinal plants and microbes (*Streptomyces* spp.-releasing antimicrobial compounds). Other than these, the use of antimicrobial peptides and use of live bacteria as predators against pathogens (probiotics) (e.g., use of *Bdellovibrio* spp. against the gram-negative fish pathogens) can also be good alternatives.

24.2   Common Antibiotics Used in Aquaculture

In low- and middle-income countries due to lack of rules and regulations there is extensive use of antimicrobial agents in aquaculture (Watts et al., 2017). Chile is the second largest farmed salmon producer and that growth is accompanied by extensive use of antibiotics (Miranda et al., 2018). Intensive use of florfenicol and oxytetracycline mainly used to treat *Piscirickettsia salmonis* in the past has now become the major threat to the salmon industries in Chile due to development of resistance in bacterial pathogens (Lozano et al., 2018). There are many other narrow and broad-spectrum antibiotics that are generally used for food animals like macrolides, penicillin G and aminoglycosides, tetracyclines, and sulfonamides. Tetracyclines, macrolides, carbapenems, quinolines, and aminoglycosides are declared as "critically important antibiotics" by the WHO for treatment of human infectious diseases, with some

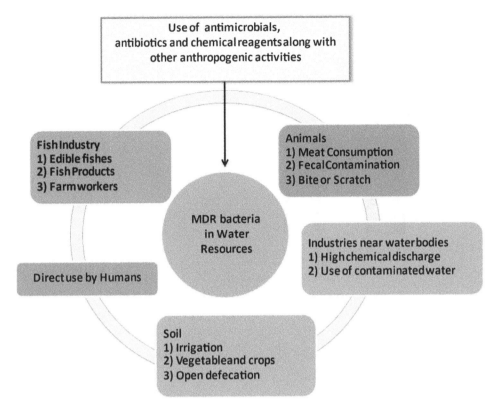

FIGURE 24.2 Diagrammatic representation of various pathways of water resources through which humans can be contaminated with MDR bacteria.

of them approved for veterinary use. Amikacin, macrolide tylosin, and nalidixic acid belong to various critical antibiotics classes and are used as growth promoters for animals (Angulo et al., 2009; Liu et al., 2017). Using these drugs can potentially increase resistant human pathogens, which is a matter of concern for public health (Liu et al., 2017). Erythromycin, sulfadiazine, and trimethoprim along with other antibiotics have been used in fish and shellfish aquaculture farms as growth promoters and for treatment of diseases in Bangladesh (Ali et al., 2016).

Various pathogenic species isolated from aquaculture-reported resistance against antibiotics have been used for human beings. *Salmonella* spp. isolated from food products in China were multidrug resistant against the antibiotics tetracycline, ampicillin, chloramphenicol, sulfisoxazole, and streptomycin, etc., commonly used for humans (Zhang et al., 2015). *Shewanella* algae and *Vibrio* spp. strains isolated from aquaculture farms in Italy were resistant against tetracycline, fosfomycin, cephalothin, amoxicillin, and multiple antimicrobials (Zago et al., 2020). *Vibrio parahaemolyticus* and *Staphylococcus aureus* (MRSA) are infectious MDR bacteria found in fish that enter the human body on raw food consumption thus causing gastrointestinal problems and food poisoning (Fri et al., 2020; Lee et al., 2018). Metals such as copper, zinc, and arsenic supplemented along with animal feed above the concentrations needed to complete the minimum nutrition requirements for disease prevention and growth promoter induce metal resistance in the community (Zhao et al., 2019).

24.3 Mechanisms Involved in Multidrug Resistance of Bacteria

Antimicrobial drugs can affect nucleotide synthesis that leads to DNA, RNA, or protein synthesis inhibition, interruption of cell membrane, and competition with enzyme substrates involved in synthesis of cell

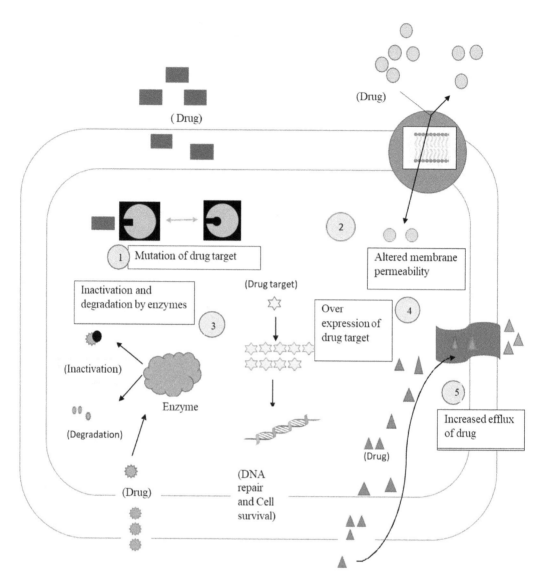

FIGURE 24.3 Mechanisms for multidrug resistance.

wall (Chethana et al., 2013). Microbes have evolved and developed an array of mechanisms to overcome the effectiveness of drugs and thus enduring exposure to drugs (Figure 24.3).

24.3.1 Enzyme Degradation

One of the main causes of MDR involves enzymatic degradation or inactivation of antimicrobials by hydrolysis of bonds (amide or ester), alteration by hydroxylation, acetylation, adenylation, phosphorylation, and glycosylation (Alekshun et al., 2007; Chethana et al., 2013).

Antibiotics like aminoglycosides (e.g., amikacin, tobramycin, and kanamycin) are deactivated by aminoglycoside phosphoryltransferase (phosphorylation), aminoglycoside acetyltransferase (acetylation), or by aminoglycoside adenyltransferase (adenylation). These can be deactivated by changes that lower the positive charge on them (Davies and Wright, 1997; Ramirez and Tolmasky, 2010). Many enzymes have been reported to modify aminoglycosides such as APH (3′)-I, AAC (3)-II, AAC (3)-II (Benveniste and Davies, 1973; Shaw et al., 1993).

β-lactams (e.g., penicillins, carbapenems, and cephalosporins) can be deactivated by β-lactamases through hydrolysis (Nikaido, 2009). Resistance can be easily acquired by the genes coding for inactivating enzymes as added genetic components on plasmids. Under β-lactamases, classes A and C resemble serine proteases in their mechanism, whereas Class B enzymes are metalloenzymes that can capably perform the function of carbapenems hydrolysis. To slow down resistance of β-lactam, numerous β-lactams have been developed. While first- and third-generation cephalosporins were prone to hydrolysis by AmpC enzyme, cephalosporins (IV generation) are more impervious to AmpC enzyme hydrolysis. ESBL (extended spectrum β-lactamases) have resulted from constant selective pressure that can now result in third- and even fourth-generation cephalosporins. (Jacoby and Medeiros, 1991).

24.3.2 Mutation at Binding Site or Target Protein

Binding of antibiotics to their targets is highly specific and with great affinity resulting in prevention of the target activity. When the target structure is altered but still manages to carry out its normal function, then resistance can be conferred. Diverse population is present during the course of an infection, so if gene coding for an antibiotic target undergoes a single-point mutation, it can confer antibiotic resistance and strains with this mutation can then multiply (Blair et al., 2015).

The process of transformation can result in resistance by modifying target protein by the formation of 'mosaic' genes. For instance, in *S. pneumoniae*, penicillin resistance is conferred by mosaic penicillin-binding protein (*pbp*) genes that code for enzymes that are insensitive to penicillin (Blair et al., 2015; Unemo et al., 2012). Recombination with DNA has given rise to these mosaic alleles from close neighbour *Streptococcus mitis*. In MRSA (methicillin-resistant *S. aureus*) resistance to methicillin is conferred by acquirement of the staphylococcal cassette chromosome *mec* (SCC*mec*) element. Protection by alteration of the target can serve as means of antibiotic resistance whereas change caused by mutation in the target molecules encoding genes is not required. It is an appropriate mechanism to gain resistance for various significant antibiotics. The ERM family (erythromycin ribosome methylase) does 16S rRNA methylation that leads to changes in drug-binding site, thus inhibiting the binding of lincosamines, macrolides, and streptogramins (Alekshun and Levy, 2007).

24.3.3 Downregulation of Outer Membrane

Cell wall plays a vital role in survival of both bacteria and fungi. By binding with the peptidoglycan layer in bacteria, drugs inhibit cell wall synthesis, therefore inhibiting growth and division of the cell (He et al., 2014). Some chromosomal mutations or horizontal gene transfer can result in changes and alterations in the cell membrane composition leading to lowered permeability and drugs uptake into the cell (Alekshun and Levy, 2007; Loeffler and Stevens, 2003). Altered membrane composition results in deficiency of active target sites for the drugs to bind (He et al., 2014). If mutation occurs in genes coding for the target, it can further lead to changes at the molecular level and preserve cell function by lowering vulnerability towards inhibition (Chethana et al., 2013; Džidić, Šušković, and Kos, 2008). Essentially, there are two main pathways taken by antibiotics through the outer membrane: (i) Lipid-mediated pathway (hydrophobic antibiotics) and (ii) diffusion porins (hydrophilic antibiotics).

The outer membrane's protein and lipid compositions have an effect on the sensitivity of bacteria to various antibiotics (Delcour, 2009). As compared to Gram-positive bacteria, Gram-negative bacteria's outer membrane has internally low permeability to many antibiotics (Kojima and Nikaido, 2013; Vargiu and Nikaido, 2012). Antibiotics that are hydrophilic in nature cross the outer membrane by getting diffused through porin proteins. Thus, by downregulation of porins, outer membrane permeability can be reduced and thus result in restricted antibiotic entry into the bacterial cell. However, in some cases of *Pseudomonas* spp, *Enterobacteriaceae*, and *Acinetobacter* spp., lowering in expression of porin considerably adds to resistance to newer drugs like carbapenems and cephalosporins, to which resistance is usually facilitated by enzymatic degradation (Wozniak and Waldor, 2010).

24.3.4 Horizontal Gene Transfer

Horizontal gene transfer (HGT) is a process that involves exchange of genetic material among "contemporary" bacteria, serving as a means by which resistance can be attained. Plasmids carry several antibiotic resistance genes that can be transferred to other members of the same or different bacterial species. Antibiotic resistance can be transmitted from one species to another species of bacteria through different methods of horizontal gene transfer and consequently arming the antibiotic-resistant genes in the recipient. The following are brief descriptions of HGT methods:

A) **Transformation** is the process of uptake of short naked DNA fragments by naturally transformable bacteria. Living donor cell is not required, only the presence of persistent DNA in the environment is needed.

B) **Transduction** involves the use of bacteriophages to transfer DNA from one bacterium to another. Viruses called bacteriophages are able to infect bacterial cells and use them as hosts to make more viruses.

C) **Conjugation** includes the use of sexual pilus for transfer of DNA and requires cell contact. Conjugation is a multi-step process involving mating pair formation, conjugal DNA synthesis and DNA transfer.

Fragments of DNA that encode resistance genes carried by drug-resistant donors (antibiotic resistant bacteria) can turn formerly susceptible bacteria to express resistance coded by these newly acquired resistance genes. R plasmids that are very small and lack the genes needed for mating-pair formation complex can be mobilized and transferred efficiently into recipient cells. Conjugational transfer of plasmids has been the prime method utilised for the evolution of several bacterial groups and is not a unique mechanism intended for multidrug resistance (Ochman et al., 2000). Bacteriophages and plasmids are also known to serve as vehicles for mechanism of horizontal gene transfer. Events of this kind of gene transfer can be categorized as a) acquirement of novel genes; b) acquirement of already existing genes paralogs; and (c) xenolog displacement of gene. Examples include isoleucyl-tRNA synthetase in eukaryotes whose acquirement in many bacteria has resulted in antibiotic resistance and parasites (e.g., *Chlamydia*-acquired ATP/ADP translocases from plants that may have implications in its pathogenesis) (Koonin et al., 2001).

24.3.5 Efflux Pumps

The process of pumping out of a solute of a cell is known as efflux. Efflux pumps are present in both antibiotic-susceptible and -resistant bacteria. When appropriate substrates are present, by some system induction, the susceptible strain can overproduce a pump and thus become resistant.

In the case of efflux mutation, antimicrobial resistance is due to either (a) increase in expression of the efflux pump protein or (b) an amino acid substitution (s) in pump protein making it more efficient at export. In both cases, the organism becomes less susceptible to that agent as the intracellular concentration of the substrate antimicrobial is lowered (Piddock, 2006). Multidrug resistance is facilitated by drug efflux pumps remains the predominant mechanism. Antibiotics are actively transported out of the cell by efflux pumps, and thus contribute to the intrinsic resistance of Gram-negative bacteria to various drugs. But when these pumps are overexpressed, they can confer a high degree of resistance to previously clinically useful antibiotics. Some efflux pumps have constricted substrate specificity (such as the Tet pumps), but many have a broad range of structurally different substrates and are known as MDR efflux pumps.

A subset of several genes coding for efflux pumps of all types confers multidrug resistance (Saier Jr and Paulsen, 2001). It is known that genome size is imitated in the number of pump genes, that is, large genomes have a higher number of pump genes, which in turn is known to be dependent on bacterial ecological behaviour (Ren and Paulsen, 2005). Every so often, multiple MDR efflux pumps can be possessed by a single organism (such as Acr systems of the *Enterobacteriaceae*; Mex systems in *Pseudomonas aeruginosa*). There are five different families of efflux pump proteins with regard to bacterial MDR efflux:

1. RND family (resistance nodulation division)
2. MFS (major facilitator superfamily)
3. SMR (staphylococcal multiresistance) and
4. MATE (multidrug and toxic compound extrusion)
5. ABC (ATP binding cassette)

These MDR efflux pumps can aid antibiotic resistance in bacteria in various means: (a) innate resistance to an entire class of agents in gram-negative bacteria, (b) inherent resistance to specific agents of some species of gram-negative bacteria, and (c) resistance by efflux pump overexpression in clinically significant bacteria.

Genes encoding for ATP-binding cassette (ABC) transporter membrane proteins can overexpress (Alekshun and Levy, 2007; Li and Nikaido, 2009), resulting in multidrug resistance and enduring normal cellular functions without any intervention. In species such as *Leishmania and Entamoeba*, MRP (multidrug-resistant protein) overexpression alters the permeability and fluidity, leading to an efflux (ATP-dependent) of the antimicrobials and therefore lowering their intracellular concentration (Bansal et al., 2006; Orozco et al., 2002).

24.4 Antimicrobial Resistance in Aquaculture

The uncontrolled use of antibiotics as growth promoters and/or to treat bacterial and fungal infections leads to their persistence in the aquatic environment. It could be directly applied as in water or indirectly through feed and immersions (Heuer et al., 2009). Depending on biodegradability, the initial concentration of the antibiotic and other physical and chemical forms, it could be retained in undigested food and faeces (Burridge et al., 2010). This causes the selection pressure on the bacterial populations and emergence of antimicrobial-resistant determinants because the susceptible biodiversity is replaced with these resistant communities and this resistance then persists even in the absence of responsible antibiotics (Chiew et al., 1998). Aquaculture and hospital environments serve as possible reservoirs for dissemination of AMR genes to fish and human pathogens mediated by plasmids, transposons, and integrons (Gao et al., 2012; Rhodes et al., 2000). These mobile genetic elements are responsible for horizontal gene transfer (HGT) and along with clonal selection caused due to antibiotic selective pressure are the main factors responsible for AMR (Schmidt et al., 2001). This indicates transfer of AMR genes from other niches. Integrated fish farming plays a major role in transfer of AMR globally. There have been reports of spread of AMR through integrated fish farming in Asia and Africa (Watts et al., 2017). Petersen et al. (2002) reported increased incidence of AMR from 5% to 100% among *Acinetobacter* spp. towards oxytetracycline and sulfamethoazole in integrated chicken-fish farms. Integrated fish farming was also responsible for development of resistant strains of *Enterococcus* and *Aeromonas* species in the gut of cultured fish (Petersen and Dalsgaard, 2003). The AMR has also been observed in massive catfish industries (Sarter et al., 2007).

Today, the antibiotic sensitivity is a topic for concern for scientists all over the world. Many researchers have worked on antibiotic-resistant bacteria associated within aquaculture. Investigation of antibiotic resistance in the gut metagenome of endangered fish *Tor putitora* revealed the presence of antibiotic resistance genes (ARGs). The identified ARGs encoded for beta-lactamases, efflux pumps, multidrug transporters, polymyxins, vancomycin, and tetracycline resistance. *Klebsiella pneumoniae* exhibited the highest relative abundance of beta-lactamase and *Escherichia coli* showed the highest relative abundance of efflux pumps (Khurana et al., 2020). Thus, fish gut microbiome serves as possible reservoir for dissemination of antibiotic-resistant genes to commensal or mutualistic bacteria, which may pose a serious threat to other fish and human beings. This is because the beneficial bacteria would also be converted into potential pathogens (Khurana et al., 2020). Gufe et al. (2019) implemented a study in Zimbabwe on antibiotic sensitivity of eight bacterial isolates of market fish against 10 antibiotics. This study ascertained the presence of the different levels of antibiotic sensitivity pattern in all eight isolates among which seven were highly resistance to at least three or more drugs. Another study isolated MDR bacteria from fish and fish handlers and found resistance against tetracycline with susceptibility to few other antibiotics (Grema et al., 2015). Ogbonna and Inana (2018) isolated 54 species of *Acinetobacter* in edible snow crabs and analyzed the presence of antibiotic resistance in almost 60% of species. Lee et al. (2018) collected 240 fish samples from different markets of Selangor and found the presence of 88% resistance against ampicillin, 50% against kanamycin, and 64% against amikacinin isolates of *V. parahaemolyticus*. Recently, Fri et al. (2020) found high antibiotic resistance in *Staphylococcus aureus* (MRSA) isolates from healthy and edible marine fish. The same study also found 100% antibiotic susceptibility to chloramphenicol and imipenem. Rabia et al. (2017) found 21% of multidrug resistance in *Staphylococcus aureus* isolates of fish samples meant for ready-to-eat food in Tanzania. Even the ornamental fish associated with aquaculture can lead to disease outbreak. In a study of commercial farm goldfish, *Carassius auratus*, Sahoo et al. (2016) found out the association of MDR *Aeromonas hydrophila* with Cyprinid herpes virus-2, further pointing out the greater risk of infections in fish and their transfer to humans while handling.

Uses of antibiotics in different river systems to kill various bacteria and virus have also affected antimicrobial resistance. Chakraborty et al. (2018) found the presence of common antibiotic-resistant bacteria and superbugs with high resistance against multiple drugs were detected from water resources of Ganga in Kolkata. Falgenhauer et al. (2019) sampled water bodies from northern Germany and found 58% MDR bacterial isolates along with the presence of *Pseudomonas aeruginosa*, which has a tendency to cause serious lung infections in humans including cystic fibrosis. A study of the rivers of Nigeria identified seven bacterial isolates from fish with skin lesions from pond aquaculture and found high antibiotic resistance against Tetracycline, Ceftazidine, Cetriaxone, Cephalexin, Cefotaxine, and Ciproflaxacin (Ogbonna and Inana, 2018). Thus, wastewater, especially those with antimicrobial treatment, has become a major hotspot for the development of MDR bacteria.

The unreasonable and limitless use of antibiotics can result in the development of MDR bacteria in hospital waste leading to dangerous infectious diseases (Rabbani et al., 2017). Adesoji et al. (2015) observed transferrable tetracycline resistance genes in 29 out of 105 multi-drug-resistant bacteria with high prevalence of *tet*(A) in genus *Alcaligenes* from untreated water in southwest Nigeria dams indicating that these genes can easily be transferred to other pathogenic bacteria. Wastewater samples from two hospitals of Dhaka city were used to isolate *Escherichia coli* and *Klebsiella pneumonia*, which showed high levels of resistance against 10 commonly used antibiotics (Rabbani et al., 2017).

Various researchers have done studies on fish cultivation and edible fish bacteria and their response against drugs in India. In Navi Mumbai, isolates of *Escherichia coli, faecal Streptococci* and sulphite-reducing *Clostridia* were obtained from water samples of retail outlets used for fish processing and cultivation. The study found high levels of antibiotic resistance against 20 antibiotics especially for Augmentin and Colistin (Visnuvinayagam et al., 2019). Sivaraman et al. (2017) isolated MDR *E.coli* samples from 238 fish samples of fishery outlets of Gujarat and found maximum resistance against ampicillin. A recent study showed the presence of high resistance against streptomycin, trimethoprim, and other antibiotics in isolates of *E. coli, Salmonella* spp. and *S. aureus* from fish fecal samples obtained from Rajasthan, India (Saharan et al., 2020). Asla, et al. (2016) isolated gut bacteria from two ornamental fish (i.e., *E. maculatus* and *A. lineatus)* from which 50% bacterial isolates of *E. maculatus* showed high resistance against multiple drugs whereas bacterial isolates of *A. lineatus* showed only 38.41% resistance against drugs. Visnuvinayagam et al. (2015) studied *S. aureus* in Cochin and Mumbai coast retail fishery outlets and found resistance against 20 drugs with maximum resistance to erythromycin. Sivalingam et al. (2019) reviewed the prevalence of the most dangerous pathogen CRE (*carbapenem resistance enterobacteriaceae*) in India and studied its resistance and spread in different environments. A recent study done on fish of West Bengal by Malick et al. (2020) found the presence of resistance against multiple drugs in *Acinetobacter* spp., which is responsible for high fish mortality.

Aquaculture products tested positive for antimicrobial resistance that is carried in *Salmonella* probably by the exposure to contaminated water and food processing practices. After examining the 730 samples of aquatic animals sampled from market and retailers in Shanghai, China, 217 tested positive with different *Salmonella* serovars among which *Salmonella Aberdeen* were the most abundant. In fact, 43.3% of the *Salmonella* isolates were found to be multidrug resistant (Zhang et al., 2015). *Shewanella* algae and *Vibrio* spp. strains isolated from aquaculture farms in Italy were found as reservoirs for antibiotic-resistant genes like beta-lactam and many of them were positive for other antibiotics as well (Zago et al., 2020). Oxolinic acid treatment in an integrated aquaculture system led to the resistance in *Vibrio* species spanned in the intestine of fish, but in bivalves a clear evolution was not determined for resistance (Giraud et al., 2006). Several bacterial strains isolated from the sediment, water, fish, and shrimps collected from aquaculture farms located at districts of Sarawak, Malaysian Borneo. Among the 94 identified strains and 17 genera, 63.8% of bacteria were resistant to multiple antibiotics, and *Chryseobacterium* spp. was resistant to 12 out of 19 tested antibiotics, which was the highest among the 17 tested genera (Kathleen et al., 2016). Integrated fish farming practices is another reason for high yield with low input. The manure from terrestrial animal farms is directly administered to fish ponds and becomes a mediator of transferring multidrug resistance to the fish and hence increases the risk of antimicrobial resistance in the aquatic system. Because of antimicrobial agents, growth promoters are generally used for therapeutic and prophylactic purposes for farming animals that ultimately reach aquatic organisms through direct transfer of manure for fish feeding which further becomes the source for antimicrobial-resistant bacteria in addition to residual antimicrobials (Monteiro et al., 2018). *Acinetobacter* spp. and *Enterococcus* spp. isolated from the ponds of integrated farm developed significant increase towards antimicrobial resistance within 2 months (Petersen et al., 2002). *Vibrio* strains isolated from different fish ponds in Benin city, Nigeria showed antimicrobial resistance profile against 20 antimicrobial agents. Out of 167 isolates 67.6% were multidrug resistance, which indicates that these isolates were exposed to high risk of contamination sources with frequent use of antibiotic history (Igbinosa, 2016). The inappropriate use of antimicrobial agents for long term in aquaculture increases the susceptibility of acquiring resistance to multiple drugs by bacteria and enhances the chances of transfer to others. These aquaculture reservoirs should not be underestimated as they are a big risk to public and environmental health as can be transferred to humans and environment by various means (Figure 24.1). Manure from farmlands used as fertilizer in agriculture can become a reason for transmission of AMR and can enter the food chain (Founou et al., 2016; Han et al., 2018). AMR can also be transmitted via aquaculture that can easily contaminate our water resources (Cabello et al., 2016). The exchange of genetic material between the AMR genes harbouring bacteria to another bacteria can lead to transmission of infection in humans and other animals quite easily (Figure 24.2) (Cabello et al., 2013; Von Wintersdorff et al., 2016). Moreover, the workers that handle the animals in farmhouse and slaughterhouse and later are at high risk of being infected by antimicrobial-resistant bacteria and can spread infection to other public places (Larsen et al., 2015; Reynaga et al., 2016).

23.5 Mitigation

Selective reduction in consumption of antibiotics both in livestock and integrated farms can significantly reduce the chances of dissemination of antibiotic-resistant genes (Levy, 2014) and the susceptible ones can outcompete the resistant ones over time. Prebiotics, probiotics, and derivatives from medicinal plants can be used as alternatives to antibiotics that could reduce the development of resistance in animals (Gaggìa et al., 2010). Antimicrobial peptides are another alternative, and are efficient in antimicrobial properties and offer reduced chances of resistance ability (Han et al., 2018). The search for AMPs became necessary with the widespread use of antibiotics in aquaculture, which resulted in the development of antibiotic-resistant strains of bacteria leading to diseased state in fish. These peptides constitute 12–100 amino acid residues. More than 3900 AMPs have been identified from plant and animal sources. Identification of AMPs is necessary for the production of new antibiotics as they are effective against microbes and induce only weak resistance (Dong et al., 2017). Composting of manure before further application can significantly destroy the residues of antimicrobials in manure and reduce the chances of selection of antimicrobial resistance genes (Liao et al., 2018; Selvam and Wong, 2017). Treating wastewater from livestock farms and aquaculture before entry into other water bodies can efficiently control dissemination of antimicrobial genes and MDRs (An et al., 2018; He et al., 2020). Awareness of antimicrobial resistance among researchers, farmworkers, farm stakeholders, general public, and policy makers is necessary. Along with all the other measures, powerful models and planning are required to screen for the use of chemicals and antimicrobials among livestock and aquaculture to build up a base for the protection of animals and humans from various infectious diseases. Improvement in current regulations for implementation of antimicrobial agents in farm industries and necessary improvements should be applied.

Education about dissemination of ARGs and knowledge about alternative sustainable approaches are needed to change the current situation.

REFERENCES

An, X-L., Su, J-Q., Li, B., Ouyang, W-Y., Zhao, Y., Chen, Q-L., et al. 2018. Tracking antibiotic resistome during wastewater treatment using high throughput quantitative PCR. *Environment International* 117:146–153.

Adesoji, A.T., Ogunjobi, A.A., Olatoye, I.O., Douglas, D.R. 2015. Prevalence of tetracycline resistance genes among multi-drug resistant bacteria from selected water distribution systems in southwestern Nigeria. *Annals of Clinical Microbiology and Antimicrobials* 14:35.

Alekshun, M.N., Levy, S.B. 2007. Molecular mechanisms of antibacterial multidrug resistance. *Cell* 128:1037–1050.

Ali, H., Rico, A., Murshed-e-Jahan, K., Belton, B. 2016. An assessment of chemical and biological product use in aquaculture in Bangladesh. *Aquaculture* 454:199–209.

Aly, S. M., Albutti, A. 2014. Antimicrobials use in aquaculture and their public health impact. *Journal of Aquaculture Research and Development* 5:1.

Angulo, F. J., Collignon, P., Powers, J. H., Chiller, T. M., Aidara-Kane, A., Aarestrup, F. M. 2009. World Health Organization ranking of antimicrobials according to their importance in human medicine: a critical step for developing risk management strategies for the use of antimicrobials in food production animals. *Clinical Infectious Diseases* 49:132–141.

Asla, V., Neethu, K., Athira, V., Nashad, M., Mohamed, H. 2016. Prevalence of antibiotic resistance among the gut associated bacteria of indigenous freshwater fish *aplocheilus lineatus* and *etroplus maculatus*. *International Journal of Aquaculture* 6.

Bansal, D., Sehgal, R., Chawla, Y., Malla, N., Mahajan, R. 2006. Multidrug resistance in amoebiasis patients. *Indian Journal of Medical Research* 124:189.

Benveniste, R., Davies, J. 1973. Aminoglycoside antibiotic-inactivating enzymes in actinomycetes similar to those present in clinical isolates of antibiotic-resistant bacteria. *Proceedings of the National Academy of Sciences* 70:2276–2280.

Blair, J.M., Webber, M.A., Baylay, A.J., Ogbolu, D.O., Piddock, L.J. 2015. Molecular mechanisms of antibiotic resistance. *Nature Reviews Microbiology* 13:42–51.

Burridge, L., Weis, J.S., Cabello, F., Pizarro, J., Bostick, K. 2010. Chemical use in salmon aquaculture: a review of current practices and possible environmental effects. *Aquaculture* 306:7–23.

Cabello, F.C., Godfrey, H.P., Buschmann, A.H., Dölz, H.J. 2016. Aquaculture as yet another environmental gateway to the development and globalisation of antimicrobial resistance. *The Lancet Infectious Diseases* 16:e127–e133.

Cabello, F.C., Godfrey, H.P., Tomova, A., Ivanova, L., Dölz, H., Millanao, A., Buschmann, A.H. 2013. Antimicrobial use in aquaculture re-examined: its relevance to antimicrobial resistance and to animal and human health. *Environmental Microbiology* 15:1917–1942.

Chakraborty, A., Poira, K., Saha, D., Halder, C., Das, S. 2018. Multidrug-resistant bacteria with activated and diversified MDR genes in Kolkata water: ganga action plan and heterogeneous phyto-antibiotics tackling superbug spread in India. *American Journal of Drug Delivery and Therapeutics* 5:1–9.

Chethana, G., Venkatesh, K., Mirzaei, F., Gopinath, S. 2013. Review on multidrug resistant bacteria and its implication in medical sciences. *Journal of Biological and Scientific Opinion* 1:32–37.

Chiew, Y-F., Yeo, S-F., Hall, L., Livermore, D.M. 1998. Can susceptibility to an antimicrobial be restored by halting its use? The case of streptomycin versus *Enterobacteriaceae*. *The Journal of Antimicrobial Chemotherapy* 41:247–251.

Čížek, A., Dolejská, M., Sochorová, R., Strachotová, K., Piačková, V., Veselý, T. 2010. Antimicrobial resistance and its genetic determinants in aeromonads isolated in ornamental (koi) carp (*Cyprinus carpio* koi) and common carp (*Cyprinus carpio*). *Veterinary Microbiology* 142:435–439.

Davies, J., Wright, G.D. 1997. Bacterial resistance to aminoglycoside antibiotics. *Trends in Microbiology* 5:234–240.

Delcour, A.H. 2009. Outer membrane permeability and antibiotic resistance. *Biochimica et Biophysica Acta (BBA) - Proteins and Proteomics* 1794:808–816.

Dong, B., Yi, Y., Liang, L., Shi, Q. 2017. High throughput identification of antimicrobial peptides from fish gastrointestinal microbiota. *Toxins* 9:266.

Džidić, S., Šušković, J., Kos, B. 2008. Antibiotic resistance mechanisms in bacteria: biochemical and genetic aspects. *Food Technology and Biotechnology* 46 (1).

Falgenhauer, L., Schwengers, O., Schmiedel, J., Baars, C., Lambrecht, O., Heß, S., et al. 2019. Multidrug-resistant, clinically relevant Gram-negative bacteria are present in German surface water samples. *Frontiers in Microbiology* 10:2779.

Fleming, A. 1929. On the antibacterial action of cultures of a penicillium, with special reference to their use in the isolation of *B. influenzae*. *British Journal of Experimental Pathology* 10:226.

Founou, L.L., Founou, R.C., Essack, S.Y. 2016. Antibiotic resistance in the food chain: a developing country-perspective. *Frontiers in Microbiology* 7:1881.

Fri, J., Njom, H.A., Ateba, C.N., Ndip, R.N. 2020. Antibiotic resistance and virulence gene characteristics of methicillin-resistant *staphylococcus aureus* (MRSA) isolated from healthy edible marine fish. *International Journal of Microbiology* 2020.

Gaggìa, F., Mattarelli, P., Biavati, B. 2010. Probiotics and prebiotics in animal feeding for safe food production. *International Journal of Food Microbiology* 141:S15–S28.

Gao, P., Mao, D., Luo, Y., Wang, L., Xu, B., Xu, L. 2012. Occurrence of sulfonamide and tetracycline-resistant bacteria and resistance genes in aquaculture environment. *Water Research* 46:2355–2364.

Giraud, E., Douet, D-G., Le Bris, H., Bouju-Albert, A., Donnay-Moreno, C., Thorin, C., Pouliquen, H. 2006. Survey of antibiotic resistance in an integrated marine aquaculture system under oxolinic acid treatment. *FEMS Microbiology Ecology* 55:439–448.

Grema, H.A., Geidam, Y.A., Suleiman, A., Gulani, I.A., Birma, R.B. 2015. Multi-drug resistant bacteria isolated from fish and fish handlers in Maiduguri, Nigeria. *International Journal of Animal and Veterinary Advances* 7:49–54.

Gufe, C., Canaan Hodobo, T., Mbonjani, B., Majonga, O., Marumure, J., Musari, S., et al. 2019. Antimicrobial profiling of bacteria isolated from fish sold at informal market in Mufakose, Zimbabwe. *International Journal of Microbiology*.

Han, X-M., Hu, H-W., Chen, Q-L., Yang, L-Y., Li, H-L., Zhu, Y-G., et al. 2018. Antibiotic resistance genes and associated bacterial communities in agricultural soils amended with different sources of animal manures. *Soil Biology and Biochemistry* 126:91–102.

He, X., Li, S., Kaminskyj, S.G. 2014. Using aspergillus nidulans to identify antifungal drug resistance mutations. *Eukaryotic Cell* 13:288–294.

He, Y., Yuan, Q., Mathieu, J., Stadler, L., Senehi, N., Sun, R., Alvarez, P.J. 2020. Antibiotic resistance genes from livestock waste: occurrence, dissemination, and treatment. *npj Clean Water* 3:1—11.

Heuer, O.E., Kruse, H., Grave, K., Collignon, P., Karunasagar, I., Angulo, F.J. 2009. Human health consequences of use of antimicrobial agents in aquaculture. *Clinical Infectious Diseases* 49:1248–1253.

Igbinosa, E.O. 2016. Detection and antimicrobial resistance of Vibrio isolates in aquaculture environments: implications for public health. *Microbial Drug Resistance* 22:238–245.

Jacoby, G.A., Medeiros, A.A. 1991. More extended-spectrum β-lactamases. *Antimicrob Agents Chemother* 35:1697-1704

Kathleen, M., Samuel, L., Felecia, C., Reagan, E., Kasing, A., Lesley, M., Toh, S. 2016. Antibiotic resistance of diverse bacteria from aquaculture in Borneo. *International Journal of Microbiology* 2016;2016:2164761. doi: 10.1155/2016/2164761

Khurana, H., Singh, D.N., Singh, A., Singh, Y., Lal, R., Negi, R.K. 2020. Gut microbiome of endangered *Tor putitora* (Ham.) as a reservoir of antibiotic resistance genes and pathogens associated with fish health. *BMC Microbiology* 20:1–18.

Kojima, S., Nikaido, H. 2013. Permeation rates of penicillins indicate that Escherichia coli porins function principally as nonspecific channels. *Proceedings of the National Academy of Sciences* 110:629–634.

Koonin, E.V., Makarova, K.S., Aravind, L. 2001. Horizontal gene transfer in prokaryotes: quantification and classification. *Annual Reviews in Microbiology* 55:709–742.

Larsen, J., Petersen, A., Sørum, M., Stegger, M., van Alphen, L., Valentiner-Branth, P., et al. 2015. Meticillin-resistant *Staphylococcus aureus* CC398 is an increasing cause of disease in people with no livestock contact in Denmark, 1999 to 2011. *Euro Surveill* 20:30021.

Laxminarayan, R., Duse, A., Wattal, C., Zaidi, A. K., Wertheim, H. F., Sumpradit, N., et al. 2013. Antibiotic resistance – the need for global solutions. *The Lancet Infectious Diseases* 13:1057–1098.

Lee, L-H., Ab Mutalib, N-S., Law, JW-F., Wong, S.H., Letchumanan, V. 2018. Discovery on antibiotic resistance patterns of *Vibrio parahaemolyticus* in Selangor reveals carbapenemase producing *Vibrio parahaemolyticus* in marine and freshwater fish. *Frontiers in Microbiology* 9:2513.

Lee, L.-H., Raghunath, P. 2018. Vibrionaceae diversity, multidrug resistance and management. *Frontiers in Microbiology* 9:563.

Levy, S. 2014. Reduced antibiotic use in livestock: how Denmark tackled resistance. *Environ Health Perspect.* 122(6): A160–A165. doi: 10.1289/ehp.122-A160

Li, X-Z., Nikaido, H. 2009. Efflux-mediated drug resistance in bacteria. *Drugs* 69:1555–1623.

Liao, H., Lu, X., Rensing, C., Friman, V.P., Geisen, S., Chen, Z., et al. 2018. Hyperthermophilic composting accelerates the removal of antibiotic resistance genes and mobile genetic elements in sewage sludge. *Environmental Science and Technology* 52:266–276.

Liu, X., Steele, J. C., Meng, X-Z. 2017. Usage, residue, and human health risk of antibiotics in Chinese aquaculture: a review. *Environmental Pollution* 223:161–169.

Loeffler, J., Stevens, D.A. 2003. Antifungal drug resistance. *Clinical Infectious Diseases* 36 (Supplement 1):31–41.

Lozano, I., Díaz, N. F., Muñoz, S., Riquelme, C. 2018. Antibiotics in Chilean aquaculture: a review. *Antibiotic Use in Animals* 3:25–44.

Malick, R.C., Bera, A.K., Chowdhury, H., Bhattacharya, M., Abdulla, T., Swain, H.S., et al. 2020. Identification and pathogenicity study of emerging fish pathogens *Acinetobacter junii* and *Acinetobacter pittii* recovered from a disease outbreak in *Labeo catla* (Hamilton, 1822) and *Hypophthalmichthys molitrix* (Valenciennes, 1844) of freshwater wetland in West Bengal, India. *Aquaculture Research* 51:2410–2420.

Miranda, C. D., Godoy, F. A., Lee, M. R. 2018. Current status of the use of antibiotics and the antimicrobial resistance in the Chilean salmon farms. *Frontiers in Microbiology* 9:1284.

Monteiro, S., Andrade, G., Garcia, F., Pilarski, F. 2018 Antibiotic residues and resistant bacteria in aquaculture. *The Pharmaceutical and Chemical Journal* 5:127–147.

Monteiro, S., Francisco, J., Campion, T., Pimpinato, R., Andrade, G. M., Garcia, F., Tornisielo, V. 2015. Multiresidue antimicrobial determination in Nile tilapia (*Oreochromis Niloticus*) cage farming by liquid chromatography tandem mass spectrometry. *Aquaculture* 447:37–43.

Nikaido, H. 2009. Multidrug resistance in bacteria. *Annual Review of Biochemistry* 78:119–146.

Ochman, H., Lawrence, J.G., Groisman, E.A. 2000. Lateral gene transfer and the nature of bacterial innovation. *Nature* 405:299–304.

Ogbonna, D.N., Inana, M.E. 2018. Characterization and multiple antibiotic resistance of bacterial isolates associated with fish aquaculture in ponds and rivers in Port Harcourt, Nigeria. *Journal of Advances in Microbiology* 1–14.

Orozco, E., Lopez, C., Gomez, C., Perez, D., Marchat, L., Banuelos, C., Delgadillo, D. 2002. Multidrug resistance in the protozoan parasite *Entamoeba histolytica*. *Parasitology International* 51:353–359.

Petersen, A., Andersen, J.S., Kaewmak, T., Somsiri, T., Dalsgaard, A. 2002. Impact of integrated fish farming on antimicrobial resistance in a pond environment. *Applied and Environmental Microbiology* 68:6036–6042.

Petersen, A., Dalsgaard, A. 2003. Antimicrobial resistance of intestinal *Aeromonas* spp. and *Enterococcus* spp. in fish cultured in integrated broiler-fish farms in Thailand. *Aquaculture* 219:71–82.

Piddock, L.J. 2006. Clinically relevant chromosomally encoded multidrug resistance efflux pumps in bacteria. *Clinical Microbiology Reviews* 19:382–402.

Preena, P.G., Swaminathan, T.R., Kumar, V.J.R., Singh, I.S.B. 2020. Antimicrobial resistance in aquaculture: a crisis for concern. *Biologia* 1–21.

Rabbani, M., Howlader, M.Z.H., Kabir, Y. 2017. Detection of multidrug resistant (MDR) bacteria in untreated waste water disposals of hospitals in Dhaka City, Bangladesh. *Journal of Global Antimicrobial Resistance* 10:120–125.

Rabia, A., Wambura, P., Kimera, S., Mdegela, R., Mzula, A. 2017. Potential public health risks of pathogenic bacteria contaminating marine fish in value chain in Zanzibar, Tanzania. *Microbiology Research Journal International* 1–11.

Ramirez, M.S. and Tolmasky, M.E. 2010. Aminoglycoside modifying enzymes. *Drug Resistance Updates* 13:151–171.

Ren, Q., Paulsen, I.T. 2005. Comparative analyses of fundamental differences in membrane transport capabilities in prokaryotes and eukaryotes. *PLoS Computational Biology* 1:e27.

Reverter, M., Sarter, S., Caruso, D., Avarre, J-C., Combe, M., Pepey, E., et al. 2020. Aquaculture at the crossroads of global warming and antimicrobial resistance. *Nature Communications* 11:1–8.

Reynaga, E., Navarro, M., Vilamala, A., Roure, P., Quintana, M., Garcia-Nuñez, M.,et al. 2016. Prevalence of colonization by methicillin-resistant *Staphylococcus aureus* ST398 in pigs and pig farm workers in an area of Catalonia, Spain. *BMC Infectious Diseases* 16:716.

Rhodes, G., Huys, G., Swings, J., Mcgann, P., Hiney, M., Smith, P., Pickup, R.W. 2000. Distribution of oxytetracycline resistance plasmids between aeromonads in hospital and aquaculture environments: implication of Tn1721 in dissemination of the tetracycline resistance determinant Tet A. *Applied and Environmental Microbiology* 66:3883–3890.

Saharan, V.V., Verma, P., Singh, A.P. 2020. High prevalence of antimicrobial resistance in *Escherichia coli*, *Salmonella* spp. and *Staphylococcus aureus* isolated from fish samples in India. *Aquaculture Research* 51:1200–1210.

Sahoo, P., Swaminathan, T.R., Abraham, T.J., Kumar, R., Pattanayak, S., Mohapatra, A., et al. 2016. Detection of goldfish haematopoietic necrosis herpes virus (Cyprinid herpesvirus-2) with multi-drug resistant *Aeromonas hydrophila* infection in goldfish: First evidence of any viral disease outbreak in ornamental freshwater aquaculture farms in India. *Acta Tropica* 161:8–17.

Saier Jr, M.H., Paulsen, I.T. 2001. Phylogeny of multidrug transporters. In: Seminars in cell and developmental biology, vol 3. *Elsevier* 205–213.

Santos, L., Ramos, F. 2018. Antimicrobial resistance in aquaculture: current knowledge and alternatives to tackle the problem. *International Journal of Antimicrobial Agents* 52:135–143.

Sarter, S., Nguyen, H.N.K., Lazard, J., Montet, D. 2007. Antibiotic resistance in Gram-negative bacteria isolated from farmed catfish. *Food Control* 18:1391–1396.

Schmidt, A.S., Bruun, M.S., Larsen, J.L., Dalsgaard, I. 2001. Characterization of class 1 integrons associated with R-plasmids in clinical *Aeromonas salmonicida* isolates from various geographical areas. *Journal of Antimicrobial Chemotherapy* 47:735–743.

Selvam, A., Wong, J. 2017. Degradation of antibiotics in livestock manure during composting. In Current Developments In Biotechnology And Bioengineering. *Elsevier*, pp. 267–292.

Shaw, K., Rather, P., Hare, R., Miller, G. 1993. Molecular genetics of aminoglycoside resistance genes and familial relationships of the aminoglycoside-modifying enzymes. *Microbiology and Molecular Biology Reviews* 57:138–163.

Sivalingam, P., Poté, J., Prabakar, K. 2019. Environmental prevalence of carbapenem resistance Enterobacteriaceae (CRE) in a tropical ecosystem in India: Human health perspectives and future directives. *Pathogens* 8:174.

Sivaraman, G., Prasad, M., Jha, A., Visnuvinayagam, S., Renuka, V., Remya, S., et al. 2017. Prevalence of extended-spectrum β-lactamase producing *Escherichia coli* in seafood from the retail fishery outlets of Veraval, Gujarat, India. *Journal of Environmental Biology* 38(4):523–526. doi:10.22438/jeb/38/4/MRN-366

Thornber, K., Verner-Jeffreys, D., Hinchliffe, S., Rahman, M.M., Bass, D., Tyler, C.R. 2020. Evaluating antimicrobial resistance in the global shrimp industry. *Reviews in Aquaculture* 12:966–986.

Unemo, M., Golparian, D., Nicholas, R., Ohnishi, M., Gallay, A., Sednaoui, P. 2012. High-level cefixime-and ceftriaxone-resistant *Neisseria gonorrhoeae* in France: novel penA mosaic allele in a successful international clone causes treatment failure. *Antimicrobial Agents and Chemotherapy* 56:1273–1280.

Vargiu, A.V., Nikaido, H. 2012. Multidrug binding properties of the AcrB efflux pump characterized by molecular dynamics simulations. *Proceedings of the National Academy of Sciences* 109:20637–20642.

Visnuvinayagam, S., Joseph, T.C., Murugadas, V., Chakrabarti, R., Lalitha, K. 2015. Status on methicillin resistant and multiple drug resistant *Staphylococcus aureus* in fish of Cochin and Mumbai coast, India. *Journal of Environmental Biology* 36:571.

Visnuvinayagam, S., Murthy, L., Parvathy, U., Jeyakumari, A., Adiga, T.G., Sivaraman, G. 2019. Detection of multi drug resistant bacteria in retail fish market water samples of Vashi, Navi Mumbai. *Proceedings of the National Academy of Sciences, India Section B: Biological Sciences* 89:559–564.

Von Wintersdorff C.J., Penders, J., Van Niekerk, J.M., Mills, N.D., Majumder, S., Van Alphen, L.B., et al. 2016. Dissemination of antimicrobial resistance in microbial ecosystems through horizontal gene transfer. *Frontiers in Microbiology* 7:173.

Watts, J. E., Schreier, H. J., Lanska, L., Hale, M. S. 2017. The rising tide of antimicrobial resistance in aquaculture: sources, sinks and solutions. *Marine drugs* 15:158.

Wozniak, R.A., Waldor, M.K. 2010. Integrative and conjugative elements: mosaic mobile genetic elements enabling dynamic lateral gene flow. *Nature Reviews Microbiology* 8:552–563.

Zago, V., Veschetti, L., Patuzzo, C., Malerba, G., Lleo, M.M. 2020. *Shewanella* algae and *Vibrio* spp. strains isolated in Italian aquaculture farms are reservoirs of antibiotic resistant genes that might constitute a risk for human health. *Marine Pollution Bulletin* 154:111057.

Zhang, J., Yang, X., Kuang, D., Shi, X., Xiao, W., Zhang, J., et al. 2015. Prevalence of antimicrobial resistance of non-typhoidal *Salmonella* serovars in retail aquaculture products. *International Journal of Food Microbiology* 210:47–52.

Zhao, Y., Cocerva, T., Cox, S., Tardif, S., Su, J-Q., Zhu, Y-G., Brandt, K.K. 2019. Evidence for co-selection of antibiotic resistance genes and mobile genetic elements in metal polluted urban soils. *Science of The Total Environment* 656:512–520.

25

Role of Probiotics in the Prevention and Management of Obesity: What Have We Learned So Far?

Tajpreet Kaur
Department of Pharmacology, Khalsa College of Pharmacy, Amritsar, India

Ashwani Kumar Sharma, Balbir Singh, and Amrit Pal Singh
Department of Pharmaceutical Sciences, Guru Nanak Dev University, Amritsar, India

Harpal S. Buttar
Department of Pathology & Laboratory Medicine, University of Ottawa, Ottawa, Canada

Abbreviations

AMPK	Adenosine adenosine monophosphate-activated protein kinase
FIAF	Fasting-induced adipose factor
FXR	Farnesoid X receptor
GLP-1	Glucagon Like Peptide-1
IL-1, IL-6	Interleukins-1 and 6
JNK-c	Jun N-Terminal kinase
LPL	Lipoprotein lipase
LPS	Lipopolysaccaride
NFκB	Nuclear factor kappalight-chainenhancer of activated B cells
PYY	Peptide YY
SCFA	Short-chain fatty acid
TG	Triglycerides

25.1 Introduction

The term "obesity" refers to the excessive accumulation of white adipose tissue in the body, especially in the abdomen, which causes health issues in human beings. Primarily, obesity is the consequence of imbalanced energy intake and expenditure. As per the World Health Organization (WHO), body mass index (BMI) serves as the basis of defining overweight (BMI $\geq$ 25) and obesity (BMI $\geq$ 30). Since 1975, a three-fold increase in the number of obese people has been reported. Around 13% of the world's population (men 11% and women 15%) is obese (WHO, 2020). The data suggests that 650 million and 1.9 billion adults are obese and overweight, respectively. Obesity in children is increasing at an alarming rate. It is projected that over 38 million children under 5 are obese, whereas more than 340 million children and adolescents (5–19 years) are overweight/obese (WHO, 2020). Obesity is major health challenge in the developed world and growing at an alarming pace in developing nations. Obesity has been reported to induce and aggravate cardiovascular disorders, stroke, diabetes mellitus, and cancer.

25.2 Environment and Obesity

Hippocrates (the Father of Medicine -ca. 460–370 BC) was the first to highlight the impact of environmental factors on health and advocated a harmonic relation between individual and environment (Hobbs & Radley, 2020). The deteriorating natural environment and increasing air pollution has been suggested to be the root cause of various diseases in humans. The chemicals, including pesticides, biphenyls, heavy metals, phthaltes, and solvents, have been found to disturb weight regulation mechanisms by inducing adipocyte hyperplasia, mimicking lipophilic hormones, and interfering with appetite and satiety pathways (Burgio et al., 2015). The WHO listed obesity and air pollution among the top 10 threats affecting human health. Interestingly, a decent interplay between the two has been suggested. Obese people are more prone to inflammatory disorders like asthma. On the contrary, pollution compels individuals to stay indoors, which reduces energy expenditure and causes obesity. In various studies, poor air quality has been positively co-related with BMI (Yang et al., 2019). Rats exposed to polluted air demonstrated activation of toll-like receptors, intrusion of polymorphonuclear cells in adipose tissues, systemic inflammation, and highlighted non-diet-induced body weight gain (Wei et al., 2016). Apart from natural environment, the social and built environments have been noted to contribute towards obesity. Our built environment including walkability, availability of green spaces, supermarket density, and density of junk food outlets affects calorie intake and energy expenditure. Recently a cohort study "Studying Lifecourse Obesity PrEdiction, SLOPE" highlighted the impact of built environment and childhood obesity (Wilding et al., 2020).

25.3 Current Therapeutic Strategies for Treating Obesity and Their Limitations

Dietary therapy is mainly employed for treating obesity in humans, which includes calorie restriction, changes in dietary styles, and meal replacement (Ruban et al., 2019). Calorie restriction elicits health benefits and extends lifespan (Wang et al., 2018). Apart from management of obesity, calorie restriction reduces the risk of diabetes mellitus, atherosclerosis, and cancer (Griffin et al., 2017). Meal replacement involves low-calorie substitutes for daily meals, and offers a convenient method for restriction of calorie intake. The Mediterranean diet is comprised of increased intake of fruits and vegetables and moderate amount of cheese, yogurt, and poultry has been identified as an effective methodology to prevent obesity and associated diseases (D'Innocenzo et al., 2019).

The US Food and Drug Administration (FDA) has approved Lorcaserin, a centrally acting serotonin agonist and appetite suppressant for treating obesity. Lorcaserin facilitates weight loss without increasing the risk of CVDs (Bohula et al., 2018). Orlistat prevents pancreatic lipases-mediated conversion of dietary fat into fatty acids and consequently discourages fat absorption in the body (Ruban et al., 2019; Seo et al., 2019). The combination of phentermine (a centrally acting appetite suppressant) and topiramate (an anti-epileptic) has been noted to promote weight reduction by increasing energy utilisation in the body (Lonneman et al., 2013; Saunders et al., 2018). Liraglutide is an effective therapy in obese subjects having dyslipidemia, hypertension, and diabetes mellitus. Naltrexone is an opioid antagonist used clinically for opium withdrawal. Bupropion inhibits catecholamine uptake and is used for smoking cessation. Combination of naltrexone and bupropion has been noted to alleviate obesity by suppressing appetite and inhibiting triglyceride hydrolysis and fatty acid absorption in patients (Hall &Kahan, 2018; Canuto et al., 2021). Apart from diet management and drug therapy for obesity, bariatric surgery is another choice available for weight reduction and remission of co-morbid conditions.

Existing drug therapy for obesity has been reported to potentiate risk of breast cancer, depression, cardiac valvulopathy, vitamin A, D, E, and K deficiency, metabolic acidosis, acute pancreatitis, gallbladder disease, and renal impairment (Allison et al., 2012; Zembutsu, 2015; Patel & Stanford, 2018; Pilitsi et al., 2019; Canuto et al., 2021). Bariatric surgery has limitations of significant mortality after discharge and increased prevalence of infection, arrhythmias, anastomotic leaks, and pulmonary emboli. Therefore, it is of paramount interest to explore novel therapeutic options for safe treatment of obese patients.

25.4 Role of Gut Microbiota in the Human Body

Gut microbiota or microbiome is a complex system of micro-organisms residing in the human digestive system and playing a crucial role in managing the host's health. It is estimated that our gastro-intestinal tract comprises more than 10^{14}-10^{15} micro-organisms, which is 10-fold higher than human body cells (Sender et al., 2016). Primarily, gut microbiota are comprised of three major classes: Bacteroidetes (*Bacteroides*, *Prevotella*, *Porphyromonas*), Firmicutes (*Lactobacillus*, *Clostridium*, *Eubacteria*, *Ruminococcus*), and Actinobacteria (*Bifidobacteria*), with maximum representation by *Bacteroides* and *Bifidobacterium* (Scheithauer et al., 2016). Gut microbiota finds its involvement in removal of dietary toxins, micronutrient synthesis, fermentation of indigestible food, and absorption of electrolytes and trace minerals. In addition, gut microbiota affect enterocyte growth by regulating production of short-chain fatty acids (Mozaffarian et al., 2011; Cani et al., 2012). In the host, gut microbiome induces hepatic lipogenesis by regulating carbohydrate response element-binding protein and hepatic sterol response element-binding protein type-1 (Bäckhed et al., 2005). Gut microbiota provocates energy production from dietary constituents and regulate genes controlling energy storage (Go et al., 2013).

25.5 Diet-Induced Alterations in Gut Microbiota and Their Relationship with Obesity

It has been reported that diet alters gut microbiota and subsequently leads to obesity (Yatsunenko et al., 2012). High-fat diet is reported to produce disbalance between firmicutes and bacteroidetes thereby causing "dysbiosis" and consequent obesity. A link between diet-induced obesity and increased growth of firmicutes has been demonstrated in experimental animals. High-fat diet, artificial sweeteners, an dincreased calorie intake make the gut environment acidic by promoting release of bile acids, which further causes expansion of firmicutes causing obesity (Wang & Donovan, 2015). Another contributing factor affecting gut microbial alteration is the fasting period. Experiments on rodents revealed that fasted mice had increased number of bacteroidetes in comparison to unfasted mice with the same body fat. Physical activity has a favourable effect on gut microbiome and maintains a stable ratio between certain bacterial genera, including bacteroidetes and firmicutes (Aitman et al., 2016). Animal studies suggest that microbes in the gut play a vital role in host nutrient acquisition and energy regulation. Of note, in obese vs. lean animals and humans, the composition of gut microbiota is different (DiBaise et al., 2008; Allen et al., 2018). Metabolic activity of gut microbiota facilitates calorie extraction from ingested food and helps its storage in adipose tissues for future use (Angelakis et al., 2012). Gut flora of obese rodents and humans witness more firmicutes and fewer bacteroidetes as compared to their slim counterparts (Crovesy et al., 2020). The increased number of bacteroidetes and *Staphylococcus aureus* has been noted in normal weight women but excessive weight gain during pregnancy is corroborated with increase in bacteriodetes (Santacruz et al., 2010). Modulation of the gut microbiota is suggested to serve as a novel strategy for managing obesity and allied problems. The number and proportion of various microbes such as *Eubacterium dolichum*, *Actinobacteria*, *Clostridium innocuum*, *Catenibacteriummitsuokai*, *Lactobacillussakei*, *Lactobacillus reuteri*, and *Archaea* bacteria like *Methanobrevibactersmithii* have been noted to vary in obesity. Various studies have explored the mechanisms of crosstalk between obesity and gut microbiota (Muscogiuri et al., 2019). Intestinal microbiota-derived lipopolysaccharide has been noted to trigger inflammation in metabolic diseases including obesity (Annalisa et al., 2014). Microhabitat alterations such as changes in oxygen level, pH, and availability of nutrients affect the specific number and bacterial type in gastro-intestinal tract (Donaldson et al., 2016).

Diet-induced alteration in microbiotacauses obesity through excessive accumulation of lipids, insulin resistance, and chronic inflammation (Wiciński et al., 2020). Short-chain fatty acids (SCFA) are monocarboxylic acids having upto six carbon atom chain, which are produced in large intestine during anaerobic fermentation of indigestible fibres and resistant starch by the microbiota (Silva et al., 2020). For intestinal epithelial cells, SCFAs serve as fuel and are noted to uplift the functioning of gut barrier. Abundance of bacteroidetes in gut has been noted to be directly associated with fecal concentrations of

SCFAs (Gérard, 2016). SCFA signalling involves G-protein coupled receptors like GPR41 and GPR43 to control immune functions (Parada Venegas et al., 2019). In obese individuals, alteration in the levels of SCFAs has been reported (Scott et al., 2013). The GPR43 and GPR41 are predominantly present in colon as well as small intestine (Ang & Ding, 2016). The GPR43 genetically deficient mice are obese even on normal diet, whereas GPR43 overexpressing mice are protected against obesity (Kimura et al., 2013). The SCFAs affect plasma glucose levels by enhancing the secretion of pancreatic polypeptide YY and glucagon-like peptide-1, which induce satiety and reduce food intake. Both, pancreatic polypeptide YY and glucagon-like peptide-1, deject the passage of food in intestine, and facilitate the absorption of nutrients (Tremaroli & Bäckhed, 2012). Dysbiosis led to decreased stimulation of GPR 41/43 receptors, which decreases leptin secretion and lipolysis in adipose tissue thereby causing obesity (Wiciński et al., 2020). Adenosine monophosphate kinase (AMPK) is primarily expressed in skeletal muscles and liver, and takes part in maintaining energy homeostasis of the cell (Bonfili et al., 2020). Decreased AMPK expression causes deactivation of carnitine palmitoyl transferase, which ultimately leads to decreased β-oxidation in liver and muscles as well as increases cholesterol and triglyceride synthesis (Jeon, 2016). Gut dysbiosis alters AMPK activity, thereby increasing fatty acid oxidation and increasing susceptibility towards obesity. Diet-induced altered microbiota decreases fasting-induced adipose factor levels that causes increased fat storage in white adipose tissue (Bäckhed et al., 2004). Microbiota activates the gut endocannabinoid system, which increases gut permeability, plasma lipopolysaccharides levels, and aggravates gut barrier disruption. Interestingly, the activated endocannabinoid system and increased lipopolysaccharide levels promote adipogenesis (Giovanna et al., 2019). Gut microbiota regulates bile acid homeostasis through farnesoid X receptor (Zheng et al., 2017). High-fat diet-induced bile acid secretion serves as a driving force in changing the composition of intestinal microflora. Of note, cholic acid-fed rats demonstrate a decrease in bacteroidetes and increase in firmicutes, which mimick the gut microbial alteration similar to that of obesity (Islam et al., 2011). Various mechanisms of high-fat diet-induced dysbiosis and consequent obesity are summarized in Figure 25.1.

25.6 Emergence of Probiotics and Definitions

Probiotics are viable microbial species that when consumed cause alteration of gastrointestinal flora and provide health benefits. The term "probiotic" comes from tje Greek word meaning "for life" (Khalighi et al., 2016). The modern concept of probiotics was introduced by Nobel laureate Elie Metchnikoff in 1907, who suggested the possibility to modify gut microbe composition. He suggested that replacing harmful microbes with useful ones could demonstrate health benefits (Cavaillon & Legout, 2016). Elie Metchnikoff demonstrated the benefit of lactic acid bacteria in fermented milk on the longevity of Bulgarian population (Tang & Zhao, 2019). Later, Rettger and Cheplin's experiments using *Lactobacillus acidophilus* demonstrated health benefits in rodents and human subjects with disappearance of *Balantidium coli* and other gas-producing bacteria (Swathi, 2016). Clinical trials using *Lactobacillus acidophilus* witnessed encouraging results related to amelioration of chronic constipation. The current definition of probiotics by the Food and Agriculture Organization of the United Nations and WHO is "the live microorganisms conferring health benefits to host, when given in adequate amounts" (Sánchez et al., 2017). The European Food and Feed Cultures Association define probiotic as "a live microbial food ingredient conferring health benefits and live microorganisms providing proven health benefits, when consumed in appropriate amount and number, respectively" (Vandenplas et al., 2015).

25.7 Probiotics as Medicines

Probiotics are well recognized as therapeutic agents for metabolic disorders (Sivamaruthi et al., 2019). Studies have shown that *Bifidobacterium* and *Lactobacillus* strains have strong probiotic properties and are reported to improve lactose intolerance and indigestion problems (Fijan, 2014). Various studies suggest that probiotics improve immune response and reduce allergies (Ouwehand et al., 2002; Plaza-Díaz et al., 2018). Various studies have demonstrated the role of probiotics in preventing allergies such as allergic

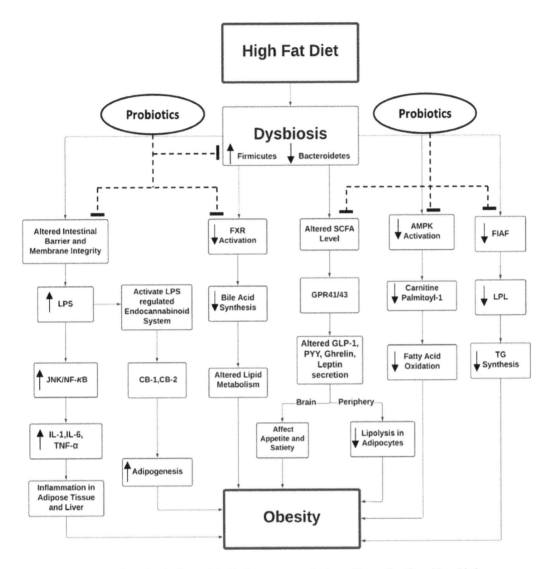

FIGURE 25.1 Role of high-fat diet-induced dysbiosis, consequent obesity and its amelioration with probiotics.

rhinitis, atopic dermatitis, *Clostridium*-associated diarrhoea, antibiotic-linked diarrhoea, irritable as well as inflammatory bowel disease (Moayyedi et al., 2010; Hempel et al., 2012; Saez-Lara et al., 2015; Rather et al., 2016; Berings et al., 2017; Goldenberg et al., 2017). Probiotics involving various micro-organisms have been reported to ameliorate insulin resistance, diabetes mellitus, and obesity (Salles et al., 2020).

25.8 Probiotics in the Management of Obesity: Lessons Learned from Animal Studies and Clinical Trials

The role of probiotics in managing obesity has been tried in various animal species. Of note, the species and strains used for evaluation of probiotics in experimental obesity include golden Syrian hamster (Avolio et al., 2019), rabbits (Bouaziz et al., 2021), piglets (Shin et al., 2019), zebrafish (Falcinelli et al., 2017), guinea fowls (Yeboah et al., 2020), broiler chicken (Zhang et al., 2020), mice (Li et al., 2016; Balolong et al.,2017; Cao et al., 2019), and rats (Karlsson et al., 2011; Carreras et al., 2018; Chunchai et al., 2018). Most of the animal studies made use of either *Lactobacillus* or *Bifidobacterium* alone or in combination with different strains. In the majority of studies, probiotic treatment led to decrease in weight gain/fat accumulation and decreased the level of pathogenic bacteria. A summary of various species and strains employed in evaluation of probiotics against obesity in various animal species is given in Table 25.1. The clinical trials involving use of probiotics in obese and overweight human subjects and their outcomes are presented in Table 25.2.

TABLE 25.1

Summary of Preclinical Studies Involving Use of Probiotics for Treating Obesity and Associated Metabolic Disorders

Species	Probiotics Used	Dose of Probiotics (colony forming units)	Study duration (in weeks)	Gender	Study outcomes	References
Goldensyrian hamsters	*Bifidobacterium lactis* (CNCM I-2494) *Lactobacillus acidophilus* *L. plantarum* *L.reuteri* (DSM 17938) *L. bulgaricus* (CNCM I-1632) *Lactococcus lactis* subsp. *Lactis* (CNCM I-1631) *Streptococcus thermophilus* (CNCM I-1630)	1.5×10^{10}	4 weeks	Male	Decrease in body weight as well as reduction in food consumption was observed.	Avolio et al., 2019
Piglets	*Lactobacillusplantarum* JDFM LP11	2.5×10^{7}	4 weeks	Female	Probiotics conferred beneficial effect on swine gut health and immune system	Shin et al., 2019
Rabbits	*BifidobacteriumanimalisBB-12* *Lactobacillus plantarum* 299v	1×10^{9} 1×10^{10}	14 weeks	Both	Probiotics exerted beneficial effects against obesity and metabolic syndrome.	Bouazizet al., 2021
Zebrafish	*Lactobacillus rhamnosus* IMC 501	1×10^{6}	4 weeks	Both	Probioticattenuated obesity and-related metabolic disorders.	Falcinelliet al., 2017
Guinea fowls	RE3™ probiotic containing *Lactobacilli, Bacillus, Saccharomyces cerevisiae*	1×10^{8} 1×10^{12} 1×10^{5}	12 weeks	Both	Probiotic supplementation increased growth rate and final body weight in guinea fowls.	Yeboah et al., 2020
Broiler chickens	*Bifidobacterium animalis* *Clostridium butyrate* *Lactococcus faecalis* *Lactobacillus plantarum*	2×10^{5} 4×10^{5} 2×10^{5} 2×10^{5}	6 weeks	Male	Probiotics decreased the pathogenic bacteria andimproved overall gut microbiota health.	Zhang et al., 2020
C57BL/6J mice	*Bifidobacterium licheniformis* *Bifidobacteriumsubtilis*	1×10^{8} 1×10^{8}	8 weeks	Male	Probiotic decreased body weight, improved glucose tolerance and reduced fat deposition in mouse liver.	Cao et al., 2019

TABLE 25.1 (Continued)

Summary of Preclinical Studies Involving Use of Probiotics for Treating Obesity and Associated Metabolic Disorders

Species	Probiotics Used	Dose of Probiotics (colony forming units)	Study duration (in weeks)	Gender	Study outcomes	References
Sprague-Dawley rats	*Lactobacillus mali* APS1 *L.mali* HFL *L.mali* HFM	5×10^7 5×10^8 5×10^9	12 weeks	Male	Probiotic regulated lipid metabolism, glucose homeostasis, suppressed progression of hepatic steatosis.	Chen et al., 2018
Sprague-Dawley rats	*Lactobacillus plantarum*	1×10^9	26 weeks	Female	*Lactobacillus* treated animals demonstrated decrease in adipose tissues, body weight, and lower plasma leptin level.	Karlsson et al., 2011
Zücker fatty rats	*Bifidobacterium animalis* subsp.*lactis* CECT 8145	1×10^{10}	12 weeks	Male	Probiotic improved the cholesterol level and decreased oxidative stress and inflammatory response.	Carreras et al., 2018
Wistar rats	*Lactobacillus paracasei*	1×10^8	12 weeks	Male	Decrease in fat mass, body weight, cholesterol along with improvement in insulin resistance was noted.	Chunchai et al., 2018
BALB/c mice	*Lactobacillus coryniformis* subsp. *Torquens* T3 *L. paracasei* subsp. Paracase *i*M5 *L. paracasei* subsp. *paracase* iX12	1×10^9 1×10^8	6 weeks	Male	Reduction in body weight was observed with probiotic treatment.	Song et al., 2016
BALB/c mice	*Bifidobacterium animalis VKB* *B.animalis VKL* *Lactobacillus casei* IMV B-7280 *L.delbrueckii* subsp. *bulgaricus* IMV B-7281	1×10^6	4 weeks	Female	Reduction in body weight was seen in probiotic treated groups.	Bubnov et al., 2017
ICR mice	*Bifidobacterium bifidum* BGN4 *B. longum* BORI *Lactobacillus acidophilus* AD031 *L. case i*IBS04	5×10^8	8 weeks	Male	Suppression in weight gain and liver fat deposition in mice.	Li et al., 2016
ICR mice	*Lactobacillus fermentum* 4B1	5×10^8	3 weeks	Female	Probiotic reduced body weight in mice.	Balolong et al., 2017
KK/Ta Mice	*Lactobacillus plantarum*	1×10^8	10 weeks	Male	*Lactobacillus* prevented insulin resistance in mice.	Okubo et al., 2013

TABLE 25.2

Summary of Clinical Trials Related to Usage of Probiotics in Obese/Overweight Human Subjects

Sr. No.	Probiotics Used	Form/dose of Probiotics (colony forming units)	No. of Participants Probiotic/Total Participants	Study Design and duration (in weeks)	Age/Sex	Clinical outcomes	References
1	*Bifidobacterium bifidum* CUL20 *Lactobacillus acidophilus* CUL21 *L. plantarum* CUL66 *L. acidophilus* CUL60	Capsule/ 5×10^{10}	110/220	Randomized, double-blind, placebo-controlled (26 weeks)	30-65 years. (M/F)	Supplementation with probiotic significantly reduced weight and improved small dense LDL-cholesterol and quality of life.	Michael et al., 2020
2	*Lactobacillus plantarum* CBT LP3	Capsule/ 15×10^{9}	25/50	Randomized, double-blind, placebo-controlled (12 weeks)	20-60 years. (M/F)	Probiotics corrected the obesity markers in obese subjects.	Song et al., 2020
3	*Bifidobacterium animalis* subspecies *lactis, Lactobacillus rhamnosus*	Capsule/ 1×10^{9}	207/411	Randomized, double-blind (20 weeks of gestation to delivery)	> 18 years, F	Probiotics did not resist gestational diabetes mellitus in obese pregnant women.	Callaway et al., 2019
4	Probiotic freeze-dried *Lactobacillus rhamnosus* GG	Capsule/ 1.6×10^{9}	22/44	Randomized controlled trial (12 weeks)	(M/F)	Probiotics improved cholesterol and LDL-cholesterol without affecting other lipid parameters. Probiotics supplementations decreased risk of CVDs as compared to only weight loss.	Moludi et al., 2019
5	*Bifidobacterium pseudocatenulatum* CECT 7765	Capsule/ $1\times10^{9\text{-}10}$	23/60	Prospective intervention study (13 weeks)	10-15 years, (M/F)	Beneficial effects of intervention on lipid profile and decreased inflammation in obese children.	Sanchis-Chordà et al., 2019
6	*Bifidobacterium animalis* subsp. *lactis* CECT 8145	Capsule/ 1×10^{10}	86/126	Double-blind, placebo-controlled (13 weeks)	> 18 years. (F)	Probiotic supplementation improved adiposity biomarkers in obese individuals.	Pedret et al., 2019

No.	Probiotic strains	Form/dose	Sample	Study design	Age/Sex	Outcome	Reference
7	Lactobacillus acidophilus W37, L. brevis W63, L. caseiW56, L. lactis W19, L. lactis W58, L.salivariusW24, Bifidobacterium bifidum W23, B. lactis W51, B. lactis W52	Sachet/ HD 1×10^{10} LD 2.5×10^{9}	47/71	Double-blind, placebo-controlled (12 weeks)	45-70 years, (F)	Probiotics supplementation demonstrated beneficial effect onmetabolic parameters in obese post-menopausal women.	Szulinska et al., 2018
8	Fortified yogurtwith whey protein, calcium,vitamin D, fiber, probiotic with Bifidobacterium lactis BB-12,Lactobacillus bulgaricus Streptococcus thermophilus	Yogurt/ 1×10^{7}	87/150	Randomized, double-blind trial (10 weeks)	20-65 years, (M/F)	Consumption offortified yogurt-improved metabolic parameters and body composition in overweight/obese patients.	Mohammadi-Sartang et al., 2018
9	Lactobacillus gasseriBNR17	Capsule/ LD 1×10^{9} HD 1×10^{10}	60/90	Double-blind, placebo-controlled (12 weeks)	20-25 years (M/F)	Daily consumption of probiotic decreased visceral fat in obese subjects.	Kim et al., 2018
10	Bifidobacterium lactis BL-4, B. bifidum BB-06, Lactobacillus acidophilus LA-14, L. caseiLC-11, L.lactisLL-23	Sachet/ 2×10^{10}	21/43	Double-blind, placebo-controlled (8 weeks)	20-59 years. (F)	Probiotic supplementation decreased abdominal adiposity and increased antioxidant enzyme activity.	Gomes et al., 2017
11	Lactobacillus curvatusHY7601, L. plantarum KY1032	Powder/ 5×10^{9}	32/66	Double-blind, placebo-controlled (12 weeks)	(M/F)	Weight loss and decrease in adiposity with probiotic supplementation in overweight individuals.	Kim et al., 2017
12	Lactobacillus rhamnosusCGMCC1.3724	Capsule/ 1.6×10^{8}	62/125	Double-blind, placebo-controlled (12 weeks)	18-55 years. (M/F)	Probiotic supplementation resulted in weight loss and decreased craving for food. And improved appetite control.	Sanchez et al., 2017
13	Bifidobacterium bifidum, Lactobacillus acidophilus, L.casei	Capsule/ 2×10^{9}	30/60	Randomized, double-blind, placebo-controlled (12 weeks)	40-85 years. (M/F)	Probiotic supplementation witnessedpositive effects on levels of insulin and HDL-cholesterol in diabetic patients.	Tajabadi-Ebrahimi et al., 2017

(continued)

TABLE 25.2 (Continued)

Summary of Clinical Trials Related to Usage of Probiotics in Obese/Overweight Human Subjects

Sr. No.	Probiotics Used	Form/dose of Probiotics (colony forming units)	No. of Participants Probiotic/Total Participants	Study Design and duration (in weeks)	Age/Sex	Clinical outcomes	References
14	*Bifidobacterium animalis* subspecies *Lactis* 420	Sachet/ 1×10^{10}	56/134	Double-blind, placebo-controlled (26 weeks)	18-65 years. (M/F)	Probiotic controlled the body fat mass, decreased food intake and waist circumference.	Stenman et al., 2016
15	*Pediococcus pentosaceus* LP28	Powder/ 1×10^{11}	42/62	Double-blind, placebo-controlled (12 weeks)	20-70 years, (M/F)	Probiotic demonstrated anti-obesity effect.	Higashikawa et al., 2016
16	*Bifidobacterium lactis* BB12 *Lactobacillus acidophilus* LA5	Yogurt/ 1×10^{7}	45/89	Double-blind, placebo-controlled (12 weeks)	18-50 years. (F)	Probiotic yogurt improved lipid profiles and insulin sensitivity.	Madjdet al., 2016
17	*Lactobacillus curvatus* HY7601 *L. plantarum* KY1032	Powder/ 2.5×10^{9}	49/95	Double-blind, placebo-controlled (12 weeks)	(M/F)	Probiotic-induced weight loss was observed.	Jung et al., 2015
18	*Bifidobacterium breve* *B. longum* *Lactobacillus acidophilus* *L. bulgaricus* *L.casei* *L.rhamnosus* *Streptococcus thermophilus*	Capsule/ 2×10^{8}	29/56	Randomized, triple-masked controlled trial (8 weeks)	6-18 years, (M/F)	Probiotic supplementation decreased inflammation factors and led to weight loss in overweight children.	Kelishadi et al., 2014
19	*Bifidobacterium lactis* BB12 *Lactobacillus acidophilus* La5 *L.casei*DN001	Yogurt/ 1×10^{8}	50/75	Double-blind, placebo-controlled (8 weeks)	20-50 years. (M/F)	Probiotic supplementation reduced body mass index, fat percentage, and leptin levels.	Zarrati et al., 2014
20	*Lactobacillus gasseri*SBT2055	Fermented milk/ 1×10^{7} 1×10^{6}	69/105	Double-blind, placebo-controlled (12 weeks)	35-62 years, (M/F)	Probiotic consumption lowered abdominal adiposity.	Kadooka et al., 2013

The best non-surgical approach for management of obesity in human subjects includes change in diet, physical activity, and making use of our inbuilt biological systems such as gut microbiota for maintaining energy balance and preventing energy excess in body (Ruban et al., 2019). Obesity is linked with intestinal dysbiosis and low-grade inflammation. Recent studies endorse the correction that altered microbial gut composition could serve as a novel approach in treating obesity (Boulangéet al., 2016; Sivamaruthi et al., 2019). Various bacterial strains and microorganisms such as *Bifidobacterium, Lactobacillus, Enterococcus, Saccharomyces,* and *Streptococcus* help in the management of obesity as well as boost the immune system (Morelli & Capurso, 2012). Ingestion of dietary fibres along with probiotics serve as an effective approach for appetite control, to help in breakdown of certain macromolecules, and to maintain body weight (Parnell et al., 2012). The relation between impaired gut microbiota and obesity has been established in animal models and clinical studies. Studies have reported a comprehensive reduction in bacteroidetes and an increase in firmicutes in obese animals (Ley et al., 2005). Various studies on human subjects have reported an analogical trend of bacteroidetes and firmicutes in people with obesity in contrast to lean controls (Crovesy et al., 2020). Probiotics use improves the antioxidant system and reduces obesity-associated complications (Wang et al., 2017). The beneficial impact of probiotics in obese people depends on the nature and composition of probiotic strain (single/multiple strains), dose, and duration of use as well as aided activities including dietary restrictions and weight loss medications (Wiciński et al., 2020). Probiotic supplementation exhibits anti-obesity effect by remodelling energy metabolism and altering expression of gene expression involved in glucose and lipid metabolism. In addition to the probiotic increase in intestinal permeability and decrease in endotoxin release and inflammation (Ejtahed et al., 2019). Probiotics modifying the composition of gut microbiota (by increasing load of *Lactobacillus, Bifidobacterium, Bacteroidetes,* and decreasing *firmicutes, Clostridium,* and *Actinobacteria*) exhibited anti-obesity effect in animals and human subjects (Abenavoli et al., 2019). The intact intestinal epithelial barrier serves as an important defence system for the host (L Madsen, 2012). In the case of compromised integrity of intestinal epithelial barrier, the antigens invade submucosa and trigger a profound inflammatory response. Altered gut epithelial integrity is associated with progression of various disorders ranging from inflammatory bowel disease to obesity (Hooper et al., 2001). Probiotic administration improves the intestinal barrier function (Anderson et al., 2010). Probiotics encourage mucous secretion as well as gut barrier function and promote exclusion of pathogens (Caballero-Franco et al., 2007; Bermudez-Brito et al., 2012). Based on the existing literature, the probiotic-induced anti-obesity effect is compiled and presented in Figure 25.1.

25.9 Commercial Formulations of Probiotics

Various systems including food-based approaches and pharmaceutical supplements are available for delivery of probiotics (Khedkar et al., 2017). Fermented foods account for majority of probiotic formulations and could be categorized intodairy productsincluding cheeses, yogurt, milk, cream and non-dairy products such as meat, bread, fibre snacks, fruit juice, and chocolates (Eor et al., 2019; Tenore et al., 2019). Pharmaceutical supplements in the form of powder, tablet, or capsule dosage form generally contain lyophilized bacteria. Of note, the pharmaceutical preparations are said to be much more effective than commercial food-based products (Putta et al., 2018). The lyophilizedprobiotic formulations are more concentrated than probiotics containing fermented products. Enteric-coated tablets reported more survival rates than non-enteric coated tablets (Millette et al., 2013). Patient-related factors also affect the choice of dosage forms. For instance, yogurts or fermented products cannot be given to lactose-intolerant individuals. However, for clinical efficacy, probiotics must provide a sufficient number of live organisms to exert therapeutic effects (Millette et al., 2013; Tenore et al., 2019).

25.10 Summary and Conclusions

Existing pharmacotherapy for treating obesity has numerous side effects. The gut microbiota serve as a key regulator of energy homeostasis. Environmental factors and diet have been noted to affect composition and functioning of gut microbiota thereby causing obesity and related metabolic disorders. The composition of obese individuals is different from their lean counterparts with more firmicutes and fewer bacteridetes. Animals and human studies revealed that diet-induced alteration in gut microbiota leads to obesity and metabolic disorders. Probiotic supplementation (mainly *Lactobacillus* and/ or *Bifidobacterium*) has demonstrated health benefits along with attenuation of obesity in pre-clinical and clinical set up. Probiotic supplementation has been suggested as an excellent tool to combat obesity and associated co-morbidities without any major side effects. A limited number of clinical trials has been conducted to assess the role of probiotics in obese subjects to determine the effectiveness but these trials find limitation of small sample size and do not study the aftereffects of probiotic supplementation. Further clinical trials with comprehensive sample size are required to further strengthen our information regarding long-term safety and efficacy of probiotics for treating obesity and other metabolic disorders.

Acknowledgments

The authors thank Mr. Arshdeep Singh and Mr. Rajanpreet Singh from the Department of Pharmaceutical Sciences, Guru Nanak Dev University, and Amritsar for their help in preparing Figure 25.1 of this book chapter.

REFERENCES

Abenavoli L, Scarpellini E, Colica C, Boccuto L, Salehi B, Sharifi-Rad J, et al. (2019). Gut microbiota and obesity: a role for probiotics. *Nutrients* 11(11):2690.

Aitman T, Dhillon P, Geurts AM (2016). A RATional choice for translational research? *Dis Model Mech* 9(10):1069–1072.

Allen JM, Mailing LJ, Niemiro GM, Moore R, Cook MD, White BA, et al. (2018). Exercise alters gut microbiota composition and function in lean and obesehumans. *Med Sci Sports Exerc* 50(4):747–757.

Allison DB, Gadde KM, Garvey WT, Peterson CA, Schwiers ML, Najarian T, et al. (2012). Controlled-release phentermine/topiramate in severely obese adults: a randomized controlled trial (EQUIP). *Obesity* 20(2):330–342.

Anderson RC, Cookson AL, McNabb WC, Park Z, McCann MJ, Kelly WJ, Roy NC (2010). Lactobacillus plantarum MB452 enhances the function of the intestinal barrier byincreasing the expression levels of genes involved in tight junction formation. *BMC Microbiol* 10(1):1–11.

Ang Z, Ding JL (2016). GPR41 and GPR43 in obesity and inflammation – protective or causative? *Front Immunol* 7:28.

Angelakis E, Armougom F, Million M, Raoult D (2012). The relationship between gut microbiota and weight gain in humans. *Future Microbiol* 7(1):91–109.

Annalisa N, Alessio T, Claudette TD, Erald V, Antonino DL, Nicola DD (2014). Gut microbioma population: an indicator really sensible to any change in age, diet, metabolic syndrome, and life-style. *Mediators Inflamm* 2014:901308.

Avolio E, Fazzari G, Zizza M, De Lorenzo A, Di Renzo L, Alò R, Facciolo RM, Canonaco M (2019). Probiotics modify body weight together with anxiety states via pro-inflammatory factors in HFD-treated Syrian golden hamster. *Behav BrainRes* 356:390–399.

Bäckhed F, Ding H, Wang T, Hooper LV, Koh GY, Nagy A, et al. (2004). The gut microbiota as an environmental factor that regulates fat storage. *ProcNatl Acad Sci* 101(44):15718–15723.

Bäckhed F, Ley RE, Sonnenburg JL, Peterson DA, Gordon JI (2005). Host-bacterialmutualism in the human intestine. *Science* 307(5717):1915–1920.

Balolong MP, Bautista RLS, Ecarma NCA, Balolong Jr EC, Hallare AV, Elegado FB (2017). Evaluating the anti-obesity potential of *Lactobacillus fermentum* 4B1, a probioticstrain isolated from balao-balao, a traditional Philippine fermented food. *Int Food Res J* 24(2):819–824.

Berings M, Karaaslan C, Altunbulakli C, Gevaert P, Akdis M, Bachert C, Akdis CA (2017). Advances and highlights in allergen immunotherapy: on the way to sustained clinicaland immunologic tolerance. *J Allergy Clin Immunol* 140(5):1250–1267.

Bermudez-Brito M, Plaza-Díaz J, Muñoz-Quezada S, Gómez-Llorente C, Gil A (2012). Probiotic mechanisms of action. *Ann NutrMetab* 61(2):160–174.

Bohula EA, Wiviott SD, McGuire DK, Inzucchi SE, Kuder J, Im K, et al. (2018). Cardiovascular safety of lorcaserin inoverweight or obese patients. *N Engl J Med* 379(12):1107–1117.

Bonfili L, Cecarini V, Gogoi O, Berardi S, Scarpona S, Angeletti M, et al. (2020). Gut microbiota manipulation through probiotics oral administration restoresglucose homeostasis in a mouse model of Alzheimer's disease. *Neurobiol Aging* 87:35–43.

Bouaziz A, Dib AL, Lakhdara N, Kadja L, Espigares E, Moreno E, et al. (2021). Study of probiotic effects of Bifidobacterium animalis subsp. lactis BB-12and Lactobacillus plantarum 299v strains on biochemical and morphometricparameters of rabbits after obesity induction. *Biology* 10(2):131.

Boulangé CL, Neves AL, Chilloux J, Nicholson JK, Dumas ME (2016). Impact of the gutmicrobiota on inflammation, obesity, and metabolic disease. *Genome Med* 8(1):1–12.

Bubnov RV, Babenko LP, Lazarenko LM, Mokrozub VV, Demchenko OA, Nechypurenko OV, Spivak MY (2017). Comparative study of probiotic effects of Lactobacillus and Bifidobacteria strains on cholesterol levels, liver morphology and the gut microbiota in obese mice. *EPMA J* 8(4):357–376.

Burgio E, Lopomo A, Migliore L (2015). Obesity and diabetes: from genetics to epigenetics. *Mol Biol Rep* 42(4):799–818.

Caballero-Franco C, Keller K, De Simone C, Chadee K (2007). The VSL# 3 probiotic formula induces mucin gene expression and secretion in colonic epithelial cells. *Am J Physiol Gastrointest Liver Physiol* 292(1):G315–G322.

Callaway LK, McIntyre HD, Barrett HL, Foxcroft K, Tremellen A, Lingwood BE, et al. (2019) Probiotics for the prevention of gestational diabetes mellitus in overweight and obese women: findingsfrom the SPRING double-blind randomized controlled trial. *Diabetes Care* 42(3): 364–371.

Cani PD, Osto M, Geurts L, Everard A (2012). Involvement of gut microbiota in the development of low-grade inflammation and type 2 diabetes associated with obesity. *Gut Microbes* 3(4):279–288.

Canuto R, Garcez A, de Souza RV, Kac G, Olint MTA (2021). Nutritional intervention strategies for the management of overweight and obesity in primary health care: A systematic review with meta-analysis. *Obes Rev* 22(3):e13143.

Cao GT, Dai B, Wang KL, Yan Y, Xu YL, Wang YX, Yang CM (2019). Bacilluslicheniformis, a potential probiotic, inhibits obesity by modulating colonic microflorain C57BL/6J mice model. *J Appl Microbiol* 127(3):880–888.

Carreras NL, Martorell P, Chenoll E, Genovés S, Ramón D, Aleixandre A (2018). Anti-obesity properties of the strain Bifidobacterium animalis subsp. lactis CECT 8145 in Zücker fatty rats. *Benef Microbes* 9(4):629–641.

Cavaillon JM, Legout S (2016). Centenary of the death of Elie Metchnikoff: a visionary and an outstanding team leader. *Microbes Infect* 18(10):577–594.

Chen YT, Lin YC, Lin JS, Yang NS, Chen MJ (2018). Sugary kefir strain lactobacillus maliAPS1 ameliorated hepatic steatosis by regulation of SIRT-1/Nrf-2 and gut microbiotain rats. *Mol Nutr Food Res* 62(8):e1700903.

Chunchai T, Thunapong W, Yasom S, Wanchai K, Eaimworawuthikul S, Metzler G, et al. (2018). Decreased microglial activation through gut-brain axis by prebiotics, probiotics, or synbiotics effectively restored cognitive function in obese-insulin resistant rats. *J Neuroinflammation* 15(1):1–15.

Crovesy L, Masterson D, Rosado EL (2020). Profile of the gut microbiota of adults with obesity: a systematic review. *Eur J Clin Nutr* 74(9):1251–1262.

D'Innocenzo S, Biagi C, Lanari M (2019). Obesity and the mediterranean diet: a review of evidence of the role and sustainability of the mediterranean diet. *Nutrients* 11(6):1306.

DiBaise JK, Zhang H, Crowell MD, Krajmalnik-Brown R, Decker GA, Rittmann BE (2008). Gut microbiota and its possible relationship with obesity. *Mayo Clin Proc* 83(4):460–469.

Donaldson GP, Lee SM and Mazmanian SK (2016). Gut biogeography of the bacterial microbiota. *Nat Rev Microbiol* 14(1):20–32.

Ejtahed HS, Angoorani P, Soroush AR, Atlasi R, Hasani-Ranjbar S, Mortazavian AM, Larijani B (2019). Probiotics supplementation for the obesity management; A systematic review of animal studies and clinical trials. *J Funct Foods* 52:228–242.

Eor JY, Tan PL, Lim SM, Choi DH, Yoon SM, Yang SY, Kim SH (2019). Laxative effect of probiotic chocolate on loperamide-induced constipation in rats. *Food Res Int* 116:1173–1182.

Falcinelli S, Rodiles A, Hatef A, Picchietti S, Cossignani L, Merrifield DL, et al. (2017). Dietary lipid content reorganizes gut microbiota and probiotic L.rhamnosus attenuates obesity and enhances catabolic hormonal milieu inzebrafish. *Sci Rep* 7(1):1–15.

Fijan S (2014). Microorganisms with claimed probiotic properties: an overview of recentliterature. *Int J Environ Res Public Health* 11(5):4745–4767.

Gérard P (2016). Gut microbiota and obesity. *Cell Mol Life Sci* 73(1):147–162.

Giovanna M, Cantone E, Sara C, Dario T, Luigi B, Savastano S, Annamaria C (2019). Gutmicrobiota: a new path to treat obesity. *Int J Obes Suppl* 9(1):10–19.

Go GW, Oh S, Park M, Gang G, McLean D, Yang HS, et al. (2013). t10, c12conjugated linoleic acid upregulates hepatic de novo lipogenesis and triglyceridesynthesis via mTOR pathway activation. *J Microbiol Biotechnol* 23(11):1569–1576.

Goldenberg JZ, Yap C, Lytvyn L, Lo CKF, Beardsley J, Mertz D, Johnston BC (2017) Probiotics for the prevention of Clostridium difficile-associated diarrhoea in adults and children. *Cochrane Database Syst Rev* (12):CD006095. doi: 10.1002/14651858.CD006095.pub4

Gomes AC, de Sousa RGM, Botelho PB, Gomes TLN, Prada PO, Mota JF (2017). The additional effects of a probiotic mix on abdominal adiposity and antioxidant Status: a double-blind, randomized trial. *Obesity* 25(1):30–38.

Griffin NW, Ahern PP, Cheng J, Heath AC, Ilkayeva O, Newgard CB, et al. (2017) Prior dietary practices and connections to a human gut microbialmetacommunity alter responses to diet interventions. *Cell Host Microbe* 21(1):84–96.

Hall KD, Kahan S (2018). Maintenance of lost weight and long-term management of obesity. *Med Clin North Am* 102(1):183–197.

Hempel S, Newberry SJ, Maher AR, Wang Z, Miles JN, Shanman R, et al. (2012). Probiotics for the prevention and treatment of antibiotic-associated diarrhoea: asystematic review and meta-analysis. *JAMA* 307(18):1959–1969.

Higashikawa F, Noda M, Awaya T, Danshiitsoodol N, Matoba Y, Kumagai T, Sugiyama M (2016). Antiobesity effect of *Pediococcus pentosaceus* LP28 on overweight subjects: a randomized, double-blind, placebo-controlled clinical trial. *Eur J Clin Nutr* 70(5):582–587.

Hobbs M, Radley D (2020). Obesogenic environments and obesity: A comment on 'Are environmental area characteristics at birth associated with overweight and obesity in school-aged children? Findings from the SLOPE (Studying Lifecourse Obesity PrEdictors) population-based cohort in the south of England'. *BMC Med* 18(1):1–3.

Hooper LV, Wong MH, Thelin A, Hansson L, Falk PG, Gordon JI (2001). Molecular analysis of commensal host-microbial relationships in the intestine. *Science* 291(5505):881–884.

Islam KS, Fukiya S, Hagio M, Fujii N, Ishizuka S, Ooka T, et al. (2011). Bile acid is a host factor that regulates the composition of the cecal microbiotain rats. *Gastroenterology* 141(5):1773–1781.

Jeon SM (2016). Regulation and function of AMPK in physiology and diseases. *Exp Mol Med* 48(7):e245–e245.

Jung S, Lee YJ, Kim M, Kim M, Kwak JH, Lee JW, et al. (2015). Supplementation with two probiotic strains, Lactobacillus curvatus HY7601 and Lactobacillus plantarum KY1032, reduced body adiposity and Lp-PLA2 activity inoverweight subjects. *J Funct Foods* 19:744–752.

Kadooka Y, Sato M, Ogawa A, Miyoshi M, Uenishi H, Ogawa H, et al. (2013). Effect of Lactobacillus gasseri SBT2055 in fermented milk on abdominal adiposity in adults in a randomised controlled trial. *Br J Nutr* 110(9):1696–1703.

Karlsson CL, Molin G, Fåk F, Hagslätt MLJ, Jakesevic M, Håkansson Å, et al. (2011). Effects on weight gain and gut microbiota in rats givenbacterial supplements and a high-energy-dense diet from fetal life through to 6months of age. *Br J Nutr* 106(6):887–895.

Kelishadi R, Farajian S, Safavi M, Mirlohi M, Hashemipour M (2014). A randomized triple-masked controlled trial on the effects of synbiotics on inflammation markers inoverweight children. *J Pediatr* 90(2):161–167.

Khalighi A, Behdani R, Kouhestani S (2016). Probiotics: A comprehensive review oftheir classification, mode of action and role in human nutrition. In *Probiotics and Prebiotics in Human Nutrition and Health*. Rao V and Rao LG (Eds.). doi:10.5772/63646.

Khedkar S, Carraresi L and Bröring S (2017). Food or pharmaceuticals? Consumers' perception of health-related borderline products. *Pharma Nutrition* 5(4):133–140.

Kim J, Yun JM, Kim MK, Kwon O, Cho B (2018). Lactobacillus gasseri NR17supplementation reduces the visceral fat accumulation and waist circumference in obese adults: a randomized, double-blind, placebo-controlled trial. *J Med Food* 21(5):454–461.

Kim M, Kim M, Kang M, Yoo HJ, Kim MS, Ahn YT, et al. (2017). Effects of weight loss using supplementation with Lactobacillus strains on body fatand medium-chain acylcarnitines in overweight individuals. *Food Funct* 8(1):250–261.

Kimura I, Ozawa K, Inoue D, Imamura T, Kimura K, Maeda T, et al. (2013). The gut microbiota suppresses insulin-mediated fat accumulation via the short-chainfatty acid receptor GPR43. *Nat Commun* 4(1):1–12.

Ley RE, Bäckhed F, Turnbaugh P, Lozupone CA, Knight RD, Gordon JI (2005). Obesity alters gut microbial ecology. *Proc Natl Acad Sci* 102(31):11070–11075.

Li Z, Jin H, Oh SY, Ji GE (2016). Anti-obese effects of two Lactobacilli and two Bifidobacteria on ICR mice fed on a high fat diet. *Biochem Biophys Res Commun* 480(2):222–227.

Lonneman Jr DJ, Rey JA, McKee BD (2013). Phentermine/Topiramate extended-releasecapsules (qsymia) for weight loss. *P T* 38(8):446–452.

Madjd A, Taylor MA, Mousavi N, Delavari A, Malekzadeh R, Macdonald IA, Farshchi HR (2016). Comparison of the effect of daily consumption of probiotic compared withlow-fat conventional yogurt on weight loss in healthy obese women following anenergy-restricted diet: a randomized controlled trial. *Am J Clin Nutr* 103(2):323–329.

L Madsen K (2012). Enhancement of epithelial barrier function by probiotics. *J Epithel Biol Pharmacol* 5(1):55–59.

Michael DR, Jack AA, Masetti G, Davies TS, Loxley KE, Kerry-Smith J, et al. (2020). A randomised controlled study shows supplementation of overweight and obese adults with lactobacilli and bifidobacteria reduces bodyweight and improves well-being. *Sci Rep* 10(1):1–12.

Millette M, Nguyen A, Amine KM, Lacroix M (2013). Gastrointestinal survival of bacteria incommercial probiotic products. *Int J Probiotics Prebiotics* 8(4):149–156.

Moayyedi P, Ford AC, Talley NJ, Cremonini F, Foxx-Orenstein AE, Brandt LJ, Quigley EM (2010). The efficacy of probiotics in the treatment of irritable bowel syndrome: asystematic review. *Gut* 59(3):325–332.

Mohammadi-Sartang M, Bellissimo N, de Zepetnek JT, Brett NR, Mazloomi SM, Fararouie M, et al. (2018). The effect of daily fortified yogurt consumption on weight loss in adults with metabolic syndrome: A 10-week randomized controlled trial. *Nutr Metab Cardiovasc Dis* 28(6):565–574.

Moludi J, Alizadeh M, Behrooz M, Maleki V, Seyed Mohammadzad MH, Golmohammadi A (2019). Interactive effect of probiotics supplementation and weight loss diet onmetabolic syndrome features in patients with coronary artery diseases: a double-blind, placebo-controlled, randomized clinical trial. *Am J Lifestyle Med* 15(6):653–663. doi: 10.1177/1559827619843833

Morelli L, Capurso L (2012). FAO/WHO guidelines on probiotics: 10 years later. *J Clin Gastroenterol* 46:S1–S2.

Mozaffarian D, Hao T, Rimm EB, Willett WC, Hu FB (2011). Changes in diet and lifestyleand long-term weight gain in women and men. *N Engl J Med* 364(25):2392–2404.

Muscogiuri G, Cantone E, Cassarano S, Tuccinardi D, Barrea L, Savastano S, Colao A (2019). Gut microbiota: a new path to treat obesity. *Int J Obes Suppl* 9(1):10–19.

Okubo T, Takemura N, Yoshida A, Sonoyama K (2013). KK/Ta mice administered Lactobacillus plantarum strain no. 14 have lower adiposity and higher insulinsensitivity. *Biosci Microbiota Food Health* 32(3):93–100.

Ouwehand AC, Salminen S, Isolauri E (2002). Probiotics: an overview of beneficialeffects. *Antonie Van Leeuwenhoek* 82(1-4):279–289.

Parada Venegas D, De la Fuente MK, Landskron G, González MJ, Quera R, Dijkstra G, et al. (2019). Short chain fatty acids (SCFAs)-mediated gut epithelial and immune regulation and its relevance for inflammatorybowel diseases. *Front Immunol* 10:277.

Parnell JA, Raman M, Rioux KP, Reimer RA (2012). The potential role of prebiotic fibre fortreatment and management of non-alcoholic fatty liver disease and associated obesityand insulin resistance. *Liver Int* 32(5):701–711.

Patel DK, Stanford FC (2018). Safety and tolerability of new-generation anti-obesitymedications: a narrative review. *Postgrad Med* 130(2):173–182.

Pedret A, Valls RM, Calderón-Pérez L, Llauradó E, Companys J, Pla-Pagà L, et al. (2019). Effects of daily consumption of theprobiotic Bifidobacterium animalis subsp. lactis CECT 8145 on anthropometricadiposity biomarkers in abdominally obese subjects: a randomized controlled trial. *Int J Obes* 43(9):1863–1868.

Pilitsi E, Farr OM, Polyzos SA, Perakakis N, Nolen-Doerr E, Papathanasiou AE, Mantzoros CS (2019). Pharmacotherapy of obesity: available medications and drugs underinvestigation. *Metabolism* 92:170–192.

Plaza-Díaz J, Ruiz-Ojeda FJ, Gil-Campos M, Gil A (2018). Immune-mediated mechanismsof action of probiotics and synbiotics in treating pediatric intestinaldiseases. *Nutrients* 10(1):42.

Putta S, Yarla NS, Lakkappa DB, Imandi SB, Malla RR, Chaitanya AK, et al. (2018). Probiotics: Supplements, food, pharmaceutical industry. In *Therapeutic, Probiotic, and Unconventional Foods*. Grumezescu A, Holban AM (Eds.). Academic Press 15–25.

Rather IA, Bajpai VK, Kumar S, Lim J, Paek WK, Park YH (2016). Probiotics and atopic dermatitis: an overview. *Front Microbiol* 7:507.

Ruban A, Stoenchev K, Ashrafian H, Teare J (2019). Current treatments for obesity. *ClinMed* 19(3):205–212.

Saez-Lara MJ, Gomez-Llorente C, Plaza-Diaz J, Gil A (2015). The role of probiotic lactic acid bacteria and bifido bacteria in the prevention and treatment of inflammatory bowel disease and other related diseases: a systematic review of randomized human clinical trials. *Bio Med Res Int* 2015:505878. doi:10.1155/2015/505878

Salles BIM, Cioffi D and Ferreira SRG (2020). Probiotics supplementation and insulinresistance: a systematic review. *Diabetol Metab Syndr* 12(1):1–24.

Sánchez B, Delgado S, Blanco-Míguez A, Lourenço A, Gueimonde M, Margolles A (2017). Probiotics, gut microbiota, and their influence on host health and disease. *Mol Nutr Food Res* 61(1):1600240.

Sanchez M, Darimont C, Panahi S, Drapeau V, Marette A, Taylor VH, et al. (2017). Effects of a diet-based weight-reducing program with probioticsupplementation on satiety efficiency, eating behaviour traits, and psychosocialbehaviours in obese individuals. *Nutrients* 9(3):284.

Sanchis-Chordà J, Del Pulgar EMG, Carrasco-Luna J, Benítez-Páez A, Sanz Y, Codoñer-Franch P (2019). Bifidobacterium pseudocatenulatum CECT 7765 supplementation improves inflammatory status in insulin-resistant obese children. *Eur J Nutr* 58(7):2789–2800.

Santacruz A, Collado MC, Garcia-Valdes L, Segura MT, Martin-Lagos JA, Anjos T, et al. (2010). Gut microbiotacomposition is associated with body weight, weight gain and biochemical parametersin pregnant women. *Br J Nutr* 104(1):83–92.

Saunders KH, Umashanker D, Igel LI, Kumar RB, Aronne LJ (2018). Obesity Pharmacotherapy. *Med Clin* 102(1):135–148.

Scheithauer TP, Dallinga-Thie GM, de Vos WM, Nieuwdorp M, van Raalte DH (2016). Causality of small and large intestinal microbiota in weight regulation and insulin resistance. *Mol Metab* 5(9):759–770.

Scott KP, Gratz SW, Sheridan PO, Flint HJ, Duncan SH (2013). The influence of diet on thegut microbiota. *Pharmacol Res* 69(1):52–60.

Sender R, Fuchs S, Milo R (2016). Are we really vastly outnumbered? Revisiting the ratio of bacterial to host cells in humans. *Cell* 164(3):337–340.

Seo MH, Lee WY, Kim SS, Kang JH, Kang JH, Kim KK, et al. (2019). 2018 Korean society for the study of obesity guideline for the management of obesity in Korea. *J Obes Metab Syndr* 28(1):40–45.

Shin D, Chang SY, Bogere P, Won K, Choi JY, Choi YJ, et al. (2019). Beneficial roles of probiotics on the modulation of gut microbiota andimmune response in pigs. *PloS One* 14(8):e0220843.

Silva YP, Bernardi A, Frozza RL (2020). The role of short-chain fatty acids from gut microbiota in gut-brain communication. *Front Endocrinol* 11:25.

Sivamaruthi BS, Kesika P, Suganthy N, Chaiyasut C (2019). A review on role of microbiomein obesity and antiobesity properties of probiotic supplements. *Bio Med Res Int* 2019:3291367.

Song EJ, Han K, Lim TJ, Lim S, Chung MJ, Nam MH, et al. (2020). Effect of probiotics on obesity-related markers per enterotype: a double-blind, placebo-controlled, randomized clinical trial. *EPMA J* 11(1):31–51.

Song W, Song C, Shan Y, Lu W, Zhang J, Hu P, et al. (2016). The antioxidative effects of three lactobacilli on high-fat diet induced obese mice. *RSC Adv* 6(70):65808–65815.

Stenman LK, Lehtinen MJ, Meland N, Christensen JE, Yeung N, Saarinen MT, et al. (2016). Probiotic with or without fiber controls body fat mass, associatedwith serum zonulin, in overweight and obese adults-randomized controlled trial. *EBio Medicine* 13:190–200.

Swathi KV (2016). Probiotics – A Human Friendly Bacteria. *Res J Pharm Technol* 9(8):1260.

Szulińska M, Łoniewski I, Van Hemert S, Sobieska M, Bogdański P (2018). Dose-dependenteffects of multispecies probiotic supplementation on the lipopolysaccharide (LPS)level and cardiometabolic profile in obese postmenopausal women: A 12-weekrandomized clinical trial. *Nutrients* 10(6):773.

Tajabadi-Ebrahimi M, Sharifi N, Farrokhian A, Raygan F, Karamali F, Razzaghi R, et al. (2017). A randomized controlled clinical trial investigating the effect ofsynbiotic administration on markers of insulin metabolism and lipid profiles inoverweight type 2 diabetic patients with coronary heart disease. *Exp Clin Endocrinol Diabetes* 125(1):21–27.

Tang X, Zhao J (2019). Commercial strains of lactic acid bacteria with health benefits. In *Lactic Acid Bacteria, Omics and Functional Evaluation,* Chen W (Ed.), Springer: Singapore. pp. 297–369.

Tenore GC, Caruso D, Buonomo G, D'Avino M, Ciampaglia R, Maisto M, et al. (2019). Lactofermented Annurca apple puree as a functional food indicated for the control of plasma lipid and oxidative amine levels: Results from a randomised clinical trial. *Nutrients* 11(1):122.

Tremaroli V, Bäckhed F (2012). Functional interactions between the gut microbiota and host metabolism. *Nature* 489(7415):242–249.

Vandenplas Y, Huys G, Daube G (2015). Probiotics: an update. *J Pediatr* 91(1):6–21.

Wang M, Donovan SM (2015). Human microbiota-associated swine: current progress andfuture opportunities. *ILAR J* 56(1):63–73.

Wang S, Huang M, You X, Zhao J, Chen L, Wang L, et al. (2018). Gut microbiotamediates the anti-obesity effect of calorie restriction in mice. *Sci Rep* 8(1):1–14.

Wang Y, Wu Y, Wang Y, Xu H, Mei X, Yu D, et al. (2017). Antioxidant propertiesof probiotic bacteria. *Nutrients* 9(5):521.

Wei Y, Zhang J, Li Z, Gow A, Chung KF, Hu M, et al. (2016). Chronic exposure to air pollution particles increases the risk ofobesity and metabolic syndrome: findings from a natural experiment in Beijing. *FASEBJ* 30(6): 2115–2122.

Wiciński M, Gębalski J, Gołębiewski J, Malinowski B (2020). Probiotics for the treatment of overweight and obesity in humans – A review of clinical trials. *Microorganisms* 8(8):1148.

Wilding S, Ziauddeen N, Smith D, Roderick P, Chase D, Alwan NA (2020). Are environmental area characteristics at birth associated with overweight and obesity in school-aged children? Findings from the SLOPE (Studying Lifecourse Obesity PrEdictors) population-based cohort in the south of England. *BMC Med* 18(1):1–13.

World Health Organization (2020). Obesity and overweight. www.who.int/news-room/fact-sheets/detail/obesity-and-overweight

Yang Z, Song Q, Li J., Zhang Y (2019). Air pollution as a cause of obesity: micro-levelevidence from Chinese cities. *Int J Environ Res Public Health* 16(21):4296.

Yatsunenko T, Rey FE, Manary MJ, Trehan I, Dominguez-Bello MG, Contreras M, et al. (2012). Human gut microbiome viewed across age and geography. *Nature* 486(7402):222–227.

Yeboah P, Odoi FNA, Teye M, Yangtul T (2020). Assessment of Growth and CarcassParameters of Guinea Fowls (Numida meleagris) Fed Diets with Re3™ Probiotics. *J Anim Plant Sci* 44(2):7609–7620.

Zarrati M, Salehi E, Nourijelyani K, Mofid V, Zadeh MJH, Najafi F, et al. (2014). Effects of probiotic yogurt on fatdistribution and gene expression of proinflammatory factors in peripheral bloodmononuclear cells in overweight and obese people with or without weight-loss diet. *J Am Coll Nutr* 33(6):417–425.

Zembutsu H (2015). Pharmacogenomics toward personalized tamoxifen therapy for breastcancer. *Pharmacogenomics* 16(3):287–296.

Zhang JM, Liu XY, Gu W, Xu HY, Jiao HC, Zhao JP, et al. (2020). Different effects of probiotics and antibiotics on the composition of microbiota, SCFAs Concentrations and FFAR2/3 mRNA expression in broiler chickens. *J Appl Microbiol* DOI: 10.1111/jam.14953.

Zheng X, Huang F, Zhao A, Lei S, Zhang Y, Xie G, et al. (2017). Bile acid is a significant host factor shaping the gut microbiome of diet-induced obese mice. *BMC Biol* 15(1):1–15.

Section III

Therapeutics and Novel Approaches

26

Protease Inhibitors of Marine Origin: Promising Anticancer and HIV Therapies

Maushmi S. Kumar, Yashodhara Dalal, and Sahil Khan
Shobhaben Pratapbhai Patel School of Pharmacy and Technology Management, SVKM's NMIMS, Mumbai, India

Harpal S. Buttar
Department of Pathology & Laboratory Medicine, University of Ottawa, Ottawa, Canada

26.1 Introduction

Proteases or proteolytic enzymes are a category of enzymes that help to digest different kinds of proteins. They play multifunctional roles in the normal physiological functions of the body and disease conditions. Some proteases are found in foods, and some are produced by pathogenic bacteria, and some by healthy microbiota in the gastrointestinal tract. They are thought to have evolved as proteinaceous destructive enzymes. From an evolutionary point of view, the major mechanism of action of these enzymes was directed towards protein catabolism and amino acid generation in primitive organisms. Proteases are known to hold a vital position in the biological world due to their synthetic and biodegradation functions. They play a very important role in carcinogenesis, which involves the uncontrolled growth of abnormal cells termed as cancer or tumor cells and their metastasis (Ruiz-Torres et al., 2017). Many steps are involved in the growth and proliferation of malignant tumors such as proliferation, apoptosis, angiogenesis, invasion, and circulation of tumor cells in the systemic circulation, as well as extravasations (where tumor cells escape from the blood vessels), and growth of secondary tumors at a new site due to metastasis. The balance between cell division and apoptosis (programmed cell death) is impaired in tumor cells (Gupta et al., 2010; Jedinák and Maliar, 2005). Proteases are considered to play a very crucial role in the metastasis process of tumorigenesis. They help in digesting the extracellular matrix (ECM) to provide entry to cancerous cells in the systemic circulation (Jedinák and Maliar, 2005). Some of the ECM-destroying enzymes also plays a pivotal role in the development of new blood vessels or angiogenesis. These newly formed blood vessels provide oxygen and nutrition and remove waste products of cancer cells (DeClerck et al., 2004). A wide variety of protease-like matrix, including matrix metalloproteinases (MMPs), serine proteases plasmin and urokinase plasminogen activator (uPA), cysteine proteases cathepsins L and B, and aspartic protease cathepsin D help in the biodegradation of ECM and migration of tumor cells (Jedinák and Maliar, 2005). In view of these observations, the protease inhibitors (PIs) are the prime therapeutic targets for anticancer activities.

Currently, the PIs have formed a new arena for treating different cancer types, and their diverse anticancer molecules now form the prime hub of cancer research. These molecules include serine inhibitors, matrix metalloproteinase inhibitors, and cysteine inhibitors, which are not only restricted to treating cancer in humans, but may also be used for treating other chronic ailments (Castro-Guillen et al., 2010). Although the mechanisms of the main PIs are partially understood, the target-specific PIs including HIV-1 PIs remain unknown (Huang et al., 2012). The hepatitis C virus (HCV) NS3/4A PIs (Qin et al., 2017), Glycine max PI (Vasudev and Sohal, 2016), Bowman-Birk PI, Kunitz Trypsin PI, Bikunin, hepatocyte growth factor inhibitor type-1, Serpins, Maspins, Pigment Epithelium-derived Factor, and Secretory Leukocyte PI require further supplementary scrutiny and analysis (Castro-Guillen et al., 2010). The majority of the currently marketed PIs originate from terrestrial plants and animals. Some PIs have been isolated from marine sources like Norwegian spring-spawning herring (Christopeit et al., 2013), sponges, cone snail, molluscs, and tunicate (Mayer et al., 2010; Jordan et al., 2005; Olivera et al., 1987; D'Incalci et al., 2014; Newland et al., 2013). The major inhibitory target of PIs is the catabolism process of proteolysis. In vitro and in vivo carcinogenesis studies have revealed suppression of signalling pathways as an important mode in cancer growth inhibition (Kennedy and Little, 1978; Troll et al., 1984; Messadi et al., 1986; Kennedy 1998). Research in marine-derived compounds has portrayed antitumor mechanisms that involve the incorporation of the bioactive molecules into the DNA strands, thus modifying or leading to the inhibition of DNA topoisomerase. Furthermore, this mechanism was found to affect the polymerization of microtubules, which interferes and prevents the completion of the cell cycle (Song et al., 2018). Such bioactivities are not only restricted to the cancerous cell but also cause the death of normal cells. Rakashanda and Amin (2017) summarized studies suggesting that the PIs are mainly effective during the initiation and promotion stages of carcinogenesis, whereas they are ineffective against the final transformed cancerous cells.

This chapter focuses on the therapeutic potential of PIs for treating cancer in humans. We will discuss the ability of PIs to destroy the cancerous cells through their potent cytotoxic mechanisms such as autophagy, endoplasmic reticulum stress induction, MMP inhibition, proteasome activity inhibition, AKT phosphorylation, angiogenesis inhibition, and HIV-PIs.

26.2 Role of Proteases in Cancer Progression

Proteases play a central role in cancer signalling pathways, due to which they are potential drug targets. Several cell surface-associated proteases (MMPs, cathepsins B and L, cathepsin D, plasmin, and uPA) facilitate the process of tumor cell migration and invasion of surrounding ECM. This process can be inhibited by natural and synthetic low-molecular-weight inhibitors, which will eventually result in inhibition of tumor growth. Therefore, it appears to be a promising anticancer therapy (Jedinak and Maliar, 2005).

26.2.1 Matrix Metalloproteinases

It has been reported that the expression of MMPs is recurrent in malignant tumor as it plays a crucial role in the degradation of many substrates (Kessenbrock et al., 2010). There are 25 types of different MMPs, which are differentiated by catalytic domains, specific conserved peptide, and an active site that contain a zinc ion (Overall and Kleifeld, 2006). They can inactivate chemokine, degrade cell surface receptors, and can cause the release of apoptosis mediators. They can process bioactive molecules and can cleave all types of ECM proteins (Van Lint and Libert, 2007). They also play a very crucial role in cell differentiation, proliferation, angiogenesis, migration, and apoptosis. MMP-9 and MMP-2 are the main MMPs involved in metastasis (Trezza et al., 2020). These endopeptidases are classified into four subfamilies: gelatinases (exhibit higher activity against type IV collagen and gelatin), collagenases (break down fibrillar collagens), membrane-bound MMP (break down ECM proteins), and stromelysins (Khasigov et al., 2001). Tissue inhibitors of metalloproteinases (TIMPs) and α2 macroglobulin are endogenous inhibitors involved in controlling MMPs (Gomez et al., 1997). MMPs are also associated with the extravasation of tumor cells along with the degradation of the basal lamina of blood capillaries (Voura et al., 2013). As they have an important role in cancer metastasis, a wide range of MMP-PIs have been investigated. These MMP inhibitors are known to target MMP 1, 2, 3, 7, 8, 9, 13, and 14, but the inhibitors identified for the same were cancelled during phase 3 trials due to high levels of toxicity including musculoskeletal syndrome, GI disturbance, and CVD. These inhibitors were categorized as zinc chelators (Winer et al., 2018). The clinical trials showed inhibition of tumor progression in mice but not in humans because of a few hypothesized theories like the difference in biology (Wojtowicz-Praga et al.,1997), localization, progressive nature of the tumor as well as the specificity of the MMP-PIs. Most likely, a bolus of the tumor was used for metastasis in preclinical studies, which was responsible for the failure of the clinical trials. Even though such failures have been observed, the activity of MMP and MMP-PIs are still being investigated and explored for anticancer activities.

26.2.2 Urokinase-Type Plasminogen Activator

Two protease systems are modulated by tumor and stromal cells: Urokinase-type plasminogen activator (uPA) and MMPs (Eatemadi et al., 2017). Urokinase belongs to the class of serine protease found in humans and other organisms (Degryse, 2011). The system includes one substrate (plasminogen), uPA enzyme, two receptors (plasminogen receptor and uPA receptor (uPAR), and inhibitors (protease nexin 1, plasminogen activator inhibitors PAI-1, PAI-2) (Wang, 2001). uPA is produced by normal cells (i.e., phagocytic cells, keratinocytes, trophoblasts, kidney tubule cells, pneumocytes, fibroblasts) and cancer cells (Schmitt et al., 2000). It activates the enzyme plasminogen, which is also a serine protease. Plasmin as a result stimulates proteolytic cascades, which are responsible for thrombolysis in vascular disease and ECM degradation in cancer (Tang and Han, 2013). They are also responsible for the stimulation of angiogenesis for feeding cancerous cells (Trezza et al., 2020).

26.2.3 Apoptosis and Caspases

Cancer cells bypass programmed cell death to progress towards malignancy. Caspases are the most important proteases that play a crucial role in inflammation and programmed cell death; 2, 8, 9, and 10 are the initiator caspases that are involved at the beginning of apoptosis. These caspases have cysteine protease activity (Li and Yuan, 2008; Siegel, 2006). These initiator caspases cleave their prodomains to activate 3, 6, and 7 effector caspases directly or indirectly. These effector caspases then trigger apoptosis by cleavage of various biochemical compounds (Trezza et al., 2020). Caspase 8 is a metastasis suppressor gene. Caspase 8 along with integrins controls the invasive capacity and survival of neuroblastoma cells. Loss of initiator caspase 8 can lead to metastasis due to which it plays an important role in cancer progression (Stupack et al., 2006).

26.2.4 Lysosomal Proteases

They are also known as cathepsins, which are involved in many physiological processes like antigen presentation, bone resorption, bulk proteolysis, chronic inflammation, etc. (Blasi and Stoppelli, 1999). Among all the cathepsins, cathepsin B is a widely studied cysteine protease (Turk and Guncar, 2003). During cancer, the secretion of cathepsin B is enhanced. Cathepsin B has ECM-degrading activity and hence helps in tumor growth and metastasis (Bromme and Kaleta, 2002; Krepela, 2001). Various MMPS and receptor-bound uPA are also activated by cathepsins B (Kobayashi et al., 1993; Kobayashi et al., 1991), which can further degrade various components of ECM. Cathepsin B also plays an important role in other beneficial processes of tumor cells like catabolism and autophagy (Fais, 2007). Cathepsin D is involved in metastasis and invasion of breast cancer (Ahmad and Hart, 1997). Cathepsin D acts on autocrine mitogen and does not degrade ECM to promote metastasis of cancer cells. It reduces contact inhibition and increases the growth of cancer cells (Levicar et al., 2002).

26.2.5 Serine Protease

Disease like cancer can be caused due to abnormal regulation of these proteases (DeClerck et al., 2004). It has a characteristic Ser residue at its active site (Hedstrom, 2002). These proteases are known to have various catalytic triads and dyads like Asp-His-Ser, His-Ser-His, Ser-His-Glu, Ser-Lys/His, and N-terminal Ser (Dodson and Wlodawer, 1998). Trypsin is one of the well-characterized serine proteases, which play a crucial role in various pathological conditions such as atherosclerosis, inflammation, and cancer (DeClerck et al., 2004).

26.3 Protease Inhibitors of Marine Origin with Potent Anticancer Properties

Protease inhibitors are ideally known to work on oncogenes and carcinogens. They are segregated based on their activity and target. As previously mentioned, these PIs work on DNA, RNA, proteins, microtubules, and their related inhibitors and kinases (Ruiz et al., 2017). Many of the marine-derived PIs are still in clinical trials and a few of them have been approved in the market due to their potent anticancer properties. Ecteinascidin 743 (Yondelis®) is approved for the treatment of soft tissue sarcoma in European markets. Cytarabine, Ara-C (Cytosar-U®) has also been approved for market use due to its DNA polymerase inhibitory effect (Mayer et al., 2010). LAF389, a Bengamide B derivative, is obtained from *Jaspidae* sponges and is in phase 1 clinical trials. It exhibits both antiangiogenic and antiproliferative properties. It has potent antitumor activity, but at escalated dose, it can cause unpredictable cardiac problems (Dumez et al., 2007). HT1286 (Hemiasterlin derivative) is a peptide-like molecule obtained from marine sponges. It blocks the polymerization of tubulin, degrades the organization of microtubule in the cell, triggers apoptosis as well as mitotic arrest. It is a potent proliferation inhibitor and is in phase 1 clinical trial (Loganzo et al., 2003). E7974 is a cytotoxic peptide obtained from marine sponges *Auletta sp.*, *Cymbastela sp.*, and *Hemiasterella minor* (Yamashita et al., 2004). It is an antitumor molecule that prevents the polymerization of Tubulin. It activates caspase 3 and cleaves poly ADP ribose polymerase, which are biomarkers of apoptosis. Even after a long period of administration and low blood levels, it shows antitumor effects for a longer duration of time (Kuznetsov et al., 2009). Discodermolide is a polypeptide obtained from marine sponge *Discodermia dissoluta* and is tested for its anticancer properties. It interferes with microtubule organization and assembling. It is in phase 1 of clinical trials (Bhatnagar and Kim, 2010; Shaw, 2008). Two novel polyketides, PM060184 and PM050489, obtained from marine sponge *Lithoplocamialithistoides* showed antitubulin and antimitotic activity in human cancer cell lines. Out of these novel molecules, PM060184 is in phase 1 of clinical trials (NCT01299636) (Newman and Cragg, 2014). Glycoprotein NMB (gpNMB) is a transmembrane protein that is overexpressed and promotes metastasis in breast cancer. Glembatumumab vedotin is an anti-gpNMB monoclonal antibody used against it. It has a good safety profile. In phase 1 studies it was found that Glembatumumab vedotin has a maximum tolerated dose of 1.88mg/kg once every 3 weeks and was recommended as a phase 2 dose (Bendell et al., 2014). Elisidepsin a synthetic cyclodepsi peptide that is isolated from *Elysia rufescens*, a sacoglossan sea slug species. It is in phase 2 of clinical trials due to its potent antitumor activity. It rapidly inserts itself into the plasma membrane of cancer cells, impairing its membrane integrity and causing necrotic death. Glycosylceramides present in the plasma membrane of tumor cells are its main target (Molina-Guijarro et al., 2015). PM00104 (Zalypsis®), a synthetic tetrahydroisoquinolone alkaloid, is another PI that is in phase 2 of clinical trials to treat urothelial carcinoma, cervical cancer, multiple myeloma, and Ewing sarcoma (Petek and Jones, 2014). It is a natural alkaloid isolated from the mucus and skin of Pacific *nudibranch Jorunnafunebris* and also from tunicates and sponges (Fontana et al., 2000; Oku et al., 2003). It resembles various marine compounds like renieramycins, jorumycin, ecteinascidins, saframycins, and safracins. It inhibits transcription and can cause breakage of DNA (Petek and Jones, 2014). Bryostatin-1 is a macrolide that is highly oxygenated and has a distinct poly acetate backbone. It is obtained from *Bugula neritina* L. (Bugulidae). The mechanism of action of bryostatin is mainly associated with the diacylglycerol (DAG) binding site of C-26, C-19, and C-1 domain of protein kinase C. Bryostatin is a protein kinase C agonist (Kollár et al., 2014). It can prevent the development of multidrug resistance by regulating PKC and can also inhibit angiogenesis, tumor invasion, and cell adhesion (Nezhat et al., 2004). Gemcitabine is a deoxycytidine analog that has potent cytotoxic activity. It is a very effective drug against nonsmall cell lung cancer, bladder cancer, pancreatic cancer, and ovarian cancer. It replaces cytidine during DNA replication and causes chain termination. Its most commonly administered dose is 1000 mg/m^2 per week intravenously for 3 weeks followed by a 1-week rest (Toschi et al., 2005). Pinatuzumab vedotin is a conjugate of an antibody and a drug. It involves conjugation of anti-CD22 antibody and monomethyl auristatin E (MMAE) by a linker, which can be cleaved by a protease. It is a potent antimicrotubule PI. It is used for the treatment of Non-Hodgkin lymphoma and leukemia (Advani et al., 2017). NVP-LAQ824 is a derivative of hydroxamic acid, which inhibits histone deacetylase. It acts against multiple myeloma cell lines by inducing apoptosis. It controls

TABLE 26.1

Summary of Protease Inhibitors Isolated from Different Marine Sources and Their Purported Anticancer Mechanisms

Compound Name	Chemical Class	Source	Disease area	Mechanism	Reference
Bengamide B derivative (LAF389) (I)	Peptide	Sponge	Anticancer	Inhibition of methionine aminopeptidase	Bhatnagar and Kim, 2010
PM-060184 (I)	Polyketide	Sponge	Anticancer	Interferes withmicrotubule assembly	Newman and Cragg, 2014
HT1286 (Hemiasterlin derivative) (I)	Tripeptide	Sponge	Anticancer	Interferes with microtubule assembly	Bhatnagar and Kim, 2010
NVP-LAQ824 (Psammaplin derivative, Dacinostat) (I)	Miscellaneous	Sponge	Anticancer	Inhibition of histone deacetylase (HDAC) and DNA methyl transferases (DNMT)	Catley et al., 2003
E7974 (Hemiasterlin) (I)	Tripeptide	Sponge	Anticancer	Interferes with microtubule assembly	Bhatnagar and Kim 2010; Yamashita et al., 2004
HuMax® -TFADC (Tisotumab Vedotin) (I)	Antibody drug amalgamation	Mollusk	Endometrium, ovarian, prostate, and cervix	Antineoplastic Drug conjugate and monoclonal antibodies Immunotoxin	Kim et al., 2007
Bryostatin 1 (I)	Polyketide	Bryozoa	Anticancer	Protein kinase C	Kollár et al., 2014
Pinatuzumab vedotin (I)	Antibody drug amalgamation	Mollusk	Leukemia, Non-Hodgkin lymphoma	Apoptosis stimulant Mitosis and tubulin inhibitor	Advani et al., 2017
Discodermolide (I/II)	Polyketide	Sponge	Anticancer	Interferes with microtubule assembly	Bhatnagar and Kim, 2010; Shaw, 2008
PM-1004 (Zalypsis®) (I/II)	Alkaloid	Sponge	Anticancer	Inhibition of transcription	Petek and Jones, 2014; Fontana et al., 2000; Oku et al., 2003
Glembatumumab vedotin (II)	Conjugation of antibody drug	Mollusk	Breast melanoma	Target's glycoprotein NMB (a protein overexpressed by multiple tumor types)	Bendall et al., 2014
Elisidepsin (II)	Depsipetide	Mollusk	Anticancer	Antineoplastic agent Modification of lipids from cell membrane	Molina-Guijarro et al., 2015
Gemcitabine (GEM) (Gemzar) (III)	Nucleoside	Sponge	Anticancer	Ribonucleotide reductase inhibitor Replaces cytidine during DNA replication	Toschi et al., 2005
Plitidepsin (III)	Depsipetide	Tunicate	Anticancer	Causes apoptosis or cell cycle arrest	Leisch et al., 2018

(I) – Phase 1 trials; (I/II) – Phase ½ trials; (II) – Phase 2 trials; (III) – Phase 3 trials

the growth of multiple myeloma cell in a time-dependent and dose-dependent manner. It was found that treatment of multiple myeloma cells with NVP-LAQ824 also inhibits proteasome chymotrypsin-like activity (Catley et al., 2003). Plitidepsin is an anticancer agent that is derived from Mediterranean tunicate *Applidium albicans*. It binds to eEF1A2 gene and alters its translation. This leads to induction

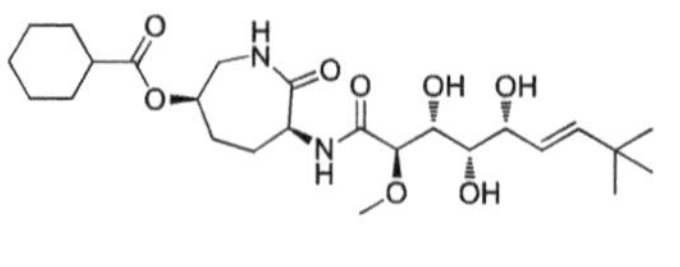

Bengamide B derivative (LAF389) [1]

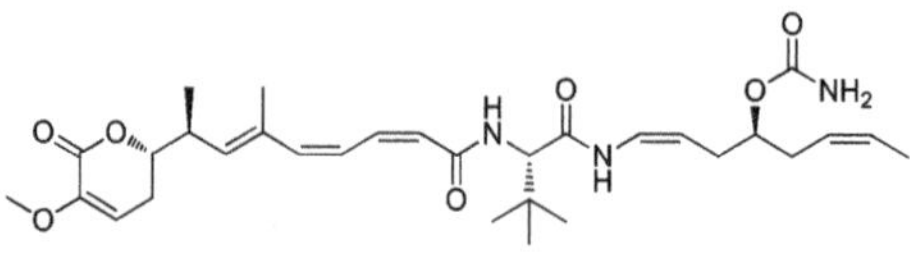

PM-060184 [1]

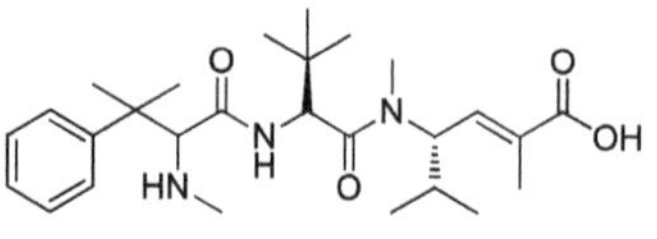

HT1286 (Hemiasterlin derivative) [1]

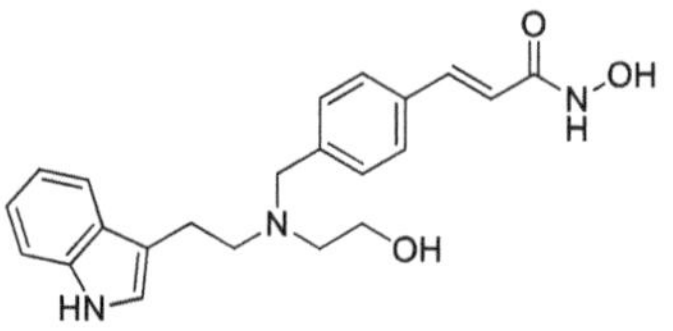

NVP-LAQ824 (Psammaplin derivative, Dacinostat) [1]

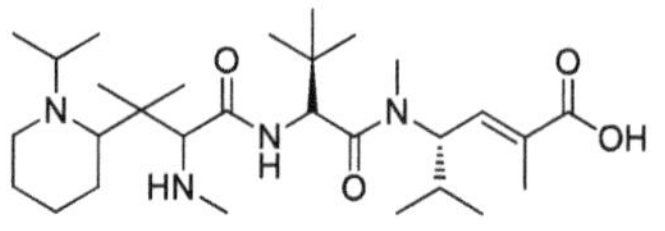

E7974 (Hemiasterlin) [1]

FIGURE 26.1 Chemical structures of major anticancer bioactive PIs isolated from marine origin.

of apoptosis, inhibition of growth, and cell-cycle arrest by alteration of various pathways. It is currently in phase 3 of the clinical trial and is tested against multiple myeloma (Leisch et al., 2018). The detailed sources and mechanisms are given in Table 26.1. The chemical structures of major anticancer bioactive PIs isolated from marine origin are shown in Figure 26.1.

26.4 Recent Developments on HIV-PIs Towards Malignant Cancers

Various HIV-PIs have shown positive results in inhibiting the growth of malignant tumors. Three inhibitors, namely nelfinavir, ritonavir, and saquinavir, out of all HIV-PIs showed maximum tumor-inhibiting activity. These three inhibitors inhibited the growth of nonsmall-cell lung carcinoma (NSCLC) cells. They inhibited the growth of all the cells in the NCI-60 cell line. This NCI-60 cell lines panel consists of 60 cancer lines that are prominent in humans. The National Cancer Institute (NCI) investigates the activity and potential of all new anticancer molecules against these cell lines (Gills et al., 2007).

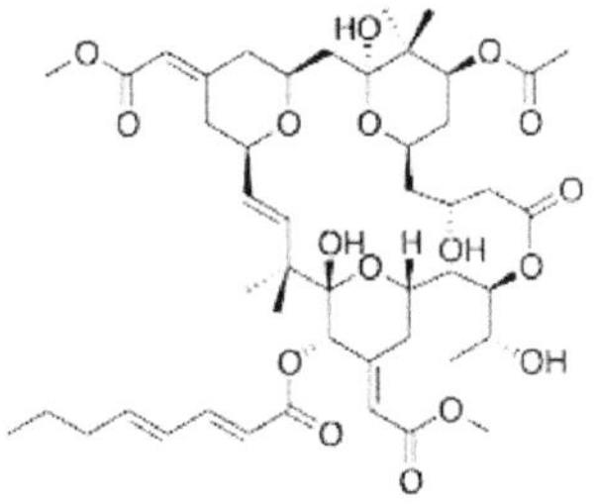

Bryostatin-1 [(I)]

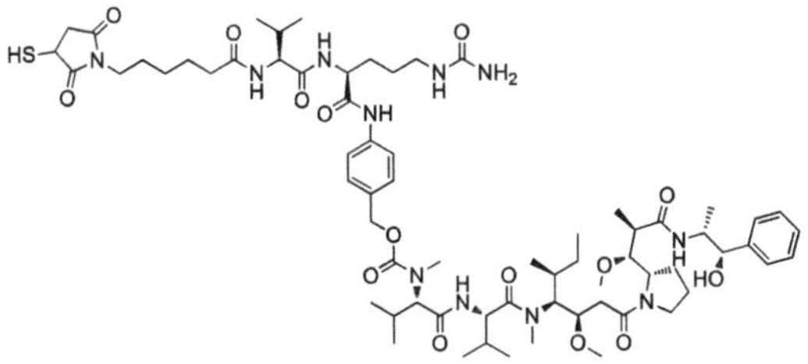

Pinatuzumabvedotin (I)

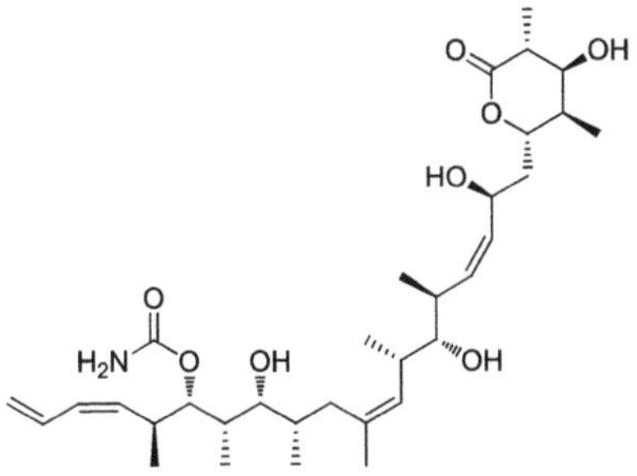

Discodermolide (I/II)

FIGURE 26.1 (Continued)

26.5 Different Pathways Targeted by HIV-PIs

HIV-PIs are known to work on several pathways to prevent the activity of cancer. The blocking of these pathways aids in the futuristic approach towards novel anticancer drugs. The mechanism of action of HIV-PIs, in particular, are MMP inhibition, autophagy, endoplasmic reticulum stress induction, proteasome activity inhibition, AKT phosphorylation, and angiogenesis inhibition, which are discussed below.

26.5.1 AKT Pathways

It was reported that HIV-PI acted on various other proteases rather than HIV protease. These reports were supported by insulin resistance and lipodystrophy (Bernstein and Dennis, 2008). They block the release of insulin from pancreatic cells (Schutt et al., 2004) and also make adipocytes, skeletal muscle cells, and hepatocytes insensitive to insulin. This insulin resistance is caused due to blockage of isoforms of protein kinase C and Akt by HIV PIs (Ben-Romano et al., 2004; Ben-Romano et al., 2003). It is also caused due to blockage of Glut4 and Glut1 (Ben-Romano et al., 2003; Murata et al., 2000). The AKT pathway is stimulated by the activation of phosphatidylinositol-3-kinase (PI3K). After activation of

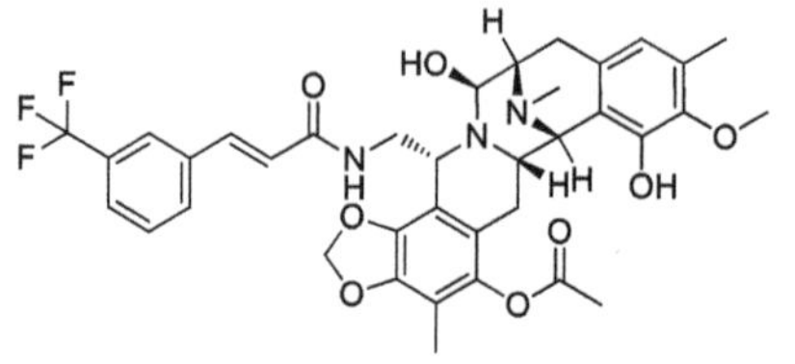

PM1004 (II)/ PM-10450 (Zalypsis®) (I/II)

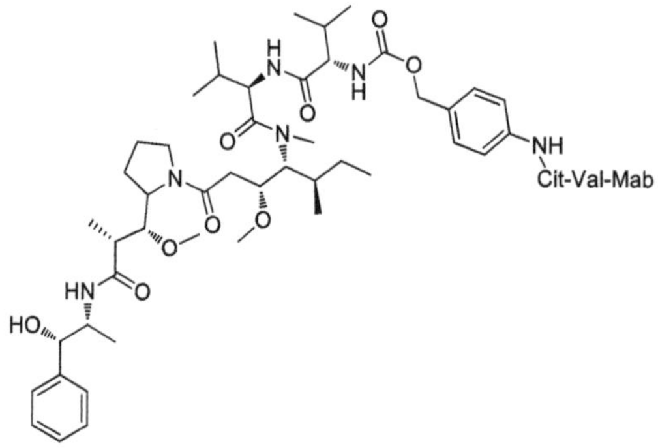

Glembatumumabvedotin (II)

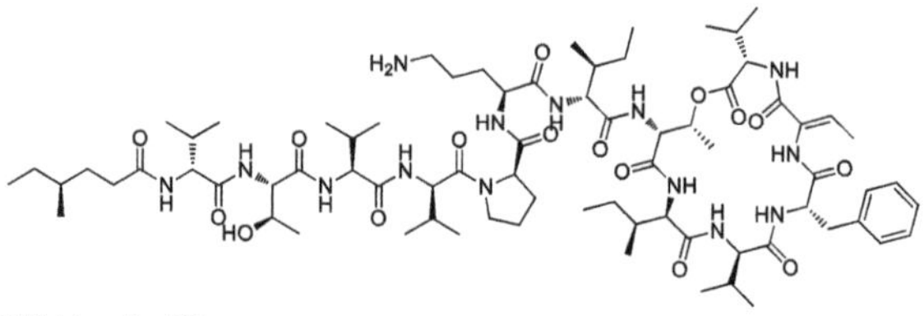

Elisidepsin (II)

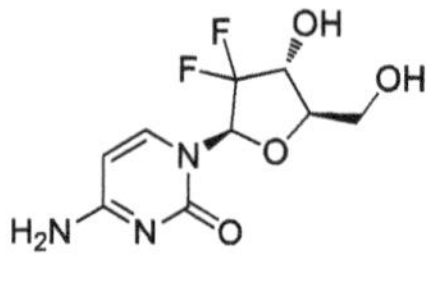

Gemcitabine (GEM) (Gemzar) (III)

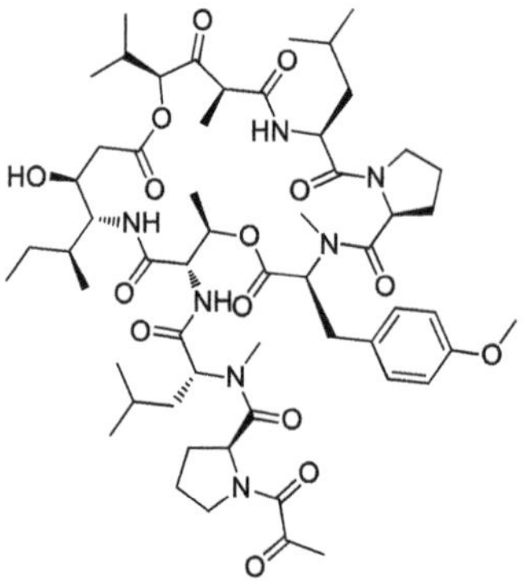

Plitidepsin (III)

FIGURE 26.1   (Continued)

P13K, cross-linking of growth factor take place on receptors located on the cell surface. The activation of PI3K phosphorylates the phosphoinositides, which are bound to the membranes. These phosphorylated phosphoinositides further bind to the AKT, which results in the translocation of the same into the inner cell surface where it may undergo phosphorylation through different mechanisms. (Thompson and Thompson, 2004; Bernstein and Dennis, 2008). The activation of the AKT pathway activates substrates, which aid in apoptosis, transcription, translation, and cell progression (Thompson and Thompson, 2004; LoPiccolo et al., 2008). The AKT pathway is responsible for major cellular changes like cellular proliferation and transformation of tumor cells. The AKT pathway is known to resist the activity of chemo and radiotherapy, due to which the inhibition of this pathway is mandatory for the treatment of cancers (Tsurutani et al., 2006).

There are various theories or hypotheses of the mechanisms by which HIV-PIs inhibit the AKT pathway. Several investigators have reported that HIV-PIs act by inhibiting activation of AKT by P13K. These groups of investigators proved that the sensitivity towards radio and chemotherapy is increased by reducing the phosphorylation of AKT (Yang et al., 2006; Gupta et al., 2005; Cuneo et al., 2007; Jiang et al., 2007). The AKT pathway can also be inhibited indirectly. For example, inhibition of the AKT pathway is reported in a few studies after the arrest of the cell cycle without apoptosis (Cuneo et al., 2007; Pore et al., 2006; Gills et al., 2007), arrest of cell cycle with apoptosis (Gaedicke et al., 2002; Ikezoe et al., 2004; Yang et al., 2006; Srirangam et al., 2006; Chow et al., 2006; Gills et al., 2007; Jiang et al., 2007) and only apoptosis (Gupta et al., 2007; Pyrko et al., 2007). Similarly, other groups of investigators suggested that the inhibitory activity of HIV PIs is due to blocking of Hsp 90 chaperone function (Srirangam et al., 2006), blocking expression of various factors like hypoxia-inducible factor-1a (HIF-1a), and vascular endothelial growth factor (VEGF) (which could be secondary to AKT inactivation) (Pore et al., 2006).

26.5.2 ER Stress

The endoplasmic reticulum regulates multiple cellular responses. Any alteration in the homeostasis of the ER and its related functionality may result in the signalling event of unfolded protein response (UPR), which is commonly known as the ER stress response. The different stress pathways of ER may be classified as UPR, IRE1 pathway, PERK pathway, and ATF6 pathway (Limonta et al., 2019). Prolong persistence of the UPR system may trigger apoptosis, which may aid in anticancer treatment. ER stress may cause a large setback to the human body as the cell death pathway may get activated during extreme stress conditions (Maurel et al., 2015). The mechanism of ER stress with anticancer activity is highly complex and usually determined with respect to the pathway. The final result of the mechanism is observed to be apoptosis.

Accumulation of abnormal proteins activates UPR. Activation of UPR leads to removal of an intron (256 nucleotides) from precursor mRNA of HAC-1p transcription factor. Active HAC-1p is then produced from the resulting mature mRNA HAC-1p. Transcription of chaperones like GRP78 is promoted by the HAC-1p transcription factor. These chaperones help in removing abnormal proteins from ER and then dispose them through ubiquitin-proteasome pathway. Nelfinavir induces ER stress by the accumulation of abnormal or misfolded proteins. Chaperones then bind to the misfolded proteins and activate protein kinase cascades, which blocks translation, reverses translocation, and activates ubiquitination enzymes, which induce autophagy. They can even induce apoptosis in extreme stressful conditions (Koltai, 2015).

There aer various proposed mechanisms by which ER stress exhibits antitumor activity. It inhibits AKT pathway. It is involved in dephosphorylation of AKT by protein phosphatase 1 (Gupta et al., 2007) further decreasing the synthesis of proteins. Cells can directly undergo apoptosis or survive through autophagy if they do not recover from ER stress (Bernstein and Dennis, 2008). Pyrko et al. (2007) observed that ER stress and ER dilation are important activities shown by PI when he treated glioma cell lines with atazanavir and nelfinavir. Gills et al. (2007) suspected that events in ER appear much before other cellular responses. Activating transcription factor 3 (ATF3) and phosphorylation of eIF2a are the two markers associated with ER stress. Transmission electron microscopy showed that the expression of these two markers increases within a few hours of treatment with nelfinavir.

26.5.3 Autophagy

Autophagy is a major catabolism mechanism that focuses on the degradation of cellular components. Similar to the MMP pathway, autophagy has a complex mechanism due to its dual nature of working for and against cancerous activity therefore providing an opening to chemotherapeutic treatments that engage in autophagy (Fulda, 2017). The cytoprotective nature of autophagy is a proposed theory based on data stating that the knockdown of the core elements of autophagy signaling pathway like BECN1 may increase the malignant glioma cell sensitivity, which shows important activity for the reduction of TMZ-related colony formation post-TMZ treatment (Katayama et al., 2007). Although extensive research and investigation has been conducted towards the further mechanism of TMZ-related ACD and autophagy, evidence has yet to be provided for the triggering of apoptosis (Knizhnik et. al., 2013)

There are various hypotheses related to the induction of autophagy by HIV PIs. Autophagy can be triggered by ER stress and UPR (Gills et al., 2008). ER stress through calcium signaling, JNK, or eIF2a can trigger autophagy for degradation of aggregated or misfolded proteins (Hoyer-Hansen and Jaattela, 2007). ER stress and UPR are caused by nelfinavir (Gills et al., 2008). Agents that activate eEF2K can cause autophagy (Wu et al., 2006) and it was found that nelfinavir was involved in the phosphorylation of eEF2. eEF2K causes autophagy by calcium and AMPK activation (Browne et al., 2004; Bagaglio et al., 1993). Nelfinavir can also induce autophagy by mimicking nutrient starvation by inhibiting receptor signaling of growth factor. Nelfinavir blocks downstream activation of AKT by inhibiting activation of cognate receptors by IGF-I and EGF (Schutt et al., 2004; Ben-Romano et al., 2004). Nelfinavir also induces autophagy independent of Beclin 1 (Zhu et al., 2007). Another major marker that is involved in the induction of autophagy is LC3-II. Aggregation and expression of LC3-II are enhanced by nelfinavir and the autophagosomes so produced were detected by electron microscopy (Gills et al., 2008).

26.5.4 Proteasome

Proteasomes are eukaryotic catalytic complexes found in abundance in the nucleus and cytoplasm. Proteasomes are known to degrade intracellular proteins including mediators of apoptosis and cell-cycle progression. Proteasomes inhibitors are usually categorized into five categories, namely peptide vinyl sulfones, peptide aldehydes, peptide epoxy ketones (eponomycin and epoxomicin), peptide boronates, and β-lactones (lactacystin and its derivatives). This categorization is based on the pharmacophore, which react with threonine residue of proteasomes (Kisselev and Goldberg, 2001). The inhibition of proteasomes has also proved to be valuable to the study of anticancer as they bypass or reverse the previously occurred mutation, which leads to tumorigenesis. The proteasome inhibitors also improve the sensitivity of cells towards chemo- and radiotherapy. For example, bortezomib has been clinically proven to treat relapsed and refractory multiple myeloma (Adams, 2004a). A few other activities have been observed to affect the activity of the proteasome including oncogene transformation, which degrades the C-fos, C-jun, and N-myc proteins (Adams, 2002; Almond and Cohen, 2002); protein turnover, which affects approximately 80% of the cellular proteins; and tumor suppression (Adams, 2004b; Adams, 2002). Further, they are known to cause apoptosis of Bax proteins (Li and Dou, 2000), pro-angiogenesis (Sunwoo et al., 2001), and ER stress (Lee et al., 2003).

The major mechanisms of action of HIV-PIs for anticancer activity are represented in Figure 26.2.

26.6 HIV PIs with Potent Antitumor Activity

FDA-approved HIV-PIs include nelfinavir, ritonavir, indinavir, atazanavir, and lopinavir (Maksimovic-Ivanic et al., 2017). The major role of this PI is to block the active site where the protease molecule shows ideal cohesion. The HIV-Pis are recognized as broad-spectrum inhibitors of cell proliferation as well as are responsible for stimulating apoptosis in cancerous cells. They have been tested for dose-dependent activity on different cell lines. The combination of Pis with previously existing cytotoxic chemotherapies and targeted therapies has set the platform for HIV-PI as future anticancer drugs (Ikezoe et al., 2004;

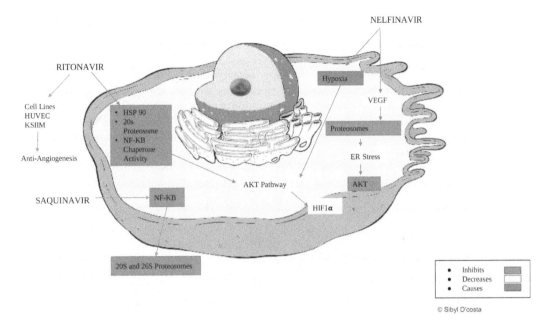

FIGURE 26.2 Mechanism of action of HIV-PIs for anticancer activity.

Gupta et al., 2007;Yang et al., 2006). HIV-PI includes drugs such as ritonavir, indinavir, atazanavir, nelfinavir, saquinavir, fosamprenavir, darunavir, and tipranavir (Watson and Carter, 2019).

26.6.1 Nelfinavir

Out of all the HIV-Pis nelfinavir was repositioned by FDA as an antitumor PI due to its potent pleiotropic anticancer activity. It induces autophagy and ER stress, which causes cell death in two ways: caspase-independent death and caspase-dependent apoptosis. Moreover, it has good bioavailability and a broad spectrum of activity (Gills et al., 2007). In preclinical studies, it showed anticancer activity in prostate cancer, liposarcoma, glioblastoma, multiple myeloma, breast cancer, lung cancer, cervical cancer, thyroid cancer, and head and neck cancer (Maksimovic-Ivanic et al., 2017). The major mechanism of action included AKT inhibition, STAT3 inhibition, ERK ½ inhibition, decrease MMP2/9, and inhibition of SREBP1as a cause of ER stress (Koltai, 2015).

26.6.2 Lopinavir/Ritonavir

Lopinavir (LPV) along with ritonavir (RIT) (booster) is used for the treatment of HIV. LPV is an aspartate PI of HIV. It binds to the catalytic site and thereby prevents the cleavage of viral polyprotein precursors into mature proteins that are required for viral assembly and replication. RIT in small doses is usually given in combination with LPV as it improves the pharmacokinetics of LPV by reducing its hepatic metabolism by inhibiting enzyme cytochrome P450 3A4. The standard recommended dosage of LPV in adults is 800 mg daily in combination with 200 mg of ritonavir, usually in two divided doses (Meini et al., 2020).

RIT has been identified to inhibit the chaperone function of Hsp90, 20S proteasome as well as NF-κB activity (Srirangam et al., 2006; Gaedicke et al., 2002; Pati et al., 2002). Furthermore, it was observed to show antiangiogenesis activity in certain cell lines like HUVEC and KSIIM (Pati et al., 2002). RIT is also known to reduce p-AKT (Srirangam et al., 2006). It has shown promising results in prostate cancer, multiple myeloma, cervical cancer, and breast cancer (Maksimovic-Ivanic et al., 2017).

26.6.3 Saquinavir

In preclinical studies it showed anticancer activity in prostate cancer, leukemia, cervical cancer, liver cancer, colon cancer, multiple myeloma, breast cancer, kaposi sarcoma, and lung cancer (Maksimovic-Ivanic et al., 2017). It was reported to show inhibitory activity towards the activity of NF-κB and the levels of the 20S and 26S proteasome. These major mechanisms were accompanied by apoptosis. It has also shown good anticancer activities through the inactivation of cell lines, CYP3A4, and AKT pathways alongside the major mechanisms (Bernstein and Dennis, 2008). There are different saquinavir derivatives developed for anticancer use through modifications to reduce its side effects. These derivatives have been attempted for modifications by attachment of different ligands, transporters, folic acid conjugated nanoparticles, and nitric oxide (NO) derivatives. One of its derivative is Saquinavir-NO, which shows a significantly strong antineoplastic effect with lower toxicity than that of the drug alone.

26.6.4 Indinavir

It showed promising results in preclinical trials for the treatment of leukemia, colon cancer, kaposi sarcoma, lung cancer, and breast cancer. Currently, three trials on indinavir are in progress; (1) NCT01067690, studying the activity of indinavir along with vinblastine ± bleomycin in patients suffering from HIV associated KS; (2) NCT00637637 a phase 2 clinical trial testing the effect of beam radiation therapy along with the combination of indinavir and ritonavir in patients suffering from brain metastases; and (3) phase 2 trial of NCT00362310, testing the effect of indinavir in non-HIV-related KS (Maksimovic-Ivanic et al., 2017).

Although PIs are not as potent as other anticancer drugs their wide spectrum activity leaves a large scope of untreated cancers for exploration. The above PIs are known to show side effects like cerebrovascular and cardiovascular disease as well as metabolic syndrome like insulin-resistance, lipoatrophy, and dyslipidemia. Marine sources have been researched upon and produce compounds portraying the same chemical structure and mechanism with lower possibilities of side effects (Bozzette et al., 2003; Hruz, 2008; Kotler, 2008). The anti-HIV mechanisms of PIs are compiled in Table 26.2.

26.7 Discussion and Future Directions

This review summarized all the PIs derived from marine sources along with their mechanism of action. Significant attention was given to HIV-PIs due to their potent antitumor activity. They inhibit tumor cell metastasis by inhibiting various proteases like MMPs, uPA, caspases, cathepsins, etc. The main mechanisms involved are AKT pathway inhibition, induction of ER stress, proteasome inhibition, and autophagy. HIV-PIs when used in combination with proteasome inhibitors produce synergistic activity by inducing ER stress and cytotoxicity in multiple myeloma, thus limiting the resistance built up due to proteasome inhibitor in preclinical models. Bortezomib/nelfinavir/dexamethasone is the most active drug combination tested in phase 2 clinical trials. (Mendez-Lopez et al., 2019). Tanomastat is a MMP inhibitor that is used for the treatment of cancer.

When we look for recent marine originated PIs, many studies have been reported. There have been past failures due to broad-spectrum PIs, which have drawn scientist's attention towards the importance of targeted approaches and responsible pharmacological activity. Marshall et al. (2015) studied therapeutic antibodies specific to activated proteases like MMP9 in an orthotopic colorectal cancer mouse model where they reduced tumor and metastasis. Kromann-Hansen et al. (2016) suggested variants (e.g., camelids) and antibody-like molecules (e.g., knottins), which could be further useful in this direction. There are various antibody conjugates like Pinatuzumabvedotin, Tisotumab vedotin, and Glembatumumab vedotin, which are in clinical trials for their potent anticancer activity. Therapeutics like these could uniquely target extracellular signaling and processing.

Marine organisms have proven to be a diverse source of anticancer compounds. It would be interesting to explore these cytotoxic compounds for their PI activity. The research of anticancer drugs has led to an opening of a wide scope of novel approaches. Marine sources have been previously proved to show

TABLE 26.2

Anticancer Mechanisms of HIV-Pis in Different Cancer Types

Drug Name	Cancer in focus	Cell lines	Mechanism	References
Nelfinavir	Multiple myeloma	MM1S,LP1, U266, RPMI8226, OPM2, 293T, ARH77.	↓AKT, STAT3 and ERK1/2	Ikezoe et al.,2004, Bono et al., 2012
			↓Mcl-1 ↑PERK phosphorylation	
	Prostate cancer	LNCap	AKT signalling and ↓AR-induced STAT3	Yang et al., 2005
	Breast cancer	MCF-7, HCC38,/ HCC1143, HCC1395, HCC1937, HCC1954, HCC2218, BT474	↓HSP90	Shim et al., 2012
	Lung cancer	A549	↓VEGF/HIF1alpha	Pore et al., 2006
	Liposarcoma	LiSa2 and SW872	Arrest cell cycle via↓ SREBP1, ↑ apoptosis	Chow et al., 2006
	Cervical cancer	Hela, CaSki and SiHa	↑Apoptosis, cell cycle arrest ↑Mitochondrial ROS	Xiang et al., 2015
Ritonavir	Prostate cancer	DU145	↓binding activity of NFkB	Ikezoe et al., 2004
	Cervical cancer	primary cells	↓MMP-2, MMP-9	Barillari et al., 2012
	Multiple myeloma	RPMI8226, U266	↓ AKT, ERK1/2, STAT3	McBrayer et al., 2012
			↓Mcl-1 ↓GLUT4	
	Breast cancer	MDA-MB-231, MDA-MB-436, MCF7, T47D	↓HSP90	Srirangam et al., 2006
			↓ AKT ↑Cell cycle arrest	
Saquinavir	Prostate cancer	DU-145, LNCap, PC3	↓26s Proteasome ↑Apoptosis ↓NFkB	Pajonk et al., 2002
	Lung cancer	A549	↓MMPs ↓Angiogenesis	Toschi et al., 2011
	Breast cancer	MDA-MB-468	↓MMPs ↓Angiogenesis	Toschi et al., 2011
	Kaposi sarcoma	Primary cells	↓MMPs ↓Angiogenesis	Sgadari et al., 2002
	Colon cance	SW480	↓MMPs ↓Angiogenesis	Toschi et al., 2011
	Liver cancer	SK-HEP-1	↓MMPs ↓Angiogenesis	Toschi et al., 2011
	Cervical cancer	Primary cells	↓MMP-2, MMP-9	Barillari et al., 2012
	Multiple myeloma	RPMI8226, U266, ARH77	↓ AKT, ERK1/2, STAT3	Ikezoe et al., 2004
			↓Mcl-1	

(continued)

TABLE 26.2 (Continued)

Anticancer Mechanisms of HIV-PIs in Different Cancer Types

Drug Name	Cancer in focus	Cell lines	Mechanism	References
Indinavir	Lung cancer	A549	↓MMPs ↓Angiogenesis	Toschi et al., 2011
	Breast cancer	MDA-MB-468	↓MMPs ↓Angiogenesis	Toschi et al., 2011
	Leukemia	Jurkat	↑ activity of telomerase	Adamo et al., 2013
	Colon cancer	SW480	↓MMPs ↓Angiogenesis	Toschi et al., 2011
	Kaposi sarcoma	primary cells	↓MMPs ↓Angiogenesis	Sgadari et al., 2002
Amprenavir	Prostate tumor	LNCaP	Prevents cleavage of androgen receptors, which is involved in ↑ apoptosis	Libertini et al., 2007
	Breast cancer	MCF-7	Inhibit ERK2 ↑apoptosis	Jiang et al., 2017
	Liver carcinoma	Huh-7	inhibit MMP proteolytic activation	Esposito et al., 2013
Lopinavir Indinavir	Cervical carcinoma	SiHa C33A, C33AE6 Nontransformed N1H/3T3 cells CaSki	Arrestation of P53 degradation	Hampson et al., 2006

Amprenavir
  Saquinavir
  Nelfinavir
	Lung cancer	T24
		A549
		SQ20B
		MIAPACA2
			Inhibition of phosphatidylinositol 3-kinase of the Akt signalling pathway causes tumor cell viability to reduce	Gupta et al., 2005

Nelfinavir Atazanavir	Malignant Glioma	LN229 U251	Stimulation of pro apoptotic caspase-4 (ER stress response associated)	Pyrko et al., 2007

good activity against various diseases and thus are highly recommended for marine PIs. The mechanism of action is partially known due to its complex nature, but further adequate analysis of the known and unknown binding is needed to improve the selectivity and specificity of the isolated compounds.

26.8 Conclusion

Protein inhibitors from various marine sources have been found to actively inhibit tumor enhancing and supporting cells and proteases. Although many PIs are yet under trial, quite a few have been developed, specifically as HIV-PIs to act against malignant cancers. Through the different pathways like AKT pathways, ER stress, autophagy, and proteasome, we have been able to understand and have a better view of the mechanism of action of HIV-PIs and their potent antitumor properties through drugs Nelfinavir, Lopinavir/Ritonavir, Saquinavir, and Indinavir. Furthermore, this field of marine-derived anticancer drugs has a wide availability of potent activities and novel approaches and future technologies can aid in the further development and advancement of the same.

Acknowledgements

The authors thank Ms Sibyl D'costa and Ms Tanuja Yadav for helping us with artwork and chemical structures. We remain grateful to our home institution SVKM's NMIMS for all the support.

REFERENCES

Adamo R, Comandini A, Aquino A, Bonmassar L, Guglielmi L, Bonmassar E, Franzese O (2013). The antiretroviral agent saquinavir enhances hTERT expression and telomerase activity in human T leukaemia cells in vitro. *J Exp Clin Cancer Res* 32(1):38.

Adams J (2002). Development of the proteasome inhibitor. *Oncologist* 7(1):9–16.

Adams J (2004a). The development of proteasome inhibitors as anticancer drugs. *Cancer Cell* 5(5):417–421.

Adams J (2004b). The proteasome: A suitable antineoplastic target. *Nat Rev Cancer* 4(5):349–360.

Advani R H et al (2017). Phase I study of the anti-CD22 antibody-drug conjugate pinatuzumab vedotin with/without rituximab in patients with relapsed/refractory B-cell non-Hodgkin's lymphoma. *Clin Cancer Res* 23(5):1167–1176.

Ahmad A and Hart IR (1997). Mechanisms of metastasis. *Crit Rev Oncol Hematol* 26(3):163–173.

Almond, JB and Cohen GM (2002).The proteasome A novel target for cancer chemotherapy. *Leukemia* 16(4):433–443.

Bagaglio DM, Cheng EH, Gorelick FS, Mitsui K, Nairn AC, Hait WN (1993). Phosphorylation of elongation factor 2 in normal and malignant rat glial cells. *Cancer Res* 53:2260-2264.

Barillari G, Iovane A, Bacigalupo I, Palladino C, Bellino S, Leone P, et al (2012). Ritonavir or saquinavir impairs the invasion of cervical intraepithelial neoplasia cells via a reduction of MMP expression and activity. *AIDS* 2012 May 15;26(8):909–919.

Bendell J et al (2014). Phase I/II study of the antibody-drug conjugate glembatumumab vedotin in patients with locally advanced or metastatic breast cancer. *J Clin Oncol* 32(32):3619–3625.

Ben-Romano R, Rudich A, Tirosh A, Potashnik R, Sasaoka T, Riesenberg K, et al (2004). Nelfinavir-induced insulin resistance is associated with impaired plasma membrane recruitment of the PI 3-kinase effectors Akt/PKB and PKC-zeta. *Diabetologia* 47(6):1107-1117.

Ben-Romano R, Rudich A, Török D, Vanounou S, Riesenberg K, Schlaeffer F, et al (2003). Agent and cell-type specificity in the induction of insulin resistance by HIV protease inhibitors. *AIDS* 17(1):23–32.

Bernstein WB and Dennis PA (2008). Repositioning HIV protease inhibitors as cancer therapeutics. *Curr Opin HIV AIDS* 3(6):666–675.

Bhatnagar I and Kim S-K (2010). Marine antitumor drugs: status, shortfalls and strategies. *Mar Drugs* 8(10):2702–2720.

Blasi F and Stoppelli MP (1999). Proteases and cancer invasion: from belief to certainty. AACR meeting on proteases and protease inhibitors in cancer, Nyborg, Denmark, 14–18 June 1998. *Biochimica et Biophysica Acta* 1423(1):35–44.

Bono C et al (2012). The human immunodeficiency virus-1 protease inhibitor nelfinavir impairs proteasome activity and inhibits the proliferation of multiple myeloma cells in vitro and in vivo. *Haematologica* 97(7):1101–1109.

Bozzette, SA, Ake CF, Tam HK, Chang SW, Louis TA (2003). Cardiovascular and cerebrovascular events in patients treated for Human immunodeficiency virus infection. *N Engl J Med* 348(8):702–710.

Brömme D and Kaleta J (2002). Thiol-dependent cathepsins: pathophysiological implications and recent advances in inhibitor design. *Curr Pharm Des* 8(18):1639–1658.

Browne GJ, Finn SG and Proud CG (2004). Stimulation of the AMP-activated protein kinase leads to activation of eukaryotic elongation factor 2 kinase and to its phosphorylation at a novel site, serine 398. *J Biol Chem* 279(13):12220-12231.

Castro GJL, Garcia-Gasca T, Blanco-Labra A (2010). Chapter V. Protease inhibitors as anticancer agents. In *New Approaches in Treatment of Cancer*, ed: Dra Ma. Del Carmen Mejia Vazquez, Samuel Navarro. Nova Science Publishers, Inc. pp. 91–124.

Catley L et al (2003). NVP-LAQ824 is a potent novel histone deacetylase inhibitor with significant activity against multiple myeloma. *BLOOD* 102(7):2615–2622.

Chow WA, Guo S and Valdes-Albini F (2006). Nelfinavir induces liposarcoma apoptosis and cell cycle arrest by upregulating sterol regulatory element binding protein-1. *Anticancer Drugs* 17(8):891–903.

Christopeit T, Øverbø K, Danielson UH, Nilsen IW (2013). Efficient screening of marine extracts for protease inhibitors by combining FRET based activity assays and surface plasmon resonance spectroscopy based binding assays. *Mar Drugs* 11(11):4279–4293.

Cuneo KC, Tu T, Geng L, Fu A, Hallahan DE, Willey CD (2007). HIV protease inhibitors enhance the efficacy of irradiation. *Cancer Res* 67(10):4886–4893.

D'Incalci M, Badri N, Galmarini CM, Allavena P (2014). Trabectedin, a drug acting on both cancer cells and the tumour microenvironment. *Br J Cancer* 111(4):646– 650.

DeClerck YA et al (2004). Proteases, extracellular matrix, and cancer: a workshop of the path B study section. *Am J Pathol* 164(4):1131–1139.

Degryse B (2011). The urokinase receptor system as strategic therapeutic target: challenges for the 21st century. *Curr Pharm Des* 17(19):1872–1873.

Dodson G and Wlodawer A (1998). Catalytic triads and their relatives. *Trends Biochem Sci* 23(9):347–352.

Dumez H, Gall H, Capdeville R, Dutreix C, Van Oosterom AT, Giaccone G (2007). A phase 1 and pharmacokinetic study of LAF389 administered to patients with advanced cancer. *Anticancer Drugs* 18(2):219–225.

Eatemadi A, Aiyelabegan HT, Negahdari B, Mazlomi MA, Daraee H, Daraee N, et sl (2017). Role of protease and protease inhibitors in cancer pathogenesis and treatment. *BiomedPharmacother* 86:221–231.

Fais S (2007) Cannibalism: a way to feed on metastatic tumors. Cancer Lett 258(2):155–164. https://doi.org/10.1016/j.canlet.2007.09.014

Fontana A, Cavaliere P, Wahidulla S, Naik CG, Cimino G (2000). A new antitumor isoquinoline alkaloid from the marine nudibranch *Jorunnafunebris*. *Tetrahedron* 56(37):7305–7308.

Fulda S (2017). Autophagy in cancer therapy. *Front Oncol* 7:128

Gaedicke S, Firat-Geier E, Constantiniu O, Lucchiari-Hartz M, Freudenberg M, Galanos C, Niederman G (2002). Antitumor effect of the human immunodeficiency virus protease inhibitor ritonavir: induction of tumor-cell apoptosis associated with perturbation of proteasomal proteolysis. *Cancer Res* 62(23):6901–6908.

Gills JJ et al (2007). Nelfinavir, a lead HIV protease inhibitor, is a broad-spectrum, anticancer agent that induces endoplasmic reticulum stress, autophagy, and apoptosis in vitro and in vivo. *Clin Cancer Res* 13(17):5183–5194.

Gills JJ, LoPiccolo J and Dennis PA (2008). Nelfinavir, a new anti-cancer drug with pleiotropic effects and many paths to autophagy. *Autophagy* 4(1):107-109.

Gomez DE, Alonso DF, Yoshiji H, Thorgeirsson UP (1997). Tissue inhibitors of metalloproteinases: structure, regulation andbiologicalfunctions. *Eur J Cel lBiol* 74(2):111–122.

Gupta AK, Li B, Cerniglia GJ, Ahmed MS, Hahn M, Maity A (2007). The HIV protease inhibitor nelfinavir downregulates Akt phosphorylation by inhibiting proteasomal activity and inducing the unfolded protein response. *Neoplasia* 9(4):271–278.

Gupta AK, Cerniglia GJ, Mick R, McKenna WG, Muschel RJ (2005). HIV protease inhibitors block Akt signaling and radiosensitize tumor cells both in vitro and in vivo. *Cancer Res* 65(18):8256–8265.

Gupta SC, Hye Kim J, Prasad S, Aggarwal B (2010). Regulation of survival, proliferation, invasion, angiogenesis, and metastasis of tumor cells through modulation of inflammatory pathways by nutraceuticals. *Cancer Metastasis Rev* 29(3):405–434.

Gupta V, Samuelson CG, Su S, Chen TC (2007). Nelfinavir potentiation of imatinib cytotoxicity in meningioma cells via surviving inhibition. *Neurosurg Focus* 23(4):E9.

Hampson L, Kitchener HC, Hampson IN (2006). Specific HIV protease inhibitors inhibit the ability of HPV16 E6 to degrade p53 and selective kill E6-dependent cervical carcinoma cells in vitro. *AntivirTher* 11(6):813–825

Hedstrom L (2002). Serine protease mechanism and specificity.*Chem Rev* 102(12):4501–4524.

Hoyer-Hansen M and Jaattela M (2007). Connecting endoplasmic reticulum stress to autophagy by unfolded protein response and calcium. *Cell Death Differ* 14(9):1576-1582.

Hruz PW (2008). HIV protease inhibitors and insulin resistance: lessons from in vitro, rodent and healthy human volunteer models. *Curr Opin HIV AIDS* 3(6):660–665.

Huang Q, Jin H, Liu Q, Wu Q, Kang H, Cao Z, Zhu R (2012).Proteochemometric modeling of the bioactivity spectra of HIV-1 protease inhibitors by introducing protein-ligand interaction fingerprint. *PLoS ONE* 7(7): e41698.

Ikezoe T, Hisatake Y, Takeuchi T, Ohtsuki Y, Yang Y, Said JW, et al (2004). HIV-1 Protease Inhibitor, Ritonavir: A potent inhibitor of CYP3A4, enhanced the anticancer effects of Docetaxel in androgen-independent prostate cancer cells in vitro and in vivo. *Cancer Res* 64(20):7426–7431.

Ikezoe T, Saito T, Bandobashi K, Yang Y, Koeffler HP, Taguchi H (2004). HIV-1 protease inhibitor induces growth arrest and apoptosis of human multiple myeloma cells via inactivation of signal transducer and activator of transcription 3 and extracellular signal-regulated kinase 1/2. *Mol CancerTher* 3(4):473–479.

Jedinak A and Maliar T (2005). Inhibitors of proteases as anticancer drugs. *Neoplasma* 52(3):185–192.

Jiang W et al (2017). Repositioning of amprenavir as a novel extracellular signal-regulated kinase-2 inhibitor and apoptosis inducer in MCF-7 human breast cancer. *Int J Oncol* 50(3):823–834.

Jiang W, Mikochik PJ, Ra JH, Lei H, Flaherty KT, Winkler JD, Spitz FR (2007). HIV protease inhibitor nelfinavir inhibits growth of human melanoma cells by induction of cell cycle arrest. *Cancer Res* 67(3):1221–1227.

Jiang Z, Pore N, Cerniglia GJ, Mick R, Georgescu M–M, Bernhard EJ, et al (2007). Phosphatase and tensin homologue deficiency in glioblastoma confers resistance to radiation and temozolomide that is reversed by the protease inhibitor nelfinavir. *Cancer Res* 67(9):4467–4473.

Jordan MA, Kamath K, Manna T, Okouneva T, Miller HP, Davis C, et al (2005). The primary antimitotic mechanism of action of the synthetic halichondrin E7389 is suppression of microtubule growth. *Mol. CancerTher* 4(7):1086–1095.

Katayama M, Kawaguchi T, Berger MS, Pieper RO (2007). DNA damaging agentinduced autophagy produces a cytoprotective adenosine triphosphate surge in malignant glioma cells. *Cell Death Differ* 14(3):548–558.

Kennedy AR (1998). Chemopreventive agents: Protease inhibitors. *Pharmacol Ther* 78(3):167–209.

Kennedy AR and Little JB (1978). Protease inhibitors suppress radiation-induced malignant transformation in vitro. *Nature* 276(5690):825–826.

Kessenbrock K, Plaks V andWerb, Z (2010). Matrix metalloproteinases: regulators of the tumor microenvironment. *Cell* 141(1):52–67.

Khasigov PZ, Podobed OV, Ktzoeva SA, Gatagonova TM, Grachev SV, Shishkin SS, Berezov TT (2001). Matrix metalloproteinases of normal human tissues. *Biochemistry (Mosc)* 66(2):130–140.

Kim YH et al (2007). Clinical efficacy of zanolimumab (HuMax-CD4): two phase 2 studies in refractory cutaneous T-cell lymphoma. *Blood* 109(11):4655–4662.

Kisselev AF and Goldberg AL (2001). Proteasome inhibitors. *Chem Biol* 8:739–758

Knizhnik AV, Roos WP, Nikolova T, Quiros S, Tomaszowski K-H, Christmann M, Kania B (2013). Survival and death strategies in glioma cells: autophagy, senescence and apoptosis triggered by a single type of temozolomide-induced dna damage. *PLoS ONE* 8(1): e55665.

Kobayashi H, Moniwa N, Sugimura M, Shinohara H, Ohi H, Terao T (1993). Effects of membrane-associated cathepsin B on the activation of receptor-bound prourokinase and subsequent invasion of reconstituted basement membranes. *Biochimica et Biophysica Acta* 1178(1):55–62.

Kobayashi H, Schmitt M, Goretzki L, Chucholowski N, Calvete J, Kramer M, et al (1991) Cathepsin B efficiently activates the soluble and the tumor cell receptor-bound form of the proenzyme urokinase-type plasminogen activator (Pro-uPA). *J Biol Chem* 266(8):5147–5152.

Kollár P, Rajchard J, Balounová Z, Pazourek J (2014). Marine natural products: Bryostatins in preclinical and clinical studies. *Pharm Biol* 52(2):237—242.

Koltai T (2015).Nelfinavir and other protease inhibitors in cancer: mechanisms involved in anticancer activity. *Version 2. F1000Research* 4:9.

Kotler DP (2008). HIV and antiretroviral therapy: lipid abnormalities and associated cardiovascular risk in HIV-infected patients. *J Acquir Immune Defic Syndr* 1:49(Suppl 2):S79–85.

Krepela E (2001). Cysteine proteinases in tumor cell growth and apoptosis. *Neoplasma* 48(5):332–349.

Kromann-Hansen T, Oldenburg E, Yung KW, Ghassabeh GH, Muyldermans S, Declerck PJ, et al (2016). A camelid derived antibody fragment targeting the active site of a serine protease balances between inhibitor and substrate behavior. *J Biol Chem* 291(29):15156–15168.

Kuznetsov G et al (2009). Tubulin-based antimitotic mechanism of E7974, a novel analogue of the marine sponge natural product hemiasterlin. *Mol Cancer Ther* 8(10):2852–2860.

Lee AH, Iwakoshi NN, Anderson KC, Glimcher LH (2003). Proteasome inhibitors disrupt the unfolded protein response in myeloma cells. *Proc Natl Acad Sci USA* 100(17):9946–9951.

Leisch M, Egle A, Greil R (2018). Plitidepsin: a potential new treatment for relapsed/refractory multiple myeloma. *Future Oncol* 15(2):109–120.

Levicar N, Strojnik T, Kos J, Dewey RA, Pilkington GJ, Lah TT (2002). Lysosomal enzymes, cathepsins in brain tumour invasion. *J Neuro-Oncol* 58(1):21–32.

Li B and Dou QP (2000). Bax degradation by the ubiquitin/proteasome-dependent pathway involvement in tumor survival and progression. *Proc Natl Acad Sci USA* 97(8):3850–3855.

Li J and Yuan J (2008). Caspases in apoptosis and beyond. *Oncogene* 27(48):6194–6206.

Libertini SJ, Tepper CG, Rodriguez V, Asmuth DM, Kung HJ, Mudryj M (2007). Evidence for calpain-mediated androgen receptor cleavage as a mechanism for androgen independence. *Cancer Res* 67(19):9001–9005.

Limonta P, Moretti RM, Marzagalli M, Fontana F, Raimondi M, Marcella MM (2019). Role of endoplasmic reticulum stress in the anticancer activity of natural compounds. *Int J Mol Sci* 20(4):961.

Loganzo F et al (2003). HTI-286, a synthetic analogue of the tripeptide hemiasterlin, is a potent antimicrotubule agent that circumvents p-glycoprotein-mediated resistance in vitro and in vivo. *Cancer Res* 63(8):1838–1845.

LoPiccolo J, Blumenthal GM, Bernstein WB, Dennis PA (2008). Targeting the PI3K/Akt/mTOR pathway: Effective combinations and clinical considerations. *Drug Resist Updat* 11(1–2):32–50.

Maksimovic-Ivanic D, Fagone P, McCubrey J, Bendtzen K, Mijatovic S, Nicoletti F (2017). HIV- protease inhibitors for the treatment of cancer: Repositioning HIV protease inhibitors while developing more potent NO- hybridized derivatives? *Int J Cancer* 140(8):1713–1726.

Marshall DC et al (2015). Selective allosteric inhibition of MMP9 is efficacious in preclinical models of ulcerative colitis and colorectal cancer. *PLOS ONE* 10(5): e0127063.

Maurel M, McGrath EP, Mnich K, Healy S, Chevet E, Samali A (2015). Controlling the unfolded protein response-mediated life and death decisions in cancer. *Semin Cancer Biol* 33:57–66.

Mayer AMS, Glaser KB, Cuevas C, Jacobs RS, Kem W, Little RD, et al (2010). The odyssey of marine pharmaceuticals: a current pipeline perspective. *Trends Pharmacol Sci* 31(6):255–265.

McBrayer SK, Cheng JC, Singhal S, Krett NL, Rosen ST, Shanmugam M (2012). Multiple myeloma exhibits novel dependence on GLUT4, GLUT8, and GLUT11: implications for glucose transporter-directed therapy. *Blood* 119:4686–4697.

Meini S, Pagotto A, Longo B, Vendramin I, Pecori D, Tascini C (2020). Role of lopinavir/ritonavir in the treatment of covid-19: a review of current evidence, guideline recommendations, and perspectives. *J Clin Med* 9(7):2050.

Mendez-Lopez M, Sutter T, Driessen C, Besse L (2019). HIV protease inhibitors for the treatment of multiple myeloma. *Clin Adv Hematol Oncol* 17(11):615–623.

Messadi DV, Billings P, Shklar G, Kennedy AR (1986). Inhibition of oral carcinogenesis by a protease inhibitor. *J Natl Cancer Inst* 76(3):447–452.

Molina-Guijarro JM et al (2015). Elisidepsin interacts directly with glycosylceramides in the plasma membrane of tumor cells to induce necrotic cell death. *Plos one* 10(10): e0140782.

Murata H, Hruz PW and Mueckler M (2000).The mechanism of insulin resistance caused by HIV protease inhibitor therapy. *J Biol Chem* 275(27):20251–20254.

Newland AM, Li JX, Wasco LE, Aziz MT, Lowe DK (2013). Brentuximab Vedotin: a CD30-directed antibody-cytotoxic drug conjugate. *Pharmacotherapy* 33(1):93–104.

Newman DJ and Cragg GM (2014). Marine-sourced anticancer and cancer pain control agents in clinical and late preclinical development. *Mar Drugs* 12(1):255–278.

Nezhat F, Wadler S, Muggia F, Mandeli J, Goldberg G, Rahaman J, et al (2004). Phase II trial of the combination of bryostatin-1 and cisplatin in advanced or recurrent carcinoma of the cervix: A New York Gynecologic Oncology Group study. *Gynecol Oncol* 93(1):144–148.

Oku N, Matsunaga S, Van Soest RWM, Fusetani N (2003). Renieramycin J, a highly cytotoxic tetrahydroisoquinoline alkaloid, from a marine sponge *Neopetrosia sp. J Nat Prod* 66:1136–1139.

Olivera BM, Cruz LJ, De Santos V, LeCheminant G, Griffin D, Zeikus R, Rivier J (1987). Neuronal calcium channel antagonists. Discrimination between calcium channel subtypes usingomega-conotoxin from Conus magus venom. *Biochemistry* 26(8):2086–2090.

Overall CM and Kleifeld O (2006). Tumour microenvironment—opinion: validating matrix metalloproteinase as drug targets and anti-targets for cancer therapy. *Nat Rev Cancer* 6(3):227–239.

Pajonk F, Himmelsbach J, Riess K, Somner A, Mcbride WH (2002). The human immunodeficiency virus (HIV)21 protease inhibitor saquinavir inhibits proteasome function and causes apoptosis and radio sensitization in non-HIV-associated human cancer cells. *Cancer Res* 62(18):5230–5235.

Pati S, Pelser CB, Dufraine J, Bryant JL, Reitz MS, Weichold FF (2002). Antitumorigenic effects of HIV protease inhibitor ritonavir: inhibition of Kaposi sarcoma. *Blood* 99(10):3771–3779.

Petek BJ and Jones RL (2014). PM00104 (Zalypsis®): a marine derived alkylating agent. *Molecules* 19(8):12328–12335.

Pore N, Gupta AK, Cerniglia GJ, Jiang Z, Bernhard EJ, Evans SM, et al (2006). Nelfinavir down-regulates hypoxia-inducible factor 1α and VEGF expression and increases tumor oxygenation: implications for radiotherapy. *Cancer Res* 66(18):9252–9259.

Pyrko P, Kardosh A, Wang W, Xiong W, Schönthal AH, Chen TC (2007). HIV-1 protease inhibitors nelfinavir and atazanavir induce malignant glioma death by triggering endoplasmic reticulum stress. *Cancer Res* 67(22):10920–10928.

Qin Z, Wang M, Yan A (2017). QSAR studies of the bioactivity of hepatitis C virus (HCV) NS3/4A protease inhibitors by multiple linear regression (MLR) and support vector machine (SVM). *Bioorg Med Chem Lett* 27(13):2931–2938.

Rakashanda S and Amin S (2017). Proteases as targets in anticancer therapy using their inhibitors. *Biotechnol Genet Eng* 33(2):133–138.

Ruiz-Torres V, Encinar JA, Herranz-López M, Pérez-Sánchez A, Galiano V, Barrajón-Catalán E, Micol V (2017). An updated review on marine anticancer compounds: the use of virtual screening for the discovery of small-molecule cancer drugs. *Molecules* 22(7):1037.

Schmitt M et al (2000). The urokinase plasminogen activator system as a novel target for tumour therapy. *Fibrinol Proteol* 14(2–3):114–132.

Schutt M, Zhou J, Meier M, Klein HH (2004). Long-term effects of HIV-1 protease inhibitors on insulin secretion and insulin signaling in INS-1 beta cells. *J Endocrinol* 183(3):445–454.

Sgadari C et al (2002). HIV protease inhibitors are potent anti-angiogenic molecules and promote regression of Kaposi sarcoma. *Nat Med* 8(3):225–232.

Shaw SJ (2008). The structure activity relationship of discodermolide analogues. *Mini Rev Med Chem* 8(3):276–284.

Shim JS, Rao R, Beebe K, Neckers L, Han I, Nahta R, Liu JO (2012). Selective inhibition of HER2-positive breast cancer cells by the HIV protease inhibitor nelfinavir. *J Natl Cancer Inst* 104(20):1576–1590.

Siegel RM (2006). Caspases at the crossroads of immune-cell life and death. *Nat Rev Immunol* 6(4):308–317.

Song X, Xiong Y, Qi X, Tang W, Dai J, Gu Q, Li J (2018).Moleculartargets of active anticancer compounds derived from marine sources. *Mar Drugs* 16(5):175.

Srirangam A et al (2006). Effects of HIV protease inhibitor ritonavir on akt-regulated cell proliferation in breast cancer. *Clin Cancer Res* 12(6):1883–1896.

Srirangam A et al (2011). The human immunodeficiency virus protease inhibitor ritonavir inhibits lung cancer cells, in part, by inhibition of surviving. *J Thorax Oncol* 6(4):661–670.

Stupack DG, Teitz T, Potter MD, Mikolon D, Houghton PJ, Kidd VJ, et al (2006). Potentiation of neuroblastoma metastasis by loss of caspase-8. *Nature* 439(7072):95–99.

Sunwoo JB, Chen Z, Dong G, Yeh N, Bancroft CC, Sausville E, et al (2001). Novel proteasome inhibitor PS-341 inhibits activation of nuclear factor-κB, cell survival, tumor growth, and angiogenesis in squamous cell carcinoma. *Clin Cancer Res* 7(5):1419–1428

Tang L and Han X (2013). The urokinase plasminogen activator system in breast cancer invasion and metastasis. *Biomed Pharmacother* 67(2):179–182.

Thompson JE and Thompson CB (2004). Putting the rap on Akt. *J Clin Oncol* 22(20):4217–4226.

Toschi E et al (2011). Human immunodeficiency virus protease inhibitors reduce the growth of human tumors via a proteasome-independent block of angiogenesis and matrix metalloproteinases. *Int J Cancer* 128(1):82–93.

Toschi L, Finocchiaro G, Bartolini S, Gioia V, Cappuzzo F (2005). Role of gemcitabine in cancer therapy. *Future oncology* 1(1):7–17.

Trezza A, Cicaloni V, Spiga O (2020). Chapter 2: Potential roles of protease inhibitors in anticancer therapy. In Cancer-Leading Proteases: Structures, Functions and Inhibition, 1st Edition,13–49. Elsevier.

Troll W, Frenkel K and Wiesner R (1984). Protease inhibitors as anticarcinogens. *J Natl Cancer Inst* 73(6):1245–1250.

Tsurutani J, Fukuoka J, Tsurutani H, Shih JH, Hewitt SM, Travis WD, et al (2006). Evaluation of two phosphorylation sites improves the prognostic significance of Akt activation in non–small-cell lung cancer tumors. *J Clin Oncol* 24(2):306–314.

Turk D and Guncar G (2003). Lysosomal cysteine proteases (cathepsins): promising drug targets. *Acta Crystallogr D Biol Crystallogr* 59(Pt 2):203–213.

Van Lint P and Libert C (2007). Chemokine and cytokine processing by matrix metalloproteinases and its effect on leukocyte migration and inflammation. *J Leukoc Biol* 82(6):1375–1381.

Vasudev A and Sohail SK (2016). Partially purified Glycine max proteinase inhibitors: potential bioactive compounds against tobacco cutworm, *Spodoptera litura* (Fabricius, 1775) (Lepidoptera: Noctuidae). *Turk J Zool* 40(3):379–387.

Voura EB, English JL, Yu H-YE, Ho AT, Subarsky P, Hill RP, et al (2013). Proteolysis during tumor cell extravasation in vitro: Metalloproteinase involvement across tumor cell types. *Plos one* 8(10): e78413.

Wang Y (2001). The role and regulation of urokinase-type plasminogen activator receptor gene expression in cancer invasion and metastasis. *Med Res Rev* 21(2):146–170.

Watson S, and Carter A (2019). HIV: Guide to protease inhibitors. www.healthline.com/health/hiv-aids/protease-inhibitors (accessed 16th December 2019).

Winer A, Adams S and Mignatti P (2018). Matrix metalloproteinase inhibitors in cancer therapy: Turning past failures into future successes. *Mol Cancer Ther* 17(6):1147–1155.

Wojtowicz-Praga, SM, Dickson RB and Hawkins MJ (1997). Matrix metalloproteinase inhibitors. *Invest New Drugs* 15(1):61–17.

Wu H, Yang JM, Jin S, Zhang H, Hait WN (2006). Elongation factor-2 kinase regulates autophagy in human glioblastoma cells. *Cancer Res* 66(6):3015–3023.

Xiang T, Du L, Pham P, Zhu B, Jiang S (2015). Nelfinavir, an HIV protease inhibitor, induces apoptosis and cell cycle arrest in human cervical cancer cells via the ROS-dependent mitochondrial pathway. *Cancer Lett* 364(1):79–88.

Yamashita A et al (2004). Synthesis and activity of novel analogs of hemiasterlin as inhibitors of tubulin polymerization: Modification of a segment. *Bioorg Med Chem Lett* 14(21):5317–5322.

Yang Y, Ikezoe T, Nishioka C, Bandobashi K, Takeuchi T, Adachi Y, et al (2006). NFV, an HIV-1 protease inhibitor, induces growth arrest, reduced Akt signalling, apoptosis and docetaxel sensitisation in NSCLC cell lines. *Br J Cancer* 95(12):1653–1662.

Yang Y, Ikezoe T, Takeuchi T, Adachi Y, Ohtsuki Y, Takeuchi S, et al (2005). HIV-1 protease inhibitor induces growth arrest and apoptosis of human prostate cancer LNCaP cells in vitro and in vivo in conjunction with blockade of androgen receptor STAT3 and AKT signaling. *Cancer Sci* 96(7):425–433.

Zhu JH, Horbinski C, Guo F, Watkins S, Uchiyama Y, Chu CT (2007). Regulation of autophagy by extracellular signal-regulated protein kinases during 1-methyl-4-phenylpyridinium-induced cell death. *Am J Pathol* 170(1):75-86.

27

Skin Stem Cells: Therapeutic Potential in Vitiligo

Harjot Kaur, Naveed Pervaiz, and Ravinder Kumar
Department of Zoology, Panjab University, Chandigarh, India

Davinder Parsad
Department of Dermatology, PGIMER, Chandigarh, India

27.1 Introduction

Skin is the externalmost layer that covers the whole of the body and integrates all the crucial support systems of the body (i.e., blood, nerves, muscles within itself). Continuous exposure of skin to solar, mechanical, thermal energies, and to hostile environmental factors like microorganisms justifies its strategic location as a blockade between the inner milieu and the outer environment (Slominski, 2005). Ultraviolet radiation detection, immunological competence, and endocrine functions together partake in maintaining the homeostasis of skin as well as regulating the homeostasis of entire mammalian body (Tobin, 2017).

The epidermis is the outer layer of skin followed by the dermis; both the layers of skin are heavily populated by various cell populations (Figure 27.1). The outermost epidermis largely comprises keratinocytes. Other than actively participating in the barrier formation keratinocytes also play active roles at the forefront in immunity (Klicznik et al., 2018). They initiate an immune reaction leading to activation of langerhanscells, which further amplify the response by migrating to the lymph nodes to recruit T lymphocytes to the skin (Kimber and Cumberbatch, 1992).

Another kind of cells present in epidermis are melanocytes, responsible for synthesis of melanin and skin color (Zhu et al., 2020). Melanin synthesis is actually a defense mechanism against photodamage caused to DNA by ultraviolet radiation. Melanogenesis protects the skin from chronic photoaging, acute photodamage, and cancer development.

The inner layer of skin known as the dermis mainly constitute fibroblasts population. Fibroblasts display a great dynamic in maintaining melanogenesis by regulating pigmentation via signal cross-talk between epidermal keratinocytes and melanocytes (Wang et al., 2017). Recent evidence has shown that fibroblasts play a role in pathogenesis of many diseases, including cancer (Kalluri and Zeisberg, 2006; Sorrell and Caplan, 2009), skin aging (Tigges et al., 2014; Korosec et al., 2019), and wound healing (Stunova and Vistejnova, 2018), and can be readily reprogrammed into induced pluripotent stem cells (Lowry et al., 2008; Nakagawa et al., 2008).

Hyper or hypo-functioning of melanocytes leads to incidences of pigmentary disorders, thus signifying the importance of mechanisms of melanocyte development with clear relevance to understanding human pigmentary disease in the field of developmental and stem cell biology (Mort et al., 2015). Vitiligo is one such hypomelanotic disorder in which significant loss of melanocytes leads to lesions and patches all over the body. Therapies like the use of corticosteroids, narrow band ultraviolet B (NBUVB), and monobenzone creams are currently in use, but complex pathogenesis is the reason behind their limited success in inducing repigmentation.

DOI: 10.1201/9781003220404-30

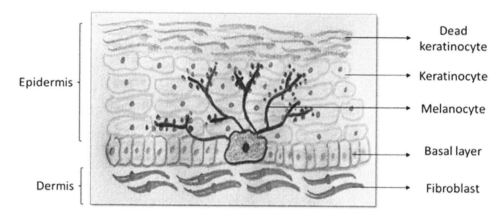

FIGURE 27.1   Skin diagram depicting epidermal keratinocytes, melanocytes, and dermal fibroblasts.

27.2 Stem Cell Niches in Skin

Adult stem cells require spatially distinct microenvironments to reside in for their maintenance and functioning. Skin harbors several diverse populations of adult stem cells (Hsu et al., 2014). Interfollicular epidermal stem cells, dermal stem cells, hair follicle stem cells, and sebaceous gland stem cells are among various subtypes of stem cells present in skin (Shi et al., 2006).

Epidermal stem cells are evenly distributed throughoutbasal layer of the interfollicular epidermis, forming functionally independent compartments known as epidermal proliferative units (Niezgoda et al.,2017). The progenitor cells function to replenish basal layer, and also generate the outer layers of terminally differentiated, dead stratum corneum cells, thus continuously replacing the epidermal layer (Vasioukhin et al.,1999).

Dermis acts as home to adult dermal stem cells also known as skin-derived progenitor cells. These cells are capable of synthesizing fibronectin, vimentin, and nestin showing their potential to differentiate into several lineages (multipotency) such as mesodermal lineage cells, like chondrocytes, adipocytes and osteoblasts, ectodermal nerve cells and endodermal liver cells (Toma et al., 2001; Biernaskie et al., 2006). Dermal stem cells play a significant role in the maintenance of skin homeostasis and in replacement of damaged dermis (Vishnubalaji et al.,2012; Shim et al., 2013).

Hair follicles are rooted deep in the dermis from where hair shafts extend via basement membrane beyond the epidermal layer. Numerous stem cell populations combinedly known as hair follicle stem cells (HFSCs) such as mesenchymal stem cells and bulge melanocyte stem cells (MSCs) originate from hair follicles (Figure 27.2). Hair follicles, unlike epidermis, which is regularly renewed, undergo distinct phases of growth (anagen), rest (telogen) and degeneration (catagen). Multipotent stem cells in hair follicles have differentiation capacity to generate multiple cell lineages.

Hair follicle epithelial stem cells were the first population of cells to be discovered through label retaining technique (Cotsarelis et al., 1990), where rapidly and transiently amplifying cells tend to eventually lose the label but slow cycling stem cells tend to retain the label for a prolonged time (Ceder et al., 2017). These stem cells are located in the bulge area of hair follicle, positioned beneath pilosebaceous unit and in the dermal papilla at the base of hair follicle (Blanpain et al., 2004). Hair follicle epithelial stem cells have a dual role to play: under normal physiological conditions, they maintain and replenish the epithelium of hair follicle, while upon stimulation of skin either by wounding or under conditions of trauma, they tend to completely regenerate the lost epidermis (Ito et al., 2005).

Another subtype of precursor cell belonging to the dermal papilla of hair follicle are mesenchymal stem cells. These stem cells support the remodeling of connective tissue sheath as well as dermal papilla itself during anagen phase of hair follicle (Tobin et al., 2003). Previously, both in vitro and in vivo studies have evidenced the supporting differentiation of these stem cells into not only fibroblasts, but also adipocytes, chondrocytes, hematopoietic, and neuronal precursors (Jahoda et al., 2003).

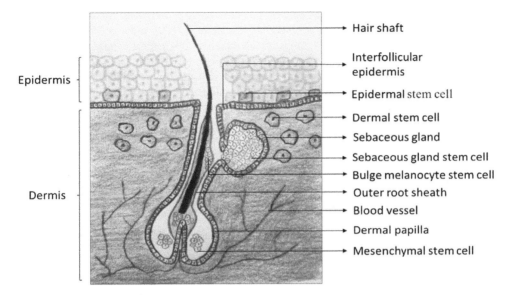

FIGURE 27.2 Schematic representation of hair follicle in human skin showing stem cell niches in epidermis, dermis, and hair follicle.

A separate population of stem cells is responsible for providing pigmentation to hair shaft, thus melanocyte stem cells form the hair follicle pigmentary unit. These cells are derived from neural crest and resideinouter sheath region of hair follicle (Nishimura et al., 2002; Peters et al., 2002). Hair greying is observed with aging because melanocyte stem cells in hair follicles tend to lose their self-renewal capacity unlike skin melanocytes in the epidermis, which retain a lifelong proliferative potential (Tobin and Paus, 2001). In the human body sebaceous glands are responsible for holocrine sebum secretion into the sheath of a hair follicle (Ghazizadeh and Taichman, 2001). A unipotent stem cell population called sebaceous gland stem cells is sited along the periphery of sebaceous gland acting as a continuous source to maintain the homeostasis of the gland (Niemann et al., 2003). Interdependence of sebaceous gland and the hair follicle is such that when one organ is lost the other one often collapses (Selleri et al., 2006).

27.3 Stem Cells in Treatment of Vitiligo

Stem cells in the field of dermatology have been and continue to be a breakthrough in treatment of various diseases, vitiligo being one of them. Multipotent stem cells in skin do not express melanocyte differentiation markers; therefore, they can escape the autoimmune destruction mechanisms and provide differentiated melanocytes for repigmentation (Osawa et al., 2005).

27.3.1 Hair Follicle Melanocyte Stem Cells

The presence of hair follicle melanocyte stem cells called amelanotic melanocytes were shown in outer root sheath of hair follicle by Staricco in 1959 for the first time. While dopa-positive melanin-producing active melanocytes in epidermis are targeted for destruction in vitiligo the inactive melanocytes in the hair follicle remain unaffected indicating hair follicle melanocyte stem cells have a substantial role to play in the repigmentation of the vitiliginous lesion. The identification of melanocyte stem cell population among other hair follicle populations showed the presence of dopachrometautomerase (DCT) and paired box gene (Pax)-3, but absence of SRY-box transcription factor (SOX)-10, microphthalmia-associated transcription factor (MITF), and tyrosinase (TYR) gene markers (Ortonne et al., 1979). During the repigmentation process, active melanocytes in the epidermis mature from inactive melanocytes in hair follicle as the number of inactive melanocytes increases significantly in the outer root sheaths of hair follicle indicating their proliferation, maturation, and migration to epidermis (Cui et al., 1991). Ultraviolet radiation stimulates pigmentation as a protective measure in response to DNA damage by chemically modifying melanin and spatial redistribution of melanosomes in keratinocytes and melanocytes (Routaboul et al., 1999) signifying the use of ultraviolet radiation as a treatment strategy. Activation of amelanotic melanocyte population in the hair follicle after subsequent exposure to ultraviolet radiations (Staricco and Miller-Milinska, 1962; Chau et al., 2013) and NBUVB treatment has been shown to stimulate the melanocyte stem cells and their migration to lesional skin resulting in repigmentation of the vitiligo lesions (Yamada et al., 2013; Goldstein et al., 2015).

Hair follicle melanocyte stem cell population gives rise to both hair bulb melanocytes responsible for hair pigmentation and epidermal melanocytes and the melanocortin 1 receptor (MC1R) pathway particularly promotes the epidermal fate of follicular melanocyte stem cells (Chau et al., 2013). These various studies firmly established the part played by hair follicle melanocyte stem cells in epidermal pigmentation.

27.3.2 Other Stem Cell Populations in Vitiligo

How multipotent stem cells control the outcome to a distinct phenotype remains unknown to an extent; however, several in vitro studies indicate the differentiation to a particular phenotype is regulated by stem-cell-intrinsic differences in the relative sensitivity and timing of responses to growth factors (Shah and Anderson, 1997). Dermal stem cells segregated from human dermis have been shown to express characteristic neural crest marker nerve growth factor receptor (NGFRp)-75 and an embryonic stem cell marker octamer-binding transcription factor (OCT) 4. These dermal stem cells isolated from foreskin region lacking hair follicles have been shown to differentiate into HMB45-positive melanocytes in dermis followed by their migration to basal layer of epidermis (Li et al., 2010). These dermal stem cells are negative for both E-cadherin and N-cadherin, which explain their migration to epidermis. After reaching epidermis these dermal melanocytes become more functionally mature and start expressing E-cadherin upon contact with the adjacent keratinocytes.

Significant infiltration of cytotoxic CD8$^+$ T lymphocytes has been seen in the perilesional area of vitiligo patients undergoing melanocyte transplantation signifying efficiency of the treatment is intimately related to skin-homing capacity of CD8$^+$ T cell activities (Zhou et al., 2013). Dermal stem cells were shown to hinder the proliferation of CD8$^+$ T cells, induce their apoptosis and also regulated production of cytokines and chemokines. These stem cells inhibited secretion of the pro-inflammatory cytokines tumor necrosis factor (TNF)-α, interleukin (IL)-1α, and IL-12; cytokines associated with T helper cells such as interferon (IFN)-γ, IL-13, and macrophage inflammatory protein (MIP)-1 and immune regulatory cytokines like transforming growth factor (TGF)-β. These results established the role of dermal stem cells as supporting agents, which may assist in improving the efficacy of melanocytes transplantation. Induced pluripotent stem cells have been generated from dermal fibroblasts using either four (Octamer-binding transcription factor (OCT) 3/4, SRY-box transcription factor (SOX) 2, kruppel-like factor (KLF) 4, c-MYC), or three (without c-MYC) Yamanaka factors and these induced pluripotent stem cells were then shown to differentiate in vitro into melanocytes using Wnt3, stem cell factor, endothelin 3, and (cyclic adenosine monophosphate) cAMP inducers (cholera toxin) in melanocyte differentiation medium (Ohta et al., 2011). The growth factors (i.e., wingless-related integration site (Wnt)3, stem cell factor, cAMP, and endothelin 3) regulate MITF promotor through downstream transcription factors PAX3, SOX10, lymphoid enhancer-binding factor (LEF) 1, and cAMP response element-binding protein (CREB); therefore, it is believed that the differentiation conditions biased melanocyte differentiation through a combinatorial activation of MITF. MITF mediates melanocytic lineage by triggering the activation of pigment-producing genes such as DCTand TYR, and contributes to their survival by upregulating anti-apoptotic genes such as B-cell lymphoma(Bcl)-2 and Bcl-XL (Lin and Fisher, 2007). Evolving such mechanisms for differentiation of multipotent stem cells into human melanocyte could be of paramount importance for patients with various pigmentary disorders such as vitiligo.

27.3.3 Surgical Methods Employing Stem Cell Populations

Surgical therapies are of the utmost importance in treating vitiligo when the vitiligo lesions have been stable for at least a couple of years and reluctant to non-surgical methods (Mohanty et al., 2011; Rao et al., 2012). Hair follicles are now an established and efficient source of melanocyte precursor cells and are therefore employed in the treatment of vitiligo.

Follicular unit transplantation is one such surgical procedure where an incision is made in occipital scalp and then from a larger donor graft multiple small grafts with single hair are cut (Kumaresan, 2011; Thakur et al., 2015). Single hair grafts are transplanted into the recipient site after which the grafted melanocytes spread to the depigmented area (Malakar and Dhar, 1999; Sardi, 2001; Chen et al., 2020). Sometimes additional therapies like psoralen and ultraviolet A (PUVA) or topical corticosteroid therapy are given along with transplantation in order to enhance the rate of repigmentation (Chouhan et al., 2013; Ezz-Eldawla et al., 2019). Some of the advantages of this method are a single hair has a greater number of melanocytes than the epidermal graft, the method can be performed in the angle of the mouth or eyelash area where other surgical methods are hard to perform, and the colour match is much more satisfactory compared to other surgical modalities, but the method is a laborious, tedious, and delicate procedure to follow (Na et al., 1998; Mapar et al., 2014).

Extraction of outer root sheath cell suspension from hair follicle has emerged as another method to treat vitiliginous lesions where outer root sheath cells are isolated from hair follicle by trypsinization (Kumar et al., 2013; Vinay et al., 2015; Kumar et al., 2018). The single-cell suspension is then transplanted onto dermabraded recipient site (Vanscheidt and Hunziker, 2009; Mohanty et al., 2011; Shah et al., 2016). Comparisons have been studied between epidermal melanocyte transfer and extracted outer root sheath solution in treatment of vitiligo with non-cultured epidermal solution showing better efficacy than extracted outer root sheath solution without achieving a statistical significance (Singh et al., 2013; Donaparthi and Chopra, 2016).

Keratinocytes regulate pigmentation process by providing essential factors such as stem cell factor, basic fibroblast growth factor, and endothelin-1, therefore extracted hair follicle outer root sheath cell suspension is being used in combination with non-cultured epidermal cell suspension (Razmi et al., 2018). A better and faster rate of repigmentation was observed with non-cultured epidermal cell suspension and follicular cell suspension (ECS + FCS) in comparison to epidermal cell suspension (ECS) alone owing to: a) higher ratio of melanocyte to keratinocyte (1:5) in the follicles in contrast to skin where the melanocyte to keratinocyte ratio is 1:36; b) keratinocyte growth factors like stem cell factor and basic fibroblast growth factor (bFGF) facilitating expression of stem cells in follicular cell suspension in ECS + FCS (Razmi et al., 2017).

27.4 Conclusions

With concern for evolutionary adaptation of life on an ultraviolet radiation-soaked terrestrial planet, skin-based diseases to date rank fourth in terms of leading causes of non-fatal disease burden (Tobin, 2017). Skin stem cell research first started in the 1970s. Initial experiments on the proliferation of mouse epidermal cells demonstrated the presence of slow-cycling cells that were either in a dormant state or in a tremendously slow cell cycle state in basal layer of epidermis (Akamatsu et al., 2016). In recent times, numerous stem cells have been found in other layers of skin such as dermis, bulge, outer root sheath, and secondary germ area of hair follicle in addition to the basal layer of the epidermis. Other than maintaining skin homeostasis these stem cells are thought to be the new era of treatment for skin disorders (Zouboulis et al., 2008). Though in recent times various studies have employed the potential of stem cells in vitiligo their vast potential remains unexplored in treatment of vitiligo patients. Proliferation, differentiation, and migration of melanocyte stem cells in the outer root sheath region of hair follicle can deliver an enormous supply of melanocytes. Recent advances in the field of skin stem cell research have made the future prospect of vitiligo treatment encouraging and optimistic.

REFERENCES

Akamatsu H, Hasegawa S, Yamada T, Mizutani H, Nakata S, Yagami A and Matsunaga K (2016). Age-related decrease in CD 271+ cells in human skin. *J Dermatol* 43(3):311–313.

Biernaskie JA, McKenzie IA, Toma JG and Miller FD (2006). Isolation of skin-derived precursors (SKPs) and differentiation and enrichment of their Schwann cell progeny. *Nat Protoc* 1(6):2803–2812.

Blanpain C, Lowry WE, Geoghegan A, Polak L and Fuchs E (2004). Self-renewal, multipotency, and the existence of two cell populations within an epithelial stem cell niche. *Cell* 118(5):635–648.

Ceder JA, Aalders TW and Schalken JA (2017). Label retention and stem cell marker expression in the developing and adult prostate identifies basal and luminal epithelial stem cell subpopulations. *Stem Cell Res Ther* 8(1):1–12.

Chen Y, Yan J, Chen X, Gan L, Song M, Wang J, et al. (2020). Comparative study between follicular unit transplantation with intact and unintact hair bulb in treatment for stable vitiligo. *J Dermatolog Treat* 1–16.

Chou WC, Takeo M, Rabbani P, Hu H, Lee W, Chung YR, et al. (2013). Direct migration of follicular melanocyte stem cells to the epidermis after wounding or UVB irradiation is dependent on Mc1r signaling. *Nat Med* 19(7):924–929.

Chouhan K, Kumar A and Kanwar AJ (2013). Body hair transplantation in vitiligo. *J Cutan Aesthet Surg* 6(2):111–112.

Cotsarelis G, Sun TT and Lavker RM (1990). Label-retaining cells reside in the bulge area of pilosebaceous unit: implications for follicular stem cells, hair cycle, and skin carcinogenesis. *Cell* 61(7):1329–1337.

Cui J, Shen LY and Wang GC (1991). Role of hair follicles in the repigmentation of vitiligo. *J Invest Dermatol* 97(3):410–416.

Donaparthi N and Chopra A (2016). Comparative study of efficacy of epidermal melanocyte transfer versus hair follicular melanocyte transfer in stable vitiligo. *Indian J Dermatol* 61(6):640–644.

Ezz-Eldawla R, Abu El-Hamd M, Saied SM and Hassanien SH (2019). A comparative study between suction blistering graft, mini punch graft, and hair follicle transplant in treatment of patients with stable vitiligo. *J Dermatolog Treat* 30(5):492–497.

Ghazizadeh S and Taichman LB (2001). Multiple classes of stem cells in cutaneous epithelium: a lineage analysis of adult mouse skin. *EMBO J* 20(6):1215–1222.

Goldstein NB, Koster MI, Hoaglin LG, Spoelstra NS, Kechris KJ, Robinson SE, et al. (2015). Narrow band ultraviolet B treatment for human vitiligo is associated with proliferation, migration, and differentiation of melanocyte precursors. *J Invest Dermatol* 135(8):2068–2076.

Hsu YC, Li L and Fuchs E (2014). Emerging interactions between skin stem cells and their niches. *Nat Med* 20(8):847–856.

Ito M, Liu Y, Yang Z, Nguyen J, Liang F, Morris RJ and Cotsarelis G (2005). Stem cells in the hair follicle bulge contribute to wound repair but not to homeostasis of the epidermis. *Nat Med* 11(12):1351–1354.

Jahoda CA, Whitehouse J, Reynolds AJ and Hole N (2003). Hair follicle dermal cells differentiate into adipogenic and osteogenic lineages. *Exp Dermatol* 12(6):849–859.

Kalluri R and Zeisberg M (2006). Fibroblasts in cancer. *Nat Rev Cancer* 6(5):392–401.

Kimber I and Cumberbatch M (1992). Stimulation of Langerhans cell migration by tumor necrosis factor alpha (TNF-alpha). *J Invest Dermatol* 99(5):48S-50S.

Klicznik MM, Szenes-Nagy AB, Campbell DJ and Gratz IK (2018). Taking the lead-how keratinocytes orchestrate skin T cell immunity. *Immunol Lett* 200:43–51.

Korosec A, Frech S, Gesslbauer B, Vierhapper M, Radtke C, Petzelbauer P and Lichtenberger BM (2019). Lineage identity and location within the dermis determine the function of papillary and reticular fibroblasts in human skin. *J Invest Dermatol* 139(2):342–351.

Kumar A, Mohanty S, Sahni K, Kumar R and Gupta S (2013). Extracted hair follicle outer root sheath cell suspension for pigment cell restoration in vitiligo. *J Cutan Aesthet Surg* 6(2):121–125.

Kumar P, Bhari N, Tembhre MK, Mohanty S, Arava S, Sharma VK and Gupta S (2018). Study of efficacy and safety of noncultured, extracted follicular outer root sheath cell suspension transplantation in the management of stable vitiligo. *Int J Dermatol* 57(2):245–249.

Kumaresan M (2011). Single-hair follicular unit transplant for stable vitiligo. *J Cutan Aesthet Surg* 4(1):41–43.

Li L, Fukunaga-Kalabis M, Yu H, Xu X, Kong J, Lee JT and Herlyn M (2010). Human dermal stem cells differentiate into functional epidermal melanocytes. *J Cell Sci* 123(Pt 6):853–860.

Lin JY and Fisher DE (2007). Melanocyte biology and skin pigmentation. *Nature* 445(7130):843–850.

Lowry WE, Richter L, Yachechko R, Pyle AD, Tchieu J, Sridharan R, et al. (2008).Generation of human induced pluripotent stem cells from dermal fibroblasts. *Proc Natl Acad Sci USA* 105(8):2883–2888.

Malakar S and Dhar S (1999). Repigmentation of vitiligo patches by transplantation of hair follicles. *Int J Dermatol* 38(3):237–238.

Mapar MA, Safarpour M, Mapar M and Haghighizadeh MH (2014). A comparative study of the mini-punch grafting and hair follicle transplantation in the treatment of refractory and stable vitiligo. *J Am Acad Dermatol* 70(4):743–747.

Mohanty S, Kumar A, Dhawan J, Sreenivas V and Gupta S (2011). Non-cultured extracted hair follicle outer root sheath cell suspension for transplantation in vitiligo. *Br J Dermatol* 164:1241–1246.

Mort RL, Jackson IJ and Patton EE (2015). The melanocyte lineage in development and disease. *Development* 142(7):1387.

Na GY, Seo SK and Choi SK (1998). Single hair grafting for the treatment of vitiligo. *J Am Acad Dermatol* 38(4):580–584.

Nakagawa M, Koyanagi M, Tanabe K, Takahashi K, Ichisaka T, Aoi T, et al. (2008). Generation of induced pluripotent stem cells without Myc from mouse and human fibroblasts. *Nat Biotechnol* 26(1):101–106.

Niemann C, Unden AB, Lyle S, Zouboulis CC, Toftgard R and Watt FM (2003). Indian hedgehog and beta-catenin signaling: role in the sebaceous lineage of normal and neoplastic mammalian epidermis. *Proc Natl Acad Sci USA* 100(Suppl 1):11873–11880.

Niezgoda A, Niezgoda P, Nowowiejska L, Białecka A, Męcińska-Jundziłł K, Adamska U and Czajkowski R (2017). Properties of skin stem cells and their potential clinical applications in modern dermatology. *Eur J Dermatol* 27(3):227–236.

Nishimura EK, Jordan SA, Oshima H, Yoshida H, Osawa M, Moriyama M, et al. (2002). Dominant role of the niche in melanocyte stem-cell fate determination. *Nature* 416(6883):854–860.

Ohta S, Imaizumi Y, Okada Y, Akamatsu W, Kuwahara R, Ohyama M, et al. (2011). Generation of human melanocytes from induced pluripotent stem cells. *PLoSOne* 6(1):e16182.

Ortonne JP, MacDonald DM, Micoud A and Thivolet J (1979). PUVA-induced repigmentation of vitiligo: a histochemical (split-DOPA) and ultrastructural study. *Br J Dermatol* 101(1):1–12.

Osawa M, Egawa G, Mak SS, Moriyama M, Freter R, Yonetani S, et al. (2005). Molecular characterization of melanocyte stem cells in their niche. *Development* 132(24):5589–5599.

Peters EM, Tobin DJ, Botchkareva N, Maurer M and Paus R (2002). Migration of melanoblasts into the developing murine hair follicle is accompanied by transient c-Kit expression. *J Histochem Cytochem* 50(6):751–766.

Rao A, Gupta S, Dinda AK, Sharma A, Sharma VK, Kumar G, et al. (2012). Study of clinical, biochemical and immunological factors determining stability of disease in patients with generalized vitiligo undergoing melanocyte transplantation. *Br J Dermatol* 166(6):1230–1236.

Razmi TM, Kumar R, Rani S, Kumaran SM, Tanwar S and Parsad D (2018). Combination of follicular and epidermal cell suspension as a novel surgical approach in difficult-to-treat vitiligo: a randomized clinical trial. *JAMA Dermatol* 154(3):301–308.

Razmi TM, Parsad D and Kumaran SM (2017). Combined epidermal and follicular cell suspension as a novel surgical approach for acral vitiligo. *J Am Acad Dermatol* 76(3):564–567.

Routaboul C, Denis A and Vinche A (1999). Immediate pigment darkening: description, kinetic and biological function. *Eur J Dermatol* 9(2):95–99.

Sardi JR (2001) Surgical treatment for vitiligo through hair follicle grafting: how to make it easy. *Dermatol Surg* 27(7):685–686.

Selleri S, Seltmann H, Gariboldi S, Shirai YF, Balsari A, Zouboulis CC and Rumio C (2006). Doxorubicin-induced alopecia is associated with sebaceous gland degeneration. *J Invest Dermatol* 126(4):711–720.

Shah AN, Marfatia RK and Saikia SS (2016). A study of noncultured extracted hair follicle outer root sheath cell suspension for transplantation in vitiligo. *Int J Trichology* 8(2):67–72.

Shah NM and Anderson DJ (1997). Integration of multiple instructive cues by neural crest stem cells reveals cell-intrinsic biases in relative growth factor responsiveness. *Proc Natl Acad Sci USA* 94(21):11369–11374.

Shi C, Zhu Y, Su Y and Cheng T (2006). Stem cells and their applications in skin-cell therapy. *Trends Biotechnol* 24(1):48–52.

Shim JH, Lee TR and Shin DW (2013). Novel in vitro culture condition improves the stemness of human dermal stem/progenitor cells. *Mol Cells* 36(6):556–563.

Singh C, Parsad D, Kanwar AJ, Dogra S and Kumar R (2013). Comparison between autologous noncultured extracted hair follicle outer root sheath cell suspension and autologous noncultured epidermal cell suspension in the treatment of stable vitiligo: a randomized study. *Br J Dermatol* 169(2):287–293.

Slominski A (2005). Neuroendocrine system of the skin. *Dermatology* 211(3):199–208.

Sorrell JM and Caplan AI (2009). Fibroblasts-a diverse population at the center of it all. *Int Rev Cell Mol Biol* 276:161–214.

Staricco RG and Miller-Milinska A (1962). Activation of the amelanotic melanocytes in the outer root sheath of the hair follicle following ultra violet rays exposure. *J Invest Dermatol* 39:163–164.

Staricco RG (1959). Amelanotic melanocytes in the outer sheath of the human hair follicle. *J Invest Dermatol* 33:295–297.

Stunova A andVistejnova L (2018). Dermal fibroblasts-A heterogeneous population with regulatory function in wound healing. *Cytokine Growth Factor Rev* 39:137–150.

Thakur P, Sacchidanand S, Nataraj HV and Savitha AS (2015). A study of hair follicular transplantation as a treatment option for vitiligo. *J Cutan Aesthet Surg* 8(4):211–217.

Tigges J, Krutmann J, Fritsche E, Haendeler J, Schaal H, Fischer JW, et al. (2014). The hallmarks of fibroblast ageing. *Mech Ageing Dev* 138:26–44.

Tobin DJ, Gunin A, Magerl M and Paus R (2003). Plasticity and cytokinetic dynamics of the hair follicle mesenchyme during the hair growth cycle: implications for growth control and hair follicle transformations. *J Investig Dermatol Symp Proc* 8(1):80–86.

Tobin DJ and Paus R (2001). Graying: gerontobiology of the hair follicle pigmentary unit. *Exp Gerontol* 36(3):591–592.

Tobin DJ (2017). Introduction to skin aging. *J Tissue Viability* 26(1):37–46.

Toma JG, Akhavan M, Fernandes KJ, Barnabé-Heider F, Sadikot A, Kaplan DR and Miller FD (2001). Isolation of multipotent adult stem cells from the dermis of mammalian skin. *Nat Cell Biol* 3(9):778–784.

Vanscheidt W and Hunziker T (2009). Repigmentation by outer-root-sheath-derived melanocytes: proof of concept in vitiligo and leucoderma. *Dermatology* 218(4):342–343.

Vasioukhin V, Degenstein L, Wise B and Fuchs E (1999). The magical touch: genome targeting in epidermal stem cells induced by tamoxifen application to mouse skin. *Proc Natl Acad Sci USA* 96(15):8551–8556.

Vinay K, Dogra S, Parsad D, Kanwar AJ, Kumar R, Minz RW and Saikia UN (2015). Clinical and treatment characteristics determining therapeutic outcome in patients undergoing autologous non-cultured outer root sheath hair follicle cell suspension for treatment of stable vitiligo. *J Eur Acad Dermatol Venereo* l29(1):31–37.

Vishnubalaji R, Al-Nbaheen M, Kadalmani B, Aldahmash A and Ramesh T (2012). Skin-derived multipotent stromal cells-an archrival for mesenchymal stem cells. *Cell Tissue Res* 350(1):1–12.

Wang Y, Viennet C, Robin S, Berthon JY, He L and Humbert P (2017). Precise role of dermal fibroblasts on melanocyte pigmentation. *J Dermatol Sci* 88(2):159–166.

Yamada T, Hasegawa S, Inoue Y, Date Y, Yamamoto N, Mizutani H, et al. (2013). Wnt/β-catenin and kit signaling sequentially regulate melanocyte stem cell differentiation in UVB-induced epidermal pigmentation. *J Invest Dermatol* 133(12):2753–2762.

Zhou MN, Zhang ZQ, Wu JL, Lin FQ, Fu LF, Wang SQ, et al. (2013). Dermal mesenchymal stem cells (DMSCs) inhibit skin-homing CD8+ T cell activity, a determining factor of vitiligo patients' autologous melanocytes transplantation efficiency. *PLoS One* 8(4):e60254.

Zhu JW, Ni YJ, Tong XY, Guo X and Wu XP (2020). Activation of VEGF receptors in response to UVB promotes cell proliferation and melanogenesis of normal human melanocytes. *Exp Cell Res* 387(2):111798.

Zouboulis CC, Adjaye J, Akamatsu H, Moe-Behrens G and Niemann C (2008). Human skin stem cells and the ageing process. *Exp Gerontol* 43(11):986–997.

28

Interplay of Cancer-Associated Fibroblasts (CAFs) and Tumor-Associated Macrophages (TAMs) in Metastasis and Their Potential for Therapeutic Interventions

Indu Sharma and Anuradha Sharma
Department of Zoology, Panjab University, Chandigarh, India

28.1 Introduction

The concept of cancer being a non-healing wound is deep rooted in our society. Cancer tissue is composed of both carcinoma cells and stromal cells. The fibroblasts, adipocytes, inflammatory cells (lymphocytes and macrophages), and lymphatic as well as blood capillaries together make up the intra-tumoral stroma. In the early days, based on primitive knowledge cancer was misinterpreted to be confined only to the occurrence of genetic mutation and unstoppable cell growth. But now the increasing advancements of study have shed light on the role of the neighboring stromal cells that also secrete different growth factors and cytokines and thus promote tumorigenesis and metastasis (Xing et al., 2010). Recently, the cell–cell communications have also caught the attention of the researchers and play an important role in cancer initiation, promotion, and progression.

28.2 Cancer-Associated Fibroblasts

In particular, cancer-associated fibroblasts (CAFs) are the intra-tumoral fibroblasts and the key component of the tumor micro-environment, which differ from normal fibroblasts in the means of promoting cancer progression through the cytokine signals. The presence of mesenchymal markers (alpha-smooth muscle actin-ASMA, vimentin, paladin 4Ig, podoplanin) and absence of epithelial (cytokeratin), endothelial (CD31) and fully differentiated smooth muscle (smoothelin) markers have been used to define myofibroblasts as a population of morphologically similar cells in the peri-tumoral microenvironment that does not express all these markers yet shares certain functional and lineage traits with CAFs (Serini and Gabbiani, 1999; Eyden, 2008). However, none of these markers by themselves is unique to CAFs. In addition to the circumstantial evidence, these cells constitute a substantial volume of the tumor mass in certain epithelial tumors such as pancreatic, gastric, and breast cancers, as much as 50–70% (Desmouliere et al., 2004).

Although many discrete features of morphology and physiology of CAFs have been identified, CAFs owe their high heterogeneity to their different origins. It has become quite evident now that the cross-talk between the cancer cells and the CAFs mediate the proliferation of cancer cells, and therefore targeting this mutual interaction between the two would eventually pave the way for cancer treatment (Xing et al., 2010). Considering all the normal stromal components, fibroblasts are indispensible for the production and deposition of the extracellular matrix (ECM) as they produce a variety of collagens and fibronectin. The paracrine and autocrine growth factors known to regulate the growth of themselves, and the neighboring cells are also supplied by these fibroblasts (Nakamura et al., 1997).

Interestingly, fibroblasts do not only tether to the wear and tear of the ECM and basement membrane, they can also regulate the integrity of ECM through the proteases such as matrix metalloproteinases (MMPs). These proteases are capable of disrupting the ECM through various mechanisms (Simian et al., 2001). Wound healing is another application of fibroblasts where they provide a scaffold for tissue regeneration in the form of ECM. During this process they get converted into the specific type called myofibroblasts, which have higher capability of ECM synthesis. These myofibroblasts regain their phenotype after some time through unknown mechanisms (Hanahan and Weinburg, 2000).

An alarming number of CAFs morphologically similar to the myofibroblasts (associated with wound healing) form the stromal component of the cancerous tissue along with the fibrin deposition. The tumor cells are capable of modulating the surrounding stroma as per their need. This theory has been validated by a study in which approximately 80% of the fibroblasts were found to be activated in breast cancer (Sappino et al., 1988). Unlike the normal fibroblasts and the myofibroblasts involved in wound healing, CAFs are everlastingly activated, which means that they neither revert back to their normal phenotype nor undergo apoptosis (Li et al., 2007).

28.2.1 Different Origins of CAFs

28.2.1.1 Normal Fibroblasts

Not only the CAFs are sensitive to the ECM including growth factors and cytokines, but they are also susceptible to the genetic alterations (Tsellou and Kiaris, 2008). In a study, it was observed that cancer-promoting characteristics of CAFs do not exclusively depend upon the exposure of cancer cells, but can be stably maintained even in a normal environment. These observations indicate that the cancer stroma may have undergone some genetic or epigenetic changes independent of the original tumor (Littlepage et al., 2005). The epithelium of breast carcinoma continuously undergoes various somatic mutations of the two genes obligatory to cell cycle arrest (i.e., P53 and PTEN). It is already well-known that their malfunction directly leads to cancer progression. Interestingly, the CAFs surrounding the cancer regions possess the inactivation of these two genes (Mayo et al., 2002).

28.2.1.2 Epithelial Cells Through Epithelial-Mesenchymal Transition

Epithelial-mesenchymal transition (EMT) is a process in which the epithelial cells having tight junctions get converted into mesenchymal cells with a loose cell-cell adhesion. The special case of EMT occurs when the myofibroblasts are transdifferentiated from the epithelial cells, which produce CAFs only rather than tumor cells (Forino et al., 2006). It may be estimated that under favorable conditions, the breast cancer cells may give rise to CAFs through myofibroblasts as the intermediate products (Petersen et al., 2001). The CAFs generated through EMT enhance the cancer growth and metastasis considerably. Genetic evidence has also been obtained that supports the origin of CAFs found in human breast cancer biopsies from the epithelial tumor cells (Petersen et al., 2003).

28.2.1.3 Mesenchymal Cells

It has been reported that bone marrow is associated with the myofibroblasts and fibroblasts of the desmoplastic response along with the tumor angiogenesis (Direkze and Alison, 2006). Recent evidence also claimed that there is a selective proliferation of mesenchymal stem cells (MSC) in tumor areas wherein they contribute to the CAF formation. In another study by Mishra and co-workers it was found that when the mesenchymal stem cells isolated from human bone marrow (hMSCs) were exposed to tumor-conditioned medium (TCM) of human breast cancer cell line (MDA-MB231) for an extensive time period, the cells showed functional similarity to CAFs along with the expression of SDF-1 (Mishra et al., 2008).

28.2.2 Role of CAF in Tumorigenesis And Metastasis

28.2.2.1 Support Primary Tumor Growth

Tumor cells employ supportive stromal cells for the sake of unhindered growth and propagation at metastatic sites. CAFs are responsible for releasing various growth factors and cytokines like TGF-beta, hepatocyte growth factor (HGF), and fibroblast secreted protein-1 (FSP1) into adjacent cancer cells. In a study, it was found that tumor formation is rare when metastatic cancer cells are transplanted into FSP1 knockout mice. On the other hand, simultaneously injecting fibroblasts with high expression of FSP1 with the same tumor cells initiates tumor formation (Grum-Schwensen et al., 2005). The results revealed that the FSP1 produced by CAFs mold the tumor microenvironment in order to make it favorable for cancer growth. Furthermore, tumorigenic ability is also greatly enhanced by the CAFs as the reactive oxygen species (ROS) produced by CAFs under low pH and hypoxia serve as a mutagen for the surrounding cells (Yuan and Glazer, 1998).

Furthermore, various types of cancer tissues have been found to highly express TGF-beta such as colon (Tsushima et al., 1996) and breast cancers (Serra and Crowley, 2003). TGF-beta is the only growth factor identified to be involved in the transdifferentiation of fibroblasts into CAFs (Ronnov-Jessen and Petersen, 1993). Moreover, TGF-beta serves as a potent chemo-attractant for human dermal fibroblasts, which employs the fibroblasts outside of the tumor region (Postlethwaite et al., 1987). Since present in abundance, the CAFs also mediate the metabolic pathways in cancer cells and thus affect the cancer growth (Figure 28.1). They preferably switch to anaerobic glycolysis even in the presence of oxygen. They also instigate some complementary metabolic pathways dealing with the reprocessing of products of anaerobic metabolism, which in turn promotes the cancer cell growth (Koukourakis et al., 2006).

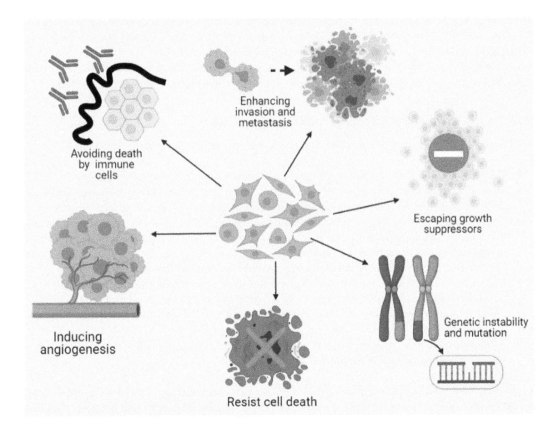

FIGURE 28.1 Role of CAFs in cancer progression.

28.2.2.2 Sustaining Invasion and Metastasis of Tumor Cells

CAFs found in the vicinity of cancer cells not only promote cancer cell growth but also upsurge their power to invade through cell-cell interactions (Powell et al., 1999). CAFs initiate the invasive growth by means of cell-cell communication and paracrine signaling. The cancer cells and CAFs interact with each other to modulate the adjacent ECM and basement membrane. It is already known that the disruption of basement membrane initiates the intravasation of cancer cells into the circulatory system. CAFs have also been reported to serve as the guiding element for the relocation of cancer cells.

In an experiment where different cell types were co-cultured with cancer cells, it was found that the most prominent cells to invade were of stromal origin, and they disrupted the ECM and basement membrane in order to enhance the cancer cell metastasis (Gaggioli et al., 2007). As already discussed, the MMPs are responsible for regulating the integrity of the ECM and hence are important for the cancer proliferation and metastasis. Therefore, it becomes necessary to maintain the balance between the MMPs and their inhibitors under normal conditions. For example, urokinase-type plasminogen activator (uPA) activates the matrix-degrading proteases by cleaving the MMPs, and this enhanced MMP activity causes significant ECM disruption, leading to angiogenesis and metastasis (Lu et al., 2011).

28.2.2.3 Induce Inflammation in Cancer Regions

Cancer cells are known to secrete the pro-inflammatory cytokines around them and CAFs recruit excessive immune cells like macrophages, neutrophils, and lymphocytes in the area. Macrophages release a number of factors that influence the endothelial cell behavior like VEGF, HGF, MMP2, and IL-8. Once recruited in the tumor region, the macrophages get transformed into tumor-associated macrophages (TAMs) (Leek and Harris, 2002). Stromal cells contribute to create a unique environment of chronic inflammation and immune tolerance for the survival and proliferation of cancer cells (Swann and Smyth, 2007) (Figure 28.2). Thrombospondin-1 (TSP-1) is produced by the stromal cells and poses both positive and negative feedback on angiogenesis and interaction with immune cells (Li et al., 2007). As mentioned previously, CAFs excessively secrete MMPs, which on cleaving produce fibronectin and collagen, which attract leukocytes, and thus modulate the proliferation of the immune cells (Brundula et al., 2002).

28.2.3 CAFs as Potential Targets of Anti-Cancer Therapy

Targeting the CAFs may make the anti-cancer therapy more efficient because of the following features:

1. CAFs are known to support tumor epithelial proliferation, angiogenesis, and invasion.
2. Stromal cells are less prone to *de novo* acquisition of genetic mutations than malignant epithelial cells, so CAFs may be less susceptible to escape or resistance to therapy via genomic instability.
3. Current cancer therapy (both chemo- and radiation therapy) often results in residual fibrosis and it has been pointed out recently that adjuvant therapy may need to target this fibrosis as well as residual tumor embedded within it (Harless, 2009).
4. CAF-derived factors may interfere with anti-cancer therapies (Crawford et al., 2009).
5. CAF-derived factors can contribute to the recruitment of bone-marrow derived cells (BMDCs), commonly called endothelial progenitor cells, to tumor micro-environment (Orimo et al., 2005).
6. Tumor stroma may prevent effective immune surveillance or anti-tumor immune response (Zhang, 2008).
7. A negative correlation may exist between the magnitude of the desmoplastic stromal reaction and survival in certain cancers (Maeshima et al., 2002).

However, the wound healing or fibrosis that follows surgery, chemotherapy, and radiation therapy may also be a source of factors that can support recurrence and metastasis and thus stromal therapies may also emerge as important in the adjuvant setting. As the differentiation into an activated CAF is increasingly viewed as a key carcinogenic event, inhibition of differentiation has become another attractive therapeutic target.

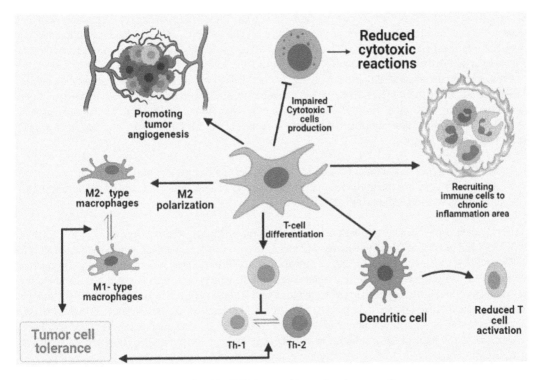

FIGURE 28.2 Immune-suppression mediated by CAFs by recruiting various immune cells.

While not yet done in a cancer system, myofibroblast differentiation from hepatic stellate cells was halted by inhibition of DNMT1 by 5-aza-2-deoxycytidine (5aza-dC) (Mann et al., 2007). Especially in the context of the importance of epigenetic regulations in myofibroblast function, this finding may be particularly of relevance. In addition, certain epithelial cell-derived MMPs (i.e. MMP7) may have a role in myofibroblast differentiation and can be targeted in therapy (Hemers et al., 2005; McCaig et al., 2006).

The recognition of the active role that CAFs play in carcinogenesis adds a new level of complexity to cancer biology but also brings an opportunity for new therapeutic strategies. Understanding the genetics and epigenetics of this stromal compartment will be especially important in order to differentiate CAFs as therapeutic targets. Altered DNA methylation in CAFs has been a common finding across several recent animal and human studies and as this epigenetic mark can be targeted by available drugs epigenetic therapy against CAFs will be an interesting avenue for future research.

28.3 Tumor-Associated Macrophages

Metastasis is the main reason for the mortality caused by cancer. It depends on the intrinsic genetic alterations as well as the mutual interaction between the tumor cells and their neighboring extracellular components. Macrophages that infiltrate the tumor tissue are called TAMs. These TAMs play a crucial role in growth, angiogenesis, and metastasis, and in regulating the chemo-resistance in the cancer cells. They also function to design an immune-suppressive environment for tumor cells by secreting various cytokines, chemokines, etc., and also stimulate the T-cells to release inhibitory immune proteins (Lin et al., 2019). Accordingly, in many but not all human tumors, a high frequency of infiltrating TAM leads to poor prognosis.

Usually, the metastasis of tumor cells undergoes multiple stages in a cyclic manner, which starts from the invasion at primary sites and ends at growth and division at the metastatic sites (Scully et al., 2012; Fidler and Kripke, 2015). TAMs being the prominent promoters of the tumor micro-environment mediate all the cascade steps of this cyclic progression. Therefore, TAMs have been explored as the potential target for designing therapeutic strategies against cancer. The occurrence of TAM-derived inflammatory cytokines interleukin (IL)-23 and IL-17 have been shown to trigger the inflammation stimulated by tumor cells, which in turn drives tumor growth (Grivennikov et al., 2012).

Another study demonstrated that the high expression of IL-6 stimulated by TAM further exaggerates the inflammation and through STAT3 signalling facilitates the initiation and proliferation of hepatocellular carcinoma mediated (Kong et al., 2016). Further, the transformation of TAMs into M2 phenotype acts as a key step for the tumor development and metastasis (Laoui et al., 2011). The activated macrophages fall under two distinct classes:

1. M1, which generate the inflammation response against pathogens and tumor cells and
2. M2, which carry out the immune-suppressive role and enhance the tissue repair and tumor proliferation (Biswas and Mantovani, 2010).

M1 macrophages secrete pro-inflammatory cytokines (IL-12, tumor necrosis factor (TNF)-α, CXCL-10, and interferon (IFN)-γ) whereas M2 macrophages secrete anti-inflammatory cytokines (IL-10, IL-13, and IL-4) (Qian and Pollard, 2010; Movahed et al., 2010). These two phenotypes get converted to one another in response to micro-environmental stimuli, which may include cytokines, chemokines, growth factors, and other signals derived from tumor and stromal cells (Qian and Pollard, 2010), and this process is called "macrophage polarization" (Figure 28.3). Most researchers consider TAMs to be M2 phenotype (Laoui et al., 2011). A powerful pro-tumor factor vascular endothelial growth factor A (VEGF-A) (Ferrara, 2009) induces TAM infiltration and M2 conversion in the presence of IL-4 and IL-10 (Linde et al., 2012).

Hypoxia is a common characteristic of majority of carcinomas (Vaupel and Harrison, 2004). It favors the tumor growth and proliferation by allowing escape from immune system-enhancing glycolysis, promoting dedifferentiation and reducing the efficiency of therapeutics (Chae et al., 2016; Zhang and Sadek, 2014). It also allows the tumor cells to overpower the nutritive scarcity and makes the TME favorable to the cancer cell growth. The TAMs migrate to the hypoxic sites under the influence of chemokines like CCL2, CCL5, CSF-1, VEGF, semaphorin 3A (SEMA3A), endothelin, stromal cell-derived factor (SDF)-1α, etc. (Henze and Mazzone, 2016) (Figure 28.4).

Cancer is one of the most life-threatening diseases and holds an extremely high rate of incidence and mortality globally. TAMs account for one of the most crucial components of the tumor microenvironment and play a key role in the cancer development and proliferation. Therefore, it will be extremely beneficial to design therapeutic strategies for cancer targeting TAMs. Briefly these strategies may be based on stopping TAM infiltration and suppressing macrophage polarization, and thus reducing the number of TAMs overall.

However, it must also be noted that TAMs do not function individually to promote metastasis but in collaboration with the network of other cells present in tumor microenvironment, which include fibroblasts, neutrophils, mesenchymal stem cells, etc. (Joyce and Pollard, 2009). Therefore, while designing the therapeutic strategies against cancer, one must take into consideration the flexibility and versatility of this collaboration failing, which may jeopardize the efficiency of valid research.

28.4 Conclusions

Carcinoma cell lines help us in better understanding the dynamics of cancer cell biology. Numerous researchers have used these carcinoma cell lines as a single- or mono-culture. But it should also be kept in mind that the mono-culture system is not sufficient to evaluate the interactions between carcinoma and intra-tumoral stromal cells. Therefore, the co-culture of two different types of cancer tissues (i.e., cancerous cell lines and fibroblasts, macrophages, and other cell types) can be employed in order to evaluate cell–cell interactions in this cancer micro-environment. Despite many critical obstacles still lying ahead, TAMs and CAFs represent novel and worthy candidates, which may pave the way for new therapeutic

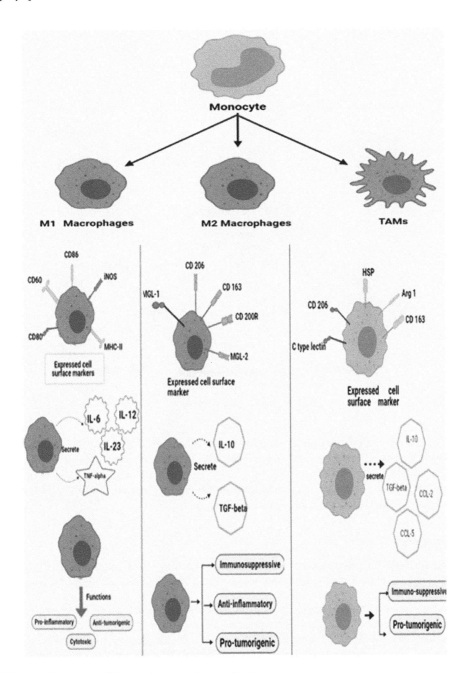

FIGURE 28.3 Macrophage differentiation and their respective functions.

approaches to be employed for the cure of cancer in future. This co-culture system provides an advantage of evaluating cell-cell interactions of cancer micro-environment and enables us:

- To understand the mechanisms by which cancer cells communicate with surrounding normal cells and enlist their help in promoting tumor growth by evaluating cell proliferation, migration, gene expression, and receptor expression.
- To elucidate how cells and tissues in different organs interact with cancer cells to prevent or promote metastasis (spread).

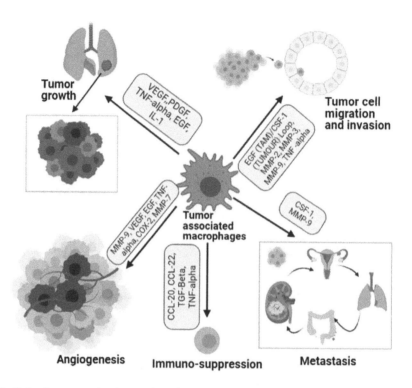

FIGURE 28.4   Role of tumor-associated macrophages in cancer progression.

- To characterize the components of the tumor microenvironment including the cancer cells and connective tissue cells (fibroblasts) and immune cells to determine their individual and collective influences on tumor progression.
- To understand the genetic and epigenetic changes that give rise to cancer as well as how genes are abnormally regulated metabolically via stress response.

REFERENCES

Barcellos-Hoff (1993) Radiation-induced transforming growth factor beta and subsequent extracellular matrix reorganization in murine mammary gland. Cancer Res 53:3880–3886. https://doi.org/10.1038/nrc1735

Biswas SK, Mantovani A (2010) Macrophage plasticity and interaction with lymphocyte subsets: cancer as a paradigm. Nat Immunol 11(10):889–896. https://doi.org/10.1038/ni.1937

Brundula V, Rewcastle NB, Metz LM, Bernard CC, Yong VW (2002) Targeting leukocyte MMPs and transmigration: minocycline as a potential therapy for multiple sclerosis. Brain 125:1297–1308. https://doi.org/10.1093/brain/awf133

Chae YC, Vaira V, Caino MC, Tang HY, Seo JH, Kossenkov AV, et al. (2016) Mitochondrial akt regulation of hypoxic tumor reprogramming. Cancer Cell 30(2):257–272. https://doi.org/10.1016/j.ccell.2016.07.004

Crawford Y, Kasman I, Yu L, Zhong C, Wu X, Modrusan Z, et al. (2009) PDGF-C mediates the angiogenic and tumorigenic properties of fibroblasts associated with tumors refractory to anti-VEGF treatment. Cancer Cell 15 (1):21–34. https://doi.org/10.1016/j.ccr.2008.12.004

Desmouliere A, Guyot C, Gabbiani G (2004) The stroma reaction myofibroblast: a key player in the control of tumor cell behavior. Int J Dev Biol 48(5-6): 509–517. https://doi.org/10.1387/ijdb.041802ad

Direkze NC, Alison MR (2006) Bone marrow and tumour stroma: an intimate relationship. Hematol Oncol 24:189–195. https://doi.org/10.1002/hon.788

Eyden, B (2008) The myofibroblast: phenotypic characterization as a prerequisite to understanding its functions in translational medicine. J Cell Mol Med 12(1): 22–37. https://doi.org/10.1111/j.1582-4934.2007.00213.x

Fidler IJ, Kripke ML (2015) The challenge of targeting metastasis. Cancer Metastasis Rev 34(4):635–641. https://doi.org/10.1007/s10555-015-9586-9

Forino M, Torregrossa R, Ceol M, Murer L, Della Vella M, Del Prete D, et al. (2006) TGF beta1 induces epithelial-mesenchymal transition, but not myofibroblast transdifferentiation of human kidney tubular epithelial cells in primary culture. Int J Exp Pathol 87:197–208. https://doi.org/10.1111/j.1365-2613.2006.00479.x

Gaggioli C, Hooper S, Hidalgo-Carcedo C, Grosse R, Marshall JF, Harrington K, Sahai E (2007) Fibroblast-led collective invasion of carcinoma cells with differing roles for RhoGTPases in leading and following cells. Nat Cell Biol 9:1392–1400. https://doi.org/10.1038/ncb1658

Grivennikov SI, Wang K, Mucida D, Stewart CA, Schnabl B, Jauch D, et al. (2012) Adenoma-linked barrier defects and microbial products drive IL-23/IL-17-mediated tumour growth. Nature 491(7423):254–258. https://doi.org/10.1038/nature11465

Grum-Schwensen B, Klingelhofer J, Berg CH, El-Naaman C, Grigorian M, Lukanidin E, Ambartsumian N (2005) Suppression of tumor development and metastasis formation in mice lacking the S100A4(mts1) gene. Cancer Res 65:3772–3780. https://doi.org/10.1158/0008-5472.CAN-04-4510

Hanahan D, Weinberg RA (2000) The hallmarks of cancer. Cell 100(1): 57–70. https://doi.org/10.1016/S0092-8674(00)81683-9

Harless WW (2009) Revisiting perioperative chemotherapy: the critical importance of targeting residual cancer prior to wound healing. BMC Cancer 9(1):118. https://doi.org/10.1186/1471-2407-9-1181186/1471-2407-9

Hemers E, Duval C, McCaig C, Handley M, Dockray GJ, Varro A (2005) Insulin-like growth factor binding protein-5 is a target of matrix metalloproteinase-7: implications for epithelial mesenchymal signaling. Cancer Res 65(16):7363–7369. https://doi.org/10.1158/0008-5472.CAN-05-0157

Henze AT, Mazzone M (2016) The impact of hypoxia on tumor-associated macrophages. J Clin Invest 126(10):3672–3679. https://doi.org/10.1172/JCI84427

Joyce JA, Pollard JW (2009) Microenvironmental regulation of metastasis. Nat Rev Cancer 9(4):239–252. https://doi.org/10.1038/nrc2618

Koukourakis MI, Giatromanolaki A, Harris AL, Sivridis E (2006) Comparison of metabolic pathways between cancer cells and stromal cells in colorectal carcinomas: a metabolic survival role for tumor-associated stroma. Cancer Res 66:632–637. https://doi.org/10.1158/0008-5472.CAN-05-3260

Laoui D, Movahedi K, Van Overmeire E, Van den Bossche J, Schouppe E, Mommer C, et al. (2011) Tumor-associated macrophages in breast cancer: distinct subsets, distinct functions. Int J Dev Biol 55(7-9):861–867. https://doi.org/10.1387/ijdb.113371dl.

Leek RD, Harris AL (2002) Tumor-associated macrophages in breast cancer. J Mammary Gland Biol Neoplasia 7:177–189. https://doi.org/10.1023/A:1020304003704

Li H, Fan X, Houghton J (2007) Tumor microenvironment: the role of the tumor stroma in cancer. J Cell Biochem 101(4), 805–815. https://doi.org/10.1002/jcb.21159

Lin Y, Xu J, Lan H (2019) Tumor-associated macrophages in tumor metastasis: biological roles and clinical therapeutic applications. J Hematol Oncol 12(1), 76. https://doi.org/10.1186/s13045-019-0760-3

Linde N, Lederle W, Depner S, van Rooijen N, Gutschalk CM, Mueller MM (2012) Vascular endothelial growth factor-induced skin carcinogenesis depends on recruitment and alternative activation of macrophages. J Pathol 227(1): 17–28. https://doi.org/10.1002/path.3989

Littlepage LE, Egeblad M, Werb Z (2005) Coevolution of cancer and stromal cellular responses. Cancer Cell 7:499–500. https://doi.org/10.1016/j.ccr.2005.05.019

Lu P, Takai K, Weaver VM, Werb Z (2011) Extracellular matrix degradation and remodeling in development and disease. Cold Spring Harb Perspect Biol 3(12): a005058. https://doi.org/10.1101/cshperspect.a005058.

Maeshima AM, Niki T, Maeshima A, Yamada T, Kondo H, Matsuno Y (2002) Modified scar grade: a prognostic indicator in small peripheral lung adenocarcinoma. Cancer 95(12):2546–54. https://doi.org/10.1002/cncr.11006

Mann J, Oakley F, Akiboye F, Elsharkawy A, Thorne AW, Mann DA (2007) Regulation of myofibroblast transdifferentiation by DNA methylation and MeCP2: implications for wound healing and fibrogenesis. Cell Death Differ 14(2):275–85. https://doi.org/10.1038/sj.cdd.4401979

Mayo LD, Dixon JE, Durden DL, Tonks NK, Donner DB (2002) PTEN protects p53 from Mdm2 and sensitizes cancer cells to chemotherapy. J Biol Chem 277:5484–5489. https://doi.org/10.1074/jbc.M108302200

McCaig C, Duval C, Hemers E, Steele I, Pritchard DM, Przemeck S, et al. (2006) The role of matrix metalloproteinase-7 in redefining the gastric microenvironment in response to Helicobacter pylori. Gastroenterology 130(6):1754–1763. http://doi.org/10.1053/j.gastro.2006.02.031

Mishra PJ, Mishra PJ, Humeniuk R, Medina DJ, Alexe G, Mesirov JP, et al. (2008) Carcinoma-associated fibroblast-like differentiation of human mesenchymal stem cells. Cancer Res 68:4331–4339. https://doi.org/10.1158/0008-5472.CAN-08-0943

Movahedi K, Laoui D, Gysemans C, Baeten M, Stange G, Van den Bossche J, et al. (2010) Different tumor microenvironments contain functionally distinct subsets of macrophages derived from Ly6C(high) monocytes. Cancer Res 70(14):5728–5739. https://doi.org/10.1158/0008-5472.CAN-09-4672

Nakamura T, Matsumoto K, Kiritoshi, A, Tano Y (1997) Induction of hepatocyte growth factor in fibroblasts by tumor-derived factors affects invasive growth of tumor cells: in vitro analysis of tumor-stromal interactions. Cancer Res 57(15), 3305–3313. https://pubmed.ncbi.nlm.nih.gov/9242465/

Orimo A, Gupta PB, Sgroi DC, Arenzana-Seisdedos F, Delaunay T, Naeem R, et al. (2005) Stromal fibroblasts present in invasive human breast carcinomas promote tumor growth and angiogenesis through elevated SDF-1/CXCL12 secretion. Cell 121:335–48. https://doi.org/10.1016/j.cell.2005.02.034

Petersen OW, Lind Nielsen H, Gudjonsson T, Villadsen R, Ronnov-Jessen L, Bissell MJ (2001) The plasticity of human breast carcinoma cells is more than epithelial to mesenchymal conversion. Breast Cancer Res 3:213–217. https://doi.org/10.1186/bcr298

Petersen OW, Nielsen HL, Gudjonsson T, Villadsen R, Rank F, Niebuhr E, et al. (2003) Epithelial to mesenchymal transition in human breast cancer can provide a nonmalignant stroma. Am J Pathol 162:391–402. https://doi.org/10.1016/S0002-9440(10)63834-5

Postlethwaite AE, Keski-Oja J, Moses HL, Kang AH (1987) Stimulation of the chemotactic migration of human fibroblasts by transforming growth factor beta. J Exp Med 165:251–256. https://doi.org/10.1084/jem.165.1.251

Powell DW, Mifflin RC, Valentich JD, Crowe SE, Saada JI, West AB (1999) Myofibroblasts. I. Paracrine cells important in health and disease. Am J Physiol 277:C1–C9. https://doi.org/10.1152/ajpcell.1999.277.1.C1

Qian BZ, Pollard JW (2010) Macrophage diversity enhances tumor progression and metastasis. Cell 141(1):39–51. https://doi.org/10.1016/j.cell.2010.03.014

Ronnov-Jessen L, Petersen OW (1993) Induction of alpha-smooth muscle actin by transforming growth factor-beta 1 in quiescent human breast gland fibroblasts. Implications for myofibroblast generation in breast neoplasia. Lab Invest 68:696–707. https://pubmed.ncbi.nlm.nih.gov/8515656/

Sappino AP, Skalli O, Jackson B, Schurch W, Gabbiani G (1988) Smooth-muscle differentiation in stromal cells of malignant and non-malignant breast tissues. Int J Cancer 41(5): 707–712. https://doi.org/10.1002/ijc.2910410512

Scully OJ, Bay BH, Yip G, Yu YN (2012) Breast cancer metastasis. Cancer Genomics Proteomics 9 (5):311–20. https://pubmed.ncbi.nlm.nih.gov/22990110/

Serini G, Gabbiani G (1999) Mechanisms of myofibroblast activity and phenotypic modulation. Exp Cell Res 250(2): 273–283. https://doi.org/10.1006/excr.1999.4543

Serra R, Crowley MR (2003) TGF-beta in mammary gland development and breast cancer. Breast Dis 18:61–73. https://doi.org/10.3233/bd-2003-18107

Simian M, Hirai Y, Navre M, Werb Z, Lochter A, Bissell MJ (2001) The interplay of matrix metalloproteinases, morphogens and growth factors is necessary for branching of mammary epithelial cells. Development 128(16): 3117–3131. https://www.ncbi.nlm.nih.gov/pmc/articles/PMC2785713/

Swann JB, Smyth MJ (2007) Immune surveillance of tumors. J Clin Invest 117:1137–1146. https://doi.org/10.1172/JCI31405

Tsellou E, Kiaris H (2008) Fibroblast independency in tumors: implications in cancer therapy. Future Oncol 4(3): 427–432. https://doi.org/10.2217/14796694.4.3.427

Tsushima H, Kawata S, Tamura S, Ito N, Shirai Y, Kiso S, et al. (1996) High levels of transforming growth factor beta 1 in patients with colorectal cancer: association with disease progression. Gastroenterology 110:375–382. https://doi.org/10.1053/gast.1996.v110.pm8566583

Vaupel P, Harrison L (2004) Tumor hypoxia: causative factors, compensatory mechanisms, and cellular response. Oncologist 9:4–9. https://doi.org/10.1634/theoncologist.9-90005-4

Xing F, Saidou J, Watabe K (2010) Cancer associated fibroblasts (CAFs) in tumor microenvironment. Frontiers in bioscience (Landmark edition) 15:166–179. https://doi.org/10.2741/3613

Yuan J, Glazer PM (1998) Mutagenesis induced by the tumor microenvironment. Mutat Res 400:439–446. https://doi.org/10.1016/s0027-5107(98)00042-6

Zhang B (2008) Targeting the stroma by T cells to limit tumor growth. Cancer Res 68(23):9570–9573. https://doi.org/10.1158/0008-5472.CAN-08-2414

Zhang CC, Sadek HA (2014) Hypoxia and metabolic properties of hematopoietic stem cells. Antioxidants and Redox Signalling 20(12):1891–901. https://doi.org/10.1089/ars.2012.5019.

29

Lantibiotics: Strengthening Our Armor Against Antibiotic-Resistant Pathogens

Shweta Kishen, Mangal Singh, and Dipti Sareen
Department of Biochemistry, Panjab University, Chandigarh, India

29.1 Introduction

29.1.1 Antimicrobial Natural Products

Production of antimicrobial compounds is a part of innate immune systems in all the life forms, from bacteria to plants and animals. Bacteria employs antibiotics and antimicrobial peptides to target specific bacteria that might compete for the same resources. These antimicrobials are a part of the battery of natural products (NPs) produced by bacteria, which also include the terpenoids and alkaloids (Arnison et al., 2013). Since the discovery of penicillin in 1928 by Alexander Fleming, many classes of antibiotics have been discovered and used in treatment of bacterial infections. In the initial phase of antibiotic discovery, many new classes of antibiotics were discovered and within a year or less of the introduction of antibiotics in therapeutics, antibiotic-resistant strains developed (Mishra et al., 2012), thus posing a need for the identification of novel antibiotics. More potent drugs are being developed by modifying the existing drug, which act on an established target and also drugs are being explored that can act on targets alternative to these (Khan and Khan, 2016).

The initial phase of antibiotic discovery was fast enough to discover many classes of antibiotics, which later ceased with various cases of rediscoveries, after a resource-hungry screening process (Baltz, 2007; Sandiford, 2017). The later years saw an upsurgence in the discovery of antibiotics with the advancing sequencing technologies, faster computing, and development of bioinformatic tools (Baltz, 2014; Medema and Fischbach, 2015). This enhancement reduced the risk of rediscovery and a pool of unexplored natural products were identified within the bacterial genomes, from where antibiotics were already discovered. Most antibiotics in use today are non-ribosomal natural products, synthesized by mega-synthases known as polyketide synthases (PKSs) and non-ribosomal peptide synthetases (NRPSs) (Singh et al., 2017). The examples include the polyketides like erythromycin, nystatin, rifamycin, etc., synthesized by PKSs and non-ribosomal peptide antibiotics like actinomycin, chloramphenicol, cyclosporine, pristinamycin, etc., synthesized by NRPSs. Although non-ribosomal antibiotics are high in number, the need of the hour is to discover novel antibiotics that can treat the drug-resistant pathogens.

Bacteria produce peptides and proteins of ribosomal origin that inhibit growth of other related bacteria known as bacteriocins. One class of bacteriocins includes ribosomally synthesized and post-translationally modified peptides (RiPPs), known as lantibiotics. These are antimicrobial peptides containing unique lanthionine rings or thioether bridges. Lantibiotics, owing to their unique mode of action, have been found active against drug-resistant pathogenic bacteria like vancomycin-resistant *Enterococci* (VRE) and *Staphylococcus aureus* (VRSA), *methicillin-resistant Staphylococcus aureus* (MRSA), etc. (Begley et al., 2009; Delves-Broughton et al., 1996). Besides the antimicrobial activity, lantibiotics have also shown antiviral, antiallodynic, antinociceptive and antidiabetic activity (Van Staden et al., 2021). Both ribosomally synthesized and non-ribosomally synthesized antibiotics are macrocyclized to generate a peptide diversity that leads to diverse activities, which is not possible at the ribosomal level. A comparison of ribosomal and non-ribosomal route of natural product synthesis is given in Figure 29.1.

DOI: 10.1201/9781003220404-32

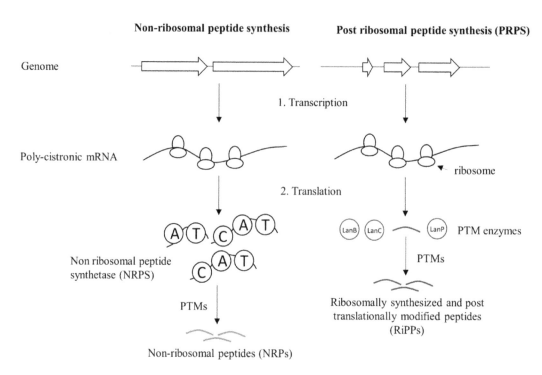

FIGURE 29.1   A comparison of the two routes of natural product synthesis. Non-ribosomal peptides (NRP) are synthesized by enzymes known as NRPS, instead of ribosomes and hence known as non-ribosomal peptide synthesis. NRPs undergo posttranslational modification either by the domains of NRPS (not shown) in *cis* or other genome-encoded enzymes in *trans*. Post-ribosomal peptide synthesis (PRPS) involves PTMs of a ribosomally synthesized peptide by co-translated PTM enzymes.

29.1.2 Ribosomally Synthesized and Post-Translationally Modified Peptides

A majority of peptide natural products are ribosomally synthesized, which undergo extensive post-translational modifications. Historically, these were classified depending upon the producer organisms, like the *microcins* produced by Gram-negative bacteria or their biological activities like the *bacteriocins*. In a recent classification, these are termed as RiPPs with a size limit of 10 kDa to differentiate from the post-translationally modified proteins. The biosynthetic pathway of RiPPs is termed as PRPS opposed to the non-ribosomal peptide synthesis of NRPS (Figure 29.1).

29.1.3 Lantibiotics

Lantibiotics are antimicrobial peptides containing lanthionine bridges. These bridges or rings are responsible for restricting the conformational flexibility of the peptide for its bioactivity and stability. A ribosomally synthesized peptide of ~20–110 amino acid residues undergoes a two-step post-translational modification in the C-terminal core-peptide region for introduction of these bridges (Figure 29.2). The first step involves dehydration of some serine and threonine residues to form 2,3-didehydroalanine (Dha) and 2,3-didehydrobutyrine (Dhb), respectively (Figure 29.3). In the second step, these dehydrated residues undergo Michael type addition with neighbouring intra-peptide cysteine residues, leading to generation of thioether bridged lanthionine (lan) and/or (methyl)lanthionine (MeLan) rings (Figure 29.4). The serine and threonine residues are dehydrated to

form electrophilic centres for the enzymatic attack of the nucleophilic sulfhydryl group (Okeley et al., 2003). The amino acid encoded in the precursor peptide are all L-amino acids but the Lan and MeLan show DL configuration. The cysteine half being L and serine/threonine half as D (i.e., lanthionine formation

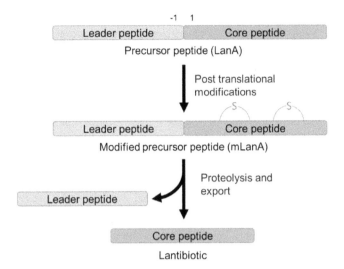

FIGURE 29.2   Lantibiotic synthesis. The leader and the core peptide region comprise the precursor peptide. PTMs occur in the C-terminal core-peptide region and leader and are removed for bioactive lantibiotic formation. The position of amino acid residues in leader are numbered in negative. Modification in the core peptide is depicted with thioether bridge formation, whose number can vary.

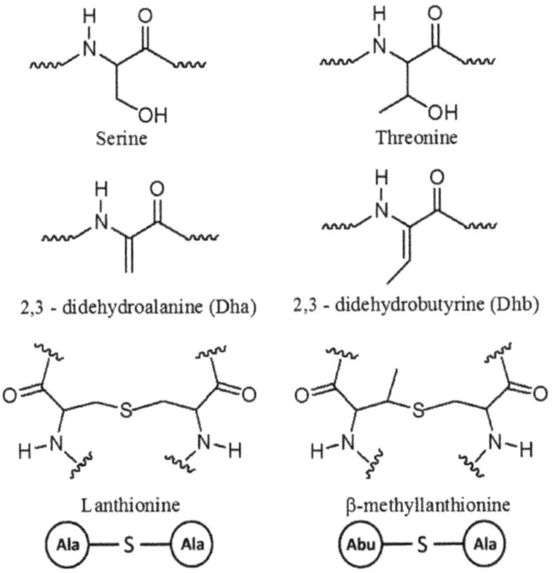

FIGURE 29.3   Lanthionine and (methyl)lanthionine moieties. Serine and threonine residues are dehydrated to Dha and Dhb to form lanthionine and β-(methyl)lanthionine by addition of cysteine. Thioether links two alanine (Ala) in lanthionine rings and aminobutyrine (Abu) and alanine in the case of β-(methyl)lanthionine (MeLan).

leads to inversion of chirality of the serine and threonine alpha carbon). There are also unusual examples of MeLan where LL stereochemistry is observed when Dhx-Dhx-Xxx-Xxx-Cys motif is present (Lohans et al., 2014; Zhao and van der Donk, 2016). The peptide after thioether bridge formation undergoes a proteolytic cleavage to remove the N-terminal leader sequence, only after which it becomes antimicrobial (Figure 29.4). The lanthionine rings are responsible for a conformationally constrained peptide structure

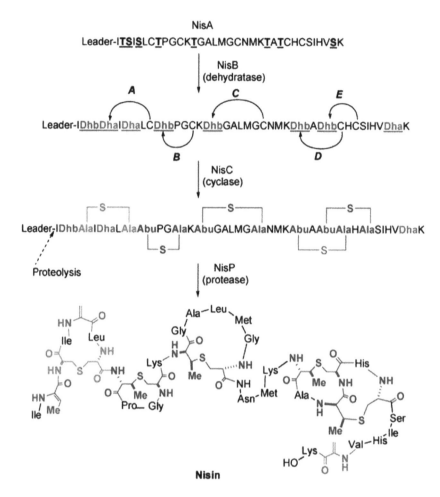

FIGURE 29.4 Biosynthesis of nisin. A typical lantibiotic biosynthesis with dehydration and cyclization (thioether bridge formation) reactions followed by proteolytic cleavage. Class II lanthipeptides are synthesized by a single lanthionine synthetase LanM for both these reactions. (adopted from Chatterjee et al., 2005).

that can penetrate the bacterial membrane (Figure 29.4), are resistant to proteolytic cleavage, are highly thermostable, and target specific.

29.1.4 Gene organization

The genes for lantibiotic biosynthesis are clustered and represented with generic locus symbol "*lan*." These cluster contains one or more genes for the structural/precursor peptide (*lanA*), modification enzymes (*lanB, lanC, lanM, LanD, LanO*, etc.), transport (*lanT*), transcriptional regulation (*lanR, lanK*), proteolytic processing (*lanP*), and immunity genes (*lanFEG, lanI*). For a specific lantibiotic the designation for locus is changed to specify the particular BGC, like *nis* for nisin, *lct* for lacticin, etc. The biosynthetic gene clusters of lantibiotics are found on chromosomal DNA (e.g., subtilin), plasmids (e.g., lacticin 481), and conjugative transposable genetic elements (e.g., nisin) (Chatterjee et al., 2005). Lantibiotics have been classified into four classes in a recent classification scheme given by Arnison et al., on the basis of the enzyme involved in thioether crosslink formation (Arnison et al., 2013) (Figure 29.5). Class I lantibiotics have separate enzymes for dehydration and cyclization to form lanthionine rings (Figures 29.4 & 29.5), while classes II, III, and IV have a bifunctional single lanthionine synthetase.

A typical BGC for class I lantibiotic nisin is given in Figure 29.7 and the detailed biosynthetic genes for each class are given under individual headings.

29.2 Genome Mining Studies for Discovery of Novel Lantibiotics

The conventional methods of lantibiotic discovery employ bioactivity-based screening of producers, which are time-consuming and resource-hungry. The availability of worldwide identified and sequenced bacterial genomes on protein and nucleotide sequence database have opened the gate for screening of thousands of strains for their novel lantibiotics. The precursor peptide coding gene sequence is often present in vicinity of the gene encoding biosynthetic proteins responsible for lantibiotic production. This feature, with the ability of BLAST search to identify novel homologs, has been exploited for genome mining studies aimed at identification of novel clusters of all the four classes of lantibiotics and their characterization. The diversity in the lantibiotic precursor peptides and their small size makes it difficult to identify novel lanthipeptides by homology search with the precursor peptide. Thus, various in silico mining strategies utilized larger biosynthetic proteins like lanthionine dehydratase LanB (Walsh et al., 2017) lanthionine cyclase LanC (Marsh et al., 2010), lanthionine synthetase LanM (Begley et al., 2009; O'Sullivan et al., 2011), and the bifunctional transporter, LanT (Wang et al., 2011; Singh and Sareen, 2014). These genome mining studies identified widespread occurrence of lantibiotic clusters among the bacterial classes outnumbering the known lanthipeptides. Genome mining studies also aimed at particular niches, like the human gastrointestinal tract based on the human microbiome project's reference genome database (Donia et al., 2014; Walsh et al., 2015) and ruminal bacteria (Azevedo et al., 2015) for ribosomal and non-ribosomal natural products. Screening of human oral and gut microbiome with different strategies of LanB HMM profile, pfam search, and BLAST yielded a remarkable 2007 unique class I lantibiotic gene clusters indicating a vast reservoir of therapeutic compounds in the human microbiota (Walsh et al., 2017). There are many tools available for genome mining of RiPPs, including the antiSMASH6.0 (Blin et al., 2013) and BAGEL4 (van Heel et al., 2018) based on HMM profile, and/or integrated ORF identification and output in the form of a graphical presentation of the BGC. Both antiSMASH6.0 and BAGEL4 also work as a database of the known lantibiotics. The RiPPs discovery efforts in our lab were also targeted for the novel class I and II lantibiotics, following a genome mining approach. As the bifunctional transporter protein LanT is exclusive to this class, the other classes were filtered out in the initial homology search for the transporter (Singh and Sareen, 2014). A preliminary homology search for the lantibiotic transporter gene on bacterial genomes led to 24 novel lantibiotic clusters spread among representatives of different phyla (Singh and Sareen, 2014).

One of the clusters identified by this genome mining study led us to an actinomycete, *Streptomyces filamentosus* (old *roseosporus*) NRRL 11379, encoding a putative lantibiotic cluster with two unique novel precursor peptides, a lanthionine synthetase, a bifunctional transporter, putative immunity genes, and one transcriptional regulator. The precursor peptide had a high number of modifiable cysteine, serine, and threonine residues that are involved in lanthionine ring formation, indicating that a highly conformationally strained lantibiotic is produced. As *Streptomyces* sp. is known to produce many other ribosomal and non-ribosomal natural products like the antibiotic daptomycin, arylomycin, stenothricin, and a AmfS like class III lanthipeptide (Ueda et al., 2002; Kersten et al., 2011; Krug and Müller, 2010), which would hinder in its isolation (Dischinger et al., 2009), the *Streptomyces filamentosus*'s lantibiotic gene cluster was taken up for further study by heterologous production of the two lanthipeptides in *E. coli*. This work of our lab led to development of a novel bacteriocin (specifically a lantibiotic) named Roseocin (Singh et al., 2020), for the first time from an Actinomycete, *Streptomyces roseosporus* NRRL 11379, comprising two peptides (RosA2α and RosA1β) that show synergistic antimicrobial activity. The bacteriocin was produced by heterologous overexpression of the genes in *E. coli* followed by in vitro reconstitution for functional characterization. The constituent peptides displayed antimicrobial activity against Gram-positive bacteria of clinical importance including *L. monocytogenes,* MRSA, and VRE. Multiple sequence alignment, cysteine alkylation, and structural analysis of the two peptides with MALDI TOF MS/MS confirmed that the peptides have a unique conformationally constrained structure, with an indispensable disulphide bond which differs from the currently known two-component lantibiotics (all isolated from firmicutes). Hence, Roseocin has been recognized as a novel two-component lantibiotic from a non-*firmicute,* developed and characterized in our lab by heterologous production and semi in vitro reconstitution (Singh et al., 2020). The characterization of Roseocin from the wild-type host *Streptomyces roseosporus* was unsuccessful in an earlier study by Kersten et al. (2011) as both peptides could not be detected from the wild-type culture and hence it remained uncharacterized.

Thus, genome mining coupled with experimental work can harness the unexplored "cryptic" gene clusters while minimizing the rate of rediscovery of known metabolites and expand the molecular diversity of NPs with medicinal potential. Employing the genome mining approach using a series of freely available bioinformatics tools (Russell and Truman, 2020), we have recently identified eight novel putative thiopeptide encoding biosynthetic gene clusters (BGCs) from different bacterial genomes, most of which belong to the class Actinobacteria (Aggarwal et al., 2021). Our results provide confidence in the newly identified BGCs to proceed with wet-bench experiments and discover novel thiopeptide(s).

29.2.1 Class I Lantibiotics

Class I lantibiotics involve the synthesis of lanthionine rings by combined action of two separate enzymes for dehydration and cyclization activity, respectively (Figures 29.4 & 29.5). The precursor peptide of class I lantibiotics like NisA (or LanA) contains a conserved FNLD motif in the leader peptide region, which is absent in other classes and a conserved proline at -2 position (McAuliffe et al., 2001). The most common bacteriocin nisin is a class I lantibiotic, processed by NisB and NisC enzymes for lanthionine formation (Figure 29.4). The selective serine and threonine residues are dehydrated by lanthionine dehydratase followed by enzymatic cyclization by lanthionine cyclase (Figure 29.4). These enzymes form a complex with the precursor peptide to install thioether bridges and act simultaneously in introducing lanthionine rings by alternating dehydration and cyclization reactions. In vitro reconstitution of the biosynthesis of class II–IV lanthipeptides was tried (Arnison et al., 2013), but reconstitution of class I biosynthesis had proven recalcitrant. The reason for this problem became clear when it was revealed that dehydration by the LanB dehydratases (InterPro families IPR006827 and IPR023809)

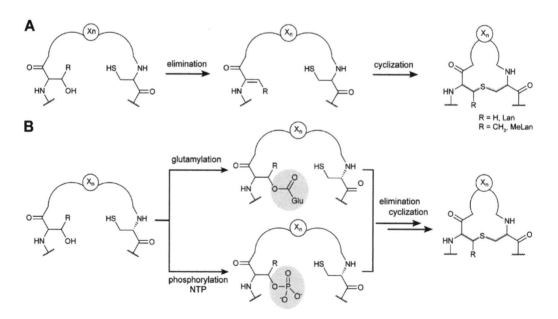

FIGURE 29.5 A) Post-translational modifications resulting in lanthionine and (methyl)lanthionines from Ser/Thr and Cys. B) Two different mechanisms for dehydration utilizing either Glu-tRNA or NTP for activation of the Ser/Thr side-chain hydroxyl groups prior to elimination of Glu/phosphate.

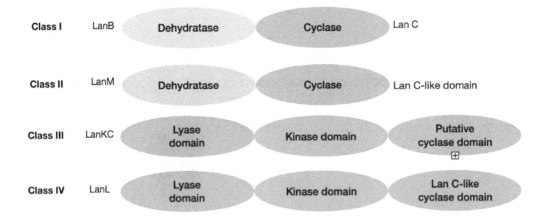

FIGURE 29.6 Recommended universal classification of lanthipeptides. Four classes of lanthipeptides are defined by the biosynthetic enzyme that installs lanthionine rings.

during class I lanthipeptide biosynthesis requires glutamyl-tRNA, a co-substrate that was not anticipated (Figure 29.5 B).

Moreover, employing the two enzymes for thioether ring formation, there are some other genes encoded in the lantibiotic BGC (Figure 29.7). Lanthionine ring formation in nisin is followed by extracellular transport of the lanthipeptide by a transporter NisT (or LanT) and subsequent extracellular cleavage of the leader peptide by a dedicated S8 or subtilisin-like serine protease NisP (or LanP) (van der Meer et al., 1993). The cleavage of the leader is very specific at the cleavage site marked by the presence of a conserved Pro residue at -2 position. The activation of the lanthipeptide by extracellular proteolytic cleavage of the leader is a strategic event that prevents suicidal action. To further prevent the lantibiotic action on the producer, the cluster also encodes immunity genes (i.e., NisF, NisE, NisG, and NisI (Stein et al., 2003). The first three are ATP binding cassette (ABC) transporters, which pump the lantibiotic extracellularly, and the NisI is a lipoprotein, which prevents the direct interaction of nisin to the membrane by decreasing nisin titre (Stein et al., 2003). The *lanFEG* are more commonly found in the lantibiotic biosynthetic clusters than the *lanI*. Nisin controls its own production with quorum sensing which is used by bacteria for cell density-dependent gene expression. It involves a two-component NisRK regulatory system, comprising of histidine kinase sensor (LanK) and a response regulator (LanR), both of which regulate the biosynthesis of all the genes at optimum level (Kleerebezem et al., 1997). The histidine kinase sensor is a membrane bound protein that senses the presence of an extracellular lantibiotic and autophosphorylates a His residue and transfers it to the Asp residue of the response regulator which then acts a transcriptional regulator for expression of the biosynthetic genes.

Class I lantibiotic nisin is being used worldwide in food preservation for more than 50 years (Delves-Broughton et al., 1996) without development of any significant resistance owing to its mode of action (de Kruijff et al., 2008) and is also under clinical trials for treatment of bovine mastitis (Garg et al., 2012).

29.2.1.1 Mode of Action of Class I Lantibiotics

Most of the lantibiotics target the lipid II component of the peptidoglycan layer of bacterial membrane. This is also apparent from the fact that the majority of lantibiotics do not act on Gram-negative bacteria, where the peptidoglycan layer is protected by an outer membrane, unless weakened artificially (Stevens et al., 1991). Peptidoglycan is synthesized from lipid II monomers (Figure 29.8A), which are synthesized from two nucleotide precursors, UDP-N-acetylglucosamine (UDP-GlcNAc) and UDP-N-acetylmuramic acid-pentapeptide (UDP-MurNAc-pentapeptide), synthesized in the cytoplasm (Barreteau et al., 2008). Cytoplasmic membrane-associated enzyme MraY catalyzes the transfer of MurNAc-pentapeptide from UDP to bactoprenyl-phosphate carrier to yield lipid I. The bactoprenyl phosphate (C_{55}-P) or polyisoprenoid

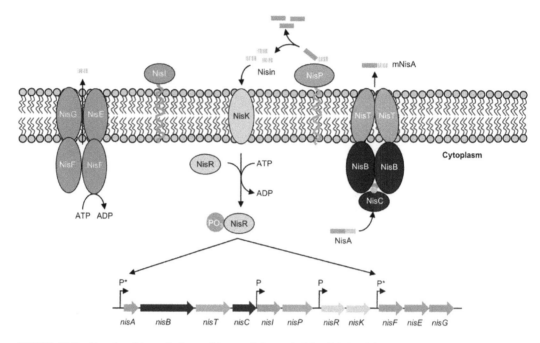

FIGURE 29.7 Complete biosynthetic machinery of the typical lantibiotic nisin. All the nisin biosynthetic genes are clustered together in multiple operons. Nisin precursor peptide NisA is synthesized ribosomally and the lanthionine dehydratase NisB and cyclase NisC introduce thioether rings in the core peptide (mNisA) followed by extracellular transport by NisT. The extaceullur membrane bound protease NisP cleaves the leader peptide to form active nisin. Nisin acts as a ligand for the receptor histidine kinase sensor NisK, which autophosphorylates a His residue and subsequently transfers the phosphate to the Asp of cytoplasmic response regulator NisR. NisR then acts as a transcriptional regulator for the expression for *nisABTCPRK* and *nisFEG* genes (adopted and modified from Chatterjee et al., 2005).

is a 55 carbon lipid chain formed from 11 isoprene units. Next, coupling of the UDP-GlcNAc by the membrane-associated MurG yields lipid II (Bouhss et al., 2008). Finally, lipid II is translocated for pep-tidoglycan synthesis and the lipid carrier bactoprenyl phosphate is recycled for next round of lipid II syn-thesis. In a bacteria, there are only a limited number of bactoprenyl phosphate units, which are recycled, limiting the synthesis of lipid II and making them an ideal target for antibiotics (Breukink and Kruijff, 2006). The non-ribosomal glycopeptide antibiotic, vancomycin, also acts by targeting lipid II, specific-ally the D-Ala-D-Ala of the pentapeptide chain attached to lipid II (Figure 29.8A), thereby hindering cell wall biosynthesis. The lantibiotic nisin, sequester lipid II molecule (Brötz et al., 1998b), making it unavailable (1) for cell wall synthesis and (2) bactoprenyl phosphate recycling for delivering new lipid II molecules and also leads to loss of membrane potential by making permanent pores using lipid II. The cationic nature of nisin drives its initial interaction with anionic membrane phospholipids. Nisin contains a total of five lanthionine rings (Figure 29.4) with three separate rings at the N-terminal and two over-lapped rings at the C-terminal separated by a flexible hinge region (Wiedemann et al., 2001). The NMR structure of nisin-lipid II complex revealed that the first N-terminal two rings of nisin capture the lipid II molecule forming a pyrophosphate cage structure for holding the pyrophosphate moiety of lipid II and interact with some part of MurNAc and first isoprene unit (Figure 29.8C) (Hsu et al., 2004). The two N-terminal amino acid bend inwards making a further hold and the lanthionine ring amide backbone makes hydrogen bonds with pyrophosphate. All other lipid II targeting lantibiotics show a conservation in these two rings like the epidermin and subtilin (Breukink and Kruijff, 2006). As was evident from the NMR structure of pyrophosphate cage, nisin does not interact with the pentapeptide of lipid II and that is why it is active against vancomycin-resistant bacterial strains, which mutated the pentapeptide N-terminal D-Ala to D-Lac (Arthur and Courvalin, 1993), making the vancomycin target unavailable. Following binding of nisin to lipid II, nisin bends from the hinge region in a transmembrane orientation and form

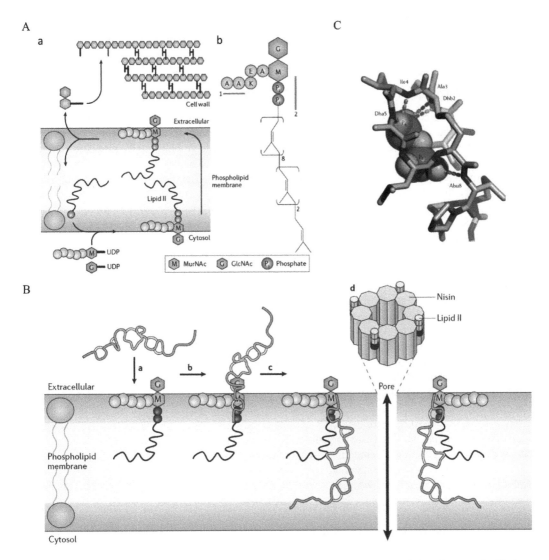

FIGURE 29.8 Mode of action of lipid II-targeting antibiotics. A) Lipid II is (a) assembled on the cytosolic side from UDP-activated precursors, UDP-GlcNAc and UDP-MurNAc-pentapeptide and a polyisoprenoid lipid carrier. Then it is translocated to extracellular side to feed up the peptidoglycan synthesis and polyisoprenoid carrier is released back for next cycle of lipid II synthesis. (b) Structure of lipid II with the highlighted binding site (red bars) for glycopeptide antibiotics (1) and nisin (2). B) Mechanism of pore formation of nisin. C) Pyrophosphate cage of nisin formed by the two N-terminal residues and rings A and B. The hydrogen bonds formed by backbone amides of lanthionine rings are presented in yellow and thioether sulphurs are shown in orange.

a stable pore complex with eight nisin and four lipid II molecules (Figure 29.8B) (Breukink and Kruijff, 2006). Despite, the widespread use of nisin for more than 50 years, negligible resistance developed against it. It is tough for bacteria to alter a basic wall components like lipid II, which is synthesized in ten steps (Schneider and Sahl, 2010) than to acquire an other mode of resistance. The known mechanism of resistance involves modification in the cell wall composition (increasing D-ala content to reduce anionic charge of lipotechoic acid) (Neuhaus and Badilley, 2003), biofilm formation, acquiring resistance providing ABC transporters, and resistance protein such as NSR, which cleaves nisin and reduce its activity. NSR protein is a S41 protease produced by *Lactococcus lactis* subsp. *diacetylactis*

(Froseth and McKay, 1991) and some other species comprising many human pathogenic strains (Khosa et al., 2013; Kawada-Matsuo et al., 2013). It is encoded by an operon comprising of five genes, which encode for NSR, a two-component regulatory system (NsrRK), and an ABC transporter (NsrFP). This operons resemble the self-immunity systems found in lantibiotic producers, which hinder lantibiotic interaction to bacterial membrane and provide immunity to nisin (Khosa et al., 2016).

29.2.1.2 Heterologous Production of Class I Lantibiotics

Various methods for induction of lantibiotic production in vivo and antimicrobial activity analysis include co-culturing, media alteration, and growth in unfavourable conditions. In co-culturing the producer and suspected indicator strains are grown on solid media to induce antimicrobial activity, observed as zone of inhibited growth. A common problem associated with activity-based natural product discovery is finding the environmental trigger for production. Wild-type bacteria produce lantibiotics in amounts sufficient to its need when required, and sometimes not produce the lantibiotic at all under the laboratory conditions. Heterologous production of many lantibiotics have been done, mostly for class II lantibiotics but some class I have also been produced, which not only provided the insight into the biosynthesis but biocatalysts to generate novel therapeutic peptides, and enzymes for biosynthetic applications. Heterologous production of class I lantibiotic is a bit cumbersome, in comparison to the other three classes, due to the involvement of two separate enzymes required for installation of lanthionine rings (Figure 29.4), which are also believed to be membrane associated (Figure 29.6) (Xie et al., 2004). The typical class I lantibiotic, nisin, was produced successfully in the heterologous host *E. coli,* in inactive form (Shi et al., 2011) and reconstituted in vitro. The strategy involved cloning of the genes for precursor peptide *nisA*, dehydratase enzyme *nis*B, and cyclase enzyme *nisC* in the three of the four MCS sites (two MCS in each) of plasmid vector pRSFDuet-1 and pACYC, followed by co-overexpression of the three genes in *E. coli* BL21(DE3). This led to the installation of five lanthionine rings (Figure 29.5) by NisB and NisC, on the hexahistidine tagged NisA, with the leader peptide still attached (inactive nisin). The leader peptide with tag was removed in vitro using trypsin, instead of the native membrane-associated NisP protease (Figure 29.6). Most recently a genome mining strategy identified a nisin analog, geobacillin I from thermophilic bacterium *Geobacillus thermodenitrificans* NG80-2, which was found to be more potent than nisin against *Streptococcus dysgalactiae,* the casual organism for bovine mastitis and more stable than at pH 7. Nisin displays limited stability at pH 7 hindering its application as food preservative at neutral pH (Davies et al., 1998). Geobacillin with seven lanthionine rings was found to be more heat stable than nisin (with five lanthionine rings). Geobacillin I was also produced heterologously in *E. coli* using a similar strategy as nisin production by the same group (Garg et al., 2012).

The discovery of the requirement of glutamyl-tRNA was foreshadowed by targeted mutagenesis of the NisB enzyme, the LanB involved in nisin biosynthesis, which resulted in glutamylation of Ser and Thr residues in the precursor peptide, NisA, during heterologous expression in *Escherichia coli.* Reconstitution of the dehydration activity of NisB in vitro, required the macromolecular fraction of *E. coli* cell extract, and the activity was lost upon treatment with RNAse, suggesting the role of RNA in the mechanism. Subsequent in vitro biochemical studies confirmed the requirement of glutamyl-tRNA^{Glu} synthesized *in situ* by GluRS (glutamyl-tRNA synthetase) for NisB to dehydrate NisA and illustrated that NisB cannot use uncharged tRNA^{Glu}.

A crystal structure of the dehydratase NisB bound to the leader peptide (LP) of its substrate NisA (Protein Databank, PDB: 4WD9) demonstrated the enzyme contained three domains (Figure 29.9) (Ortega et al., 2015). One domain (InterPro family IPR006827) catalyzes the transfer of glutamate from the tRNA to the peptide substrate. Then, the glutamylated peptide is translocated to another domain (InterPro family IPR023809) in which the glutamate is eliminated to form Dha/Dhb.

A ping-pong type mechanism in which the glutamyl group is first transferred from the glutamyl-tRNA to the enzyme, prior to transfer of the glutamyl moiety to the Ser/Thr in NisA, was ruled out by mutagenesis. The LP binding domain in NisB (Ortega et al., 2015) was termed as the RiPP precursor recognition element (RRE) (Burkhart et al., 2015). Structure elucidation with a non-reactive analog of glutamylated NisA (PDB: 6M7Y) identified the elimination active site of NisB, while the glutamyl transfer active site is inferred based on a structure of a biosynthetic enzyme that carries out Glu-tRNA-dependent glutamylation of Ser residues during thiopeptide (another member of RiPPs) biosynthesis (Bothwell et al., 2019). Covalent attachment of the LP to the RRE demonstrated that catalysis can take place with

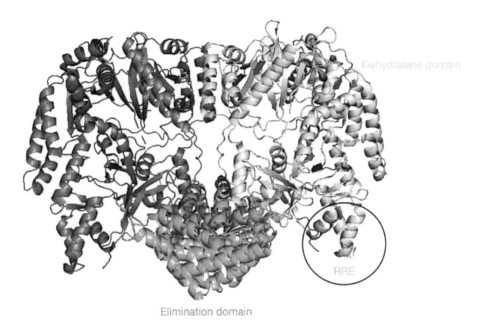

FIGURE 29.9 Crystal structure of the NisB (PDB: 4WD9).

the LP occupying only a single-binding site and also ruling out models in which the LP needs to move during catalysis (Repka et al., 2018). Studies with LanB enzymes from different bacterial phyla have shown that the nucleotide sequence in the acceptor stem of the $tRNA^{Glu}$ is critical for the enzyme to accept the cognate glutamyl-tRNA as substrate (Acedo et al., 2019), an observation that explains difficulties in heterologous expression of many class I lanthipeptides. Some RiPP BGCs such as those of the antifungal pinensins (Mohr et al., 2015) or the thiopeptides (Hudson et al., 2015) contain split LanB dehydratases (Montalba´n-Lopez et al., 2021) in which glutamylation and elimination are carried out by separate polypeptides. Compared to advances in understanding the mechanism of dehydration and LP recognition, the mechanism of cyclization in class I lanthipeptides by LanC enzymes (InterPro family: IPR033889) remains to be investigated in detail. The nisin lanthionine synthetase complex comprises NisB, NisC, and the precursor peptide NisA in a stoichiometric ratio of 2:1:1 (Reiners et al., 2017). The complex is formed in the presence of the unmodified precursor peptide and dissociates upon complete installation of the thioether bridges, which due to conformational constraint, destabilizes the complex. The leader sequence of the precursor peptide is required for recognition by the modification enzymes (van der Meer et al., 1994) and finally cleaved off by the protease LanP to produce active lantibiotic. A lanthionine-containing peptide without antimicrobial activity is known as a lanthipeptide.

A recent report by Bothwell et al. (2021) on structural analysis of class I lanthipeptides from the Bacteroidetes, *Pedobacter lusitanus* NL19, well supported with biochemical and biophysical data, describes several new findings, which are significant advancements in the current understanding of the biosynthesis of lanthipeptide class of natural products in general and will assist in characterization of such clusters. The work describes the essentiality of $tRNA^{Glu}$ and GluRS genes and a method for in vitro reconstitution of this novel lanthipeptide from this Gram-negative bacterium, along with the functional characterization of a first lantibiotic cyclase, which is devoid of the conventional catalytic zinc-binding residues. Structural characterization of the thioether bonds also revealed an unusual LL-stereochemistry.

29.2.2 Class II Lantibiotics

This class is considered more evolved than the class I lantibiotics, as the function of four genes is performed by only two (Zhang et al., 2012). The dehydration and cyclization reactions for lanthionine ring formation is performed by a single bifunctional enzyme LanM and the extracellular transport and proteolytic removal of leader peptide is performed by a single bifunctional transporter LanT. Reduction in the number of post-translational modification enzymes makes these lantibiotics preferable for heterologous expression in *E. coli* for mechanistic studies and characterization. The bifunctional lanthionine synthetase LanM is a protein of approximately ~1000 amino acid residues and contains an N-terminal dehydratase and a C-terminal cyclase domain. The cyclase domain shows homology with class I cyclase enzyme but the N-terminal is not homologous to LanB (Li et al., 2005). The encoded precursor peptides show marked differences in the motifs from class I lantibiotics. The FNLD motif is absent and the protease cleavage site is marked by double glycine motif (Håvarstein et al., 1995), where a glycine residue is highly conserved at -2 position instead of proline of class I lantibiotics. Although the glycine at -2 position is highly conserved, the -1 position has been found varying (GG to GA, GS and AG) from the initially observed glycine at this position, hence conventionally termed as double glycine motif.

Some of the Type II lantibiotic clusters encode two or more peptides with a promiscuous lanthionine synthetase, LanM. For example, a single ProcM encoded in prochlorosin gene cluster is able to process more than 17 different precursor peptides (Li et al., 2010). However, the two-peptide lantibiotic haloduracin is processed by two different HalM dedicated to each of the two HalA peptides, showing no promiscuity (McClerren et al., 2006). Class II lantibiotics are of two types depending upon the constituent peptides and their bioactivity. There are single-component lantibiotics with peptide(s) that display antimicrobial activity in isolation (Wang et al., 2014b) (e.g., lacticin 481, mersacidin), and the two-component lantibiotics that constitute two different variety of peptides that show synergistic antimicrobial activity (Lawton et al., 2007) (e.g., cytolysin, lacticin 3147, haloduracin, staphylococcin C55, lichenicidin, plantaricin W, bicereucin, flavecins, Smb, Bht-A, carnolysins, etc.) (Table 29.1; Figure 29.10). Although only alpha peptides of the two-component lantibiotics are shown in Figure 29.10, single-peptide class II lantibiotics (i.e., lacticin and mersacidin) also show conservation in this motif, like the two-component class II lantibiotics (Field et al., 2013). Understanding of genetic organization of lantibiotic-encoding BGCs has led to the discovery of novel lantibiotics by combinatorial approach of genome mining, activity-based screening of the thus identified potential producers, and/or in vitro reconstitution of BGCs from the native producers (Begley et al., 2009; McClerren et al., 2006). In our previous genome mining study, we identified multiple two-component lantibiotic clusters in actinomycetes, with two precursor peptides and two LanMs (Singh & Sareen, 2014). In addition, a cluster was identified in *S. roseosporus* NRRL 11379 with a single LanM and two precursor peptides. To date, since all the two-component lantibiotics have been isolated from firmicutes (Zhang et al., 2015), we wanted to analyze whether this actinomycete BGC produces peptides with synergistic bioactivity, as in two-component lantibiotics, or produces peptides with additive antimicrobial activity. Additionally, the presence of six cysteine residues in each of these two peptides led us to speculate that they might form a highly constrained structure, and display worthier bioactivity than the existing lantibiotics. Hence, this cluster was undertaken for characterization by a semi in vitro reconstitution approach, involving heterologous expression of the lanthipeptides in *E. coli* (Singh et al., 2020).

Most of the two-component lantibiotics have a lipid II-binding α-peptide, which acts in synergy with β-peptide, thereby enhancing the antimicrobial activity by manyfold (Breukink & Kruijff, 2006). While

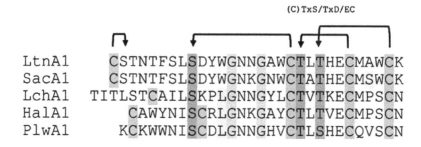

FIGURE 29.10 Lipid II-binding motif present in class II lantibiotics. Shown here is the multiple alignment of alpha peptides of two component lantibiotic of class II, with highlighted conserved lipid II-binding motif (C)TxS/TxD/EC and the lanthionine bridging pattern. Lacticin 3147 (LtnA1); staphylococcin C55 (SacA1); plantaricin W (PlwA1).

TABLE 29.1

Examples of Class II Lanthipeptides: Class II lantibiotics comprise both single- and two-component lantibiotics (synergistic activity) with alpha and beta peptide(s). Usually two-component lantibiotics have two LanM for the processing of *two* peptides. The exceptions to this rule are cytolysin and bicereucin, which being two-component are processed by a single LanM and flavecins with 12 precursor peptides processed by two LanMs

Lanthipeptide	Component/ peptides	LanM	Source	Reference
Roseocin	Two/2	1	*Streptomyces roseosporus* NRRL 11379	(Singh et al., 2019)
Mersacidin	Single/1	1	*Bacillus sp. strain HIL Y-85,54728*	(Chatterjee et al., 1991)
Plantaricin W	Two/2	2	*Lactobacillus plantarum* LMG 2379	(Holo et al., 2001)
Smb	Two/2	2	*Streptococcus mutans*	(Yonezawa and Kuramitsu, 2005)
Bht-A	Two/2	2	*Streptococcus rattus* BHT	(Hyink et al., 2005)
Lacticin 3147	Two/2	2	*Lactococcus lactis* subsp. *Lactis* DPC3147	(Martinet al., 2004)
Cytolysin	Two/2	1	*Enterococcus faecalis*	(Cox et al., 2005)
Lacticin 481	Single/1	1	*Lactococcus lactis*	(Xie et al., 2004)
Haloduracin	Two/2	2	*Bacillus halodurans* C-125	(McClerren et al., 2006)
Prochlorosins	Single/29	1	*Prochlorococcus marinus MIT9313*	(Li et al., 2010)
Lichenicidin	Two/2	2	*Bacillus licheniformis ATCC 14580*	(Dischinger et al., 2009; Begley et al., 2009; Caetano et al., 2011a)
Geobacillin II	Single/1	1	*Geobacillus thermodenitrificans* NG80-2	(Garg et al., 2012)
Carnolysin	Two/2	2	*Carnobacterium maltaromaticum C2*	(Lohans et al., 2014)
Bicereucin	Two/1	1	*Bacillus cereus* SJ1	(Singh and Sareen, 2014; Huo and van der Donk, 2016)
Bovicin	Single/1	1	*Streptococcus bovis HJ50*	(Xiao, 2004; Wang et al., 2016)
Flavecins	Two/12	2	*Ruminococcus flavefaciens* FD-1	(Singh and Sareen, 2014; Zhao and van der Donk, 2016)

there are many examples of characterized and putative two-component lantibiotics synthesized by two LanMs (Begley et al., 2009; Singh & Sareen, 2014; Zhang et al., 2015), only three are known to be processed by a single LanM (i.e., carnolysin and cytolysin), which are homologs (Booth et al., 1996; Lohans et al., 2014), and bicereucin having D-amino acids as the major post-translational modification (PTM) in comparison to lanthionine (Huo & van der Donk, 2016). The cloning and purification of individual genes for production of a complete lantibiotic heterologously provides an approach for expression of silent lantibiotic clusters and enhancing the yield. In a previous study, to interrogate the biosynthetic capacity of the potential producers, Kersten et al. executed a mass spectrometry-guided genome mining approach for natural product peptidogenomics in eight different *Streptomyces* strains, which are the known producers of various antimicrobial natural products (Kersten et al., 2011). They provided enormous MS data of *S. roseosporus* NRRL 15998 along with the in silico analysis of the genome and mentioned an identical cluster to Roseocin, with two precursor peptides (73 a.a. and 80 a.a. residues, respectively) without the identification of immunity genes of this BGC. This previous study did not focus on the bioactivity analysis of the lanthipeptides, and only one of the two RosA gene products carrying nine dehydrations was detected (*m/z* 3,108.43) from the n-butanolic extract of *S. roseosporus* (Kersten et al., 2011). Hence, it could not be studied further due to the absence of the second gene product. Though attempts were not made to characterize Roseocin from *S. roseosporus* NRRL 11379, heterologous production of the two modified RosA peptides and in vitro leader peptide removal for generation of bioactive lanthipeptides led to the bioactivity evaluation and partial structural analysis of the encoded two-component lantibiotic, Roseocin.

The biosynthetic clusters of this class have also been found to encode multiple precursor peptides with a diversity in the structures (Begley et al., 2009; Li et al., 2010; Singh and Sareen, 2014; Zhao and van der Donk, 2016). The lanthipeptide cluster of prochlorosins constitutes a total of 29 precursor peptides, which show a high level of conservation in the N-terminal leader sequence and a high variability in the core peptide region. All 29 peptides were found to be modified by a highly promiscuous lanthionine synthetase ProcM (Li et al., 2010). It was concluded that, as the leader peptide was conserved, a single promiscuous LanM was able to install the lanthionine rings in the variable core-peptide region of all of the precursor peptides tested of the 29 peptides. Similarly, the two FlvM present in the two-component lantibiotic flavecin could modify multiple alpha and beta peptides (Zhao and van der Donk, 2016). This promiscuous behaviour could be exploited for lanthionine synthesis in non-native substrates, as promiscuous LanM recognizes the leader region of the precursor peptide for modification and when ligated with a non-native core peptide region (peptide chimera) leads to the installation of the complex lanthionine moieties on non-native core-peptide. The lanthionine synthetase BovM of bovicin biosynthetic cluster was successfully used for modifying the core peptide of suicin and lacticin 481 by fusing these with bovicin leader peptide (Wang et al., 2016, 2014a).

The modified precursor peptide, after introduction of lanthionine rings, is exported via a bifunctional transporter LanT. The N-terminal 150 residues of LanT encode a peptidase (C39 peptidase) that cleaves next to the double glycine motif of the precursor peptide, concomitant with the extracellular transport by the C-terminal ABC transporter domain (Håvarstein et al., 1995). C39 is a family of endopeptidases present in clan CA, the largest clan of cysteine proteases. While in most of the lantibiotics of class II, lanthipeptide is activated by C39 protease-mediated leader cleavage, in some cases, a second cleavage is required to remove additional N-terminal residues by S8 or subtilin like serine protease LanP (Tang et al., 2015). To date, LanP protease is observed in class II lantibiotic clusters discovered in firmicutes only. For example, LicP of lichenicidin (Caetano et al., 2011a), CerP of cerecidin (Wang et al., 2014b), BsjP of bicereucin (Huo and van der Donk, 2016), and CylA from Cytolysin (Booth et al., 1996) have all been discovered in representatives of firmicutes only. The in silico-identified lantibiotic clusters with LanP also belong to the firmicutes (Singh and Sareen, 2014).

29.2.2.1 Mode of Action of Class II Lantibiotics

Mostly, the α-peptide of the two-component lantibiotics binds with lipid-II precursor of the peptidoglycan making a complex that serves as a dock for β-peptide for pore formation, thereby enhancing the bioactivity of the compound (Breukink & Kruijff, 2006; Martin et al., 2004). The precursor peptides are found to contain a conserved lipid II-binding motif (Figure 29.10) that indicates their mode of action by interacting with lipid II (Breukink and Kruijff, 2006; Cotter et al., 2006). The class II lantibiotic mersacidin and alpha component of two-component lantibiotics target lipid II molecules (Brötz et al., 1998a). The interaction of mersacidin spans a larger binding site on lipid II then nisin (discussed in mode of action) including the GlcNAc moiety of lipid II (Brötz et al., 1998b). One of the unorthodox features of the alpha peptide of Roseocin, RosA2α, (Singh et al., 2020) is the lack of lipid II-binding motif, CTxTxEC, which is found in the α-component of all the haloduracin-related two-component lantibiotics. This is quite perplexing, in light of its importance for interaction with lipid II and its conservation in all the known α-peptides. Hence, it will indeed be very interesting to find its possible molecular target and mode of action.

29.2.2.2 Heterologous Production of Class II Lantibiotic

Many class II lantibiotics have been heterologously produced in *E. coli*, for increasing yield, mechanistic studies, and to provide enzymatic tools for synthetic biology applications (Table 29.2). The class II lantibiotics like lacticin 481, haloduracin, bovicin, flavecins, geobacillin II, prochlorosins, lichenicidin, and carnolysin have been successfully produced in *E. coli*. Only the prochlorosins identified from a cyanobacteria have not been found to be antimicrobial and were considered to serve other purposes in this organism (Li et al., 2010). Such peptides that contain lanthionine moiety are termed as lanthipeptides and if antimicrobial as lantibiotics. The first of the examples include the in vitro reconstitution of lacticin 481, by heterologous expression of the structural gene lctA and the lanthionine synthetase lctM in *E. coli*

TABLE 29.2

Enzymes Obtained from Study on Heterologous Expression Studies on Lantibiotics

Enzyme	Class	Synthetic biological application	Reference
EpiD, GdmD	I	Oxidative decarboxylation of peptides containing C-terminal sequence (V/I/L/M/F/Y/W)-(A/S/V/T/C/I/L)-C.	(Van Heel et al., 2013; Ortega et al., 2017)
LicP	II	Application as a sequence-specific protease for traceless removal of leader peptides and MBP expression tag.	(Tang et al., 2015)
LanM	II	Installation of lanthionine rings in peptides	(Wang et al., 2016).

BL21(DE3) employing a plasmid vector, to produce hexa-histidine tagged unmodified lacticin precursor peptide and hexa-histidine-tagged LctM (Xie et al., 2004). Both proteins were purified by metal affinity chromatography and incubated together in the presence of ATP and Mg^{2+} for introducing lanthionine rings in the precursor peptide. The leader peptide along with the tag was cleaved with a commercial protease LysC, instead of the protease native to the cluster. The native C39 protease (also known as LctT150 for N-terminal 150 residues) is a domain of the ABC transporter, which is membrane associated. Although the cytosolic domain was cloned and used for in vitro reconstitution in another work by the same group (Ihnken et al., 2009) in both the lantibiotic production strategy of GluC and Lct150 treatment, in vitro reconstitution strategy was adopted in order to avoid the cytotoxic effects of active lantibiotic to *E. coli*. LctA mutants were created and studied for dehydration and cyclization activity by LctM (Xie et al., 2004). This strategy of lanthipeptide generation in vitro with the precursor peptide in hand and activation by a purified or commercial protease overcame the problem associated with the in vivo site-directed mutagenesis studies for novel lantibiotics, which sometimes leads to loss of lantibiotic production (Kuipers et al., 1995), and hence cannot be obtained for characterization.

Another study established the first complete heterologous production of the lantibiotic lichenicidin in a Gram-negative culture (Caetano et al., 2011b). A library of the entire genome of wild-type lichenicidin producer *B. licheniformis* I89 was constructed in *E. coli* EPI300™ and screened for bioactivity against *Micrococcus luteus* ATCC 9341. Mass corresponding to lichenicidin alpha and beta peptide was detected in isopropanol cell wash and culture supernatant of *E. coli*, indicating that it is able to synthesize fully bioactive lantibiotic. The positive clones encoded the entire lichenicidin biosynthetic cluster consisting of 14 ORFs including that of the precursor peptide (BliA1, BliA2), modification (BliM1, BliM2), transport and proteolytic cleavage (BliT), additional cleavage (BliP), regulation (BliR, BliY), and lichenicidin immunity (BliF, BliE, BliG, BliH, BliI).

The most recent of the lantibiotic production strategy in *E. coli* led to the successful production of a fully processed and secreted lantibiotic bovicin HJ50 (Wang et al., 2016), in the absence of the bovicin immunity proteins, unlike the heterologous production of lichenicidin with immunity genes. An insignificant level of bovicin cytotoxicity was observed on *E. coli*, without hampering its production. While the previous heterologous production strategies involved a final in vitro reconstitution step (lacticin 481) or with the native regulatory elements for a complete lantibiotic (as in lichenicidin), the strategy employed cloning and co-expression of all the required genes *bovA*, *bovM*, and for first the time *bovT* in *E. coli* C43(DE3) under the control of T7 promoter. Also, an enzyme chimera of peptidase domain BovT150 and BovM was constructed to perform dual function of precursor peptide modification and cleavage. Adding to the argument of Xie et al., 2004 (for mutant screening) that this chimera generation will further ease the study and production of mutant lanthipeptides.

29.2.3 Class III Lantibiotics

For classes III & IV lanthipeptides, a single lanthionine synthetase is utilized for dehydration and cyclization. The dehydrations are carried out by a distinct mechanism that involves combined action of its central kinase domain and N-terminal phosphoSer/Thr lyase domain, while cyclization is carried out by C-terminal cyclization domain. The Ser/Thr residues present in the precursor peptides are phosphorylated

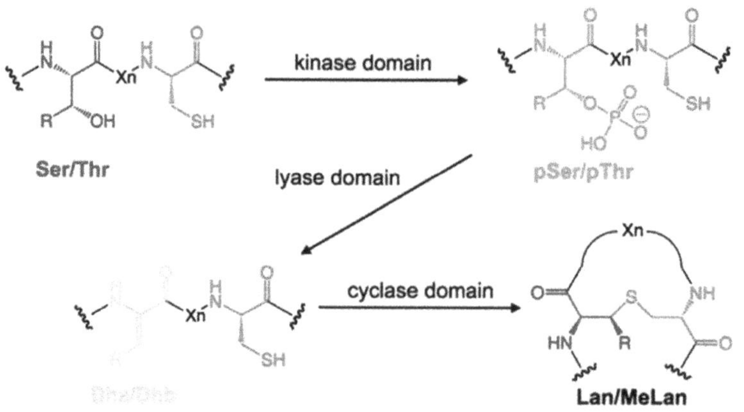

FIGURE 29.11   Mechanism of PTMs by class III and class IV enzymes. The central kinase domain phosphorylates Ser/Thr residues, which are then eliminated by the N-terminal lyase domain and the cyclization by a LanC-like cyclase domain that catalyze the nucleophilic attack of cysteines residues to form lanthionine or a labionin ring (adopted from Goto et al., 2010).

by the kinase domain and then removed by lyase domain for Dha and Dhb formation, followed by thioether ring formation by C-terminal cyclase domain (Figure 29.11). The three zinc ligands present in the cyclization domain of the classes I, II, and IV lanthionine synthetases (Figure 29.6) are absent in class III enzymes.

Class III enzyme LanKC forms a carbon-carbon crosslink, known as labionin (Lab), named as such as they were initially found in labyrinthopeptins (Meindl et al., 2010). A cysteine thiol attacks the dehydrated Dha to generate an enolate intermediate, which further attacks a second Dha forming a labionin ring (Figure 29.12A) (Müller et al., 2010). Besides the PTM LanKC and structural peptide, the class III BGC comprises genes for lantibiotic transporter and rarely a protease (Iorio et al., 2014), which is often encoded elsewhere in the genome (Kodani et al., 2004; Meindl et al., 2010; Krawczyk et al., 2012; Wang and van der Donk, 2012; Jungmann et al., 2016). The precursor peptide contains a conserved LLELQ motif (Müller et al., 2011). The first class III lantibiotic cluster identified was for a morphogen, SapB, which is required for aerial mycelium formation in filamentous bacterium *Streptomyces coelicolor* (Kodani et al., 2004). Since then many more such examples have been identified (Table 29.3). *ramS* is the structural gene for SapB. The peptide-encoded therefrom (ramS) is post-translationally modified by installation of lanthionine rings by the class III enzyme, RamC. Although LabKC andRamC homologous (43% identity), the products formed by these enzymes, labyrinthopeptins and SapB, respectively, are quite different in structure and functional groups (Figure 29.12 B) (Wang and van der Donk, 2012). Labyrinthopeptin A2 contains two labionin groups and SapB contains two lanthionine rings, both moieties synthesized from Ser, Thr, and Cys residues from a common Ser(Xxx)$_2$Ser(Xxx)$_3$Cys motif (Wang and van der Donk, 2012). Other class III lantibiotics, stackepeptin and erythreapeptin, have been found with both labionin and lanthionine structures (Völler et al., 2012; Jungmann et al., 2016), indicating their modification enzymes to be promiscuous in installation of two different types of rings. Promiscuity is also observed for the phosphate donor co-substrate as discussed ahead. Class III lanthipeptide have been found displaying an array of activities like morphogenetic for filamentous *Streptomyces*, antibacterial, antiviral, and antinociceptive in formalin-induced pain mice model (Iorio et al., 2014), and antiallodynic activity in a nerve injury mouse model of neuropathic pain (Meindl et al., 2010) (Table 29.3).

29.2.3.1 Heterologous Production of Class III Lanthipeptides

Multiple in vitro reconstitution studies have been done on class III lantibiotics, eased with requisite of a single PTM enzyme for lanthipeptide maturation. Although found in the culture extracts, the antiviral and antiallodyniclabyrinthopeptin was reconstituted in vitro for first mechanistic insights into the

TABLE 29.3

Discovered Class III Lanthipeptides and Their Bioactivities

Lanthipeptide	Source	Bioactivity	Reference
AmfS	*Streptomyces griseus*	Morphogen	(Ueda et al., 2002)
SapB	*Streptomyces coelicolor* A3	Morphogen	(Kodani et al., 2004)
SapT	*Streptomyces tendae* Tü901/8c	Limited antibacterial activity, Morphogen	(Kodani et al., 2005)
Labyrinthopeptins	*Actinomadura namibiensis* DSM 6313	Antiviral activity against Herpes Simplex virus (HSV) and Human Immunodeficiency virus (HIV) and antiallodynic effects (or antineuropathic pain activity)	(Meindl et al., 2010) (Férir et al., 2013)
Erythreapeptin,	*Saccharopolyspora erythraea* NRRL 2338	Not mentioned	(Völler et al., 2012)
Avermipeptin	*Streptomyces avermitilis* DSM 46492	Not mentioned	(Völler et al., 2012)
Griseopeptin	Streptomyces griseus DSM 40236	Not mentioned	(Völler et al., 2012)
Catenulipeptin	Catenulispora acidiphilia DSM 44928	Probable morphogen	(Wang and van der Donk, 2012)
Curvopeptin	Thermomonospora curvata DSM43183	Not mentioned	(Krawczyk et al., 2012)
NAI-112	Actinoplanes sp. DSM24059	Weakly antibacterial, antinociceptive activity (or antipain activity)	(Iorio et al., 2014)
Stackepeptin	Stackebrandtia nassauensis DSM-44728	Not mentioned	(Jungmann et al., 2016)

biosynthesis of these molecules (Müller et al., 2011). A hexahistidine-tagged LabKC was amplified from a cosmid library, cloned and purified from *E. coli* for activity analysis with synthetic peptide (synthesized by SPPS) substrates. The observation made were similar to the other lantibiotic, like the requirement of leader peptide for PTMs and the important hydrophobic patch (LLELQ motif) present in the leader, required for PTMs by LabKC. Similarly, catenulipeptin was produced by co-incubation of purified hexahistidine-tagged precursor peptide AciA (with triple lysine as a linker for increasing solubility) and AciKC from *E. coli*. The enzymes did not require Zn for activity, as was evident from the absence of Zn ligands in these enzymes. While LabKC uses GTP as a co-substrate (Müller et al., 2011) or phosphate donor, AciKC displayed promiscuity by utilizing any of the NTPs (ATP, GTP, CTP, or TTP) as phosphate donor (Wang and van der Donk, 2012). A thermostable CurKC (stable upto ~55°C) produced from *E. coli* for curvopeptin biosynthesis was also able to utilize all the NTPs as co-substrates, with a preference for purine nucleotides (ATP/dATP, GTP/dGTP). In another heterologously produced class III enzyme, EryKC, ATP was identified as the co-substrate, although the enzyme could not be fully reconstituted, owing to the added solubility-enhancing SUMO tag, which was speculated to interfere with its activity (Völler et al., 2012). The labyrinthopeptins were heterologously produced in *S. lividans* (and *S. albus*) using a shuttle vector (for *E. coli* and *Streptomyces*) for cloning of the whole BGC under the control of *ErmE** promoter (Krawczyk et al., 2013). This resulted in ring topologies in labyrinthopeptins the same as the wild type, but the leader processing was incomplete, due to the fact that the leader peptide cleavage is dependent upon the original host proteases and not present in the heterologous hosts. Although desired cleavage was obtained by leader peptide optimization and mutating -1 position to methionine for CNBr-mediated cleavage of the leader (Krawczyk et al., 2013). In the most recent examples, stackepeptins were identified with three labionin rings instead of the usual two (hence termed supersized) and no lanthionine rings formed from the three conserved Ser(Xxx)$_2$Ser(Xxx)$_3$Cys motif (Jungmann et al., 2016). In contrast to three labionin rings in vitro synthesized stackepeptin had a lanthionine and labionin ring installed by

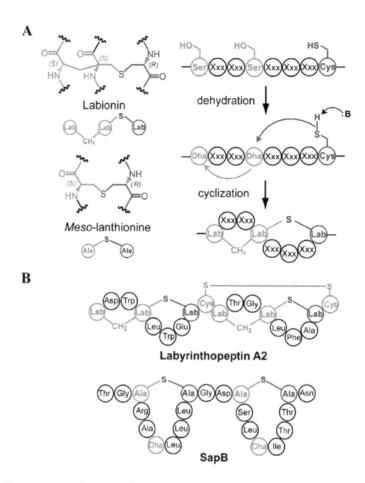

FIGURE 29.12   Structural comparison of labyrinthopeptin A2 and SapB. A) A labionine structure links three amino acid residues (i.e., two Dha in C-C link and one Cys with thioether link), while a lanthionine links only two amino acid residues with a thioether link. Mechanism of labionin formation. B) Labyrinthopeptin A2 contains two labionin rings and a disulphide linkage, while SapB contains two lanthionine rings. Both are formed from a common Ser(Xxx)$_2$Ser(Xxx)$_3$Cys motif (adopted from Wang and van der Donk, 2012).

the enzyme His$_6$-StaKC, which was heterologously produced in *E. coli* with GroEL and GroES chaperonin system (Jungmann et al., 2016).

29.2.4 Class IV lantibiotics

As already discussed, similar to class III, a single tri-domain lanthionine synthetase installs lanthionine rings in the structural peptide. The only difference is the presence of Zn-binding ligands common to class I LanC and class II LanM (Figure 29.6). A class IV BGC contains gene for structural peptide (LanA), modification enzyme (LanL), and putative ABC transporters (LanT and LanH), but a protease is absent. To date, only two class IV lantibiotics have been characterized, although many homologous gene clusters have been identified by genome mining (Goto et al., 2010). The first was venezuelin from *Streptomyces venezuelae*, for which neither any bioactivity was identified (Goto et al., 2010) nor it was detected from the wild-type culture. The most recently discovered class IV lanthipeptide streptocollin from *Streptomyces collinus* Tü 365 was isolated from the wild culture and found to be a potent lead for developing anti-diabetic and anti-obesity drugs, as it inhibited protein tyrosine phosphatase1B (PTB1B) activity (Iftime et al., 2015). PTP1B is a negative regulator of insulin and leptin signalling pathways and its inhibitors increase the action of insulin and leptin and hence are therapeutic for Type 2 diabetes and obesity (Combs, 2010).

29.2.4.1 Heterologous Production of Class IV Lanthipeptides

The product of the first discovered class IV lanthipeptide BGC for *venezuelin* was not identified in the extracts of *Streptomyces venezuelae* and was rather confirmed by the heterologous expression of the structural gene *venA* for venezuelin and the unique lanthionine synthetase gene termed *venL*. VenA was tagged both with a maltose-binding protein (MBP) and a hexa-histidine (His_6) to increase solubility and assist in purification by IMAC, respectively. Like other lantibiotic classes, VenL also required the presence of ATP, Mg^{2+} and a reducing agent for its lanthionine synthetase activity. The proposed tri-domain structure of the lanthionine synthetase, LanL with N-terminal phosphoSer/Thr lyase, central kinase, and C-terminal cyclase domain was proposed by in silico analysis and was then confirmed by creation of truncated versions of VenL with activity analysis for each domain. The kinase domain alone was able to phosphorylate Ser and Thr residues in VenA (precursor peptide) and the lyase domain alone was able to perform β-elimination of these phosphates for formation of dehydrated residues Dha and Dhb, as confirmed by the alterations in mass of His_6-VenA (precursor peptide) by MS analysis. The study was not able to detect or establish the role of venezuelin in the wild-type organism under the labora-tory conditions or from heterologous host, *Streptomyces lividans*. The lanthipeptide streptocollin is the first example of class IV lanthipeptide isolated from wild-type culture (1.8 mg/L). Its expression was enhanced (3 mg/L) by inserting a constitutive promoter *ermE** upstream of the streptocollin BGC in place of its own promoter (Iftime et al., 2015). This cluster was also expressed in the heterologous host using a cosmid in *S. coelicolor* A3(2) strain M1146 and strain M1152 to further increase the yield of streptocollin (5.5 mg/L and 10 mg/L, respectively). This way the initial 1.8 mg/L yield was enhanced to 10 mg/L, for a potent antidiabetic, antiobesity lanthipeptide streptocollin (Iftime et al., 2015).

29.2.5 Lanthidins, Class V Lanthipeptides

The antibiotic cacaoidin (Figure 29.13) is the first reported member of the lanthidins, a new RiPP sub-family with structural elements found in lanthipeptides and linaridins (Ortiz-López et al., 2020). Cacaoidin displayed potent antibacterial activity against Gram-positive pathogens including *Clostridium difficile*. This natural product was isolated from *Streptomyces cacaoi* CA-170360 and bears an unprecedented N,N-dimethyl lanthionine (N-Me₂Lan) that is not found in known lanthipeptides (Ortiz-López et al., 2020). Though N-terminal bis-N-methylation has been reported for linaridins and LAPs (Montalba′n-Lopez et al., 2021), these RiPP families lack lanthionines. The molecule also combines other unusual structural features, such as O-glycosylation of Tyr with a 6-deoxygulopyranosyl-(rhamnopyranose) disaccharide, and several D-amino acids including D-2-aminobutyric acid (Abu) (Figure 29.13).

The cacaoidin BGC could not be identified by any bioinformatics prediction software tool and was mapped in the region adjacent to the core peptide structural gene (Montalba′n-Lopez et al., 2021). The cluster shows low homology with those of other lanthipeptides or linaridins and suggests an alternative RiPP biosynthetic pathway. Since linaridins are characterized by dehydrobutyrine (Dhb) residues (see Figure 29.3), which are not present in cacaoidin, but rather has lanthionine rings, which is a character-istic of lanthipeptides, we have proposed in a RiPP scientific community review (Montalba′n-Lopez et al., 2021) that cacaoidin is the founding member of lanthidins, a new RiPP subfamily (i.e., class V lanthipeptides). These peptides are made via a biosynthetically distinct pathway since the BGC does not contain genes for class I-IV lanthionine synthases.

Very recent genome mining efforts have also identified additional class V lanthipeptides (Kloosterman et al., 2020; Xu et al., 2020). Cacaoidin BGC was only found in the genomes of all publicly available *Streptomyces cacaoi* subsp. *cacaoi* strains and not in any other species, suggesting that this cluster may be a species-specific trait. Undoubtedly, cacaoidin BGC has an unprecedented genetic organization, com-pletely different from any other previously described RiPP cluster. Moreover, the detection of similar putative lanthidin homologous clusters opens the door to the study of a new exciting family of RiPPs.

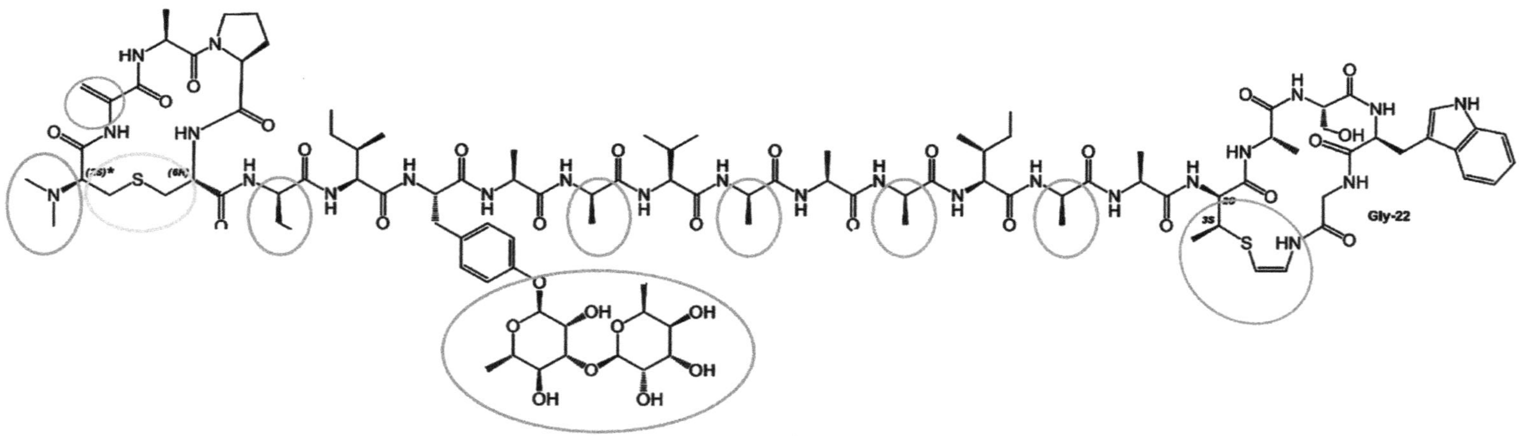

FIGURE 29.13 Structure of the class V lanthipeptide, cacaoidin. The stereochemistry of the lanthionine is proposed. The class-defining PTMs are encircled in yellow. Secondary PTMs are encircled in cyan.

29.2.4.1 Heterologous Production of Class V Lanthipeptides

In a recent study, Hurtado et al., 2021 reported the first ever heterologous production of a class V lanthipeptide, where they have described the complete identification, cloning, and heterologous expression of the cacaoidin biosynthetic gene cluster, which shows unique RiPP genes whose functions could not be predicted by any bioinformatics tool.

Cacaoidin BGC was obtained from the wild-type *S. cacaoi* CA-170360 genome sequence, with a combination of de novo PacBio and Illumina approaches, yielding two contigs of 5,971,081 bp and 2,704,105 bp. The genome sequence was analyzed with antiSMASH, BAGEL4, and PRISM, but none of these tools could help in predicting the BGC responsible for cacaoidin biosynthesis. The C-terminal sequence of the earlier isolated and identified cacaoidin (Thr-Ala-Ser-Trp-Gly-Cys; Ortiz-López et al., 2020) was used as the query in a tBLASTn using the whole genome sequence. A 162 bp Open Reading Frame (ORF) was found to encode this sequence and helped to elucidate the final structure of cacaoidin structural gene *caoA*, which encodes a 23-amino acid C-terminal core peptide (SSAPCTIYASVSASISATASWGC) following a predicted 30-amino acid N-terminal leader peptide (MGEVVEMVAGFDTYADVEELNQI AVGEAPE). Neither the leader nor the core peptide sequences showed high-sequence similarity with any other lanthipeptide or linaridin. To confirm that the genes included in the putative 30 kb cao cluster (having 27 ORFs) were sufficient for biosynthesis of the antibiotic, cloning and heterologous expression of the cacaoidin BGC in the genetically amenable host *Streptomyces albus* J1074 was done. For the purpose, the CATCH method (Cas-9-assisted targeting of chromosome) was followed and a 40 kb region containing the cao BGC was cloned into the pCAP01 vector, yielding the plamid pCAO. pCAO was then introduced into NEB-10-beta *E. coli* ET12567 cells via electroporation and a triparental conjugation was carried out to obtain *S. albus* J1074. The transconjugants obtained were genetically verified via PCR amplification of the selected cao genes. Five positive transconjugants were selected and grown for acetone extraction of the cultures, and the extracts were analyzed by LC-HRESIMS(+)-TOF and MS/MS.

29.3 Structure-Activity Relationship Studies

Structure activity relationship (SAR) is the relation between chemical structure and biological activity of a molecule. SAR enables the determination of the chemical group responsible for expressing a target biological effect in the lantibiotics. The development of methods to produce new lantibiotic variants has enabled the investigation of the structure activity relationships of these compounds and hence an evaluation of this hitherto underexploited class of natural products as a source of potential therapeutic drug candidates. Restriction in the use of lantibiotics is due to the factors like low yield, insolubility, and instability at physiological pH. To tackle these problems, various techniques have been employed for creating enhanced variants of the lantibiotics like site-saturation mutagenesis (Healy et al., 2013), site-directed mutagenesis, suitable heterologous expression systems, and efficient bioactivity assay techniques (such as antagonistic deferred bioassay; Barbosa et al., 2019). However, not every alteration leads to enhanced activity and can also decrease or can completely knock it down, which makes understanding SAR even more crucial. The study of two-peptide lantibiotics represents a relatively new field and consequently is less exploited for SAR studies.

29.3.1 Impact of Altering Bonds and Bridges

Maturation of the lantibiotics takes place after PTM where formation of the rings is one of the main steps. While they differ in sequences and in their conformational arrangement, the common structural motif present in all lantibiotics is the uncommon moiety lanthionine, consisting of two alanine residues crosslinked via a thioether linkage. Apart from general modifications (mentioned in Section 29.1.1) there are further modifications like addition of neighbouring sulfhydryl groups to form thioethers and formation of lysinoalanine bridges, which can be seen in cinnamycin-containing lysinoalanine (Lal) bridge present between lysine 19 and a Ser6 (Figure 29.14) (Ökesli et al., 2011)

a.

(2S,9S)-Lysinoalanine

b.

dehydroalanine   dehydrobutyrine   2-oxobutyryl   D-alanine

FIGURE 29.14   a) The structure of cinnamycin. In red and blue are Lan and MeLan, respectively. Lal is shown in purple (Ökesli et al., 2011). b) Structures of some unusual amino acids found in lantibiotics.

Formation of novel N-terminal blocking groups and oxidative decarboxylation of a C-terminalcysteine also takes place in class I lantibiotics (like Mutacin1140). These PTMs not only determine the three-dimensional structure of the peptides but are also critical for their biological activity (Cooper et al., 2010; Ruiz et al., 2018).

The conformation of lanthipeptides is not only governed by the sequence of amino acid but also by the presence of these rings at the specific sites (Yoganathan and Vederas, 2008). In order to know the structural importance of the rings researchers have performed various experiments.

Lacticin 3147: Alanine-scanning and random mutagenesis have been applied to the genes encoding the precursor peptides of lacticin 3147, resulting in a large amount of valuable data (Cotter et al., 2006; Field et al., 2013). However, the absence of bioactivity of several of the mutants involving the thioether rings resulted from abolished production and hence provided no direct information regarding their importance for activity. A single variant in lacticin 3147 Ltnα in which the histidine at position 23 was substituted with a serine had an increase in activity against a pathogenic strain of *S. aureus* (Field et al., 2013).

Lichenicidin: *Bacillus licheniformis* I89, a bacteria isolated from a hot spring in the Azores islands, produces the two-peptide lantibiotic, lichenicidin. The lichenicidin spectrum of activity includes several pathogens such as *S. aureus* (including MRSA), *Enterococcus faecium, Haemophilus influenza,* and *Listeria monocytogenes.* Lichenicidin was the first lantibiotic of its class to be produced totally in vivo using the Gram-negative *E. coli* (Caetano et al., 2011a). This was a major breakthrough, since the system allows the manipulation of lantibiotic peptides using simpler and less time-consuming procedures. For instance, the system enabled the production in vivo of some variants harbouring noncanonical amino acids and helped exploring the aspects necessary to understand the structure-activity function relationship of two peptide lantibiotics and also explore their bioengineering. Barbosa et al. (2019) performed the rational site-directed mutagenesis of lichenicidin lanthipeptides, based on the extensive bibliographical search available for other lantibiotics. They studied the structure-activity relationship in lichenicidin by disrupting the rings by inter-substituting threonine and serine involved in ring formation. It was observed that Dha11Dhb variant of Bliα showed significant decrease in bioactivity (Figure 29.17). It has been recognized that not all the rings present in a lantibiotic are important for its antimicrobial activity (Appleyard et al., 2009; Barbosa et al., 2019; Cooper et al., 2008; van Kraaij et al., 2000; Geng et al., 2018; Khosa et al., 2016).

Haloduracin: The structural features essential for biological activity of haloduracin were investigated using a recently developed in vitro biosynthetic system (McClerren et al., 2006). A number of haloduracin analogues were constructed and the impact of the alterations on antibiotic activity was assessed. The thioether rings in lantibiotics are believed to be the basis for their biological activity and in general disruption of a ring results in abolishment of the antimicrobial activity (Bierbaum et al., 1996; Chatterjee et al., 2005; Kuipers et al., 1995; van Kraaij et al., 2000). A comprehensive examination of the importance of each (methyl)lanthionine in haloduracin (Figure 29.15) for biological activity was performed, taking advantage of its in vitro reconstituted biosynthesis. These experiments show that mutation of Cys17, Cys23, and Cys27 resulted in Halα analogues in which the A-, B-, and C-rings were disrupted, respectively.

The qualitative antimicrobial activity of these mutants shows that the C-ring of Halα is essential for activity. The retention of bioactivity upon disrupting the B-ring of Halα was surprising given its high level of conservation in comparison with mersacidin (C-ring) actagardine (B-ring), and lacticin 3147 A1 (C-ring). These three lantibiotics bind to the peptidoglycan precursor lipid II (Brötz et al., 1998a; Wiedemann et al., 2006b; Zimmermann and Jung, 1997) and the CTLTXEC motif encompassing the conserved rings is believed to be important for this activity.

The qualitative SAR studies on Halβ resulted in removal of its A–D-rings. For the mutants disrupting the A-, C-, and D-rings, the rings not targeted by mutagenesis were still formed by HalM2 according to the p-hydroxymercuribenzoate data, but mutation of Cys15 resulted in disruption of cyclization for other rings in addition to the B-ring. These findings illustrate the danger of reaching conclusions regarding the importance of certain residues for bioactivity on the basis of mutagenesis studies, without confirming that the mutation did not interfere with ring formation.

This study also provides some additional insights into proteolytic processing of haloduracin. Interestingly, when Halα was first reduced, opening the disulfide ring at its N-terminus, followed by alkylation of Cys1 and Cys5 with IAA, it too became susceptible to additional N-terminal proteolysis. Since the disulfide is shown not to be important for antimicrobial activity in haloduracin or in plantaricin W (Holo et al., 2001; McClerren et al., 2006), it may be conserved to protect the peptide from such degradation in the extracellular environment. Similarly, the N-terminal lanthionine in lacticin 3147 A1, which is also not required for antimicrobial activity (Cotter et al., 2006), may protect this compound from proteolyis.

Study of these lantibiotic analogs suggests the importance of particular amino acid residues for activity and also points towards the possibility of other function of the rings apart from providing proteolytic stabilityto lantibiotics (Yoganathan and Vederas, 2008).

Roseocin: A two-component lantibiotic, identified in genome of *Streptomyces roseosporus* is the first two-component lantibiotic from a non-firmicute (Walker et al., 2020). Its two components RosA1β and RosA2α contain six and four thioether bridges, respectively, along with a disulphide bond present in α-peptide between Cys13 & Cys33 (Figure 29.16). Singh et al., in order to evaluate the significance of this disulphide bond, reduced it by chemically modifying it with iodoacetamide. Further it was checked for activity with the β-component against *L. monocytogenes*, MRSA, and VRE but zone of inhibition was not observed as it was with disulphide bond containing α-component, confirming that this disulphide bond is indispensable and plays an important structural role (Singh et al., 2020).

Cytolysin: Enterococcal cytolysin in a two-component lanthipeptide produced by pathogenic strains of *Enterococcus faecalis*. Cytolysin subunits, CylL$_L$" and CylL$_S$", (heterologously expressed in *E.coli* and

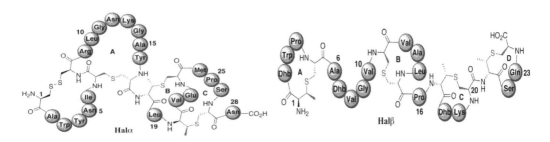

FIGURE 29.15 Detailed structure of haloduracin components (Yoganathan and Vederas, 2008).

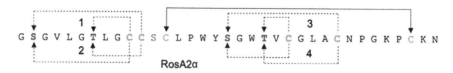

FIGURE 29.16   Possible ring patterns and unique disulphide bond position (Singh et al., 2020).

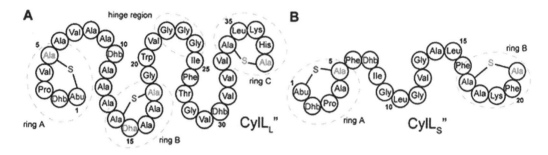

FIGURE 29.17   Structure of CylL$_L$ with rings A−C and hinge region highlighted in dashed ellipses. (B) Structure of CylL$_s$ with A and B rings highlighted in dashed ellipses (Rahman et al., 2021).

TABLE 29.4

Minimum Inhibitory Concentration Against *L.Lactis* and Values > Two Dilutions of the MIC of wt Cytolysin. Peptides in Bold are Residues Involved in Ring Formation (Rahman et al., 2021).

Peptide	MIC (nM)	Peptide	MIC (nM)
CylLL-Thr2	> 256	**CylL$_S$-T1A**	> 256
CylLL-Gly24	> 256	**CylL$_S$C5A**	> 256
CylLL-T1A	> 256	**CylL$_S$-S17A**	> 256
CylLL-C5A	> 256	**CylL$_S$-C21A**	> 256
CylLL-S14A	> 256		
CylLL-C18A	> 256		
CylLL-S34A	> 256		
CylLL-C38A	128		

post-translationally modified by CylM and hence labelled as " ; structures shown in Figure 29.17), work synergistically to lyse both bacterial and mammalian cells. Cytolysin possesss not only a unique stereo-chemistry but also an unusual lytic activity against mammalian cells (Mukherjee et al., 2016)

In a recent study, alanine substitution in both the components was done in order to identify the key residues responsible for overall activity (Rahman et al., 2021). The ring-forming residues in both the components (**CylL$_L$**"-T1A, C5A, S14A, C18A, S34A, C38A and **CylL$_S$**"-T1A, C5A, S17A, C18A) when substituted with alanine were not only essential for bioactivity but also for hemolytic activity, as mutants showed no bioactivity against *L. lactis sp.* cremoris unlike the wild type (MIC 32nM). It was observed that when Ser34 was substituted with Ala, the formation of the C-ring was prevented due to which no activity was seen. Hence, all five rings in the two peptides proved to be crucial for both antibacterial and cytolytic activity. In addition two non-ring-forming residues, CylLL-Thr2 and CylLL-Gly24, also appeared to be crucial for both biological activities (Table 29.4). The role of Thr2 was important because after dehydration to Dhb, it plays a vital role in driving stereochemistry of the A-ring (Rahman et al.,

2021). Hinge region flexibility turned out to be important for cytotoxic activity. As both bioactivities after alanine substitution in CylL$_L$"-G24A were terminated.

29.3.2 Substitution of Aromatic Amino Acid

Aromatic amino acids are important to promote hydrophobic interactions between antibacterial peptides and the cytoplasmic membrane at the lipid–water interface (Jing et al., 2003, Sanderson & Whelan; 2004). Barbosa et al. (2019) using site-directed mutagenesis created some enhanced variants of lichenicidin. From their study it was found that substitution of tyrosine in Bliα and tryptophan in Bliß with corresponding aromatic amino acid but comparatively of smaller size resulted in enhanced antimicrobial activity (Figure 29.19). It was also suggested by various studies such as of lacticin 3147 that the activity of lantibiotics can be inversely related to the size of their aromatic amino acids: Trp > Tyr > Phe (Cotter et al., 2006; Field et al., 2013).

Nisin is the most studied lantibiotic and contains no tryptophan residues (Zhou et al., 2016). Tryptophan and its three analogues (5-fluoroTrp (5FW), 5-hydroxyTrp (5HW), and 5-methylTrp (5MeW)) were integrated at four different positions of nisin (I1W, I4W, M17W, and V32W) following Petrović et al, (2013). The antimicrobial activity of both I1W and its 5FW analogue against the indicator strain L. *lactis* MG1363 decreased two times in comparison to nisin, while that of 5HW analogue decreased four times (Figure 29.18). Additionally, the tryptophan mutants (I4W and V32W) were also seen to affect the dehydration efficiency of serines or threonines.

29.3.3 Substitution of Charged Amino Acid

For generating improved variants, charged amino acids seem to play a significant role (Deegan et al., 2010; Field et al., 2013). In lichenicidin, lysine substitution in Bliα with the same charge (i.e., K12H) resulted in increased productivity and almost the same bioactivity as that of wild type. In Bliß component, mutations at K27H, K27E, and K27Q resulted in slight increase in bioactivity in comparison to the wild type.

Proline is known to influence structural conformation of peptides and glycine is also reported to do the same. Therefore, proline was substituted by Ala and Gly, which did not result in enhancement of bioactivity in Bliα; however, in Bliß proline substituted with alanine (P3A and P24A) showed enhanced bioactivity (Figure 29.19).

Molloy et al. (2013) performed saturation mutagenesis of the lysine codon at position 12 of nisA. The bioactivity was found to be significantly increased in the case of K12A, K12S, K12T, and K12P (> 125% in comparison to the wild-type). Although bioactivity was significantly enhanced against most Gram-positive strains tested, it is important to note that the level of enhanced activity shown by each derivative was strain variable. The K12A derivative consistently showed the greatest bioactivity.

29.3.4 Other Sites

In bovicin, putative lipid-II binding residue L21 when substituted with Meth and Val retained the bioactivity. Targeting variable ring B residues in bovicin N15A and A17G showed significant increase in bioactivity. The C-terminal variables were also targeted, among those A27, which was highly tolerant to change and yielded greater number of bioactive variants (A27R, A27S) (Field et al., 2013).

29.4 Conclusion and Future Prospects

As new antibiotic discovery has come to saturation, lantibiotics have proven to have great potential against antibiotic-resistant strains. The rings and bridges provide conformational flexibility and stability to the peptides, which masks them from proteolytic degradation, making them highly stable in order to penetrate bacterial membrane. Various in silico mining tools such as antiSMASH6.0 and BAGEL4 based on

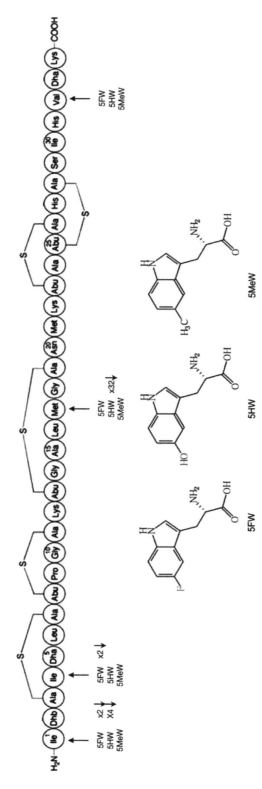

FIGURE 29.18 Insertion of tryptophan analogues in Nisin A. The arrows show the fold decrease in the bioactivity of the analogue containing variants against *L. lactisin* comparison to Nisin A.

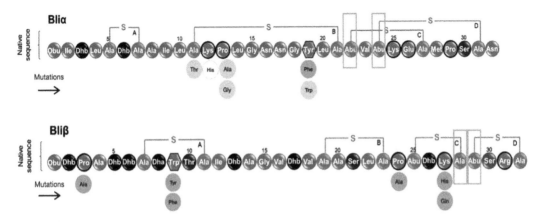

FIGURE 29.19 Mutation in Bliα and Bliβ components of lichenicidin, amino acid residues in blues indicates increase in activity, yellow indicates decrease in activity, and no color indicates no change. Amino acids vital for activity are enclosed in the box.

HMM profile and/or integrated ORF identification helped uncovering many novel lantibiotic biosynthetic gene clusters including Roseocin's. Lanthipeptides identified are not always readily produced by the native producer and hence an appropriate heterologous expression system, including appropriate modification enzyme according to their class and nature, is important. Moreover, these expression systems can also be used for vast fundamental studies including gene function, structure-function relationships, and gene expression regulation. Lantibiotics are particularly active against Gram-positive bacteria. Sequence homology coupled with experimental work, in order to tap in the potential of bioengineered lantibiotics, can further expand the antibiotic armaments against Gram-negative pathogens.

Lantibiotics, being a promising alternative to antibiotics, can be used as prophylactics and in probiotics as well. Lantibiotics serve as bactericidal barriers, which can help to reduce the levels of contaminating bacteria that might be present in packaging areas in food industries. In addition to this, their modification machinery opens the possibility to produce improved synthetic lanthipetides, which can also be used as adjuvants or additives, in relieving neuropathic pain, and even act as immune regulators apart from performing known functions like being antifungal and antiviral.

REFERENCES

Acedo JZ, Bothwell IR, An L, Trouth A, Frazier C, van der Donk WA (2019) O-Methyltransferase-Mediated Incorporation of a β-Amino Acid in Lanthipeptides. J Am Chem Soc 141: 16790–16801.

Aggarwal E, Chauhan S, Sareen D (2021) Thiopeptides encoding biosynthetic gene clusters mined from bacterial genomes. Journal of Biosciences 46: 36.

Appleyard AN, Choi S, Read DM, Lightfoot A, Boakes S, Hoffmann A, et al. (2009) Dissecting structural and functional diversity of the lantibiotic Mersacidin. Chemistry & Biology 16: 490–498.

Arnison PG, Bibb MJ, Bierbaum G, Bowers AA, Bugni TS, Bulaj G, et al. (2013) Ribosomally synthesized and post-translationally modified peptide natural products: overview and recommendations for a universal nomenclature. Nat Prod Rep 30: 108–160.

Arthur M, Courvalin P (1993) Genetics and mechanisms of glycopeptide resistance in enterococci. Antimicrob Agents Chemother. 37: 1563–1571.

Azevedo AC, Bento CBP, Ruiz JC, Queiroz MV, Mantovani HC (2015) Distribution and genetic diversity of bacteriocin gene clusters in rumen microbial genomes. Appl Environ Microbiol 81: 7290–7304.

Barbosa J, Caetano T, Mösker E, Süssmuth R, Mendo S. (2019) Lichenicidin rational site-directed mutagenesis library: A tool to generate bioengineered lantibiotics. Biotechnol Bioeng 116: 3053–3062.

Baltz RH (2007) Antimicrobials from actinomycetes: Back to the future. Microbe 2: 125–131.

Baltz RH (2014) MbtH homology codes to identify gifted microbes for genome mining. J Ind Microbiol Biotechnol 41: 357–369.

Barreteau H, Kovač A, Boniface A, Sova M, Gobec S, Blanot D (2008) Cytoplasmic steps of peptidoglycan biosynthesis. FEMS Microbiol. Rev. 32:168–207.

Begley M, Cotter PD, Hill C, Ross RP (2009) Identification of a novel two-peptide lantibiotic, lichenicidin, following rational genome mining for LanM proteins. Appl Environ Microbiol 75: 5451–5460.

Bierbaum G, Götz F, Peschel A, Kupke T, Van de kamp M, Sahl GH (1996) The biosynthesis of the lantibiotics epidermin, gallidermin, Pep5 and epilancin K7. Antonie van Leeuwenhoek 69, 119–127

Blin K, Medema MH, Kazempour D, Fischbach MA, Breitling R, Takano E, Weber T (2013) antiSMASH 2.0 – a versatile platform for genome mining of secondary metabolite producers. Nucleic Acids Res 41: 204–212.

Booth MC, Bogie CP, Sahl HG, Siezen RJ, Hatter KL, Gilmore MS (1996) Structural analysis and proteolytic activation of *Enterococcus faecalis* cytolysin, a novel lantibiotic. Mol Microbiol 21: 1175–1184.

Bothwell IR, Caetano T, Sarksian R, Mendo S, van der Donk WA (2021) Structural analysis of class I lanthipeptides from *Pedobacter lusitanus* NL19 reveals an unusual ring pattern. ACS Chem Biol 16: 1019–1029.

Bothwell IR, Cogan DP, Kim T, Reinhardt CJ, van der Donk WA, Nair SK (2019) Characterization of glutamyl-tRNA-dependent dehydratases using nonreactive substrate mimics. Proc Natl Acad Sci 116: 17245–17250.

Bouhss A, Trunkfield AE, Bugg TD, Mengin-Lecreulx D (2008) The biosynthesis of peptidoglycan lipid-linked intermediates. FEMS Microbiol. Rev. 32: 208–233.

Breukink E, Kruijff BD (2006) Lipid II as a target for antibiotics. Nat Rev Drug Discov 5: 1–12.

Brötz H, Bierbaum G, Leopold K, Reynolds PE, Sahl HG (1998a) The lantibiotic mersacidin inhibits peptidoglycan synthesis by targeting lipid II. Antimicrob Agents Chemother 42: 154–160.

Brötz H, Josten M, Wiedemann I, Schneider U, Götz F, Bierbaum G, Sahl HG (1998b) Role of lipid-bound peptidoglycan precursors in the formation of pores by nisin, epidermin and other lantibiotics. Mol Microbiol 30: 317–327.

Burkhart BJ, Hudson GA, Dunbar KL, Mitchell DA (2015). A prevalent peptide-binding domain guides ribosomal natural product biosynthesis. Nature Chemical Biology 11(8): 564–570. DOI: 10.1038/nchembio.1856.

Caetano T, Krawczyk JM, Mösker E, Süssmuth RD, Mendo S (2011a) Lichenicidin biosynthesis in *Escherichia coli*: licFGEHI immunity genes are not essential for lantibiotic production or self-protection. Appl Environ Microbiol 77: 5023–5026.

Caetano T, Krawczyk JM, Mösker E, Süssmuth RD, Mendo S (2011b) Heterologous expression, biosynthesis, mutagenesis of type II lantibiotics from *Bacillus licheniformis* in *Escherichia coli*. ChemBiol 18: 90–100.

Chatterjee C, Paul M, Xie L, van der Donk, WA (2005) Biosynthesis and mode of action of lantibiotics. ChemRev 105: 633–684.

Chatterjee S, Chatterjee D, Jani R, Blumbach J, Ganguli B, Klesel N, et al. (1991) Mersacidin, a new antibiotic from bacillus in vitro and in vivo antibacterial activity. J Antibiot (Tokyo) 45: 839–845

Combs AP (2010) Recent advances in the discovery of competitive protein tyrosine phosphatase 1B inhibitors for the treatment of diabetes, obesity, and cancer. J Med Chem 53: 2333–2344.

Cooper LE, Li B & van der Donk WA (2010) Biosynthesis and mode of action of lantibiotics. In Comprehensive Natural Products II: Chemistry and Biology, Elsevier Ltd 5: 217–256.

Cotter PD, Deegan LH, Lawton EM, Draper LA, O'Connor PM, Hill C, Ross RP (2006) Complete alanine scanning of the two-component lantibiotic lacticin 3147: Generating a blueprint for rational drug design. Mol Microbiol 62: 735–747.

Cox CR, Coburn PS, Gilmore MS (2005) Enterococcal cytolysin: a novel two component peptide system that serves as a bacterial defense against eukaryotic and prokaryotic cells. Curr Protein Pept Sci 6: 77–84.

Davies EA, Bevis HE, Potter R, Harris J, Williams GC, Delves-Broughton J (1998) Research note: The effect of pH on the stability of nisin solution during autoclaving. Lett Appl Microbiol 27: 186–187.

Deegan LH, Suda S, Lawton EM, Draper LA, Hugenholtz F, Peschel A, et al. (2010) Manipulation of charged residues within the two-peptide lantibiotic lacticin 3147. Microbial Biotechnology 3: 222–234.

De Kruijff B, van Dam V, Breukink E (2008) Lipid II: A central component in bacterial cell wall synthesis and a target for antibiotics. Prostaglandins Leukot Essent Fatty Acids 79: 117–121

Delves-Broughton J, Blackburn P, Evans RJ, Hugenholtz J (1996) Application of bacteriocin nisin. Antonie Van Leeuwenhoek 69: 193–202.

Dischinger J, Josten M, Szekat C, Sahl HG, Bierbaum G (2009) Production of the novel two-peptide lantibiotic lichenicidin by *Bacillus licheniformis* DSM 13. PLoS One 4: e6788.

Donia MS, Cimermancic P, Schulze C, Brown L, Martin J, Mitreva M, et al. (2014) A systematic analysis of biosynthetic gene clusters in the human microbiome reveals a common family of antibiotics. Cell 158: 1402–1414.

Férir G, Petrova MI, Andrei G, Huskens D, Hoorelbeke B, Snoeck R, et al. (2013) The lantibiotic peptide labyrinthopeptin A1 demonstrates broad anti-HIV and anti-HSV Activity with Potential for Microbicidal Applications. *PLoS One* 8(5): e64010.

Field D, Molloy EM, Iancu C, Draper LA, O'Connor PM, Cotter PD, Hill C, Ross RP (2013) Saturation mutagenesis of selected residues of the a-peptide of the lantibiotic lacticin 3147 yields a derivative with enhanced antimicrobial activity. Microb Biotechnol 6: 564–575.

Froseth, B. R., McKay, L. L. (1991). Molecular characterization of the nisin resistance region of Lactococcus lactis subsp. lactis biovar diacetylactis DRC3. Applied and Environmental microbiology *57*: 804–811.

Garg N, Tang W, Goto Y, Nair SK, van der Donk WA (2012) Lantibiotics from *Geobacillus thermodenitrificans*. Proc Natl Acad Sci U S A 109: 5241–5246.

Geng M, Smith L (2018) Modifying the lantibiotic mutacin 1140 for increased yield, activity, and stability. Appl Environ Microbiol 84:e00830–18.

Goto, Y, Li, B, Claesen, J, Shi, Y, Bibb, M.J, van der Donk WA (2010) Discovery of unique lanthionine synthetases reveals new mechanistic and evolutionary insights. PLoS Biol 8: 4–13.

Håvarstein LS, Diep DB, Nes IF (1995) A family of bacteriocin ABC transporters carry out proteolytic processing of their substrates concomitant with export. Mol Microbiol 16: 229–240.

Healy B, Field D, O'Connor PM, Hill C, Cotter PD, et al. (2013) Intensive mutagenesis of the nisin hinge leads to the rational design of enhanced derivatives. PLoS ONE 8(11): e79563. doi:10.1371/journal. pone.0079563.

Holo H, Jeknic Z, Daeschel M, Stevanovic S, Nes IF (2001) Plantaricin W from *Lactobacillus plantarum* belongs to a new family of two-peptide lantibiotics. Microbiology 147: 643–651.

Hsu ST, Breukink E, Tischenko E, Lutters MA, de Kruijff B, Kaptein R, Bonvin AM, van Nuland NA (2004) The nisin-lipid II complex reveals a pyrophosphate cage that provides a blueprint for novel antibiotics. NatStructMolBiol 11: 963–967.

Hudson GA, Zhang Z, Tietz JI, Mitchell DA, van der Donk WA (2015) In vitro biosynthesis of the core scaffold of the thiopeptide thiomuracin. JAmChemSoc 137:16012.

Huo L, van der Donk WA (2016) Discovery and characterization of bicereucin, an unusual D-amino acid-containing mixed two-component lantibiotic. JAmChemSoc 138: 5254–7.

Hyink O, Balakrishnan M, Tagg JR (2005) Streptococcusrattus strain BHT produces both a class I two-component lantibiotic and a class II bacteriocin. FEMSMicrobiolLett 252: 235–41.

Iftime D, Jasyk M, Kulik A, Imhoff JF, Stegmann E, Wohlleben W, et al. (2015) Streptocollin, a type IV lanthipeptide produced by *Streptomyces collinus* Tü 365. ChemBioChem 16: 2615–2623.

Ihnken LA, Chatterjee C, van der Donk WA (2009) In vitro reconstitution and substrate specificity of lantibiotic protease. Biochemistry 47: 7352–7363.

Iorio M, Sasso O, Maffioli SI, Bertorelli R, Monciardini P, Sosio M, et al. (2014) A glycosylated, labionin-containing lanthipeptide with marked antinociceptive activity. ACS Chem Biol 9: 398–404.

Jing W, Hunter HN, Hagel J, Vogel HJ (2003) The structure of the antimicrobial peptide Ac-RRWWRF-NH2 bound to micelles and its interactions with phospholipid bilayers. The Journal of Peptide Research 61: 219–229.

Jungmann NA, van Herwerden EF, Hügelland M, Süssmuth RD (2016) The supersized class III lanthipeptide stackepeptin displays motif multiplication in the core peptide. ACSChemBiol 11: 69–76.

Kawada-Matsuo M, Yoshida Y, Zendo T, Nagao J, Oogai Y, et al. (2013) Three distinct two-component systems are involved in resistance to the class I bacteriocins, nukacin ISK-1 and nisin A, in *Staphylococcus aureus*. PLoSOne 8: e69455.

Kersten RD, Yang YL, Xu Y, Cimermancic P, Nam SJ, Fenical W, Fischbach MA, Moore BS, Dorrestein PC (2011) A mass spectrometry-guided genome mining approach for natural product peptidogenomics. NatChemBiol 7: 794–802.

Khan SN, Khan AU (2016) Breaking the spell: Combating multidrug resistant "superbugs." FrontMicrobiol 7: 174.

Khosa S, Alkhatib Z, Smits SH (2013) NSR from *Streptococcus agalactiae* confers resistance against nisin and is encoded by a conserved *nsr* operon. BiolChem 394: 1543–1549.

Khosa S, Frieg B, Mulnaes D, Kleinschrodt D, Hoeppner A, Gohlke H, Smits SHJ (2016) Structural basis of lantibiotic recognition by the nisin resistance protein from *Streptococcus agalactiae*. SciRep 6: 18679.

Kleerebezem M, Quadri LE, Kuipers OP, Vos de WM (1997) Quorum sensing by peptide pheromones and two-component signal-transduction systems in Gram-positive bacteria. MolMicrobiol 24: 895–904.

KloostermanA M, Cimermancic P, Elsayed S S, Du C, Hadjithomas M, Donia M S, Fischbach M A, van Wezel G P, Medema H M (2020) Expansion of RiPP biosynthetic space through integration of pan-genomics and machine learning uncovers a novel class of lanthipeptides. Plos Biology 18(12): e3001026. https://doi.org/10.1371/journal.pbio.3001026.

Kodani S, Hudson ME, Durrant MC, Buttner MJ, Nodwell JR, Willey JM (2004) The SapB morphogen is a lantibiotic-like peptide derived from the product of the developmental gene ramS in *Streptomyces coelicolor*. ProcNatlAcadSciUSA 101: 11448–53.

Kodani S, Lodato MA, Durrant MC, Picart F, Willey JM (2005) SapT, a lanthionine-containing peptide involved in aerial hyphae formation in the *streptomycetes*. MolMicrobiol 58: 1368–1380.

Krawczyk B, Völler GH, Völler J, Ensle P, Süssmuth RD (2012) Curvopeptin: a new lanthionine-containing class III lantibiotic and its co-substrate promiscuous synthetase. ChemBioChem 13: 2065–2071.

Krawczyk JM, Völler GH, Krawczyk B, Kretz J, Brönstrup M, Süssmuth RD (2013) Heterologous expression and engineering studies of labyrinthopeptins, class III lantibiotics from *Actinomadura namibiensis*. ChemBiol 20: 111–122.

Krug D, Müller R (2014) Secondary metabolomics: the impact of mass spectrometry-based approaches on the discovery and characterization of microbial natural products. NatProdRep 31: 768–83.

Kuipers OP, Beerthuyzen MM, Ruyter PG de, Luesink EJ, Vos WM de (1995) Autoregulation of nisin biosynthesis in *Lactococcus lactis* by signal transduction. JBiolChem 270: 27299–27304.

Lawton, EM, Ross, RP, Hill, C, Cotter, PD (2007) Two-peptide lantibiotics: a medical perspective. MiniRevMedChem 7: 1236–1247

Li B, Sher D, Kelly L, Shi Y, Huang K, Knerr PJ (2010) Catalytic promiscuity in the biosynthesis of cyclic peptide secondary metabolites in planktonic marine cyanobacteria. ProcNatlAcadSciUSA 107: 10430–1435.

Li B, Yu JP, Brunzelle JS, Moll GN, van der Donk WA (2005) Structure and mechanism of the lantibiotic cyclase involved in nisin biosynthesis. Science 311: 1464–1467.

Lohans, CT, Li, JL, Vederas, JC (2014) Structure and biosynthesis of carnolysin, a homologue of enterococcal cytolysin with D-amino acids. JAmChemSoc 136: 13150–13153.

Martin NI, Sprules T, Carpenter MR, Cotter PD, Hill C, Ross RP, Vederas, JC (2004) Structural characterization of Lacticin 3147, A two-peptide lantibiotic with synergistic activity. Biochemistry 43: 3049–3056.

Marsh, AJ, O'Sullivan, O, Ross, RP, Cotter, PD, Hill, C (2010) *In silico* analysis highlights the frequency and diversity of type 1 lantibiotic gene clusters in genome sequenced bacteria. BMC Genomics 11: 679.

McAuliffe, O, Ross, R, Hill, C (2001) lantibiotics: Biosynthesis and mode of action. ChemRev 105: 633–683.

McClerren, AL, Cooper, LE, Quan, C, Thomas, PM, Kelleher, NL, van der Donk, W A (2006) Suppl Discovery and in vitro biosynthesis of haloduracin, a two-component lantibiotic. Proc Natl Acad Sci USA 103: 17243–17248.

Medema MH, Fischbach MA (2015) Computational approaches to natural product discovery. Nat Chem Biol 11: 639–648.

Meindl K, Schmiederer T, Schneider K, Reicke A, Butz D, Keller S, et al. (2010) Labyrinthopeptins: a new class of carbacyclic lantibiotics. Angew Chem Int Ed Engl 49: 1151–1154.

Mishra RPN, Oviedo-Orta E, Prachi P, Rappuoli R, Bagnoli F (2012) Vaccines and antibiotic resistance. CurrOpinMicrobiol 15: 596–602.

Mohr KI, Volz C, Jansen R, Wray V, Hoffmann J, Bernecker S, et al. (2015) Pinensins: the first antifungal lantibiotics. Angew Chem Int Ed Engl 54:11254–8.

Molloy EM, Field D, O' Connor PM, Cotter PD, Hill C, et al. (2013) Saturation mutagenesis of lysine 12 leads to the identification of derivatives of nisin a with enhanced antimicrobial activity. PLoS ONE 8: e58530

Montalbán-López M, Scott TA, Ramesh S, Rahman IR, van Heel AJ, Viel JH, et al. (2021) New developments in RiPP discovery, enzymology and engineering. Natural Products Reports 38: 130–239.

Mukherjee S, Huo L, Thibodeaux G, van der Donk WA (2016) Synthesis and bioactivity of diastereomers of the virulence lanthipeptide cytolysin. Org Lett 18(23): 6188–6191.

Müller, WM, Ensle, P, Krawczyk, B, Süssmuth, RD (2011) Leader peptide-directed processing of labyrinthopeptin A2 precursor peptide by the modifying enzyme LabKC. Biochemistry 50: 8362–8373.

Müller WM, Schmiederer T, Ensle P, Süssmuth RD (2010) In vitro biosynthesis of the prepeptide of Type-III lantibiotic labyrinthopeptin A2 including formation of a C-C bond as a post-translational modification. Angew Chemie Int Ed 49: 2436–2440.

Neuhaus FC, Baddiley J (2003) A continuum of anionic charge: Structures and function of D-alanyl-Teichoic acids in Gram-positive bacteria. Microb Mol Bio Rev 67: 686–723.

O'Sullivan O, Begley M, Ross RP, Cotter PD, Hill C (2011) Further identification of novel lantibiotic operons using LanM-based genome mining. Probiotics Antimicrob Proteins 3: 27–40.

Okeley, NM, Paul, M, Stasser, JP, Blackburn N, van der Donk WA (2003) SpaC and NisC, the cyclases involved in subtilin and nisin biosynthesis, are zinc proteins. Biochemistry 42: 13613–13624.

Ökesli A, Cooper LE, Fogle EJ, van der Donk WA. (2011) Nine post-translational modifications during the biosynthesis of cinnamycin. J Am Chem Soc. 133: 13753–13760.

Ortega, MA, Cogan, DP, Mukherjee, S, Garg, N, Li, B, Thibodeaux, GN, et al. (2017) Two flavoenzymes catalyze the post-translational generation of 5-Chlorotryptophan and 2-aminovinyl-cysteine during NAI-107 biosynthesis. ACS Chem Biol 12: 548–557.

Ortega MA, Hao Y, Zhang Q, Walker MC, van der Donk WA, Nair SK (2015) Structure and mechanism of the tRNA-dependent lantibiotic dehydratase NisB. Nature 517: 509–12

Ortiz-López FJ, Carretero-Molina D, Sánchez-Hidalgo M, Martín J, González I, Román-Hurtado F, et al. (2020) First member of the new lanthidin RiPP Family. Angew Chem Int Ed Engl 59: 12654–12658.

Petrović DM, Leenhouts K, van Roosmalen ML, Broos J (2013) An expression system for the efficient incorporation of an expanded set of tryptophan analogues. Amino Acids 44: 1329–1336.

Rahman IR, Sanchez A, Tang W, van der Donk WA. (2021) Structure-activity relationships of the enterococcal cytolysin. ACS Infect Dis. https://doi.org/10.1021/acsinfecdis.1c00197.

Reiners J, Abts A, Clemens R, Smits SHJ, Schmitt L (2017) Stoichiometry and structure of a lantibiotic maturation complex. Sci Rep 7: 42163.

Repka LM, Hetrick KJ, Chee SH, van der Donk WA (2018) Characterization of Leader Peptide Binding During Catalysis by the Nisin Dehydratase NisB. J Am Chem Soc 140: 4200–4203

Román-Hurtado F, Sánchez-Hidalgo M, Martín J, Ortiz-López FJ, Genilloud O (2021) Biosynthesis and heterologous expression of cacaoidin, the first member of the lanthidin family of RiPPs. Antibiotics (Basel) 10:403.

Russell AH, Truman AW (2020) Genome mining strategies for ribosomally synthesised and post-translationally modified peptides. Comput Struct Biotechnol J 18:1838–1851.

Sanderson JM, Whelan EJ (2004) Characterisation of the interactions of aromatic amino acids with diacetyl phosphatidylcholine. Phys Chem Chem Phys 6: 1012–1017.

Sandiford SK (2017) Genome database mining for the discovery of novel lantibiotics. Expert Op in Drug Discov 12: 489–495.

Schneider T, Sahl HG (2010) Lipid II and other bactoprenol-bound cell wall precursors as drug targets. Curr Op in Investig Drugs 11: 157–164.

Shi Y, Yang X, Garg N, van der Donk WA (2011) Production of lantipeptides in *Escherichia coli*. J Am Chem Soc 133: 2338–2341.

Singh M, Chaudhary S, Sareen D (2017) Non-ribosomal peptide synthetases: Identifying the cryptic gene clusters and decoding the natural product. J Biosci 42: 175–187.

Singh M, Chaudhary S, Sareen D (2020) Roseocin, a novel two-component lantibiotic from an actinomycete. Mol Microbiol 113: 326–337.

Singh M, Sareen D (2014) Novel LanT associated lantibiotic clusters identified by genome database mining. PLoS One 9: e91352.

Stevens KA, Sheldon BW, Klapes NA, Klaenhammer TR (1991) Nisin treatment for inactivation of *Salmonella* species and other Gram-negative bacteria. Appl Environ Microbiol 57: 3613–3615.

Stein T, Heinzmann S, Solovieva I, Entian KD (2003) Function of *Lactococcus lactis* nisin immunity genes nisI and nisFEG after coordinated expression in the surrogate host *Bacillus subtilis*. J Biol Chem 278: 89–94.

Tang W, Dong S-H, Repka LM, He C, Nair SK, van der Donk WA (2015) Applications of the class II lanthipeptide protease LicP for sequence-specific, traceless peptide bond cleavage. Chem Sci 6: 6270–6279.

Ueda K, Oinuma KI, Ikeda G, Hosono K, Ohnishi Y, Horinouchi S, Beppu T (2002) AmfS, an extracellular peptidic morphogen in *Streptomyces griseus*. J Bacteriol 184: 1488–1492.

van der Meer JR, Polman, J, Beerthuyzen MM, Siezen RJ, Kuipers OP, de Vos WM (1993) Characterization of the *Lactococcus lactis* nisin A operon genes nisP, encoding a subtilisin-like serine protease involved in precursor processing, and nisR, encoding a regulatory protein involved in nisin biosynthesis. J Bacteriol 175:2578–2588.

van der Meer JR, Harry S, Rollema S, Siezen RJ, Beerthuyzen MM, Kuipers OP, de Vos WM (1994) Influence of amino acid substitutions in the nisin leader peptide on biosynthesis and secretion of nisin by lactococcus lactis. J Biol Chem 5: 3555-3562.

Van Heel AJ, de Jong A, Song C, Viel JH, Kok J, Kuipers OP (2018) BAGEL4: A user-friendly web server to thoroughly mine RiPPs and bacteriocins. Nucleic Acids Res 46: 278–281.

Van Kraaij C, Breukink E, Rollema HS, Bongers RS, Kosters HA, de Kruijff B, Kuipers OP (2000) Engineering a disulfide bond and free thiols in the lantibiotic nisin Z. Eur J Biochem 267: 901–909.

Van Staden ADP, van Zyl WF, Trindade M, Dicks LMT, Smith C (2021) Therapeutic application of lantibiotics and other lanthipeptides: Old and new findings. Appl Environ Microbiol. 87: e0018621.

Völler, GH, Krawczyk, JM, Pesic, A, Krawczyk, B, Nachtigall, J, Süssmuth, RD (2012) Characterization of new class III lantibiotics-erythreapeptin, avermipeptin and griseopeptin from *Saccharopolyspora erythraea*, *Streptomyces avermitilis* and *Streptomyces griseus* demonstrates stepwise N-terminal leader processing. Chem Bio Chem 13: 1174–1183.

Walker MC, Eslami SM, Hetrick KJ, Ackenhusen SE, Mitchell DA, van der Donk WA (2020) Precursor peptide-targeted mining of more than one hundred thousand genomes expands the lanthipeptide natural product family. BMC Genomics. 21: 387. https://doi.org/10.1186/s12864-020-06785-7.

Walsh CJ, Guinane CM, Hill C, Ross RP, O'Toole PW, Cotter PD (2015) *In silico* identification of bacteriocin gene clusters in the gastrointestinal tract, based on the Human Microbiome Project's reference genome database. BMC Microbiol 15: 183.

Walsh CJ, Guinane CM, O' Toole, PW Cotter, PD (2017) A Profile Hidden Markov Model to investigate the distribution and frequency of LanB-encoding lantibiotic modification genes in the human oral and gut microbiome. Peer J 5: e3254.

Wang H, van der Donk WA (2012) Biosynthesis of the class III lantipeptide catenulipeptin. ACS Chem Biol 7: 1529–1535.

Wang H, Fewer DP, Sivonen K (2011) Genome mining demonstrates the widespread occurrence of gene clusters encoding bacteriocins in cyanobacteria. PLoS One 6: e22384.

Wang J Ge, X Zhang L, Teng K, Zhong J (2016) One-pot synthesis of class II lanthipeptide bovicin HJ50 via an engineered lanthipeptide synthetase. Sci Rep 6: 38630.

Wang J, Ma H, Ge X, Zhang J, Teng K, Sun Z, Zhong J (2014a) Bovicin HJ50-like lantibiotics, a novel sub-group of lantibiotics featured by an indispensable disulfide bridge. PLoS One 9: 1–11.

Wang J, Zhang L, Teng K, Sun S, Sun Z, Zhong J (2014b) Cerecidins, novel lantibiotics from *Bacillus cereus* with potent antimicrobial activity. Appl Environ Microbiol 80: 2633–2643.

Wiedemann I, Breukink E, Kraaij C van, Kuipers OP, Bierbaum G, Kruijff B de, Sahl HG (2001) Specific binding of nisin to the peptidoglycan precursor lipid II combines pore formation and inhibition of cell wall biosynthesis for potent antibiotic activity. J Biol Chem 276: 1772–1779.

Xiao H (2004) Bovicin HJ50, a novel lantibiotic produced by *Streptococcus bovis* HJ50. Microbiology 150: 103–108.

Xie L, Miller LM, Chatterjee C, Averin O, Kelleher NL, van der Donk W (2004) Lacticin 481: in vitro reconstitution of lantibiotic synthetase activity. Science 303: 679–681.

Xu M, Zhang F, Cheng Z, Bashiri G, Wang J, et al. (2020) Functional genome mining reveals a class V lanthipeptide containing a d-amino acid introduced by an F420 H2-dependent reductase. Angew Chem Int Ed Engl 59:18029–18035.

Yoganathan S, & Vederas JC (2008) Fracturing rings to understand lantibiotics. Chemistry & Biology 15: 999–1001.

Yonezawa H, Kuramitsu HK (2005) Genetic analysis of a unique bacteriocin, Smb, produced by *Streptococcus mutans* GS5. Antimicrob Agents Chemother 49: 541–548.

Zhang Q, Doroghazi JR, Zhao X, Walker, MC, van der Donk WA (2015) Expanded natural product diversity revealed by analysis of lanthipeptide-like gene clusters in Actinobacteria. Appl Environ Microbiol 18: 4339–4358.

Zhang Q, Yu Y, Velasquez JE, van der Donk WA (2012) Evolution of lanthipeptide synthetases. Proc Natl Acad Sci 109: 18361–18366.

Zhao X, van der Donk WA (2016) Structural characterization and bioactivity analysis of the two-component lantibiotic *flv* system from a ruminant bacterium. Cell Chem Biol 23: 1–11

Zhou L, Shao J, Li Q, van Heel AJ, de Vries MP, Broos J, Kuipers OP (2016) Incorporation of tryptophan analogues into the lantibiotic nisin. Amino Acids 48:1309–1318.

Zimmermann N, Jung G (1997) The three-dimensional solution structure of the lantibiotic murein-biosynthesis-inhibitor actagardine determined by NMR. Eur J Biochem 246: 809–819.

30

Traditional Medicines for the Control of Leishmaniasis: Experimental Studies

Jyoti Joshi
Goswami Ganesh Dutta Sanatan Dharma College, Chandigarh, India

Rupinder Kaur
Khalsa College for Women, Civil Lines, Ludhiana, India

Sukhbir Kaur
Department of Zoology, Panjab University, Chandigarh, India

30.1 Introduction

Leishmaniasis includes a broad array of diseases infecting humans and other mammals (Ramirez et al., 2016). It is a neglected tropical disease (WHO, 2010) prevalent in 98 countries of the world and more than 350 million people are at risk globally (Herrera et al., 2020). The disease is estimated with 7 lakh-10 lakh new cases (WHO, 2020) and 20,000 to 30,000 deaths occurring annually (WHO, 2017). Among the various forms of leishmaniasis, the highest endemicity of visceral leishmaniasis (VL) is found in the East Africa and Indian subcontinent. According to the World Health Organization, in 2018, more than 95% of new cases were reported in 10 countries: Brazil, China, Ethiopia, India, Iraq, Kenya, Nepal, Somalia, South Sudan, and Sudan (WHO, 2020). In India, leishmaniasis is found endemic in the states of Bihar, Uttar Pradesh, Jharkhand, and West Bengal (Gupta et al., 2017).

30.1.1 Vaccines

Leishmaniasis is considered as one of the few parasitic diseases likely to be controlled by vaccination. The long-lasting effect of vaccines and the fact that resistant cases will not occur makes them more profitable over chemotherapy. The earliest vaccination procedures included the use of live parasites called leishmanization (Joshi et al., 2014) later followed by killed or live attenuated *Leishmania* parasites (first-generation vaccines). More recent approaches include second-generation subunit and recombinant *Leishmania* proteins and DNA encoding third-generation vaccines (Nagill and Kaur, 2011). Though many scientists are investigating the possibility of vaccination, no human vaccine is available against this fatal disease (Thakur et al., 2020; Singh et al., 2012).

30.1.2 Chemotherapy

It is well known that leishmaniasis is a disease that can be treated and cured (WHO, 2016). The treatment depends on several factors like type of disease and the causative species, associated pathogenesis, and geographic location. Chemotherapy is the main control strategy for leishmaniasis, and pentavalent antimonials (SbV) were the first-line drugs used (Arevalo et al., 2007) as shown in Table 30.1. Nevertheless, these antimonials have drawbacks and side effects including anorexia, emesis, giddiness, muscles and joint pain, fever, parenteral administration, high cost, and long course therapy (Fernandez

TABLE 30.1

Drugs Used for the Cure of Leishmaniasis (Source: WHO, 2017)

Drugs	Dosing	Regions	Limitations
Pentavalent Antimonials: Sodium stibogluconate, Meglumine antimoniate	> 30 days, Intramuscular or Intravenous injections or 17 days in combination with paromomycin ointment	All endemic regions Used in East Africa	Toxic, and drug resistance is common
Liposomal amphotericin B (L-AmB)	1 to 5 days, intravenous injections	First-line treatment: Indian subcontinent Second-line treatment: East Africa	IV injection limits its use in peripheral settings; requires cold chain
Miltefosine	28 days, oral	In India since 2003	Few limitations, include diarrhoea or vomiting; cannot be given to women in child-bearing age without contraception (teratogenic); adherence to 28 days treatment is an issue; high price, limited availability
Paromomycin	17 days, Intramuscular injection	First-line treatment: East Africa (in combination with antimonials)	

et al., 2014; Gamboa-Leon et al., 2014). Moreover, the increasing parasite resistance and treatment failure pose major constraints to successful therapy of the disease (Jain and Jain, 2015). Amphotericin B deoxycholate (AmB-D) was recommended as the second-line drug with more than 90% efficacy in Indian VL patients. However, prolonged hospitalization and other side effects like nephrotoxicity, hypokalemia, and infusion-related fever and chills do not suggest the use of conventional amphotericin B over antimonials for use outside India (Pavli and Maltezou, 2010). To ameliorate the side effects, different lipid complexes replacing the conventional lipids of amphotericin B were prepared that facilitated the target delivery in specified tissues and reduced the toxicities (Sundar and Chakravarty, 2015). Thus, L-AmB is the drug of choice but the high cost and varied dose requirements due to the geographical variations limits its use in various parts of the world (Sundar and Chakravarty, 2015). The discovery of miltefosine was considered as a new hope against the standard antileishmanial therapy as for the first time, an oral drug was identified. However, the teratogenic nature of miltefosine strongly prohibits its use in pregnant women (Coelho, 2016). Thus, none of the anti-leishmanials discovered so far can circumvent the limitations making it more necessary to find alternatives for the cure of the disease (Pavli and Maltezou, 2010).

30.1.3 Immunology

The battle between susceptibility to leishmaniasis and eradication of disease depends upon the type of immune response elicited by the host immune system against the parasite. Components of the immune system involved in this process are innate and adaptive immune responses (Gupta et al., 2013). Earlier studies have revealed that complement systems play a leading role in the elimination of parasite from the blood stream. But later studies reported that the eradication of promastigotes is dependent upon the concentration of serum-complement components (Evans-Osses et al., 2013). However, the amastigote form and metacyclic promastigotes have been found more resistant to complement lysis as compared to procyclic promastigotes (Gupta et al., 2013). A clear dichotomy between protection and disease

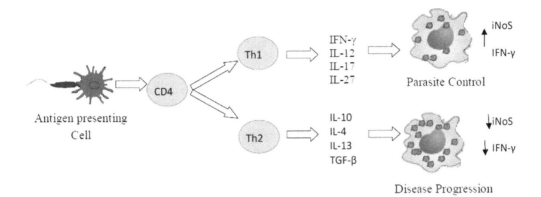

FIGURE 30.1   Immune response in leishmaniasis.

progression through Th1 or Th2 immune responses has been well demonstrated in experimental cutaneous leishmaniasis (Cummings et al., 2010). However, this dichotomy is not that clear in murine visceral leishmaniasis and even more complicated in human visceral leishmaniasis (Rodrigues et al., 2016). IFN-γ and IL-10 are, respectively, identified as counter regulatory Th1 and Th2 cytokines promoting resistance and susceptibility to infection (de Freitas et al., 2016). In canine visceral leishmaniasis, the central target organs (i.e., liver and spleen) present a mixed cytokine immune response in early infection. However, IFN-γ and IL-2 are upregulated in chronic stages of infection (Rodriguez-Cortés et al., 2016). In some studies, during acute visceral leishmaniasis in humans and elevated levels of IFN-γ and TGF-β have been observed in serum samples along with increased expression of IFN-γ mRNA in lymphoid organs. Whereas in PBMC (peripheral blood mononuclear cells) supernatants, the IL-12 has been found to be absent along with negligible or no levels of IFN-γ and IL-2 (Goto and Prianti, 2009). The absence of Th1 type of immune responses in the PBMC from VL patients is correlated with the progression of disease (Nylen and Sacks, 2007). IL-12 augments the Th1 type of immune response in naturally infected and experimentally infected dogs by enhancing the lymphocytic proliferation and IFN-γ production by PBMC (Strauss-Ayali et al., 2005; Rodríguez-Cortés et al., 2016). IL-17, another inflammatory cytokine, also acts synergistically with IFN-γ in providing protection against infection with *L. infantum* as demonstrated by increased NO production in the infected macrophages (Pitta et al., 2009).

Th1 type of immune responses are limited by the action of Th2 type of immune responses via IL-10 and IL-4 cytokines, which suppress the activation of macrophages and help in survival of intracellular amastigotes and development of disease (Awasthi et al., 2004) as shown in Figure 30.1. Experimental studies have established that IL-10 plays a crucial role in the progression of VL (Mutiso et al., 2013). The BALB/c mice lacking the gene for IL-10 became highly resistant to VL, which was followed by increased IFN-γ and NO production (Faleiro et al., 2014). The blockage of IL-10 receptor by monoclonal Ab in experimental murine VL markedly enhanced IL-12 and IFN-γ in serum samples and tissue-inducible NO synthase expression (Murray et al., 2003). CD8+ T cells also play a decisive role in the control of VL in non-self-cure mice (i.e., BALB/c mice by exhibiting perforin-dependent cytotoxicity and secretion of IFN-γ and CC chemokines) (Tsagozis et al., 2003; Kaushal et al., 2014). During chronic *L. donovani* infection, bystander CD8+ T cells expanded for the enhanced production of IFN-γ and provide heterologous immunity (Polley et al., 2005; Stager and Rafati, 2012).

30.2 Traditional Medicines

It is well advocated that during *Leishmania* infection, the immune system is suppressed. During the onset of disease, the levels of Th2 type of cytokines like IL-4, IL-10, and IL-13 are elevated while Th1 type

(IFN-γ, IL-12, and IL-17) are lowered. Thus, in the search for an effective antileishmanial agent, an ideal approach is to explore those compounds that can modulate Th2 type of immune response towards Th1 type via restoration of requisite signaling between macrophages and T cells, thus helping in resolution of the disease.

Hence, identification of novel antileishmanial drugs with good immunomodulatory property is the priority area of ongoing research. Many medicinal plants are available in the nature that help in curing our daily health problems and promote positive health by maintaining organic resistance against infections.

Ayurveda is one of the oldest traditional system of Indian medicine, is based on plants and their byproducts. It involves a holistic approach to healing that includes our life, mind, body and spirit. The ethno-medicines in ayurveda works through modulation of immune responses without causing an imbalance in overall physiology (Kumar et al., 2014; Vayalil et al., 2002). Various studies have proved the antiparasitic potential of different plant extracts. These extracts are used either in crude form or as purified components and are increasingly becoming potential sources of newer drug candidates against a variety of parasites (Passero et al., 2014; Kayser and Kiderlen, 2001). A range of different plant species have been screened that possess the antileishmanial and immunomodulatory potential to cure life-threatening and disfiguring leishmaniasis (Chan-Bacab and Peña-Rodríguez, 2001).

30.2.1 *In Vitro* Antileishmanial Activity of Plant Extracts

The first step in screening an antileishmanial compound is testing its efficacy *in vitro* and finding if the drug/extract used is toxic to the cell or not. A lot of research work has been carried out on different plant extracts. For instance, El-on et al. (2009) evaluated the *in vitro* antileishmanial potential of 41 Israeli plants (methanolic extracts) against *Leishmania major*. Of all the plants, *Nuphar lutea* and *Withania somnifera* were most effective, while other plants (i.e., *Pteris vittata, Smyrnium olusatrum, Trifolium clypeatum, Erodium malacoides, Hyparrhenia hirta, Thymelaea hirsute,* and *Pulicaria crispa)* were moderate to marginally effective against the parasite. In a similar study conducted by Mesquita et al. (2005) about 31 extracts of 13 medicinal plants from Brazil were evaluated for their antiprotozoal activity against promastigotes of *L. donovani.* Fifteen extracts, particularly those of *Annona crassiflora, Guarea kunthiana, Himatanthu sobovatus, Serjania lethalis,* and *Cupania vernalis,* were found to be active with inhibitory concentration ranging between 0.1 to10 µg/ml. Iranian plants such as *Hyssopus officinalis, Tussilago farfara,* and *Carum copticum* were also found to have significant antileishmanial efficacy against promastigotes (Tabatabaie et al., 2014). The n-hexane fraction of *Achillea wilhelmsii* crude extract was found active against *Leishmania major* promastigotes (IC50:58.27 ± 0.52 µg/mL) and consisted of 66 compounds as analyzed by GC-MS (Achakzai et al., 2019). Similarly, it was observed that out of 22 different extracts prepared from 7 plant species, the ethanolic extract prepared form the leaves from *Dyospiros hispida* (IC50 55.48 ± 2.77 µg/mL and IC50 80.63 ± 13.17 µg/mL, respectively) and the EtOAc extract from the stems of *Aspidosperma tomentosum* (IC50: 9.70±2.82 µg/mL and IC50:15.88±1.53 µg/mL, respectively) were found most active against both the promastigote and amastigote forms of *L. infantum.* Further, TLC and HPLC detected the presence of anthraquinones, terpenes, and saponins in the *Dyospiros hispida* while, alkaloids, and flavonoids in *Aspidosperma tomentosum*, respectively, which were considered the reason for growth inhibition of these parasites (de Paula et al., 2019). The methanolic and chloroform extracts of roots of "Indian Valerian" *Valeriana wallichii* have shown significant antileishmanial activity against promastigotes of *L. donovani* and both promastigotes and amastigotes of *L. major* (Ghosh et al., 2011). The two fractions, Fab4 and Fab5, of *Agaricusblazei* water extract have shown significant inhibition of the parasite viability in vitro, with IC50 values of 15.8 ± 1.2 and 13.0 ± 1.3 µg/mL, respectively. These fractions were also found to significantly reduce the liver and spleen parasite load in therapeutic and chemoprophylactic animals (Valadares et al., 2012). The fatty acid-rich fraction of *Arrabidaeachica*hexanic extract has shown significant inhibition of promastigotes of *L. amazonensis* and *L. infantum* at IC50 of 37.2 and 18.6 µg/mL, respectively. It was found that the inhibition could be due to mitochondrion damage and peptidase inhibition of both the species (Rodrigues et al., 2014). The isolation of an essential oil and its major constituent 7-hydroxycalamenene of *Croton cajucara* has shown MIC (minimum inhibitory concentration) of 250 and 15.6 µg/mL, respectively, against

L. chagasi promastigotes by causing cell membranes perforation and disruption of membrane polysaccharides, fatty acids, and phospholipids, leading to serious cell damage (Rodrigues et al., 2013). *Cinnamomum cassia* dichloromethane fraction (CBD) exhibited significant antipromastigote activity (IC50) of 33.6 µg/ml as evident by increased proportion of cells in sub-G_0-G_1 phase, increase ROS production, Phosphatidyl serine externalization and DNA fragmentation (Afrin et al., 2019). In another study, alcoholic extracts of *Delonix regia* and *Sida acuta* significantly inhibited promastigote growth at concentrations ranging from 10 to 100 µg/ml against SSG responsive and unresponsive strains of *Leishmania donovani* and showed negligible cytotoxicity against HeLa cells (Ganeti et al., 2015) showing that the plant extract can be beneficial for those cases where resistance has been reported to the standard drugs. The hexane extract of *Warburgia ugandensis* has been found most effective against *L. major* promastigotes and amastigotes amongst various other solvents used with IC50 value of 9.95 µg/mL for promastigotes and 8.65 µg/mL for amastigotes and minimum inhibitory concentrations of 62.5 µg/mL (Ngure et al., 2009). It has been well documented that the antileishmanial efficacy of the plant extract is due to the presence of secondary metabolites present in them. Be it alkaloids, terpenes, saponins, glycosides, essential oil, etc. These secondary metabolites work alone or as synergist/antagonist with the other compound and work like a combination therapy in the plant extracts. Thus, isolating these compounds and evaluating them for the antileishmanial potential is a growing area of research interest. The three quinoline alkaloids (i.e., chimanine-B, chimanine-D, and 2-n-propylquinoline) isolated from *Galipea longiflora* exhibited significant antileishmanial activity (i.e., IC90 of 25, 25 µg/mL, and 50, respectively, against *L. braziliensis* promastigotes). The four alkaloids (i.e., lysicamine, trivalvone, palmatine, and jatrorrhizine) obtained from *Annickiakummeriae* have shown moderate leishmanicidal activity with minimum inhibitory concentration ranging from 2.7±0.001 to 20.4±0.003 µg/mL and selectivity index 1.7–15.6 against *L. donovani* (Malebo et al., 2013). The alkaloids and acetogenins isolated from two *Annonacea* species have been examined against promastigotes and amastigotes of *L. chagasi,* which exhibited an IC50 of 23.3 µg/mL ranging from 25.9 to 37.6 µg/mL and 3.5 to 28.7 µg/mL, respectively (Vila-Nova et al., 2011). The semi-synthetic derivatives of natural biflavonoids obtained from the ethyl acetate extract of fruit epicarps of *Garcinia brasiliensis* (i.e., morelloflavone-7,4',7'',3''',4'''-penta-O-butanoyl, morelloflavone-7,4',7'',3''',4'''-penta-O-methyl and Morelloflavone-7,4',7'',3''',4'''-penta-O-acetyl) have shown significant leishmanicidal activity against the promastigotes of *L.amazonensis* with IC50 values of 0.0189, 0.0403, and 0.0147 µM, respectively (Gontijo et al., 2012). In a similar study, a bioflavonoid fukugetin derived from ethyl acetate extract of pericarp of this plant was found to be a significant (50%) protease inhibitor of 3.2±0.5 µM/mL against *Leishmania* by inhibiting its proteases but exhibited no activity against leishmanial cells (Pereira et al., 2011). However, flavonones from *Baccharis retusa* exhibited significant activity against cutaneous leishmaniasis species (GreccoSdos et al., 2012). A flavonol methyl ether compound isolated from methanolic leaf extract of *Vitex peduncularis* Wall was found to show better leishmanicidal activity than SAG having IC50 values for promastigote, 2.4 and 58.5 µM and for amastigotes, 0.93 and 36.2 µM, respectively. This flavonol enhanced the production of NO and increased the inducible nitric oxide synthase activity in parasite-infested macrophages in order to suppress the disease (Rudrapaul et al., 2014). Arginase is an enzyme that is central to *Leishmania* polyamine biosynthesis. The glucoside flavonoid Orientin (luteolin-8-C-glucoside) isolated from the ethanol extract of *Cecropia pachystachya* was evaluated for survival/proliferation and arginase activity of *L. amazonensis* promastigotes and was found to inhibit the arginase with IC50 of 15.9 mM. The ethyl acetate fraction was found to be non-cytotoxic to splenocytes at 200 µg/mL concentration and also inhibited the growth of *L. amazonensis* promastigotes with IC50 of 53.3 ± 6.4 µg/mL by altering mitochondrial DNA arrangement and inhibiting arginase (Cruz Ede et al., 2013). The two triterpenic acids (i.e., oleanolic and maslinic acids fractioned from Tunisian olive leaf extract) were examined for their effect on promastigotes of *L. infantum* and *L. amazonensis* and showed activity with 50% inhibitory concentration of 12.5±1.25 and 9.3±1.65 µg/mL, respectively. They significantly inhibited the parasite growth by inhibiting the mitochondrial membrane potential concomitant with reduction in ATP levels in promastigotes (Sifaoui et al., 2014). *Musa paradisiaca* fruit peel consisisting of triterpenes, cycloeucalenone and 24-methylene-cicloartanol, showed antileishmanial activity similar to amphotericin B against amastigotes (Silva et al., 2014). Interestingly, the two diterpenes (i.e., pinifolic and kaurenoic acid) were isolated from copaiba oil of *Copaifera officinales* and found to possess significant antiamastigote activity with IC50 of 3.5 and 4.0 µg/mL, respectively. It was demonstrated that significant mitochondrial alterations led to amastigote apoptosis (Santos et al., 2013). A sesquiterpene lactone isolated from *Tithonia diversifolia* leaves extract was checked for its anti-promastigote activity against *L. braziliensis* promastigotes and showed IC50 of 1.5±0.50 µg/mL (de Toledo et al., 2014). Likewise, a dichloromethane fraction enriched in sesquiterpene lactone isolated from the plant *Tanacetum parthenium* (L.) aerial parts revealed IC50 of 2.40±0.76 µg/mL against promastigotes and 1.76±0.25 µg/mL against axenic amastigotes of *L. amazonensis* (Rabito et al., 2014). Sesquiterpene lactones have shown activity against *L. donovani* parasites (Trossini et al., 2014). Similarly, when infected mice were treated with a triterpenic fraction purified from *Baccharis uncinella* leaves, an improvement in Th1 type of protective immune response and parasite reduction in liver and spleen was observed (Yamamoto et al., 2014). Hypnophilin and panepoxydone, terpenoids isolated from *Lentinus strigosus*, have 67% inhibitory activity against *L. amazonensis* at a concentration of 1.25 µg/mL, but panepoxydone was found to be cytotoxic (Souza-Fagundes et al., 2010). Iridoid glucoside, arbortristoside A, isolated from the traditional plant *Nyctanthes arbortristis*, has also shown antileishmanial activity against amastigotes by 79.68±1.68% in macrophage cultures and at a dosage of 100 mg/kg body wt. exhibited 57% inhibition of parasites in hamsters (Tandon et al., 1991). This compound caused increased production of ROS by inhibiting the enzymatic activity of an important enzyme of redox system (i.e., trypanothione reductase), which causes an oxidative burst, cell membrane disintegration, and programmed cell death of *Leishmania* species (Shukla et al., 2011; 2012). Quinovic acid glycosides and cadambine acid isolated from *Nauclea diderrichii* were examined for their leishmanicidal activities against intracellular amastigotes of *L. infantum* and it was noticed that four quinovic acid glycosides and cadambine acid possessed strong antileishmanial activity with IC50 of 1 µM by inhibiting parasite internalization and NO production in macrophages (Di Giorgio et al., 2006). The latex isolated from the Ethiopian plant *Aloe calidophila* was assessed for its leishmanicidal activity against *L. aethiopica* (IC50 of 64.05) and *L. major* (IC50 of 82.29 µg/mL). However, three anthrones (i.e., aloinoside, aloin, and microdontin) isolated from this plant demonstrated better leishmanicidal activities with IC50=1.76-6.32 µg/mL and 2.09–8.85 µg/mL against *L. aethiopica* and *L. major*, respectively (Abeje et al., 2014). A new ventiloquinone and five triterpenes were fractionated from *Parinariexcelsa* (3β)-3-hydroxyolean-12-en-28-oic acid (IC50=8.2 µM) and 3β-hydroxyolean-5,12-dien-28-oic acid (IC50=7.7 µM) were found most effective against *L. donovani* (Attioua et al., 2012). Two sterols (i.e., cholest-5,20,24-trien-3β-ol and cholest-4-en-3) were found effective against amastigotes of *L. mexicana*, whereas cholest-5,20,24-trien-3β-ol was found most effective with IC50 of 0.03 µM (Pan et al., 2012). Seventeen labdane type derivatives, 11 semisynthetic manoyl oxide, and a triterpene purified from *Cistus monspeliensis* were also screened for their antileishmanial activity against *L. donovani* promastigotes. 13-(E)-8a-hydroxylabd-13-en-15-ol 2-chloroethylcarbamate, 15,18-diacetoxy-cis-clerod-3-ene, and 18-acetoxy-cis-clerod-3-en-15-ol exhibited the highest leishmanicidal activity with IC50 values of 3.5, 3.4, and 3.3 µg/mL, respectively (Fokialakis et al., 2006). The antileishmanial potential of lupeol, a triterpenoid, arrested parasites at sub G0/G1 phase in vitro and increased the levels of NF-κB and iNOS genes leading to the parasite killing in BALB/c mice infected with *Leishmania donovani* (Kaur et al., 2019). One of the major concerns of leishmaniasis is the increasing resistance of standard antileishmanials. In this regard, certain compounds have been found to be very promising to combat this disease. Rutin (flavonoid) and salidroside (glycoside) were investigated for their antileishmanial potential against both the sensitive and resistant strains of *L. donovani*. It was observed that both the active components polarized the immune response to Th1 type with increased production of CD4+ T cells and increased proinflammatory cytokines without causing any toxicities making them a safe alternative to fight the disease (Chauhan et al., 2018; 2019).

30.2.2 *In Vivo* Antileishmanial Activity of Plant Extracts

Besides a lot of research work in vitro, there are many promising plant products with antileishmanial efficacy in animal models. For instance, many phenols such as curcuminoids (Alves et al., 2003), neolignans (Barata et al., 2000), and stilbenoids (Nakayama et al., 2009) have been found to decrease the *Leishmania* load in BALB/c mice. Similarly, terpenes like dihydroartemisinin (Ma et al., 2004) and limonene

(Arruda et al., 2009) have been found to suppress *Leishmania* growth in different animal models. 16a-Hydroxycleroda-3,13 (14)Z-dien-15,16-olide a compound isolated from *Polyalthia longifolia* was found to be active against *L. donovani* parasites (Misra et al., 2010). The withanolides purified from the ethanolic extract of *Withania somnifera* leaves have also shown significant antileishmanial property (Chandrasekaran et al., 2013). Racemoside A, purified from the fruits of *Asparagus racemosus*, was also shown to be a potent antileishmanial molecule (Dutta et al., 2007). An essential oil consisting of rans-sabinyl acetate from *Artemisia absinthium* restricted the replication of both the promastigotes and amastigotes (14.4±3.6μg/mL and 13.4±2.4μg/mL, respectively) of *L. amazonensis* and also reduced the lesion size in infected BALB/c mice at 30 mg/kg body wt. (Monzote et al., 2014). Oral administration of essential oil from *Chenopodium ambrosioides* to BALB/c mice with a dosage of 150 mg/kg was also found to significantly reduce lesion size caused by *L. amazonensis* (Monzote et al., 2009). The ethanolic extract of traditional medicinal plant *Desmodium gangeticum* and its three fractions (i.e., hexane, n-butanol, and aqueous) were evaluated prophylactically and therapeutically against VL in hamsters. The n-butanol fraction exhibited maximum inhibition of 66.7± 6.1% at dosage 250 mg/kg × 2 per day on 7 pre- and postinfection days (Singh et al., 2005). One of the major immunopathological outcomes of visceral leishmaniasis is abolishment of protective Th1 type of immune responses. The combined therapy of whole plant crude extracts of *Asparagus racemosus* and *Withania somnifera* with dose regimen of 200 mg/kg body weight significantly reduced the parasite load of *L. donovani* amastigotes in liver along with production of IL-2 and IFN-γ cytokines, which showed protective Th1 type of immune responses in BALB/c mice (Kaur et al., 2014). In another similar study, *W. somnifera* chemotypes (NMITLI-101, NMITLI-118) and pure withanolide-withaferin A were investigated against *L. donovani* infected hamsters and NMITLI-101 was found to be the most potent immunoprophylactic agent (Tripathi et al., 2014). Similarly, the essential oil from *Chenopodium ambrosioides* showed a synergic activity after incubation in conjunction with pentamidine against promastigotes of *L. amazonensis* (Monzote et al., 2007). Herbal plants not only cause immunomodulation but also help in reducing the toxicities. This is evident from the studies done in our lab where herbal plants *W. sominifera, A. racemosus,* and *T. cordifolia* in combination with cisplatin were found to ameliorate the cisplatin-induced toxicities and augment its antileishmanial activity by immunomodulation in mice (Sachdeva et al., 2013; 2014a, b). Similarly, ethanolic extracts of *Chlorophytum borivilianum* and *Bergenia ligulata* (Wall.) Engl. were found highly active against the promastigotes in vitro (IC50:28.25 μg/mL and 22.70 μg/mL, respectively) and significantly reduced the hepatic parasite load in vivo by modulating the Th2 immune response towards Th1 type (Kaur and Kaur, 2020; 2017). Methanolic extracts of *C. album* showed normal kidney and liver function tests in addition to a heightened DTH response and increased IgG2a as an indicator of protective Th1 type of immune responses (Kaur et al., 2016). The methanolic extract of *Allium sativum* was found to significantly reduce the parasite load in *L. major*-infected mice by increasing nitric oxide levels in the macrophages (Wabwoba et al., 2010). The purified compound picroliv isolated from *Picrorhiza kurroa* was found to enhance the efficacy of conventional drug miltefosine against VL infection in hamsters on different posttreatment days (Gupta et al., 2005). It has been found that proteases play crucial role in the virulence of *Leishmania* parasites. Therefore, a fraction isolated from potato tuber extract (PTEx), which inhibited the serine protease activity of parasites, was revealed to inhibit the parasite growth and intracellular amastigote parasite load with IC50 of 312.5 ± 0.1 μg/mL and 82.3 ± 0.2 μg/mL, respectively. Its activity was attributed to induced acute production of ROS and NO (Paik et al., 2014). In another study, the antileishmanial activity of different extracts from three Cuban *Pluchea*species (i.e., *P. carolinensis, P. odorata,* and *P. rosea*) was evaluated against *L. amazonensis* in BALB/c mice by Garcia et al. (2012). The intraperitoneal injection of the ethanolic extract of *P. carolinensis* at 100 mg/kg prevented the lesion development. In an identical study, the water extract of the *Agaricus blazei* was also found effective in inhibiting the growth of promastigotes and amastigotes of three different species of *Leishmania* (i.e. *amazonensis, chagasi,* and *major*) (Valadares et al., 2011). The flavonoids (quercetin and luteolin) purified from *Vitex negundo* and *Fagopyrum esculentum* have shown remarkable antileishmanial activity against *L. donovani* promastigotes and amastigotes by inhibiting DNA replication via topoisomerase II inhibition resulting in cell cycle arrest (Mittra et al., 2000). In addition, quercitin was found to exert its antileishmanial activity by interfering with iron metabolism of *L. donovani*. The combination of quercitin with serum albumin reduced the parasite burden in spleen by inhibiting the activity of ribonucleotide reductase, which is a key enzyme of DNA replication (Sen et al., 2008). The oral administration of leaf extract of *Kalanchoe pinnata* in *L. amazonensis*-infected mice showed notable reduction in parasite load without increase in delayed type hypersensitivity responses (Da Silva et al., 1995).

30.3 Conclusion and Future Implications

Extensive and exhaustive research is being conducted to find a new drug or an effective vaccine. However, no drug is available that can overcome the problem of increasing resistance and is nontoxic in nature. Thus, there is a need for discovery of new agents from natural sources. Ayurveda can provide an alternative to conventional chemotherapy for a variety of diseases, especially when the diseases cause immunosuppression. Thus, there is a need to evaluate traditional medicines for their immunomodulatory and antileishmanial property with their signaling pathways to find the target sites ultimately leading to an efficient cure for human healthcare.

REFERENCES

Abeje, F., Bisrat, D., Hailu, A., Asres K. 2014. Phytochemistry and antileishmanial activity of the leaf latex of *Aloe calidophila* Reynolds. *Phytotherapy Research*. 28: 1801–1805.

Achakzai, J.K., Panezai, M.A., Kakar, A.M. et al., 2019. In vitro antileishmanial activity and GC-MS analysis of whole plant hexane fraction of *Achillea wilhelmsii* (WHFAW). *Journal of Chemistry*. 2019: 1–26.

Afrin, F., Chouhan, G., Islamuddin, M., Want, M.Y., Ozbak, H.A., Hemeg, H.A. 2019. *Cinnamomum cassia* exhibits antileishmanial activity against *Leishmania donovani* infection in vitro and in vivo. *PLoS Neglected Tropical Diseases*. 13: e0007227.

Alves, L.V., Temporal, R.M., Cysne-Finkelstein, L., Leon, L.L. 2003. Efficacy of a diarylheptanoid derivative against *Leishmania amazonensis*. *The Memórias do Instituto Oswaldo Cruz*. 98: 553–555.

Arevalo, J., Ramirez, L., Adaui, V. et al., 2007. Influence of *Leishmania* (*Viannia*) species on the response to antimonial treatment in patients with americantegumentary leishmaniasis. *The Journal of Infectious Diseases*. 195: 1846–1851.

Arruda, D.C., Miguel, D.C., Yokoyama-Yasunaka, J.K., Katzin, A.M., Uliana, S.R. 2009. Inhibitory activity of limonene against *Leishmania* parasites in vitro and in vivo. *Biomedicine and Pharmacotherapy*. 63: 643–649.

Attioua, B., Yeo, D., Lagnika, L. et al. 2012. In vitro antileishmanial, antiplasmodial and cytotoxic activities of a new ventiloquinone and five known triterpenes from *Parinariexcelsa*. *Pharmaceutical Biology*. 50: 801–806.

Awasthi, A., Mathur, R.K., Saha, B. 2004. Immune response to *Leishmania* infection. *Indian Journal of Medical Research*. 119: 238–58.

Barata, L.E., Santos, L.S., Ferri, P.H., Phillipson, J.D., Paine, A., Croft, S.L. 2000. Anti-leishmanial activity of neolignans from *Virola* species and synthetic analogues. *Phytochemistry*. 55: 589–595.

Chan-Bacab, M.J and Peña-Rodríguez, L.M. 2001. Plant natural products with leishmanicidal activity. *Natural Products Reports*. 18: 674–688.

Chandrasekaran, S., Dayakar, A., Veronica, J., Sundar, S., Maurya, R. 2013. An in vitro study of apoptotic like death in *Leishmania donovani* promastigotes by withanolides. *Parasitology International*. 62: 253–261.

Chauhan, K., Kaur, G., Kaur, S. 2018. Activity of rutin, a potent flavonoid against SSG-sensitive and resistant *Leishmania donovani* parasites in experimental leishmaniasis. *International Immunopharmacology*. 64: 372–385.

Chauhan, K., Kaur, G., Kaur, S. 2019. Evaluation of antileishmanial efficacy of Salidroside against the SSG-sensitive and resistant strain of *Leishmania donovani*. *Parasitology International*. 72: 101298.

Coelho, A.C. 2016. Miltefosine susceptibility and resistance in *Leishmania*: from the laboratory to the field. *Journal of Tropical Diseases and Public Health*. 4: 203.

Cummings, H.E., Tuladhar, R., and Satoskar, A.R. 2010. Cytokines and their STATs in cutaneous and visceral leishmaniasis. *Journal of Biomed Biotechnology*. 2010: 294389.

da Silva, S.A., Costa, S.S., Mendonca, S.C., Silva, E.M., Moraes, V.L., Rossi-Bergmann, B. 1995. Therapeutic effect of oral *Kalanchoe pinnata* leaf extract in murine leishmaniasis. *Acta Tropica*. 60: 201–210 de Freitas, E.O, Leoratti, F.M., Freire-de-Lima, C.G., Morrot, A., Feijo, D.F. 2016. The contribution of immune evasion mechanisms to parasite persistence in visceral leishmaniasis. *Frontiers in Immunology*. 7: 153.

de Mello Cruz, E., da Silva, E.R., do Carmo Maquiaveli, C. et al. 2013. Leishmanicidal activity of *Cecropia pachystachya* flavonoids: Arginase inhibition and altered mitochondrial DNA arrangement. *Phytochemistry*. 89: 71–77

de Paula, R.C., da Silva, S.M., Faria, K.F. et al. 2019. In vitro antileishmanial activity of leaf and stem extracts of seven Brazilian plant species. *Journal of Ethnopharmacology*. 232: 155–164

de Toledo, J.S., Ambrósio, S.R., Borges, C.H. 2014. In vitro leishmanicidal activities of sesquiterpene lactones from *Tithonia diversifolia* against *Leishmania brasiliensis* promastigotes and amastigotes. *Molecules*. 19: 6070–6079

Di Giorgio, C., Lamidi, M., Delmas, F., Balansard, G., Ollivier, E. 2006. Antileishmanial activity of quinovic acid glycosides and casambine acid isolated from *Naucleadiderrichii*. *Planta Medica*. 72: 1396–1402

dos S Grecco, S., Reimão, J.Q., Tempone, A.G. 2012. In vitro antileishmanial and antitrypanosomal activities of flavanones from *Baccharis retusa* DC (Asteraceae). *Experimental Parasitology*. 130: 141–145

Dutta, A., Ghoshal, A., Mandal, D. et al. 2007. Racemoside A, an anti-leishmanial, water-soluble, natural steroidal saponin, induces programmed cell death in *Leishmania donovani*. *Journal of Medical Microbiology*. 56: 1196–1204.

El-On, J., Ozer, L., Gopas, J. et al., 2009. Antileishmanial activity in Israeli plants. *Annals of Tropical Medicine Parasitology*. 103: 297–306.

Evans-Osses, I., de Messias-Reason, I., Ramirez, M.I. 2013. The emerging role of complement lectin pathway in trypanosomatids: molecular bases in activation, genetic deficiencies, susceptibility to infection, and complement system-based therapeutics. *The Scientific World Journal*. 2013: 1–12.

Faleiro, R.J, Kumar, R., Hafner, L.M., Engwerda, C.R. 2014. Immune regulation during chronic visceral leishmaniasis. *PLoS. Neglected Tropical Diseases*. 8: e2914.

Fernández, O.L, Diaz-Toro, Y., Ovalle, C. et al., 2014. Miltefosine and antimonial drug susceptibility of *Leishmania/Viannia*species and populations in regions of high transmission in Colombia. *PLoS. Neglected Tropical Diseases*. 8: e2871.

Fokialakis, N., Kalpoutzakis, E., Tekwani, B.L., Skaltsounis, A., Duke, S.O. 2006. Antileishmanial activity of natural diterpenes from *Cistus* sp. and semisynthetic derivatives thereof. *Biological and Pharmaceutical Bulletin*. 29: 1775–1778.

Gamboa-Leon, R., Vera-Ku, M., Peraza-Sanchez, S.R., Ku-Chulim, C., Horta-Baas,A., Rosado-Vallado, M. 2014. Antileishmanial activity of a mixture of *Tridax procumbens* and *Allium sativum* in mice. *Parasites*. 21: 1–7.

Ganeti, A., Kaur, R., Kaur, J and Kaur, S. 2015. In vitro antileishmanial activity and cytotoxicity of some Indian traditional medicinal plants against sensitive and resistant strains of *Leishmania donovani*. *European Journal of Biomedical and Pharmaceutical Sciences*. 2: 1368–1382.

Garcia, M., Monzote, L., Scull, R., Herrera, P. 2012. Activity of Cuban plants extracts against *Leishmania amazonensis*. *ISRN Pharmacology*. 2012: 104540.

Ghosh, S., Debnat, S., Hazra S. et al., 2011. *Valerianawallichii* root extracts and fractions with activity against *Leishmania* spp. Parasitology Research 108: 861–871.

Gontijo, V.S., Judice, W.A., Codonho, B. et al. 2012. Leishmanicidal, antiproteolytic and antioxidant evaluation of natural biflavonoids isolated from *Garcinia brasiliensis* and their semisynthetic derivatives. *European Journal of Medicinal Chemistry*. 58: 613–623.

Goto, H., Prianti, M.G., 2009. Immunoactivation and immunopathogeny during active visceral leishmaniasis. *Revista do Instituto de Medicina Tropical de São Paulo*. 51: 241–246.

Gupta, G., Oghumu, S., Satoskar, A.R., 2013. Mechanisms of immune evasion in leishmaniasis. *Advances in Applied Microbiology*. 82: 155–184.

Gupta, N., Kant K., Mirdha, B.R. 2017. Clinical and laboratory analysis of patients with leishmaniasis: A retrospective study from a tertiary care centre in New Delhi. *Iranian Journal of Parasitology*. 12: 632–637.

Gupta, S., Ramesh, S.C., Srivastava, V.M. 2005. Efficacy of picroliv in combination with miltefosine, an orally effective antileishmanial drug against experimental visceral leishmaniasis. *Acta Tropica*. 94: 41–47.

Herrera, G., Barragán, N., Luna, N., 2020. An interactive database of *Leishmania* species distribution in the Americas. *Scientific Data*. 7: 110.

Jain, K., Jain, N.K. 2015. Vaccines for visceral leishmaniasis: A review. *Journal of Immunological Methods*. 422: 1–12.

Joshi, J., Malla, N., Kaur, S. 2014. A comparative evaluation of efficacy of chemotherapy, immunotherapy and immunochemotherapy in visceral leishmaniasis-an experimental study. *Parasitology International.* 63: 612–620.

Kaur, G., Chauhan, K., Kaur, S. 2019. Lupeol induces immunity and protective efficacy in a murine model against visceral leishmaniasis. *Parasitology.*146:1440–1450.

Kaur, R., Kaur, J., Kaur, S., Joshi, J. 2016. Evaluation of the antileishmanial efficacy of medicinal plant *Chenopodium album*linn. against experimental visceral leishmaniasis. *International Journal of Pharmacy and Pharmaceutical Sciences.* 8:1–9.

Kaur, R., Kaur, S. 2017. Evaluation of in vitro and in vivo antileishmanial potential of bergenin rich *Bergenia ligulata* (Wall.) Engl. root extract against visceral leishmaniasis in inbred BALB/c mice through immunomodulation. *Journal of Traditional and Complementary Medicine.* 8: 251–260.

Kaur, R., Kaur, S. 2020. Protective efficacy of *Chlorophytum borivilianum* root extract against murine visceral leishmaniasis by immunomodulating the host responses. *Journal of Ayurveda and Integrative Medicine.* 11: 53–61.

Kaur, S., Chauhan, K., Sachdeva, H., 2014. Protection against experimental visceral leishmaniasis by immunostimulation with herbal drugs derived from *Withania somnifera* and *Asparagus racemosus.* *Journal of Medical Microbiology.* 63: 1328–1338.

Kaushal, H., Bras-Gonçalves, R., Negi, N.S., Lemesre, J., Papierok, G., Salotra, P. 2014. Role of CD8+ T cells in protection against *Leishmania donovani* infection in healed visceral leishmaniasis individuals. *BMC Infectious Diseases.* 14: 653.

Kayser, O., Kiderlen, A.F. 2001. In vitro leishmanicidal activity of naturally occurring chalcones. *Phytotherapy Research.* 15: 148–152.

Kumar, S., Shukla, R., Rapolu, S.B., Tiwari, A. 2014. Role of rasayana in immune deficiency disease. *Pharma Science Monitor.* 5: 1–6.

Ma. Y., Lu, D.M., Lu, X.J., Liao, L., Hu, X.S. 2004. Activity of dihydroartemisinin against *Leishmania donovani* both in vitro and in vivo. *Chinese Medical Journal (Engl).* 117: 1271–1273.

Malebo, H.M., Wenzler, T., Cal, M. et al., 2013. Anti-protozoal activity of aporphine and protoberberine alkaloids from *Annickiakummeriae* (Engl. & Diels) Setten & Maas (Annonaceae). *Complementary and Alternative Medicine.* 13:48.

Mesquita, M.L., Desrivot, J., Bories, C. et al., 2005. Antileishmanial and trypanocidal activity of Brazilian Cerrado plants. *The Memórias do Instituto Oswaldo Cruz.* 100: 783–787.

Misra, P., Sashidhara, K.V., Singh, S.P. et al. 2010. 16α-Hydroxycleroda-3,13(14)Z-dien-15,16-olide from *Polyalthia longifolia*: a safe and orally active antileishmanial agent. *British Journal of Pharmacology.* 159: 1143–1150.

Mittra, B., Saha, A., Chowdhury, A.R. et al. 2000. Luteolin, an abundant dietary component is a potent anti-leishmanial agent that acts by inducing topoisomerase II-mediated kinetoplast DNA cleavage leading to apoptosis. *Molecular Medicine.* 6: 527–541.

Monzote, L, Montalvo, A.M., Scull, R., Miranda, M., Abreu, J. 2007. Combined effect of the essential oil from *Chenopodium ambrosioides* and antileishmanial drugs on promastigotes of Leishmania amazonensis. *The Revista do Instituto de Medicina Tropical de São Paulo.* 49: 257–260.

Monzote, L., García, M., Montalvo, A.M., Linares, R., Scull, R. 2009. Effect of oral treatment with the essential oil from *Chenopodium ambrosioides* against cutaneous leishmaniasis in BALB/c mice caused by *Leishmania amazonensis.* Forsch Komplementmed 16: 334–338.

Monzote, L., Pinon, A., Sculli, R., Setzer, W.N. 2014. Chemistry and leishmanicidal activity of the essential oil from *Artemisia absinthium* from Cuba. *Natural Product Communications.* 9: 1799–1804.

Murray, H.W., Moreira, A.L., Lu, C.M. et al., 2003. Determinants of response to interleukin-10 receptor blockade immunotherapy in experimental visceral leishmaniasis. *Journal of Infectious Diseases.* 188: 458–464.

Mutiso, J.M., Macharia, J.C., Kiio, M.N., Ichagichu, J.M., Rikoi, H., Gicheru, M.M. 2013. Development of *Leishmania* vaccines: predicting the future from past and present experience. *Journal of Biomedical Research.* 27: 85–102.

Nagill, R., Kaur, S. 2011. Vaccine candidates for leishmaniasis: A review. *International Immunopharmacology.* 11: 1464–1488.

Nakayama, H., Caballero. E., Maldonado, M. et al., 2009. In vivo antileishmanial efficacy of combretastatin heteroanalogues. *The Revista Latino americana de Química.* 37: 56–64.

Ngure, P.K., Nganga, Z., Ingonga, J., Rukunga, G., Tonui, W.K. 2009. In vivo efficacy of oral and intraperitoneal administration of extracts of *Warburgia ugandensis* in experimental treatment of Old World cutaneous leishmaniasis caused by *Leishmania major*. *African Journal of Traditional, Complementary and Alternate Medicine*. 6: 207–212.

Nylen, S., Sacks, D. 2007. Interleukin-10 and the pathogenesis of human visceral leishmaniasis. *Trends in Immunology*. 28: 378–84.

Paik, D., Das, P., De, T., Chakraborti, T. 2014. In vitro antileishmanial efficacy of potato tuber extract (PTEx): Leishmanial serine protease(s) as putative target. *Experimental Parasitology*. 146: 11–19.

Pan, L., Lezama-Davila, C.M., Isaac-Marquez, A.P. et al., 2012. Sterols with antileishmanial activity isolated from the roots of *Pentalinonandrieuxii*. *Phytochemistry*. 82: 128–135.

Passero, L.F., Laurenti, M.D., Santos-Gomes, G., Soares Campos, B.L., Sartorelli, P., Lago, J.H. 2014. Plants used in traditional medicine: extracts and secondary metabolites exhibiting antileishmanial activity. *Current Clinical Pharmacology*. 9: 187–204.

Pavli, A., Maltezou, H. C. 2010. Leishmaniasis, an emerging infection in travellers. *International Journal of Infectious Diseases*. 14: e1032–e1039.

Pereira, I.O., Assis, D.M, Juliano, M.A. et al., 2011. Natural products from *Garcinia brasiliensis* as *Leishmania* protease inhibitors. *Journal of Medicinal Food*. 14: 557–562.

Pitta, M.G., Romano, A., Cabantous, S. et al., 2009. IL-17 and IL-22 are associated with protection against human kala azar caused by *Leishmania donovani*. *Journal of Clinical Investigation*. 119: 2379–2387.

Polley, R., Sanos, S.L., Prickett, S., Haque, A., Kaye, P.M. 2005. Chronic *Leishmania donovani* infection promotes bystander CD8+-T-cell expansion and heterologous immunity. *Infection Immunity*. 73: 7996–8001.

Rabito, M.F., Britta, E.A., Pelegrini, B.L. et al., 2014. In vitro and in vivo antileishmanial activity of sasquiterpene lactone-rich dichloromethane fraction obtained from *Tanacetum parthenium* (L.) Schultz-Bip. *Experimental Parasitology*. 143: 18–23.

Ramirez, J.D., Hernandez, C., León, C.M., Ayala, M.S., Florez, C., Gonzalez, C. 2016. Taxonomy, diversity, temporal and geographical distribution of cutaneous leishmaniasis in Colombia: A retrospective study. *Nature Scientific Reports*. 28266:1–24.

Rodrigues, I.A., Azevedo, M.M., Chaves, F.C.M. et al. 2013. In vitro cytocidal effects of the essential oil from *Croton canucara* (red sacaca) and its major constituent 7-hydroxycalamenene against *Leishmania chagasi*. *BMC Complementary and Alternative Medicine*. 13: 249.

Rodrigues, I.A., Azevedo, M.M.B., Chaves, F.C.M., Alviano, C.S., Alviano, D.S., Vermelho, A.B. 2014. *Arrabidaeachica* hexanic extract induces mitochondrion damage and peptidase inhibition on *Leishmania* spp. *Biomedical Research International*. 2014: 985171.

Rodrigues, V., Cordeiro-da-Silva, A., Laforge, M., Silvestre, R., Estaquier, J. 2016. Regulation of immunity during visceral *Leishmania* infection. *Parasites and Vectors*. 9: 118.

Rodríguez-Cortés, A., Carrillo, E., Martorell, S. et al. 2016. Compartmentalized immune response in leishmaniasis: Changing Patterns throughout the Disease. *PLoS ONE*. 11: e0155224.

Rudrapaul, P., Sarma, I.S., Das, N., De, U.C., Bhattacharjee, S., Dinda, B. 2014. New flavonol methyl erher from the leaves or *Vitex peduncularis* exhibits potential inhibitory activity against *Leishmania donovani* through activation of iNOS expression. European *Journal of Medicinal Chemistry*. 87: 328– 33.

Sachdeva, H., Sehgal, R., Kaur, S. 2013. Studies on the protective and immunomodulatory efficacy of *Withania somnifera* along with cisplatin against experimental visceral leishmaniasis. *Parasitology Research*. 112: 2269–2280.

Sachdeva, H., Sehgal, R., Kaur, S. 2014a. *Asparagus racemosus* ameliorates cisplatin induced toxicities and augments its antileishmanial activity by immunomodulation in vivo. *Parasitology International*. 63: 21–30.

Sachdeva, H., Sehgal, R., Kaur, S. 2014b. *Tinospora cordifolia* as a protective and immunomodulatory agent in combination with cisplatin against murine visceral leishmaniasis. *Experimental Parasitology*. 137: 53–65.

Santos, A.O., Izumi, E., Ueda-Nakamura, T., Dias-Filho, B.P., Veiga-junior, V.F., Nakamura, C.V. 2013. Antileishmanial activity of diterpene acids in copaiba oil. *The Memórias do Instituto Oswaldo Cruz*. 108: 59–64.

Sen, G., Mikhopadhyay, S., Ray, M., Biswas, T. 2008. Quercetin interferes with iron metabolism in *Leishmania donovani* and targets ribonucleotide reductase to exert leishmanicidal activity. *Journal of Antimicrobial Chemotherapy*. 61: 1066–1075.

Shukla, A.K., Patra, S., Dubey, V.K. 2011. Deciphering molecular mechanism underlying antileishmanial activity of *Nyctanthes arbortristis*, an Indian medicinal plant. *Journal of Ethnopharmacology.* 134: 996–998.

Shukla, A.K., Patra, S., Dubey, V.K. 2012. Iidoid glucosides from *Nyctanthes arbortristis* result in increased reactive oxygen species and cellular redox homeostasis imbalance in *Leishmania* Parasite. *European Journal of Medicinal Chemistry.* 54: 49–58.

Sifaoui, I., López-Arencibia, A., Martín-Navarro, C.M. et al., 2014. In vitro effects of triterpenic acids from olive leaf extracts on the mitochondrial membrane potential of promastigote stage of *Leishmania* spp. *Phytomedicine.* 21: 1689–1694.

Silva, A.A., Morais, S.M., Falcão, M.J. et al. 2014. Activity of cycloartane-type triterpenes and sterols isolated from *Musa paradisiaca* fruit peel against *Leishmania infantum chagasi*. *Phytomedicine.* 21: 1419–1423.

Singh, N., Mishra, P.K., Kapil, A., Arya, K.R., Maurya, R., Dube, A. 2005. Efficacy of *Desmodium gangeticum* extract and its fractions against experimental visceral leishmaniasis. *Journal of Ethnopharmacology.* 98: 83–88.

Singh, R.P., Picado, A., Alam, S. et al.,2012. Post-kala-azar dermal leishmaniasis in visceral leishmaniasis-endemic communities in Bihar, India. *Tropical Medicine and International Health.* 17: 1345–1348.

Souza-Fagundes, E.M., Cota, B.B, Rosa, L.H. et al. 2010. In vitro activity of hypnophilin from *Lentinus strigosus*: a potential prototype for Chagas disease and leishmaniasis chemotherapy. *Brazilian Journal of Medical and Biological Research.* 43: 1054–1061.

Stäger, S and Rafati, S. 2012. CD8+ T Cells in *Leishmania* infections: friends or foes? *Frontiers in Immunology.* 3: 5.

Strauss-Ayali, D., Baneth, G., Shor, S., Okano, F., Jaffe, C.L. 2005. Interleukin-12 augments a Th1-type immune response manifested as lymphocyte proliferation and interferon gamma production in *Leishmania infantum* infected dogs. *International Journal of Parasitology.* 35: 63–73.

Sundar, S., Chakravarty, J. 2015. An update on pharmacotherapy for leishmaniasis. *Expert Opinion on Pharmacotherapy.* 16: 237–252.

Tabatabaie, F., Keighobadi, A., Golestani, M. et al. 2014. Antileishmanial activity of *Hyssopus officinalis*, *Tussilago farfara*, *Carum copticum* extracts in comparison with Glucantime in Iran. *Journal of Medicinal Plant Studies.* 2: 12–18.

Tandon, J.S., Srivastava, V., Guru, P.Y. 1991. Iridoids: a new class of Leishmanicidal agents from *Nyctanthes arboriristis*. *Journal of Natural Products.* 54: 1102–1104.

Thakur, S., Joshi, J., Kaur, S. 2020. Leishmaniasis diagnosis: an update on the use of parasitological, immunological and molecular methods. *Journal of Parasitic Diseases.* 2020: 1–20.

Tripathi, C.D., Gupta, R., Kushawaha, P.K, Mandal, C., Bhattacharya, S. M., Dube, A. 2014. Efficacy of *Withania somnifera* chemotypes NMITLI-101R, 118R and withaferin A against experimental visceral leishmaniasis. *Parasite Immunology.* 36: 253–265.

Trossini, G.H., Maltarollo, V.G., Schmidt, T.J. 2014. Hologram QSAR studies of antiprotozoal activities of sasquiterpene lactones. *Molecules.* 19: 10546–10562.

Tsagozis, P., Karagouni, E., Dotsika, E. 2003. CD8(+) T cells with parasite-specific cytotoxic activity and a Tc1 profile of cytokine and chemokine secretion develop in experimental visceral leishmaniasis. *Parasite Immunology.* 25: 569–579.

Valadares, D.G., Duarte, M.C., Oliveira, J.S. et al. 2011. Leishmanicidal activity of the *Agaricus blazei* Murill in different *Leishmania* species. *Parasitology International.* 60: 357–363.

Valadares, D.G., Duarte, M.C., Ramirez, L., Chavez-Fumagalli, M.A, Lage, P.S. 2012. Therapeutic efficacy induced by the oral administration of *Agaricus blazei* Murill against *Leishmania amazonensis*. *Parasitology Research.* 111: 1807–1816.

Vayalil, P.K., Kuttan, G., Kuttan, R. 2002. Rasayanas: evidence for the concept of prevention of diseases. *American Journal of Chinese Medicine.* 30: 155–171.

Vila-Nova, N.S., Morais, S.M, Falcão, M.J. et al., 2011. Leishmanicidal activity and cytotoxicity of compounds from two Annonacea Species cultivated in North-eastern Brazil. *Revista da Sociedade Brasileira de Medicina Tropical.* 44: 567–571.

Wabwoba, B.W., Anjili, C.O., Ngeiywa, M.M. et al. 2010. Experimental chemotherapy with *Allium sativum* methanolic extracts in rodents infected with *Leishmania major* and *Leishmania donovani*. *Journal of Vector Borne Diseases.* 47: 160–167.

World Health Organisation (WHO). 2010. Technical Report Series: Control of Leishmaniases. whqlibdoc.who.int/trs/WHO_TRS_949_eng.pdf. 949.

World Health Organisation (WHO). 2016. Media Centre Leishmaniasis Fact Sheet. www.who.int/mediacentre/factsheets/fs3 75/en/.

World Health Organisation (WHO). 2017. WHO Global Observatory on Health R&D: Preliminary Analysis for R&D for Leishmaniasis. 1–9.

World Health Organisation (WHO). 2020. Leishmaniasis Fact Sheet. www.who.int/news-room/fact-sheets/detail/leishmaniasis

Yamamoto, E.S., Campos, B.L, Laurenti, M.D. et al. 2014. Treatment with triterpenic fraction purified from *Baccharis uncinella* leaves inhibit *Leishmania amazonensis* spreading and improves Th1 response in infected mice. *Parasitology Research*. 113: 333-339.

31

Metal-Embedded Complexes: Accelerated Antimicrobial Activity Against Microorganisms

Preeti Garg, Gurpreet Kaur, and Ganga Ram Chaudhary
Department of Chemistry and Centre of Advanced Studies in Chemistry, Panjab University, Chandigarh, India

31.1 Introduction

Microbial infection in human health is a global threat ultimately leading to death. It was reported that nearly 35,000 people die each year in the United States and more than 33,000 people in Europe due to this threat. According to one estimate (2019), about 2 million people may die of antimicrobial resistance by 2050 in India (www.cdc.gov/drugresistance/pdf/threatsreport/2019-ar-threatsreport-508.pdf). To tackle this issue, a number of successful antibiotics have been developed to satisfy the clinical pipelines. However, over time, these microbes change their genetics and no longer respond to antibiotics (termed as antibiotic resistance). Moreover, the main cause of the evolution of antibiotic resistance is the misuse or overuse of antibiotics. In 2019, the World Health Organization (WHO) acknowledged 32 antibiotics in clinical development, and only 6 of these antibiotics were classified as novel structures (www.who.int/news-room/fact-sheets/detail/antimicrobialresistance). Therefore, new quality antibiotics are urgently required to develop effective biocidal or bacteriostatic activity. For several years, most of the antimicrobial agents (Saidin et al., 2021) were prepared by using organic compounds because most of the components in living organisms (i.e., DNA or proteins) are based on carbon element. However, these organic-based antibiotics represent a viable short-term solution because microbes developed resistance to these compounds.

Transition metals offer an alternative to organic drugs by incorporating into their molecular structure and exploiting the structural diversity and because of various oxidation states of metal, it has the ability to target different biochemical pathways. Transition metal complexes have access to modes of action that are difficult or even impossible to cover with organic molecules alone. Therefore, a vast variety of metal complexes have been designed and applied in the medical field from the treatment of cancer to malaria and neurodegenerative diseases (Biot et al., 2011; Monro et al., 2019; Kenny et al., 2019). Despite these applications, metal complexes have received little attention as potential antimicrobial agents. However, the number of reports on antimicrobial activity of metal complexes have increased over the last decade. They ensure sustainability for both the environment and the industry. Metal complexes may provide an exchange of ligands, redox action as well as production of reactive oxygen species, which enables them to interfere the enzyme activity, cause detrimental cell membrane, or damage DNA. The efficacy of metal complexes as antimicrobial agents is mostly dependent on the nature of the metal ions and the type of ligands because different ligands exhibit different biological properties.

In this regard, metal complex-based surfactants known as metallosurfactants are rapidly becoming a prime focus for the development of more efficacious metal-based antimicrobial entities due to their unique chemical and physical properties of adsorption and aggregation, interfacial property, cytotoxic activity, charge transfer, and selective binding. These fundamental characteristics make them useful tools for achieving exceptional arrangements including micelles, vesicles, bilayers, liquid crystals, mesoporous materials, etc. (Garg et al., 2017; Griffiths et al., 2004; García et al., 2018), which have been

DOI: 10.1201/9781003220404-34

used in biological activities. There are many reasons this approach is highly tempting or demanding. As a global leader in antibiotics, metallosurfactants undoubtedly have immense potential to further strengthen their footprint and may be able to shoulder the responsibility and help to avert an antibiotic disaster. This chapter offers a brief description of antimicrobial activity of transition metal complexes and metallosurfactants.

31.2 Overview of Microbes Present in Environment

There are three major types of microbes:

31.2.1 Bacteria

Bacteria are small microscopic cells with simple and primitive form of cellular structure, firstly termed by a German scientist C. E. Chrenberg in 1928. Their cells are neither like plants nor resemble animal form. They are divided into five groups depending upon their basic shapes: spherical (cocci), rod (bacilli), spiral (spirilla), comma (vibrios), or corkscrew (spirochaetes). Based on their cell wall, they are classified into two types: Gram-positive bacteria and Gram-negative bacteria. Gram-positive bacteria are made up of a thick peptidoglycan layer and the presence of teichoic acids and lipids while Gram-negative bacteria consist of a thin peptidoglycan layer with outer membrane containing lipopolysaccharides. For the anti-bacterial study, *Staphylococcus aureus (S. aureus) and Bacillus subtilis (B. subtilis)* from Gram-positive group of bacteria and *Escherichia coli (E. coli) and P. aeruginosa* from Gram-negative group of bacteria have been widely used. They are responsible for various disease, such as pneumonia, urinary tract infections, and tuberculosis.

31.2.2 Fungi

A fungus is a multicellular organism that lacks chlorophyll and vascular tissues. They consist of three layers; the outermost layer is comprised of glucans and cellulose, the second is the chitin layer (distinguish feature of fungus), and the third is the phospholipid membrane, which is adjacent to the cytoplasm. They exist in two main forms: yeasts and molds. Yeasts (*Candida* and *Cryptococcus*) are single-celled and reproduce by budding while molds (e.g., *Aspergillus niger* and *Penicillium* produce multicellular hyphae by apical extension).

31.2.3 Virus

A virus is a tiny infectious agent present inside living cells. It consists of genetic material (RNA or DNA) and is surrounded by a protein coat called a capsid. Viruses vary in shape such as helical, icosahedral, or more complex structures. The capsid may or may not be surrounded by a lipid membrane termed as the envelope. A simple interpretation of the structure of a virus is shown in Figure 31.1.

31.3 Role of Metals in Biomedical Chemistry

From the 1970s, metal has played a key role in the clinical development of a variety of drugs such as the most successful platinum coordinated complex [cisplatin (cis-[Pt(NH$_3$)$_2$Cl$_2$])] used for cancer therapy (Kelland et al., 2007). Gold was one of the metals used in auranofin drug for the cure of rheumatoid arthritis (Eckhardt et al., 2013a). Silver (Ag) act as an anti-inflammatory agent and the US Food and Drug Administration (FDA) approved the use of Ag(I) sulphadiazine complexes having a well-established and potent antibacterial action against burn injuries (Klasen et al., 2000). Lanthanides (Gd) and transition metals (Fe, Mn) were used as paramagnetic contrast agents for magnetic resonance imaging. The

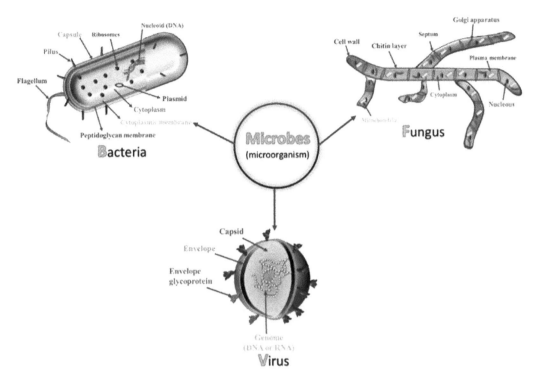

FIGURE 31.1 Diagram representation of three types of microbes.

complexes containing copper metal are employed in the treatment of Alzheimer's disease and as potential drugs to combat Parkinson's disease (Iakovidis et al., 2011). Copper is one of the vital metal that participates in various biological processes. Rhodium was also introduced as anticancer metal in the past. The complexes of osmium and rhenium have also been considered as tumor-inhibiting metal species recently (Konkankit et al., 2018).

Metals have played a historical role in antimicrobial applications such as in water disinfection and food preservation (Cu and Ag), agriculture (Cu), and medicine (Ag, Cu, Hg, Te, Mg, and As) (Lemire et al., 2013). Metals damage the cell membrane and cause injuries to microbial cells through oxidative stress or protein dysfunction. However, due to the introduction of antibiotics by Sir Alexander Fleming, the usage of metals decreases in antimicrobial applications. Currently, due to the deficiency of effective antibiotics and the growing threat of multidrug-resistant microbes, metal ions and their complexes are being strongly considered as antimicrobial agents. The organometallic complex containing arsenic was developed as the first effective treatment of syphilis (Salvarsan) by Paul Ehrlich and co-workers (Sakurai et al., 2008). Since then, researchers have discovered advanced classes of metal complexes with different ligands and metals as effective and targeted antimicrobial agents. Antibiotic compounds are often bound to metal to enhance their efficacy or to avoid drug resistance. Although a vast library of metal complexes is applied as anticancer agents, a significant amount of studies has also been employed in other fields as anti-inflammatory, antibacterial, antitubercular, antirheumatic, and antimalarial drugs.

31.4 Antimicrobial Mechanism of Metal Complexes

Various modes of microbial action by metal complexes have been envisioned (Table 31.1), and these mechanisms can be vary between different types of metal complexes.

TABLE 31.1

Different Types of Antimicrobial Mechanisms Followed by Metal Complexes

Mechanism of action	Description	Ref
Impaired cell membrane	Metal complexes interact with the lipid components of the bacterial membrane, ultimately penetrating both their outer and inner membranes and killing the bacterial cells.	Raman et al., 2008; Oladipo et al., 2013
Protein dysfunction and inhibit enzyme activity	Metal complexes interfere in protein activity, stop RNA/DNA replication, and kill the bacterial cell.	Sharma et al., 2009; Saraiva et al., 2010.
DNA cleavage	Metal complexes bind with DNA through intercalative mode and cleave DNA	Pradeep et al., 2014
Oxidative stress	Metal complexes produce destructive ROS such as superoxide, a hydroxyl radical, which can induce cell death by oxidising proteins, lipids, and DNA. They can also trigger mutations that promote antibiotic resistance.	Paez et al., 2013

31.5 Metal Complexes as Antimicrobial Agents

31.5.1 First Transition Series Metal Complexes

According to the Community for Open Antimicrobial Drug Discovery (CO-ADD), the first transition series metals represent almost 50% of all metal complexes screened as antimicrobial drugs that have been evaluated against bacterial and fungal pathogens. Metal complexes of chromium (Cr), manganese (Mn), iron (Fe), cobalt (Co), copper (Cu), and zinc (Zn) are commonly used for antimicrobial efficiency.

Cr is one of the fundamental elements associated with cysteine and histidine of cellular proteins of microbes, and their accumulation reduces changes in DNA replication and increase mutation frequency. Cr-coordinated complexes have been studied for antimicrobial activity against several pathogenic bacteria, but they have seldom shown high potency. For example, Reddy et al. (2009) studied the antimicrobial activity of macrocyclic Cr(III)-complexes containing Schiff base ligands against Gram-positive (*B. subtilis, S. aureus*) and Gram-negative bacteria (*E. coli, Klebsiella pneumonia*). They showed high antibacterial activities as compared to their parent ligand as well as antimicrobial standards, streptomycin, ampicillin, and rifampicin. It could be attributed to the chelation process that decreased the polarity of Cr-ion and enhanced its lipophilic nature, which in turn facilitated its permeation through the bacterial membrane (Reddy et al., 2009). Cr-complexes studied by Singh et al. (2009) have excellent antibacterial activity against Gram-positive bacteria and antifungal activity toward the yeast (*S. cerevisiae)* and molds (*A. niger* and *A. fumigatus*) while they were found less susceptible against Gram-negative bacteria and yeast (*C. albicans)* (Singh et al., 2009). Cr-complexes are also attributed to the deactivation of different cellular enzymes, which play a vital role in the microorganism metabolic pathways (Vlasiou et al., 2020). Cr-complexes with azo dye ligand were also screened for antifungal activity against the *C. albicans* and it was observed that free azo ligand have no fungal activity while its complexes present significant activity as compared to the standard antifungal drug (Mahmoud et al., 2016).

In 1970, Mn(II)-complexes based on 3,4,7,8-tetramethyl-phenanthroline (phen) were used for dermatological infections caused by *Candida* sp. However, these complexes showed only 50% reduction in the bacterial infection occurred due to the Gram-positive bacteria as compared to Gram-negative bacteria and hence no microbial resistance has been developed further (Cade et al., 1970). Although Mn-complexes are not used as commercialized drugs some of their antimicrobial activities have been reported. For example, Mn(II)-complexes based on quinolone (antibacterial drug) and 1,10-phen are active against Gram-positive (*B. subtilis, B. cereus, and S. aureus*) and Gram-negative bacteria (*E. coli*) (Barmpa et al., 2018). Mn(II)-complexes with hexaaza macrocycle Schiff base ligand showed promising antimicrobial activities (Arthi et al., 2015). Mn exhibited antifertility properties, which was the main issue encountered in its complexes. Jain et al. (2004) synthesized sulphonamide-coordinated Mn-complexes

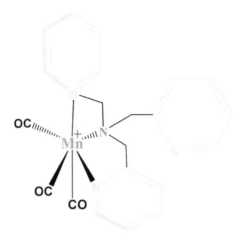

FIGURE 31.2 Chemical Structure of Mn(CO)3(tpa-k3N)]Br Complex [https://pubmed.ncbi.nlm.nih.gov/28954688/#&gid=article-figures&pid=fig-6-uid-5].

that showed two- to nine-fold higher inhibition activity against *S. aureus* than that of streptomycin. Also, they displayed antifungal activity for *A. niger* (Jain et al., 2004). Among Mn-complexes, antimicrobial activity of photoactivatable CO-releasing Mn-complexes (i.e., [Mn(CO)$_3$(tpa-k^{3}N)]Br-complex) have been extensively studied [Figure 31.2]. They are highly active towards various *E. coli* strains in the presence of light. In the absence of light, they perturb the growth of multidrug-resistant isolates of *E. coli* (Nagel et al., 2014).

As we know, iron is part of heme present in hemoglobin and performs many biological functions such as DNA replication, central metabolism, and respiration. It is also required for the growth of pathogenic bacteria and based on the process of iron acquisition, researchers developed a strategy to synthesized iron complexes coordinated with organic drugs to increase antimicrobial activity. For example, iron complex synthesized with quinoxaline derivative was found to be a more potent antibacterial (minimum inhibitory concentration (MIC = 0.78 µg/mL) against *Mycobacteria tuberculosis* (*M. tuberculosis*) than the parent quinoxaline ligand (MIC = 3.9 µg/mL). It was proposed that Fe(III) acts as a carrier of quinoxaline ligands and increases the concentration of bioactive ligand inside the mycobacterial cells (Tarallo et al., 2010). However, in some complexes, the chelation of drugs or antibiotics with metal ions is attributed to loss of the capacity of ligands to bind with microorganisms due to the already occupation of chelation sites. As observed in Fe(III)-complexes of cloxacillin and amoxicillin, antibacterial and antifungal activities of complexes decreased more than that of the corresponding parent ligands (Eze et al., 2014). Additionally, iron complexes with triazole ligands also possessed significant antimicrobial activity against different bacterial strains due to the presence of quinolones in the complexes that interfere with enzyme production (Kharadi et al., 2013). Iron complexes are also designed as bio-organometallic derivatives where metals mimic a part of the drug. Ferroquine is one of the most advanced organometallic drugs, soon to enter clinical phase III trials. Ferroquine (Figure 31.3) was synthesized by the inclusion of ferrocene molecule with antimalarial chloroquine by Biot et al. (1997). It is highly active against chloroquine-resistant parasitic strains (Biot et al., 1997).

Vitamin B$_{12}$ is an example of cobalt complex that acts as co-factor for a number of enzymes and helps in the synthesis and regulation of DNA with energy production. In 1952, the first biological study was performed with Co(III)-complexes and the results highlighted the low toxicity of Co(III) in mice. Along with this, it was also found that complexes exhibited micromolar bacteriostatic and bacteriocidal activity against *E. coli* and *S. haemolyticus* (Dwyer et al., 1952). Since then, Cu-complexes have invoked considerable interest as antibacterial, antiviral, and anticancer agents, as reviewed by Chang et al. (2010). Cobalt complexes are mainly active in Co(II) form, however, Co(III)-complexes are also known for their biological activity. For example, Co(III)-complex of [Co(acacen)(L)$_2$]$^+$ (L = 2–methylimidazole) known as Doxovir (CTC–96) is used in phase II clinical trials for the Herpes virus treatment and reached phase

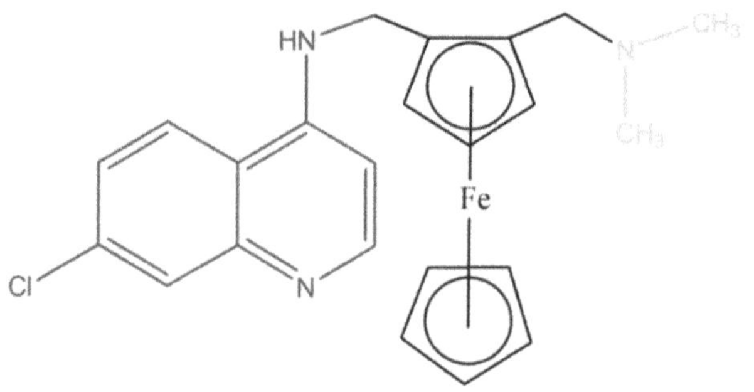

FIGURE 31.3 Chemical structure of ferroquine [www.researchgate.net/figure/Chemical-structure-of-ferroquine-Chemical-structure-of-ferroquine_fig2_233895391].

I clinical trials for the treatment of viral eye infections. The mechanism suggested for this action would be ligand exchange between histidine (His) residues of protein and labile axial ligands of complex (Schwartz et al., 2001). Cu-complexes synthesized with azide-based Schiff base (MIC values in the range of 4–18.5 µg/m) (Zhu et al., 2010), heterocyclic ligands (i.e., bipy or phen with quinolone derivative (MIC in the range of 1–2 µg/mL) (Irgi et al., 2015), and ethylenediamine (MICs = 16 µg/mL) (Turecka et al., 2018) also served as efficient antimicrobial agents. The mechanism involved in the bactericidal action by all these complexes is Overtone's concept and Tweedy's chelation theory. Coordination of metal ion with ligands leads to decrease in the polarity of the metal ion, which in turn increases the π-electrons delocalization over the chelate ring and increased the lipophilicity of the Cu-complexes (Zhu et al., 2010).

Despite the success of other metals, Ni-complexes have not been investigated much as antimicrobial agents due to their carcinogenic effect on humans. Nevertheless, there are a few reports in the literature explaining the antimicrobial activity of Ni-complexes based on Schiff base ligand (Hossain et al., 2019). For example, Raj et al. (2017) studied the antimicrobial activity of Ni(II) Schiff complex against different bacterial strains. Compared to the standard drug, ciprofloxacin, the Ni-complex showed good activity against *S. aureus* (15–30 µg/mL) and methicillin-resistant *S. aureus* (MRSA, 20–50 µg/mL) by disintegrating the cell membrane. However, the metal complexes were found to be negative for other bacteria (*P. aeruginosa and E. coli*) and fungal strains (Raj et al., 2017). Moreover, Ni has also demonstrated antibacterial activity with thiocarbamide ligand but the activity was less than that of standard antibiotics (Revathi et al., 2019). Ni was also coordinated with existing antibiotics (i.e., Ceclor and kefzol) to improve their efficacy, and it was observed that Ni-complexes have better activity against *S. pyogenes* and *E. coli* (Chohan et al., 1991). The chemical structure of Ni-complexes is shown in Figure 31.4 (a and b).

Copper (Cu) is an essential trace element that acts as co-factor in various enzymes, but their free ions have been found to be toxic for microbes. Therefore, copper is coordinated with organic molecules to enhance their antimicrobial activity. For example, Cu(I) incorporated into chelating ligands (i.e., N-methylbenzothiazole-2-thione and 4,5-bis(diphenylphosphano)-9,9-dimethylxanthene) were found to be 100-fold more active against both Gram-negative (*E. coli, X. campestris*) and Gram-positive bacteria (*B. subtilis and B. cereus*) compared to the clinical antibiotic ampicillin. This was due to the production of reactive oxygen species (ROS), which leads to damage of bacterial cell wall (Chohan et al., 2004). Cu(II) ion is also coordinated with the aromatic rings such as phthalimide ligand (IC50 = 0.0019 µg/mL) (Arif et al., 2018) and 1-phenyl-1,3-butanedione (MIC = 10.4 µg/mL) (Krishnegowda et al., 2019), and exhibited high antibacterial activity against different bacterial strains as compared to the free ligand. Moreover, Cu-complexes based on Schiff base have shown excellent antimicrobial properties. For example, Schiff base derived from ethyl 5-aminobenzofuran-2-carboxylate coordinated with Cu(II) have nearly two-fold and four-fold higher antibacterial activity against *M. Tuberculosis* (MIC = 1.6 µg/mL) than that of ciprofloxacin (MIC = 3.125 µg/mL) and streptomycin (MIC = 6.25 µg/mL), respectively (Nazirkar et al., 2019). Despite this, Cu-complexes have also been synthesized with sulfonamide ligands for their antimicrobial properties against Gram-positive and Gram-negative bacteria. Due to low lipophilicity of

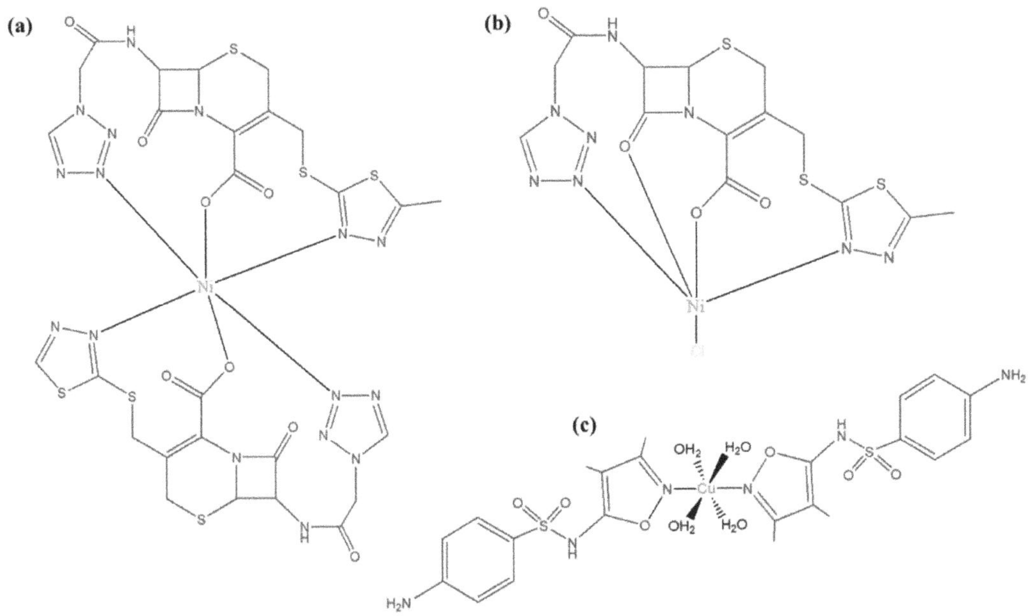

FIGURE 31.4 (a) Chemical structure of Ni(II)-Ceclor and (b) Ni(II)-kefzol complexes and (c) [Cu(sulfisoxazole)$_2$(H$_2$O)$_4$]·2H$_2$O complex [www.mdpi.com/2624-8549/2/4/56/htm].

sulphonamide, their penetration efficacy towards the bacterial membrane is low but complexation of this kind of ligand with metal ions could be one possibility to increase their lipophilicity. For instance, Kremer et al. (2006) observed that five-membered heterocyclic ring substituted Cu(II)-complexes (sulfisoxazole, sulfamethoxazole, and sulfamethizole) were more active than the free sulphonamides ligand (MIC in the range from 4 to 32 µg/mL). This may be due to the lipophilicity and superoxide dismutase-like activity of complexes (Kremer et al., 2006). The chemical structure of Cu(II)-coordinated sulfisoxazole complex is shown in Figure 31.4c. Similarly, copper complexes of mixed amino acid/phen ligand have shown high activity (IC$_{50}$ = 24.3 µg/ml) against *E. coli* as compared to free CuCl$_2$ salt (IC$_{50}$ = 120 µg/ml). This was due to the presence of phen in the complexes, which increased their lipophilicity and improved the transfer of Cu ions into the cells, causing excessive intracellular accumulation of Cu ion and induce the elevation of Cu levels (Li et al., 2011).

Zinc is the second most abundant metal ion present in the human body. Zn-complexes have been involved in many studies as part of metallodrugs for antiviral and antibacterial activities. In general, Zn^{2+} has zero ligand field splitting energy (LFSE), therefore Zn ion has no preference for any specific ligand field geometry. But it could be an advantage for Zn to make unique structural complexes that are not appropriate with other metals. It was suggested that Zn can bind with bacterial membrane, which leads to an increase in the lag phase and generation period of microbes, which delays the cell division resulting in cell death (Radke et al., 1994). In this context, Zn(II)-complexes have been synthesized with anti-inflammatory Ibuprofen drug (Figure 31.5) and heterocyclic nitrogen-based ligands, which were screened for their antibacterial activities against both Gram-positive (*M. luteus, S.aureus,* and *B. subtilis*) and Gram-negative bacteria (*E. coli, K. pneumoniae,* and *P. mirabilis*). The obtained results showed high antibacterial activities, which were strongly influenced by the concentration and geometry of the complexes (Ali et al., 2016)[54]. Zn(II)-complex with antibiotics (i.e., sulfadiazine and enrofloxacin) was also synthesized and showed high antibacterial activity (MIC = 0.5 µg/mL) against *E. coli, S. aureus* and *E. faecalis* (Boughougal et al., 2018). For antibacterial textile application, Zn(II) was coordinated with a fluorescent symmetrical benzanthrone tripod and displayed the activity against *B. cereus* (MIC= 450 µg/mL) (Staneva et al., 2019).

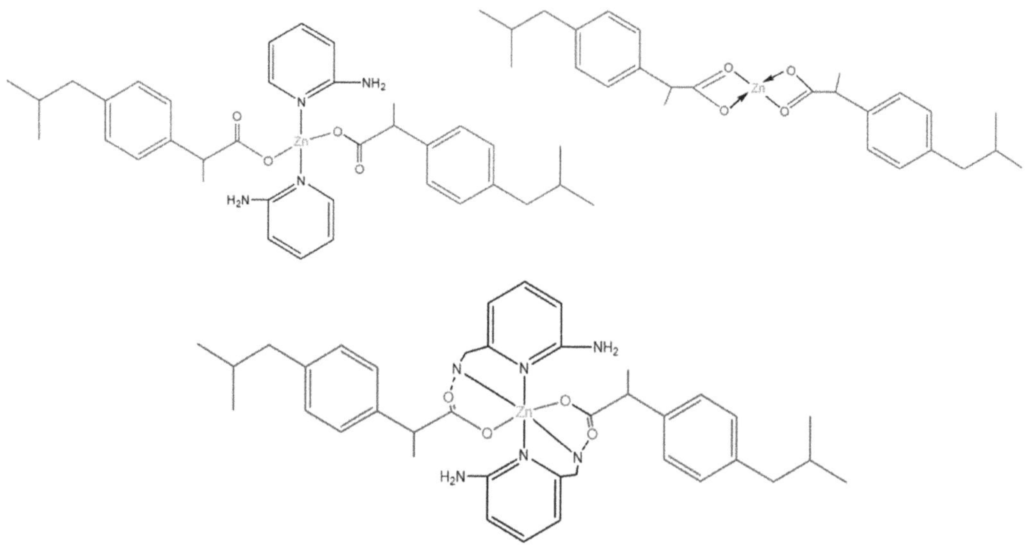

FIGURE 31.5   Chemical structure of Zn(II)-Ibuprofen complexes [www.mdpi.com/2624-8549/2/4/56/htm]

31.5.2 Second and Third Transition Series Metal Complexes

Second and third transition series metals and their complexes have shown various biological applications, especially when structurally rigid compounds are needed. They mimic their first transition series metal complexes with moderate changes of the geometrical parameters, but they show significant differences in the redox as well as kinetic properties. Ruthenium (Ru)-complexes have been widely used for anticancer activity, but in many reports, Ru was also described as central metal ion in antimicrobial agents. For example, inert polypyridylruthenium(II) complex [Ru(Me$_4$phen)$_3$]$^{2+}$showed remarkable antimicrobial activity (in vitro) against Gram-positive bacteria due to their binding ability with nucleic acids through intercalation with aromatic bases. Additionally, there was electrostatic interactions between positively charged Ru-complex and negatively charged phosphate groups (Li et al., 2015). Similarly, mononuclear Ru-complex, [Ru(2,9-Me$_2$phen)$_2$(dppz)]$^{2+}$ exhibited antibacterial activity through DNA binding ability against Gram-positive bacteria (*B. subtilis and S. aureus*, MIC = 2–8 µg/mL) in vitro and in vivo. But the metal complex was not active for Gram-negative bacteria (*E. coli*) (Bolhuis et al., 2011). Antimicrobial activity was observed by non-symmetric dinuclear polypyridylruthenium(II) complexes (Li et al., 2016), which contained one inert and one labile metal center, linked through bis[4(4'-methyl-2,2'-bipyridyl)]-1,n-alkane ligand. Complexes showed higher and lower activity against Gram-positive bacteria (MRSA) and Gram-positive bacteria (*E. coli*), respectively. Several examples of Ru-complexes as antimicrobial agents have been reviewed (Li et al., 2015).

Silver has been documented in various medical applications in the 18th and 19th centuries when silver nitrate was used as ointment for burn wounds and colloidal silver for wound antisepsis. In the early 20th century, the use of silver has declined, but still its complexes actively participate in medicinal areas due to their low toxicity and high activity at low concentration. They have been given more attention because their easy participation in ligand exchange reactions, ROS generation and direct target to DNA, RNA, or proteins. The main mechanism of Ag(I)-complexes was not clearly known. However, it was suggested that Ag(I) ions release via a dissociative process, interact with proteins, and damage the cell membrane. Therefore, several silver complexes have been synthesized that displayed antimicrobial activity against Gram-positive bacteria, Gram-negative bacteria, and fungi (Medici et al., 2016; Eckhardt et al., 2013b).

A few complexes of Iridium (Ir) and Rhodium (Rh) were also reported as significant antimicrobial agents. For example, Lu et al. synthesized and evaluated the antibacterial activity of kinetically inert cyclometallated Ir (III)-complexes. The results showed that Ir-complex exhibited prominent antibacterial effect against *S. aureus* (MIC=3.60 µM), and it was the first example of the kinetically inert organo-metallic complex from group 9 used as a direct inhibitor for *S. aureus* (Lu et al., 2015). Pandrala et al. reported the antibacterial activity of chlorido-substituted Ir(II) polypyridyl complexes and compared it with analogs Ru (II)-complexes. Interestingly, it was observed that Ir(III)-complexes (+4 charge) showed bacteriostatic inhibitory effect as compared to bactericidal effects like Ru (II)-complexes (+2 charge). It may depend upon the high charge on the Ir(III)-complexes, which prevent their entry into the bacterial cell. Moreover, Ir(III)-complexes possessed chloride anions that were found to be more labile than for the Ru(II)-complexes, which might also affect their accumulation within the bacteria, and thereby their bactericidal activity (Pandrala et al., 2013). Lapasam and group tested the antimicrobial activity of Rh(III) and Ir(III) arene complexes comprising hydrazone ligands (Lapsam et al., 2019a) and pyridyl azine Schiff base ligands (Lapsam et al., 2019b). The former complexes showed an inactive effect against *S. aureus* and *E. coli* while later complexes exhibited potent antibacterial activities. Ir (II) metal ion was also found to bind with various biguanide derivatives, including the antidiabetic drug metformin, which leads to formation of organoiridium cyclopentadienyl complexes. Most of these complexes showed significantly more activity against both Gram-negative and Gram-positive bacteria including MRSA (MICs values < 0.125 µg/mL) than the clinically used antibiotic vancomycin. Moreover, they exhibited low cytotoxicity toward mammalian cells and were highly stable in broth medium. Additionally, a few complexes also displayed high antifungal activity against the fungal strains *C. albicans* and *C. neoformans* (MICs values < 0.25 µg/mL), as compared to the standard fluconazole. Interestingly, it was found that biguanide ligand on its own had no antimicrobial effect (Chen et al., 2018).

After the discovery of cisplatin, various Pt-complexes have been synthesized and tested for antimicrobial activity. Some complexes have shown improved antibacterial activity while others show less effect on bacterial cells. For instance, in vitro antibacterial activity of Pt(IV) dithiocarbamato complexes were studied by Manav et al., where it was observed that complexes showed less activity against *E. coli, B. subtilis, P. aeruginosa,* and *Z. mobilis* bacterial strains (Manav et al., 2006). Solmaz et al. carried out the antimicrobial activity of *N,N*-Di-®-*N'*-(4-chlorobenzoyl)thiourea platinum(II) complexes against different bacterial and fungal strains. They were mainly effective against *S. pneumonia, P. aeruginosa,* and *A. baumannii* (MIC value = 3.90 µg/mL) while moderately active against *S. aureus, E. coli,* and *C. albicans* (MIC value = 15.62 µg/mL) (Solmaz et al., 2018). A few more Pt-complexes have been synthesized, and it was reportedtha t their antimicrobial activities had significant results (Odularu et al., 2019). Similar to platinum metal ions, palladium (Pd) (II)-complexes have also been highlighted as antimicrobial agents

TABLE 31.2

Antimicrobial Activity of Some Metal Complexes Belonging to the Second and Third Transition Series

Metal complexes	Test organism	Antimicrobial action	Ref
Bi(III) thiosemicarbazone complexes	*S. aureus*	15 to 64 times higher activity than free ligand (MIC$_{(complex)}$ = 5.5–6.1 µM)	Lessa et al., 2012
Ranitidine bismuth citrate	*Severe acute respiratory syndrome coronavirus*	Inhibited the SARS-coronavirus helicase (enzyme) and block virus replication	Yang et al., 2007
Au(I) alkynyl complexes	*MSSA* and *MRSA S. aureus*	Higher activity against *S. aureus* (MIC in the range of 2-32 µg/mL)	Hikisz et al., 2015
Au(I) bis-N-heterocyclic carbene complexes	*E. faecium, E. coli, P. aeruginosa, Acinetobacter baumannii, K. pneumonia and MRSA.*	Good antibacterial activity but not as effective as auranofin (MIC = 1.7–2.3 µM)	Schmidt et al., 2017
Gallium protoporphyrin IX	*Acinetobacter. Baumannii, P. aeruginosa*	Disrupt different pathways of bacterial ion acquisition (MIC = 31.7 µM) and targeting Cytochromes	Arivett et al., 2015; Hijazi et al., 2017

because of their high solubility and lipophilicity with low toxicity effects (Abu-Dief et al., 2020). For example, Pd(II)-complexes containing *N*-heterocycle carbene and triphenylphosphine showed significant in vitro antibacterial activity against Gram-positive (*M. luteus, S. aureus* and *L. monocytogenes*) and Gram-negative (*S. typhimurium* and *P. aeruginosa*) bacteria (Boubakri et al., 218)[71]. Pd(II) complexes with the biologically active Schiff base ligands derived from 3-amino-2-methyl-4(3H)-quinazolinone were tested for antibacterial activity. The results showed higher activity of metal complexes as compared to ligands due to chelation with metal ion (Prasad et al., 2013). Recently, 2-pyrral amino acid Schiff base Pd(II)-complexes were investigated for the antibacterial activity against Gram-positive (*S. aureus,* MRSA, *S. epidermidis,* and *S. pyogenes*) and Gram-negative (*P. aeruginosa* and *K. pneumonia)* bacteria. The authors found that complexes showed higher activity than ligands. Moreover, metal complexes comprising the imidazole and indole tail amino acids were more active against the bacteria strains than metal complexes containing an aliphatic sulfur group amino acid (Nyawade et al., 2020).

31.6 Metallosurfactant as Antimicrobial

Metallosurfactants are one of the most successful metal complexes that provide interfacial surfactant models associated with metal ion functionality (i.e., magnetism, redox variety, catalytic properties, higher electronic contrast, etc.) and which would be highly desirable due to their amphiphilic character. Due to their amphiphilic nature, they bind to the hydrophobic cell membrane and hydrophilic non-membrane proteins (Figure 31.6). Therefore, metallosurfactants are rapidly becoming a prime focus for the development of more efficacious metal-based drugs that possess antibacterial, anticancer, antiproliferative, or anthelmintic activity (Veeralakshmi et al., 2015; Riyasdeen et al., 2014). Until now, mostly research has been done on the antimicrobial activity of metallosurfactants.

31.6.1 Metallosurfactants with Metal Ions in Hydrophilic Head

In these metallosurfactants, a metal ion with its primary coordinated sphere forms the part of a head group and an alkyl chain of surfactant acts as the hydrophobic part of the metallosurfactant. Several articles have reported on their synthesis and their antibacterial activity against several pathogens. For example, Cr(III) metallosurfactants containing chelate ligands with amine surfactants (dodecylamine or cetylamine) have higher antibacterial and antifungal activity than that of standard ciprofloxacin (for

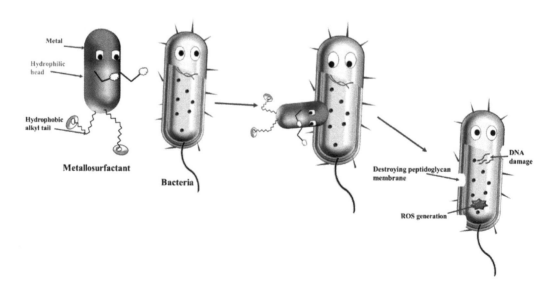

FIGURE 31.6 Metallosurfactant-damaged action on bacteria.

bacteria) and clotrimazole (for fungus) drugs. Moreover, the number of alkyl chains (i.e., hydrophobicity) of a metallosurfactant influence the activity against the microbes. They have shown high activity with double alkyl chain as compared to the single alkyl chain (Kumaraguru and Santhakumar, 2009).

The antibiotic activity of Co(III) metallosurfactants (i.e., cis-[CoX$_2$(C$_{14}$H$_{29}$NH$_2$)Cl]$^{2+}$) made up of N,N-donor ligands (X = en, bpy, phen or X$_2$ = trien) and a long-chain amine ligand were described by the Arunachalam and co-workers. The complexes showed higher activity against Gram-positive (*S. aureus and B. subtilis*) than Gram-negative bacteria (*E. coli* and *P. aeruginosa*). This was due to the diffusion of metallosurfactants inside the bacterial cells. Moreover, Co(III) metallosurfactant containing trien ligand showed higher performance as compared to other ligands, which may be due to its high hydrophobicity (Kumar and Arunachalam, 2008). Similar activities were observed in another article reported for Co(III) metallosurfactant, cis-[CoX$_2$(C$_{11}$H$_{23}$NH$_2$)$_2$]$^{3+}$, made up of the same ligand as above. The results showed that metallosurfactant with en and trien ligand have better activity as compared to bpy and phen for all pathogens (Sasikala and Arunachalam, 2013). Chander et al. synthesized cobalt(III) metallosurfactants with hexadecylamine and bidentate ligand (i.e., dimethyl glyoxime) and studied their antimicrobial activity. They were found to be very effective when tested on bacteria. In the case of fungus, they showed more fungistatic effect on *C. albicans* and less effect on *A. niger* and *Penicillium spp* (Chandar et al., 2011). The same group used Schiff base Co (III) metallosurfactant for antibacterial activity against Gram-positive and Gram-negative bacteria as well as fungi. An acceptable reason for the increase in activity may be the chelation process, which decreases the metal polarity and enhances its permeability across the cell membranes (Chandar et al., 2009).

The biocide activity of Ni and Cu metallosurfactants prepared from cationic surfactant (termed as alkyl acetate benzyl diphenyl ammonium salt) was investigated on bacterial and fungal strains. As expected, they showed significant activity toward the tested microbes. This may be due to the electrostatic interactions between the positively charged head group and oppositely charged centers on the cellular membrane. Additionally, hydrophobic chains also penetrated the cell membrane due to similarities in their chemical structure. These interactions modulate the selective permeability of cell membranes, which in turn disturbs the metabolic mechanism within the cytoplasm. Moreover, it was also observed that Cu-metallosurfactant has higher activity than that of Ni-metallosurfactant because of lower electronegativity and larger volume of the Cu ion, which reflects its high molecular area and enhanced biocidal activity (Adawy and Khowdiary, 2013). Cu^{2+} metal ion is an electrophile that employs microbiological toxicity through various biochemical routes such as reactive oxygen species (ROS) formation, oxidation of cellular protein thiols, and the displacement of similar transition metal ions (e.g., Fe^{3+}) from another binding site in bacteria. Metallosurfactants of Cu(II) with dodecylamine and cetylamine were potent antibacterial and antifungal agents as compared to the standard drugs, ciprofloxacin and fluconazole, respectively. The higher activity may be due to interaction or an efficient diffusion of the metallosurfactants into the bacterial/fungal cells. Moreover, they exhibited higher activity against Gram-positive bacteria (*S. aureus* and *B. subtilis*) than Gram-negative bacteria (*E. coli* and *P. aeruginosa*) (Sasikala and Arunachalam, 2012). The biological potential of Pd(II) metallosurfactant comprising long-chain amine surfactant was investigated against *B. cereus, K. pneumoniae, and Curvularia lunata*. Their activity was higher than that of the respective parent surfactant. Along with antibacterial activity, cytotoxicity of Pd(II) metallosurfactant was studied in Vero cells (healthy), and was found to be 10 mg/mL (i.e., IC$_{50}$) (Chaudhary et al., 2015).

Natural polysaccharide carbohydrate-derived cationic sodium alginate surfactant was tested for the antimicrobial activity against both Gram-positive (*B. subtilis, S. aureus*) and Gram-negative bacteria (*E. coli, P. aeruginosa*). The metal ions, Co (II), Cu (II), and Zn (II), coordinated with the surfactant showed higher antibacterial activity than the free alginate cationic surfactant. The action of mechanism was the adsorption of the positively charged metallosurfactant on the lipoteichoic acid layer of Gram-positive and non-polar lipid layer of Gram-negative bacteria that causes disturbance in the selective permeability of bacterial membrane and biological reactions. Chelation process also takes part in the antibacterial mechanism. Moreover, the counter ion (i.e., halogen atoms (Br$^-$)) of metallosurfactant also participate to increase the potent action when penetrating the cells (Tawfik et al., 2016).

As discussed above, Ru-complexes are significantly active in biological processes. Nehru et al. synthesized various Ru-metallosurfactants by substituting the precursor Ru(II)-complexes, [Ru(bpy)2Cl2] and [Ru(phen)2Cl2], with hexadecylamine or dodecylamine surfactants. The authors observed that the metallosurfactant showed more prominent effect against the *K. pneumoniae* and *MRSA* as compared to the precursor. This was mainly due to the hydrophobicity of the metallosurfactants, which is responsible for the penetration in bacterial membrane. Moreover, metallosurfactants decrease the viability of lung cancer cell lines (Nehru et al., 2020). Ru-metallosurfactant comprised of 2,9-dimethyl[1,10]phenanthroline and cetyl amine surfactant possessed good bacteriostatic against the bacterial species. At low concentrations, Ru(II) metallosurfactants showed high cytotoxicity towards the cervical cancer cell lines. This may be due to the decrease in the energy value in tumor cells because of Ru(II) metallosurfactants. This deficiency affects cellular functions, which may lead to cell death (Suganthidevi and Kumaraguru, 2020).

31.6.2 Metallosurfactants with Metallic Counter Ion

The presence of metallic ions as counter ions with surfactant head groups represents the different classes of metallosurfactants. As antibacterial agents, these metallosurfactants showed high antimicrobial activities as compared to parent surfactants. For example, a series of cationic ferrosurfactants (Aiad et al., 2012) were developed to study the antimicrobial activity against bacteria (*E. coli, B. sutilus*) and fungus *(A. Nigar, C. albicans)*. They adsorb at interface of microbial cells. This adsorption increases their permeability towards the other components that interfere in the biochemical reactions inside the cell. This leads to inhibition of the growth of tested microbes. Pyrazolium derivative surfactants and their metallosurfactants with Sn (II) and Cu (II) ions were synthesized by Negm et al. Surfactants possessed moderate antibacterial activity against Gram-positive and Gram-negative bacteria as well as fungi. However, on complexation with metal ions, the antibacterial activity was considerably increased (Sn(II) > Cu(II)). These results correlated with charge formation on the metallosurfactants. The metal complexation of the cationic surfactants reduced the positive charge on the nitrogen atom, which facilitated its adsorption at the cellular membrane and enhanced the activity of metallosurfactants. Moreover, Sn(II) metallosurfactants had higher antibacterial activity, which was due to the higher electronegativity (EN) (1.96) of Sn(II) than that of Cu(II) (1.90). They also showed increased antifungal activity upon complaxation against fungus *C. albicans* and *A. flavus* (Negm et al., 2010a).

A similar study was carried out for cationic Mn, Co, and Cu metallosurfactants containing Schiff base having fatty amines. The synthesized metallosurfactants showed higher activity than that of free Schiff base surfactants due to their high hydrophobicity, which facilitates their adsorption to cell walls. Cu metallosurfactants seem to be more effective than Co and Mn metallosurfactants due to high EN and atomic radii of Cu (II) ion. Moreover, the results reported that long alkyl-chain complexes exhibited less antibacterial activity due to the early formation of micelles and less availability to interact with the cellular membrane (Negm et al., 2010b). Metallosurfactants synthesized from non-ionic Schiff bases are also considered as antibacterial and antifungal agents. It was reported that the antibacterial activity of these surfactants was enhanced after complaxation with Cu(II) and Fe(III). Moreover, metallosurfactants with short alkyl chains have higher activity than long alkyl-chain metallosurfactants (Negm et al., 2008).

Quaternary ammonium-based metallosurfactants have also been explored as potent antibacterial agents. In this case, Kaur and her group tested the antimicrobial activity of double-chain cationic metallosurfactants (M= Fe, Co and Ni) using hexadecylpyridinium chloride (CPC) surfactant (Kaur et al., 2019). The results showed that Fe(II) metallosurfactant was less effective and Ni(II) show comparable activity as parent surfactant. Co(II) metallosurfactants were more active against Gram-positive and Gram-negative bacteria. Additionally, a similar trend was observed with single-chain metallosurfactants prepared by using the same combination of metal salts and ligand in 1:1 molar ratio. Haemolysis assay was performed for their biocompatibility study, where metallosurfactants showed high toxicity (Fe > Ni > Co) at premicellar concentration but low toxicity at postmicellar concentration. Similarly, Cu-based single- and double-chain metallosurfactants (Kaur et al., 2016) were synthesized and evaluated for antimicrobial activity. They were found to be highly effective against bacteria, but not for the fungus. However, both metallosurfactants showed nearly equal antibacterial activity. ut in haemolysis assay, Cu metallosurfactant with double alkyl chain was more biocompatible than its single-chain analog. Interestingly, Pt-CPC metallosurfactant showed less antibacterial activity than CPC surfactant as studied by Sharma et al. This may be due to the weak interaction between Pt metal ion and CPC. In contrast, the anticancer activity of CPC was increased after coordination with Pt metal ion against human breast cancer lines (Sharma et al., 2018).

Metallosurfactant with hexadecyltrimethyl ammonium chloride (CTAC) surfactant (M = Fe, Co, Ni, and Cu) was synthesized and the antibacterial activity was evaluated. As expected, high antibacterial activity was observed against both the bacterial cells (Garg et al., 2020). Similarly, Pd metallosurfactant showed dual action towards cancer cells and microorganisms (Kaur et al., 2016). However, they were found to be more active against bacteria than fungus. Badawi et al. explored the antimicrobial activity of copper cetyl trimethylammonium bromide (Cu-CTAB) and the results showecthat Cu-CTAB had 35% higher activity than CTAB. This might be due to the action of quaternary ammonium surfactant on the phospholipid components of the bacterial membrane, which distort the membrane and cause leakage of intracellular components. These complexes were also employed for anticancer activity by loading it with cyclodextrin nanoparticles (Badawi et al., 2009). Complexes of benzyl triphenyl phosphonium tri-chloro cupprate and tetra-chloroferrate were designed into metallosurfactants by interacting with dodecyl amine and CPC. They were screened against major food pathogens such as *E. coli*, *P. aeruginosa*, *S. faecalis*, and *S. aureus*. All synthesized metallosurfactants exhibited higher activity than parent ligand. Generally, the cytoplasmic membrane of bacteria is the target site for surfactants. Therefore, the interaction of metallosurfactants with cytoplasmic bacterial membrane facilitates the interpretation of metallosurfactants on membranes and solubilizes the inner components of cytoplasmic membranes, resulting in the death of bacterial cells. It was also observed that Fe-metallosurfactant with dodecyl amine was less effective among metallosurfactants (Hafiz et al., 2008).

31.7 Conclusion

This chapter provided a concise overview of potential metal-based complexes of first, second, and third transition series for their antimicrobial applications. They offer a great prospective for therapeutic and diagnostic purposes owing to their various redox potentials, diverse coordination number, and geometries. All metal complexes have multiple mechanisms of action against different microbes. Various factors such as the nature of ligand and their chelation effect, charge on the metal complexes, and metal center affects the antimicrobial property of metal complexes. However, the antimicrobial metal toxicity is still hindered due to limited in vivo experiments available for metal complexes. Therefore, it becomes necessary to perform further work to better understand in vivo activities of metal complexes. Apart from metal complexes, amphiphilic metallosurfactants have untapped potential for antimicrobial activities. They possessed dual functionality of metal and that of surfactant, which bring some unique advantages. They have also shown very promising results in terms of their easier interaction with biomolecules, higher bioactive moieties released, and better selectivity. The recent developments of metallosurfactants will increase the chances of reaching clinical trials.

REFERENCES

Abu-Dief AM, Abdel-Rahman LH, Abdel-Mawgoud AAH (2020). A robust in vitro anticancer, antioxidant and antimicrobial agents based on new metal-azomethine chelates incorporating Ag(I), Pd(II) and VO(II) cations: Probing the aspects of DNA interaction. *Appl. Organomet. Chem.* 34:5373.

Adawy AI, Khowdiary MM (2013). Structure and biological behaviors of some metallo cationic surfactants. *J. Surfact. Deterg.* 16:709–715.

Aiad I, Ahmed MHM, Hessein A, Ali Md. (2012). Preparation, surface, and biological activities of some novel metallosurfactants. *J. Dispers. Sci. Technol.* 33(8), 144–1153

Ali HA, Omar SN, Darawsheh MD (2016). H. Fares. Synthesis, characterization and antimicrobial activity of zinc(II) ibuprofen complexes with nitrogen-based ligands. *J. Coord. Chem.* 69:1110–1122.

Arif R, Nayab PS, Ansari IA, Shahid M, Irfan M, Alam S, Abid M (2018). Synthesis, molecular docking and DNA binding studies of phthalimide-based copper(II) complex: In vitro antibacterial, hemolytic and antioxidant assessment. *J. Mol. Struct.* 1160:142–153

Arthi P, Shobana S, Srinivasan P, Prabhu D, Arulvasu C, Rahiman AK (2015). Dinuclear manganese(II) complexes of hexaazamacrocycles bearing N-benzoylated pendant separated by aromatic spacers: Antibacterial, DNA interaction, cytotoxic and molecular docking studies. *J. Photoch. Photobio. B* 153:247–260.

Arivett BA, Fiester SE, Ohneck EJ, Penwell WF, Kaufman CM, Relich RF, Actis LA, Antimicrobial activity of gallium protoporphyrin IX against acinetobacter baumannii strains displaying different antibiotic resistance phenotypes. *Antimicrob. Agents Chemother.* 59:7657–7665 (2015).

Badawi AM, Zakhary NI, Morsy SMI, Sabry GM, Mohamed Md. R, Mousa AM (2009). Copper (II)-surfactant complex and its nano analog as potential antitumor agents. *J. Dispers. Sci. Technol.* 30:1303–1309.

Barmpa A, Frousiou O, Kalogiannis S, Perdih F, Turel I, Psomas G (2018). Manganese(II) complexes of the quinolone family member flumequine: Structure, antimicrobial activity and affinity for albumins and calf-thymus DNA. *Polyhedron* 145:166–175.

Biot C, Nosten F, Fraisse L, Ter-Minassian D, Khalife J, Dive D (2011). The antimalarial ferroquine: From bench to clinic. *Parasite* 18:207–214.

Biot C, Glorian G, Maciejewski LA, Brocard JS, Domarle O, Blampain G, Millet P, Georges AJ, Abessolo H, Dive D (1997). Synthesis and antimalarial activity in vitro and in vivo of a new ferrocene–chloroquine analogue. *J. Med. Chem.* 40:3715–3718.

Boubakri L, Mansour L, Harrath AH, Ozdemir I, Yaşar S, Hamdi N (2018). N-Heterocyclic carbene-Pd(II)-PPh_3 complexes as a new highly efficient catalyst system for the Sonogashira cross-coupling reaction: Synthesis, characterization and biological activities. *J. Coord. Chem.* 71:183–199.

Boughougal A, Cherchali FZ, Messai A, Attik N, Decoret D, Hologne M, Sanglar C, Pilet G, Tommasino JB, Luneau D (2018). New model of metalloantibiotic: Synthesis, structure and biological activity of a zinc(II) mononuclear complex carrying two enrofloxacin and sulfadiazine antibiotics. *New J. Chem.* 42:15346–15352.

Bolhuis A, Hand L, Marshall JE, Richards AD, Rodger A, Wright JA (2011). Antimicrobial Activity of Ruthenium-Based Intercalators. *Eur. J. Pharm. Sci.* 42, 313–317.

Cade G, Shankly KH, Shulman A, Wright RD, Stahle IO, Macgibbon CB, Lew-Sang E (1970). The treatment of dermatological infections with a manganese phenanthroline chelate. A controlled clinical trial. *Med. J. Aust.* 2:304–309.

Chang EL, Simmers C, Knight DA (2010). Cobalt complexes as antiviral and antibacterial agents. *Pharmaceuticals* 3:1711–1728.

Chandar SCN, Sangeetha D, Arumugham MN (2011). Synthesis, structure, CMC values, thermodynamics of micellization, steady-state photolysis and biological activities of hexadecylamine cobalt (III) dimethyl glyoximato complexes. *Transition Met. Chem.* 36:211–216.

Chandar SCN, Santhakumar K, Arumugham MN (2009). Metallosurfactant Schiff base cobalt (III) coordination complexes. Synthesis, characterization, determination of CMC values and biological activities. *Transition Met. Chem.* 34:841–848.

Chaudhary GR, Singh P, Kaur G, Mehta SK, Kumar S, Dilbaghi N (2015), Multifaceted approach for the fabrication of metallomicelles and metallic nanoparticles using solvophobic bisdodecylaminepalladium (II) chloride as precursor. *Inorg. Chem.* 54, 9002–9012.

Chen F, Moat J, McFeely D, Clarkson G, Hands-Portman IJ, Furner-Pardoe JP, Harrison F, Dowson CG, Sadler PJ (2018). Biguanide iridium (III) complexes with potent antimicrobial activity. *J. Med. Chem.* 61:7330–7344.

Chohan ZH (1991). Synthesis of cobalt (II) and nickel (II) complexes of Ceclor (Cefaclor) and preliminary experiments on their antibacterial character. *Chem. Pharm. Bull.* 39:1578–1580.

Chohan ZH, Supuran CT, Scozzafava A (2004). Metalloantibiotics: Synthesis and antibacterial activity of cobalt (II), copper(II), nickel(II) and zinc(II) complexes of kefzol.

Dwyer FP, Gyarfas EC, Rogers WP, Koch JH (1952). Biological activity of complex ions. *Nature* 170:190–191.

Eckhardt S, Brunetto PS, Gagnon J, Priebe M, Giese B, Fromm KM(2013a). Nanobio silver: Its interactions with peptides and bacteria, and its uses in medicine. *Chem. Rev.* 113:4708–4754

Eckhardt S, Brunetto PS, Gagnon J, Priebe M, Giese B, Fromm KM (2013b). Silver: its interactions with peptides and bacteria, and its uses in medicine. *Chem. Rev.* 113:4708–4754.

Eze FI, Ajali U, Ukoha PO (2014). Synthesis, physicochemical properties, and antimicrobial studies of iron (III) complexes of ciprofloxacin, cloxacillin, and amoxicillin, *Int J Med.* 2014:735602.

Garg P, Kaur B, Kaur G, Saini S, Chaudhary GR (2020). A study of the spectral behaviour of Eosin dye in three states of metallosurfactants: Monomeric, micelles and metallosomes. *Colloids Surf. A Physicochem. Eng.* 610:125697.

Garg P, Kaur G, Chaudhary GR, Gawali SL, Hassan PA (2017). Fabrication of metalosomes (metal containing cationic liposomes) using single chain surfactants as a precursor via formation of inorganic organic hybrids. *Phys. Chem. Chem. Phys.* 37:25764–25773.

Griffiths PC, Fallis IA, Willock DJ, Paul A, Barrie CL, Griffiths PM, G.M. Williams GM, King SM, Heenan RK, Görgl R (2004).The structure of metallomicelles. *Chem-A Eur J.* 10:2022–2028. 43.

Hafiz AA (2008). Crystal structure of benzyl triphenyl phosphonium chlorometallate: Some surface and biological properties of their metallosurfactant derivatives. *J. Iran. Chem. Soc.* 5:106–114.

Hijazi S, Visca P, Frangipani E (2017). Gallium-protoporphyrin IX inhibits pseudomonas aeruginosa growth by targeting cytochromes. *Front. Cell. Infect. Microbiol.* 7:12.

Hikisz P, Szczupak L, Koceva-Chyla A, Gu Spiel A, Oehninger L, Ott I, Therrien B, Solecka J, Kowalski K (2015). Anticancer and antibacterial activity studies of gold(I)-alkynyl chromones. *Molecules* 20:19699–19718.

Hossain Md. S, Islam HMT, Khan Md. N, Sarker AC, Chaki BM, Latif A, Uddin N, Alam Md. A, Zakaria Md. C, Zahan Md. KE (2019). A short review on antimicrobial activity study on transition metal complexes of Ni incorporating schiff bases. *Appl. Chem.* 2:1–16.

Iakovidis I, Delimaris I, Piperakis SM (2011). Copper and its complexes in medicine: a biochemical approach. *Mol. Biol. Int.* 2011:594529–42.

Irgi EP, Geromichalos GD, Balala S, Kljun J, Kalogiannis S, Papadopoulos A, Turel I, Psomas G (2015). Cobalt(II) complexes with the quinolone antimicrobial drug oxolinic acid: Structure and biological perspectives. *RSC Adv.* 5:36353–36367.

Jain M, Gaur S, Diwedi SC, Joshi SC, Singh RV, Bansal A (2004). Nematicidal, insecticidal, antifertility, antifungal and antibacterial activities of salicylanilide sulphathiazole and its manganese, silicon and tin complexes. *Phosphorus Sulfur Silicon Relat. Elem.* 179:1517–1537.

Kaur G, Garg P, Kaur B, Chaudhary GR, Kumar S, Dilbaghi N, Hassan PA, Aswal VK (2019). Synthesis, thermal and surface activity of cationic single chain metal hybrid surfactants and their interaction with microbes and proteins. *Soft Matter.* 15:2348.

Kaur G, Kumar S, Dilbaghi N, Bhanjana G, Guru SK, Bhushan S, Jaglan S, Hassan PA, Aswal VK (2016). Hybrid surfactants decorated with copper ions: aggregation behavior, antimicrobial activity and antiproliferative effect. *Phys. Chem. Chem. Phys.* 18: 23961.

Kaur G, Kumar S, Dilbaghi N, Kaur B, Kant R, Guru SK, Bhushan S, Jaglan S (2016). Evaluation of bishexadecyltrimethyl ammonium palladium tetrachloride based dual functional colloidal carrier as an antimicrobial and anticancer agent, *Dalton Trans.* 45:6582–91.

Kharadi GJ, Antioxidant, tautomerism and antibacterial studies of Fe (III)-1,2,4-triazole based complexes (2013). *Spectrochim. Acta Part. A Mol. Biomol. Spectrosc.* 110:311–316.

Kelland L et al. (2007). The resurgence of platinum-based cancer chemotherapy. *Nat. Rev. Cancer.* 7:573–584

Klasen HJ et al. (2000). A historical review of the use of silver in the treatment of burns. II. Renewed interest for silver. *Burns.* 26:131–138.

Kenny RG, Marmion CJ (2019). Toward multi-targeted platinum and ruthenium drugs-a new paradigm in cancer drug treatment regimens. *Chem. Rev.* 119:1058–1137

Konkankit CC, Marker SC, Knopfa KM, Wilson JJ (2018). Anticancer activity of complexes of the third row transition metals, rhenium, osmium, and iridium, *Dalton Trans.* 47:9934–9974.

Krishnegowda HM, Karthik CS, Marichannegowda MH, Kumara K, Kudigana PJ, Lingappa M, Mallu P, Neratur LK (2019). Synthesis and structural studies of 1-phenyl-1,3-butanedione copper(II) complexes as an excellent antimicrobial agent against methicillin-resistant Staphylococcus aureus. *Inorganica Chim. Acta* 484:227–236.

Kremer E, Facchin G, Estévez E, Alborés P, Baran EJ, Ellena J, Torre MH (2006). Copper complexes with heterocyclic sulfonamides: Synthesis, spectroscopic characterization, microbiological and SOD-like activities: Crystal structure of [Cu(Sulfisoxazole)2(H2O)4].2H2O. *J. Inorg. Biochem.* 100: 1167–1175.

Kumaraguru N, Santhakumar K (2009). Synthesis, characterization, critical micelle concentration determination, and antimicrobial studies of some complexes of chromium (III) metallosurfactants. *J. Coord. Chem.* 62:3500–3511.

Kumar RS, Arunachalam S (2008). Synthesis, micellar properties, DNA binding and antimicrobial studies of some surfactant–cobalt (III) complexes. *Biophysical Chem.* 136:136–144.

Lapasam A, Banothu V, Addepally U, Kollipara MR (2019a). Antimicrobial selectivity of ruthenium, rhodium, and iridium half sandwich complexes containing phenyl hydrazone schiff base ligands towards B. Thuringiensis and P. Aeruginosa bacteria. *Inorg. Chim. Acta* 484:255–263

Lapasam A, Banothu V, Addepally U, Kollipara MR (2019b). Synthesis, structural and antimicrobial studies of half-sandwich ruthenium, rhodium and iridium complexes containing nitrogen donor Schiff-base ligands. *J. Mol. Struct.* 1191:314–312.

Lemire JA, Harrison JJ, Turner RJ (2013). Antimicrobial activity of metals: mechanisms, molecular targets and applications. *Nat. Rev. Microbiol.* 11:371–384.

Lessa JA, Reis DC, Da Silva JG, Paradizzi LT, Da Silva NF, de Fátima A, Carvalho M, Siqueira SA, Beraldo H (2012). Coordination of thiosemicarbazones and bis(thiosemicarbazones) to bismuth(III) as a strategy for the design of metal-based antibacterial agents. *Chem. Biodiverse.* 9:1955–1966.

Li F, Collins JG, Keene FR (2015). Ruthenium complexes as antimicrobial agents. *Chem. Soc. Rev.* 44:2529–2542.

Li X, Zhang Z, Wang C, Zhang T, He K, Deng F (2011). Synthesis, crystal structure and action on Escherichia coli by microcalorimetry of copper complexes with 1,10-phenanthroline and amino acid. *J. Inorg. Biochem.* 105:23–30.

Li X, Heimann K, Li F, Warner JM, Keene FR, Collins JG (2016). Dinuclear ruthenium (II) complexes containing one inert metal centre and one coordinatively-labile metal centre: Syntheses and biological activities. *Dalton Trans.* 45:4017–402.

Lu L, Liu LJ, Chao WC, Zhong HJ, Wang M, Chen XP, Lu JJ, Li RN, Ma DL, Leung CH (2015). Identification of an iridium(III) complex with anti-bacterial and anti-cancer activity. *Sci. Rep.* 5:14544.

Manav N, Mishra AK, Kaushik NK (2006). In vitro antitumour and antibacterial studies of some Pt(IV) dithiocarbamate complexes, *Spectrochimica Acta Part A.* 65:32–35.

Mbese JZ, Odularu AT, Ajibade PA, Oyedeji OO (2019). Developments in platinum-group metals as dual anti-bacterial and anticancer agents, *Chem. J.* 2019:1–18.

Mahmoud WH, Sayed FN, Mohamed GG (2016). Synthesis, characterization and in vitro antimicrobial and anti-breast cancer activity studies of metal complexes of novel pentadentate azo dye ligand. *Appl. Organomet. Chem.* 30:959–973.

Marín-García M, Benseny-Cases N, Camacho M, Perrie Y, Suades J, Barnadas-Rodríguez R(2018). Metallosomes for biomedical applications by mixing molybdenum carbonyl metallosurfactants and phospholipids. *Dalton Trans.* 47:14293–303.

Medici S, Peana M, Crisponi G, Nurchi V, Lachowicz JI, Remelli M, Zoroddu MA (2016). Silver coordination compounds: A new horizon in medicine. *Coord. Chem. Rev.* 327:349–359.

Monro S, Colón KL, Yin H, Roque J, Konda P, Gujar S, Thummel RP, Lilge L, Cameron CG, McFarland SA (2019). Transition metal complexes and photodynamic therapy from a tumor-centered approach: Challenges, opportunities, and highlights from the development of TLD1433. *Chem. Rev.* 119:797–828.

Nagel C, McLean S, Poole RK, Braunschweig H, Kramer T, Schatzschneider U (2014). Introducing [Mn(CO)3(tpa-k3N)]+ as a novel photoactivatable CO-releasing molecule with well-defined iCORM intermediates–synthesis, spectroscopy, and antibacterial activity. *Dalton Trans.* 43:9986–9997.

Nazirkar B, Mandewale M, Yamgar R (2019). Synthesis, characterization and antibacterial activity of Cu(II) and Zn(II) complexes of 5-aminobenzofuran-2-carboxylate Schiff base ligands. *J. Taibah Univ. Sci.* 13:440–449.

Negm NA, Said MM, Morsy SMI (2010). Pyrazole derived cationic surfactants and their tin and copper complexes: Synthesis, surface activity, antibacterial and antifungal efficacy. *J. Surfact. Deterg.* 13:521–528.

Negm NA, Zaki Md. F, Salem MAI (2010). Cationic schiff base amphiphiles and their metal complexes: Surface and biocidal activities against bacteria and fungi. Colloids Surf. B 77:96–103

Negm NA, Zaki Md. F, Structural and biological behaviors of some nonionic Schiff base amphiphiles and their Cu(II) and Fe(III) metal complexes. *Colloids Surf. B* 64, 179–183 (2008).

Nehru S, Veeralakshmi S, Kalaiselvam S, David SPS, Sandhya J, Arunachalam S (2020). DNA binding, antibacterial, hemolytic and anticancer studies of some fluorescent emissive surfactant-ruthenium(II) complexes. *J. Biomol. Struct. Dyn.* 39:2242–2256.

Nyawade EA, Onani MO, Meyer S, Dube P (2020). Synthesis, characterization and antibacterial activity studies of new 2-pyrral-L-amino acid Schiff base palladium (II) complexes. *Chem. Pap.* 74:3705–3715.

Odularu AT, Ajibade PA, Mbese JZ, Oyedeji OO (2019). Developments in platinum-group metals as dual antibacterial and anticancer agents. *J. Chem.* 2019:18.

Oladipo MA, Olaoye OJ (2013). Antimicrobial, DNA cleavage and antitumoral properties of some transition metal complexes of 1, 10-phenanthroline and 2, 2'-bipyridine: a review. *Int. J. Res. Pharm. Biomed. Sci.* 4:1160–1171.

Paez PL, Bazán CM, Bongiovanni ME, Toneatto J, Albesa I, Becerra MC, Argüello GA (2013). Oxidative stress and antimicrobial activity of chromium(III) and ruthenium(II) complexes on Staphylococcus aureus and Escherichia coli. *Biomed. Res. Int.* 2013:1–7.

Pandrala M, Li F, Feterl M, Mulyana Y, Warner JM, Wallace L, Keene FR, Collins JG (2013). Chlorido-containing ruthenium(ii) and iridium(iii) complexes as antimicrobial agents. *Dalton Trans.* 42:4686.

Prasad KS, Kumar LS, Chandan S, Kumar RMN, Revanasiddappa HD (2013). Palladium(II) complexes as biologically potent metallo-drugs: Synthesis, spectral characterization, DNA interaction studies and antibacterial activity, *Spectrochim. Acta A* 107: 108–116.

Pradeep I, Megarajan S, Arunachalam S, Dhivya R, Vinothkanna A, Akbarshab MA, Sekar S (2014). Ferrocenyl methylene units and copper(II) phenanthroline complex units anchored on branched poly(ethyleneimine)-DNA binding, antimicrobial and anticancer activity. *New J. Chem.* 38:4204–4211.

Radke LL, Hahn BL, Wagner DK, Sohnle PG (1994). *Clin. Immunol. Immunopathol.* 73:344.

Raj P, Singh A, Singh A, Singh N (2017). Syntheses and photophysical properties of schiff base Ni(II) complexes: Application for sustainable antibacterial activity and cytotoxicity. *ACS Sustain. Chem. Eng.* 5:6070–6080.

Raman N, Raja JD, Sakthive A, Synthesis, spectral characterization of Schiff base transition metal complexes: DNA cleavage and antimicrobial activity studies (2007). *J. Chem. Sci.* 119:303–310.

Reddy PM, Shanker K, Rohini R, Ravinder V (2009). Antibacterial active tetraaza macrocyclic complexes of Chromium (III) with their spectroscopic approach, *Int. J. Chem. Tech. Res.* 1:367–372

Revathi V, Karthik K (2019). Physico-chemical properties and antibacterial activity of Hexakis (Thiocarbamide) Nickel(II) nitrate single crystal. *Chem. Data Collect.* 21:100229.

Riyasdeen A, Senthilkumar R, Subbarayan V, Periasamy, Preethy P, Suresh S, Zeeshan Md., Krishnamurthy H, Arunachalam S, Akbarsh Md. A (2014). Antiproliferative and apoptosis-induction studies of a metallosurfactant in human breast cancer cell MCF-7. *RSC Adv.* 4:49953–49959.

Saidin S, Jumat MA, Md. Amin NAA, Al-Hammadi ASS (2021). Organic and inorganic antibacterial approaches in combating bacterial infection for biomedical application. *Mater. Sci. Eng. C* 118:111382.

Sasikala K, Arunachalam S (2013). Antimicrobial activity, spectral studies and micellar properties of some surfactant-cobalt (III) complexes. *Chem. Sci. Trans.* 2:157–166.

Sasikala K and Arunachalam S (2012). Antimicrobial activity, Spectral studies and CMC determination of some surfactant-copper (II) complexes. *J. Chem. Biol. Phys. Sci.* 2:708–718.

Staneva D, Tonkova EV, Grabchev I (2019). A new bioactive complex between Zn(II) and a fluorescent symmetrical benzanthrone tripod for an antibacterial textile. *Materials.* 12:3473.

Solmaz U, Gumus I, Binzet G, Celik O, Balci GK, Dogen A, Arslan H (2018). Synthesis, characterization, crystal structure, and antimicrobial studies of novel thiourea derivative ligands and their platinum complexes. *J. Coord. Chem.* 71:200–218.

Schmidt C, Karge B, Misgeld R, Prokop A, Brönstrup M, Ott I (2017)., Biscarbene gold(I) complexes: Structure–activity-relationships regarding antibacterial effects, cytotoxicity, TrxR inhibition and cellular bioavailability. *Med. Chem. Commun.* 8:1681–1689.

Sakurai H, Yoshikawa Y, Yasui H (2008). Current state for the development of metallopharmaceutics and antidiabetic metal complexes. *Chem. Soc. Rev.* 37:2383–2392.

Saraiva R, Lopes S, Ferreira M, Novais F, Pereira E, Feio MJ, Gameiro P (2010). Solution and biological behaviour of enrofloxacin metalloantibiotics: a route to counteract bacterial resistance. *J. Inorg. Biochem.* 104:843–850.

Schwartz JA, Lium EK, Silverstein SJ (2001). Herpes simplex virus type 1 entry is inhibited by the cobalt chelate complex CTC-96. *J. Virol.* 75:4117–4128.

Sharma A, Sharma S, Khuller GK, Kanwar AJ, In vitro and ex vivo activity of peptide deformylase inhibitors against Mycobacterium tuberculosis H37Rv. *Int. J. Antimicrob. Agents.* 34, 226–230 (2009).

Sharma NK, Singh M (2018). New class of Platinum based metallosurfactant: Synthesis, micellization, surface, thermal modelling and in vitro biological properties. *J. Mol. Liq.* 268: 55–65.

Singh DP, Kumar K, Sharma C (2009). Antimicrobial active macrocyclic complexes of Cr(III), Mn(III) and Fe(III) with their spectroscopic approach. *Eur. J. Med. Chem.* 44:3299–3304.

Suganthidevi R, Kumaraguru N (2020). Interaction of CT-DNA with ruthenium(ii) metallosurfactant complexes: synthesis, cmc determination, antitumour and antimicrobial activities. *Asian J. Chem.* 32:665–677.

Tawfik SM, Hefni HH (2016). Synthesis and antimicrobial activity of polysaccharide alginate derived cationic surfactant–metal(II) complexes. *Int. J. Biol. Macromol.* 82:562–572.

Tarallo MB, Urquiola C, Monge A, Costa BP, Ribeiro RR, Costa-Filho AJ, Mercader RC, Pavan FR, Leite CQF, Torre MH (2010). Design of novel iron compounds as potential therapeutic agents against tuberculosis. *J. Inorg. Biochem.* 104:1164–1170.

Turecka K, Chylewska A, Kawiak A, Waleron KF (2018). Antifungal activity and mechanism of action of the Co(III) coordination complexes with diamine chelate ligands against reference and clinical strains of candida spp. *Front. Microbiol.* 9:1594.

Veeralakshmi S, Nehru S, Sabapathi G, Arunachalam S, Venuvanalingam P, Kumar P, Anushad C, Ravikumar V (2015). Single and double chain surfactant–cobalt(III) complexes: the impact of hydrophobicity on the interaction with calf thymus DNA, and their biological activities. *RSC Adv.* 5:31746–31758.

Vlasiou MC, Pafiti KS (2020). Chromium coordination compounds with antimicrobial activity: Synthetic routes, structural characteristics, and antibacterial activity. *Open J. Med. Chem.* 14:1–25.

Yang N, Tanner JA, Zheng BJ, Watt RM, He ML, Lu LY, Jiang JQ, Shum KT, Lin YP, Wong KL (2007). Bismuth complexes inhibit the SARS coronavirus. *Angew. Chem. Int. Ed.* 46:6464–6468.

Zhu Y, Li W-H (2010). Syntheses, crystal structures and antibacterial activities of azido-bridged cobalt(III) complexes with Schiff bases. *Transition Met. Chem.* 35:745–749.

Section IV

Drugs and Delivery Systems

32

Stem Cells: Emerging Novel Approaches to Drug Research and Disease Therapeutics

Shiv Bharadwaj
Department of Biotechnology, Yeungnam University, College of Life and Applied Sciences, Gyeongsan, Republic of Korea

Nikhil Kirtipal
Department of Science, MIT, Rishikesh, India

Meena Bharti
School of Life and Environmental Sciences, Deakin University, Warrnambool, Australia

R.C. Sobti
Department of Biotechnology, Panjab University, Chandigarh, India

32.1 Introduction

Cell, in biology, is defined as the basic membrane-bound unit that comprises the fundamental molecules of life. A single cell can exist as a complete organism in itself, such as bacterium or yeast. The fundamental architect of all the cells is same, however, certain cells have special functions upon maturation. These various cells collaborate with other dedicated cells and become building blocks of multicellular organisms, such as humans. Hence, the body of mammalians (human beings and other animals) is a very complicated structure containing various types of cells with unique functions. In fact, matured cells or somatic cells are basically originated from the non-mature special types of cells, named stem cells, and are responsible for the multi-cellular level of organization in the human body (Korkusuz, Kose et al., 2016). Thus, principally a stem cell represents an undifferentiated cell of the multicellular organism, and holds the ability to divide and produce, via a cellular process called mitotic division, into various types of somatic cells in the body and new stem cells. By definition, stem cells are defined as unspecialized cells that are capable of becoming specialized cells, with self-renewal and differentiation ability to build different types of mammalian cells (Chaudhury, Raborn et al., 2012). The ability of stem cell to divide and transform into different types of cells is known as stem cell plasticity (Krause, Theise et al., 2001; Mountford 2008). This process helps the human body regenerate damaged cells or tissues; for instance, cells in the blood and epithelia divide rapidly and are replaced by newly regenerated cells throughout life, while cells in most other tissues turn over slowly and respond only to specific biological signals (Krebsbach and Robey, 2002). The identity of the powerful cells that allow humans to regenerate some tissues was first discovered when experiments with bone marrow in the 1950s established the existence of stem cells in our bodies (Bhat, Shetty et al., 2019). The first stem cells studied by researchers were derived from adult tissues, and more recently, scientific breakthroughs have permitted research on stem cells that are removed from one of the earliest human cellular formations, such as the blastocyst (stem cells are basic cells of all multicellular organisms with the potency to differentiate into a wide

DOI: 10.1201/9781003220404-36

range of adult cells) (Kalra, Tomar et al., 2014). Hence, the distinctive characteristics of regeneration and pliable nature of stem cells assist in the formation of a new range of cells in the form of stem cell-based therapy (Krause, Theise et al., 2001; Mountford 2008).

32.2 Classification of Stem Cells and Their Applications in Medicine

In the last few decades, the significance of stem cell technology has remained noticeably recognized, and extensive work has been done to determine their role in numerous human diseases and physiological conditions (Burns and Thapar, 2014).

Because of the distinctive ability to convert into other cells, stem cell technology has been formulated as regenerative medicine or tissue regeneration (Zhou, E Grottkau et al., 2016), such as for regeneration of heart, lung, pancreas, skin, nerve tissue, etc. Additionally, stem cell-based therapy was also found useful in central nervous system (CNS) disorders and its derivatives were suggested to act as neuroprotective agents and induced neuronal growth in neurodegenerative diseases (Ouyang, Goldberg et al., 2016). Stem cell-based therapy therefore offers a promising therapeutic approach in the treatment of several degenerative disorders, organ/tissue damage, or injury as well as in cancer treatment for which no or insufficient treatments are available (Hardikar, Lees et al., 2006).

32.2.1 Classification of Stem Cells

During the developmental process in all the mammals, including humans, distinct types of stem cells grow and differentiate into specialized cells.

These specialized cells conduct specific functions in different parts of the body. Hence, based on the site of origin, proliferation, and differentiation ability, stem cells are divided into the following different classes (also as shown in Figure 32.1).

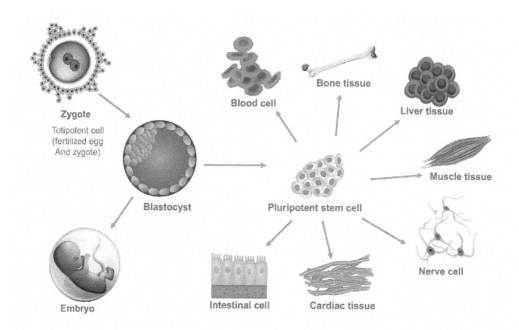

FIGURE 32.1 Classification of stem cells from zygote (totipotent) to adult stem cells, such as nerve cell, blood cells, bone tissue, muscle tissue, etc.

32.2.1.1 Classification I

Initially, based on the site of origin or source of isolation, stem cells are broadly classified into two types: (i) embryonic stem cells (ESCs) and (ii) adult or somatic stem cells. However, more precisely, there is another type of stem cell called a fetal stem cell (Agrawal, Alexander et al., 2019). A brief discussion on each class of stem cells is given below.

Embryonic Stem Cell

The fertilized egg or zygote, the primordial cell that originates a new life, is the first stem cell with the capability to create both the embryonic and extra embryonic tissue.

Additionally, this cell holds the potential to produce all types of cells of the mammalian or human body. Such ability of differentiation and proliferation of the zygote is defined as totipotency (Gage, 2000). Moreover, during the process of embryonic growth, a constant cell division occurs that results in the transformation of zygote into a blastocyst. Hence, a blastocyst consists of two different types of cells: A trophoblast forms the outer cellular layer and other is the inner cell mass (Jyoti and Tandon, 2015). The trophoblast cells lead to generation of extra embryonic tissue while the inner cells are responsible for the production of different types of tissues, including the developing embryo. Thus, the cells extracted and in vitro cultured from the inner cell mass of the blastocyst are defined as embryonic stem cells (ESCs). Of note, these cells further differentiate into all types of body cells called pluripotent stem cells (PSCs) (Smith, 2001, Draper and Fox, 2003). ESCs were first isolated from the mice and grown as in vitro culture in 1981 (Evans and Kaufman, 1981; Kingham and Oreffo, 2013). After that, in 1998, Thomson and colleagues derived human embryonic stem cells (hESCs) (Thomson, Itskovitz-Eldor et al., 1998).

Somatic/Adult Stem Cell

After birth, stem cells are essentially required in the process of growth, constant body maintenance and repair process, and recovery from physical injury or disease condition throughout the life. In this context, the stem cells present in the body to complete such tasks after development are known as somatic stem cells or adult stem cells. A typical role of somatic stem cell is to replace the dead, damaged, or diseased cells with the new cells. Hence, these cells exhibit multipotent differentiation behavior and produce cells with identical anatomical and functional properties (Nancarrow-Lei, Mafi et al., 2017).

Furthermore, these cells can be differentiated or categorized from each other based on their source of origin and features, such as a hematopoietic stem cell, neural stem cell, bone marrow stem cell adipose tissue, muscle tissue, ocular stem cell, dental pulp stem cell, etc. (Bulgin, 2015; Adak, Mukherjee et al., 2017).

Fetal Stem Cell

Fetal stem cells are typically originate from the fetus body where these cells are extracted from the fetus bone marrow, blood, or other organ such as kidney, liver, and nerve cells. Moreover, fetal stem cells may be collected from proper fetal cells after abortion or from extraembryonic fetal membrane and umbilical cord after birth (Lu, Liu et al., 2006). These stem cells are non-immortal in nature and hold greater differentiation potential in comparison to the adult/somatic stem cells. The fetal stem cells are a promising therapeutic and analytical tool to study the substantial traits of cell biology, cell/organ transplantation, and in gene therapy. However, further experimental studies are required to establish a proper procedure for propagation, engraftment, and in vivo differentiation of fetal stem cells (O'Donoghue and Fisk. 2004).

32.2.1.2 Classification II

Another classification of stem cell is based on the differentiation and proliferation capability of the cells; a brief discussion on each type of stem cell is given below. By proliferation and differentiation ability the stem cells are divided into following categories (Agrawal, Alexander et al., 2019).

Totipotent Stem Cell

The totipotent stem cells are represented as an essential type of stem cell, which originated with the imitation of the life. These cells can differentiate and proliferate into other types of cells in the human body and include extraembryonic and placental cells. In this context, the first embryo/fertilized egg/zygote is the only cell that holds the characteristic property totipotency (Gage, 2000).

Pluripotent Stem Cell

Following zygote or preliminary embryo formation, further cell division occurs, which produces more similar totipotent cells; after four days of fertilization, the formed zygote remains transformed into blastocyst with the assistance of some specific cell function. This main blastocyst mass holds the potential to form all the body cells, except extraembryonic and placental cells; these ESCs are known as pluripotent stem cells (Alateeq, RJ Fortuna et al., 2015). These stem cells have the unique potential to grow into various progenies of daughter cells, which are similar to mother cells but with different characteristic features. Following differentiation and proliferation, pluripotent cells produce three cell linings (i.e., endoderm, mesoderm, and ectoderm) of the an embryo, which further develop into various tissues of the body (Kingham and Oreffo, 2013; Zhang et al., 2015). Hence, to maintain the pluripotent nature of pluripotent stem cells, a standard method involves isolation of the cells and culturing in a controlled environment, which simplifies the unlimited proliferation without undergoing differentiation cycle. This process by which stem cells produce more stem cells and perpetuate indefinitely is called self-renewal (Williams, Hilton et al., 1988; S Wilson et al., 2015; Zhang, Huang et al., 2015).

Induced Pluripotent Stem Cell

The induced pluripotent stem cells (iPSCs) are pluripotent stem cells that are produced from the adult cells using genetically engineered reprogramming at the particular environmental conditions to induce pluripotent behavior (Figure 32.2) (Zhang, Huang et al., 2015). This type of stem cell is mostly employed

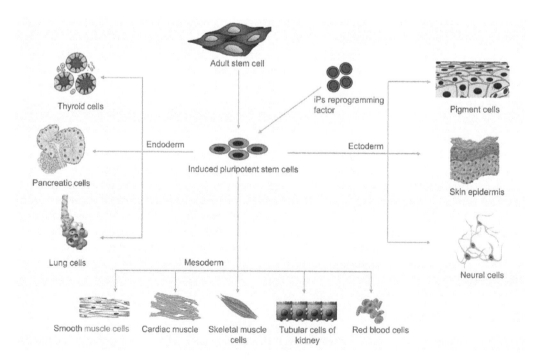

FIGURE 32.2 Reprogramming of iPSCs from adult stem cell and differentiation into different cell layers: mesoderm, endoderm, and ectoderm.

in stem cell-based therapy and molecular or cellular biology to fulfill the demands required in new technology or research and development (Rosner, Schipany et al., 2014). The major benefit of iPSCs is that there are no ethical issues associated with them; instead, the restrictions relate to safety and efficacy of the generated stem cells.

32.2.1.3 Multipotent Stem Cell

Like all the other stem cells, a multipotent stem cell is marked as an undifferentiated cell, which has the ability of self-renewal and differentiation into specialized cells linked with limited characteristics (Chaudhury, Raborn et al., 2012). For instance, the hematopoietic cell can generate all types of blood cells while multipotent neural cells can only produce nerve cells. In fact, most adult stem cells or somatic stem cells can pursue multipotent traits due to their ability to produce a specific group of cells or limited to a particular cell line (Eun, 2014). Moreover, mesenchymal stem cells (MSCs) are a type of multipotent stem cell that can differentiate into various types of cells, such as bone, cartilage, muscle, fat, and other related tissues.

32.2.1.4 Unipotent Stem Cell

Unipotent stem cells are a type of stem cell that can only generate its progeny and differentiate into a singular cell lineage like stem cells originated from the dermis of the skin. However, unipotent stem cells have a limited differentiation ability compared to totipotent and pluripotent stem cells; hence, they possess limited clinical applications (Gage, 2000). For instance, these stem cells are strongly used in the treatment of several disorders and replacement therapy such as skin-derived stem cells are employed in skin replacement, plastic surgery, skin disorder, etc.

32.2.2 Clinical Applications of Stem Cells

In the last decade, stem cell therapy has gained popularity in medical research, and researchers are constantly working in the development of advanced therapeutics using stem cell-based strategies against several life-threatening disorders. For instance, stem cell-based therapy is being established for the development of new promising therapeutic approaches in the treatment of various chronic disorders, such as wound healing, skin repair and regeneration, organ replacement or regeneration, bone regeneration, etc. (Morelli, Salerno et al., 2016) (Figure 32.3). Thus, based on the available clinical applications and investigations conducted on stem cells for medical use, they can be mainly divided into four major classes: (i) Human embryonic stem cells; (ii) fetal stem cells (stem cells are extracted from the amniotic fluid and placenta); (iii) induced pluripotent stem cells or genetically reprogrammed stem cells; (iv) and mesenchymal or adult stem cells.

The therapeutic efficacy of stem cell-based treatment is primarily explained by three underlying mechanisms (Tran and Damaser, 2015). The first approach includes the replacement of stem cells at the site of injury to the particular area of injury by chemical gradient after the systemic administration; this process is defined as "homing" of stem cell (Tran and Damaser, 2015). Secondly, differentiation of stem cells into required type of cells at the site of injury to recover the area with new cells. And thirdly, the release of bioactive molecules to assist the replacement therapy by altering various physiological responses at the area of injury (Tran and Damaser, 2015). The primary advantage of stem cell therapy is it eliminates the painful and tedious surgical procedure and also minimizes the risk of donor site morbidity (in organ trans-plantation therapy) (Eun, 2014). Various clinical applications of stem cell therapy in different chronic pathological condition are discussed below.

32.2.2.1 ESCs in Regenerative Medicine

Human ESCs (hESCs) were isolated for the first time by Thomson in 1998 (Thomson, Itskovitz-Eldor et al., 1998). hESCs have the pluripotent property and divide into more than 200 types of cells with promising applications in the treatment of many kind of diseases (Thomson, Itskovitz-Eldor et al.,

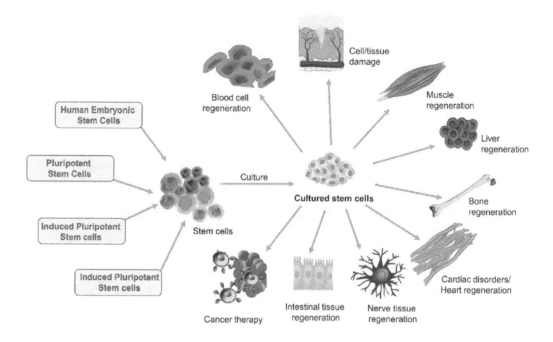

FIGURE 32.3   Therapeutic applications of stem cells.

1998). Of note, the pluripotency nature of ESCs is mediated by functional dynamics of specific transcription factors, including Octamer-binding transcription factor 4 (OCT4), sex-determining region Y-box transcription factor 2 (SOX2), and NANOG, commonly called pluripotency factors. The diverse lineage of ESCs represents an ideal model in regeneration therapeutic applications against diseases and tissue anomalies (Mahla, 2016). Thus, in the last decade, various attempts have been made to discover the approach to repair the injured spinal cords in experimental models, which may provide a novel therapeutic application in humans. In this context, a few examples of ESC-based therapy using animal models of diseases haven been reported with encouraging and promising results. For instance, ESCs were also suggested to be utilized as an in vitro system to study cell differentiation as well as to evaluate the effects of new drugs and identification of drug target genes/proteins for therapeutic applications (He, Li et al., 2003). Recently, it was reported that developmentally relevant signaling factors can induce mouse ESC differentiation into functional motoneurons, which repopulate the embryonic spinal cord, extend axons, and form synapses with target muscles (Wichterle, Lieberam et al., 2002). Moreover, transplantation of ESCs into adult rat spinal cord following chemical demyelination or in myelin-deficient mutant mice, the stem cells successfully differentiated into mature oligodendrocytes, generated myelin, and myelinated host axons (Liu, Qu et al., 2000).

Also, severe infection, cancer, and accidents that can induce spinal card injuries (SCIs) were suggested to improve by the transplantation of hESCs in paraplegic or quadriplegic SCI patients to improve body control, balance, sensation, and limbal movements (Shroff and Gupta, 2015). Furthermore, transplantation of the inert biomaterial encapsulated hESCs-derived pancreatic progenitors (CD24+, CD49+, and CD133+) were noted for differentiation into β-cells, reducing high-fat diet-stimulated glycemic and obesity consequences in mice (Bruin, Saber et al., 2015). Interestingly, addition of antidiabetic drugs into transdifferentiation regime were suggested to boost the ESCs transformation into β-cells (Bruin, Saber et al., 2015), which ideally can cure permanently Type 2 Diabetes (Bruin, Saber et al., 2015). ESCs can be distinguished precisely into insulin secreting β-cells (marked with GLUT2, INS1, GCK, and PDX1), which can be accomplished via PDX1-mediated epigenetic reprogramming (Salguero-Aranda, Tapia-Limonchi et al., 2016). Also, the reliability of ESCs to incorporate and distinguish into electro-physiologically active cells delivers a means for natural management of heart rhythm as biological pacemaker. Coaxing of ESCs into inert biomaterial and division in defined culture conditions leads to transdifferentiation of ESCs to grow to be sinoatrial node (SAN) pacemaker cells (PCs) (Vedantham, 2015). Transplantation of PCs was reporte to restore pacemaker functions in an ailing heart (Vedantham, 2015).

Conclusively, ESCs can be transdifferentiated into any type of cell demonstrating three germ layers of the body and are considered as the most promising source of regenerative medicine in tissue engineering and disease therapy. However, ethical matters restrict the applications of ESCs, where guidelines need to be followed for therapeutic application (Mahla, 2016).

32.2.2.2 TSPSCs in Regenerative Medicine

The role of TSPSCs is to sustain the tissue homeostasis via continuous cell division; however, unlike ESCs, TSPSCs carry the stem cell plasticity and differentiation in a tissue-specific manner that give rises to a few types of cells. This results in undersized population of TSPSCs in total number of cell population, hence, extraction and in vitro manipulation of such cells for therapeutic scale is a really tricky task (Greggio, De Franceschi et al., 2013). The human body is the result of various types of TSPSCs; for instance, pancreatic progenitor cells (PPCs), dental pulp stem cells (DPSCs), inner ear stem cells (IESCs), intestinal progenitor cells (IPCs), limbal progenitor stem cells (LPSCs), epithelial progenitor stem cells (EPSCs), mesangioblasts (MABs), spermatogonia stem cells (SSCs), skin-derived precursors (SKPs), and adipose-derived stem cells (AdSCs).

For example, in the process of embryogenesis, PPCs differentiate into insulin-producing β-cells and are negatively mediated by insulin (Ye, Robertson et al., 2016). While PPCs need active FGF and NOTCH signaling and rapidly grow in community rather than in single-cell populations these factors suggest the functional role of niche effect in transdifferentiation and self-renewal processes. For instance, mice embryo-derived PPCs grown on 3D-scaffold culture system exhibit hollow organoid spheres and eventually differentiate into insulin-producing β-cell clusters (Greggio, De Franceschi et al., 2013). Another example, DPSCs, which are essentially required to maintain teeth health and can be obtained from deciduous teeth, apical papilla, periodontal ligaments, and dental follicle, have emerged as potential regenerative medicine candidate for the treatment of several kinds of diseases, including restoration neurogenic functions in teeth (Ellis, O'Carroll et al., 2014; Potdar and Jethmalani, 2015). One of the most important tissue-specific stem cells, male germline stem cells or spermatogonial stem cells (SSCs), which generate spermatogenic lineage via mesenchymal and epithets cells (Simon, Ekman et al., 2009), have a niche effect on other cells. Of note, in vivo transplantation of SSCs with skin, prostate, and uterine mesenchyme differentiated into epithelia of the tissue of origin (Simon, Ekman et al., 2009). The newly generated tissues display all the chief physical and physiological features of prostate and skin, and the physical characteristics of skin, prostate, and uterus, express tissue-specific markers. These observations suggest the role of factors secreted from SSCs that lead to lineage conservation and define the importance of niche effects in regenerative medicine (Simon, Ekman et al., 2009). Moreover, other kinds of stem cells have been reported for therapeutic potential in regenerative medicine, such as to repair eye defects (Mead, Berry et al., 2015) and Fallopian tubes flaws (Kessler, Hoffmann et al., 2015). Likewise, subcutaneous visceral tissue-specific cardiac adipose (CA)-derived stem cells (AdSCs) were reported to have the potential to differentiate into cardiovascular tissue (Nagata, Ii et al., 2016).

In summary, TSPSCs are potentiated with tissue regeneration, where advancement in organoid culture methods have established the importance of niche effect in tissue regeneration and therapeutic outcomes of ex vivo expanded stem cells (Mahla, 2016).

32.2.2.3 MSCs/Stromal Cells in Regenerative Medicine

MSCs, the multilineage stem cells, solely differentiate into the tissue of mesodermal origin, including tendons, bone, cartilage, ligaments, muscles, and neurons (Dominici, Le Blanc et al., 2006). MSCs specially express the combination of markers (i.e., CD73$^+$, CD90$^+$, CD105$^+$, CD11b$^-$, CD14$^-$, CD19$^-$, CD34$^-$, CD45$^-$, CD79a$^-$, and HLA-DR) (Dominici, Le Blanc et al., 2006). Thus, potential applications of MSCs in regenerative medicine can be generalized from ongoing clinical trials and clinical phases at different stages of completion (Squillaro, Peluso et al., 2016). For instance, MSCs have been studied with the potential to regenerate liver tissue and treat liver cirrhosis (Volarevic, Nurkovic et al., 2014). The regenerative medical application of MSCs used the cells in two formats, as direct transplantation or first transdifferentiation followed by transplantation; ex vivo transdifferentiation of MSCs deploys a retroviral delivery system that can cause an oncogenic effect on cells. Moreover, nonviral, nanoscript technology, using transcription factor (TF) functionalized gold nanoparticles (AuNPs), can target a specific regulatory site in the genome effectively and direct differentiation of MSCs into another type of cell; such events depend on the regime of TFs. For instance, myogenic regulatory factor containing nanoscript-MRF transforms the adipose tissue-derived MSCs into muscle cells (Patel, Yin et al., 2015). The multipotency features signify MSCs as encouraging candidates for attaining stable tissue constructs via coaxed 3D organoid culture; however, heterogeneous distribution of MSCs slows down cell proliferation, and renders therapeutic applications of MSCs. Therefore, adopting a two-step culture system for MSCs can be used to produce the homogeneous distribution of MSCs in biomaterial scaffolds. For instance, cultured fetal-MSCs coaxed on biomaterial in rotating bioreactor when transferred to static culture yield homogeneous distribution of MSCs in ECM components (Leferink, Chng et al., 2015). Moreover, in vitro chondrogenic, osteogenic, and audiogenic potential of MSCs suggests therapeutic applications of MSDs in orthopedic injuries (Csaki, Matis et al., 2007). Conclusively, the multilineage differentiation potential of MSCs and adoption of the next-generation organoid culture systems purposes MSCs as an ideal regenerative medical candidate.

32.2.2.4 UCSCs in Regenerative Medicine

Umbilical cord, commonly thrown away at the time of childbirth, is the best-known resource of stem cells, which are acquired in a noninvasive manner with fewer ethical constraints compard to ESCs. The umbilical cord is a rich supplier of hematopoietic stem cells (HSCs) and MSCs, which retain enormous regeneration potential (Shahrokhi, Menaa et al., 2012). The HSCs of cord blood are responsible for constant restoration of all types of blood cells and defensive immune cells. The proliferation of HSCs is regulated by Musashi-2 protein-mediated attenuation of Aryl hydrocarbon receptor (AHR) signaling in the stem cells (Rentas, Holzapfel et al., 2016). UCSCs can be cryopreserved at stem cell banks operated by both private and public sector organizations. The public stem cell banks operate on donation formats and conduct rigorous screening for HLA typing while donated UCSCs remain available to anyone who needs them; however, private stem cell bank operation is more personalized, availing the cells according to donor consent. Even then, stem cell banking is not common in developed countries. A recent survey estimates that educated women are more keen to donate UCSCs but the willingness for donation deceases with subsequent deliveries because of associated expenses and safety concerns for preservation (Lu, Chen et al., 2015). Of note, the FDA has approved five HSCs for the treatment of blood and other immunological complications (Rosemann, 2014). UCSCs are the best alternatives for those patients who lack donors with fully matched HLA typing for peripheral blood and PBMCs and bone marrow (Gluckman, Koegler et al., 2005). One major issue with UCSCs is the number of cells in transplant, since fewer cells in transplant require more time for engraftment to mature, and there are also risks of infection and mortality; in such cases, ex vivo propagation of UCSCs can fulfill the demand of required outcomes. A diverse number of protocols has been studied for the ex vivo expansion of UCSCs (Mehta, Rezvani et al., 2015).

For instance, amniotic fluid stem cells (AFSCs) coaxed to fibrin hydrogel and PEG supplemented with vascular endothelial growth factor (VEGF) results in production of vascularized tissue upon grafting on mice, suggesting the most promising application of UCSCs to generate biocompatible tissue patches as treatment for infants born with congenital heart defects (Benavides, Brooks et al., 2015).

Moreover, in stem cell therapeutics, UCSC transplantation can be performed in either autologous or allogenic nature. However, on some occasions, autologous UCSCs transplants are not effective to combat tumor relapse, as observed in Hodgkin's lymphoma (HL), which might require a second dose replacement of allogenic stem cells. Herein, it is important to monitor the efficacy and tolerance of stem cells at the site of tumor replacement. For instance, a case study demonstrated that a second dose of allogenic transplants of UCSCs was effective for HL patients, who had a heavy dose in a prior transplant and increased long-term persistence chances by 30% (Thompson, Perera et al., 2016).

32.2.2.5 BMSCs in Regenerative Medicine

Bone marrow present in the soft spongy bones produce all the blood cells, including HSCs (for generating blood cells) and stromal cells (producing fat, cartilage, and bones) (Travlos, 2006). Since 1980, bone marrow replacement has been routinely accepted as one of the potent treatments for cancer (Gschweng, De Oliveira et al., 2014). To avoid graft rejection, HLA typing of donors is used as a standard method while absolute matches are limited to family members, which restricts the allogenic transplantation applications. As matching of all HLA antigen is not a critical requirement in bone marrow transplantation, characterizing the essential antigens for a haploidentical allogenic donor for a patient, who cannot find a fully matched donor, might alleviate donor constraints. Hence, haploidentical HLA matching protocol is major for minorities and others who do not have access to matched donor (Gaballa, Palmisiano et al., 2016). For instance, hepatitis C virus (HCV) infection can cause liver cirrhosis and deterioration of hepatic tissue. Under these circumstances, the intraparenchymal transplantation of bone marrow mononuclear cells (BMMNCs) into liver tissue was shown to decrease aspartate aminotransferase (AST), alanine transaminase (ALT), bilirubin, CD34, and α-SMA, suggesting the administration of BMSCs assisted in the restoration of hepatic function via the regeneration of hepatic tissues (Lukashyk, Tsyrkunov et al., 2014). Thus, to fulfil the increasing demand for stem cell transplantation therapy, donor encouragement is always considered as the primary requirement (Gubareva, Sjöqvist et al., 2016).

32.2.3 Applications in Other Medical Disorders

32.2.3.1 In Neurodegeneration and Brain or Spinal Cord Injury

Sometimes injuries and pathologies result in the degeneration of the nervous system. However, few curative measurements and therapeutic interventions have been developed and become available to repair or treat damage in the nervous system. In this context, the therapeutic effect of stem cells and their derived extracellular vehicles (EVs) have been investigated with significant effects on the nervous system (neurons and nerves). For example, EVs extracted from MSCs enriched in miRNA-133b were demonstrated to stimulate neural cells to produce neurite outgrowth (Merianos, Heaton et al., 2008). The beneficial efficiency of human MSC-EV was recently elucidated in preclinical models against several diseases and injuries (Gowen, Shahjin et al., 2020). EV derived from the human adipose tissue-derived MSCs (hAMSCs) have also been shown to possess therapeutic potential in neurodegenerative disorders, including Huntington's disease and Alzheimer's disease (AD). Moreover, hAMSC-derived EVs have been shown to ameliorate the progression of beta-amyloid-induced neuronal death in vitro AD mouse model (Lee, Ban et al., 2018). Also, the investigation of the therapeutic effects of hAMSC-derived exosomes on in vitro Huntington's model demonstrated neuroprotective effects while Huntington's disease phenotype was amended via mediation of mutant Huntington aggregates' mitochondrial and apoptotic functions (Lee, Liu et al., 2016). Interestingly, this neuroprotective property appears to manipulate the neurodevelopment of the fetal brain; application of human bone marrow (hBMMSC)-derived EV was demonstrated to protect the fetal brain development afflicted with hypoxia (Ophelders, Wolfs et al., 2016).

Moreover, regenerative and anti-inflammatory properties of the MSC-EV have been studied in animal models of traumatic brain injury (Kim, Nishida et al., 2016; Das, Mayilsamy et al., 2019; Ni, Yang et al., 2019), stroke (Doeppner, Herz et al., 2015; Bang and Kim, 2019, Dabrowska, Andrzejewska et al., 2019), wound healing (Zhang, Guan et al., 2015), and perinatal brain injury (Thomi, Surbek et al., 2019). Altogether the future of MSCs has been long anticipated with an increase in the number of clinical trials; however, the ability of EVs to operate similar to MSCs and holding no substantial drawbacks in cell-based therapies suggest they are a unique niche in medical therapeutics.

32.2.3.2 In Frailty Syndrome

Chronic diseases and degenerative environments are strongly connected with the geriatric syndrome of frailty and share a disproportionate percentage of healthcare budgets.

Frailty increases the risk of falls, hospitalization, institutionalization, disability, and death. By definition, frailty syndrome is typified by decreases in lean body mass, strength, endurance, balance, gait speed, activity and energy levels, and organ physiologic reserve (Schulman, Balkan et al., 2018). Collectively, these alterations lead to the loss of homeostasis and the capability to withstand stressors and results in serious susceptibilities. There is a strong association between frailty, inflammation, and the impaired capacity to repair tissue injury due to drops in endogenous stem cell production (Schulman, Balkan et al., 2018). In frailty, aging-related changes decrease the stem cell self-renewal, maintenance, and recovery potential. With regard to frailty, reformed and dysfunctional stem cell niches have been implicated in frailty syndrome (López-Otín, Blasco et al., 2013; Golpanian, DiFede et al., 2016). As such, it has been proposed that a regenerative medicine therapeutic approach has the potential to enhance or reverse the signs and symptoms of frailty (Kanapuru and Ershler, 2009; Raggi and Berardi, 2012). Interestingly, there are specific features of frailty syndrome that sustain the potential role of MSCs to improve or ameliorate frailty; MSCs drawn at the sites of injuries were noted to reduce inflammation and promote cellular repair (Bagno, Hatzistergos et al., 2018). Notably, MSCs were also observed to amend the cardiovascular outcomes in patients with acute myocardial infraction (Hare, Traverse et al., 2009), ischemic (Hare, Fishman et al., 2012), and non-ischemic cardiomyopathy (Hare, DiFede et al., 2017), decreased the levels of TNF-α and C-reactive protein (CRP), and were reliable activities in all patients irrespective of age (Golpanian, El-Khorazaty et al., 2015; Bagno, Hatzistergos et al., 2018).

32.2.3.3 In Cardiovascular Disease

Coronary heart disorders result in insufficient oxygen allocation to the myocardial muscles, which may further lead to cardiac necrosis, myocardial infarction, or cardiac arrest (Effat, 1995; Calin, Stan et al., 2013; Dixit and Katare, 2015; Chen, Zeng et al., 2017). Cardiac muscles have poor regeneration ability and thus damage may lead to severe, life-threatening conditions (Chi and Karliner, 2004; Frangogiannis, 2015). Stem cell regeneration therapy advances new hope for such cardiac conditions. Conservatively, heart transplant is a standard approach to treat the ischemic heart or injured heart; however, this treatment is very tedious and a challenging process to procure a healthy replaceable heart, typically from a brain-dead body. This process is almost out of reach in many cases. Therefore, stem cell therapy offers an advantage by comparison to heart replacement by competently regenerating the heart tissues (Lemon, Sjoqvist et al., 2016). Recently, several clinical and preclinical studies on ESCs, iPSCs, bone marrow stem cells, skeletal myoblasts, and MSCs have suggested endogenous cardiac stem cells as suitable therapy for differentiation of myocardial lineage (Calin, Stan et al., 2013; Preda and Valen, 2013; Dixit and Katare, 2015).

32.2.3.4 In Blood-Cell Formation

The initiation of human-induced pluripotent stem cell (iPSC) technology over 10 years ago provided investigators with an essential tool in the field of cellular therapeutics (Takahashi, Tanabe et al., 2007; Borst, Sim et al., 2017). One goal in the hematopoietic field has been to produce donor-independent platelets to complement current transfusion results. Platelets derived from megakaryocytes play a significant role in hemostasis and thrombus development and facilitate aspects of immunity, inflammation, and angiogenesis (Semple, Italiano et al., 2011; Ware, Corken et al., 2013; Golebiewska and Poole, 2015; Jenne and Kubes, 2015; Walsh, Metharom et al., 2015).

Even though shortage of donors has not been a recurrent problem to date, the number of transfusions in developed countries has been progressively enhanced due to improved lifespan and increases in hematologic malignancies (Whitaker, Rajbhandary et al., 2016). The advantages of using iPSCs to produce platelets is linked with their amenability for genetic manipulation. Hence, this creates a drive to build donor-independent sources of platelets for transfusions.

Although significant progress has been made, much work still needs to be done to bring in vitro-derived megakaryocytes and platelets to the clinic. However, efforts are being made by numerous laboratories to increase the quality and yield of iPSC-derived megakaryocytes and platelets.

In vitro bioreactors are being utilized to closely mimic the in vivo environment by incorporating ECM components, endothelial cells, and applying a flow to induce shear stress (Figure 32.6E) (Thon,

Dykstra et al., 2017). These in vitro bioreactors yield approximately 30 platelets per megakaryocyte, which is well below the in vivo yield of > 2000 (Feng, Shabrani et al., 2014). One potential explanation for low platelet yield is that these bioreactors are mainly plastic-based; it is possible that silk bioreactors or lung mini-chip bioreactors would help to increase yields. Alternatively, iPSC-derived megakaryocytes could be infused directly into patients to obtain maximal platelet release (Borst, Sim et al., 2017).

32.2.3.5 *In Regrowing Teeth*

Dental stem cells are a trivial population of MSCs that exist in specialized dental tissues, including periodontium, apical papilla, dental pulp, and dental follicle (Shuai, Ma et al., 2018). Several types of stem cells have been identified from the various teeth and tooth supporting tissues that share common in vitro properties by comparison to bone marrow mesenchymal stem cells (BMMSCs) like periodontal ligament stem cells (PDLSCs), stem cells from apical papilla (SCAPs), dental pulp stem cells (DPSCs), and dental follicle cells (DFCs) (Sharpe, 2016; Shuai, Ma et al., 2018). Although dental stem cells hold colony formation, propagation, and multipotent differentiation ability to produce osteogenic, adipogenic, and chondrogenic lineages in vitro cultures like BMMSCs under specific conditions, these cells also exhibit distinct regenerative potential by comparison to each other in an in vivo model, suggesting the application of tissue-specific stem cells as an optimal approach for self-tissue restoration and rejuvenation (Shuai, Ma et al., 2018). In this context, basic research and clinical pilot studies have reported the promising application of dental stem cell-dependent translational medicine in regenerative treatments (Shuai, Ma et al., 2018). Moreover, dental stem cells were noted for good regeneration of dental tissues, but a long process of tooth extraction, primary culture, and in vitro cell development limits their conventional application at the time of clinical requirements. Hence, long-term storage and timely utilization of dental stem cells remain to be settled. Recently, dental stem cell banking, such as StoreA-ToothTM (Lexington, USA, www.storea-tooth.com), BioEDEN (Austin, USA, www.bioeden.com), Teeth Bank Co., Ltd. (Hiroshima, Japan, www.teethbank.jp), Advanced Center for Tissue Engineering Ltd. (Tokyo, Japan, www.acte-group.com), and Stemade Biotech Pvt. Ltd. (Mumbai, India, www.stemade.com) emerged for cryo-preservation of dental stem cells, which emphasizes the potential to achieve a novel methodology to sustain large-scale dental stem cell-based regenerative medicine (Shuai, Ma et al., 2018). Moreover, apart from the therapeutic effects of dental stem cell evaluation on tooth regeneration, it is crucial to formulate legislation, industry standards, bio-insurance, quality control, checks and audits for dental stem cell banking development.

32.2.3.6 *In Cochlear Hair Cell Regrowth*

In the present scenario, differentiation of stem cell offers an immensely popular field to restore hearing ability, but so far only moderate results have been obtained using this therapeutic approach in patients (Hu and Ulfendahl, 2013; Géléoc and Holt, 2014; Mittal, Nguyen et al., 2017). Stem cells have the ability to restore and repair inner ear sensory structures and respective sensory ganglia. Moreover, therapeutic application of stem cells was also noticed for providing protection through direct integration into the scratched receptor or ganglion for subsequent replacement of neuronal cell types or sensory hairs (Mittal, Nguyen et al., 2017). Moreover, a series of experiments using sphere culture methods demonstrated that both neonatal cochlear and vestibular tissues comprise endogenous stem cells. Such cells have shown the ability to generate hair cell-like cells, but only vestibular tissue collected from adult animals possessed the potential to form hair cell-like cells in the respective cultures (Oshima, Grimm et al., 2007; Oshima, Senn et al., 2009).

Another study using murine ESCs in vitro culture showed their capability to induce a stepwise differentiation of both neurons and inner ear hair cells (Koehler, Mikosz et al., 2013). The differentiated hair cells from these ESCs exhibited functional characteristics of hair cells in the 3D cultures (Koehler, Mikosz et al., 2013). Additionally, these cells in 3D cultures also differentiated into specialized synaptic contacts with the sensory neurons (Koehler, Mikosz et al., 2013). Furthermore, stringent molecular pathway analysis of ESCs in 3D culture revealed that the modulation of Wnt signaling via potent Wnt agonist can enhance the process of differentiation of culture cells into inner ear sensory tissues (DeJonge, Liu et al., 2016).

An admirable resource for human MSCs for promising stem cell therapy to repair and restore inner ear sensory receptors and ganglia damage are stem cells collected from human umbilical cord: namely, Wharton's Jelly cells, also called human umbilical cord mesenchymal stromal cells (hUCMSCs) (Mellott, Detamore et al., 2016). One of the major advantages of using hUCMSCs is that they hold the ability to differentiate into multiple cell types evolving from all three embryonic germ layers (Mellott, Detamore et al., 2016). These hUCMSCs treated with Atoh 1 expression vector demonstrated differentiation into hair cell-like cells that expressed hair-cell-specific markers (Devarajan, Forrest et al., 2013), suggesting them as a promising candidate for the treatment of both hearing loss and balance disorders. Hence, stem cell application has been speculated for future medical applications for ex vivo expansion of patient-derived cells and re-transplant at the site of damage such as spiral ganglion.

32.2.3.7 In Disorders of Pancreatic Beta Cells

Diabetes mellitus, a chronic autoimmune disorder, is exemplified by its self-destruction ability. This disorder imitates the progressive destruction of β-cells in the pancreas, which results in altered glucose metabolism in the body via decreased secretion of insulin (Van Belle, Coppieters et al., 2011; Chhabra and Brayman, 2013). While no permanent treatment is available for this degenerative disorder applied treatment methods include to halt the autoimmune response of the body and other repairment of damaged pancreatic cells to recover the normal metabolic function (Eisenbarth, 1986; Sherry, Tsai et al., 2005; Tsai, Sherry et al., 2006). In this context, stem cell therapy has been demonstrated to repair and restore the function in several preclinical and clinical investigations for the treatment of diabetes mellitus (Reddi, Kothari et al., 2015). Also, various types of stem cells originated from different sources, such as ESCs, iPSCs, bone marrow-derived hematopoietic stem cell, adipose tissue-derived multipotent stem cell, and umbilical cord-generated stem cell (Harris, 2013), etc., were noted as ideal candidates to repair and replace damage tissue, prevent autoimmunity, and re-establish the β-cells to secrete insulin (Muir, Lima et al., 2014; Masoud, Qasim et al., 2017).

32.3 Challenges Facing Stem Cell Therapy

Along with such prospective therapeutic applications, there are some problems linked with stem cell therapy in the context of its safety and the accuracy. The primary hazard connected with stem cell replacement therapy is loss of differentiation ability into required cell type. Such faults result in tumor formation because of aggregation of the undifferentiated cell (Knoepfler, 2009). Another essential factor taken into consideration is the native immune response of the body. Hence, stem cell therapy has to be performed with high accuracy and precision to avoid immunological rejection of the transplanted cells or tissues or organs (Caplan, 2017). Since the human body, for the most part, treats stem cell as a foreign body and instigates a severe autoimmune reaction to kill it, application of immuno-suppression is suggested to be injected at the time of stem cell replacement therapy. Moreover, in vitro stem cell cultures may gain mutations, which tend to form stem cells of undesired traits. Such changes can also induce harmful effects such as cell cycle arrest, unwanted immune response, cancer, etc. (Närvä, Autio et al., 2010; Herberts, Kwa et al., 2011; Jilkine and Gutenkunst, 2014).

32.4 Conclusions

Modern medical science has gained advancements with highly refined, patient-friendly technologies and treatment approaches. Under the umbrella of modern medical science, even a cure for several lethal and chronic disorders is available for patients. For instance, it is possible to detect a disease precisely and treat it accordingly like never before.

In this sequence, stem cell therapy has evolved as a magical tool with an ability to cure a wide range of physiological conditions when medication is not effectively available or inconvenient. These cell lines have the ability to convert into any body tissue and regenerate or heal damaged tissues and organs of the body to their respective basic function. Thus, a large number of clinical studies are underway to advance stem cell therapy and overcome its limitations. If all the investigation results are positive as expected, in the future, stem cell therapy will bring in a new era of therapeutic applications in the medical industry.

REFERENCES

Adak, S., S. Mukherjee and D. Sen (2017). Mesenchymal stem cell as a potential therapeutic for inflammatory bowel disease-myth or reality? Current Stem Cell Research Therapy 12(8): 644–657.

Agrawal, M., A. Alexander, J. Khan, T. K. Giri, S. Siddique, S. K. Dubey, et al. (2019). Recent Biomedical Applications on Stem Cell Therapy: A Brief Overview. Curr Stem Cell Res Ther 14(2): 127–136.

Alateeq, S., P. R. J. Fortuna and E. Wolvetang (2015). Advances in reprogramming to pluripotency. Current Stem Cell Research Therapy 10(3): 193–207.

Bagno, L., K. E. Hatzistergos, W. Balkan and J. M. Hare (2018). Mesenchymal stem cell-based therapy for cardiovascular disease: progress and challenges. Mol Ther 26(7): 1610–1623.

Bang, O. Y. and E. H. Kim (2019). Mesenchymal stem cell-derived extracellular vesicle therapy for stroke: challenges and progress. Front Neurol 10: 211.

Benavides, O. M., A. R. Brooks, S. K. Cho, J. Petsche Connell, R. Ruano and J. G. Jacot (2015). In situ vascularization of injectable fibrin/poly (ethylene glycol) hydrogels by human amniotic fluid-derived stem cells. Journal of Biomedical Materials Research Part A 103(8): 2645–2653.

Bhat, M., P. Shetty, S. Shetty, F. A. Khan, S. Rahman and M. Ragher (2019). Stem cells and their application in dentistry: A review. J Pharm Bioallied Sci 11(Suppl 2): S82.

Borst, S., X. Sim, M. Poncz, D. L. French and P. Gadue (2017). Induced pluripotent stem cell-derived megakaryocytes and platelets for disease modeling and future clinical applications. Arteriosclerosis, Thrombosis, and Vascular Biology 37(11): 2007–2013.

Bruin, J. E., N. Saber, N. Braun, J. K. Fox, M. Mojibian, A. Asadi, et al. (2015). Treating diet-induced diabetes and obesity with human embryonic stem cell-derived pancreatic progenitor cells and antidiabetic drugs. Stem Cell Reports 4(4): 605–620.

Bulgin, D. (2015). Therapeutic angiogenesis in ischemic tissues by growth factors and bone marrow mononuclear cells administration: biological foundation and clinical prospects. Current Stem Cell Research Therapy 10(6): 509–522.

Burns, A. J. and N. Thapar (2014). Neural stem cell therapies for enteric nervous system disorders. Nature Reviews: Gastroenterology Hepatology 11(5): 317.

Calin, M., D. Stan and V. Simion (2013). Stem cell regenerative potential combined with nanotechnology and tissue engineering for myocardial regeneration. Current Stem Cell Research Therapy 8(4): 292–303.

Caplan, A. I. (2017). Mesenchymal stem cells: time to change the name! Stem Cells Translational Medicine 6(6): 1445–1451.

Chaudhury, H., E. Raborn, L. C. Goldie and K. K. Hirschi (2012). Stem cell-derived vascular endothelial cells and their potential application in regenerative medicine. Cells Tissues Organs 195(1–2): 41–47.

Chen, Z., C. Zeng and W. E. Wang (2017). Progress of stem cell transplantation for treating myocardial infarction. Current Stem Cell Research Therapy 12(8): 624–636.

Cheng, L., Y. Zhang, Y. Nan and L. Qiao (2015). Induced pluripotent stem cells (iPSCs) in the modeling of hepatitis C virus infection. Current Stem Cell Research Therapy 10(3): 216–219.

Chhabra, P. and K. L. Brayman (2013). Stem cell therapy to cure type 1 diabetes: from hype to hope. Stem Cells Translational Medicine 2(5): 328–336.

Chi, N. C. and J. S. Karliner (2004). Molecular determinants of responses to myocardial ischemia/reperfusion injury: focus on hypoxia-inducible and heat shock factors. Cardiovascular Research 61(3): 437–447.

Csaki, C., U. Matis, A. Mobasheri, H. Ye and M. Shakibaei (2007). Chondrogenesis, osteogenesis and adipogenesis of canine mesenchymal stem cells: a biochemical, morphological and ultrastructural study. Histochemistry Cell Biology 128(6): 507–520.

Dabrowska, S., A. Andrzejewska, B. Lukomska and M. Janowski (2019). Neuroinflammation as a target for treatment of stroke using mesenchymal stem cells and extracellular vesicles. J Neuroinflammation 16(1): 178.

Das, M., K. Mayilsamy, S. S. Mohapatra and S. Mohapatra (2019). Mesenchymal stem cell therapy for the treatment of traumatic brain injury: progress and prospects. Rev Neurosci 30(8): 839–855.

DeJonge, R. E., X-P. Liu, C. R. Deig, S. Heller, K. R. Koehler and E. Hashino (2016). Modulation of Wnt signaling enhances inner ear organoid development in 3D Culture: PloS One 11(9): e0162508.

Devarajan, K., M. L. Forrest, M. S. Detamore and H. Staecker (2013). Adenovector-mediated gene delivery to human umbilical cord mesenchymal stromal cells induces inner ear cell phenotype. Cellular Reprogramming 15(1): 43–54.

Dixit, P. and R. Katare (2015). Challenges in identifying the best source of stem cells for cardiac regeneration therapy. Stem Cell Res Ther 6(1): 26.

Doeppner, T. R., J. Herz, A. Görgens, J. Schlechter, A. K. Ludwig, S. Radtke, et al. (2015). Extracellular vesicles improve post-stroke neuroregeneration and prevent postischemic immunosuppression. Stem Cells Transl Med 4(10): 1131–1143.

Dominici, M., K. Le Blanc, I. Mueller, I. Slaper-Cortenbach, F. Marini, D. Krause, et al. (2006). Minimal criteria for defining multipotent mesenchymal stromal cells. The International Society for Cellular Therapy position statement. Cytotherapy 8(4): 315–317.

Draper, J. S. and V. Fox (2003). Human embryonic stem cells: multilineage differentiation and mechanisms of self-renewal. Archives of Medical Research 34(6): 558–564.

Effat, M. A. (1995). Pathophysiology of ischemic heart disease: an overview. AACN Advanced Critical Care 6(3): 369–374.

Eisenbarth, G. S. (1986). Type I diabetes mellitus. A chronic autoimmune disease. N Engl J Med 314(21): 1360–1368.

Ellis, K. M., D. C. O'Carroll, M. D. Lewis, G. Y. Rychkov and S. A. Koblar (2014). Neurogenic potential of dental pulp stem cells isolated from murine incisors. Stem Cell Research Therapy 5(1): 1–13.

Eun, S-C. (2014). Stem cell and research in plastic surgery. Journal of Korean Medical Science 29 (Suppl 3): S167–S169.

Evans, M. J. and M. H. Kaufman (1981). Establishment in culture of pluripotential cells from mouse embryos. Nature 292(5819): 154–156.

Feng, Q., N. Shabrani, J. N. Thon, H. Huo, A. Thiel, and K. R. Machlus (2014). Scalable generation of universal platelets from human induced pluripotent stem cells. Stem Cell Reports 3(5): 817–831.

Frangogiannis, N. G. (2015). Inflammation in cardiac injury, repair and regeneration. Current Opinion in Cardiology 30(3): 240.

Gaballa, S., N. Palmisiano, O. Alpdogan, M. Carabasi, J. Filicko-O'Hara, M. Kasner, et al. (2016). A two-step haploidentical versus a two-step matched related allogeneic myeloablative peripheral blood stem cell transplantation. Biology of Blood and Marrow Transplantation 22(1): 141–148.

Gage, F. H. (2000). Mammalian neural stem cells. Science 287(5457): 1433–1438.

Géléoc, G. S. and J. R. Holt (2014). Sound strategies for hearing restoration. Science 344(6184).

Gluckman, E., G. Koegler and V. Rocha (2005). Human leukocyte antigen matching in cord blood transplantation. Seminars In Hematology. Elsevier.

Golebiewska, E. M. and A. W. Poole (2015). Platelet secretion: From haemostasis to wound healing and beyond. Blood Reviews 29(3): 153–162.

Golpanian, S., D. L. DiFede, M. V. Pujol, M. H. Lowery, S. Levis-Dusseau, B. J. Goldstein, et al. (2016). Rationale and design of the allogeneic human mesenchymal stem cells (hMSC) in patients with aging frailty via intravenous delivery (CRATUS) study: A phase I/II, randomized, blinded and placebo controlled trial to evaluate the safety and potential efficacy of allogeneic human mesenchymal stem cell infusion in patients with aging frailty. Oncotarget 7(11): 11899–11912.

Golpanian, S., J. El-Khorazaty, A. Mendizabal, D. L. DiFede, V. Y. Suncion, V. Karantalis, et al. (2015). Effect of aging on human mesenchymal stem cell therapy in ischemic cardiomyopathy patients. J Am Coll Cardiol 65(2): 125–132.

Gowen, A., F. Shahjin, S. Chand, K. E. Odegaard and S. V. Yelamanchili (2020). Mesenchymal stem cell-derived extracellular vesicles: Challenges in clinical applications. Frontiers in Cell and Developmental Biology 8: 149.

Greggio, C., F. De Franceschi, M. Figueiredo-Larsen, S. Gobaa, A. Ranga, H. Semb, et al. (2013). Artificial three-dimensional niches deconstruct pancreas development in vitro. Development 140(21): 4452–4462.

Gschweng, E., S. De Oliveira and D. B. Kohn (2014). Hematopoietic stem cells for cancer immunotherapy. Immunological Reviews 257(1): 237–249.

Gubareva, E. A., S. Sjöqvist, I. V. Gilevich, A. S. Sotnichenko, E. V. Kuevda, M. L. Lim, et al. (2016). Orthotopic transplantation of a tissue engineered diaphragm in rats. Biomaterials 77: 320–335.

Hardikar, A. A., J. G. Lees, K. S. Sidhu, E. Colvin, and B. E. Tuch (2006). Stem-cell therapy for diabetes cure: how close are we? Current Stem Cell Research 1(3): 425–436.

Hare, J. M., D. L. DiFede, A. C. Rieger, V. Florea, A. M. Landin, J. El-Khorazaty, et al. (2017). Randomized comparison of allogeneic versus autologous mesenchymal stem cells for nonischemic dilated cardiomyopathy: POSEIDON-DCM trial. J Am Coll Cardiol 69(5): 526–537.

Hare, J. M., J. E. Fishman, G. Gerstenblith, D. L. DiFede Velazquez, J. P. Zambrano, V. Y. Suncion, et al. (2012). Comparison of allogeneic vs autologous bone marrow–derived mesenchymal stem cells delivered by transendocardial injection in patients with ischemic cardiomyopathy: the POSEIDON randomized trial. Jama 308(22): 2369–2379.

Hare, J. M., J. H. Traverse, T. D. Henry, N. Dib, R. K. Strumpf, S. P. Schulman, et al. (2009). A randomized, double-blind, placebo-controlled, dose-escalation study of intravenous adult human mesenchymal stem cells (prochymal) after acute myocardial infarction. J Am Coll Cardiol 54(24): 2277–2286.

He, Q., J. Li, E. Bettiol and M. E. Jaconi (2003). Embryonic stem cells: new possible therapy for degenerative diseases that affect elderly people. The Journals of Gerontology: Series A58(3): M279–M287.

Herberts, C. A., M. S. Kwa and H. P. Hermsen (2011). Risk factors in the development of stem cell therapy. Journal Of Translational Medicine 9(1): 29.

Hu, Z. and M. Ulfendahl (2013). The potential of stem cells for the restoration of auditory function in humans. Regenerative Medicine 8(3): 309–318.

Jenne, C. N. and P. Kubes (2015). Platelets in inflammation and infection. Platelets 26(4): 286–292.

Jilkine, A. and R. N. Gutenkunst (2014). Effect of dedifferentiation on time to mutation acquisition in stem cell-driven cancers. PLoS Comput Biol 10(3): e1003481.

Jyoti, S. and S. Tandon (2015). Chemical and physical factors influencing the dynamics of differentiation in embryonic stem cells. Curr Stem Cell Res Ther 10(6): 477–491.

Kalra, K. and P. C. Tomar (2014). Stem cell: basics, classification and applications. Am Jour of Phytomed & Clinical Therapeut 2(7): 919–930.

Kanapuru, B. and W. B. Ershler (2009). Inflammation, coagulation, and the pathway to frailty. Am J Med 122(7): 605–613.

Kessler, M., K. Hoffmann, V. Brinkmann, O. Thieck, S. Jackisch, B. Toelle, et al (2015). The Notch and Wnt pathways regulate stemness and differentiation in human fallopian tube organoids. Nature Communications 6(1): 1–11.

Kim, D. K., H. Nishida, S. Y. An, A. K. Shetty, T. J. Bartosh and D. J. Prockop (2016). Chromatographically isolated CD63+CD81+ extracellular vesicles from mesenchymal stromal cells rescue cognitive impairments after TBI. Proc Natl Acad Sci U S A 113(1): 170–175.

Kingham, E. and R. O. Oreffo (2013). Embryonic and induced pluripotent stem cells: understanding, creating, and exploiting the nano-niche for regenerative medicine. ACS Nano 7(3): 1867–1881.

Knoepfler, P. S. (2009). Deconstructing stem cell tumorigenicity: a roadmap to safe regenerative medicine. Stem Cells 27(5): 1050–1056.

Koehler, K. R., A. M. Mikosz, A. I. Molosh, D. Patel and E. Hashino (2013). Generation of inner ear sensory epithelia from pluripotent stem cells in 3D culture. Nature 500(7461): 217–221.

Korkusuz, P., S. Kose and C. Z. Kopru (2016). Biomaterial and Stem Cell Interactions: Histological Biocompatibility. Curr Stem Cell Res Ther 11(6): 475–486.

Krause, D. S., N. D. Theise, M. I. Collector, O. Henegariu, S. Hwang, R. Gardner, et al. (2001). Multi-organ, multi-lineage engraftment by a single bone marrow-derived stem cell. Cell 105(3): 369–377.

Krebsbach, P. H. and P. G. Robey (2002). Dental and skeletal stem cells: potential cellular therapeutics for craniofacial regeneration. J Dent Educ 66(6): 766–773.

Lee, M., J. J. Ban, S. Yang, W. Im and M. Kim (2018). The exosome of adipose-derived stem cells reduces β-amyloid pathology and apoptosis of neuronal cells derived from the transgenic mouse model of Alzheimer's disease. Brain Res 1691: 87–93.

Lee, M., T. Liu, W. Im and M. Kim (2016). Exosomes from adipose-derived stem cells ameliorate phenotype of Huntington's disease in vitro model. Eur J Neurosci 44(4): 2114–2119.

Leferink, A. M., Y.-C. Chng, C. A. van Blitterswijk and L. Moroni (2015). Distribution and viability of fetal and adult human bone marrow stromal cells in a biaxial rotating vessel bioreactor after seeding on polymeric 3D additive manufactured scaffolds. Frontiers in bioengineering biotechnology 3: 169.

Lemon, G., S. Sjoqvist, M. Ling Lim, N. Feliu, A. B. Firsova, R. Amin, et al. (2016). The use of mathematical modelling for improving the tissue engineering of organs and stem cell therapy. Current Stem Cell Research 11(8): 666–675.

Liu, S., Y. Qu, T. J. Stewart, M. J. Howard, S. Chakrabortty, T. F. Holekamp and J. W. McDonald (2000). Embryonic stem cells differentiate into oligodendrocytes and myelinate in culture and after spinal cord transplantation. Proc Natl Acad Sci USA 97(11): 6126–6131.

López-Otín, C., M. A. Blasco, L. Partridge, M. Serrano and G. Kroemer (2013). The hallmarks of aging. Cell 153(6): 1194–1217.

Lu, H., Y. Chen, Q. Lan, H. Liao, J. Wu, H. Xiao, et al. (2015). Factors that influence a mother's willingness to preserve umbilical cord blood: a survey of 5120 Chinese mothers. PLoS One 10(12): e0144001.

Lu, L.-L., Y.-J. Liu, S.-G. Yang, Q.-J. Zhao, X. Wang, W. Gong, et al. (2006). Isolation and characterization of human umbilical cord mesenchymal stem cells with hematopoiesis-supportive function and other potentials. Haematologica 91(8): 1017–1026.

Lukashyk, S. P., V. M. Tsyrkunov, Y. I. Isaykina, O. N. Romanova, A. T. Shymanskiy, O. V. Aleynikova and R. I. Kravchuk (2014). Mesenchymal bone marrow-derived stem cells transplantation in patients with HCV related liver cirrhosis. Journal Of Clinical and Translational Hepatology 2(4): 217.

Mahla, R. S. (2016). Stem Cells Applications in Regenerative Medicine and Disease Therapeutics. International Journal of Cell Biology 2016: 6940283.

Masoud, M. S., M. Qasim and M. U. Ali (2017). Translating the potential of stem cells for diabetes mellitus: challenges and opportunities. Current Stem Cell Research Therapy 12(8): 611–623.

Mead, B., M. Berry, A. Logan, R. A. Scott, W. Leadbeater and B. A. Scheven (2015). Stem cell treatment of degenerative eye disease. Stem Cell Research 14(3): 243–257.

Mehta, R. S., K. Rezvani, A. Olson, B. Oran, C. Hosing, N. Shah, et, al. (2015). Novel techniques for ex vivo expansion of cord blood: clinical trials. Frontiers in Medicine 2: 89.

Mellott, A. J., M. S. Detamore and H. Staecker (2016). The use of human Wharton's jelly cells for cochlear tissue engineering. Auditory and Vestibular Research. Springer. pp. 319–345.

Merianos, D., T. Heaton and A. W. Flake (2008). In utero hematopoietic stem cell transplantation: progress toward clinical application. Biol Blood Marrow Transplant 14(7): 729–740.

Mittal, R., D. Nguyen, A. P. Patel, L. H. Debs, J. Mittal, D. Yan, et al. (2017). Recent advancements in the regeneration of auditory hair cells and hearing restoration. Front Mol Neurosci 10(236).

Morelli, S., S. Salerno, H. Mohamed Magdy Ahmed, A. Piscioneri and L. De Bartolo (2016). Recent strategies combining biomaterials and stem cells for bone, liver and skin regeneration. Current Stem Cell Research Therapy 11(8): 676–691.

Mountford, J. (2008). Human embryonic stem cells: origins, characteristics and potential for regenerative therapy. Transfusion Medicine 18(1): 1–12.

Muir, K. R., M. J. Lima, H. M. Docherty and K. Docherty (2014). Cell therapy for type 1 diabetes. QJM: An International Journal of Medicine 107(4): 253–259.

Nagata, H., M. Ii, E. Kohbayashi, M. Hoshiga, T. Hanafusa and M. Asahi (2016). Cardiac adipose-derived stem cells exhibit high differentiation potential to cardiovascular cells in C57BL/6 mice. Stem Cells Translational Medicine 5(2): 141–151.

Nancarrow-Lei, R., P. Mafi, R. Mafi and W. Khan (2017). A systemic review of adult mesenchymal stem cell sources and their multilineage differentiation potential relevant to musculoskeletal tissue repair and regeneration. Current Stem Cell Research Therapy 12(8): 601–610.

Närvä, E., R. Autio, N. Rahkonen, L. Kong, N. Harrison, D. Kitsberg, et al. (2010). High-resolution DNA analysis of human embryonic stem cell lines reveals culture-induced copy number changes and loss of heterozygosity. Nature Biotechnology 28(4): 371–377.

Ni, H., S. Yang, F. Siaw-Debrah, J. Hu, K. Wu, Z. He, et al. (2019). Exosomes derived from bone mesenchymal stem cells ameliorate early inflammatory responses following traumatic brain injury. Front Neurosci 13: 14.

O'Donoghue, K. and N. M. Fisk (2004). Fetal stem cells. Best Practice Research Clinical Obstetrics Gynaecology 18(6): 853–875.

Ophelders, D. R., T. G. Wolfs, R. K. Jellema, A. Zwanenburg, P. Andriessen, T. Delhaas, et al. (2016). Mesenchymal stromal cell-derived extracellular vesicles protect the fetal brain after hypoxia-ischemia. Stem Cells Transl Med 5(6): 754–763.

Oshima, K., C. M. Grimm, C. E. Corrales, P. Senn, R. M. Monedero, G. S. Géléoc, et al. (2007). Differential distribution of stem cells in the auditory and vestibular organs of the inner ear. Journal of the Association for Research in Otolaryngology 8(1): 18–31.

Oshima, K., P. Senn and S. Heller (2009). Isolation of sphere-forming stem cells from the mouse inner ear. Auditory and Vestibular Research. Springer. pp. 141–162.

Ouyang, H., J. L. Goldberg, S. Chen, W. Li, G.-T. Xu, K. Zhang, et al. (2016). Ocular stem cell research from basic science to clinical application: a report from Zhongshan Ophthalmic Center Ocular Stem Cell Symposium. International Journal Of Molecular Sciences 17(3): 415.

Patel, S., P. T. Yin, H. Sugiyama and K.-B. Lee (2015). Inducing stem cell myogenesis using nanoscript. ACS Nano 9(7): 6909–6917.

Potdar, P. D. and Y. D. Jethmalani (2015). Human dental pulp stem cells: Applications in future regenerative medicine. World Journal Of Stem Cells 7(5): 839.

Preda, M. B. and G. Valen (2013). Evaluation of gene and cell-based therapies for cardiac regeneration. Current Stem Cell Research Therapy 8(4): 304–312.

Raggi, C. and A. C. Berardi (2012). Mesenchymal stem cells, aging and regenerative medicine. Muscles Ligaments Tendons J2(3): 239–242.

Rentas, S., N. T. Holzapfel, M. S. Belew, G. A. Pratt, V. Voisin, B. T. Wilhelm, et al. (2016). Musashi-2 attenuates AHR signalling to expand human haematopoietic stem cells. Nature 532(7600): 508–511.

Rosemann, A. (2014). Why regenerative stem cell medicine progresses slower than expected. Journal of Cellular Biochemistry 115(12): 2073–2076.

Rosner, M., K. Schipany and M. Hengstschläger (2014). The decision on the "optimal" human pluripotent stem cell. Stem Cells Translational Medicine 3(5): 553–559.

S Reddi, A., N. Kothari, K. Kuppasani and N. Ende (2015). Human umbilical cord blood cells and diabetes mellitus: recent advances. Current Stem Cell Research Therapy 10(3): 266-270.

Salguero-Aranda, C., R. Tapia-Limonchi, G. M. Cahuana, A. B. Hitos, I. Diaz, A. Hmadcha, et al. (2016). Differentiation of mouse embryonic stem cells toward functional pancreatic β-cell surrogates through epigenetic regulation of Pdx1 by nitric oxide. Cell Transplantation 25(10): 1879–1892.

Schulman, I. H., W. Balkan and J. M. Hare (2018). Mesenchymal stem cell therapy for aging frailty. Frontiers in Nutrition 5: 108–108.

Semple, J. W., J. E. Italiano and J. Freedman (2011). Platelets and the immune continuum. Nature Reviews Immunology 11(4): 264–274.

Shahrokhi, S., F. Menaa, K. Alimoghaddam, C. McGuckin and M. Ebtekar (2012). Insights and hopes in umbilical cord blood stem cell transplantations. Journal of Biomedicine Biotechnology 2012.

Sharpe, P. T. (2016). Dental mesenchymal stem cells. Development 143(13): 2273–2280.

Sherry, N. A., E. B. Tsai and K. C. Herold (2005). Natural history of β-cell function in type 1 diabetes. Diabetes 54(suppl 2): S32–S39.

Shroff, G. and R. Gupta (2015). Human embryonic stem cells in the treatment of patients with spinal cord injury. Annals of Neurosciences 22(4): 208.

Shuai, Y., Y. Ma, T. Guo, L. Zhang, R. Yang, M. Qi, et al. (2018). Dental stem cells and tooth regeneration. Adv Exp Med Biol 1107: 41–52.

Simon, L., G. C. Ekman, N. Kostereva, Z. Zhang, R. A. Hess, M. C. Hofmann and P. S. Cooke (2009). Direct transdifferentiation of stem/progenitor spermatogonia into reproductive and nonreproductive tissues of all germ layers. Stem Cells 27(7): 1666–1675.

Smith, A. G. (2001). Embryo-derived stem cells: of mice and men. Annual Review Of Cell Developmental Biology 17(1): 435–462.

Squillaro, T., G. Peluso and U. Galderisi (2016). Clinical trials with mesenchymal stem cells: an update. Cell Transplantation 25(5): 829–848.

Sun, C., G. S Wilson, J.-G. Fan and L. Qiao (2015). Potential applications of induced pluripotent stem cells (iPSCs) in hepatology research. Current Stem Cell Research Therapy 10(3): 208–215.

T Harris, D. (2013). Umbilical cord tissue mesenchymal stem cells: characterization and clinical applications. Current Stem Cell Research Therapy 8(5): 394–399.

Takahashi, K., K. Tanabe, M. Ohnuki, M. Narita, T. Ichisaka, K. Tomoda and S. Yamanaka (2007). Induction of pluripotent stem cells from adult human fibroblasts by defined factors. Cell 131(5): 861–872.

Thomi, G., D. Surbek, V. Haesler, M. Joerger-Messerli and A. Schoeberlein (2019). Exosomes derived from umbilical cord mesenchymal stem cells reduce microglia-mediated neuroinflammation in perinatal brain injury. Stem Cell Res Ther 10(1): 105.

Thompson, P. A., T. Perera, D. Marin, B. Oran, U. Popat, M. Qazilbash, et al. (2016). Double umbilical cord blood transplant is effective therapy for relapsed or refractory Hodgkin lymphoma. Leukemia & Lymphoma 57(7): 1607–1615.

Thomson, J. A., J. Itskovitz-Eldor, S. S. Shapiro, M. A. Waknitz, J. J. Swiergiel, V. S. Marshall and J. M. Jones (1998). Embryonic stem cell lines derived from human blastocysts. Science 282(5391): 1145–1147.

Thon, J. N., B. J. Dykstra and L. M. Beaulieu (2017). Platelet bioreactor: accelerated evolution of design and manufacture. Platelets 28(5): 472–477.

Tran, C. and M. S. Damaser (2015). Stem cells as drug delivery methods: application of stem cell secretome for regeneration. Advanced Drug Delivery Reviews 82: 1–11.

Travlos, G. S. (2006). Normal structure, function, and histology of the bone marrow. Toxicologic Pathology 34(5): 548–565.

Tsai, E. B., N. A. Sherry, J. P. Palmer and K. C. Herold (2006). The rise and fall of insulin secretion in type 1 diabetes mellitus. Diabetologia 49(2): 261–270.

Van Belle, T. L., K. T. Coppieters and M. G. Von Herrath (2011). Type 1 diabetes: etiology, immunology, and therapeutic strategies. Physiological Reviews 91(1): 79–118.

Vedantham, V. (2015). New approaches to biological pacemakers: links to sinoatrial node development. Trends in Molecular Medicine 21(12): 749–761.

Volarevic, V., J. Nurkovic, N. Arsenijevic and M. Stojkovic (2014). Concise review: therapeutic potential of mesenchymal stem cells for the treatment of acute liver failure and cirrhosis. Stem Cells 32(11): 2818–2823.

Walsh, T. G., P. Metharom and M. C. Berndt (2015). The functional role of platelets in the regulation of angiogenesis. Platelets 26(3): 199–211.

Ware, J., A. Corken and R. Khetpal (2013). Platelet function beyond hemostasis and thrombosis. Current Opinion In Hematology 20(5).

Whitaker, B., S. Rajbhandary, S. Kleinman, A. Harris and N. Kamani (2016). Trends in United States blood collection and transfusion: results from the 2013 AABB blood collection, utilization, and patient blood management survey. Transfusion 56(9): 2173–2183.

Wichterle, H., I. Lieberam, J. A. Porter and T. M. Jessell (2002). Directed differentiation of embryonic stem cells into motor neurons. Cell 110(3): 385–397.

Williams, R. L., D. J. Hilton, S. Pease, T. A. Willson, C. L. Stewart, D. P. Gearing, et al. (1988). Myeloid leukaemia inhibitory factor maintains the developmental potential of embryonic stem cells. Nature 336(6200): 684–687.

Ye, L., M. A. Robertson, T. L. Mastracci and R. M. Anderson (2016). An insulin signaling feedback loop regulates pancreas progenitor cell differentiation during islet development and regeneration. Developmental Biology 409(2): 354–369.

Zhang, J., J. Guan, X. Niu, G. Hu, S. Guo, Q. Li, Z., et. al. (2015). Exosomes released from human induced pluripotent stem cells-derived MSCs facilitate cutaneous wound healing by promoting collagen synthesis and angiogenesis. J Transl Med 13: 49.

Zhang, Z., B. Huang, F. Gao and R. Zhang (2015). Impact of immune response on the use of iPSCs in disease modeling. Current Stem Cell Research Therapy 10(3): 236–244.

Zhou, C., B. E Grottkau and S. Zou (2016). Regulators of stem cells proliferation in tissue regeneration. Current Stem Cell Research 11(3): 177–187.

33

Bioinformatics Review in miRNA System Biology and Drug Discovery

Ankita Sethia
Bioinformatics Infrastructure Facility Centre of DBT (Govt. of India), India

Swati Srivastava
Department of Bioscience, Integral University, Lucknow, India

Vijay Laxmi Saxena
Sir Asutosh Mookerjee Fellow, Indian Science Congress Association, Kolkata, India
Bioinformatics Infrastructure Facility Centre of DBT (Govt. of India), India
Department of Zoology DG (PG) College, Kanpur, India

33.1 Introduction

In recent years, the bioinformatics field has rapidly developed into an essential aid for genomic data analysis and powerful bioinformatics tools have been developed, many of them publicly available through the web. High-throughput data such as genomic, proteomic, epigenetic, transcriptomic, and genome architecture data have all made significant contributions to mechanism-based drug discovery. Molecular modelling, structure-based drug design, structure-based virtual screening, ligand-based modelling, and molecular dynamics methods are used as powerful tools to understand pharmacokinetic and pharmacodynamics properties and structural activity relationships of ligands with targets. miRNAs are small non-coding RNAs with an average 22 nucleotides in length. Most miRNAs are transcribed from DNA sequences into primary miRNAs (pri-miRNAs) and processed into precursor miRNAs (pre-miRNAs) and mature miRNAs. In most cases, miRNAs interact with the 3′ UTR of target mRNAs to suppress expression. miRNA play essential roles in several biological and pathological mechanisms in the human system (Paul et. al., 2020). miRNAs derive from longer transcripts and encode in plants, animals, and virus genomes. miRNAs regulate gene expression of post-transcription and regulate the expression of target genes depending on the binding capacity of their transcripts. According to recent reports, occurrence of miRNA is also found in a single-celled eukaryotes (Saxena et. al., 2016). According to recent research in system biology, network biology has become a powerful tool to research complex biological activity (Zheng et. al., 2018). System biology is a combination of versatile knowledge and has caused the advent of big-data biology and network biology. System biology also facilitates system-level understanding of cellular components. (Altaf-Ul-Amin et. al., 2014). In this chapter, we summarize and describe the basic bioinformatics tools for genomic research, drug design, and tools for ab initio gene prediction, recent advancements of miRNAs, and system biology deciphering the regulatory mechanisms and also discussing tools involved in system biology.

DOI: 10.1201/9781003220404-37

33.2 miRNA

miRNAs belong to a major class of small noncoding RNAs with a single strand of 18–25 nucleotide interference of transcriptional, translational, or epigenetics process and are also involved in regulation of multiple target genes at the post-transcriptional level (Chen et al., 2019; Walayat et al., 2018). miRNA is an evolutionarily ancient component of gene regulation, which is well conserved in both plants and animals. Usually, miRNA derives from RNA transcript regions in short hairpin formations, whereas siRNAs are derived from longer regions of double-standard RNA (Srivastava et. al., 2018). According to a study, more than one third of human genes are regulated by miRNAs, and are involved in various cellular processes such as differentiation, cell purification, apoptosis, and immunological response (Paul et al., 2020). Currently, 38,589 miRNAs are available in which 2,675 human mature miRNAs have been annotated in the miRBase miRNA database (Release 22.1, March 22, 2018). miRNA plays significant roles in various regulatory mechanisms during developmental timing and host-pathogen interactions as well as cell differentiation, proliferation, apoptosis, and tumorigenesis in organisms (Cai et al., 2009). miRNAs are intergenic components of gene regulation, and are either produced by introns or produced from own genes; they are also involved in regulation of gene expression through recognition of cognate sequences.

33.3 Target Prediction in miRNAs

For the study of miRNA, miRNA target prediction is probably the most important part of the computational way to predict miRNA function. Target prediction tools are based on seed matching, which is combined with thermodynamic stability through requirement of co-expression with target genes. According to an observational study, potential miRNA predicted the different types of target sites in human gene and these target sites of the genes contain different conserved regions or conserved information. miRNA play a vital role as a biomarker for the diagnosis of several diseases. For miRNA structure analysis, target prediction, and discovery of new miRNA predication there are various computational tools available. These target sites of miRNA are predicted with the help of the DIANA web server, which predicts all different types of target sites of miRNA (Chen et al., 2019; Srivastava et al., 2018).

33.4 miRNA Biogenesis and Function

A functional study of miRNA revealed the importance of miRNAs in various biological functions such as cell development timings, embryogenesis, metabolism, cell differentiation, and apoptosis (Saliminejad et al., 2019). miRNAs are involved in various developmental cell processes and pathways such as metabolism, apoptosis, cell proliferation, and in diseases including cancer (Saxena V. L. et al., 2018).

In canonical pathway of miRNA biogenesis, there are genetic alterations involved. Synthesis of miRNA initiates in the nucleus and completes in the cytosol. In the nucleus, DROSHA cleaves Pri-miRNA into pre-miRNAs, and this cleavage is substituted with splicing. In the cytoplasm, dicer cleaves two pre-miRNAs into small double-standard RNAs. Then, RISC complex mediates the recognition of the targeted mRNA. Through the spliceosome machinery Pri-miRNAs are processed to pre-miRNAs and enzymes to generate double-standard loop structures. This continues with the canonical pathway, and the RNA product of splicing adopts a pre-miRNA-like form, and transforms to cytoplasm by Exportin5.

33.5 Tools for miRNA Biogenesis and Functional Analysis

miRNA identification tools are also important. Various tools have been designed for this purpose. MiRscan is a user-friendly tool for identification of conserved miRNAs. miRNAFold is an ab initio method for miRNA prediction at a large scale in the genome. There are several other tools available that identify miRNAs based on next-generation sequencing (NGS) data. GenMAPP (Paraskevopoulou et al., 2013) is used for predicting miRNA target via paired mRNA/miRNA expression data. More ways continually become available to study miRNA as the technology develops with the help of bioinformatics tools.

33.6 System Biology

The origins of modern system biology emerged in the middle of the last century. The major feature of system biology is the use of mathematical and computational models, which are essential for analysis of inherent complexity of biological systems. From the diversity of components, the complexity arises with the high selectivity of their interactions and also non-linear nature of these interactions. System biology considers the interaction results of multiple biological molecules with each other; not just the results of a single gene or protein. System biology can help us explore the underlying mechanisms of biological processes and understand the process of biological function (Zheng et al., 2018). The main purpose of this field is to understand organisms or function of cells on various levels in cellular mechanism. System biology faces new challenges of analyzing big data due to availability of a large amount of molecular data and various huge biological networks (Altaf-Ul-Amin et al., 2014).

33.7 Tools Used for Network Analysis in System Biology

The rapidly increasing number of publications provide evidence of the gaining momentum in system biology. Bioinformatics provide various tools to handle increasingly large amounts of biological data, increasingly merging and contributing to systems approaches. The main bioinformatics tools for system biology research are visualization tools of structures of networks such as Cystoscope (Shannon et al., 2003) and Pathway Tool Omics Viewer. Another highly useful tool in system biology is Cell Designer (Funahashi et al., 2007), a Java-based program for constructing and editing of a biochemical network. In Cell Designer, models can connect to external simulators or alternatively be simulated with a built-in simulator. Systems Biology Markup Language (SBML) is a well-defined format that different software tools can use for the exchange of biological models (Likić et al., 2010). For analyzing these computational network results in disease in both human and animals, we used MCODE (Busk et al., 2014) and Cluster Viz (Wang et al., 2014) to understand the mechanism of Alexander disease. These tools feature various clustering algorithms, user-friendly topology, and intuitive visualization of clustering results (Saxena et al., 2016).

33.8 Pathway and Network Analysis

Network biology provides powerful tools for the study of complex diseases. The network-based pathway analysis method is used in a constructed network for analysis of disease-related pathways. There are two ways to construct pathways: protein-protein interaction (PPI) network information and gene expression profile data and integrated genes GO information into pathway to calculate the correlation between the pathways (Zheng et al., 2018). According to reports, over 80% of proteins do not operate alone but in complexes. Protein-protein and miRNA-mRNA interactions are regulated by several mechanisms as well as larger cellular networks of the human body. These large cellular networks are built up by highly connected protein nodes, which receive inputs and generate one or more specific outputs in the form of computational units. A dysregulated miRNA target network can be constructed with significant deregulated scores of miRNA-mRNA pairs, which predict cancer risk miRNAs from the dysregulated target network (Cai et al., 2009). The study of a miRNA and protein co-expression network is necessary for prediction of linkage association between protein and diseases, which exploit the source of information and define the physical interaction networks and linkage intervals through a class of computational approaches. There are new research challenges raised in system biology due to big data, not only size but also complexity. Big-data science is mainly supported by advances in high-throughput experimental technologies (Altaf-Ul-Amin et al., 2014).

33.9 Drug Design

Computational approaches play a tremendous role in drug discovery and are also useful for drug design. There are mainly two types of computational-aided drug discovery: structure-based drug design and ligand-based drug design. Structure-based drug design (SBDD) is based on the analysis of three-dimensional structure information of macromolecules such proteins or RNA to identify key sites and interactions that are important for their respective biological functions. This information can be useful for drug design and can compete with essential interactions involving the target and thus interrupt the biological pathways essential for survival of the microorganism(s). Ligand-based drug design (LBDD) strategies center around known anti-toxin ligands for an objective to build up a connection between their physiochemical properties and anti-microbial exercises, alluded to as a construction movement relationship (SAR), data that can be utilized for enhancement of known medications or guide the plan of new medications with improved action (Funahashi et. al., 2007).

33.10 Structure-Based Drug Design

SBDD plays a vital role in drug discovery; it is a multi-field, irritative process that is well established in the Academic Foundation and drug industry. There are several registered drugs in the market such as zamamivir, nelfinavir, and aleglitazar that were designed with the help of SBDD. Conversely, structure-based planning is generally new in the agrochemical business and as of now no items on the market were

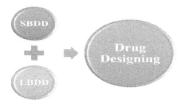

FIGURE 33.1   Types of computer-aided drug design.

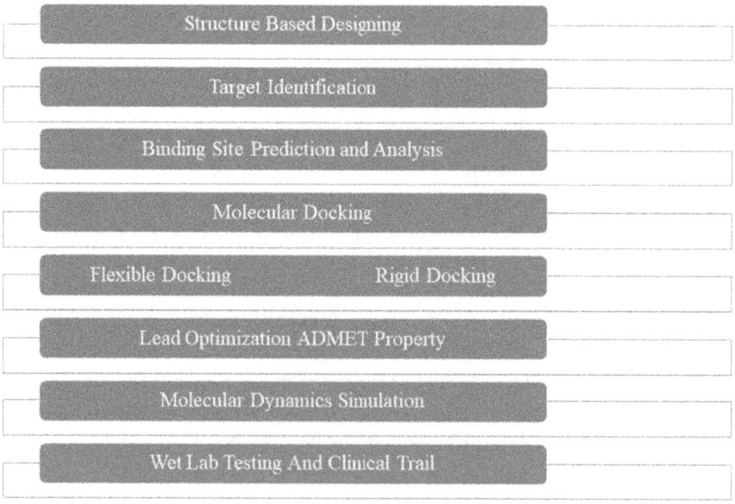

Structure Based Designing

Target Identification

Binding Site Prediction and Analysis

Molecular Docking

Flexible Docking   Rigid Docking

Lead Optimization ADMET Property

Molecular Dynamics Simulation

Wet Lab Testing And Clinical Trail

FIGURE 33.2   Systematic flow chart of structure-based drug discovery.

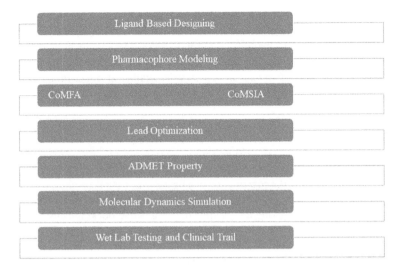

FIGURE 33.3 Systematic flow chart of ligand-based drug discovery.

TABLE 33.2

Chemical Compound Databases

S. no.	Database	Description	Availability
1.	DrugBank	DrugBank is a database that contains information regarding drugs and their compounds.	www.drugbank.com
2.	ChemSpider	ChemSpider is a chemical structure database	www.chemspider.com
3.	ChEMBL	ChEMBL is a database that contains small molecule information relating to ADMET	www.ebi.ac.uk
4.	PubChem	PubChem is a database that contains information regarding small chemical molecules and their biological activities.	www.nih.gov
5.	ZINC	ZINC database contains information that is commercially available regarding compounds for molecular docking and virtual screening.	www.docking.org

straightforwardly examined with this methodology. However, there are several databases used for drug discovery, which are listed in Table 33.2.

33.11 Target Identification

The first step of drug discovery is identification and validation of the drug target. The majority of drug targets are found in the organism, i.e., protein (enzyme), nucleic (DNA & RNA), carbohydrates, and lipid. These macromolecules are tremendous drug targets in human disease. Most medications accessible on the market are routed to proteins. However, nucleic acids could acquire large significance as a drug target for future drug discovery due to the disentangling of a few genomes of microorganisms (Gashaw et al., 2012).

33.12 Binding Site Prediction

Binding sites are the regions of proteins where drugs can bind and finding these regions is a crucial step in the design of new drugs. Binding site prediction of the receptor molecule is not an easy task;

researchers have proposed various selection criteria for binding sites. Research is being conducted into whether the highly conserved cluster of amino acid residues found in the binding site pocket controls the functional activity of any protein. The majority of currently accessible techniques are based on molecular surface similarity searches for functional site databases such as PDB, which offer information on protein structures that have been thoroughly examined and experimentally validated. In addition, a number of other models, including HMM, SVM, and CASP9, are used to build some of the methods (Pathak et al., 2021).

33.13 Molecular Docking

Docking means to unequivocally fit the construction of a ligand inside the necessities of a receptor binding site and to precisely assess the strength of the binding (Adrian-Scotto and Vasilescu, 2008). There are two main types of docking: rigid docking and flexible docking. Rigid docking is used when the internal geometry of both ligand and receptor is fixed (de Ruyck et. al., 2016). In the case of flexible docking, the ligand and receptor molecule are both flexible to each other. For induced fit docking, the primary chain is additionally moved to incorporate the conformational changes of the receptor upon ligand restricting (Yuriev and Ramsland, 2013; Rana et al., 2019; Dwivedi and Saxena, 2013; Arya et al., 2019). A summary of the molecular docking programs used in drug design is given in Table 33.3.

33.14 A Case Study: Computational Repositioning of Ethno Medicine-Elucidated Anti-Harper Drug Target E6

The human papillomavirus family includes more than 100 viruses, and 40% of them are easily transmitted through sexual contact, from the mucus and skin membrane of diseased individuals. Specifically, HPV's E6 protein functions as an oncoprotein by manipulating the numerous essential regulatory proteins in the host cell. The main objective of this research was to investigate natural inhibitors against the E6 protein. 28 inhibitors were found through literature and chosen for research. A molecular description was examined and Lipinski's rule of five was used to choose just drug likeness ligands, leaving 12 inhibitors. Molecular docking was done using AutoDock Vina. Curcumin's docking score is -7.7 binding energy (Kcal/mol) and the amino acids involved in the hydrogen bonding between receptor-ligand complex are GLY 795, VAL 794, and SER 739. Diospyrin's docking score is -7.6 binding energy (Kcal/

TABLE 33.3

Types of Docking Software

S. No	Programs	Description	Availability
1	Molecular operating environment (MOE)	It is used for molecular modeling and computer-aided drug discovery	Chemical Computing Group (CCG) | Computer-Aided Molecular Design (chemcomp.com)
2	Hex	Docking studies	Hex Protein Docking (loria.fr)
3	Glide Schrodinger	Molecular modelling and computer-aided drug discovery (CADD)	Schrödinger | The scientific innovator behind the creation of cutting-edge chemical simulation software for use in the study of pharmaceuticals, materials and biotechnology.
4	AutoDock Vina	Virtual screening and molecular docking	AutoDock Vina – molecular docking and virtual screening program (scripps.edu)
5	Discovery Studio	This software uses protein modeling, molecular docking, and molecular dynamics and simulation	www.3ds.com/products-services/biovia/products/molecular-modeling-simulation/biovia-discovery-studio/

TABLE 33.4

Docking Score for E6 Protein of HPV Against Natural Compound

S. No	Ligand	Binding energy (Kcal/mol)	Interacted Residues	Distances A0
1	Curcumin	-7.7	GLY 795, VAL 794, SER 739	3.001 3.0
2	Diospyrin	-7.6	LEU 734, ASN 741, GLY 795, VAL 794, SER 739, ARG 740.	3.75 3.55
3	Daphnoretin	-7.5	ARG 728, GLY 795, SER 739, LEU 734, VAL 794.	3.05 2.72
4	6-methoxygossypol	-7.5	VAL 794, SER 739, ALA 792, GLY 795	3.04 3.24

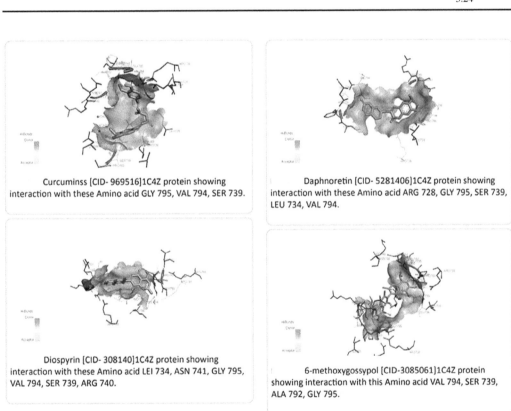

Curcuminss [CID- 969516]1C4Z protein showing interaction with these Amino acid GLY 795, VAL 794, SER 739.

Daphnoretin [CID- 5281406]1C4Z protein showing interaction with these Amino acid ARG 728, GLY 795, SER 739, LEU 734, VAL 794.

Diospyrin [CID- 308140]1C4Z protein showing interaction with these Amino acid LEI 734, ASN 741, GLY 795, VAL 794, SER 739, ARG 740.

6-methoxygossypol [CID-3085061]1C4Z protein showing interaction with this Amino acid VAL 794, SER 739, ALA 792, GLY 795.

FIGURE 33.4 Molecular interaction between receptor and ligand complex.

mol) and the amino acids involved in the hydrogen bonding between receptor-ligand complex are LEU 734, ASN 741, GLY 795, VAL 794, SER 739, and ARG 740. Daphnoreti's docking score is -7.5 binding energy (Kcal/mol) and the amino acids involved in the hydrogen bonding between receptor-ligand complex are ARG 728, GLY 795, SER 739, LEU 734, and VAL 794. 6-methoxygossypol's docking score is -7.5 binding energy (Kcal/mol) and the amino acids involved in the hydrogen bonding between receptor-ligand complex are VAL 794, SER 739, ALA 792, and GLY 795. Table 33.3 and Figures 33.1–33.4 shows the docking score of E6 protein of HPV against natural compound and their amino acids involved in protein-ligand complex. Dihydroisocoumarin and curcumin attach most strongly to the target protein. Consequently, the results of the current investigation could lead to a new drug compound (Saxena V. L. et al., 2018).

33.15 Conclusion

In this chapter we discussed computational approaches at the genomics and proteomics levels. miRNA is a non-condoning RNA and is used for full gene silencing. In silco approaches follow several steps of miRNA prediction. System biology approaches are very helpful for understanding biological network biology and how to interact one molecule with another molecule in a biological system. Computational drug discovery is a low-cost and less time-consuming process and is helpful in drug development.

Acknowledgments

This work was supported by the Indian Science Congress Association, Kolkata, India and Department of Biotechnology, Ministry of Science and Technology, Govt. of India.

REFERENCES

Adrian-Scotto M., Vasilescu D. 2008. Quantum molecular modeling of glycyl-adenylate. *J Biomol Struct Dyn* 25(6):697–708

Agarwal, V., Bell, G. W., Nam, J. W., & Bartel, D. P. 2015. Predicting effective microRNA target sites in mammalian mRNAs. *Elife*, *4*, e05005.

Altaf-Ul-Amin, M., Afendi, F. M., Kiboi, S. K., & Kanaya, S. 2014. Systems biology in the context of big data and networks. *BioMed Research International*, 2014.

An, J., Lai, J., Lehman, M. L., & Nelson, C. C. 2013. miRDeep*: an integrated application tool for miRNA identification from RNA sequencing data. *Nucleic Acids Research*, *41*(2), 727–737.

Arya K., Gupta R., Verma H., Pal G. K., Saxena V. L. 2019. Drug designing to combat MDR bacteria using potential bioactive compounds from medicinal plant. *Trends Bioinform* 12: 7–19.

Busk, P. K. 2014. A tool for design of primers for microRNA-specific quantitative RT-qPCR. *BMC Bioinformatics*, *15*(1), 1-9.

Cai, Y., Yu, X., Hu, S., & Yu, J. 2009. A brief review on the mechanisms of miRNA regulation. *Genomics, Proteomics & Bioinformatics*, *7*(4), 147–154.

Chen, L., Heikkinen, L., Wang, C., Yang, Y., Sun, H., & Wong, G. 2019. Trends in the development of miRNA bioinformatics tools. *Briefings in Bioinformatics*, *20*(5), 1836–1852.

Cho, S., Jang, I., Jun, Y., Yoon, S., Ko, M., Kwon, Y., & Lee, S. 2012. MiRGator v3. 0: a microRNA portal for deep sequencing, expression profiling and mRNA targeting. *Nucleic Acids Research*, *41*(D1), D252–D257.

de Ruyck J., Brysbaert G., Blossey R., Lensink M. F. 2016. Molecular docking as a popular tool in drug design, an in silico travel. *Adv Appl Bioinforma Chem* 9:1–11

Du, X., Li, Q., Cao, Q., Wang, S., Liu, H., & Li, Q. 2019. Integrated analysis of miRNA-mRNA interaction network in porcine granulosa cells undergoing oxidative stress. *Oxidative Medicine and Cellular Longevity*, 2019.

Dwivedi A., Saxena, V. L. 2013. In silico drug designing of protease inhibitors to find the potential drug candidate for HIV1. *Computational Biology and Bioinformatics* 1(3): 10–14. doi: 10.11648/j.cbb.20130103.11

Funahashi, A., Tanimura, N., Morohashi, M., & Kitano, H. 2007. Cell Designer. *Systems Biology Institute* www.systems-biology.org/002.

Gashaw I., Ellinghaus P., Sommer A., Asadullah K. 2012. What makes a good drug target? *Drug Discov Today* 17(Suppl): S24–S30

Hackenberg, M., Rodríguez-Ezpeleta, N., & Aransay, A. M. 2011. miRanalyzer: an update on the detection and analysis of microRNAs in high-throughput sequencing experiments. *Nucleic Acids Research*, *39*(suppl_2), W132–W138.

Hsu, S. D., Chu, C. H., Tsou, A. P., Chen, S. J., Chen, H. C., Hsu, P. W. C., & Huang, H. D. 2007. miRNAMap 2.0: genomic maps of microRNAs in metazoan genomes. *Nucleic Acids Research*, *36*(suppl_1), D165–D169.

Huang H. J., Yu H. W., Chen C. Y., Hsu C. H., Chen H. Y., Lee K. J., et al. 2010 Current developments of computer-aided drug design. *J Taiwan Inst Chem Eng* 41(6):623–635

Huang, T. H., Fan, B., Rothschild, M. F., Hu, Z. L., Li, K., & Zhao, S. H. 2007. MiRFinder: an improved approach and software implementation for genome-wide fast microRNA precursor scans. *BMC Bioinformatics*, 8(1), 1–10.

Jiang, Q., Wang, Y., Hao, Y., Juan, L., Teng, M., Zhang, X., & Liu, Y. 2009. miR2Disease: a manually curated database for microRNA deregulation in human disease. *Nucleic Acids Research*, 37(suppl_1), D98–D104.

Kalvari, I., Nawrocki, E. P., Ontiveros-Palacios, N., Argasinska, J., Lamkiewicz, K., Marz, M., & Petrov, A. I. 2021. Rfam 14: expanded coverage of metagenomic, viral and microRNA families. *Nucleic Acids Research*, 49(D1), D192–D200.

Karagkouni, D., Paraskevopoulou, M. D., Chatzopoulos, S., Vlachos, I. S., Tastsoglou, S., Kanellos, I., & Hatzigeorgiou, A. G. 2018. DIANA-TarBase v8: a decade-long collection of experimentally supported miRNA–gene interactions. *Nucleic Acids Research*, 46(D1), D239–D245.

Kozomara, A., Birgaoanu, M., & Griffiths-Jones, S. 2019. miRBase: from microRNA sequences to function. *Nucleic Acids Research*, 47(D1), D155-D162.

Li, J. H., Liu, S., Zhou, H., Qu, L. H., & Yang, J. H. 2014. StarBase v2. 0: decoding miRNA-ceRNA, miRNA-ncRNA and protein–RNA interaction networks from large-scale CLIP-Seq data. *Nucleic Acids Research*, 42(D1), D92–D97.

Likić, V. A., McConville, M. J., Lithgow, T., & Bacic, A. 2010. Systems biology: the next frontier for bioinformatics. *Advances in Bioinformatics*, 2010.

Lorenz, R., Bernhart, S. H., Zu Siederdissen, C. H., Tafer, H., Flamm, C., Stadler, P. F., & Hofacker, I. L. 2011. ViennaRNA Package 2.0. *Algorithms for Molecular Biology*, 6(1), 1–14.

Paraskevopoulou, M. D., Georgakilas, G., Kostoulas, N., Vlachos, I. S., Vergoulis, T., Reczko, M., & Hatzigeorgiou, A. G. 2013. DIANA-microT web server v5. 0: service integration into miRNA functional analysis workflows. *Nucleic Acids Research*, 41(W1), W169–W173.

Pathak, R. K., et al. 2021. *Computer-Aided Drug Design*. Springer: Singapore, 2020.

Paul, S., Bravo Vázquez, L. A., Pérez Uribe, S., Roxana Reyes-Pérez, P., & Sharma, A. 2020. Current status of microRNA-based therapeutic approaches in neurodegenerative disorders. *Cells*, 9(7), 1698.

Peng, Y. & Croce, C. M. 2016. The role of MicroRNAs in human cancer. *Signal Transduction and Targeted Therapy*, 1(1), 1–9.

Rana G., Pathak R. K., Shukla R., Baunthiyal M. 2019. In silico identification of mimicking molecule (s) triggering von Willebrand factor in human: a molecular drug target for regulating coagulation pathway. *J Biomol Struct Dyn* 38:124–136

Saliminejad, K., Khorram Khorshid, H. R., Soleymani Fard, S., & Ghaffari, S. H. 2019. An overview of microRNAs: biology, functions, therapeutics, and analysis methods. *Journal of Cellular Physiology*, 234(5), 5451–5465.

Salomonis, N., Hanspers, K., Zambon, A. C., Vranizan, K., Lawlor, S. C., Dahlquist, K. D., & Pico, A. R. 2007. GenMAPP 2: new features and resources for pathway analysis. *BMC Bioinformatics*, 8(1), 1–12.

Saxena, A. K., Saxena, V. L., & Dixit, S. 2016. Mapping of protein-protein interaction network of Alexander disease. *Cellular and Molecular Biology*, 62(6), 17–21.

Saxena, V. L., Chaturvedi, P., & Fatima, K. 2018. Insilico identification of microrna (mirnas) and their target prediction from colorado tick fever virus from complete genome. *Asian J. Exp. Sci.,* 32(1) 45–50.

Shannon, P., Markiel, A., Ozier, O., Baliga, N. S., Wang, J. T., Ramage, D. & Ideker, T. 2003. Cytoscape: a software environment for integrated models of biomolecular interaction networks. *Genome Research*, 13(11), 2498–2504.

Srivastava, S., Saxena, A. K., Farooqui, A., Hashmi, M. A., Srivastava, K., & Saxena, V. L. 2018. In silico identification of mirna and their target prediction from bolivian haemorrhagic fever virus (machupo virus). *Research Journal of Life Sciences, Bioinformatics, Pharmaceutical and Chemical Sciences.*

Tav, C., Tempel, S., Poligny, L., & Tahi, F. 2016. miRNAFold: a web server for fast miRNA precursor prediction in genomes. *Nucleic Acids Research*, 44(W1), W181–W184.

Vishnoi, A., & Rani, S. 2017. MiRNA biogenesis and regulation of diseases: an overview. *MicroRNA Profiling*, 1–10.

Walayat, A., Yang, M., & Xiao, D. 2018. Therapeutic implication of miRNA in human disease. In *Antisense Therapy*. IntechOpen.

Wang, D., Gu, J., Wang, T., & Ding, Z. 2014. OncomiRDB: a database for the experimentally verified onco-genic and tumor-suppressive microRNAs. *Bioinformatics*, *30*(15), 2237–2238.

Wang, J., Zhong, J., Chen, G., Li, M., Wu, F. X., & Pan, Y. 2014. ClusterViz: a cytoscape APP for cluster ana-lysis of biological network. *IEEE/ACM Transactions on Computational Biology and Bioinformatics*, *12*(4), 815–822.

Wang, W. C., Lin, F. M., Chang, W. C., Lin, K. Y., Huang, H. D., & Lin, N. S. 2009. miRExpress: ana-lyzing high-throughput sequencing data for profiling microRNA expression. *BMC Bioinformatics*, *10* (1), 1-13.

Xiao, F., Zuo, Z., Cai, G., Kang, S., Gao, X., & Li, T. 2009. miRecords: an integrated resource for microRNA – target interactions. *Nucleic Acids Research*, *37*(suppl_1), D105–D110.

Yu, W. & MacKerell, A. D. *Computer-Aided Drug Design Methods. in Antibiotics* (ed. Sass, P.) Springer: New York, 2017. vol. 1520, 85–106.

Yuan, C., Meng, X., Li, X., Illing, N., Ingle, R. A., Wang, J., & Chen, M. 2017. PceRBase: a database of plant competing endogenous RNA. *Nucleic Acids Research*, *45*(D1), D1009–D1014.

Yuriev E., Ramsland P. A. 2013. Latest developments in molecular docking: 2010–2011 in review. *J Mol Recognit* 26(5):215–239

Zheng, F., Wei, L., Zhao, L., & Ni, F. 2018. Pathway network analysis of complex diseases based on multiple biological networks. *BioMed Research International*, *2018*.

34

Biomaterial-Based Nanofibers for Drug Delivery Applications

Sneha Anand, P.S. Rajinikanth, Prashant Pandey, Payal Deepak, Sunita Thakur, Dilip Kumar Arya, and Shweta Jaiswal
Department of Pharmaceutical Sciences, Babasaheb Bhimrao Ambedkar University, Lucknow, India

34.1 Nanofibers

The nanomaterials world comprises a wide range of materials having unique characteristics with physical and chemical properties. These include nanoparticles, quantum dots, nanowires, nanorods, nanotubes, nanosheets, and nanofibers. The best nanomaterial is the nanofiber due to its great potential in a variety of applications. Nanofibers are defined as fibers with a diameter less than 50–500 nanometers. The National Science Foundation (NSF) defines nanofibers as having at least one dimension of 100 nanometers or less. Nanofibers can be generated from different polymers and hence have different properties and application potentials (Lim, 2017).

34.1.1 History of Nanofibers

William Gilbert was the first person to describe the process in which electric charge can deform a liquid droplet after ejection when an electrically charged amber piece approaches it. Nanofibers were first produced via electrospinning more than four centuries ago. In 1887, British physicist Charles Vernon Boys (1855–1944) published a manuscript about nanofiber development and production by constructing an electrospinning apparatus having a small dish connected with an electrical machine. In 1900, American inventor John Francis Cooley (1861–1903) filed the first modern electrospinning patent and William James Morton followed in 1902. Anton Formhals was the first person to attempt nanofiber production between 1934 and 1944 and applied for 22 patents describing the experimental production of nanofibers (Wu, 2020). In 1966, Harold Simons published a patent for a device that could produce thin and light nanofiber fabrics with diverse motifs. The theoretical procedure of electrospinning was first described by Sir Geoffrey Ingram Taylor who developed a mathematical model for analyzing the shape of the deformation cone formed by the liquid droplet due to an applied electric field. This deformation zone is now known as the "Taylor cone." (Taylor, 1964). D.H. Reneker popularized the electrospinning name. Since the 1990s, electrospinning theoretical and application research has been increasing exponentially every year.

34.1.2 Characteristics of Nanofibers

- Nanofibers are very small, which gives them unique physical and chemical properties and allows them to be used in very small places.
- Nanofibers have a high surface area, which makes them suitable for smaller chemical reactions to occur and speed up.

- Nanofibers exhibit low density, large surface area to mass, diameter range 50–1000 nm.
- Nanofibers have high pore volume and tight pore size, which make the nonwoven nanofiber appropriate for a wide range of filtration applications.
- Nanofibers have been electrospun onto a variety of substrates, including glass polyester, nylon, and cellulose filter media substrates.

34.2 Types of Methods for Producing Nanofibers

34.2.1 Self-Assembly Method

This method involves the arrangement of macromolecules and components into an ordered system without any complication into desired structures like superlattices, monolayers, tubes, fibers, and microporous films. The self-assembly of preparing nanofibers is mainly for three types of polymers: PEO, PAN, and PVA. The self-assembly mechanism only occurs at low concentrations and in a fluid state. This method only depends on the two phenomena-surface tension and electrostatic repulsion (Yan, 2011).

34.2.2 Centrifugal Spinning Method

This method is also known as rotary spinning or rotational jet spinning. This is the stretching process that requires no high voltage. Small inner diameter needles are used for better centrifugal force and spinnability. This force requires chain overlapping and entanglement. The nanofibers produced by this method are aligned vertically and have a uniform diameter.

34.2.3 Freeze-Drying Method

In this method no high temperature and leaching are necessary. It produces porous structures whose sizes can be controlled. It also not needs structure-directing additives. This process starts freezing solution, dispersion, or emulsion by excluding interstitial spaces and completes by the following sublimation.

34.2.4 Electrospinning Method

Electrospinning is the most common method for the production of nanofibers and also for fabricating nanofibers because of its versatility, cost-efficiency, simplicity, and adaptability. It was developed in 1934 by the patent of Formhals and explored in the 1960s by Sir Geoffrey Ingram Taylor who named the iconic electrospinning cone the "Taylor Cone." In this process, the liquid polymer is ejected to the grounded collector from the spinneret as a continuous jet strand after applying a high electric field to it. Due to

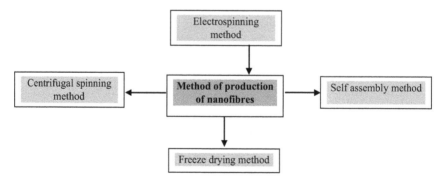

FIGURE 34.1   Types of the method for producing nanofibers.

surface tension, the polymer droplet elongates and forms a cone known as the Taylor cone, which is extruded and forms a fiber jet from which solvent is evaporated and solid fibers are collected in the collector (Xue, 2019).

Based on the preparation of polymer, the electrospinning process is classified into two groups: solution electrospinning and melt electrospinning. The drawbacks of solution electrospinning are that it requires toxic solvent and has low productivity due to extra solvent extraction. Melt electrospinning has also drawbacks due to issues like high viscosity of melting polymer, finer fiber formation, and electrical discharge due to high voltage.

34.2.4.1 Types of Electrospinning

Uniaxial electrospinning (one-nozzle configuration): The drug-polymer solution in the desired ratio is prepared to obtain ideal viscosity or conductivity. The solution is extruded from a syringe tube with a suitable force. The technique uses the Taylor cone, which refers to a cone-like extrusive solution under extremely high voltage supply on the nozzle. As the solution moves with a predefined rate, the solvent is volatilized or evaporated immediately and the nanofibers are collected on a metal collector.

Coaxial electrospinning (two concentric nozzle configuration): The fundamental principle is similar to uniaxial electrospinning, but it comprises two concentric and separate spinnerets. The drug can either be dissolved in core or shell solution, and is transported to the relevant spinneret layers forming the core-shell architectural nanofibers (Ramos, 2021).

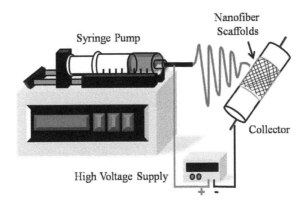

FIGURE 34.2 Schematic diagram of uniaxial electrospinning.

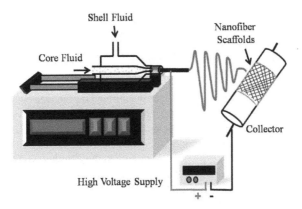

FIGURE 34.3 Schematic diagram of coaxial electrospinning.

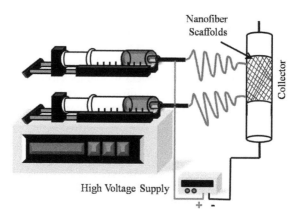

FIGURE 34.4 Schematic diagram of side-by-side electrospinning.

To obtain higher productivity from electrospinning, the following techniques are applied (Nayak, 2012):

- Side-by-side electrospinning
  Side-by-side electrospinning enables the simultaneous electrospinning of two polymer solutions. It similar to a bicomponent system that combines the mechanical strength of one component and the desired chemical functionality from the other. The important process parameters for this electrospinning are the viscosity and conductivity of each solution (Gupta, 2003).
- Multijet from single-needle electrospinning
  Two mechanisms are involved in getting multiple jets from single-needle electrospinning: solution blockage at needle tip and discrepancy in the distribution of the electric field. The researcher Vaseashta uses a curved collector to obtain this and another method to split the jet path into two subjets. Before infusing, the polymer matrix and filler are mixed well for uniform distribution.
- Multijet from multineedle electrospinning
  This technique involves fiber fabrication from polymers that are not easily solvent dissolved. To obtain multijet from multineedle, the number of needles and gauges can be optimized and the needle can also be arranged in one or two-dimensionally configurations like triangular, square, elliptical, hexagonal, and circular. It improves process stability and has higher productivity.
- Multijet from needleless system
  Multijet requires optimization of needles, big space, and jet repulsion, therefore needleless electrospinning is used in which various polymeric jets are produced from the free large liquid surface area on applying an electric field. Its mass production is higher than any other multijet technique.

34.2.4.2 Recent Advances in Electrospinning

- Bubble electrospinning
  In bubble electrospinning controllable bubbles are formed on the free surface of polymer solution after slowing of the gas pump. These bubbles change into a conical shape and multiple polymer jets are ejected from them. The number of bubbles is reduced according to the tube diameter. Another type is blown bubble spinning in which blowing air is used to produce fiber in place of electronic force. Lastly there is electroblowing in which electronic force and an air blow sheath are simultaneously applied (Alghoraibi et al., 2018).
- Porous hollow-tube electrospinning
  In this process porous polytetrafluoroethylene (PTFE) tubes were used by Varabhas et al., having 0.5 diameter holes spaced 1 cm apart. In the frame of the PVC pipe, this tube was suspended 12–15 cm above the collector. After adding solution, jets are produced by each hole-forming coil (Nayak, 2012).

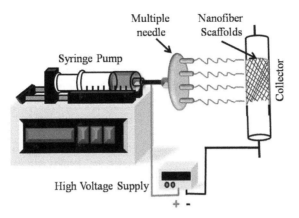

FIGURE 34.5 Schematic diagram of multijet electrospinning.

- Microfluidic manifold electrospinning

  A microfluidic device was prepared by Srivastava et al., which fabricates multicomponent nanofibers. This device is multilayered and based on polydimethylsiloxane spins many hollow fibres. Two bottom layers of microchannels flow sheath polymer solution and bottom layers of microchannels flow core material. The jets are repulsed through the Columbia repulsion. This method includes advantages like a single device having parallel electrospinning, ease of fabrication, and rapid prototyping (Srivastava, 2007).

- Roller electrospinning

  This method contains a roller electrospinning setup consisting of a rotating cylinder that spins nanofibres from the solution directly. A rotating roller made up of aluminum is immersed partially in the solution and high voltage is applied to this. Lukas et al. first described the mechanism of forming Taylor cones on the roller surface. Spinnability is affected by molecular weight and throughput by the concentration of the solution. Surface tension and electrical conductivity do not affect nanofibers (Jirsák, 2005).

- Melt electrospinning

  This is the same as solution electrospinning except for the melting polymer. The melting is performed by many heating devices and methods like electric heating, heating oven, laser melting devices, and heat guns. It produces micrometer- and nanometer-scale fibers. Its advantages include high throughput rate and toxic solvent removal, as there is no mass loss, ease of fabrication, and polymer suitability. The disadvantages of it are the need for high temperature, the problem of electric discharge, and melt low conductivity (Larrondo et al., 1981).

34.3 Biomaterials for Nanofibers

The term biomaterials refers to materials or polymers of natural origin. They are found in nature in large amounts and can be derived from biological systems. They are formed during the growth cycles of living organisms in natural conditions. They are versatile carriers because they are non-toxic, biodegradable, stable, environmentally friendly, and biocompatible. Economically also they have the advantage of being renewable and cheap. Their functional efficiency depends on their composition, structural features, and physicochemical properties. The use of biomaterials in drug delivery is a smart move by researchers. It is an emerging technological advancement that has various applications (Sharma, 2017).

The biomaterials consist of two types:

Polysaccharides derived from plants like alginate and chitosan.

- Proteins originated from animals like gelatin, silk, albumin, keratin, and collagen.

34.3.1 Alginate

Alginates are water-soluble, naturally occurring anionic, linear, and unbranched polysaccharide polymers. They are extracted and isolated from kelp species or brown seaweed algae including *Laminaria hyperborean, Ascophyllumnodosum*, and *Macrocysispyrifera* (Smidsrod and Skjak-Braek, 1990). The advantages of alginate include its easy abundance, excellent gelling properties, mucoadhesiveness, biocompatibility, cheapness, biodegradability, and nontoxicity. However, it has also some drawbacks like poor dimensional stability, low mechanical strength, high biomolecule leakage, large pore size, and too messy to work with them.

Alginate-based wound dressings include sponges, hydrogels, and electrospun mats, which have many advantages like forming gel on absorbing wound exudates and hemostatic capability. It also features properties like good water absorptivity, mild antiseptic properties, and optimal water vapor transmission rate with nontoxicity and biodegradability. Alginate wound dressings heal wounds by maintaining a moist microenvironment and minimizing bacterial infections required by wounds (Tønnesen et al., 2002).

34.3.2 Chitosan

Chitosan is a unique positively charged polysaccharide family and is found in the exoskeleton of crustaceans. It cannot be directly obtained from natural resources as it is not widely present in nature. It is the primary derivative of chitin obtained by the alkaline deacetylation by enzymatic hydrolysis at high temperatures under alkali conditions. It can easily blend with other polymers because of its reactive amino and hydroxyl functional groups and also induces inter-molecular or intra-molecular crosslinking in the matrix of polymer to improve its functional properties. The one disadvantage of chitosan-based materials is their weak mechanical strength.

It is the most popular biopolymer for the development of drug delivery systems. Its mucoadhesive nature and an ability to open epithelial tight junctions make it a delivery vehicle and helpful in delivering drugs across various well-organized epithelia. It can easily bind with proteins, cholesterol, fats, and metal ions and is used as a chelating agent. It has various remarkable activities like analgesic due to its polycationic nature and antifungal, hemostatic, and strong antibacterial activity in low-molecular weight chitosan. These properties sometimes alter drug encapsulation efficiency by affecting the aqueous solubility and hydrophobicity of chitosan (Jiang et al., 2014).

34.3.3 Collagen

Collagen represents 30% of all chief structural proteins of vertebrates. It deposits during an accelerated growth period and its synthesis rate declines with age. Collagen is resistant to the attacks of neutral proteases because it is the primary structural protein of the body. The properties of collagen, which make it beneficial for use in drug delivery are low-toxicity, adequate biocompatibility, low-antigenicity, high mechanical strength, cross-linking ability, and water uptake features. It is insoluble in organic solvents but water-soluble collagen gives only a small amount of total collagen and also depends on the animal age and type of tissue extracted (Friess et al., 1998).

34.3.4 Gelatin

Gelatin is a natural soluble biopolymer and single-stranded protein derived from collagen by its hydrolytic degradation. It is a multifunctional biopolymer and is a translucent, colorless, and tasteless powder. It is also an optically active material in the random coil and helical states. It is widely used in food, cosmetic, pharmaceutical, and medical applications because of its unique mechanical and technological properties like biodegradability, biocompatibility, low immunogenicity, adhesiveness, plasticity, cost economy, and ability to form transparent gels (Foox et al., 2015).

Gelatin exploits as a drug carrier due to its unique chemical and physical properties. The advantages like alteration in gelling property by chemical crosslinking and drug loading into the gelatin matrix under mild conditions can also be used for controlled drug release delivery systems. Crosslinked gelatin has thermal and mechanical stability and lower degradation in vivo. The properties of gelatin can be adjusted to increase the drug-loading efficiency. The hydrophilic nature of gelatin facilitates the diffusion-mediated release of bioactive molecules by increasing the penetration of body fluids into the particles. By changing the degree of crosslinking, gelatin source, and molecular weight of gelatin the release profiles of drug can be optimized. Gelatin as a carrier is used for cancer therapy, angiogenesis, inflammatory drugs, antineoplastic agents, antibacterial agents, nucleic acids, and hydrophobic materials.

The large-diameter gelatin fibers are produced by several methods such as wet spinning, melt spinning, dry spinning, or gel spinning. The fabrication of these nanofibers is done by solution/melt blow spinning, electrospinning, and centrifugal. The electrospun nanofibers have a porous network with controllable pore size and high porosity. Their high surface-area-to-volume ratio increases the drug solubility in the aqueous solution and also enhances its efficiency. The nanofiber morphology and the drug release rate are influenced by parameters like temperature, humidity, and solution properties (Laha et al., 2016).

34.3.5 Albumin

Albumin is one of the most abundant and endogenous plasma proteins in human blood (35–50 g/L human serum). It is synthesized by liver hepatocytes and ~ 10–15 g of albumin is produced and released in the bloodstream. It is of three types: ovalbumin, human serum albumin, and bovine serum albumin.

Albumin-based systems for drug delivery are approved for marketing, which increases the interest of researchers for their use in the pharmaceutical industry. It is a multipurpose tool for drug delivery that is used for formulations like nanoparticles, conjugates, and complexes loaded with antibodies, drugs, or peptides (Tan et al., 2018). Ovalbumin is mainly used in controlled drug delivery because of its many features like ease of availability, low cost, gelling ability, emulsion stabilization, and sensitivity of pH and temperature. Bovine serum albumin is best for drug delivery because of its medical importance, low cost, the amount in nature, easy purification, and ligand-binding features. Human serum albumin is used for drug delivery due to its inertness, biodegradability, ease of availability, and availability uptaken by the tumor and tissues in which inflammation occurs. Drugs and their metabolites bind albumin covalently by the glucuronidation of drugs. The carboxylic acid group present in drugs results in acid glucuronides, which bind covalently to human serum albumin. This covalent binding affects the metabolism and clearance of drugs. Multiple ligand-binding sites, cellular interactions, natural transport function, and ability to bind covalently or non-covalently give many design options and provide a rationale for using albumin in drug delivery (Larsen et al., 2016).

34.3.6 Silk Proteins

Silks are protein polymers that are present in the glands of silkworms, spiders, mites, scorpions, and bees, and are spun into fibers during their metamorphosis. All obtained silks are different in composition, structure, and properties. But in recent years, silk from Bombyxmori (silkworm) has been extensively studied due to its biocompatibility, ease of processing, robust mechanical performance, sufficient supply, tunable degradation, and ease of acquisition. Silk has no cytotoxicity and also does not induce an uncontrolled immune response (Leal-Egana and Scheibel, 2012). It is composed of a fibrous core of protein silk fibroin (70–80%) and silk sericin (20–30%). With these proteins, there are other impurities present such as wax, color pigments, and inorganic components. Silk sericin is present in three layers, outer, middle, and inner layer, containing 15%, 10.5%, and 4.5% sericin, respectively, covering silk fibroin. Three layers of silk sericin are available in the silk cocoon. These proteins are obtained by the degumming process of silk cocoons, which is accomplished by acid, alkali, and enzyme (Nagal et al., 2013).

34.3.6.1 Silk Sericin

Silk sericin is a natural, hydrophilic, macromolecular, globular glycoprotein derived from *Bombyxmori* silk cocoon. It is stored as an aqueous solution and synthesized in the middle silk gland of silkworms. It also plays an important role in the spinning process in the construction of a cocoon shell by the silkworm. Sericin is insoluble in cold water but soluble in hot water. Sericin is rich in serine (32%), aspartic acid (16.8%), and glycine (8.8%), and has a high concentration of hydroxyl groups. Sericin contains 20–30% of the total cocoon mass [6]. It has 18 different types of amino acids that display its physical and biological properties like antioxidant, antityrosinase, anti-inflammatory, antitumoural, antiaging, antiwrinkle, UV-resistant, antimicrobial, moisture absorption, biocompatibility, and promoting collagen production (Khan et al., 2013).

34.3.6.2 Silk Fibroin

Silk fibroin is a protein-based biomacromolecule that has repetitive hydrophobic domains interrupted by small hydrophilic groups. The primary structure is composed of glycine (43%), alanine (30%), and serine (12%). Silk fibroin has promising applications due to its excellent physicochemical properties like mechanical properties, biodegradability, good biocompatibility, and the versatility of structure. It is a semi-crystalline biopolymer and its crystalline part has two structures (i.e., the silk I and silk II). Silk I is obtained from spinning dope, which is unstable and water-soluble. During the spinning process when silk I transform to silk II, it becomes more stable. Its properties like high strength, low elasticity, low extensibility, and resistance to chemicals and micro-organisms are derived from its crystalline structure.

The main advantage of using silk fibroin as a drug carrier is performing mild all-aqueous processes for loadings of sensitive drugs like protein and nucleic acid, which provides good resistance to dissolution, thermal, and enzymatic degradation. The degummed silk fibroin is dissolved in a highly concentrated salt solution and after desalination, the liquid silk fibroin solution can be converted into various forms of biomaterials depending on its application like powder, fiber, film, porous matrix, 3D scaffold, and hydrogel. Silk fibroin is used to generate fibrous membranes of silk by electrospinning. Their increased surface area is good for cell adhesion. Silk sericin can also be processed in different forms like films, hydrogels, 3D porous scaffolds, and fibers by wet spinning or electrospinning (Zhao et al., 2015).

34.3.7 Silk Fibroin Nanofibers

Silk fibroin is best for the development of nanofibrous structures. They are produced by the electrospinning process by using hexafluoroisopropanol solvent in which a high electric field is subjected to the polymer solution. The surface tension of polymer is overcome by this field and it ejects, stretches, and deposits a nanofibrous mat. This process is similar to the silkworm spinning process. Electrospun fibers have advantages like high specific surface area and high porosity, which is best for cell attachment and good biocompatibility. The concentration of fibroin and pH of the solution has a significant role in the morphology of these nanofibers. It is important to do a post-treatment of nanofibers with organic solutions to change their random coil conformation to β-sheet, which is more stable and water-insoluble (Yukseloglu et al., 2015).

34.4 Applications in Drug Delivery

Nanofiber drug delivery is based on a principle of increased drug dissolution rate due to increased surface area of the drug and the carrier. Nanofibers act as a controlled drug delivery system due to the drug molecule's entrapment in the polymer structure. Nanofibers incorporated with the drug can be applied to the skin, which helps in wound healing by systemic or local therapeutic action. Various applications of pharmaceutical agents for skin are a big concern, so nanofiber formulations show promise.

34.4.1 Wound Healing

A wound is a defect or breakage in which the dermis area is damaged due to a cut or puncture in the skin barrier as a physical or thermal stimuli consequence or through any medical or pathological

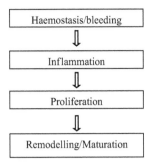

FIGURE 34.6 Stages in the wound healing process.

condition. Generally, there are two types of wounds: acute wounds, which heal in a short duration because of a well-organized process, and chronic wounds, which have prolonged inflammation, frequent infection, and sometimes failure of the dermal and epidermal cells in which recovery may not be complete. Thus, appropriate wound care is needeed for recovery from the injury. An ideal wound dressing must be an appropriate barrier and should absorb the wound exudates. As compared to traditional bandages, fibrous bandages provide more wound care as they mimic the native extracellular matrix (ECM) structure. Nanofiber-based drug delivery systems offer several advantages for wound dressing application. Their highly porous nature helps in cellular respiration and gas permeation and also prevents the infiltration of microbial particles. Their high surface area facilitates fluid absorption and the moisture under it creates ideal surroundings and promotes regeneration of skin tissue to aid wound healing (Kirsner et al., 1993).

34.4.2 Diabetic Wound Healing

The diabetic wound is the most common and dangerous complication of diabetes. Due to impaired leukocyte function, diabetic patients are more prone to wound infection. Diabetic wounds fall into three categories: neuropathic, ischemic, and neuroischemic. In diabetic wound healing pro-inflammatory cytokines, proteases, and ROS levels are elevated with cellular dysfunctions. Due to excessive production of ROS, defective phagocytic and chemotactic activities of granulocytes, and poor blood glucose level, the immune system weakens, and structural elements of ECM are damaged (Brem et al., 2007).

34.5 Conclusions

Nanofiber applications are progressing at an incredibly fast pace in research and academic studies and there is no sign of it slowing down. Due to increasing demand and use in several fields, the development of many nanofiber manufacturing technologies has progressed rapidly. Electrospinning is a common, attractive, and widely used technique for the fabrication of nanofibers. There are many electrospinning techniques based on collector shape, number of needles used (single-needle electrospinning, multiple-needle electrospinning, needleless electrospinning), and needle arrangement (standard electrospinning, coaxial electrospinning). There are also many non-electrospinning techniques such as drawing, freeze-drying, phase separation, etc. Many natural and synthetic polymers are used for their fabrication. Natural polymers easily stimulate cell growth and regulation and have high biocompatibility. Synthetic polymers provide mechanical durability to support wound healing and regeneration of skin.

The electrospun nanofibers have beneficial properties such as mechanical stability, high surface area-to-volume ratio, and high porosity, which promotes favorable cell attachment and allows the exchange of water, oxygen, and nutrient. They imitate and mimic the native ECM structure and its functionality to recapitulate the wound healing process. The wound healing process is one of the most elaborate

TABLE 34.1

Nanofibers for Wound Healing and Diabetic Wound Healing

Polymer-based Nanofibers	Drug	References
Gelatin	Silver nitrate	Rujitanaroj et al., 2008
Polyvinyl alcohol (polyvinyl alcohol)	Ciprofloxacin hydrochloride	Jannesari et al., 2011
PLA and PEVA	Tetracycline hydrochloride	Kenawy et al., 2002
Gellan and PVA	Amoxicillin	Vashisth et al., 2016
PLGA (polylactic glycolic acid)	Fusidic acid	Said et al., 2011
Silk and PEO	Epidermal growth factor	Schneider et al., 2009
Silk protein	Fenugreek	Selvaraj et al., 2017
Polylactide	Doxycycline	Cui et al., 2019
PCL and PEO	Hyaluronic acid and keratin	Su et al., 2021
Chitosan	Neurotensin	Moura et al., 2014
PCL (poly caprolactone)	Curcumin	Merrell et al., 2009
PCL-PEG	rhEGF	Choi et al., 2008
Cellulose acetate	Sesamol	Liu et al., 2020
PCL	Bixin	Pinzón-García et al., 2017
Polyurethane/carboxymethylcellulose	*Malvasylvestris*	Almasian et al., 2020
PCL, PVA and silk	Curcumin	Agarwal et al., 2021
Gelatin and PVA	Cephradine	Razzaq et al., 2021
Chitosan and PVA	Zinc oxide	Ahmed et al., 2018
HPMC and PEO	Beta glucan	Grip et al., 2018
PLGA	Curcumin	Liao et al., 2021
Cellulose and gelatin	Glybenclamide and metformin	Cam et al., 2020
Cellulose acetate	Silver nitrate	Shalaby et al., 2015
Eudragit	Gentamicin sulfate	Dwivedi et al., 2018
PLGA and PCL	Calcium phosphate	Jiang et al., 2019
PLA and PEG	Retinol	Müller et al., 2015
PLGA and Aloevera extract	rhEGF	Garcia-Orue et al., 2017
PLGA	Insulin	Lee et al., 2020

phenomena in the human body and it also fulfills a key role in body homeostasis. Nanofibers enhance many skin cell processes such as differentiation, migration, proliferation, and regeneration by infusing with the epidermal cells and growth factors to promote wound healing.

Modification of electrospinning processes and using controllable and effective approaches like the incorporation of drugs, growth factors, and antibacterial agents can prevent infections during the wound recovery process. Therefore, many researchers are developing multifunctional smart scaffolds, which provide better wound healing outcomes. Despite various nanofiber manufacturing methods, electrospinning is still considered the most potent method due to its simplicity and applicability over a wide range of materials, low cost, and ease of commercial production. Thus, the properties explored in this chapter show that the electrospun nanofiber approach has a very bright future and is beneficial and crucial in wound healing and management.

TABLE 34.2

A Summary of Polymeric Nanofibers for Chemotherapy

Nanofibers	Drug	Cancer types	Drug release mechanism	Ref
PCL/poly(glycerol monostearate-co-ε-caprolactone)(PGC-C18)	Camptothecin-11(CPT-11) and 7-ethyl-10-hydroxycamptothecin (SN-38)	Human colorectal cancer HT-29 cells	Diffusion	Yohi et al., 2012
Poly-L-lactide	5-fluorouracil (5-FU)	Human colorectal cancer HCT-116 cells	Diffusion	Li et al., 2013
Poly(L-lactic acid)	Titanocene dichloride	Human lung cancer spc-a-1 cells	Degradation of the polymeric matrix	Chen et al., 2010
Poly(ε-caprolactone)(PCL)/ gelatin (GT)	7-ethyl-10-hydroxy camptothecin (SN-38)	Human glioblastoma 251 and U87 cells	Diffusion and anomalous transport	Zhu et al., 2015
Poly(D,L-lactide-co-glycolide)/polyethylene oxide (PLGA/PEO)	Ferulic acid	Human breast carcinoma MCF-7 cells	Diffusion and degradation of a polymeric matrix	Vashisth et al., 2015
Polylactide (PLA)	5-fluorouracil and oxaliplatin	Human colorectal cancer HCT-8 cells and mouse colorectal cancer CT-26 cells	Diffusion	Zhang et al., 2016
Poly(ethylene glycol)–poly(L-lactic acid) (PEG–PLLA)	1,3-bis(2-chloroethyl)-1-nitrosourea (BCNU)	Rat glioma C6 cells	Diffusion	Xu et al., 2006
Polyvinyl alcohol (PVA)/ Chitosan (CS)	Curcumin	Human breast MCF-7 cancer cells, human liver carcinoma HepG2 cells	Diffusion and degradation of a polymeric matrix	Sedghi et al., 2017
Poly-(D,L-lactide-co-glycolide) (PLGA)	Paclitaxel	Rat C6 glioma cells	Degradation of a polymeric matrix	Ranganath et al., 2008
Poly(L-actide) (PLA)/poly(D,L-lactide-co-glucolic acid) (PLGA)	Cisplatin	Rat C6 glioma cells	Diffusion	Xie et al., 2008
Poly(ε-caprolactone)(PCL)	Camptothecin	Mouse myoblast C2C12 cells	Diffusion	Amna et al., 2013
Polycaprolactone (PCL)/silk fibroin (SF)	Titanocene dichloride	Human breast cancer MCF-7 cells	The degradation of the matrix	Laiva et al., 2015
Poly (D,L-lactic-co-glycolic) acid (PLGA)	Curcumin	Skin cancer A431 cells	Diffusion and erosion	Sampath et al., 2014
Poly(ethylene glycol)-b-poly(L-lactic acid) PEG-PLA	DOX	Human hepatocarcinoma SMMC-7721cells	Diffusion and degradation of the fiber matrix	Lu et al., 2012
Poly(L-lactide-co-D,L-lactide) (coPLA)	DOX	Human cervical cancer HeLa cells	Diffusion	Toshkova et al., 2010
Poly(ε-caprolactone) (PCL) and gelatin (GEL)	Piperine	Human cervical cancer HeLa cells and human breast MCF-7 cancer cells	Hydrolytic degradation of PCL	Jain et al., 2016
Polyvinyl pyrrolidone (PVP)	Curcumin	Murine melanoma B16 cells	Dissolution	Wang et al., 2015

(continued)

TABLE 34.2 (Continued)

A Summary of Polymeric Nanofibers for Chemotherapy

Nanofibers	Drug	Cancer types	Drug release mechanism	Ref
Polylactide (PLLA)	DOX	Secondary hepatic carcinoma SHCC cells	Diffusion and hydrolysis and degradation of PLLA	Liu et al., 2013
Chitosan (CS)/polyethylene oxide (PEO)	Paclitaxel	Prostate cancer DU145 cells	Diffusion	Ma et al., 2011
Poly(lactic-co-glycolic acid) (PLGA)	Daunorubicin	Human epidermoid carcinoma A431 cells	Diffusion and the polymer nanofiber degradation	Hu et al., 1995
Polycaprolactone (PCL)	(−)-epigallocatechin-3-O-gallate (EGCG) and caffeic acid (CA)	Human gastric cancer MKN28 cells	Diffusion and the degradation of PCL	Kim et al., 2012
Poly (L-lactic acid) (PLA)	Cisplatin	Human lung cancer Apc-a-1 cells	Diffusion and degradation of PLLA matrix	Chen et al., 2011
Poly($_{DL}$-lactic acid)–poly(ethylene glycol) (PELA)	Hydroxycamptothecin (HCPT)	Human breast cancer MCF-7 cells	Diffusion and the degradation of a polymeric matrix	Xie et al., 2010
Poly(ethylene oxide)/polylactide	Cisplatin	Murine cervical cancer U14 cells	Diffusion and frame erosion	Zong et al., 2015
Poly(ethylene glycol)-poly(L-lactic acid) (PEG–PLA)	Paclitaxel and doxorubicin hydrochloride	Murine glioma C6 cells	Diffusion	Xu et al., 2009
Poly(L-lactide) (PLA)	Oxaliplatin and cyclophosphamide	Human hepatocellular cancer HCC cells	Diffusion	Liu et al., 2015

REFERENCES

Agarwal Y., Rajinikanth P. S., Ranjan S., Tiwari U., Balasubramnaiam J., Pandey P., et al. (2021). Curcumin loaded polycaprolactone-/polyvinyl alcohol-silk fibroin based electrospunnanofibrous mat for rapid healing of diabetic wound: An in vitro and in vivo studies. *International Journal of Biological Macromolecules*, *176*, 376–386.

Ahmed, R., Tariq, M., Ali, I., Asghar, R., Khanam, P. N., Augustine, R., & Hasan, A. (2018). Novel electrospun chitosan/polyvinyl alcohol/zinc oxide nanofibrous mats with antibacterial and antioxidant properties for diabetic wound healing. *International Journal Of Biological Macromolecules*, *120*, 385–393.

Alghoraibi, I., & Alomari, S. (2018). Different methods for nanofiber design and fabrication. *Handbook of Nanofibers*, 1–46.

Almasian, A., Najafi, F., Eftekhari, M., Ardekani, M. R. S., Sharifzadeh, M., & Khanavi, M. (2020). Polyurethane/carboxymethylcellulose nanofibers containing Malvasylvestris extract for healing diabetic wounds: Preparation, characterization, in vitro and in vivo studies. *Materials Science and Engineering: C*, *114*, 111039.

Amna, T., Barakat, N. A., Hassan, M. S., Khil, M. S., & Kim, H. Y. (2013). Camptothecin loaded poly (ε-caprolactone) nanofibers via one-step electrospinning and their cytotoxicity impact. *Colloids and Surfaces A: Physicochemical and Engineering Aspects*, *431*, 1–8.

Brem, H., & Tomic-Canic, M. (2007). Cellular and molecular basis of wound healing in diabetes. *The Journal of Clinical Investigation*, *117*(5), 1219–1222.

Cam M. E., Crabbe-Mann M., Alenezi H., Hazar-Yavuz A. N., Ertas B., Ekentok C., et al. (2020). The comparison of glybenclamide and metformin-loaded bacterial cellulose/gelatin nanofibres produced by a portable electrohydrodynamic gun for diabetic wound healing. *European Polymer Journal*, *134*, 109844.

Chen, P., Wu, Q. S., Ding, Y. P., & Zhu, Z. C. (2011). Preparation of cisplatin composite micro/nanofibers and antitumor activity in vitro against human tumor spc-a-1 cells. *Nano*, *6*(04), 325–332.

Chen, P., Wu, Q. S., Ding, Y. P., Chu, M., Huang, Z. M., & Hu, W. (2010). A controlled release system of titanocene dichloride by electrospun fiber and its antitumor activity in vitro. *European Journal of Pharmaceutics and Biopharmaceutics*, *76*(3), 413–420.

Choi, J. S., Leong, K. W., & Yoo, H. S. (2008). In vivo wound healing of diabetic ulcers using electrospun nanofibers immobilized with human epidermal growth factor (EGF). *Biomaterials*, *29*(5), 587–596.

Cui, S., Sun, X., Li, K., Gou, D., Zhou, Y., Hu, J., & Liu, Y. (2019). Polylactide nanofibers delivering doxycycline for chronic wound treatment. *Materials Science and Engineering: C*, *104*, 109745.

Dwivedi C., Pandey I., Pandey H., Patil S., Mishra S. B., Pandey A. C., et al. (2018). In vivo diabetic wound healing with nanofibrous scaffolds modified with gentamicin and recombinant human epidermal growth factor. *Journal of Biomedical Materials Research Part A*, *106*(3), 641–651.

Foox, M. & Zilberman, M. (2015). Drug delivery from gelatin-based systems. *Expert Opinion on Drug Delivery*, *12*(9), 1547–1563.

Friess, W. (1998). Collagen–biomaterial for drug delivery. *European Journal of Pharmaceutics and Biopharmaceutics*, *45*(2), 113–136.

Garcia-Orue I., Gainza G., Gutierrez F. B., Aguirre J. J., Evora C., Pedraz J. L., et al. (2017). Novel nanofibrous dressings containing rhEGF and Aloe vera for wound healing applications. *International Journal of Pharmaceutics*, *523*(2), 556–566.

Grip, J., Engstad, R. E., Skjæveland, I., Škalko-Basnet, N., Isaksson, J., Basnet, P., & Holsæter, A. M. (2018). Beta-glucan-loaded nanofiber dressing improves wound healing in diabetic mice. *European Journal of Pharmaceutical Sciences*, *121*, 269–280.

Gupta, P. & Wilkes, G. L. (2003). Some investigations on the fiber formation by utilizing a side-by-side bicomponent electrospinning approach. *Polymer*, *44*(20), 6353–6359.

Hu, D. E., Hiley, C. R., Smither, R. L., Gresham, G. A., & Fan, T. P. (1995). Correlation of 133Xe clearance, blood flow and histology in the rat sponge model for angiogenesis. Further studies with angiogenic modifiers. *Laboratory Investigation; A Journal of Technical Methods and Pathology*, *72*(5), 601–610.

Jain, S., Meka, S. R. K., & Chatterjee, K. (2016). Engineering a piperine eluting nanofibrous patch for cancer treatment. *ACS Biomaterials Science & Engineering*, *2*(8), 1376–1385.

Jannesari, M., Varshosaz, J., Morshed, M., & Zamani, M. (2011). Composite poly (vinyl alcohol)/poly (vinyl acetate) electrospun nanofibrous mats as a novel wound dressing matrix for controlled release of drugs. *International Journal Of Nanomedicine*, *6*, 993.

Jiang, T., James, R., Kumbar, S. G., & Laurencin, C. T. (2014). Chitosan as a biomaterial: structure, properties, and applications in tissue engineering and drug delivery. In *Natural and Synthetic Biomedical Polymers*. Elsevier. pp. 91–113.

Jiang, Y., Han, Y., Wang, J., Lv, F., Yi, Z., Ke, Q., & Xu, H. (2019). Space-oriented nanofibrous scaffold with silicon-doped amorphous calcium phosphate nanocoating for diabetic wound healing. *ACS Applied Bio Materials*, *2*(2), 787–795.

Jirsák, O., Sanetrník, F., Lukáš, D., Kotek, V., Martinová, L., & Chaloupek, J. (2005). A method of nanofibers production from polymer solution using electrostatic spinning and a device for carrying out the method. *294274 (B6). WO, 2005024101*.

Kenawy, E. R., Bowlin, G. L., Mansfield, K., Layman, J., Simpson, D. G., Sanders, E. H., & Wnek, G. E. (2002). Release of tetracycline hydrochloride from electrospun poly (ethylene-co-vinylacetate), poly (lactic acid), and a blend. *Journal of Controlled Release*, *81*(1-2), 57–64.

Khan, M. M. R., Tsukada, M., Zhang, X., & Morikawa, H. (2013). Preparation and characterization of electrospun nanofibers based on silk sericin powders. *Journal of Materials Science*, *48*(10), 3731–3736.

Kim, Y. J., Park, M. R., Kim, M. S., & Kwon, O. H. (2012). Polyphenol-loaded polycaprolactone nanofibers for effective growth inhibition of human cancer cells. *Materials Chemistry and Physics*, *133*(2–3), 674–680.

Kirsner, R. S. & Eaglstein, W. H. (1993). The wound healing process. *Dermatologic Clinics*, *11*(4), 629–640.

Laha, A., Sharma, C. S., & Majumdar, S. (2016). Electrospun gelatin nanofibers as drug carrier: effect of crosslinking on sustained release. *Materials Today: Proceedings*, *3*(10), 3484–3491.

Laiva, A. L., Venugopal, J. R., Karuppuswamy, P., Navaneethan, B., Gora, A., & Ramakrishna, S. (2015). Controlled release oftitanocene into the hybrid nanofibrous scaffolds to prevent the proliferation of breast cancer cells. *International Journal of Pharmaceutics*, *483*(1–2), 115–123.

Larrondo, L. S. J. M. & St. John Manley, R. (1981). Electrostatic fiber spinning from polymer melts. I. Experimental observations on fiber formation and properties. *Journal of Polymer Science: Polymer Physics Edition*, *19*(6), 909–920.

Larsen, M. T., Kuhlmann, M., Hvam, M. L., & Howard, K. A. (2016). Albumin-based drug delivery: harnessing nature tocure disease. *Molecular and Cellular Therapies*, *4*(1), 1–12.

Lee C. H., Hung K. C., Hsieh M. J., Chang S. H., Juang J. H., Hsieh I. C., et al. (2020). Core-shell insulin-loadednanofibrous scaffolds for repairing diabetic wounds. *Nanomedicine: Nanotechnology, Biology and Medicine*, *24*, 102123.

Li, G., Chen, Y., Cai, Z., Li, J., Wu, X., He, et al. (2013). 5-Fluorouracil-loaded poly-l-lactide fibrous membranefor the prevention of intestinal stent restenosis. *Journal of Materials Science*, *48*(18), 6186–6193.

Liao, H. T., Lai, Y. T., Kuo, C. Y., & Chen, J. P. (2021). A bioactive multi-functional heparin-grafted aligned poly (lactide-co-glycolide)/curcuminnanofiber membrane to accelerate diabetic wound healing. *Materials Science and Engineering: C*, *120*, 111689.

Lim, C. T. (2017). Nanofiber technology: current status and emerging developments. *Progress in Polymer Science*, *70*, 1–17.

Liu S, Wang X, Zhang Z, Zhang Y, Zhou G, Huang Y, et al. (2015). Use of asymmetric multilayer polylactidenanofiber mats in controlled release of drugs and prevention of liver cancer recurrence after surgery in mice. *Nanomedicine: Nanotechnology, Biology and Medicine*, *11*(5), 1047–1056.

Liu S, Zhou G, Liu D, Xie Z, Huang Y, Wang X, et al. (2013). Inhibition of orthotopic secondary hepatic carcinoma in mice by doxorubicin-loaded electrospunpolylactidenanofibers. *Journal of Materials Chemistry B*, *1*(1), 101–109.

Liu, F., Li, X., Wang, L., Yan, X., Ma, D., Liu, Z., & Liu, X. (2020). Sesamol incorporated cellulose acetate-zein composite nanofiber membrane: An efficient strategy to accelerate diabetic wound healing. *International Journal Of Biological Macromolecules*, *149*, 627–638.

Lu, T., Jing, X., Song, X., & Wang, X. (2012). Doxorubicin-loaded ultrafine PEG-PLA fiber mats against hepatocarcinoma. *Journal of Applied Polymer Science*, *123*(1), 209–217.

Ma, G., Liu, Y., Peng, C., Fang, D., He, B., & Nie, J. (2011). Paclitaxel loaded electrospun porous nanofibers as mat potential application for chemotherapy against prostate cancer. *Carbohydrate Polymers*, *86*(2), 505–512.

Merrell, J. G., McLaughlin, S. W., Tie, L., Laurencin, C. T., Chen, A. F., & Nair, L. S. (2009). Curcumin loaded poly (ε-caprolactone) nanofibers: diabetic wound dressing with antioxidant and anti-inflammatory properties. *Clinical and Experimental Pharmacology & Physiology*, *36*(12), 1149.

Moura, L. I., Dias, A. M., Leal, E. C., Carvalho, L., de Sousa, H. C., & Carvalho, E. (2014). Chitosan-based dressings loaded withneurotensin—an efficient strategy to improve early diabetic wound healing. *Actabiomaterialia*, *10*(2), 843–857.

Müller, W. E., Tolba, E., Dorweiler, B., Schröder, H. C., Diehl-Seifert, B., & Wang, X. (2015). Electrospun bioactive mats enriched with Ca-polyphosphate/retinol nanospheres as potential wound dressing. *Biochemistry and biophysics reports*, *3* 150–160.

Nagal, A., & Singla, R. K. (2013). Applications of silk in drug delivery: Advancement in pharmaceutical dosage forms. *Indo Global Journal of Pharmaceutical Sciences*, *3*(3), 204–211.

Nayak, R., Padhye, R., Kyratzis, I. L., Truong, Y. B., & Arnold, L. (2012). Recent advances in nanofibre fabrication techniques. *Textile Research Journal*, *82*(2), 129–147.

Pinzón-García, A. D., Cassini-Vieira, P., Ribeiro, C. C., de Matos Jensen, C. E., Barcelos, L. S., Cortes, M. E., & Sinisterra, R. D. (2017). Efficient cutaneous wound healing using bixin-loaded PCL nanofibers in diabetic mice. *Journal of Biomedical Materials Research Part B: Applied Biomaterials*, *105*(7), 1938–1949.

Ramos S. D., Giaconia M. A., Assis M., Jimenez P. C., Mazzo T. M., Longo E., et al. (2021). Uniaxial and coaxial electrospinning for tailoring jussara pulp nanofibers. *Molecules*, *26*(5), 1206.

Ranganath, S. H. & Wang, C. H. (2008). Biodegradable microfiber implants delivering paclitaxel for post-surgical chemotherapy against malignant glioma. *Biomaterials*, *29*(20), 2996–3003.

Razzaq A., Khan Z. U., Saeed A., Shah K. A., Khan N. U., Menaa B., et al. (2021). Development of cephradine-loaded gelatin/polyvinyl alcohol electrospunnanofibers for effective diabetic wound healing: in vitro and in vivo assessments. *Pharmaceutics*, *13*(3), 349.

Rujitanaroj, P. O., Pimpha, N., & Supaphol, P. (2008). Wound-dressing materials with antibacterial activity from electrospun gelatin fiber mats containing silver nanoparticles. *Polymer*, *49*(21), 4723–4732.

Said, S. S., Aloufy, A. K., El-Halfawy, O. M., Boraei, N. A., & El-Khordagui, L. K. (2011). Antimicrobial PLGA ultrafine fibers: Interaction with wound bacteria. *European Journal of Pharmaceutics and Biopharmaceutics*, *79*(1), 108–118.

Sampath, M., Lakra, R., Korrapati, P., & Sengottuvelan, B. (2014). Curcumin loaded poly (lactic-co-glycolic) acid nanofiber for the treatment of carcinoma. *Colloids and Surfaces B: Biointerfaces*, *117*, 128–134.

Schneider, A., Wang, X. Y., Kaplan, D. L., Garlick, J. A., & Egles, C. (2009). Biofunctionalized electrospun silk mats as a topical bioactive dressing for accelerated wound healing. *Actabiomaterialia*, *5*(7), 2570–2578.

Sedghi, R., Shaabani, A., Mohammadi, Z., Samadi, F. Y., & Isaei, E. (2017). Biocompatible electrospinning chitosan nanofibers: a novel delivery system with superior local cancer therapy. *Carbohydrate Polymers*, *159*, 1–10.

Selvaraj, S., & Fathima, N. N. (2017). Fenugreek incorporated silk fibroin nanofibers – A potential antioxidant scaffold for enhanced wound healing. *ACS Applied Materials & Interfaces*, *9*(7), 5916–5926.

Shalaby, T. I., Fekry, N. M., Sodfy, A. S. E., Sheredy, A. G. E., & Moustafa, M. E. S. S. A. (2015). Preparation and characterisation of antibacterial silver-containing nanofibres for wound healing in diabetic mice. *International Journal of Nanoparticles*, *8*(1), 82–98.

Sharma, A. K., 2017. Biopolymers in drug delivery. Biopolymers Res 1: e101. *of*, *2*, pp. 255-263.

Srivastava, Y., Marquez, M., & Thorsen, T. (2007). Multijetelectrospinning of conducting nanofibers from microfluidic manifolds. *Journal of Applied Polymer Science*, *106*(5), 3171–3178.

Su S., Bedir T., Kalkandelen C., Başar A. O., Şaşmazel H. T., Ustundag C. B., et al. (2021). Coaxial and emulsion electrospinning of extracted hyaluronic acid and keratin based nanofibers for wound healing applications. *European Polymer Journal*, *142*, 110158.

Tan, Y. L., & Ho, H. K. (2018). Navigating albumin-based nanoparticles through various drug delivery routes. *Drug Discovery Today*, *23*(5), 1108–1114.

Taylor, G. I. (1964). Disintegration of water drops in an electric field. *Proceedings of the Royal Society of London. Series A. Mathematical and Physical Sciences*, *280*(1382), 383–397.

Tønnesen, H. H., & Karlsen, J. (2002). Alginate in drug delivery systems. *Drug Development and Industrial Pharmacy*, *28*(6), 621–630.

Toshkova, R., Manolova, N., Gardeva, E., Ignatova, M., Yossifova, L., Rashkov, I., & Alexandrov, M. (2010). Antitumor activity of quaternized chitosan-based electrospun implants against Graffi myeloid tumor. *International Journal of Pharmaceutics*, *400*(1-2), 221–233.

Vashisth, P., Sharma, M., Nikhil, K., Singh, H., Panwar, R., Pruthi, P. A., & Pruthi, V. (2015). Antiproliferative activity of ferulic acid-encapsulated electrospun PLGA/PEO nanofibers against MCF-7 human breast carcinoma cells. *3 Biotech*, *5*(3), 303–315.

Vashisth, P., Srivastava, A. K., Nagar, H., Raghuwanshi, N., Sharan, S., Nikhil, K., et al. (2016). Drug functionalized microbial polysaccharide based nanofibers as transdermal substitute. *Nanomedicine: Nanotechnology, Biology and Medicine*, *12*(5), 1375–1385.

Wang C., Ma C., Wu Z., Liang H., Yan P., Song J., et al. (2015). Enhanced bioavailability and anticancer effect of curcumin-loadedelectrospunnanofiber: in vitro and in vivo study. *Nanoscale Research Letters*, *10*(1), 1–10.

Wu T, Ding M, Shi C, Qiao Y, Wang P, Qiao R, et al. (2020). Resorbable polymer electrospunnanofibers: History, shapes and application for tissue engineering. *Chinese Chemical Letters*, *31*(3), 617–625.

Xie, C., Li, X., Luo, X., Yang, Y., Cui, W., Zou, J., & Zhou, S. (2010). Release modulation and cytotoxicity of hydroxycamptothecin-loadedelectrospun fibers with 2-hydroxypropyl-β-cyclodextrin inoculations. *International Journal of Pharmaceutics*, *391*(1-2), 55–64.

Xie, J., Tan, R. S., & Wang, C. H. (2008). Biodegradable microparticles and fiber fabrics for sustained delivery of cisplatin to treat C6 glioma in vitro. *Journal of Biomedical Materials Research Part A: An Official Journal of The Society for Biomaterials*, *85*(4), 897–908.

Xu, X., Chen, X., Wang, Z., & Jing, X. (2009). Ultrafine PEG–PLA fibers loaded with both paclitaxel and doxorubicin hydrochloride and their in vitro cytotoxicity. *European Journal of Pharmaceutics and Biopharmaceutics*, *72*(1), 18–25.

Xu, X., Chen, X., Xu, X., Lu, T., Wang, X., Yang, L., & Jing, X. (2006). BCNU-loaded PEG–PLLA ultrafine fibers and their in vitro antitumor activity against Glioma C6 cells. *Journal of Controlled Release*, *114*(3), 307–316.

Xue, J., Wu, T., Dai, Y., & Xia, Y. (2019). Electrospinning and electrospunnanofibers: Methods, materials, and applications. *Chemical Reviews*, *119*(8), 5298–5415.

Yan, G., Yu, J., Qiu, Y., Yi, X., Lu, J., Zhou, X., & Bai, X. (2011). Self-assembly of electrospun polymer nanofibers: A general phenomenon generating honeycomb-patterned nanofibrous structures. *Langmuir*, *27*(8), 4285–4289.

Yohe, S. T., Herrera, V. L., Colson, Y. L., & Grinstaff, M. W. (2012). 3D superhydrophobicelectrospun meshes as reinforcement materials for sustained local drug delivery against colorectal cancer cells. *Journal of Controlled Release*, *162*(1), 92–101.

Yukseloglu, S. M., Sokmen, N., & Canoglu, S. (2015). Biomaterial applications of silk fibroin electrospunnanofibres. *Microelectronic Engineering*, *146*, 43–47.

Zhang, J., Wang, X., Liu, T., Liu, S., & Jing, X. (2016). Antitumor activity of electrospunpolylactidenanofibers loaded with 55-fluorouracil and oxaliplatin against colorectal cancer. *Drug Delivery*, *23*(3), 784–790.

Zhao, Z., Li, Y., & Xie, M. B. (2015). Silk fibroin-based nanoparticles for drug delivery. *International Journal of Molecular Sciences*, *16*(3), 4880–4903.

Zhu X., Ni S., Xia T., Yao Q., Li H., Wang B., et al. (2015). Anti-neoplastic cytotoxicity of SN-38-loaded PCL/Gelatin electrospun composite nanofiber scaffolds against human glioblastoma cells in vitro. *Journal of Pharmaceutical Sciences*, *104*(12), 4345–4354.

Zong S., Wang X., Yang Y., Wu W., Li H., Ma Y., et al. (2015). The use of cisplatin-loaded mucoadhesivenanofibers for local chemotherapy of cervical cancers in mice. *European Journal of Pharmaceutics and Biopharmaceutics*, *93*, 127–135.

35

Therapeutic Translational Potential of Surface-Decorated Nanoparticles

Nidhi Mishra, Raquibun Nisha, Ravi Raj, Pal Alka, Priya Singh, Neelu Singh, and Shubhini Saraf
Department of Pharmaceutical Sciences, Babasaheb Bhimrao Ambedkar University, Lucknow, India

35.1 Introduction

Nanotechnology is a developing and alluring research domain that has the power to promote both targeted molecular imaging and customized therapies by facilitating the development and engineering of future multi-functional nanosystems [1]. Nanoparticles (NPs) have become a progressively practical approach for bioimaging and drug delivery recently. NPs have several exciting and peculiar characteristics due to their small dimensions. These NPs can interact on a molecular level owing to their nanometric scale. NPs are usually made up of three layers: the core (the innermost part constituting the NP's primary material); the shell layer (the middle layer, chemically distinct from the core); and the exterior layer, the outermost layer that is decorated with other particles through surface associations. Nanomaterials may be natural, synthetic, or a mix of both types of material and comprise particles in unbound forms, agglomerates, or aggregates. The external sizes range between 1 to 100 nm for almost half or more of the particles. They have been categorized based on dimensions, nature, origin, and type of material used. Nanomaterials have significant strengths over bulk counterparts in that they possess unique physical and chemical characteristics attributable to their nanoscale dimensions and elevated surface-area-to-volume ratio. Typically, nanoparticulate systems are crafted to significantly boost circulation time, address diseased cells, improve retention, and provide desired payload release at targeted sites. To achieve these goals, the NP surface is frequently altered by attaching many biological and chemical substituents, such as poly(ethylene glycol) (PEG), peptides, and smart linkers. Regardless of surface modifications, the nano-bio interface, dominated by the protein corona and opsonization, is often challenging. NPs possess improved reactivity, solubility, biomimetic properties, and the potential to be functionalized with other materials such as drugs, bioactive entities, photoactive agents, etc. [2-5]. A broad spectrum of nanopreparations formulated using natural materials (e.g., chitosan, alginate, dextran, protein), carbon-based carriers (e.g., carbon nanotubes, quantum dots), synthetic polymeric carriers (e.g., block copolymers, dendrimers, polymersomes), metallic ions, etc., have been developed for drug delivery and diagnostics to address rapid clearance rates of unmodified NPs. Despite the inherent and distinct benefits of these materials, unmodified NPs have a substantial and imprecise clearance rate. As a result, surface decoration/modification/functionalization incorporated to NPs/nanoparticle compounding materials are intended to obscure inherent NP properties or control biological interactions. Surface decoration improves the characteristics and behaviours of NPs, allowing them to play a vital role in healthcare. Due to their poor targeting and significant toxicity, NPs were feared to have minimal applications. Multi-functional NPs have been shown to transform the way molecular interactions are tracked and revealed. Without functionalization, the NPs show a non-selective distribution and are unable to cross biological barriers. For potential applications in theranostics, as well as to resolve the minor limitations that these NPs previously had, the surface attributes of NPs must be altered via surface decoration. The surface decoration of NPs is advantageous in maximizing circulation and residence time, targeting desired cell/tissue,

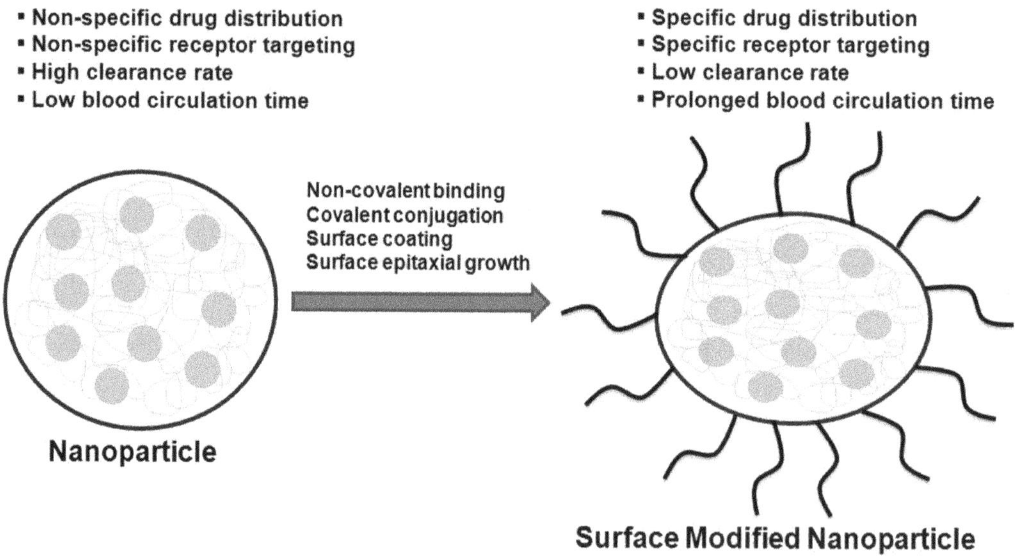

- **Non-specific drug distribution**
- **Non-specific receptor targeting**
- **High clearance rate**
- **Low blood circulation time**

- **Specific drug distribution**
- **Specific receptor targeting**
- **Low clearance rate**
- **Prolonged blood circulation time**

Non-covalent binding
Covalent conjugation
Surface coating
Surface epitaxial growth

Nanoparticle

Surface Modified Nanoparticle

FIGURE 35.1 Major advantages of surface-decorated nanoparticles over unmodified nanoparticles and common methods to surface-decorate nanoparticles.

andefficiently delivering therapeutic drug payload at the target site [6-8]. The significant advantages of surface-decorated NPs over unmodified NPs are shown in Figure 35.1.

Surface modification of NPs enables us to impart properties in NPs that we are explicitly interested in, allowing us to assist a specific therapy approach. Conjugation of molecules on the surface of the particles is needed for the functionalization of NPs. Surface decoration/functionalization is the process of conjugating chemical entities/biomolecules such as folic acid, hyaluronic acid, biotin, peptides, nucleotides, antibodies, etc., to the surface of NPs to improve their properties and target specificity. The elevated surface-to-volume ratio enables successful particle functionalization to meet our requirements. Knowing the chemistry behind the conjugation is crucial because it allows one to assess the viability of different functionalization approaches. Functionalization approaches are broadly categorized as:

1.1 Non-covalent Binding: Conjugation through non-covalent interactions involves the attachment of specific secondary ligands via $\pi-\pi$ stacking, electrostatic interaction, and adsorption of bioactive molecules in the compatible polymeric films. Affinity-based receptor-ligand systems are commonly used to execute the non-covalent conjugation of biomolecules on NPs.

1.2 Covalent Conjugation: One of the most reliable and successful methods for functionalization is direct covalent conjugation of the molecule of interest to the reactive ligands on the NP surface. This method uses a catalyst/linker to facilitate the linkage reaction, and is usually favoured over imprecise physisorption because of the acquired functionalization stability.

1.3 Surface Coating: Inorganic metallic NPs required to be coated with silica or maybe another amorphous polymer that is capable of incorporating functional groups to their surface. Surface coating gives the NP more versatility by enabling association of desired ligand/therapeutic agent.

1.4 Epitaxial Surface Growth: In the epitaxial method, an organic or inorganic overlayer is deposited on a substrate to modify the surface of NP. For example, functional composite NPs can be developed by growing iron oxide NPs epitaxially on gold to produce gold iron oxide NPs.

The functionalized NPs have excellent physical attributes as well as anti-agglomeration, anti-corrosion, and non-invasive characteristics. Functionalization of NPs has dramatically enhanced their biocompatibility and increased their applicability from imaging to theranostics, multimodal imaging, and intraoperative therapies. Surface modification can alter the solubility, biocompatibility, biodistribution, and clearance of nanosystems by influencing properties like size, shape, surface chemistry, hydrophilicity, lipophilicity, charge, etc. The nanosystems display improved biodistribution with longer circulation time and efficient cellular uptake when coated with small molecules or polymers like starch, dextran, PEG, etc. PEG-conjugated NPs show steric stabilization, prolonged in vivo blood circulation, and avoid protein absorption. Researchers are trying to develop different strategies to functionalize NPs to enrich molecular images acquired with various methodologies, both in vitro and in vivo. These functionalized nanoprobes, together with the imaging modality, may unveil the requisite structural and/or functional details. Since NP functionalization can improve both imaging and therapy at the same time, theranosticnanoprobes for tumours have become an essential subject of recent research. Due to the enhanced permeability and retention (EPR) effect, surface-modified NPs provide selective accumulation in tumour tissue, which helps to identify cells/tissues of interest for imaging and drug delivery. In contrast with healthy tissues, the tumorous tissues have more permeable vasculature, relatively poor lymphatic system, and higher levels of vascular endothelial growth factor and basic fibroblast growth factor. This distinction facilitates intensified targeting, distribution, and interaction at the molecular level. Surface decoration promotes target-specific imaging of tissues or cells to analyze a disease/tissue injury quantitatively, this can be achieved if the labelling is done with high specificity [1, 3, 6, 9].

The role of surface-decorated NPs in the imaging and treatment of diseases is discussed in the following sections.

35.2 Surface-Decorated Nanoparticles in Diagnosis of Diseases via Imaging

Surface decoration empowers the development of NPs with properties that we are primarily interested in, thus aiding a particular imaging methodology. It not only improves image quality but also expands the imaging modality's applicability and versatility. Functionalization of NPs for diagnostics has also been discovered to be done with another NP to improve its characteristics in different studies [10]. Functionalization provides NPs with multimodal features, targeted functionalities, and the potential for many intraoperative therapies. Theranostics, hybrid andmultimodal imaging, intraoperative therapies, and molecular targeting are among the other aspects relevant to molecular imaging that stand to benefit from functionalization. Figure 35.2 shows the various applications of surface-decorated NPs and common methods to surface-decorate NPs. Many in vitro and in vivo studies have shown how functionalization can improve and aid imaging techniques such asmagnetic resonance imaging (MRI), computed tomography (CT), positron emission tomography (PET), confocal microscopy, fluorescence imaging, etc. [11, 12]. Functionalized NPs tend to interact with each other as per the imaging modality, unveiling the intended functional and/or structural details.

The following are some imaging methods for disease diagnosis.

35.2.1 MRI

MRI is a well-established biomedical method among different diagnostic imaging techniques; it is a favourable diagnostic test for medicine with stronger tissue contrasts. The comparison level is hampered by the misdiagnosis of many medical conditions in other diagnostic methods, including X-rays. The peculiar magnetic properties that combine to make these excellent MRI-contrasting agents with powerful cytotoxic agents against tumours have sparked a lot of interest [13]. Contrast agents (CAs) are classified as negative (T2 weighted) or positive (T1 weighted) in MRI. NPs are preferred and substituted over CAs due to their prolonged blood circulation time advantageous for diagnosis; also, they can be surface-modified to maximize their efficiency. Examples of Negative CAs include magnetic NPs and iron oxide NPs (IONPs). However, soluble gadolinium, a T1 weighted compound can be used to capture compelling contrast images [14]. For theranostics application, NPs that are both biocompatible and biodegradable are preferred. Ratzinger et al. demonstrated that surface-functionalized PLGA NPs with Gd3+, fixed with ligands to attach reactive groups that can covalently bind with Gd3+ and other entities on the surface, turn into effective MRI CAs [15-19].

35.2.2 CT

CT, by using X-rays, can provide a 3D image, while X-rays can only provide a 2D image. The use of NPs as next-generation CT contrast agents has accelerated as CT has become one of the most widely used radiology methods in biomedical imaging. NPs are anticipated to play a prominent role in the future of medical diagnostics due to their numerous benefits over conventional contrast agents, such as extended blood circulation time, complex molecular targeting capabilities, and controlled biological clearance pathways [20]. Cole et al. established that gold NPs connected with biphosphates can detect hydroxyl apatite micro-calcifications that are undetectable when non-functionalized particles are used. As a result, through specific binding to hydroxyapatite crystals, functionalization improved image contrast. By functionalizing an involved gene with poly(2-(N,N-dimethyl amino)ethyl methacrylate), gold nanorods can be used asgene carriers as well as CT imaging agents [21-23].

35.2.3 PET

PET is a form of functional imaging that can investigate the metabolic processes and identify diseases before they become severe. PET and nanotechnology have a complex synergy that blends the sensitivity of PET with quantitative nature and the multi-functionality and tunability of nanomaterials to help solve some of the world's most pressing problems [24]. For improved and extended PET imaging, NPs are conjugated with radiotracers. Chen et al. developed stable thiol and PEG-functionalized mesoporous silica particles (mSiO2), connected with TRC105 antibody, unique to CD105 present in murine breast cancer cells to minimize opsonization. When mSiO2 NPs are functionalized with CuCl2 and connected with Cu radioisotope via a bond with NOTA ($C_{20}H_{37}N_3O_6$) chemical molecule, they become PET imaging agents [25-27].

35.2.4 Fluorescence Imaging

Fluorescence imaging has a high sensitivity for imaging and detecting molecular interactions, and it can also detect expression levels. Nanoprobes can be tuned to make the imaging device work better. Various methods based on NP functionalization have been investigated to improve fluorescence imaging. The fluorescence properties of the NPs are due to the SiO2-N. The depth of imaging is determined by the properties of the excitation light, such as transmission and focal capacity. Wang et al. demonstrated that gold nanorods functionalized with PEG became luminescent probes when excited at 1000 nm with a femtosecond laser. When excited at 760 nm, in vivo imaging of the brain is performed at a depth of 600 um, yielding high contrast images due to three-photon luminescence, while imaging at a depth of 430 um yields two-photon luminescence signals [28].

Fluorescence-based techniques such as flow cytometry and confocal microscopy are widely used to investigate the surface modification of cells with NPs or the internalization of NPs by cells. NP-specific functioning methods for fluorescent imaging are also explored via quantum dots (QDs) and silica NPs [29].

35.2.4.1 QDs

While QDs are used for efficient, bright fluorescence imaging, their application is restricted due to severe toxicity and inadequate stability. The zwitterion ligands bind to the surface of CdSe/CdS/ZnS QDs, passivating it and increasing fluorescence while lowering cytotoxicity. QDs are normally functionalized with chitosan molecules for increased stability, which then allows for additional functionality [28][30]. It is essential to visualize tumour cells and recognize the human participants inside them. Many imaging oncomarkers have overexpressed receptors on the membrane surface of tumour cells, whereas they are almost non-expressed in normal tissues [31].

35.2.4.2 Silica NPs

By attaching different functional groups, the surface of silica can be modified in many ways. Functional groups may be entrapped within mesoporous particles, protecting them from unwanted influencing factors. Vivero-Escoto et al. reported that doping silica NPs with three distinct dyes and functionalizing them with three separate aptamers by integrating biotin via PEG allows parallel multi-imaging [32]. Wang et al. identified that non-covalent interactions between silica particles and aggregation-induced emission (AIE) dyes result in increased fluorescence, but further mounting with AIE luminogens will not activate quenching. The MCF 7 cells can be targeted with higher affinity leveraging aptamer-linked functionalized particles and AIE dyes, and the accumulation of NPs induces fluorescence. False positives can be removed to eliminate ambiguities employing this strategy [33].

35.3 Surface-Decorated Nanoparticles in Treatment of Diseases via Receptor Targeting

Targeted therapy is a disease therapy strategy that involves administering sufficient quantities of therapeutic agents to the affected region of the body for an extended period. To achieve this, one of the ultimate objectives of nanomedicine is to produce safer and more proficient therapeutic NPs. Once NPs reach the bloodstream, they are susceptible to aggregation and protein opsonization. The NPs (opsonized) could be eliminated from the blood circulation via the spleen, kidney, and liver. The non-specific and rapid clearance of immune systems reduces retention time, which restricts the bioavailability. The NP's retention time can be transformed by coating them with PEG, acetyl groups, carbohydrates, or protein moieties [34]. The surface alteration, however, may affect the recognition capacity for targeted delivery. The use of long-chain polymers, including PEG, on the surface of NPs has been shown to reduce protein absorption (non-specific) onto the surface of NPs.

The use of surface-targeting ligands, which promote the binding of therapeutic molecules to their epitopes by targeting ligands to their definite receptors, is one of the most appealing approaches. As a result, developing these methods and nanotherapeutics that directly and preferentially target the desired/specific site(s)/tissues with minimal haemolytic and cytotoxicity should be prioritized [35, 36]. The overexpression of receptors at a particular site, which is essential in the biological milieu of nanomedicines, plays a crucial role in receptor-targeted bioactive delivery by the specific ligand-receptor binding affinity. Specific surface-anchored nano-carriers bind selectively with specific receptors because the receptors have specificbinding sites that allow only the specific targeting moiety with a specific orientation to be recognized [36]. Various receptors like ASGPR, CD44, Folate receptor, etc., and other targeting ligands are used for surface targeting. Figure 35.2 illustrates the representation of some of the significant receptors expressed in cells. The majorly targeted receptors via surface decoration of NPs are discussed below.

35.3.1 CD44 Targeting

CD44 (multi-functional) cell surface receptor is a glycoprotein extensively present on the surface of mammalian cells, such as epithelial cells, endothelial cells, leukocytes, fibroblasts, and keratinocytes

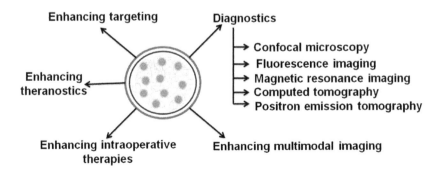

FIGURE 35.2 Applications of surface-decorated nanoparticles.

[37]. It has numerous important pharmacological and physiological functions in (cell-cell) and (cell-matrix) interactions include homing, adhesion, proliferation, haematopoiesis, migration, lymphocyte activation, and extravasation [38]. CD44 and its isoforms play essential functions in a variety of pathological settings throughout their binding to many extracellular matrix (EM) components, which includes hyaluronic acid (HA), collagens, osteopontin, and matrix metalloproteinases [39-41]. When CD44 binds to its major ligand HA, it stimulates specific signalling pathways to promote their functioning [42]. HA is a glycosaminoglycan abundantly distributed in the EM. HA regulates diverse cellular performance in this compartment like cell adhesion, cell migration, cell growth, and differentiation [43]. HA being biodegradable and biocompatible and specifically binding to the cancer cells' surface receptors has madeimmense development. It can be utilized as a nano-carrier and respond withother drugs to form surface conjugates. The cell surface conjugates have the sustained release and targeted outcome to defined pathological areas to achieve greater therapeutic efficacy [44]. It is also used in several diseases (e.g., arthritis, vascular disease, interstitial lung disease (ILD), wound healing, and infections) [37].

35.3.2 Folate Receptor

Folate receptor (FR) is a folate-binding protein that binds to the membrane with high affinity. It is a membrane glycoprotein connected to glycosylphosphatidylinositol (GPI) with an apparent molecular weight of 38–40 KDa. Its expression levels are low in healthy cells but are abundantly expressed in cancerous cells. The overexpression of FR in cancer cells makes it a possible ligand target. The folate cycle is needed for rapid cell growth and to maintainvital metabolic reactions. Exogenous reduced folates are mainly transported inside the cells in physiological situations with high-capacity, less affinity, and ubiquitously expressed reduced folate carrier. Folic acid (FA), a targeting agent (low molecular weight) that can link to the folate receptor, can be coated on NPs as a ligand. For targeting cancerous cells, FA is grafted onto the surface of NPs [45]. The surface-anchored receptor-ligand complex is transported inside the cell through receptor-mediated endocytosis for ligand release once FA binds to the FR [46].

35.3.3 Asialoglycoprotein Receptor (ASGPR)

Asialoglycoprotein is a heterooligomer (C-type lectin) receptor made up of two homologous polypeptides with a molecular mass of 41 KDa. This polypeptide is only found in the liver and is absent from the rest of the human body. This transmembrane protein is a surface receptor that can recognize the terminals of D-Galactose and is found on the hepatocytes' membranes facing the sinusoids [47]. Indeed, each hepatocyte contains around 500,000 asialoglycoproteins, glycoproteins with galactose groups, and specificity for them. This endogenous glycoprotein is overexpressed in HCC and has high binding potential,

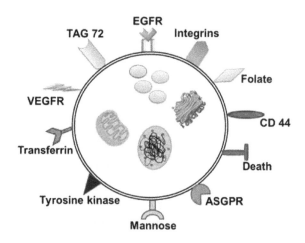

FIGURE 35.3 Some of the major receptors commonly expressed in cells.

allowing galactose ligands to be taken up efficiently by the cells. The ASGP receptors specifically recognize and attach the galactose moieties onto the surface of NPs, despite being highly overexpressed on hepatocytes [48]. The clearance of desialylated glycoproteins from circulation is its physiological role. The receptor is internalized by receptor-mediated endocytosis within minutes of ligand binding [49].

35.3.4 Epidermal Growth Factor Receptor (EGFR)

The EGFR (also known as HER1) is a transmembrane receptor with inherent tyrosine kinase activity. A gene on chromosome 7 codes for it [50]. When activated, the EGFR stimulates many downstream pathways at the cellular level, particularly those responsible for cell proliferation, viability, and anti-apoptosis [48, 49]. Squamous cell carcinoma and adenocarcinoma have higher rates of EGFR overexpression, whereas large-cell carcinoma has a lower rate. The EGFR's tyrosine kinase activity is tightly regulated in normal cells, and thus cell growth is controlled. Although the EGFR signaling cascades are complex, the tyrosine kinase in the intracellular domain of the EGFR is the core factor that triggers signaling. If tyrosine kinase activity is blocked, EGFR fails to propagate signals to the cell nucleus [50]. This may be because the wild-type EGFR usually sends a weak downstream signal that triggers the proliferation of cancer cells that depend on it, and gefitinib and erlotinib can only marginally inhibit this feeble signal [48].

35.3.5 Tumour-Associated Glycoprotein 72 (TAG 72) Receptor

TAG72 is a cell surface glycoprotein that behaves similar to mucin and is overexpressed in pancreatic cancer [51]. TAG72 overexpression is found in 88% of all stages of ovarian cancer, and there is a strong link between TAG72 expression and patient prognosis, whereas normal TAG72 expression is restricted to endometrial tissues all through the secretory stage [52]. It has been shown to be a more accurate prognostic predictor than carcinoembryonic antigen (CEA) [53]. Moreover, this, and regardless of the fact that Indium-111 satumomabpendetide, a derivative of the anti-TAG72 antibody B72.3, was the first monoclonal antibody to be approved for cancer imaging other anti-TAG72 mAb applications floundered [54]. Fortunately, novel initiatives to exploit TAG72 for prognostic assessment [55] and immunofluorescence-guided surgery are being explored [56].

35.3.6 TransferrinReceptors (TFRs)

TFR1 and TFR2 are two TFR subtypes that form a complex with iron to help cells in iron metabolism. As a result, the dysregulated expression will hinder iron metabolism in any subtype condition, leading to tumorigenesis and cancer development [57]. TFR1 is highly expressed in several cancer species, including breast, liver, pancreatic, lung, and colon cancer cells [57, 58], and hence can be used as a drug delivery target. Transferrin (Tf), a ligand of TFR1, has been commonly used in surface modification of mesoporous silica nanoparticles (MSNs) to enhance the tumour-specific distribution of MSN carriers [59]. Tf-modified MSN improves NP uptake by Panc-1 cancer cells, as demonstrated by available studies targeting TFR1 [60]. Furthermore, Quiros et al. employed MSN as a nano-vehicle adorned with Tf to provide a nano-platform for the nucleation and immobilization of silver nanoparticles (AgNPs), demonstrating that only the Tf-modified nanosystem can transport AgNPs inside Tf receptors overexpressing human hepatocarcinoma (HepG2) cells [61]. Nonetheless, Tf-decorated MSN has been used to distribute sorafenib to patients with thyroid cancer [62]. Overexpression of TFRs on brain capillary endothelial cells of the blood-brain barrier (BBB) and glioblastoma multiforme presents a channel for delivery of chemotherapeutics at the tumorous site [63]. Few study groups have developed Tf-conjugated MSN to transmit chemotherapeutic agents to glioma cells through the BBB [64, 65].

35.3.7 Tyrosine Kinase Receptors

Tyrosine kinases play a crucial function in tumorigenesis. Depending on where they are present in the cell, they are categorized into transmembrane receptor tyrosine kinases (RTK) and cytoplasmic non-receptor tyrosine kinases (NRTK). Extracellular signal molecules, such as growth factors like EGF or PDGF, activate tyrosine kinase receptor dimerization. Non-receptor tyrosine kinases, such as SRC, Abl, Fak, and Janus, differ from RTK in that they are enzymes with significant structural variability [66]. Tyrosine kinase function has been linked to the growth and progression of cancer at various levels. The stimulation of development, cell proliferation, and the inhibition of apoptosis are all functions of tyrosine kinases in cell signalling. As a result, the lack of cell growth regulation is often caused by genetic or epigenetic changes in kinase function, giving it an oncogenic nature [67]. Mutations in the genomes of tyrosine kinases such as EGFR, PI3K, ABL, FGFR1, cMer, c-Kit, and RET induce tumorigenesis in humans. In contrast, other mutations in the TK genes are frequently discovered due to the genetic instability of neo-plastic cells' uncontrolled replication and proliferation [68-77].

35.3.8 Vascular Endothelial Growth Factor Receptors (VEGFRs)

In tumour angiogenesis and metastasis, vascular endothelial growth factors (VEGFs) and their receptors (VEGFRs) are essential. VEGFR2 is the most studied of the three receptors (VEGFR1, VEGFR2, and VEGFR3) as a direct angiogenesis stimulator. In addition to its normative expression on angiogenic endo-thelial cells, VEGFR2 is overexpressed on a variety of cancer cells, including pancreatic cancer, colon cancer, breast cancer, glioblastoma, gastrointestinal cancer, liver carcinoma, adenocarcinoma, bladder cancer, ovarian cancer, osteosarcoma, etc. [78]. For the VEGFR2 target, Weibo and colleagues used VEGF121, a natural VEGFR ligand with high VEGFR2-binding affinity and strong, specific VEGF121-coated MSN surface binding in Human Umbilical Vein Endothelial Cells (HUVEC) (VEGFR+) but not in 4T1 cells (VEGFR-) [79]. Using the VEGF121 ligand to target VEGFR, the same team reported improved delivery of the MSN encapsulating the anti-cancer drug sunitinib to the U87MG tumour (glioblastoma cell line) in comparison to non-targeted delivery [80]. Furthermore, Zhang et al. found that anti-VEGFR2 targeted MSN had improved targeting capacity and retention time in anaplastic thyroid cancer tumour-bearing mice [81]. VEGF receptors have also been targeted with bevacizumab or associated antibodies.

35.3.9 Integrin Receptors

Integrin receptors are heterodimeric ($\alpha\beta$) transmembrane glycoproteins that are overexpressed on angiogenetic endothelial cells and specific tumour cells, but they are absent in pre-existing endothelial cells and healthy tissues (or found in basal levels) [82, 83]. As a consequence, integrins, particularly $\alpha\nu\beta3$ integrin receptors, are an exciting target in cancer therapy, and RGD (arginine-glycine-aspartic acid)-based peptides have been extensively used to target chemotherapeutics to tumours and tumour vasculatures via overexpressed integrin receptors [84]. Peptides containing the RGD motif have been extensively used in MSN surface decoration for cancer therapy targeting [85-90]. Pan et al. also demonstrated the effective-ness of doxorubicin-loaded MSN grafted with the RGD-motif in vivo and achieved improved accumula-tion of tumours and decreased the tumour size by coupling cell-penetrating nuclear-targeting TAT peptide and RGD to the MSNs. Treatment with RGD/TAT-MSN significantly reduced the side effects of bare MSN accumulation in the liver and spleen [91].

35.3.10 Death Receptors

Death receptors belong to the superfamily receptor TNF (tumour necrosis factor)/NGF (nerve growth factor). External killers (death ligands) binding or ligating cell surface receptors may also control apop-tosis, according to death receptors [92]. TNF-R1 (tumour necrosis factor receptor 1 (also known as CD120a), CD95 (also known as APO-1 and Fas), DR3 (also known as APO-3, LARD, TRAMP and WSL1), TRAIL-R1 (TNF-related apoptosis-inducing ligand-receptor 1 (also known as APO-2 and DR4), TRAIL-R2 (also known as DR5, KILLER, and TRICK2), and DR6 are the six members of this death receptor subfamily that have been identified so far [93-95]. Furthermore, since they contain cytoplasmic regions that resemble death domains, the ectodysplasin-A receptor (EDA-R) and the nerve growth factor receptor (NGF-R, p75, NTR) are also referred to as death receptors. On the other hand, their death domains vary significantly from the classical death domain in terms of structure and function, and no binding to fas-associated death domain (FADD) or tumor necrosis factor receptor type 1-associated death domain (TRADD) has been found. Death receptors play a critical role in preserving homeostasis by allowing toxic or undesirable cells to be eliminated without affecting liver physiology [92, 96]. Evolutionary pressure likely favoured increased death receptor expression and function in the liver to eradicate hepatotropic viruses, xenobiotic-damaged cells, and cells undergoing oncogenic transformation. The propensity of the liver to regenerate itself counterbalanced the increased sensitivity of liver cells to death receptor-mediated deletion. However, increased death receptor expression and activity is a precarious situation, as excessive activation will damage the liver in disease states. Apoptosis mediated by death receptors does facilitate hepatic inflammation and tissue destruction [97]. Mice given the Fas agonist Jo2 developed fulminant hepatitis and died within hours of injection [98]. Death receptors not only cause liver damage, but they also play a role in liver fibrosis. Hepatic fibrogenesis is inhibited by processes that block death receptor-mediated cell injury. In contrast, death receptor-mediated apoptosis of hepatic stellate cells (the cellular source of collagen in the liver) may be a possible anti-fibrogenic technique.

35.3.11 Mannose Receptor

Macrophages that are associated with tumours and that occur in the tumour microenvironment encourage tumour immunosuppression, metastasis,angiogenesis, and relapse. A successful therapeutic target for cancer treatment was suggested for tumour-associated macrophages (TAMs) expressing the multi-ligand endocytic receptor mannose receptor (CD206/MRC1) [99]. MSN combined with mannosylatedpolyethylenimine (MP) has been shown to target macrophage cells and improve transfection efficiency via receptor-mediated endocytosis through mannose receptors [100]. Furthermore, macrophages are the only cells that possess the C-type lectin receptor used to treat cancer. Recently, lectin-functionalized MSN was investigated in a model of colon cancer of the mouse [101].

Table 35.1 lists some examples of surface-decorated NPs for treatment of diseases via receptor targeting.

35.4 Patented Surface-Decorated NPs for Theranostics

Recently, surface-decorating approaches have gained increasing attention from scientists worldwide since surface-decorated NPs are precisely utilized for drug delivery and imaging applications, as well as the design of medical equipment. These functionalized particles can retain/accumulate at target sites to deliver drugs/siRNA protein or illuminate accumulated sites for diagnostic applications in a controlled manner. Also, these modified carriers deliver molecules from tissue to the cellular level. These surface-modified NPs are designed in a way that utilizes a physiological microenvironment that favours binding to specific structures. For example, for cancer conditions they offer enhanced permeability with leaky vasculature, which favours penetration and accumulations of particulate matter within the target structure [135]. Every pathological condition is associated with a modulated expression pattern of various proteins, which could be utilized for targeting, for example cancerous cells show abundant expression of the folate receptor. In this case, the folic acid-coated NP is utilized for cancer cell-specific delivery. The patents related to surface-decorated nanoformulations utilized for drug theranostic application are compiled in Table 35.2. Mannose-coated nanoparticulate suture materials that specifically bind to macrophages and inhibit their prostaglandin release were patented (KR101925442B1 South Korea) for drug delivery and coating of medical equipment.

35.5 Limitations and Perspectives

Nanotechnology has the potential to contribute to significant advancements in precision medicine in the future. The translation of scientific advancement to commercially viable products remains a challenge, and the success of developing nano-therapeutics depends on turning promising research outcomes into economically feasible technologies for stakeholders. Although numerous techniques of functionalization to enhance the properties of NPs are found and published in the mentioned domains, the majority of them

TABLE 35.1

Surface-Decorated Nanoparticles in Therapeutics via Receptor Targeting

Sr. No.	Receptors	Delivery system	Therapeutic agents	Disease	Function	References
1.	CD 44	Hyaluronic acid (HA)	Doxorubicin	Solid tumor, Breast carcinoma, Colon carcinoma, Hematological neoplasm Cancer Stem Cell (CSCs) Targeting	CD44 binds to HA present in the extracellular matrix (ECM), which helps in the attachment of CSCs to the ECM, which results in proliferation and migration of cancerous cells.	[102]
		Hyaluronic acid-fabricated gold NPs	Metformin	Hepatocellular carcinoma	HA-anchored metformin encapsulated gold NPs were fabricated through the formation of the amide bond. In vitro cytotoxicity study showed that NPs efficiently inhibited the cancer cells multiplication via active (CD44) targeting.	[103]
		PLGA NPs coated with hyaluronic acid	Paclitaxel and Salinomycin	Breast carcinoma	Surface decoration of HA enhanced (1.5-fold) uptake into the (CD44+ MDA-MB-231) cells and greater in vitro activity.	[104]
		Hyaluronic acid-coated chitosan NPs	Rifampicin	Tuberculosis (TB)	HA conjugated chitosan NPs of anti-TB agent is a promising approach to the deliver active macrophages via CD44 receptors through internalization owing to the existence of dipeptide (muramyl) onto the mycobacterium cell wall, which induces the CD44 expression.	[105]
		pH-responsive and hyaluronic acid-functionalized metal-organic frameworks	Protocatechuic acid	Osteoarthritis	HA successfully inhibited the production of IL-1β–stimulated Matrix Metallo-proteinases (MMPs) and free-radicals to save chondrocytes owing to the binding of HA to CD44 onto chondrocytes and facilitate its endurance. Surface coating provides physical protection of chondrocytes from enzyme degradation and inflammatory factors, found in an osteoarthritis environment.	[106]

	Target	NP	Drug	Disease	Description	Ref.
2	EGFR	Dual-sensitive pH/redox cationic unimolecular nanoparticle	siRNA	Breast carcinoma	An anti-EGFR peptide (GE11 peptide), was found to considerably augment the uptake of NPs in (MDA-MB) TNBC cells.	[107]
		RNA-NPs decorated with EGFR-targeting aptamer	Anti-miRNA	Breast carcinoma	In an orthotopic TNBC tumor model, significant accumulation of the NPs with diminished hepatic and renal clearance was observed.	[108]
		Lipid-encapsulated targeted superparamagnetic iron oxide (SMIO) NPs	EGFR antibody cetuximab	Glioblastoma	Conjugating cetuximab to SMIO NPs allowed specific EGFR targeting, which enhanced membrane transport ratio to cross the barrier (BBB) to recognize brain cancer tumor markers.	[109]
3	TAG 72	Regional delivery of chimeric antigen receptor-engineered T cells (CART)	CART	Peritoneal Ovarian cancer	Intraperitoneal delivery of TAG72-BBζ CAR T cells considerably decreased cancer growth and increased survival of mice. This was further enhanced with repeated CART cell infusions.	[110]
		CART	CART	Ovary tumor	TAG-72, tremendously over-expressed in ovarian tumor. In advanced-stage ovary tumor TAG-72 is an attractive candidate for CAR-T cell therapy, which binds with TAG-72 Hinge and TM regions.	[111]
4	Folate	Folate-conjugated hydrophobicity coated glycol chitosan NPs (FCHGCNPs)	Methotrexate	Rheumatoid arthritis	FCHGCNPs actively target folate receptors (FR). The internalization of folate conjugates occurred via binding of folic acid to FR through receptor-mediated endocytosis in rheumatoid arthritis therapy.	[112]
		Folate-conjugated magnetic triblock copolymer NPs	Temozolomide	Brain Glioma	Folic acid was able to transfer the highest concentration of drugs across the BBB via active targeting. With the upregulation of elevated folic acid receptor levels on glioma cancer cells, NPs enhanced the drug time. accessibility to the cancer cells.	[113]
		Folate-conjugated liposomes	Benzoporphyrin derivative	Breast cancer	The 3D (monolayer MDA-MB-231) cell model was highly approachable to the targeted nanoformulations.	[46]
		Mesoporous silica nanoparticles (MSNPs)	Cisplatin	Glioblastoma	The surface functionalization of MSNPs with folate groups can release drugs selectively with their linkage on the cell surface receptors.	[44]

(continued)

TABLE 35.1 (Continued)

Surface-Decorated Nanoparticles in Therapeutics via Receptor Targeting

Sr. No.	Receptors	Delivery system	Therapeutic agents	Disease	Function	References
5	ASGPR	Lactoferrin-modified PEGylated liquid crystalline nanoparticles (IMS-LF-LCNPs)	ImatinibMesylate	Hepatocellular carcinoma (HCC)	LCNPs modified with LF could be specially identified via ASGPR, facilitated the active drug targeting to the hepatic site for treating HCC.	[114]
		Galactosylated chitosan nanoparticles (GCNPs)	Gemcitabine to	HCC	To target the ASGPR receptor GCNPs were prepared, these GCNPs internalized into the cells through ASGPR-mediated endocytosis to treat HCC.	[44]
		Galactosylatedcarboxymethyl chitosan-magnetic iron oxide NPs	Magnetic iron oxide	Hepatocellular carcinoma	ASGPR mediated endocytosis of galactose-modified delivery system was influenced by the NP size (NP <50 nm, efficiently targeting hepatocytes and NP> 140nm were more specific for Kupffer cells)	[114]
6	Transferrin	MSNs	Gemcitabine	Pancreatic cancer	Improved uptake, inhibition of cancer cell growth	[115]
		MSNs	Doxorubicin	Cervical cancer	pH-responsive drug release, Surface-enhanced Raman scattering (SERS)–traceable characteristics and cancer cells targeting	[116]
		MSNs	Doxorubicin	Hepatic cancer	Biocompatible, site-specific system with controlled drug release	[117]
		MSNs decorated with a biocompatible protein shell (streptavidin, avidin, and biotinylated transferrin)	Doxorubicin	Exposed tumors (skin, esophagus, and stomach)	Effective photo-triggered drug delivery with high cytotoxicity in tumors	[118]
6	Tyrosine kinase	Amine-functionalized mesoporous silica nanocomposites that are surface coated with cerium oxide NPs	Sorafenib and sunitinib	Hepatocellular carcinoma	Enhanced cellular uptake, induced cell death	[119]
7	VEGFR	Poly (lactic-co-glycolic acid) NPs	-	Vascular growth (blood vessel growth)	Significant increase in total vessel volume and vessel connectivity	[120]

8	αvβ3 Integrins	Mesoporous silica-encapsulated gold nanorods	Gold	Breast cancer	Improved radio-sensitization of triple-negative breast cancer	[121]
		MSNs	Arsenic trioxide (ATO)	Breast cancer	Greater uptake in MDA-MB-231 breast cancer, enhanced concentration of NPs in in vivo studies, superior therapeutic ability of ATO-MSNs-R	[122]
		MSNs	Doxorubicin	An MMP-rich tumor (neck, head, and colorectal cancer)	Tumor-triggered targeted drug delivery, efficient inhibition of cancer cell growth	[123]
		MSNs	Doxorubicin	Cervical cancer	Facilitated active targeting and intracellular drug release	[124]
		MSNs with functional peptide-coated gold NPs	Doxorubicin	Glioblastoma	Facilitates targeting delivery, diversified multi-functional nanocomposites	[125]
		MSNs	Doxorubicin and therapeutic peptide	Glioblastoma	Tumor targeting, synergism between drug and therapeutic peptide, high cell toxicity	[126]
		MSNs	Doxorubicin	Glioblastoma	Electrostatic repulsion induced nano-valve opening and drug release, enhanced cellular association, and cell inhibition effect	[127]
		MSNs	Doxorubicin	Breast cancer	Enhanced cellular uptake, targeted drug delivery, and controlled drug release by the nano-valves	[128]
		Hollow mesoporous silica nanocapsules	Doxorubicin	Glioblastoma	Chemotherapy and photothermal therapy (PTT) together enhanced therapeutic efficacy	[129]
		Nanoparticles	Doxorubicin	Brain tumor	Remarkable increase in intratumoral drug levels	[130]
9	Death (TRAIL/DR4/Fas gene)	-	Semiprevir, Sofosbuvir, Ribavirin, Daclatasvir, Ledipasvir/Sofosbuvir	Liver cirrhosis	TRAIL 1525G/A and 1595C/T showed linkage disequilibrium, increase in AA genotype, and A allele of DR4 (683A/C)	[131]
10	Mannose	Solid lipid NPs	Gemcitabine	Lung cancer	Reduced hemolysis, significant toxicity, and greater uptake in A549 cells, by receptor-mediated endocytosis, enhanced drug concentration in lungs (in vivo studies)	[132]
		Mannan-decorated poly (D, L-lactide-co-glycolide) NPs	Tetramethyl Rhodamine Dextran (TMRD)	Dendritic cells	Highest NPs uptake was achieved by COOH terminated PLGA NPs containing covalent or adsorbed MN	[133]
		Mannose receptor-targeted and MMP-responsive gelatin NPs	Cisplatin	Lung cancer	Enhances the cancer cell-specific uptake of NPs, efficacy significantly increased against A549 cells, significantly enhanced apoptotic cell death.	[134]

TABLE 35.2

Patents Related to Theranostic Applications of Surface-Decorated Nano-Formulations

Sr. No.	Patent No.	Nano-Delivery System	Product claimed and Activity	Outcome	Reference
1	EP2436673A1	Curcumin-decorated liposome	↑ affinity for amyloid-beta1-42 peptide, ↑ physicochemical properties of curcumin	↑ Drug delivery in Alzheimer's disease and utilized for diagnosis.	[136]
2	US20180067121A1	Exosome-conjugated quantum dot NPs	Specific ligand like Glypican-1, CEA, CA19-9, mesothelin, PD-L1, telomerase binding based on the fluorescence wavelength of the quantum dot.	↑Cellular uptake and detect cancer	[137]
3	US20180133345A1	Surface-modified quantum dot nano-devices	Specific targeting EGFR (epidermal growth factor receptor) and PD-L1 (Programmed death ligand-1)	Detection and treatment of cancer	[137]
4	CN-103833871-A	The hyaluronic acid-adipodihydrazide-TQ grafted polymer	Synthesis of pH-dependent hyaluronic acid-adipodihydrazide-TQ grafted polymer for tumors specific delivery	↑ tumors targeting, pH-dependent drug release	[138]
5	DE-19844022-C1	Iron-binding glyco proteins (lactoferrin) and/or 10-hydroxy-2-decenoic acid + TQ	Treatment of AIDS and other immunodeficiency diseases via iron-binding glycoproteins and/or 10-hydroxy-2-decenoic acid in combination with TQ	↓ HIV Plaques	[139]
6	US20190192686A1	Nanodroplet micelle	Targeted nanodroplet emulsions for treating cancer	↑targeted delivery of anti-cancer drugs, ↓systemic toxicity.	[140]
7	DK2886126T3	NP conjugated to CD44-binding peptides	Specifically binds to a polypeptide encoded by exon 9 of human CD44 (CD44ex9)	Diagnosis and treatment of cancer	[141]
8	WO2017100697A1	Unmodified dextran (DNPs), DNP conjugates	Macrophage-specific DNP conjugates for imaging and therapy	Theranostic applications	[142]
9	CN102552945A	2-(methyl) acrylyl oxy-ethyl phosphocholine-modified magnetic ferric oxide NPs	Macrophage targeting, biocompatibility in aqueous medium	Diagnostic applications	[143]
10	KR101925442B1	Mannose-modified suture NPs material	Macrophage Targeting	Drug delivery and coating of medical equipment for anti-inflammation	[144]
11	US10500156B2	Multi-compartmental macrophage NPs	Macrophage targeting	Imaging and drug delivery	[145]
12	CA2735318C	Surface-modified NPs	Target antigen-presenting cells	Delivered immunotherapeutics	[146]
13	US8642787B2	Surface-modified organometallic NPs	Reduce metal toxicity	Drug delivery carrier	[147]

are not replicable identically. Even the yield reported is really little, which might require a fairly large infrastructure to scale up the product. For efficient surface modification, the functionalization processes require specific conditions. Furthermore, NP synthesis is an energy-intensive technique, and achieving even sizes is not yet a commercial possibility. Surface modification requires repetitive processing of the NPs, which reduces the yield even more because we keep losing particles across every chemical step. Aside from that, clinical translations of these techniques are also lacking, which is a huge matter of concern. The development criteria are very precise to promote different facets of NP interaction in a biological systems, and they comprise basic concepts that govern clinical translation. The crucial problems that need to be addressed while developing nanoprobes adhering to regulatory guidelines for clinical applicability are efficient targeting ability, biocompatibility, biodistribution, clearance from the body, etc. In the future, more emphasis should be placed on the development of highly consistent functionalization strategies and the integration of these nanoprobes to improve clinical applicability. By using a typical ligand/attaching chemical molecule, it should be possible to functionalize several molecules in a single step. For use as nanomedicine and nanoprobes, the size scale of NPs can be confined to a much narrower range. The scale-up process of NPs to commercial scale is also of major concern as very few lab studies can exactly be replicated to a commercial scale. Thus, focus on scaling up the processes should be given when beginning a research experiment. The multi-dimensional regulatory aspects of clinical translation are anticipated to be well addressed in future research, thanks to recently evolved effective functionalization processes and rigorous design strategies. Newer and more accurate NPs can be identified, which might translate tp more detailed medical imaging and disease diagnosis. The nano-diagnostics can be further utilized tp boost the reliability, specificity, and accuracy of diagnostic tests.

35.6 Conclusion

This chapter outlined recent and ongoing studies regarding surface-decorated NPs and how these functionalization processes can alter NP application and, as a result, improve specific therapeutic and diagnostic modalities. The surface functionalization of NP gives them multi-functional properties, which paves the way to integrate multi-disciplinary therapeutic and diagnostic applications. NPs functionalized specifically for diagnostic imaging purposes both in vitro and in vivo can significantly enhance data quality that can be analyzed and produce high-contrast distinguished images. In addition to advancing the application of NPs, surface decoration has enhanced the success of the NPs by rendering them biocompatible, improving their stability, and thereby allowing for the tracking of the concerned cells to decide the eventual fate and behavior of NPs. Despite some shortcomings regarding surface-decorated NPs, controlled functionalization processes with therapeuticallyimportant molecules can significantly impact the future of nanoscience.

REFERENCES

1. Chen, F. et al., *Functionalized upconversion nanoparticles: versatile nanoplatforms for translational research.* Current Molecular Medicine, 2013. 13(10): 613–1632.
2. Khan, I., K. Saeed, and I. Khan, *Nanoparticles: Properties, applications and toxicities.* Arabian Journal Of Chemistry, 2019. 12(7): 908–931.
3. Sanvicens, N. and M.P. Marco, *Multi-functional nanoparticles – properties and prospects for their use in human medicine.* Trends in Biotechnology, 2008. 26(8): 425–433.
4. Jeevanandam, J. et al., *Review on nanoparticles and nanostructured materials: history, sources, toxicity and regulations.* Beilstein Journal of Nanotechnology, 2018. 9(1): 1050–1074.
5. Wong, J. et al., *The potential translational applications of nanoparticles in endodontics.* International Journal of Nanomedicine, 2021. 16: 2087.
6. Shreffler, J.W. et al., *Overcoming hurdles in nanoparticle clinical translation: The influence of experimental design and surface modification.* International Journal of Molecular Sciences, 2019. 20(23): 6056.
7. De Jong, W.H. and P.J. Borm, *Drug delivery and nanoparticles: applications and hazards.* International Journal Of Nanomedicine, 2008. 3(2): 133.

8. Nie, S. et al., *Nanotechnology applications in cancer.* Annu. Rev. Biomed. Eng., 2007. 9: 257–288.

9. Peer, D. et al., *Nano-carriers as an emerging platform for cancer therapy.* Nano-Enabled Medical Applications, 2020: 61–91.

10. Hernández-Pedro, N.Y. et al., *Application of nanoparticles on diagnosis and therapy in gliomas.* BioMed Research International, 2013.

11. Tuantranont, A., Applications of Nanomaterials in Sensors and Diagnostics. Springer, Berlin, Heidelberg, 2014.

12. Kiessling, F. et al., *Nanoparticles for imaging: top or flop?* Radiology, 2014. 273(1): 10–28.

13. Gul, S. et al., *A comprehensive review of magnetic nanomaterials modern day theranostics.* Frontiers in Materials, 2019. 6: 179.

14. Herranz, F., J. Pellico, and J. ús Ruiz-Cabello, *Covalent functionalization of magnetic nanoparticles for biomedical imaging.* Resonance, 2012. 4: 6.

15. Zhu, D. et al., *Nanoparticle-based systems for T(1)-weighted magnetic resonance imaging contrast agents.* International Journal of Molecular Sciences, 2013. 14(5): 10591–10607.

16. Hernández-Hernández, A.A. et al., *Iron oxide nanoparticles: synthesis, functionalization, and applications in diagnosis and treatment of cancer.* Chemical Papers, 2020. 74(11): 3809–3824.

17. Zhao, W. et al., *Multi-functional Fe3O4@WO3@mSiO2–APTES nano-carrier for targeted drug delivery and controllable release with microwave irradiation triggered by WO3.* Materials Letters, 2016. 169: 185–188.

18. Kandasamy, G. et al., *Functionalized hydrophilic superparamagnetic iron oxide nanoparticles for magnetic fluid hyperthermia application in liver cancer treatment.* ACS Omega, 2018. 3(4): 3991–4005.

19. Ali, A. et al., *Synthesis, characterization, applications, and challenges of iron oxide nanoparticles.* Nanotechnology, Science and Applications, 2016. 9: 49.

20. Shilo, M. et al., *Nanoparticles as computed tomography contrast agents: current status and future perspectives.* Nanomedicine (Lond), 2012. 7(2): 257–269.

21. Wang, X. et al., R*henium sulfide nanoparticles as a biosafe spectral ct contrast agent for gastrointestinal tract imaging and tumor theranostics* in vivo. ACS Applied Materials & Interfaces, 2019. 11(37): 33650–33658.

22. Wang, R. et al., *Versatile functionalization of amylopectin for effective biomedical applications.* Science China Chemistry, 2015. 58(9): 1461–1470.

23. Cole, L.E., T. Vargo-Gogola, and R.K. Roeder, *Contrast-enhanced x-ray detection of microcalcifications in radiographically dense mammary tissue using targeted gold nanoparticles.* ACS Nano, 2015. 9(9): 8923–8932.

24. Goel, S. et al., *Positron emission tomography and nanotechnology: A dynamic duo for cancer theranostics.* Advanced Drug Delivery Reviews, 2017. 113: 157–176.

25. Chen, F. et al., In vivo *tumor targeting and image-guided drug delivery with antibody-conjugated, radiolabeled mesoporous silica nanoparticles.* ACS Nano, 2013. 7(10): 9027–9039.

26. Yang, Y. et al., *Facile synthesis of wormlike quantum dots-encapsulated nanoparticles and their controlled surface functionalization for effective bioapplications.* Nano Research, 2016. 9(9): 2531–2543.

27. Forte, E. et al., *Radiolabeled PET/MRI nanoparticles for tumor imaging.* Journal of Clinical Medicine, 2020. 9(1): 89.

28. Wang, S. et al., *Three-photon luminescence of gold nanorods and its applications for high contrast tissue and deep* in vivo *brain imaging.* Theranostics, 2015. 5(3): 251–266.

29. Thomsen, T. et al., *Fluorescence-based and fluorescent label-free characterization of polymer nanoparticle decorated t cells.* Biomacromolecules, 2021. 22(1): 190–200.

30. Zdobnova, T., E. Lebedenko, and S. Deyev, *Quantum dots for molecular diagnostics of tumors.* Acta Naturae, 2011. 3(1)(8).

31. Wang, X. et al., *A mini review on carbon quantum dots: preparation, properties, and electrocatalytic application.* Frontiers in Chemistry, 2019. 7(671).

32. Vivero-Escoto, J.L., R.C. Huxford-Phillips, and W. Lin, *Silica-based nanoprobes for biomedical imaging and theranostic applications.* Chem Soc Rev, 2012. 41(7): 2673–2685.

33. Wang, X. et al., *Aggregation-induced emission luminogen-embedded silica nanoparticles containing DNA aptamers for targeted cell imaging.* ACS Applied Materials & Interfaces, 2016. 8(1): 609–616.

34. Choi, S.W., W.S. Kim, and J.H. Kim, *Surface modification of functional nanoparticles for controlled drug delivery.* Journal of Dispersion Science and Technology, 2003. 24(3-4): 475–487.

35. Jain, K. et al., *A review of glycosylated carriers for drug delivery.* Biomaterials, 2012. 33(16): 4166–4186.

36. Agarwal, A. et al., *Ligand based dendritic systems for tumor targeting.* International Journal of Pharmaceutics, 2008. 350(1-2): 3–13.

37. Goodison, S., V. Urquidi, and D. Tarin, *CD44 cell adhesion molecules.* Molecular Pathology, 1999. 52(4): 189.

38. Gupta, R.C. et al., *Hyaluronic acid: Molecular mechanisms and therapeutic trajectory.* Frontiers in Veterinary Science, 2019. 6: 192.

39. Yu, Q. and I. Stamenkovic, *Cell surface-localized matrix metalloproteinase-9 proteolytically activates TGF-β and promotes tumor invasion and angiogenesis.* Genes & Development, 2000. 14(2): 163–176.

40. Misra, S. et al., *Interactions between hyaluronan and its receptors (CD44, RHAMM) regulate the activities of inflammation and cancer.* Frontiers in Immunology, 2015. 6: 201.

41. Cortes-Dericks, L. and R.A. Schmid, *CD44 and its ligand hyaluronan as potential biomarkers in malignant pleural mesothelioma: evidence and perspectives.* Respiratory Research, 2017. 18(1): 1–12.

42. Veeramani, S., K. Shanmugam, and R. Sahadevan, *Folate targeted galactomannan coated iron oxide nanoparticles as a nano-carrier for targeted drug delivery of capecitabine.* Int. J. Med. Nano. Res., 2018. 5: 25–35.

43. Ledermann, J., S. Canevari, and T. Thigpen, *Targeting the folate receptor: diagnostic and therapeutic approaches to personalize cancer treatments.* Annals of Oncology, 2015. 26(10): 2034–2043.

44. Nair, A.B. et al., *Development of asialoglycoprotein receptor-targeted nanoparticles for selective delivery of gemcitabine to hepatocellular carcinoma.* Molecules, 2019. 24(24): 4566.

45. Xue, W.J. et al., *Asialoglycoprotein receptor-magnetic dual targeting nanoparticles for delivery of RASSF1A to hepatocellular carcinoma.* Sci Rep, 2016. 6: 22149.

46. Nisha, R. et al., *Fabrication of imatinib mesylate-loaded lactoferrin-modified pegylated liquid crystalline nanoparticles for mitochondrial-dependent apoptosis in hepatocellular carcinoma.* Molecular Pharmaceutics, 2020.

47. Ioannidis, G., V. Georgoulias, and J. Souglakos, *How close are we to customizing chemotherapy in early non-small cell lung cancer?* Therapeutic Advances in Medical Oncology, 2011. 3(4): 185–205.

48. Su, K.-Y. et al., *Pretreatment epidermal growth factor receptor (EGFR) T790M mutation predicts shorter EGFR tyrosine kinase inhibitor response duration in patients with non-small-cell lung cancer.* J Clin Oncol, 2012. 30(4): 433–440.

49. Araujo, A. et al., *Genetic polymorphisms of the epidermal growth factor and related receptor in non-small cell lung cancer—a review of the literature.* The Oncologist, 2007. 12(2): 201–210.

50. Baselga, J., *Why the epidermal growth factor receptor? The rationale for cancer therapy.* The Oncologist, 2002. 7: 2–8.

51. Sheer, D.G., J. Schlom, and H.L. Cooper, *Purification and composition of the human tumor-associated glycoprotein (TAG-72) defined by monoclonal antibodies CC49 and B72. 3.* Cancer Research, 1988. 48(23): 6811–6818.

52. Minnix, M. et al., *Improved targeting of an anti-TAG-72 antibody drug conjugate for the treatment of ovarian cancer.* Cancer Medicine, 2020. 9(13): 4756–4767.

53. Louhimo, J. et al., *Serum HCGβ and CA 72-4 are stronger prognostic factors than CEA, CA 19-9 and CA 242 in pancreatic cancer.* Oncology, 2004. 66(2): 126–131.

54. Bohdiewicz, P.J., *Indium-111 satumomab pendetide: the first FDA-approved monoclonal antibody for tumor imaging.* Journal of Nuclear Medicine Technology, 1998. 26(3): 155–163.

55. Cho, J. et al., *The prognostic role of tumor associated glycoprotein 72 (TAG-72) in stage II and III colorectal adenocarcinoma.* Pathology-Research and Practice, 2019. 215(1): 171–176.

56. Gong, L. et al., *A 3E8. scFv. Cys-IR800 conjugate targeting TAG-72 in an orthotopic colorectal cancer model.* Molecular Imaging and Biology, 2018. 20(1): 47–54.

57. Daniels, T.R. et al., *The transferrin receptor and the targeted delivery of therapeutic agents against cancer.* Biochim Biophys Acta, 2012. 1820(3): 291–317.

58. Shen, Y. et al., *Transferrin receptor 1 in cancer: a new sight for cancer therapy.* Am J Cancer Res, 2018. 8(6): 916.

59. Jang, M.-H. and I. Oh, *Targeted drug delivery of Transferrin-Conjugated Mesoporous Silica Nanoparticles.* Yakhak Hoeji, 2017. 61(5): 241–247.

60. Ferris, D.P. et al., *Synthesis of biomolecule-modified mesoporous silica nanoparticles for targeted hydrophobic drug delivery to cancer cells.* Small, 2011. 7(13): 1816–1826.

61. Montalvo-Quiros, S. et al., *Cancer cell targeting and therapeutic delivery of silver nanoparticles by mesoporous silica nano-carriers: insights into the action mechanisms using quantitative proteomics.* Nanoscale, 2019. 11(10): 4531–4545.

62. Ke, Y. and C. Xiang, *Transferrin receptor-targeted HMSN for sorafenib delivery in refractory differentiated thyroid cancer therapy.* Int J Nanomedicine, 2018. 13: 8339.

63. Sun, T. et al., *Targeting transferrin receptor delivery of temozolomide for a potential glioma stem cell-mediated therapy.* Oncotarget. 2017. 8(43): 74451.

64. Luo, M. et al., *Systematic evaluation of transferrin-modified porous silicon nanoparticles for targeted delivery of doxorubicin to glioblastoma.* ACS Appl. Mater. Interfaces, 2019. 11(37): 33637–33649.

65. Sheykhzadeh, S. et al., *Transferrin-targeted porous silicon nanoparticles reduce glioblastoma cell migration across tight extracellular space.* Scientific Reports, 2020. 10(1): 1–16.

66. Paul, M.K. and A.K. Mukhopadhyay, *Tyrosine kinase – role and significance in cancer.* Int J Med Sci, 2004. 1(2): 101.

67. Valiathan, R.R. et al., *Discoidin domain receptor tyrosine kinases: new players in cancer progression.* Cancer Metastasis Rev, 2012. 31(1): 295–321.

68. Shaw, A.T. et al., *Tyrosine kinase gene rearrangements in epithelial malignancies.* Nat Rev Cancer, 2013. 13(11): 772–787.

69. Lengyel, E., K. Sawada, and R. Salgia, *Tyrosine kinase mutations in human cancer.* Curr Mol Med, 2007. 7(1): 77–84.

70. Hughes, T. et al., *Monitoring CML patients responding to treatment with tyrosine kinase inhibitors: review and recommendations for harmonizing current methodology for detecting BCR-ABL transcripts and kinase domain mutations and for expressing results.* Blood, 2006. 108(1): 28–37.

71. Mitelman, F., B. Johansson, and F. Mertens, *Fusion genes and rearranged genes as a linear function of chromosome aberrations in cancer.* Nat Genet, 2004. 36(4): 331–334.

72. McFarland, C.D. et al., *Impact of deleterious passenger mutations on cancer progression.* Proc Natl Acad Sci USA, 2013. 110(8): 2910–2915.

73. Stratton, M.R., P.J. Campbell, and PA Futreal, *The cancer genome.* Nature, 2009. 458(7239): 719–724.

74. Pon, J.R. and M.A. Marra, *Driver and passenger mutations in cancer.* Annu Rev Pathol, 2015. 10: 25–50.

75. Takeuchi, K. and F. Ito, *Receptor tyrosine kinases and targeted cancer therapeutics.* Biol Pharm Bull. 2011. 34(12): 1774–1780.

76. Torkamani, A., G. Verkhivker, and N.J. Schork, *Cancer driver mutations in protein kinase genes.* Cancer Lett, 2009. 281(2): 117–127.

77. Drake, J.M. et al., *Clinical targeting of mutated and wild-type protein tyrosine kinases in cancer.* Mol Cell Biol, 2014. 34(10): 1722–1732.

78. Costache, M. et al., *VEGF expression in pancreatic cancer and other malignancies: a review of the literature.* Rom J Intern Med, 2015. 53(3): 199–208.

79. Goel, S. et al., *VEGFR-targeted drug delivery* in vivo *with mesoporous silica nanoparticles.* ACS Appl Mater Interfaces, 2014. 55(supplement 1): 222.

80. Goel, S. et al., *VEGF121-conjugated mesoporous silica nanoparticle: a tumor targeted drug delivery system.* ACS Appl. Mater. Interfaces, 2014. 6(23): 21677–21685.

81. Zhang, R. et al., *Antitumor effect of 131 I-Labeled Anti-VEGFR2 targeted mesoporous silica nanoparticles in anaplastic thyroid cancer.* Nanoscale Res Lett, 2019. 14(1): 1–11.

82. Barui, S. et al., *Simultaneous delivery of doxorubicin and curcumin encapsulated in liposomes of pegylated RGDK-lipopeptide to tumor vasculature.* Biomaterials, 2014. 35(5): 1643–1656.

83. Barui, S. et al., *Systemic codelivery of a homoserine derived ceramide analogue and curcumin to tumor vasculature inhibits mouse tumor growth.* Mol Pharm, 2016. 13(2): 404–419.

84. Dal Corso, A. et al., *αVβ3 Integrin-targeted peptide/peptidomimetic-drug conjugates: In-depth analysis of the linker technology.* Curr Top Med Chem, 2016. 16(3): 314–329.

85. Fang, I.J. et al., *Ligand conformation dictates membrane and endosomal trafficking of arginine-glycine-aspartate (RGD)-functionalized mesoporous silica nanoparticles.* Chemistry, 2012. 18(25): 7787–7792.

86. Hu, H. et al., *The rational design of NAMI-A-loaded mesoporous silica nanoparticles as antiangiogenic nanosystems.* Journal of Materials Chemistry B, 2015. 3(30): 6338–6346.

87. Hu, H. et al., *Mesoporous silica nanoparticles functionalized with fluorescent and MRI reporters for the visualization of murine tumors overexpressing α v β 3 receptors.* Nanoscale, 2016. 8(13): 7094–7104.

88. Sun, J. et al., *A c (RGDfE) conjugated multi-functional nanomedicine delivery system for targeted pancreatic cancer therapy.* J Mater Chem B, 2015. 3(6): 1049–1058.

89. Chakravarty, R. et al., *Hollow mesoporous silica nanoparticles for tumor vasculature targeting and PET image-guided drug delivery.* Nanomedicine (Lond), 2015. 10(8): 1233–1246.

90. Mo, J. et al., *Tailoring particle size of mesoporous silica nanosystem to antagonize glioblastoma and overcome blood–brain barrier.* ACS Appl Mater Interfaces, 2016. 8(11): 6811–6825.

91. Pan, L. et al., *MSN-mediated sequential vascular-to-cell nuclear-targeted drug delivery for efficient tumor regression.* Advanced Materials, 2014. 26(39): 6742–6748.

92. Nagata, S., *Apoptosis by death factor.* Cell, 1997. 88(3): 355–365.

93. Yoon, J-H. and G.J. Gores, *Death receptor-mediated apoptosis and the liver.* J Hepatol, 2002. 37(3): 400–410.

94. Yin, X-M. and W-X. Ding, *Death receptor activation-induced hepatocyte apoptosis and liver injury.* Curr Mol Med, 2003. 3(6): 491–508.

95. Fas, SC, et al., *Death receptor signaling and its function in the immune system.* Curr Dir Autoimmun, 2006. 9: 1–17.

96. Schattenberg, J.M., P.R. Galle, and M. Schuchmann, *Apoptosis in liver disease.* Liver Int, 2006. 26(8): 904–911.

97. Canbay, A., S. Friedman, and G.J. Gores, *Apoptosis: the nexus of liver injury and fibrosis.* Hepatology, 2004. 39(2): 273–278.

98. Tanaka, M. et al., *Lethal effect of recombinant human Fas ligand in mice pretreated with Propionibacterium acnes.* J Immunol, 1997. 158(5): 2303–2309.

99. Scodeller, P. et al., *Precision targeting of tumor macrophages with a CD206 binding peptide.* Sci Rep, 2017. 7(1): 1–12.

100. Park, I.Y. et al., *Mannosylated polyethylenimine coupled mesoporous silica nanoparticles for receptor-mediated gene delivery.* Int J Pharm, 2008. 359 (1-2): 280–287.

101. Chen, N-T. et al., *Lectin-functionalized mesoporous silica nanoparticles for endoscopic detection of premalignant colonic lesions.* Nanomedicine, 2017. 13(6): 1941–1952.

102. Gao, X-M. et al., *Properties and feasibility of using cancer stem cells in clinical cancer treatment.* Cancer Biology & Medicine, 2016. 13(4): 489.

103. Muntimadugu, E. et al., *CD44 targeted chemotherapy for co-eradication of breast cancer stem cells and cancer cells using polymeric nanoparticles of salinomycin and paclitaxel.* Colloids and Surfaces B: Biointerfaces, 2016. 143: 532–546.

104. Dhamane, S.P. and S.C. Jagdale, *Development of rifampicin loaded hyaluronic acid coated chitosan nanoparticles.* European Journal of Molecular & Clinical Medicine, 2020. 7(1): 3447–3458.

105. Xiong, F. et al., *pH-responsive and hyaluronic acid-functionalized metal–organic frameworks for therapy of osteoarthritis.* Journal of Nanobiotechnology, 2020. 18(1): 1–14.

106. Chen, G. et al., *Tumor-targeted pH/redox dual-sensitive unimolecular nanoparticles for efficient siRNA delivery.* Journal of Controlled Release, 2017. 259: 105–114.

107. Chen, H-L. et al., *Identification of epidermal growth factor receptor-positive glioblastoma using lipid-encapsulated targeted superparamagnetic iron oxide nanoparticles* in vitro. Journal of Nanobiotechnology, 2017. 15(1): 1–13.

108. Murad, J.P. et al., *Effective targeting of TAG72+ peritoneal ovarian tumors via regional delivery of CAR-engineered T cells.* Frontiers in Immunology, 2018. 9: 2268.

109. Shu, R. et al., *Engineered CAR-T cells targeting TAG-72 and CD47 in ovarian cancer.* Molecular Therapy-Oncolytics, 2021. 20: 325–341.

110. Wu, Z. et al., *Folate-conjugated hydrophobicity modified glycol chitosan nanoparticles for targeted delivery of methotrexate in rheumatoid arthritis.* Journal of Applied Biomaterials & Functional Materials, 2020. 18: 2280800020962629.

111. Afzalipour, R. et al., *Dual-targeting temozolomide loaded in folate-conjugated magnetic triblock copolymer nanoparticles to improve the therapeutic efficiency of rat brain gliomas.* ACS Biomaterials Science & Engineering, 2019. 5(11): 6000–6011.

112. Sneider, A. et al., *Engineering remotely triggered liposomes to target triple negative breast cancer.* Oncomedicine, 2017. 2: 1.

113. Ortiz-Islas, E. et al., *Mesoporous silica nanoparticles functionalized with folic acid for targeted release Cis-Pt to glioblastoma cells.* Reviews on Advanced Materials Science, 2021. 60(1): 25–37.

114. Xue, W.-J. et al., *Asialoglycoprotein receptor-magnetic dual targeting nanoparticles for delivery of RASSF1A to hepatocellular carcinoma.* Scientific Reports, 2016. 6(1): 1–13.

115. Saini, K. and R. Bandyopadhyaya, *Transferrin-conjugated polymer-coated mesoporous silica nanoparticles loaded with gemcitabine for killing pancreatic cancer cells.* Applied Nano Materials, 2019. 3(1): 229–240.

116. Fang, W. et al., *pH-controllable drug carrier with SERS activity for targeting cancer cells.* Biosens Bioelectron, 2014. 57: 10–15.

117. Chen, X. et al., *Transferrin gated mesoporous silica nanoparticles for redox-responsive and targeted drug delivery B biointerfaces.* Colloids Surf B Biointerfaces, 2017. 152: 77–84.

118. Martínez-Carmona, M. et al., *Mesoporous silica nanoparticles grafted with a light-responsive protein shell for highly cytotoxic antitumoral therapy.* J Mater Chem B, 2015. 3(28): 5746–5752.

119. Sedighi, M. et al., *Controlled tyrosine kinase inhibitor delivery to liver cancer cells by gate-capped mesoporous silica nanoparticles.* ACS Appl Bio Mater, 2019. 3(1): 239–251.

120. Golub, J.S. et al., *Sustained VEGF delivery via PLGA nanoparticles promotes vascular growth.* Am J Physiol Heart Circ Physiol, 2010. 298(6): H1959–H1965.

121. Zhao, N. et al., *RGD-conjugated mesoporous silica-encapsulated gold nanorods enhance the sensitization of triple-negative breast cancer to megavoltage radiation therapy.* Int J Nanomedicine, 2016. 11: 5595.

122. Wu, X. et al., *Targeted mesoporous silica nanoparticles delivering arsenic trioxide with environment sensitive drug release for effective treatment of triple negative breast cancer.* ACS Biomater Sci Eng, 2016. 2(4): 501–507.

123. Zhang, J. et al., *Multi-functional envelope-type mesoporous silica nanoparticles for tumor-triggered targeting drug delivery.* J Am Chem Soc, 2013. 135(13): 5068–5073.

124. Cheng, Y.-J. et al., *Multifunctional peptide-amphiphile end-capped mesoporous silica nanoparticles for tumor targeting drug delivery.* ACS Appl Mater Interfaces, 2017. 9(3): 2093–2103.

125. Chen, G. et al., *Peptide-decorated gold nanoparticles as functional nano-capping agent of mesoporous silica container for targeting drug delivery.* ACS Appl Mater Interfaces, 2016. 8(18): 11204–11209.

126. Xiao, D. et al., *A redox-responsive mesoporous silica nanoparticle with a therapeutic peptide shell for tumor targeting synergistic therapy.* Nanoscale, 2016. 8(37): 16702–16709.

127. Luo, G.-F. et al., *Charge-reversal plug gate nanovalves on peptide-functionalized mesoporous silica nanoparticles for targeted drug delivery.* Journal of Materials Chemistry B, 2013. 1(41): 5723–5732.

128. Zhao, F. et al., *A facile strategy to fabricate a pH-responsive mesoporous silica nanoparticle end-capped with amphiphilic peptides by self-assembly.* Colloids Surf B Biointerfaces, 2019. 179: 352–362.

129. Li, X. et al., *An RGD-modified hollow silica@ Au core/shell nanoplatform for tumor combination therapy.* Acta Biomater, 2017. 62: 273–283.

130. Turan, O. et al., *Effect of dose and selection of two different ligands on the deposition and antitumor efficacy of targeted nanoparticles in brain tumors.* Mol Pharm, 2019. 16(10): 4352–4360.

131. Talaat, RM, et al., *TNF-related apoptosis-inducing ligand (TRAIL), death receptor (DR4) and Fas gene polymorphisms associated with liver cirrhosis in hepatitis C infected patients.* Gene Reports, 2021. 22: 101018.

132. Soni, N. et al., *Augmented delivery of gemcitabine in lung cancer cells exploring mannose anchored solid lipid nanoparticles.* J Colloid Interface Sci, 2016. 481: 107–116.

133. Ghotbi, Z. et al., *Active targeting of dendritic cells with mannan-decorated PLGA nanoparticles.* J Drug Target, 2011. 19(4): 281–292.

134. Vaghasiya, K. et al., Efficient, *Enzyme responsive and tumor receptor targeting gelatin nanoparticles decorated with concanavalin-A for site-specific and controlled drug delivery for cancer therapy.* Mater Sci Eng C Mater Biol Appl, 2021. 123: 112027.

135. Kalyane, D. et al., *Employment of enhanced permeability and retention effect (EPR): Nanoparticle-based precision tools for targeting of therapeutic and diagnostic agent in cancer.* Mater Sci Eng C Mater Biol Appl, 2019. 98: 1252–1276.

136. Antimisiari, S. et al., *Curcumin derivatives with improved physicochemical properties and nanoliposomes surface-decorated with the derivatives with very high affinity for amyloid-beta1-42 peptide.* Patent. https://patents.google.com/patent/EP2436673A1/en

137. Naasani, I., *Nano-devices for detection and treatment of cancer*. Patent. https://patents.google.com/patent/US20180133345A1/en

138. Zhou, J. et al. *Hyaluronic acid-adipodihydrazide-thymoquinone grafted polymer as well as synthesis method and application of hyaluronic acid-adipodihydrazide-thymoquinone grafted polymer*. Patent. https://patents.google.com/patent/CN104140541A/en

139. Sherif, M., and R. Sabry, *Use of iron-binding glycoproteins and/or 10-hydroxy-2-decenoic acid in combination with thymoquinone for treating immunodeficiency diseases*. 1998.

140. Malik, M.T., J.A. Kopechek, and P.J. Bates, *Targeted nanodroplet emulsions for treating cancer*. Patent. https://patents.google.com/patent/US20190192686A1/en

141. Arntz, C. & W. Greb, *Nanoparticle conjugated to CD44-binding peptides*. Patent. https://patents.google.com/patent/DK2886126T3/en

142. Weissleder, R., E.J. Keliher, & M. Nahrendorf, *Dextran nanoparticles for macrophage specific imaging and therapy*. Patent. https://patents.google.com/patent/WO2017100697A1

143. 厂克正 et al., *Surface modification method of magnetic iron oxide nanoparticles*. Patent. https://patents.google.com/patent/CN102552945A/en

144. 박지호 et al., *macrophage targeting nanoparticles, compositions for coating medical equipment containing the same, and Medical equipment for anti-inflammation*. Patent. https://patents.google.com/patent/KR101925442B1/en

145. Amiji, M.M., M. Kalariya, S. Jain, H. Attarwala, *Multi-compartmental macrophage delivery*. Patent. https://patents.google.com/patent/US10500156B2/en

146. Hubbell, J. A., C. P. O'neil, S. T. Reddy, M. A. Swartz, D. Velluto, A. Van Der Vlies, and E. Simeoni, *Nanoparticles for immunotherapy*. Patent. https://patents.google.com/patent/CA2735318C/en

147. K. Fukushima, J. L. Hedrick, A. Nelson, and D. P. Sanders, *Surface modified nanoparticles, methods of their preparation, and uses thereof for gene and drug delivery*. Patent. https://patents.google.com/patent/US8642787

Section V

Nutra-Chemistry

36

Towards Developing Biofortified Food Crops for Enhancing Nutritional Aspects and Human Health

Manu Priya and Harsh Nayyar
Department of Botany, Panjab University, Chandigarh, India

The term "biofortification" generally refers to nutritional enhancement of crops grown and produced by conventional breeding systems, new biotechnological methods, and different agronomic practices (Garg et al., 2018). It has been estimated that "hidden poverty" from micronutrient deficiencies has impacted about two billion people worldwide, or one in three individuals (FAO 2013). The prevailing cause for such deficiencies is inadequate consumption and absorption of minerals and vitamins, eventually affecting human health and development severely (Saltzman et al., 2013). Agronomic work has successfully expanded the production and availability of numerous energy-rich staple crops in developed countries (Saltzman et al., 2017). However, efforts are underway to increase production of micronutrient-rich non-staples, particularly pulses and vegetables (Bouis et al., 2011). Therefore, increasing dietary composition by planting micronutrient-rich crops would dramatically minimize micronutrient deficiencies (Bouis and Saltzman, 2016). Increased development and supply of biofortified crops will prove useful in enhancing human safety and treating these disorders (Talsma and Pachon, 2017) (Figure 36.1). Regular consumption of these crops can help meet the routine micronutrient intake requirements of individuals during their lifetime (Bouis et al., 2011). Until now, our agriculture program has mainly concentrated on increasing crop production and efficiency instead of encouraging human wellbeing (Hirschi, 2009). This strategy has seen a persistent rise in micronutrient deficiency in various food crops, triggering malnutrition among consumers (Carvalho and Vasconcelos, 2013). Now agriculture is progressively shifting from more food production to nutrient-rich food production, which will help reduce "hidden hunger," particularly in poor and developed nations where diets are deficient in micronutrients (Lyons and Cakman, 2012). While multiple nutrient supplementation initiatives have begun to provide the populace with minerals and vitamins, such programs cannot meet goals set by international health organizations because they rely solely on external funding that is not expected to be accessible year after year (Carvalho and Vasconcelos, 2013). Some other drawbacks include lack of awareness of nutrient supplements' health benefits, their high cost, and access to markets and healthcare systems (Khush et al., 2012).

The Union Ministry of Health and Family Welfare (MHFW), Government of India, conducted a survey that showed marked zinc deficiency in 19% of pre-school children and 32% of teenagers (MHFW, 2017). In their survey, 23% of pre-school infants and 37% of teenagers were found to be folate deficient. Moreover, 14–31% deficiency in vitamin A, vitamin D, and vitamin B12 was observed among teenage and pre-school children (Bhuyan, 2018). Considering this data, iron, zinc, and vitamin B6 have been identified as targeted deficits, with 41, 25, and 6% of the population theoretically falling behind estimated average requirements. Some other key micronutrients (i.e., calcium, vitamin A, B12 and folate) all indicated a widespread risk of deficiency, with 94, 89, 89, and 81% of the population facing higher risk (Ritchie et al., 2018). In India, anemia is a major public health problem. According to the National Family Health Survey (NFHS4) conducted by the Ministry of Health and Family Welfare's, the incidence of anemia was 58.6% among children aged 6–59 months, 53.1% among women aged 15–49 years, 50.4% among women aged 15–49 years, and 22.7% among men aged 15–49 years (MHFW, 2017).

36.1 Importance of Biofortification in Combating Micronutrient Deficiencies

Biofortification is the method of increasing a crop's nutritional content through traditional plant breeding or using modern biotechnology or agronomic techniques (Bouis, 2018). Plants as immobile organisms constantly transport the nutrients from the soil to the seeds and fruits (more specifically, to the edible component of the crop) and also synthesize the vitamins in the seeds before harvest (Bhuyan, 2018). While short-term, gap-filling operations are carried out at the initial points, in the long run, rising earnings and developing micronutrient-rich crops and increasing dietary diversity would significantly reduce micronutrient malnutrition (Bouis, 2018) (Figure 36.1). Near-to-medium-term utilization of biofortified crops may help address micronutrient deprivation by growing the average adequacy of people's intake of vitamins and minerals during their lifetime (Bouis, 2018). Biofortification will increase the nutritional value of staple food crops eaten daily by poor people in South Asia and other developing countries including India (Bhuyan, 2018). This is a relatively very simple, cost-effective, reliable, and a long-term way to provide more micronutrients to the vulnerable (Gorelova et al., 2017). Biofortified crops produce sufficient amounts of micronutrients, sometimes insufficient in undeveloped and emerging countries' diets (Garg et al., 2018). Biofortified crops should have no modifications in taste, smell, and other quality attributes that might contribute to customer rejection of the product (De Steur et al., 2015). A healthy reinforced diet provides improved quality for the product's unaltered rheological effects. Such biofortified products, apart from improving nutritional quality, also reduce the food's anti-nutritional aspects (Gillespie, 2016). It is time to concentrate on nutritional and micronutrient sufficiency coupled with improved growth (Mayer et al., 2008). Governments should therefore invest more in research in this specific field to boost the nutritional health of citizens living all over the world, as significant numbers of people in developing countries have restricted exposure to certain fortified foods and nutritional supplements defined by low wages, poor knowledge, and non-uniform delivery (Bouis, 2011). Thus, improving the nutritional status of staple food crops seems to be a successful way to achieve this aim of malnutrition-free developing countries in particular, and the world at large. Some examples of biofortified food crops involving various approaches are given in Table 36.1.

TABLE 36.1

Biofortified Crops Produced for Different Components Through Agronomic Approches

Crop	Component	Reference
WHEAT	Carotenoids, Iron, Anthocyanin, Phytic acid, Amylase content	Wang et al. 2014, Borg et al. 2012, Doshi et al. Bhati et al. 2016, Francesco et al. 2010
RICE	Beta-carotene, Folic acid, Iron, Zinc, Flavonoids and Antioxidants	Paine et al. 2005, Blancquaert et al. 2015, Trijatmiko et al. 2016, Masuda et al. 2013, Ogo et al. 2013
MAIZE	Vitamin E, Vitamin C, Carotenoids, Amino acids (Lysine, tryptophan and methionine), Ferritin	Cahoon et al. 2003, Chen et al.2003, Decourcelle et al. 2015, Tang et al. 2013, Huang et al. 2006, Lai and Messing 2002, Aluru et al. 2002
BARLEY	Zinc, Phytase, Lysine,	Ramesh et al. 2004, Holme et al. 2012, Ohnoutkova et al. 2012
SORGHUM	Provitamin A, Lysine,	Lipkie et al. 2013, Zhao et al. 2003
SOYBEAN	Beta-carotene, Vitamin E, Amino acids (Methionine and cysteine), Fatty acids (Linoleic acid, Stearidonic acid, Oleic acid, Arachidonic acid), Flavonoids	Kim et al. 2012, Song et al. 2013, Kim et al. 2012, Sato et al. 2004, Zhang et al. 2014, Yu et al. 2003
COMMON BEAN	Methionine	Aragao et al. 1999
LUPINES	Methionine	Molvig et al. 1997

36.2 Various Modes/Techniques of Biofortification

36.2.1 Biofortification Through Fertilizer Application

Although biofortification is easy and inexpensive, many factors complicate the application of fertilizers containing important mineral micronutrients, such as their distribution process, soil composition, mineral mobility in the plant, and accumulation site (Gould, 2017). Therefore, this strategy has been effective in only limited cases, in only some geographical locations (Qaim, 2007). Iodine and selenium are elastic in soil and plants, rendering biofortification with iodine and selenium fertilizers particularly successful. Since Zn is also mobile in soil, $ZnSO_4$ applications can also increase cereal yield and Zn concentrations (Meenakshi et al., 2010). In comparison, Fe has poor soil mobility since $FeSO_4$ is easily bound by soil particles and transformed to Fe (III), thus Fe fertilizers have not been active in biofortification efforts (Gould, 2017). Furthermore, large quantities of metals added to soils will damage plant growth and other soil species (Nestel et al., 2006). Micronutrient fertilizers often have to be distributed frequently and are both expensive and environmentally damaging (Mayer et al., 2008). Generally, these approaches refer to different crops and mineral situations, but cannot be applied universally as a method to improve food nutritional quality (Qaim, 2007).

36.2.2 Biofortification Through Traditional Plant Breeding

Plants also display genetic variation in critical nutrient content, which in turn enables breeding programs to increase mineral and vitamin rates in crops (Rhodes, 2019). For instance, specific rice genotypes display four-fold variability in iron and zinc rates and beans and peas show up to 6.6-fold variation in these nutrients (De Steur et al., 2017). Since this method utilizes a crop's inherent property to absorb the nutrients from the soil, few regulatory restrictions remain (Bouis and Saltzman, 2017). Since this technique is potentially the most expedient strategy for developing biofortified seeds, many international organizations have launched projects to increase crop nutritional content through breeding programs (Garg et al., 2018). Harvest-Plus, for example, spends $14 million annually to raise three key nutrients, vitamin A, iron, and zinc, in 12 goal crops, focusing almost entirely on conventional breeding (De Steur et al., 2017). Conventional breeding has several major disadvantages to transgenic methods as breeding techniques generally depend on the often restricted genetic variations of the gene pool (Rhodes, 2019). In some instances, this can be resolved by spreading the biofortification ability to distant relatives of the crops, and by slowly moving the trait into their commercial cultivars. Such a technique could be used to increase selenium rates in wheat, since bread wheat today shows no difference in selenium content whereas wild wheat has higher levels (Garg et al., 2018). Alternatively, mutagenesis can introduce new traits into commercial varieties and has been used to produce lysine-rich maize seeds, and is recently a trend to enhance the nutritional quality of some cereals and legumes (Garg et al., 2018) (Figure 36.1.)

36.2.3 Biofortification Through Transgenic Techniques

In the absence of genetic variation in nutrient content among various varieties, breeders find limitations in enhancing the endogenous nutrient levels in their seeds. Transgenic methods may be a legitimate option (Zhu et al., 2007). Nutritional genomics tests the genome-nutrition-health interaction (Brinch-Pedersen et al., 2007). The ability to rapidly define and classify gene activity and use these genes for engineering plant metabolism was a guiding factor in recent biofortification efforts (De Steur et al., 2017). The rapid production of whole-genome sequencing, high-throughput spatial imaging, global gene expression analysis, and metabolite profiling in a number of species (Masuda et al., 2020) rendered this possible. As stated in some studies, pathways from bacteria and other species may also be incorporated into crops to manipulate alternate metabolic engineering pathways (De Steur et al., 2017). Thus, these innovations have an effective resource unconstrained by host gene pool. Furthermore, genetic modifications can target the edible portions of commercial crops (De Steur et al., 2015). In the recent era of plant breeding and biotechnology, various crops have been genetically engineered with macronutrient and micronutrient

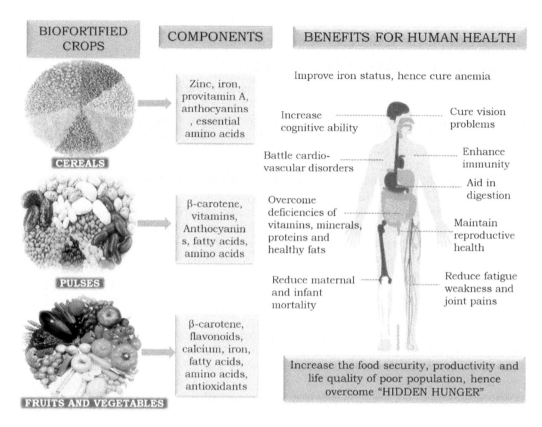

FIGURE 36.1 This image shows some biofortified crops (cereals, pulses, fruits, and vegetables) produced via enhancing various nutritional components and their role in improving human health and fighting "hidden hunger."

traits that can support consumers and domestic animals (Huang et al., 2016). Although the possibilities of transgenic methods have plant biologists hopeful, regulatory challenges associated with this technology render practical implementations challenging (Huang et al., 2012). Almost all transgenic plants have proprietary or licensed inventions; nevertheless, there was a campaign to operate beyond patents to bring biotechnology to the world's poor farmers (Hefferon, 2016). Regrettably, the new political and economic climate is not responsive to being broadly adapted to a variety of specific crops. But with these existing constraints, the ability for genetic engineering to mitigate malnutrition requires activism by both scientists and people (Hefferon, 2016).

36.3 Agronomic Approaches for Biofortification

Biofortification may be accomplished through adding soil mineral fertilizers, foliar fertilization, and soil inoculation with beneficial microorganisms (Cakmak and Kutman, 2018). Mineral fertilizers are inorganic substances comprising basic nutreints that can be added to soil to boost soil micronutrient status and therefore plant efficiency (Hefferon, 2018). The phyto-availability of minerals in soil is always low, thus to increase mineral abundance in edible plant tissues, it is important to apply mineral fertilizers with enhanced solubility and mineral mobility (Prasad et al., 2014). This approach can be used to fortify mineral-based foods, but not organic nutrients, such as enzymes, synthesized by the plant itself (Graham et al., 2007). This approach was successfully applied for Se, Fe, and Zn, as these elements have strong mobility both in soil and plant (Lyons and Cakmak, 2012). For starters, in Finland, supplementing inorganic fertilizers with sodium selenate dramatically increased Se concentration in different crops, fruits, vegetables, cereals, poultry, dairy goods, eggs, and fish (Aro et al., 1995). Therefore, sodium selenate supplementation of fertilizers has proven to be an efficient way to improve Se intake in humans (Aro et al., 1995). Similarly, plants in China and Thailand were effectively enriched with I and Zn utilizing inorganic fertilizers (Xin-Min et al., 1997); Fe fertilization, however, failed due to poor soil mobility of Fe. In field pea crops, Zn concentration was increased by either soil application of Zn fertilizer alone or coupled with foliar treatments; therefore, such approaches may theoretically be used to biofortify field peas (Poblaciones and Rengel, 2016). The biofortification fertilization strategy usually involves routine applications that may become detrimental to environmental health and may restrict certain mineral availability (Poblaciones and Rengel, 2016). However, soil quality in the particular geographical area, mineral sensitivity variations, and the propensity of anti-nutrient compounds restricting mineral bioavailability are also restrictions for the effective implementation of this strategy (Giuliano, 2017). The transfer of fertilizers directly to the leaves is by foliar fertilization, which may be effective if mineral elements are not instantly accessible in soil or not readily translocated to edible tissues (Garg et al., 2018).

36.4 Some Biofortified Crops

36.4.1 Legumes and Pulses

Biofortification of pulses and legume crops to boost their nutritional quality has gained attraction in the past decade (Rehman et al., 2019). Many experiments in pulse crops have established genetic variability for essential micronutrients in the accessible gene pools, with successful breeding lines being used in breeding, and related genotypic markers for marker-aided selection (Karakoy et al., 2012; Khazaei et al., 2017;Sharma et al., 2017). Pulse crops have been fortified with micronutrients Fe, Zn, and Se by foliar application in different studies resulting in increased rates of these micronutrients in the harvested grain. Márquez-Quiroz et al. (2015) recorded increased Fe concentration (29–32%) in cowpea seeds using this method. Similarly, increased Fe concentration (46%) in mungbeans following foliar Fe application was observed by Ali et al. (2014). Further, foliar application of Fe and Zn greatly improved these mineral concentrations along with protein in cowpea seeds (Pereira et al., 2014) and chickpeas (Upadhyaya et al., 2016). Shivay et al., 2015 observed a link between Zn uptake and chickpea grain yield after Zn foliar application, and confirmed this method was better than soil application. Likewise, Hidoto et al. (2017) tested the results of three Zn fertilization methods on five chickpea varieties and found that foliar application was an efficient Zn biofortification process with greater accumulation of Zn in grain compared to soil application and seed priming. Foliar application of Zn fertilizer was also recorded in common bean (Ram et al., 2016) and field peas (Poblaciones and Rengel, 2016). Increased Se concentration was recorded in pea seeds (Hegedüsová et al., 2015), chickpeas (Poblaciones and Rodrigo 2014), common beans (Figueiredo et al., 2017), and lentils (Thavarajah et al., 2017) after foliar application of Se fertilizers. Furthermore, improved concentration of iodine was observed by foliar application in different crops, which may avoid deficiencies in low-intake iodine human populations (Riaz et al., 2017). Some biofortified pulse and legume crops produced via various methods are discussed below.

36.4.2 Chickpea

Chickpea was targeted for mineral deficiencies, especially mineral iron, zinc, calcium, copper, manganese, and Mg, using plant-growth promoting actinobacteria (Tan et al., 2018). Chickpea has been biofortified for iron and zinc through various breeding techniques (Upadhayaya et al., 2016). Zinc and Se were also reinforced in chickpea by foliar mineral spray (Poblaciones and Rodrigo, 2014).

36.4.3 Lentil

Lentil is a primary pulse crop in many dryland countries with high protein content. ICARDA and HarvestPlus has biofortified lentils with iron and zinc through various breeding methods utilizing genetic diversity contained in gene banks (Kumar et al., 2016). Research findings have shown a positive correlation between iron and zinc production with protein synthesis, so lentil varieties with higher iron, zinc, and protein content can be produced together (ICARDA, HarvestPlus). High iron and zinc lentil types, five in Bangladesh (Barimasur-4, Barimasur-5, Barimasur-6, Barimasur-7, and Barimasur-8), seven in Nepal (ILL 7723, Khajurah-1,Khajurah-2, Shital, Sisir Shekhar, Simal), two in India (L4704, PusaVaibhav), one in Ethiopia (Alemaya), and two in Syria (Idlib-2, Idlib-3) have been raised by ICARDA and HarvestPlus (Kumar et al., 2016).

36.4.4 Beans

Breeding experiments to date have shown that the iron content of the common bean (*Phaseolus vulgaris*) may be increased by 60–80%, while the zinc content may be more moderate, possibly about 50% (Petry et al., 2015). A wide array of zinc-associated genes has been identified in common bean. HarvestPlus worked very effectively in this way and supported iron-fortified beans in several developing countries (Blair et al., 2009). They developed 10 popular biofortified bean varieties in Rwanda (RWR 2245, RWR2154, MAC 42, MAC 44, CAB 2, RWV 1129, RWV 3006, RWV 3316, RWV 3317, and RWV 2887). HarvestPlus also raised ten biofortified iron bean varieties (i.e., COD MLB 001, COD MLB 032, HM 21-7, RWR 2245, PVA 1438, COD MLV 059, VCB 81013, Nain de Kyondo, Cuarentino, Namulenga). Further, selenium-enriched soybean was developed by adding foliar selenium complex salts as fertilizers.

36.4.5 Cowpea

Cow pea, also regarded as poor man beef, was biofortified for iron content through various breeding methods. Biofortified cow pea varieties including Pant Lobia-1 (2008), Pant Lobia-2 (2010), Pant Lobia-3 (2013), and Pant Lobia-4 (2014) were raised by GB Pant University, Pantnagar, India in collaboration with HarvestPlus. Field peas are the world's second largest legume crop, often noted for their high protein content, and zinc enrichment was achieved either alone or in conjunction with soil zinc applications (Poblaciones and Rengel, 2016). An annual herbaceous bean is cultivated for edible dry grain. Beans are a good vehicle for zinc biofortification and were enriched with zinc using foliar zinc fertilizer (Ram et al., 2016; Ibrahim and Ramadan, 2015). Moreover, organic and chemical fertilizer administration has been studied to promote the absorption of N, P, K, copper, manganese, and zinc in popular bean (Westermann et al., 2011).

36.5 Cereals

Cereal plant products represent a significant part of the diet of developing-country citizens that cannot be relied on for nutritionally sufficient diets (Ortiz-Monasterio et al., 2007). Cereals play a significant role in the human diet as an essential food supply and typically produce high-quality protein and very low bioavailability of micronutrients such as magnesium, zinc, iodine, and vitamin A (Aciksoz et al., 2011). Cereal-based diets that ignore important micronutrients have detrimental impacts on human health and eventually contribute to malnutrition (Singh et al., 2017). Core micronutrients (iron, zinc, and provitamin A) are required for biological structures, and their functional and structural integrity (Ortiz-Monasterio et al., 2007). Worldwide, its failure costs billions due to weakening the immune system and hindering growth and development. To alleviate deficiency status, zinc enhancement in wheat (*Triticumaestivum* L.) varieties was achieved utilizing genetic variation in the germplasm, although it would only be necessary if the soil environment provided a sufficient zinc reservoir for absorption (Aciksoz et al., 2011). Results reported that some varieties from India (BHU 19, 17 and 1) and Pakistan (NR 421, 420, and 419) displayed a 4 to 10 ppm rise in zinc content (Singh et al., 2017). In fact, in extreme cases, an immediate increase in zinc concentration and wheat grain production was observed utilizing agronomic biofortification strategies (Singh et al., 2017). Similarly, wheat yield rose to 6.4 to 50.1% utilizing zinc as a fertilizer in soil (Velu et al., 2019). The first approach to biofortification (i.e., agronomic biofortification) may therefore be called economic, particularly when used with a fungicide depending on the existence of disease (Velu et al., 2019). Cereals are not the only material sources of selenium, but on a nutritional level they can be the major contributors of intake (Eichler et al., 2019). Agronomic biofortification with sufficient amounts of seleno-methionine can increase the nutritional value of wheat grains and may become an attractive option for improving selenium in diets (Ros et al., 2016). Sodium selenate and selenite are applied to bread wheat and durum wheat by applying 100 g/hectare of soil and foliar (Privitali et al., 2016). Average selenium content in samples ranged from 70% to 100%, and inorganic selenium was less than 5% (Privitali et al., 2016). Different findings were reported for all supplementation methods of wheat varieties.

36.5.1 Pearl Millet

After staple cereals, millets are a major source of energy, particularly in drought-prone regions and semi-arid African and Asian tropics (Velu et al., 2008). As millet grains produce significant quantities of proteins, important amino acids, vitamins, and minerals, these are considered superior nutritious grains (Mehta et al., 2017). ICRISAT, in collaboration with HarvestPlus, launched early biofortified pearl millet known as "Dhanashakti" (Vinoth and Ravindhran, 2019). People with lower nutrient intake are specifically targeted to provide them with biofortified millet to alleviate hunger (Mehta et al., 2017). Some clinical trials found that Dhanashakti's (300 gm) is adequate to fulfill 100% RDA (Recommended Dietary Allowance) content of iron (Velu et al., 2007). Restriction of food habits to a few specific cereals like rice and wheat alone does not fulfill daily requirements of essential micronutrients such as iron (Fe) and Zinc (Zn) (Haas et al., 2013). In India, pearl millet may serve as a significant source of dietary energy containing 19–63% of the Fe and 16–56% of the Zn among vast population in major parts of pearl millet growing states (Haas et al., 2013). Genetic improvement of pearl millet for adequate supply of micronutrients is relatively new area of research and is mainly focusing on improving Fe and Zn contents of grains as anemia and stunted growth are predominant across world (Mehta et al., 2017). Remarkable progress has been achieved within a short time.

36.5.2 Maize

The world's sixth largest maize producer (Zea mays) is India, which contributes about 2% of world output (Menkir et al., 2018). Maize output showed a substantial improvement of around 16% over the year 2015–2016 and projected output of 25.3 million tons in 2016–2017 (Taleon et al., 2017). Maize is the third leading cereal after wheat and rice, representing a large share of poultry feed (49%), led by human food (25%), livestock feed (12%), agricultural goods (12%), brewery (1%), and crops (1%) (Domingos et al., 2017). Just 30–40% of maize production is used for human use, and most (60–70%) is used domestically as livestock feed (Menkir et al., 2018). In India, Andhra Pradesh, Bihar, Himachal Pradesh, Karnataka, and Punjab are leading maize-growing states (Menkir et al., 2018). It is the main food for over 200 million people, offering 15% protein and 20% dietary calories. Indian maize is refined into several forms of items such as breakfast cereals, cornmeal, rice, grits, starch snacks, and tortillas (Domingos et al., 2017). Maize flour is commonly used to produce chapatis or flat bread in certain northern Indian states (Taleon et al., 2017). Consumption of 300 g cooked porridge made from yellow maize (1,2 mg β-carotene) along with added butter (20 g) and corn oil capsule (0,5 g) showed similar vitamin A behavior as retinol (0,38 mg) among eight stable Zimbabwean people (Muzingi et al., 2008). According to the RDA, it added 40–50% of adult vitamin A requirement. Daily intake of vitamin A maize has been shown to be as effective as vitamin A supplements (Listman et al., 2019). Phosphorous, potassium, and magnesium are the highly abundant minerals found in maize, accounting for approximately 85% of the kernel's mineral contents (Sawardekar et al., 2019). Considering malnutrition, zinc is an important mineral, and it has shown significant variability in maize (Maqbool and Beshir, 2018). Agronomic biofortification of maize with zinc through foliar application ($ZnSO_4$; 25kg ha^{-1}) has increased grain yield and yield attributes considerably (Kumar and Salakinkop, 2018).

36.5.3 Rice

In developed nations, biofortified rice is useful in increasing iron stores among women with low dietary iron intake (Losso et al., 2017). A study was conducted on 192 Filipino women chosen from 10 Philippine convent schools and a nine-month feeding track (Angeles-Agdeppa et al., 2008). Experimental participants received high iron rice (3.21 mg/kg Fe), while control group were fed local variety rice (0.57 mg/kg Fe) (Angeles-Agdeppa et al., 2008) and daily food intake was also reported. The results showed that biofortified rice and rice management added 1.79 mg iron per day to the diet and there was a 17% gap in overall dietary iron intake relative to regulation, contributing to a small increase in total body iron (P=.06) and serum ferritin (P=.10), but hemoglobin content did not show any change (Angeles-Agdeppa et al., 2008). A greater response for body iron and ferritin was observed in non-anemic women who took high iron rice (Angeles-Agdeppa et al., 2008).

Two German professors (Professor Ingo Potrykus, Institute of Plant Sciences, Swiss Federal Institute of Technology and Professor Peter Beyer, University of Freiburg) prepared golden rice in 1999 using genetic engineering (Garg et al., 2018). Both implanted bacteria and genes from daffodil plants to rice to create golden rice template that can contain significantly high levels of beta-carotene (Garg et al., 2018). In 2005, experts used genes from local soil micronutrients and maize to produce golden rice (current version) with approximately 20-fold extra beta carotene compared to that prepared previously in 1999. From 2006 to 2010, after choosing the key outcome of the current version, golden rice production proceeded to the next level of research and development (Datta and Datta, 2020). From 2010 to date, field trials in small and multi-location regions have helped breeders grow new varieties of golden rice that retain the same grain consistency, yield, and pest resistance (Singla and Grover, 2017). Furthermore, environmental and other data types were produced using various field tests and other estimates to help assess the productivity of golden rice (Datta and Datta, 2020). It was also proven that β-carotene in golden rice is as strong as pure β-carotene in oil and even allows children to get vitamin A. There was also a major increase in iron levels, like hemoglobin, plasma ferritin, and overall body strength, which improved the probability of overcoming iron deficiency (Hackl et al., 2019). It was hypothesized that biofortified staple food crops serve as a complementary therapy to monitor and avoid deficits in vitamin A and iron and aid enhance physiological outcomes such as brain health, cognitive efficiency, and physical activity (Hackl et al., 2019). Approximately 3 billion people consume rice as staple food all over the world, with an average consumption of 75.2 kg/capita/year (Trijatmiko et al., 2016). Further, polished rice consumption jumps up to 150 kg/capita/year in countries with medium-to-high prevalence of Fe and Zn deficiencies (Trijatmiko et al., 2016). This showed the high potential of biofortified rice to serve as a micronutrient-enriched product to decrease the severe micronutrient deficiency in rural and urban populations with limited incomes and low access to more diverse diets.

36.6 Vegetables

36.6.1 Potato

Field studies were performed to raise the concentrations of zinc in potato tubers (both flesh and tuber skin) using foliar zinc fertilizers, which significantly increased tuber zinc concentrations (Hyanes et al., 2012). Zinc oxide and zinc sulfate were also found to be more efficient than zinc nitrate as foliar fertilizers to raise tuber zinc concentrations while retaining yields (White et al., 2017). Potato tuber Se quality improved after foliar application of selenium, selenite, and selenate (Zhang et al., 2019). Foliar treatment of selenium with humic acids proved to be a good way to increase potato selenium content (Zhang et al., 2019). Potato tubers are the best sources of antioxidants in the human diet. The natural variation of seed potato germplasm comprising red and purple pigment may possibly represent potatoes contribution to the antioxidant component of human nutrition. Therefore, breeder efforts mainly focus on breeding such variants (Lachman and Hamouz, 2005). In fact, large genetic variation for micronutrients (Brown et al., 2010) occurs in potatoes that can be used for breeding to further raise iron and zinc in human diets (Burgos et al., 2007). A genetically diverse selection of South American Andean potato cultivars was collected from a set of approximately 1000 genotypes and tested as a source of antioxidants and minerals (copper, iron, manganese, and zinc) (Andre et al., 2007). Biofortified potato-targeted countries are Rwanda and Ethiopia. In Peru, the National Institute for Agrarian Innovation (INIA) Potato Program has grown the INIA 321 Kawsay variety with strong iron and zinc content.

36.6.2 Sweet Potato

Developing countries are raising 95% of the world's sweet potato production, where starvation is the biggest problem. Sweet potato was intended for vitamin A development. HarvestPlus and CIP have produced and launched many varieties of orange sweet potato with high vitamin A. There were six varieties in Uganda (Ejumula, Kakamega, Vita, Kabode, Naspot 12O, and Naspot 13O) and three in Zambia (Twatasha, Kokota and Chiwoko). Zambia Agriculture Research Institute has successfully completed 15 new varieties of reinforced sweet potatoes. HarvestPlus orange sweet potato had a significant impact on household food and nutritional welfare in sub-Saharan Africa, and for this achievement, they were recently awarded the World Food Prize-2016. Researchers have also established many sweet potato genotypes that miss or have only traces of β-amylase in their storage sources. These varieties may encourage the breeding of sweet potato for low β-amylase material, which can theoretically be used as a staple food (Kumagai et al., 1990). Increased beta-carotene in orange-fleshed sweet potato was observed with irrigation and chemical fertilizer treatments (Laurie et al., 2012).

36.6.3 Cassava

Cassava is a staple vegetable root crop in developing countries, particularly in Africa, Latin America, and the Caribbean (Bechoff et al., 2018). In the African continent, HarvestPlus, in partnership with the International Tropical Agriculture Institute, has achieved improvement in provitamin A (beta-carotene) content (Aragon et al., 2018). They have prepared six fortified varieties of cassava-rich in vitamin A in Nigeria (2011; TMS 01/1368—UMUCASS 36, TMS 01/1412—UMUCASS 37 and 2014; TMS 01/1371—UMUCASS 38 and NR 07/0220—UMUCASS 44, TMS 07/0593—UMUCASS 45, and TMS 07/539—UMUCASS 46) and one in the Democratic Republic of Congo [Kindisa (TMS 2001/1661)]. Cassava also has a wide range of genotype variations for total carotene, proteins, and minerals (iron and zinc), contributing to increased nutritional value in cassava crops (Narayanan et al., 2019; Corguinha et al., 2019).

36.6.4 Lettuce

Using KIO3 and Na2SeO4 as foliar spray and nutrient medium (Smolen et al., 2019), iodine and Se biofortification was achieved in lettuce. Se biofortification in lettuce leaves showed good results after soil agronomic biofortification with an inorganic source of selenium (Smolen et al., 2019).

36.6.5 Carrot

Carrot leaves and storage roots were supplemented with iodine and Se as fertilizers. Consumption of 100 g fresh weight of carrots fertilized with iodine and Se (KICNa2SeO3, KIO3CNa2SeO3) has been confirmed to provide 100% of the recommended daily allowance (Smolen et al., 2019).

36.6.6 Cauliflower

Brassica oleracea gene pool was tested for genetic variation in the concentration of zinc and ample natural variation was found (Singh et al., 2020). The rich orange-colored cauliflower variety (PusaBetaKesari; 800–1,000 μg/100 g) was developed by the Indian Agricultural Research Institute (IARI). The numbers of flavored cauliflower varieties are now known worldwide, with orange and purple dye abundant in beta-carotene and anthocyanin, respectively. Cornell University, USA, produced flavored cauliflower varieties, Purple Graffiti and Orange Cheddar.

36.7 FRUITS

36.7.1 Tomato

Studies have concluded that tomato is an excellent crop for biofortification programs with iron fertilizers (Landini et al., 2011). Tomato is a very useful product, an essential source of vitamins A and C. The genetically diverse wild tomato community has been intensively studied and used in tomato breeding (Raiola et al., 2014). Conventional breeding approaches have (Ilahy et al., 2018) developed biofortified tomato "Sun Black" with deep purple fruit pigmentation due to high anthocyanin content in the peel. Israel has reported another variety "Black Galaxy" generated with a similar approach (Ericsson, 2012).

36.7.2 Banana

Banana breeding is difficult and expensive, as commercial varieties are sterile triploids (3) and a high degree of cross-incompatibility may also occur among fertile classes (Amah et al., 2019). In the Democratic Republic of Congo (DRC) and Burundi, Biodiversity International (BI) in collaboration with HarvestPlus conducted a large screening of several banana germplasms to identify high levels of provitamin A (Garg et al., 2018). They prepared five varieties (Apantu, Bira, Pelipita, Lai, and To'o) rich in provitamin A in Eastern DRC and Burundi.

36.7.3 Grapes

Grapes have a strong mineral content, including high vitamins C and K, and are a natural source of antioxidants and other polyphenols, offering a variety of health benefits. Phenolic compounds and antioxidant properties of different cultivars grown in China were evaluated (Fontanella et al., 2016). An enhanced variety was developed by the Indian Agricultural Institute (i.e., PusaNavrang), which includes more complete soluble solids (i.e., carbohydrates, organic acids, proteins, fats, and minerals) and antioxidants.

36.7.4 Mango

Breeding mango provides a good source of beta-carotene, vitamin C, and essential antioxidants, but their amounts of nutrients differ with mango size. It was observed that most mango varieties provide more than recommended daily vitamin C and beta-carotene content. Mango also produces phenolics including ellagic acid, gallotannin, and mangiferin (Lauricella et al., 2017). Mexican-grown variety Ataulfo ranked highest in both vitamin C (ascorbic acid) and beta-carotene (USDA Agricultural Research Service). In India, IARI has prepared several varieties with enhanced nutritional and agronomic character.

36.8 Oilseeds

36.8.1 Mustard

Se enhancement is mainly targeted in mustard. Seas selenate was strengthened by rhizosphere bacteria from a seleniferous field (Yasin et al., 2015). Biofortified Indian mustard using high concentrations of iodine and Se represents an interesting target to improve human health (Golubkina et al., 2018). The foliar application of Se and iodine shows synergistic effects on nitrate reductase activity, increases flavonoid content in plant leaves, and also enhances the endogenous levels of of Na, Al, Co, V, B, Mn, Sr, Ca, and K (Golubkina et al., 2018).

36.8.2 Canola

Canola combined with plant-growing rhizobacteria, *Azospirillumbrasilense, Azotobactervinelandii,* and chemical fertilizers results in increased protein, oleic acid, and linoleic acid content in seeds suggesting that rhizobacteria are highly effective in increasing canola oil production and nutritional value (Nosheen et al., 2011).

36.9 Conclusions

Changing metabolic fluxes through a different pathway may influence plant growth and productivity. Changes in metal content, for example, can alter enzyme activity and metabolism. Hence, a cost-effective basic modification of plant metabolism is essential (Andersson et al., 2017). Useful biofortification activities will improve nutrient quality while maintaining low cultivation and processing costs. Advanced metabolomic and metabolic simulation techniques will, luckily, promote this research (Garg et al., 2018). The experimental criteria used to study biofortified foods will imitate clinical trials with a novel pharmacological agent (Talsma et al., 2017. Interactions with other nutrients in plant matrices, potential consumer allergic responses, and plant stress response changes are some of the parameters to be determined (Andersson et al., 2017). Interestingly, removing the anti-nutrient calcium oxalate crystals makes these modified plants more nutritious, but lowers the plant's defense to insect activity (Garg et al., 2018). Further, during these early days of genetically engineered healthy crops, the most critical challenge of the research community is to be rigorous in the protection analysis of such products before they are widely accessible to customers.

REFERENCES

Aciksoz, S. B., Yazici, A., Ozturk, L. & Cakmak, I. (2011). Biofortification of wheat with iron through soil and foliar application of nitrogen and iron fertilizers. *Plant and Soil*, *349*, 215–225.

Ali, B., Ali, A., Tahir, M. & Ali, S. (2014). Growth, Seed yield and quality of mungbean as influenced by foliar application of iron sulfate. *Pakistan Journal of Life and Social Sciences*, *12*, 20–25.

Aluru, M., Xu, Y., Guo, R., Wang, Z., Li, S., White, W. et al. (2008). Generation of transgenic maize with enhanced provitamin A content. *Journal of Experimental Botany*, *59*, 3551–3562.

Amah, D., van Biljon, A., Brown, A., Perkins-Veazie, P., Swennen, R. & Labuschagne, M. (2019). Recent advances in banana (musa spp.) biofortification to alleviate vitamin A deficiency. *Critical Reviews in Food Science and Nutrition*, *59*, 3498–3510.

Andre, C. M., Ghislain, M., Bertin, P., Oufir, M., del Rosario Herrera, M., Hoffmann, L. et al. (2007). Andean potato cultivars (Solanum tuberosum L.) as a source of antioxidant and mineral micronutrients. *Journal of Agricultural and Food Chemistry*, *55*, 366–378.

Angeles-Agdeppa, I., Capanzana, B., Florentino, R. F. & Takanashi, K. (2008). Efficacy of iron-fortified rice in reducing anemia among schoolchildren in the Philippines. *International Journal for Vitamin and Nutrition Research*, *78*, 74–86.

Aragão, F. J. L., Barros, L. M. G., De Sousa, M. V, Grossi de Sá, M. F., Almeida, E. R. P., Gander, E. S. & Rech, E. L. (1999). Expression of a methionine-rich storage albumin from the Brazil nut (Bertholletia excelsa HBK, Lecythidaceae) in transgenic bean plants (Phaseolus vulgaris L., Fabaceae). *Genetics and Molecular Biology*, *22*, 445–449.

Aragón, I. J., Ceballos, H., Dufour, D. & Ferruzzi, M. G. (2018). Pro-vitamin A carotenoids stability and bioaccessibility from elite selection of biofortified cassava roots (Manihot esculenta, Crantz) processed to traditional flours and porridges. *Food & Function*, *9*, 4822–4835.

Aro, A., Alfthan, G. & Varo, P. (1995). Effects of supplementation of fertilizers on human selenium status in Finland. *Analyst*, *120*, 841–843.

Austin-Phillips, S., Koegel, R. G., Straub, R. J. & Cook, M. (2001). *Animal feed compositions containing phytase derived from transgenic alfalfa and methods of use thereof*. The Consortium for Plant Biotechnology Research, Inc., West Lafayette, IN.

Avraham, T., Badani, H., Galili, S. & Amir, R. (2005). Enhanced levels of methionine and cysteine in transgenic alfalfa (Medicago sativa L.) plants over-expressing the Arabidopsis cystathionine γ-synthase gene. *Plant Biotechnology Journal*, *3*, 71–79.

Bechoff, A., Tomlins, K. I., Chijioke, U., Ilona, P., Westby, A. & Boy, E. (2018). Physical losses could partially explain modest carotenoid retention in dried food products from biofortified cassava. *PloS One*, *13*, 1–10.

Bhati, K. K., Alok, A., Kumar, A., Kaur, J., Tiwari, S. & Pandey, A. K. (2016). Silencing of ABCC13 transporter in wheat reveals its involvement in grain development, phytic acid accumulation and lateral root formation. *Journal of Experimental Botany, 67*, 4379–4389.

Bhuyan, U. N. (2018). Nutrition and Development of Connective Tissue: Effects of Protein and Ascorbic Acid Deficiency. In *Handbook of Nutritional Requirements in a Functional Context.* CRC Press. pp. 257–268.

Blair, M. W., Astudillo, C., Grusak, M. A., Graham, R. & Beebe, S. E. (2009). Inheritance of seed iron and zinc concentrations in common bean (Phaseolus vulgaris L.). *Molecular Breeding, 23*, 197–207.

Blancquaert, D., Van Daele, J., Strobbe, S., Kiekens, F., Storozhenko, S., De Steur, H. & Van Der Straeten, D. (2015). Improving folate (vitamin B 9) stability in biofortified rice through metabolic engineering. *Nature Biotechnology, 33*, 1076–1078.

Borg, S. (2012). Brinch-Pedersen. H., Tauris, B., Madsen, L. H., Darbani, B., Noeparvar, S., Holm, P. B., Wheat ferritins: improving the iron content of the wheat grain. *J. Cereal Sci, 56*, 204–213.

Bouis, H. (2018). Reducing mineral and vitamin deficiencies through biofortification: Progress under HarvestPlus. In *Hidden Hunger: Strategies to Improve Nutrition Quality.* Karger Publishers. Vol. 118, pp. 112–122.

Bouis, H. E., Hotz, C., McClafferty, B., Meenakshi, J. V. & Pfeiffer, W. H. (2011). Biofortification: a new tool to reduce micronutrient malnutrition. *Food and Nutrition Bulletin, 32*, S31–S40.

Bouis, H. E. & Saltzman, A. (2017). Improving nutrition through biofortification: a review of evidence from HarvestPlus, 2003 through 2016. *Global Food Security, 12*, 49–58.

Brinch-Pedersen, H., Borg, S., Tauris, B. & Holm, P. B. (2007). Molecular genetic approaches to increasing mineral availability and vitamin content of cereals. *Journal of Cereal Science, 46*, 308–326.

Brown, C. R., Haynes, K. G., Moore, M., Pavek, M. J., Hane, D. C., Love, S. L. et al. (2011). Stability and broad-sense heritability of mineral content in potato: zinc. *American Journal of Potato Research, 88*, 238–244.

Burgos, G., Amoros, W., Morote, M., Stangoulis, J. & Bonierbale, M. (2007). Iron and zinc concentration of native Andean potato cultivars from a human nutrition perspective. *Journal of the Science of Food and Agriculture, 87*, 668–675.

Cahoon, E. B., Hall, S. E., Ripp, K. G., Ganzke, T. S., Hitz, W. D. & Coughlan, S. J. (2003). Metabolic redesign of vitamin E biosynthesis in plants for tocotrienol production and increased antioxidant content. *Nature Biotechnology, 21*, 1082–1087.

Cakmak, I. & Kutman, U. B. (2018). Agronomic biofortification of cereals with zinc: a review. *European Journal of Soil Science, 69*, 172–180.

Carvalho, S. M. P. & Vasconcelos, M. W. (2013). Producing more with less: strategies and novel technologies for plant-based food biofortification. *Food Research International, 54*, 961–971.

Chen, Z., Young, T. E., Ling, J., Chang, S-C. & Gallie, D. R. (2003). Increasing vitamin C content of plants through enhanced ascorbate recycling. *Proceedings of the National Academy of Sciences, 100*, 3525–3530.

Corguinha, A. P. B., Carvalho, C. A., de Souza, G. A., de Carvalho, T. S., Vieira, E. A., Fialho, J. F. & Guilherme, L. R. G. (2019). Potential of cassava clones enriched with β-carotene and lycopene for zinc biofortification under different soil Zn conditions. *Journal of the Science of Food and Agriculture, 99*, 666–674.

Datta, S. K. & Datta, K. (2020). Golden Rice. In *The Future of Rice Demand: Quality Beyond Productivity.* Springer. pp. 135–147.

Davuluri, G. R., van Tuinen, A., Fraser, P. D., Manfredonia, A., Newman, R., Burgess, D. et al. (2005). Fruit-specific RNAi-mediated suppression of DET1 enhances tomato nutritional quality. *Nat. Biotechnol, 23*, 890–895.

de Figueiredo, M. A., Boldrin, P. F., Hart, J. J., de Andrade, M. J. B., Guilherme, L. R. G., Glahn, R. P. & Li, L. (2017). Zinc and selenium accumulation and their effect on iron bioavailability in common bean seeds. *Plant Physiology and Biochemistry, 111*, 193–202.

de La Garza, R. I. D., Gregory, J. F. & Hanson, A. D. (2007). Folate biofortification of tomato fruit. *Proceedings of the National Academy of Sciences, 104*, 4218–4222.

De Steur, H., Blancquaert, D., Strobbe, S., Lambert, W., Gellynck, X. & Van Der Straeten, D. (2015). Status and market potential of transgenic biofortified crops. *Nature Biotechnology, 33*, 25–29.

De Steur, H., Demont, M., Gellynck, X. & Stein, A. J. (2017). The social and economic impact of biofortification through genetic modification. *Current Opinion in Biotechnology, 44*, 161–168.

Deavours, B. E. & Dixon, R. A. (2005). Metabolic engineering of isoflavonoid biosynthesis in alfalfa. *Plant Physiology*, *138*, 2245–2259.

Decourcelle, M., Perez-Fons, L., Baulande, S., Steiger, S., Couvelard, L., Hem, S. Fraser, P. (2015). Combined transcript, proteome, and metabolite analysis of transgenic maize seeds engineered for enhanced carotenoid synthesis reveals pleotropic effects in core metabolism. *Journal of Experimental Botany*, *66*, 3141–3150.

Dharmapuri, S., Rosati, C., Pallara, P., Aquilani, R., Bouvier, F., Camara, B. & Giuliano, G. (2002). Metabolic engineering of xanthophyll content in tomato fruits. *Febs Letters*, *519*, 30–34.

Di, R., Kim, J. Martin, M. N., Leustek, T., Jhoo, J., Ho, C.-T. & Tumer, N. E. (2003). Enhancement of the primary flavor compound methional in potato by increasing the level of soluble methionine. *Journal of Agricultural and Food Chemistry*, *51*, 5695–5702.

Domingos, I. F. N., Baranski, M., Leifert, C., Cakmak, I., Rengel, Z., Bilsborrow, P. E. & Stewart, G. B. (2017). Protocol: Agronomic biofortification strategies to increase grain zinc concentrations for improved nutritional quality of wheat, maize and rice: a systematic review. *Campbell Systematic Reviews*, *13*, 1–16.

Doshi, K. M., Eudes, F., Laroche, A. & Gaudet, D. (2006). Transient embryo-specific expression of anthocyanin in wheat. In vitro *Cellular & Developmental Biology-Plant*, *42*, 432–438.

Eichler, K., Hess, S., Twerenbold, C., Sabatier, M., Meier, F. & Wieser, S. (2019). Health effects of micronutrient fortified dairy products and cereal food for children and adolescents: A systematic review. *PloS One*, *14*, 1–10.

Ericsson, S. (n.d.). The Antioxidant Purple Tomato. www.dailykos.com/stories/2016/8/1/1553921/-The-Antioxidant-Purple-Tomato

Falco, S. C., Guida, T., Locke, M., Mauvais, J., Sanders, C., Ward, R. T. & Webber, P. (1995). Transgenic canola and soybean seeds with increased lysine. *Bio/Technology*, *13*, 577–582.

Fontanella, M. C., D'Amato, R., Regni, L., Proietti, P., Beone, G. M. & Businelli, D. (2016). Agronomic selenium biofotification of grapes and sangiovese wine. In *6th FESTEM International Symposium*. Tecnograf srl. p. 129.

Food and Agriculture Organization [FAO] (2013): Food outlook: Biannual report on global food markets. Available at www.fao.org/giews

Francesco, S., Michela, J. & Angela, D. (2010). Increasing the amy-lose content of durum whrat through silencing of the SBE II a genes. *BMC Plant Biol*, *144*, 1–12.

Fujisawa, M., Watanabe, M., Choi, S.-K., Teramoto, M., Ohyama, K. & Misawa, N. (2008). Enrichment of carotenoids in flaxseed (Linum usitatissimum) by metabolic engineering with introduction of bacterial phytoene synthase gene crtB. *Journal of Bioscience and Bioengineering*, *105*, 636–641.

Garg, M., Sharma, N., Sharma, S., Kapoor, P., Kumar, A., Chunduri, V. & Arora, P. (2018). Biofortified crops generated by breeding, agronomy, and transgenic approaches are improving lives of millions of people around the world. *Frontiers in Nutrition*, *5*, 12.

Ghori, N. Riaz, A., Abbas, A. & Raza, S. (2017). Techniques for the Enrichment of Micronutrients in Crops through Biofortification: A Review. *Journal of Advances in Biology & Biotechnology*, *16(4)*, 1–7.

Gillespie, S., Hodge, J., Yosef, S. & Pandya-Lorch, R. (2016). Nourishing Millions.

Giuliano, G. (2017). Provitamin A biofortification of crop plants: a gold rush with many miners. *Current Opinion in Biotechnology*, *44*, 169–180.

Golubkina, N., Kekina, H. & Caruso, G. (2018). Yield, quality and antioxidant properties of Indian mustard (Brassica juncea L.) in response to foliar biofortification with selenium and iodine. *Plants*, *7*, 80.

Gorelova, V., Ambach, L., Rébeillé, F., Stove, C. & Van Der Straeten, D. (2017). Folates in plants: research advances and progress in crop biofortification. *Frontiers in Chemistry*, *5*, 21.

Goto, F., Yoshihara, T., Shigemoto, N., Toki, S. & Takaiwa, F. (1999). Iron fortification of rice seed by the soybean ferritin gene. *Nature Biotechnology*, *17*, 282–286.

Gould, J. (2017). Nutrition: A world of insecurity. *Nature*, *544*, S6–S6.

Haas, J. D., Finkelstein, J. L., Udipi, S. A., Ghugre, P. & Mehta, S. (2013). Iron biofortified pearl millet improves iron status in Indian school children: results of a feeding trial. Federation of American Societies for Experimental Biology Journal, 27, S1, 355.2

Hackl, L. S., Abizari, A.-R., Speich, C., Zungbey-Garti, H., Cercamondi, C. I., Zeder, C. et al. (2019). Micronutrient-fortified rice can be a significant source of dietary bioavailable iron in schoolchildren from rural Ghana. *Science Advances*, *5*, eaau0790.

Haynes, K. G., Yencho, G. C., Clough, M. E., Henninger, M. R. & Sterrett, S. B. (2012). Genetic variation for potato tuber micronutrient content and implications for biofortification of potatoes to reduce micronutrient malnutrition. *American Journal of Potato Research*, *89*, 192–198.

Hefferon, K. L. (2016). Can biofortified crops help attain food security? *Current Molecular Biology Reports*, *2*, 180–185.

Hefferon, K. L. (2018). Crops with improved nutritional content though agricultural biotechnology. In *Plant Micronutrient Use Efficiency*. Elsevier. pp. 279–294.

Hegedüsová, A., Mezeyová, I., Timoracká, M., Šlosár, M., Musilová J. & Juríková, T. (2015). Total polyphenol content and antioxidant capacity changes in dependence on chosen garden pea varieties. *Potravinarstvo Slovak Journal of Food Sciences*, *9*, 1–8.

Hellwege, E. M., Czapla, S., Jahnke, A., Willmitzer, L. & Heyer, A. G. (2000). Transgenic potato (Solanum tuberosum) tubers synthesize the full spectrum of inulin molecules naturally occurring in globe artichoke (Cynara scolymus) roots. *Proceedings of the National Academy of Sciences*, *97*, 8699–8704.

Hidoto, L., Tar'an, B., Worku, W. & Mohammed, H. (2017). Towards zinc biofortification in chickpea: performance of chickpea cultivars in response to soil zinc application. *Agronomy*, *7*, 11.

Hirschi, K. D. (2009). Nutrient biofortification of food crops. *Annual Review of Nutrition*, *29*, 401–421.

Holme, I. B., Dionisio, G., Brinch-Pedersen, H., Wendt, T., Madsen, C. K., Vincze, E. & Holm, P. B. (2012). Cisgenic barley with improved phytase activity. *Plant Biotechnology Journal*, *10*, 237–247.

Hong, H., Datla, N., Reed, D. W., Covello, P. S., MacKenzie, S. L. & Qiu, X. (2002). High-level production of γ-linolenic acid in Brassica juncea using a Δ6 desaturase from Pythium irregulare. *Plant Physiology*, *129*, 354–362.

Huang, Y., Yuan, L. & Yin, X. (2012). Biofortification to struggle against iron deficiency. In *Phytoremediation and Biofortification*. Springer. pp. 59–74.

Ibrahim, E. A. & Ramadan, W. A. (2015). Effect of zinc foliar spray alone and combined with humic acid or/and chitosan on growth, nutrient elements content and yield of dry bean (Phaseolus vulgaris L.) plants sown at different dates. *Scientia Horticulturae*, *184*, 101–105.

Ilahy, R., Siddiqui, M. W., Tlili, I., Hdider, C., Khamassy, N. & Lenucci, M. S. (2018). Biofortified vegetables for improved postharvest quality: Special reference to high-pigment tomatoes. In *Preharvest Modulation of Postharvest Fruit and Vegetable Quality*. Elsevier. pp. 435–454.

Karaköy, T., Erdem, H., Baloch, F. S., Toklu, F., Eker, S., Kilian, B. & Özkan, H. (2012). Diversity of macro- and micronutrients in the seeds of lentil landraces. *The Scientific World Journal*, 2012.

Khazaei, H., Podder, R., Caron, C. T., Kundu, S. S., Diapari, M., Vandenberg, A. & Bett, K. E. (2017). Marker–trait association analysis of iron and zinc concentration in lentil (Lens culinaris Medik.) seeds. *The Plant Genome*, *10*, 1–10.

Khush, G. S., Lee, S., Cho, J.-I. & Jeon, J.-S. (2012). Biofortification of crops for reducing malnutrition. *Plant Biotechnology Reports*, *6*, 195–202.

Kim, S. H., Kim, Y., Ahn, Y. O., Ahn, M., Jeong, J. C., Lee, H. & Kwak, S. (2013). Downregulation of the lycopene ε-cyclase gene increases carotenoid synthesis via the β-branch-specific pathway and enhances salt-stress tolerance in sweetpotato transgenic calli. *Physiologia Plantarum*, *147*, 432–442.

Kumagai, T., Umemura, Y., Baba, T. & Iwanaga, M. (1990). The inheritance of β-amylase null in storage roots of sweet potato, Ipomoea batatas (L.) Lam. *Theoretical and Applied Genetics*, *79*, 369–376.

Kumar, J., Gupta, D. Sen, Kumar, S., Gupta, S. & Singh, N. P. (2016). Current knowledge on genetic biofortification in lentil. *Journal of Agricultural and Food Chemistry*, *64*, 6383–6396.

Kumar, N. & Salakinkop, S. R. (2018). Agronomic biofortification of maize with zinc and iron micronutrients. *Mod Concep Dev Agrono*, *1*, 87–90.

Lachman, J., Hamouz, K., Orsák, M. & Kotíková, Z. (2016). Carotenoids in potatoes–a short overview. *Plant, Soil and Environment*, *62*, 474–481.

Lai, J. & Messing, J. (2002). Increasing maize seed methionine by mRNA stability. *The Plant Journal*, *30*, 395–402.

Landini, M., Gonzali, S. & Perata, P. (2011). Iodine biofortification in tomato. *Journal of Plant Nutrition and Soil Science*, *174*, 480–486.

Lauricella, M., Emanuele, S., Calvaruso, G., Giuliano, M. & D'Anneo, A. (2017). Multifaceted health benefits of Mangifera indica L.(Mango): the inestimable value of orchards recently planted in Sicilian rural areas. *Nutrients*, *9*, 525.

Laurie, S. M., Faber, M., Van Jaarsveld, P. J., Laurie, R. N., Du Plooy, C. P. & Modisane, P. C. (2012). β-Carotene yield and productivity of orange-fleshed sweet potato (Ipomoea batatas L. Lam.) as influenced by irrigation and fertilizer application treatments. *Scientia Horticulturae, 142,* 180–184.

Lipkie, T. E., De Moura, F. F., Zhao, Z.-Y., Albertsen, M. C., Che, P., Glassman, K. & Ferruzzi, M. G. (2013). Bioaccessibility of carotenoids from transgenic provitamin A biofortified sorghum. *Journal of Agricultural and Food Chemistry, 61,* 5764–5771.

Listman, G. M., Guzmán, C., Palacios-Rojas, N., Pfeiffer, W. H. San Vicente, F. & Govindan, V. (2019). Improving nutrition through biofortification: Preharvest and postharvest technologies. *Cereal Foods World, 64,* 1–7.

Lorenc-Kukuła, K., Wróbel-Kwiatkowska, M., Starzycki, M. & Szopa, J. (2007). Engineering flax with increased flavonoid content and thus Fusarium resistance. *Physiological and Molecular Plant Pathology, 70,* 38–48.

Losso, J. N., Karki, N., Muyonga, J., Wu, Y., Fusilier, K., Jacob, G. Greenway, F. L. (2017). Iron retention in iron-fortified rice and use of iron-fortified rice to treat women with iron deficiency: A pilot study. *BBA Clinical, 8,* 78–83.

Lu, S., Van Eck, J., Zhou, X., Lopez, A. B., O'Halloran, D. M., Cosman, K. M. et al. (2006). The cauliflower Or gene encodes a DnaJ cysteine-rich domain-containing protein that mediates high levels of β-carotene accumulation. *The Plant Cell, 18,* 3594–3605.

Lukaszewicz, M., Matysiak-Kata, I., Skala, J., Fecka, I., Cisowski, W. & Szopa, J. (2004). Antioxidant capacity manipulation in transgenic potato tuber by changes in phenolic compounds content. *Journal of Agricultural and Food Chemistry, 52,* 1526–1533.

Lyons, G. & Cakmak, I. (2012). Agronomic biofortification of food crops with micronutrients. *Fertilizing Crops to Improve Human Health: A Scientific Review, 1,* 97–122.

Maqbool, M. A. & Beshir, A. (2019). Zinc biofortification of maize (Zea mays L.): Status and challenges. *Plant Breeding, 138,* 1–28.

Márquez-Quiroz, C., De-la-Cruz-Lázaro, E., Osorio-Osorio, R. & Sánchez-Chávez, E. (2015). Biofortification of cowpea beans with iron: iron´s influence on mineral content and yield. *Journal of Soil Science and Plant Nutrition, 15,* 839–847.

Masuda, H., Aung, M. S., Kobayashi, T. & Nishizawa, N. K. (2020). Iron Biofortification: the gateway to overcoming hidden hunger. In *The Future of Rice Demand: Quality Beyond Productivity.* Springer. pp. 149–177.

Masuda, H., Kobayashi, T., Ishimaru, Y., Takahashi, M., Aung, M. S., Nakanishi, H. et al. (2013). Iron-biofortification in rice by the introduction of three barley genes participated in mugineic acid biosynthesis with soybean ferritin gene. *Frontiers in Plant Science, 4,* 132.

Mayer, J. E., Pfeiffer, W. H. & Beyer, P. (2008). Biofortified crops to alleviate micronutrient malnutrition. *Current Opinion in Plant Biology, 11,* 166–170.

Meenakshi, J. V., Johnson, N. L., Manyong, V. M., DeGroote, H., Javelosa, J., Yanggen, D. R. & Meng, E. (2010). How cost-effective is biofortification in combating micronutrient malnutrition? An ex ante assessment. *World Development, 38,* 64–75.

Mehta, S. Finkelstein, J. L., Venkatramanan, S., Huey, S. L., Udipi, S. A., Ghugre, P. & Potdar, R. D. (2017). Effect of iron and zinc-biofortified pearl millet consumption on growth and immune competence in children aged 12–18 months in India: study protocol for a randomised controlled trial. *BMJ Open, 7,* 1-10.

Menkir, A. Palacios-Rojas, N., Alamu, O., Dias Paes, M. C., Dhliwayo, T., Maziya-Dixon, B. & Pixley, K. (2018). *Vitamin A-biofortified maize: exploiting native genetic variation for nutrient enrichment.*

Ministry of Health and Family Welfare (MoHFW) (2017), Government of India, UNICEF and Population Council. Comprehensive National Nutrition Survey (CNNS). National Report New Delhi.

Molvig, L., Tabe, L. M., Eggum, B. O., Moore, A. E., Craig, S., Spencer, D. & Higgins, T. J. V. (1997). Enhanced methionine levels and increased nutritive value of seeds of transgenic lupins (Lupinus angustifolius L.) expressing a sunflower seed albumin gene. *Proceedings of the National Academy of Sciences, 94,* 8393–8398.

Morris, J., Hawthorne, K. M., Hotze, T., Abrams, S. A. & Hirschi, K. D. (2008). Nutritional impact of elevated calcium transport activity in carrots. *Proceedings of the National Academy of Sciences, 105,* 1431–1435.

Muzhingi, T., Yeum, K-J., Russell, R. M., Johnson, E. J., Qin, J. & Tang, G.. (2008). Determination of carotenoids in yellow maize, the effects of saponification and food preparations. *International Journal for Vitamin and Nutrition Research, 78,* 112–120.

Narayanan, N., Beyene, G., Chauhan, R. D., Gaitán-Solís, E., Gehan, J., Butts, P. et al. (2019). Biofortification of field-grown cassava by engineering expression of an iron transporter and ferritin. *Nature Biotechnology, 37,* 144.

Nestel, P., Bouis, H. E., Meenakshi, J. V. & Pfeiffer, W. (2006). Biofortification of staple food crops. *The Journal of Nutrition, 136,* 1064–1067.

Nosheen, A., Bano, A. & Ullah, F. (2011). Nutritive value of canola (Brassica napus L.) as affected by plant growth promoting rhizobacteria. *European Journal of Lipid Science and Technology, 113,* 1342–1346.

Ogo, Y., Ozawa, K., Ishimaru, T., Murayama, T. & Takaiwa, F. (2013). Transgenic rice seed synthesizing diverse flavonoids at high levels: a new platform for flavonoid production with associated health benefits. *Plant Biotechnology Journal, 11,* 734–746.

Ohnoutkova, L., Zitka, O., Mrizova, K., Vaskova, J., Galuszka, P., Cernei, N. et al. (2012). Electrophoretic and chromatographic evaluation of transgenic barley expressing a bacterial dihydrodipicolinate synthase. *Electrophoresis, 33,* 2365–2373.

Ortiz-Monasterio, J. I., Palacios-Rojas, N., Meng, E., Pixley, K., Trethowan, R. & Pena, R. J. (2007). Enhancing the mineral and vitamin content of wheat and maize through plant breeding. *Journal of Cereal Science, 46,* 293–307.

Paine, J. A., Shipton, C. A., Chaggar, S., Howells, R. M., Kennedy, M. J., Vernon, G. et al. Silverstone Al and Drake R (2005) A new version of Golden Rice with increased pro-vitamin A content. *Nat Biotech, 23,* 482–487.

Park, S., Kim, C.-K., Pike, L. M., Smith, R. H. & Hirschi, K. D. (2004). Increased calcium in carrots by expression of an Arabidopsis H+/Ca 2+ transporter. *Molecular Breeding, 14,* 275–282.

Pereira, E. J., Carvalho, L. M. J., Dellamora-Ortiz, G. M., Cardoso, F. S. N., Carvalho, J. L. V, Viana, D. S. et al. (2014). Effects of cooking methods on the iron and zinc contents in cowpea (Vigna unguiculata) to combat nutritional deficiencies in Brazil. *Food & Nutrition Research, 58,* 20694.

Petry, N., Boy, E., Wirth, J. P. & Hurrell, R. F. (2015). The potential of the common bean (Phaseolus vulgaris) as a vehicle for iron biofortification. *Nutrients, 7*(2), 1144–1173.

Poblaciones, M J. & Rengel, Z. (2016). Soil and foliar zinc biofortification in field pea (Pisum sativum L.): Grain accumulation and bioavailability in raw and cooked grains. *Food Chemistry, 212,* 427–433.

Poblaciones, M. J., Rodrigo, S., Santamaria, O., Chen, Y. & McGrath, S. P. (2014). Selenium accumulation and speciation in biofortified chickpea (Cicer arietinum L.) under Mediterranean conditions. *Journal of the Science of Food and Agriculture, 94*(6), 1101–1106.

Previtali, M. A., Mastromatteo, M., Conte, A., De Vita, P., Ficco, D. B. M. & Del Nobile, M. A. (2016). Optimization of durum wheat bread from a selenium-rich cultivar fortified with bran. *Journal of Food Science and Technology, 53*(2), 1319–1327.

Qaim, M., Stein, A. J. & Meenakshi, J. V. (2007). Economics of biofortification. *Agricultural Economics, 37,* 119–133.

Raiola, A., Rigano, M. M., Calafiore, R., Frusciante, L. & Barone, A. (2014). Enhancing the health-promoting effects of tomato fruit for biofortified food. *Mediators of Inflammation,* 2014:139873.

Ram, H., Rashid, A., Zhang, W., Duarte, A. P., Phattarakul, N., Simunji, S. et al. (2016). Biofortification of wheat, rice and common bean by applying foliar zinc fertilizer along with pesticides in seven countries. *Plant and Soil, 403,* 389–401.

Ramesh, S. A., Choimes, S. & Schachtman, D. P. (2004). Over-expression of an Arabidopsis zinc transporter in Hordeum vulgare increases short-term zinc uptake after zinc deprivation and seed zinc content. *Plant Molecular Biology, 54,* 373–385.

Reddy, B. V. S., Ramesh, S. & Longvah, T. (2005). Prospects of breeding for micronutrients and b-carotene-dense sorghums. *International Sorghum and Millets Newsletter, 46,* 10–14.

Rehman, H. M., Cooper, J. W., Lam, H. & Yang, S. H. (2019). Legume biofortification is an underexploited strategy for combatting hidden hunger. *Plant, Cell & Environment, 42,* 52–70.

Rhodes, D. (2019). Nutritional Genomics: Connecting Crop Improvement to Human Health. *Cereal Foods World, 64,* 1–10.

Ritchie, H., Reay, D. & Higgins, P. (2018). Sustainable food security in India – Domestic production and macronutrient availability. *PloS One, 13,* e0193766.

Römer, S., Lübeck, J., Kauder, F., Steiger, S., Adomat, C. & Sandmann, G. (2002). Genetic engineering of a zeaxanthin-rich potato by antisense inactivation and co-suppression of carotenoid epoxidation. *Metabolic Engineering, 4,* 263–272.

Ros, G. H., Van Rotterdam, A. M. D., Bussink, D. W. & Bindraban, P. S. (2016). Selenium fertilization strategies for bio-fortification of food: an agro-ecosystem approach. *Plant and Soil, 404,* 99–112.

Saltzman, A., Birol, E., Bouis, H. E., Boy, E., De Moura, F. F., Islam, Y. & Pfeiffer, W. H. (2013). Biofortification: progress toward a more nourishing future. *Global Food Security, 2,* 9–17.

Saltzman, A., Birol, E., Oparinde, A., Andersson, M. S., Asare-Marfo, D., Diressie, M. T et al. (2017). Availability, production, and consumption of crops biofortified by plant breeding: current evidence and future potential. *Annals of the New York Academy of Sciences, 1390,* 104–114.

Sato, S., Xing, A., Ye, X., Schweiger, B., Kinney, A., Graef, G. & Clemente, T. (2004). Production of γ-linolenic acid and stearidonic acid in seeds of marker-free transgenic soybean 1. *Crop Science, 44,* 646–652.

Sawardekar, S. S. & Sarkar, U. (2019). Nutritional assessment of protein content from organically grown zea mays l.(maize/corn). *International Journal of Scientific Research, 8,* 1-10.

Sharma, P., Aggarwal, P. & Kaur, A. (2017). Biofortification: A new approach to eradicate hidden hunger. *Food Reviews International, 33,* 1–21.

Shih, C-H., Chen, Y., Wang, M., Chu, I. K. & Lo, C. (2008). Accumulation of isoflavone genistin in transgenic tomato plants overexpressing a soybean isoflavone synthase gene. *Journal of Agricultural and Food Chemistry, 56,* 5655–5661.

Shivay, Y. S., Prasad, R. & Pal, M. (2015). Effects of source and method of zinc application on yield, zinc biofortification of grain, and Zn uptake and use efficiency in chickpea (Cicer arietinum L.). *Communications in Soil Science and Plant Analysis, 46,* 2191–2200.

Singh, R., Govindan, V. & Andersson, M. S. (2017). *Zinc-biofortified wheat: harnessing genetic diversity for improved nutritional quality. Science Brief: Biofortification 1*

Singh, S., Kalia, P., Meena, R. K., Mangal, M., Islam, S., Saha, S. & Tomar, B. S. (2020). Genetics and Expression Analysis of Anthocyanin Accumulation in Curd Portion of Sicilian Purple to Facilitate Biofortification of Indian Cauliflower. *Frontiers in Plant Science, 10,* 1766.

Singla, P. & Grover, K. (2017). Biofortified cereal crops: A Sustainable approach for food and nutritional security. *Current Journal of Applied Science and Technology,* 1–13.

Smoleń, S., Baranski, R., Ledwożyw-Smoleń, I., Skoczylas, Ł. & Sady, W. (2019). Combined biofortification of carrot with iodine and selenium. *Food Chemistry, 300,* 125202.

Smoleń, S., Kowalska, I., Kováčik, P., Halka, M. & Sady, W. (2019). Biofortification of six varieties of lettuce (Lactuca sativa L.) with iodine and selenium in combination with the application of salicylic acid. *Frontiers in Plant Science, 10.*

Song, S., Hou, W., Godo, I., Wu, C., Yu, Y., Matityahu, I. et al. (2013). Soybean seeds expressing feedback-insensitive cystathionine γ-synthase exhibit a higher content of methionine. *Journal of Experimental Botany, 64,* 1917–1926.

Szankowski, I., Briviba, K., Fleschhut, J., Schönherr, J., Jacobsen, H. J. & Kiesecker, H. (2003). Transformation of apple (Malus domestica Borkh.) with the stilbene synthase gene from grapevine (Vitis vinifera L.) and a PGIP gene from kiwi (Actinidia deliciosa). *Plant Cell Reports, 22,* 141–149.

Taleon, V., Mugode, L., Cabrera-Soto, L. & Palacios-Rojas, N. (2017). Carotenoid retention in biofortified maize using different post-harvest storage and packaging methods. *Food Chemistry, 232,* 60–66.

Talsma, E. F. & Pachón, H. (2017). Biofortification of crops with minerals and vitamins. World Health Organization, Rome. www.who.int/elena/titles/bbc/biofortification/en.

Tan, G. Z. H., Das Bhowmik, S. S., Hoang, T. M. L., Karbaschi, M. R., Long, H., Cheng, A. et al. (2018). Investigation of baseline iron levels in australian chickpea and evaluation of a transgenic biofortification approach. *Frontiers in Plant Science, 9,* 788.

Tang, M., He, X., Luo, Y., Ma, L., Tang, X. & Huang, K. (2013). Nutritional assessment of transgenic lysine-rich maize compared with conventional quality protein maize. *Journal of the Science of Food and Agriculture, 93*(5), 1049–1054.

Telengech, P. K., Maling'a, J. N., Nyende, A. B., Gichuki, S. T. & Wanjala, B. W. (2015). Gene expression of beta carotene genes in transgenic biofortified cassava. *3 Biotech, 5,* 465–472.

Thavarajah, D., Abare, A., Mapa, I., Coyne, C. J., Thavarajah, P. & Kumar, S. (2017). Selecting lentil accessions for global selenium biofortification. *Plants, 6,* 34.

Trijatmiko, K. R., Dueñas, C., Tsakirpaloglou, N., Torrizo, L., Arines, F. M., Adeva, C. et al. Biofortified indica rice attains iron and zinc nutrition dietary targets in the field. *Scientific Reports, 6,* 19792.

Upadhyaya, H. D, Bajaj, D., Das, S., Kumar, V., Gowda, C. L. L., Sharma, S. et al. (2016). Genetic dissection of seed-iron and zinc concentrations in chickpea. *Scientific Reports, 6,* 1–12.

Upadhyaya, H. D., Dronavalli, N., Gowda, C. L. L. & Singh, S. (2011). Identification and evaluation of chickpea germplasm for tolerance to heat stress. *Crop Science, 51*, 2079–2094.

Velu, G., Bhattacharjee, R., Rai, K. N., Sahrawat, K. L. & Longvah, T. (2008). A simple and rapid screening method for grain zinc content in pearl millet. *Journal of SAT Agricultural Research, 6*, 1–4.

Velu, G., Crespo H. L., Guzman, C., Huerta, J., Payne, T. & Singh, R. P. (2019). Assessing genetic diversity to breed competitive biofortified wheat with enhanced grain Zn and Fe concentrations. *Frontiers in Plant Science, 9*, 1971.

Vinoth, A. & Ravindhran, R. (2019). Biofortification in pearl millet: from conception to dissemination. In *Nutritional Quality Improvement in Plants*. Springer. pp. 413–428.

Waltz, E. (2014). Vitamin A Super Banana in Human Trials. Nature Publishing Group.

Wang, C., Zeng, J., Li, Y., Hu, W., Chen, L., Miao, Y. et al. (2014). Enrichment of provitamin A content in wheat (Triticum aestivum L.) by introduction of the bacterial carotenoid biosynthetic genes CrtB and CrtI. *Journal of Experimental Botany, 65*, 2545–2556.

Wei, S. H. U., Li, X., Gruber, M. Y., Li, R., Zhou, R., Zebarjadi, A. & Hannoufa, A. (2009). RNAi-mediated suppression of DET1 alters the levels of carotenoids and sinapate esters in seeds of Brassica napus. *Journal of Agricultural and Food Chemistry, 57*, 5326–5333.

Westermann, D., Terán, H., Muñoz-Perea, C. & Singh, S. (2011). Plant and seed nutrient uptake in common bean in seven organic and conventional production systems. *Canadian Journal of Plant Science, 91*, 1089–1099.

White, P. J., Thompson, J. A., Wright, G. & Rasmussen, S. K. (2017). Biofortifying Scottish potatoes with zinc. *Plant and Soil, 411*, 151–165.

Xin-Min, J., Xue-Yi, C., Ji-Yong, J., Tai, M., James, D. W., Rakeman, M. A. et al. (1997). Dynamics of environmental supplementation of iodine: four years' experience of iodination of irrigation water in Hotien, Xinjiang, China. *Archives of Environmental Health: An International Journal, 52*, 399–408.

Yasin, M., El Mehdawi, A. F., Jahn, C. E., Anwar, A., Turner, M. F. S., Faisal, M. & Pilon-Smits, E. A. H. (2015). Seleniferous soils as a source for production of selenium-enriched foods and potential of bacteria to enhance plant selenium uptake. *Plant and Soil, 386*, 385–394.

Yu, O., Shi, J., Hession, A. O., Maxwell, C. A., McGonigle, B. & Odell, J. T. (2003). Metabolic engineering to increase isoflavone biosynthesis in soybean seed. *Phytochemistry, 63*, 753–763.

Zhang, C., Liu, J., Zhang, Y., Cai, X., Gong, P., Zhang, J. et al. (2011). Overexpression of SlGMEs leads to ascorbate accumulation with enhanced oxidative stress, cold, and salt tolerance in tomato. *Plant Cell Reports, 30*, 389–398.

Zhang, H., Zhao, Z., Zhang, X., Zhang, W., Huang, L., Zhang, Z. et al. (2019). Effects of foliar application of selenate and selenite at different growth stages on Selenium accumulation and speciation in potato (Solanum tuberosum L.). *Food Chemistry, 286*, 550–556.

Zhang, L., Yang, X., Zhang, Y., Yang, J., Qi, G., Guo, D. et al. (2014). Changes in oleic acid content of transgenic soybeans by antisense RNA mediated posttranscriptional gene silencing. *International Journal of Genomics, 2014*.

Zhao, Z., Glassman, K., Sewalt, V., Wang, N., Miller, M., Chang, S. et al. (2003). Nutritionally improved transgenic sorghum. In *Plant Biotechnology 2002 and Beyond*. Springer. pp. 413–416.

Zhu, C., Naqvi, S., Gomez-Galera, S., Pelacho, A. M., Capell, T. & Christou, P. (2007). Transgenic strategies for the nutritional enhancement of plants. *Trends in Plant Science, 12*, 548–555.

37

Production of Sesquiterpene Lactones in Family Asteraceae: Structure, Biosynthesis, and Applications

Savita Bains, Vasundhara Thakur, Kashmir Singh, and Ravneet Kaur
Department of Biotechnology, Panjab University, Chandigarh, India

37.1 Introduction

The long history of medicine suggests the involvement of various plant constituents as therapeutic aids in curing a number of ailments in humans. Additionally, the plant-produced primary and secondary metabolites also assist in preventing certain disorders along with a wide range of functions. The *Asteraceae* family or the *Compositae* family is the largest family of flowering plants with around 24,000 species (Manzano et al., 2014). The vast range of metabolites obtained from *Asteraceae* plants has been a source of many bioactive constituents enriched with medicinal properties. Various bioactive compounds extracted from the *Asteraceae* plants including terpenes, saponins, flavonoids, alkaloids, phenolics, and carotenoids have proven pharmacological activities, thus revealing the pharmacological significance of the family.

The *Asteraceae* family plants are mostly herbaceous in existence while a few shrubs and rare trees also occur, most of which are employed in traditional and modern medicinal practices (Tamokou et al., 2017). These are widely distributed from the mountains to deserts and polar regions, richly found in the cold arctic, tropics, and alpine regions around the world (Manzano et al., 2014). In India, the *Asteraceae* family plants are mostly found in the higher Himalayan ranges as well as hills of western and southern India with a reported 697 species. The major plants of *Asteraceae* including *Lactuca sativa*, *Cichorium intybus*, *Cynara scolymus*, *Helianthus annuus*, *Tragopogon porrifolium*, *Carthamus tinctorius*, *Tagetes minuta*, and *Chrysanthemum coccineum* are some of the crop plants with economic importance. Most of these are consumed as vegetables and have been reported to yield various essential oils, dyes, food, and medicinal compounds (Bohm & Stuessy, 2001). The family also comprises plants with ornamental importance such as *Chrysanthemum, Cosmos, Dahlia, Zinnia, Calendula* (marigold), and *Ageratum*.

Sesquiterpene lactones (STLs) constitute one of the most widespread and biologically relevant class of plant produced secondary metabolites. These compounds are most prevalent in *Asteraceae* but are also found in several other plant families such as *Solanaceae, Cactaceae, Illiciaceae, Bombacaceae, Orchidaceae*, and *Euphorbiaceae*, with more than 5,000 reported components (Canales et al., 2005). These are synthesized mainly from the mevalonate pathway that occurs commonly among the plant families. STLs belong to the C15 terpenoids group generated from three isoprene units head-to-tail condensation and a lactone ring derived by cyclization and oxidation of one of the methanol groups (Matejić et al., 2010). The further classification of these secondary metabolites is performed on the grounds of the carbocyclic structure identifying approximately 30 subtypes of skeletals, such as eudesmanolides, germacranolides, guaianolides, heliangolides, hyptocretenolides, pseudoguaianolides, and many others. Mostly all the STLs including eudesmanolides and guaianolides are considered to be generated from a germacrene precursor, such as germacrene A as the precursor for costunolides (De Kraker et al., 1998). STLs are generally localized in the specialized secretary cells called the laticifers in the leaves and trichomes identified in many *Asteraceae* plants and are responsible for plant defense and allelopathic response. Around 90% of the identified STLs are extracted from the *Asteraceae* family; however, a plant

DOI: 10.1201/9781003220404-42

commonly manufactures a single type of STL skeletal with a dry weight in the range of 0.01% to 8%. These account for the bitter taste in plants, which prevents insects and herbivore animals from consuming the plant (Matejić et al., 2010).

The traditional system of medicine makes use of the extracts from such aromatic plants to cure a number of conditions and infections such as diarrhoea, cough, stomach pain, skin diseases, fever, cholera, paralysis, etc. (Duke & Duke, 2002). The α-methylene-γ-lactone group of the STLs is responsible for the various properties among the active constituents, including cytotoxic, anticancer, anti-inflammatory, antiviral, antimicrobial, antiprotozoal, anthelmintic, and antibacterial activities (Padilla-Gonzalez et al., 2016). Besides the α-methylene group, other modifications also occur commonly, incorporating epoxide ring and hydroxyls/esterified hydroxyls. The wide range of biological properties possessed by the STLs make them highly favourable to incorporate in number of biological applications as plant protective/defence agents as well as for medicinal use in humans. The high pharmaceutical and therapeutic value of these STLs has led to their increased demand as an anticancer component with cytotoxic properties. The anticancer activity and potential of STLs is strikingly magnificent leading to the clinical trials of some compounds such as artemisinin, parthenolide, and thapsigargin (Ghantous et al., 2010).

37.2 Structure of Sesquiterpene Lactones

STLs are prominent plant secondary metabolites, representing a large and most diversified class of sesquiterpenoids, comprising over 5,500 compounds (Rustaiyan et al., 2017). These are acrid, colorless, and lipophilic compounds. The plants species comprising the *Asteraceae* family are a rich source of bioactive compounds. The *Asteraceous* plants are considered as ubiquitous and copious source of STLs and thus are used for numerous medicinal purposes (Rodriguez et al., 1976; Zhang et al., 2005).

STLs exist in around 40 different structural types, which are well represented by germacranolides, guaianolides, eudesmanolides, and pseudoguaianolides, whereas bakkenolides, drimanolides, elemanolides, eremophilanolides, and xanthanolides are lesser known. Amongst these germacranolides, eudesmanolides, and guaianolides are considered the prominent classes. In particular, germacranolides are the most abundant type of STLs (Ludwiczuk et al., 2017; Adekenov, 2016; De Kraker et al., 2001).

Structurally, STLs comprise of 15-carbon (3 isoprene units; general formula: $C_{15}H_{24}$) basic skeleton and a lactone ring. Various STLs display different carbocyclic skeletons and appear either as hydrocarbons or oxygenated molecules like alcohols, aldehydes, ketones, and lactones. The sesquiterpene skeleton endorsing a lactone group is given a suffix "olide." Mostly, STLs contain γ-lactone ring but infrequently it can also be acyclic. The lactone ring has methylene group and carbonyl group positioned at α and β position, respectively. The γ-lactone ring with an exocyclic methylene joined to the carbonyl group is more common in STLs than the exocyclic methylene in reduced form (e.g., in artemisinin, matricin and santonin, and endocyclic double bond such as in glaucolides and hirsutinolides) (Ikezawa et al., 2011; Padilla-Gonzalez et al., 2016).

The lactone ring may be created in *cis*-configuration with regiospecificity at C6-C7 or *trans*-configurations with regiospecificity at C7-C8 position. Depending on the annulation of lactone ring STLs can be categorized into 6,12 –olide, which includes compounds such as costunolide, parthenolide, santonin, etc., and 8,12-olide, such as inunolide, alantolactone, and helenalin. The STLs are presumed to be evolutionary conserved compounds due to their extensive dominance in *Asteraceae* plants as a major secondary metabolite (Ikezawa et al., 2011).

37.2.1 Germacranolides

The germacranolides, in particular germacrenes, serve as main precursor for the biogenesis of numerous types of sesquiterpenes. It is anticipated that the lactone ring formation is followed by spontaneous cyclizations, ring fissions, and migration of methyl group to form various other STLs. The word "germacrane" is derived from "germacrone," which is isolated from *Geranium macrorrhizum*. The germacrone is a monocyclic ketone sesquiterpenoid (10-membered ring). The germacranes consist of an endocyclic double bond and depending on its position, they are designated as E,E-germacranes, Z,E-germacrenes, E,Z-germacrenes, and Z,Z-germacrenes. It is worth mentioning that E,E-germacranes are the most abundant whereas Z,Z-germacranes are less common (Adio et al., 2009a).

In germacranolides, the lactone ring is formed as a result of oxidation of three-carbon side chain and then guaianolides and eudesmanolides are derived from it (Seaman, 1982). The germacranolides, guaianolides, pseudoguaianolides, and eudesmanolides share a common structural feature (i.e., the presence of γ lactone moiety with a carbonyl group at α position).

The germacranolides carry a 10-membered ring and eudesmanolides have fused two 6-membered rings. Interestingly, guaianolides and pseudoguaianolides both have a 7- and a 5-membered ring, whereas the methyl group is present at C-4 in the former and C-5 in the latter (Chadwick et al., 2013).

37.2.2 Eudesmanolides

The *Asteraceae* family is quite enriched with structurally diverse eudesmane-12,6-olides (e.g., reynosin, santamarine, sphaeranthanolide, cichoriolide) possessing a number of biological activities, whereas eudesmane-12,8-olides, represented by compounds like gazanniolide, septuplinolide, and isoalloalantolactone, are rare (Wu et al., 2006). The majority of these compounds contain either *trans* -7,6-α,β unsaturated γ-lactone ring or its 11,13-dihydro derivatives. The compounds consist of 7,8-lactone groups exist as *cis*-and *trans*-γ-lactones. Mostly, these compounds consist of 3,4-, 4,5-, and 4,15-double bonds and derivatives of epoxide. Additionally, -OH and/or ketonic oxygen groups are characteristically present at carbon atom 1, 3, and 8 (Fischer et al., 1979).

37.2.3 Guaianolides

Guaianolides are characterized by the tricyclic skeleton along with a ring. The compounds are commonly referred to as 6,12-guaianolides (> 1400 compounds) or 8,12-guaianolides (> 170 compounds). These compounds are again more prevalent in *Asteraceae* followed by the *Apiaceae* family, despite their occurrence in a few other plant families and marine organisms. The core skeleton of guaianolides contains less than three double bonds (occasionally > three double bonds) and C-atoms are substituted with –OH group or esterified –OH group in natural compounds. The other substituents observed are epoxy groups, chlorine and hydroperoxyl groups. If C-7 is substituted with hydrogen, then it is subjected to α disposal (Simonsen et al., 2013).

37.2.4 Pseudoguaianolides

Pseudoguaianolides typically contain a lactone ring annelated in *-cis* or *-trans* conformation to the fused -7- and 5-membered rings. Pseudoguaianolides comprise ambrosanolides and helenanolides groups, the former being more prevalent than the latter subclass. Ambrosanolides are characterized by a 10-β-methyl configuration and comprised of compounds such as ambrosin, confertin, damsin, and parthenin. Helenanolide compounds such as helenalin, mexicanin, and aromatin contain a methyl group at C-10 in α configuration on the *trans*-hydroazulene nucleus. Interestingly, in these two subclasses methyl at C-7 is in β configuration (Barbero and Prandi, 2018).

37.3 Biosynthesis of STLs

Recently, tremendous advancement has been made in elucidation of structural aspects, localization, and biosynthesis of STLs. The hypothesis of STL biosynthesis via cyclization of farnesyl diphosphate to germacranolide basic skeleton and generation of diverse STLs after the rearrangement events was suggested by Herz (1977) and Fischer et al (1979) long ago. This presumption was then experimentally validated and very well supported with identification as well as characterization of quintessential genes, *germacrene A synthase*, *germacrene A oxidase*, and *costunolide synthase* isolated from *Asteraceae* plants, by several research groups (De Kraker et al., 1998; Nguyen et al., 2010; Ikezawa et al., 2011).

Several reports have proposed the biogenic route for sesquiterpenoid production. Essentially for terpenoidgeneration, five-carbon compounds, namely isopentenyl diphosphate (IPP) and dimethylallyl pyrophosphate (DMAPP), are the universal precursor molecules, supplied through cytosolic mevalonate (MVA) and plastidal methylerythritol phosphate (MEP) pathway. IPP can be generated by condensation of acetyl-CoA or derived from pyruvate and glyceraldehyde 3-phosphate (Newman et al., 1999; Eisenreich et al., 1998; Lichtenthaler et al., 1999). Subsequently, it yields different terpenes such as mono-, di-, tri-, and sesquiterpenes.

Farnesyl pyrophosphate (FPP) is produced from two molecules of IPP and one molecule of DMAPP in a reaction catalyzed by cytosolic farnesyl diphosphate synthase. FPP serves as a substrate for sterols, brassinosteroid, triterpene, and sesquiterpene compounds. IPP and DMAPP are formed in 6:1 ratio via MEP pathway (operative in plastids). One molecule of IPP and DMAPP each yield geranyl diphosphate (GPP) by GPP synthase activity, GPP thus formed results in the formation of monoterpenes. Similarly, for the production of geranyl geranyl diphosphate (GGPP), which occurs by the action of GGPP synthases, three IPP and one DMAPP molecule condenses. Further, GGPP acts as a precursor molecule for diterpene and tetraterpene synthesis (Gutensohn et al., 2013).

Farnesyl diphosphate (15-C) is produced as a result of head-to-tail fusion of IPP and DMAPP induced by FPP synthases. Terpene synthases then acts upon these prenyl phosphates, which cyclizes to produce sesquiterpenes. Further, this basic skeleton leads to formation of a wide range of terpenoid derivatives in a series of reactions catalysed by enzymes like cytochrome P450 and dehydrogenases (McGarvey et al., 1995).

Several hypothetical and proposed mechanism of STL biosynthesis are reported so far, but the major obstruction in studying these pathways lies in the fact that germacrenes are notoriously unstable and thus undergo cope rearrangement and cyclization to produce β-elemene or eudesmanes. The proton-induced emergence of α-selinene and β-selinene was also seen in chicory (De Kraker et al., 2001; De Kraker et al., 1998). Thus, a number of alternative practices are devised to study these compounds.

37.3.1 Biosynthesis of Germacranolides

Costunolide, a germacranolide, was first isolated from roots of an important medicinal plant, *Saussurea lappa* (Rao et al., 1960). The MVA pathway-derived FPP serves as the key precursor for costunolide biosynthesis.

The condensation of acetyl-CoA and acetoacetyl-CoA leads to 3-hydroxy-3-methylglutaryl-CoA production by the action of hydroxymethylglutaryl-coenzyme A synthase (HMGS). HMGS is essential for IPP production through MVA pathway, which ultimately yields metabolites such as terpene, sesquiterpene, and sterol. Hydroxymethylglutaryl-coenzyme A reductase (HMGR) induces the generation of coenzyme A and mevalonate during isoprenoid synthesis. Also, it plays pivotal role in cholesterol biosynthesis in mammals (Tabernero et al., 1999).

Subsequently, mevalonate-5-phosphate is produced from mevalonate via an ATP/divalent cation-dependent irreversible reaction catalysed by mevalonate kinase (Tchen, 1958). In the following reaction, mevalonate-5-phosphate yields mevalonate-5-diphosphate again in ATP-dependent reaction now catalysed by phosphomevalonate kinase (Garcia and Keasling, 2014). Then, IPP is generated by decarboxylation of mevalonate-5-pyrophosphate, catalysed by diphosphomevalonate decarboxylase. Finally, farnesyl di-phosphate synthase stimulates GPP or FDP synthesis, which later executes the production of mono-terpenes and di-terpenes or sesquiterpenes.

The germacrene A synthase (GAS), germacrene A oxidase (GAO), and costunolide synthase (COS) are considered as the key enzymes involved in costunolide biosynthesis. GAS catalyses the conversion of FPP into germacrene A, which is regarded as the first committed step with regard to costunolide biosynthesis. In fact, germacrene A is the main precursor for costunolide production in the majority of plants (De Kraker et al., 1998). A similar role of GAS is observed in other *Asteraceae* plants also (e.g., *Cichorium intybus, Helianthus annuus,* and *Cynara cardunculus)* (De Kraker et al., 2001; Bouwmeester et al., 2002; Gopfert et al., 2009).

It is noteworthy that two forms of sesquiterpene synthases, *CiGASsh* and *CiGASlo*, were isolated from *Cichorium intybus*, which depicted 78% similarity at protein level (Bouwmeester et al., 2002).

Interestingly, the amino acid sequence of these GAS forms is different from other sesquiterpene synthases known, which is evident from the presence of additional amino acids at the N-terminal.

The chicory-derived *germacrene A synthases* diverge from other sesquiterpene synthases such as 5-epi-cedrol and amorpha-4,11-diene synthases from *Artemisia*, which may be credited to the difference in sub-families of these plants (Bouwmeester et al., 2002). Surprisingly, GAS isolated from *Artemisia annua* is unable to form STLs unlike its homologous GASs isolated from other plants. As a consequence, the plant lacks any germacrene derivative. In contrast, *Lactuca sativa-derived* two sesquiterpene synthases (LCT1 and LCT2) are reported to have GAS activity, which points out that they may catalyse the germacrene A production from FPP (Bennett et al., 2002).

Germacrene A hydroxylase (GAO) acts on germacrene A and yield germacrene A acid. Studies revealed that the catalytic activity of GAO is evolutionary conserved in most of the *Asteraceae* subfamilies (*Asteroideae, Cichorioideae, Carduoideae*) and basal lineage *Barnedesia spinosa* (Ikezawa et al., 2011). Although sequence of germacrene A hydroxylase is not conserved in *Asteraceae*, the structural folds are believed to be significantly conserved.

In lettuce, the GAO brings out the germacrene A acid production in yeast *de novo*, whereas in *A. annua* the mutation in GAO leads to the formation of amorphadiene oxidase (AMO), whose substrate is amorphadiene. The phylogenetic studies displayed significant homology between AMO and GAOs from other plants (e.g., lettuce, chicory, and sunflower) at protein level (84.2–86.8% homology). Notably, AMO is assumed to have evolved recently as it illustrates divergence as a distinct node from rest of the GAO clade, emerging from *Barnedesia* GAO (Nguyen et al., 2010).

In *Cichorium intybus*, it was proposed that the conversion of germacrene A to gemacrene A acid requires three different enzymes (i.e., germacrene hydroxylase, germacrene alcohol dehydrogenase, and germacrene aldehyde dehydrogenase). The germacrene hydroxylase catalyze the conversion of germacrene A into germacrene A alcohol, and then dehydrogenase produces(-)-elema-1,3,11(13) -trien-12-oic acid from (-)-elema-1,3,11(13) -trien-12-ol in the presence of NADP+ and cofactor. Subsequently, the aldehyde dehydrogenase leads to the conversion of (-)-elema-1,3,11(13) -trien-12-al to (-)-elema-1,3,11(13) -trien-12-oic acid (NAD+ dependent) (De Kraker et al., 2001; 2002).

Finally, germacrene A acid undergoes lactonisation and cyclization to yield costunolide by the action of COS. De Kraker et al. (2002) was the first to report the isolation of COS from chicory roots. In *C. intybus*, COS was proved to stimulate STL-lactone ring formation in NADPH and molecular oxygen-dependent reaction. The hydroxylation of germacrene acid at C-6 followed by attack of -OH group at C-12 of carboxyl group results in lactone ring formation to produce costunolide (De Kraker et al., 2002).

The lettuce-derived COS showed close homology (more than 80%) to ESTs (expressed sequence tags) from these sub-families at amino acid level. Interestingly, the genes stored in EST database of these species also present homology to other genes of the pathway such as *GAS* and *GAO*. These findings establish the fact that biosynthesis of costunolide is exceedingly conserved in *Asteraceae* (Ikezawa et al., 2011).

Costunolide is the precursor of eudesmanolide, guaianolide, and germacranolide, which also possess medicinal properties. Importantly, costunolide is considered as the usual precursor for the production of various germacranolide STLs (Geissman et al., 1973; Fischer et al., 1979; Fischer, 1990). Earlier studies established that the formation of guaianolides and eudesmanolides occur through cyclization of costunolide via epoxidation at C4-C5 and C1-C10, respectively (Brown et al., 1975; Piet et al., 1995). The conversion of germacranolides to guaianolides may also occur by hydroxylation at C-3 (Piet et al., 1995).

37.3.2 Biosynthesis of Guaianolides, Pseudoguaianolides, and Eudesmanolides

As stated earlier, germacranolides are the so-called progenitors for biogenesis of guaianolide skeleton, which is derived from FPP molecule after series of cyclization and oxidation processes mediated by different enzymes.

In particular, the cyclization of a germacranolide-4,5-epoxide in chair-like transitional state provides the basic guaianolide skeleton. The subsequent reaction of *cis*-fused guaianolide cation with water produces guaianolide with *cis* fusion between the 5- and 7-membered rings. These types of *cis*-fused guaianolides are more pervasive with few exceptions, where *trans*-fused guaianolides are formed. On the other hand, the biosynthesis of *trans*-fused guaianolides is presumed to occur through cyclization of germacranolide-4,5-epoxide or melampolide-4,5-epoxide, which in turn supplies the *trans*-fused guaianolide cation. Then, a guaianolide skeleton with *trans*-fused 5- and 7-membered rings is formed after the reaction of *trans*-fused guaianolide cation formed in the prior step with water molecule (Alves, 2011).

The biological synthesis of ambrosanolides, a pseudoguaianolide, involves cyclization of the germacranolide-4,5-epoxide to guaianolide cation, which undergoes hydride and methyl group shift to yield the ambrosanolide skeleton. The ambrosanolides are characterized by a β-methyl group at C-10, fused-lactone ring at C6-C7 positions accompanied by C-6-β-oxygen, which is thought to help in carbo-cation rearrangement by stabilizing the centre of the cation (C-10) and permitting a hydride shift (C1 to C10) prior to attack of nucleophile, thereby assisting in guaianolide formation.

Another pseudoguaianolide, helenanolide, is also formed by a similar scheme as that of an ambrosanolide. The melampolide-4,5-epoxide as well as germacranolide 4,5-epoxide may serve as the precursor molecule and after sequential cyclization (acid-induced) carbocation formation and pre-described shifts, helenanolide skeleton is yielded. These compounds have α-methyl group at C-10, lac-tone ring at C7, and C8 position along with α/β-oxygen present at C-8. The biogenesis of ambrosanolides and helenanolides is outlined by Alves (2011).

In chicory, the guaianolide and eudesmanolide production is presumed to occur through 4,5 epoxidation and 1,10 epoxidation, respectively. For guaianolide biosynthesis to occur, costunolide acts as a precursor and undergoes 4,5 epoxidation to yield parthenolide. It is proposed that epoxide opens up to create a 3-cyclic skeleton after the intramolecular attack of the double bond (De Kraker et al., 2002; Bouwmeester et al., 2002). In the following step, the hydrogen ion abstraction of the C-atom close to carbocation (C10) results in double-bond formation (Δ1-10, Δ 9-10 or Δ10-14). On the other hand, the carbocation quenching may also occur after reacting with water and as a result C-10 alcohol can be formed.

The biosynthesis of eudesmanolide is hypothesized to take place via 1,10 epoxide as an intermediate, involving the same mechanism of intramolecular attack but yields C4 carbocation instead. Also, either the isomers with Δ4-5, Δ 3-4 or Δ4-15 double bonds are formed or an alcohol is produced at C-4 (Simonsen et al., 2013). Fischer et al. (1979) described that 1,10-epoxygermacronolides such as costunolide-1,l0-epoxide cyclizes and subsequent formation of a cation yields reynosin and santamarine.

37.4 Medicinal Properties of Various STLs

STLs are the active constituents of a number of *Asteraceae* plants, attributing to a variety of functions and thus used in curing different diseases ranging from skin diseases to major ailments and even cancer. The essential oils obtained from the aromatic plants are complex blends of such volatile STLs, enriched with pharmacological properties. Traditional medicines also appoints the usage of many STL-bearing plants in many infusions to relieve certain disorders like asthma, chronic rheumatism, diphtheria, bronchitis, gout, malaria, and leprosy (Sen & Chakraborty, 2019). Lately, the anticancer activity of many STLs has come into focus and a great deal of research work has been prompted to characterize the potential therapeutic and medical applications of STLs.

The bioactivity of STLs is attributed to the alkylation of biomolecules by Michael-type addition wherein the reaction of lactone moiety with the nucleophiles, for example thiol group (-SH), results in denaturation of various enzymes and proteins carrying cysteine residues.. For example, thiol group (-SH) results in denaturation of various enzymes and proteins carrying cysteine residues. The redox imbalance is also observed due to the reaction of lactone group and reduced glutathione present inside the cell (Rodriguez et al., 1976).

37.4.1 Anticancer and Cytotoxic Activity

Parthenolide, a germacranolide-type STL found in many medicinal plants, has been a main component to target cancer cells. The target mode of parthenolide involves the Fe (II) ions concentrated mostly in the cancer cells, which interact with parthenolide and lead to its cleavage to strongly oxidizing cytotoxic compounds, which destroy the surrounding tumor cells. It helped in the activation of c-Jun-N terminal kinase (JNK) in the tested cell lines including colorectal cancer COLO205, breast cancer MDA-MB-231, nasopharyngeal carcinoma CNE1, and cervical cancer HELA. The TNF-α-mediated NF-κB activation was inhibited by parthenolide as the IκB kinases (IKK) complex recruitment to the TNF receptor gets disrupted, blocking the further signalling events (Zhang et al., 2004). Another study revealed the sensitization of breast cancer cells HBL-100 through induction of JNK towards TNF-related apoptosis-inducing ligand (TRAIL)-induced apoptosis. The combined effect of parthenolide and TRAIL results in plasma membrane integrity loss and strongly activated apoptotic response in cancer cells (Nakshatri et al., 2004). Parthenolide has the ability to induce apoptosis in leukemia cell (pre-B acute lymphoblastic ALL leukemia) lines with t(4;11)(q21;q23) chromosomal translocation along with mitochondrial dysfunction more effective on t(4;11) lines (Zunino et al., 2007).

Costunolide, a colorless powder with crystalline structure, is a popular germacranolide series sesquiterpene lactone first isolated from the roots of *Saussurea lappa* Clarke (De Kraker et al., 2002). It has proven responses in inducing apoptosis, inhibiting metastasis and angiogenesis, inhibiting many cancer cells in vitro proliferation, and telomerase reverse transcriptase inhibition. Costunolide was observed to inhibit the Bcl-2 proteins and induce Bax proteins and cytochrome c release in many cancer cell lines including lungs, prostate, leukemia, and esophageal, while activating mitochondria-mediated apoptosis. Costunolide treatment resulted in the downregulated expression of Bcl-2, upregulation of Bax, and activated caspase-3, which led to the loss of membrane potential in mitochondria in Eca-109 cells of human esophageal cancer (Hua, Sun, et al., 2016). The human lung squamous carcinoma SK-MES-1 cells turned apoptotic on treatment with costunolide resulting from Bax and p53 expression upregulation, Bcl-2 expression downregulation, and activation of caspase-3 (Hua et al., 2016). The prostate cancer cell lines PC-3 and DU-145 were treated with costunolide, which resulted in p38 MAPK and JNK p38 MAPK, ROS generation, Bcl-2 and Bcl-xl inhibition along with Bax induction. This led to the decreased potential of mitochondrial membrane, thus releasing cytochrome c and activating caspase-3. Costunolide-induced apoptosis in mice led to the suppressed xenograft tumors of PC-3 cell growth (Chen et al., 2017). Also, the leukemia cell line K562 proliferation was inhibited by costunolide by modulating the Bcl-2 proteins levels and activating caspase-3, thus inducing mitochondrial apoptosis (Cai et al., 2018).

Cynaropicrin, a guaianolide type STL, was first isolated from *C. scolymus* L. (artichoke) in high content and responsible for approximately 80% of its bitter taste (Eljounaidi et al., 2014). Cynaropicrin obtained from *Hemisteptia lyrate* (Bunge) revealed cytotoxicity in response to human melanoma cell line LOX-IMVI, human prostate adenocarcinoma cell PC-3, human ovary adenocarcinoma cell line SK-OV-3, human breast adenocarcinoma cell MCF-7, human colorectal adenocarcinoma cell lines HCT-15, and human ovary adenocarcinoma cell lines SK-OV-3 (Ha et al., 2003). It is reported to show pro-apoptotic activity and act as a potential anticancer agent against reported leukemia cells, while inducing apoptosis and suppressing the human leukocytes cell lines proliferation in Jurkat T cells, Eol-1 and U937 (Cho et al., 2004).

Artemisinin inhibits the cell growth in A375P and A375M, the human melanoma cell lines, with accompanied growth-inhibitory and cytotoxic effects. Also, the A375M cells' ability to migrate was reduced by artemisinin as it downregulated the expression of α-V-β-3-integrin and decreased production of metalloproteinase-2 (Martínez et al., 2012). Another study revealed artemisinin being responsible for arresting G1 cell cycle in lymph node carcinoma of the human prostate cancer cell LNCaP, while protein and transcript levels of CDK2 and CDK4 were also suppressed (Willoughby et al., 2009). Along with artemisinin, its other derivatives like dihydroartemisinin, deoxoartemisinin trimer, 12-(2'-ethylthio) deoxoartemisinin dimer, dihydroartemisinin 12-benzoate, and 12-(2'-hydroxyethyl) deoxoartemisinin have also been reported to show antitumor in YD-10B, the oral squamous cancer cell line. Deoxoartemisinin trimer was observed to act more strongly against the tumor cells compared to the generally used chemotherapeutic drugs (Nam et al., 2007). Dihydroartemisinin was also reported for apoptotic activity against cultured SPC-A-1, human lung cancer cell line, by downregulating the mRNA and protein levels of survivin in the cell lines and activating apoptosis (Mu et al., 2007). These findings show the ability of artemisinin and its derivatives as potential chemotherapeutic agent with anticancer/antitumor activities.

Dehydrocostus lactone (DHE) is a naturally occurring STL obtained from various medicinal plants species like *Laurus nobilis* and *S. lappa*. It has caught the intense attention of researchers because of its promising anticancer responses against prostatic cancer, leukemias, bladder cancer, ovarian cancer, and breast cancer in various studies (Wang et al., 2017). DHE was shown to suppress various characteristics of glioblastoma cells such as the migration, proliferation, apoptotic resistance, and viability, while targeting IKKβ and inactivating NF-κB/COX-2 signalling pathway (both in vitro and in vivo). DHE also downregulated the antiapoptotic Bcl-2/BAX ratio and activated apoptosis mediated by mitochondria, which triggered the caspase signalling pathway by mitochondrial release of cytochrome c (Wang et al., 2017).

37.4.2 Anti-Inflammatory Activity

An inflammatory response is referred to as a physiological mechanism that generally helps in protection against infection and heals a tissue injury by a cascade of biological events including cellular and molecular signals (Medzhitov, 2008). The essential oils extracted from various plant species constituting surplus STLs have emerged as promising tools as anti-inflammatory agents. The NF-kB (nuclear transcription factor kappa B) pathway regulation of immune functions and inflammatory responses has been found to be responsible for the anti-inflammatory potential of STLs. The inflammation stimulus results in the activation of NF-kB, which phosphorylates its inhibitor (IκB) and generates a free NF-kB. This binds to the κB-binding sites in the target gene promoter regions located in the nucleus and causes the transcription of pro-inflammatory mediators like TNF-α (tumor necrosis factor-α), iNOS (inducible nitric oxide synthase), IL-1β, IL-6, IL-8, and COX-2 (cyclooxygenase-2) (Ghosh & Hayden, 2008).

Costunolide is isolated from a number of medicinal plants including *S. lappa* Clarke, *Aucklandia lappa* Decne, *Laurus nobilis* L., and *Vladimiria souliei* (Franch.) and has attracted great research interest due to its rich medicinal properties. Various preclinical studies reveal costunolide to possess anti-inflammatory activities, generally by the inhibition of pro-inflammatory cytokines. Costunolide treatments block the expression of iNOS, TNF-α, and COX-2 (cyclooxygenase-2) induced by 5-fluorouracil (5-FU) by inhibiting NF-kB activation in intestinal mucositis of mouse model (Chen et al., 2016). Costunolide downregulated the phosphorylation of mitogen-activated protein kinase (MAPK) and blocked the transcriptional activity of activator protein (AP-1), thus the interleukin (IL)-1β protein and mRNA expression was suppressed in lipopolysaccharide (LPS)-stimulated RAW264.7 cells (a murine macrophage cell line) (Kang et al., 2004). The toll-like signalling pathways regulate some immune responses, which are also reportedly affected by the interference of costunolide (Shin et al., 2012).

Artemisinin is an atypical STL isolated as an active principle from *Artemisia annua,* a Chinese medicinal herb and an effective antimalarial agent. In vivo studies showed immunosuppressive activity of artemisinin as it repressed the Type IV hypersensitivity against sheep blood capsule in BALB/c mice. In addition, artemisinin has also been observed to modulate NF-kB-mediated NO production in human astrocytoma cell line (Aldieri et al., 2003).

Dehydrocostus lactone, a chief sesquiterpene lactone derived from essential oil of *Aucklandia lappa,* has a reported anti-inflammatory property. The activation of LPS-induced NF-kB is inhibited by dehydrocostus lactone in RAW 264.7 cells, which suppresses the expression of proinflammatory factors like iNOS and nitric oxide (NO) production (Koo et al., 2001). Santamarin, one of the constituents extracted from *Artemisia hispanica* and *S. lappa,* showed the elicited anti-inflammatory response in LPS-stimulated RAW264.7 cells from mice pre-treated with santamarin (Choi et al., 2012). This resulted in suppressed COX-2 and iNOS expression, hence inhibiting production of NO and PGE$_2$ (prostaglandin E2), while reducing the production of TNF-α and IL-1β. The in vitro studies further revealed the increased nuclear transcription factor E2-related factor 2 (Nrf2) levels in RAW264.7 cells by santamarin. This leads to the induced expression of heme oxygenase (HO)-1 at both mRNA and protein level, which plays a cytoprotective role in response to apoptosis and inflammation (Choi et al., 2012).

Parthenolide is an essential STL naturally occurring in feverfew, and has been a source of various traditional medicines due to its enriched anti-inflammatory activity shown in several in vitro studies. Parthenolides possess great affinity to bind and suppress IκB kinase β (IKKβ), which is the mediator of cytokine-mediated signalling. The α-methylene γ-lactone moiety of parthenolide is proven to be responsible for the anti-inflammatory activity (both in vitro and in vivo) (Kwok et al., 2001). It inhibits the enzymes generating the mediators of inflammation including phosphodiesterase-4 (PDE4), phosphodiesterase-3 (PDE3), and 5-lipoxygenase (5-LOX) and also suppressed the LPS-activated production of inflammatory mediators like NO and TNF-a (Sur et al., 2009). Another study revealed that ethanolic extracts of leaves, flower, and parthenolide from *Tanacetum parthenium* showed prominent anti-inflammatory activity (Rateb et al., 2007).

Artemisolide is extracted by activity-guided fractionation method from *A. asiatica* as the inhibitor of NF-kB, along with inhibition of NO and PGE_2 production observed in LPS-stimulated macrophages RAW 264.7 cells. The simultaneous downregulation of expression of COX-2 or iNOS was also observed, thus suggesting its role as an anti-inflammatory agent (Reddy et al., 2006). Artemisolides have also been observed to inhibit the IκBα phosphorylation and thus suppress the activation of NF-kB in LPS-activated RAW 264.7 cells, along with the downregulated expression of TNF-α-dependent on NF-kB (Kim et al., 2007).

Cynaropicrin is the chemotaxonomic marker of the artichoke plants possessing great pharmaceutical potential and benefits to health (Ben Salem et al., 2015). It has also been reported to suppress the NO from interferon-γ-and LPS-activated RAW264.7 cells in a dose-dependent manner. Also, cynaropicrin inhibits IL-2, phytohemagglutinin, lipopolysaccharide, and concanavalin A-stimulated proliferation of lymphocytes from IL-2-sensitive cytotoxic T lymphocytes (CTLL-2) and splenocytes. Cynaropicrin has shown major suppressive activity on the expression of IL-1 and -6, TNF-α and NO production, suggesting it as a potential drug against chronic and acute inflammatory disorder (Elsebai et al., 2016).

Helenalin, a pseudoguaianolide type STL from *Arnica* species, has been used in traditional medicine practices to treat skin inflammations, sprains, contusions, and rheumatic diseases. Studies have shown the anti-inflammatory effects exerted by helenalin as its alkylating activity interferes with the DNA binding activity of NF-κB. Helenalin has been reported as a anti-inflammatory agent that selectively modifies the transcription factor subunit p65 and results in inhibited DNA binding. It can also inhibit the active complex of NF-κB, an important property to treat inflammation (Merfort, 2011).

37.4.3 Antimicrobial and Antibacterial Activity

Parthenolide, isolated from the aerial parts of *T. parthenium*, was revealed to possess antileishmanial activity tested against *L. amazonensis*. The promastigote growth of the microbe was inhibited by reducing its survival rate to 50% (Tiuman et al., 2005).

Vulgarone B, a component obtained from the essential oil of *A. iwayomogi*, shows antibacterial properties against specific antibiotic-resistant and susceptible bacteria. This suggests the use of vulgarone B as a favourable and safe candidate against bacterial pathogens including *Staphylococcus aureus*, *Salmonella* serotype *Typhimurium*, and *Salmonella* serotype Enteritidis. The mechanism of action was studied by treating *S. aureus* with vulgarone B extract that revealed high inhibitory action of the compound on bacteria, better than many previously studied plants (Chung et al., 2009). Dihydroartemisinin is one of the key metabolites of artemisinin and used against a number of parasites including *Plasmodium*, *Leishmania*, *Giardia lamblia*, *Toxoplasma*, *Trichomonas vaginalis*, and *Schistosoma* (Li et al., 2011).

Dehydroleucodine shows antimicrobial activity in response to *Helicobacter pylori*, which is the key factor in gastric cancer pathogenesis and the main causative agent in peptic and gastritis ulcer, suggesting it as a potential herbal component for treatment (Vega et al., 2009). Another STL obtained from *Artemisia* genus with antimicrobial activity comprises seco-tanapartholides A and B. These are the products of *A. princeps* that act on specific intestinal bacteria in humans such as *Bacteroides fragilis*, *Clostridium perfringens*, and *Staphylococcus aureus* by inhibiting their growth, without affecting the intestinal *Escherichia coli* and lactic acid-producing bacteria (Cho et al., 2003).

Costunolides have been shown to exhibit antimicrobial activity in response to *P. aeruginosa*, *E. coli*, and *S. aureus*. Also, they possess potent activity against *Helicobacter pylori*, the major pathogen responsible for peptic and gastric ulcer disease, as well as endocrine disorders and autoimmune diseases (Bruno et al., 2013).

Recently, various STLs have been isolated from *Vernonia cinerascens* Sch. Bip, which is a medicinal herb native to Africa and Tropical Asia. These include vernodalin, vernodalol, 11β,13-dihydrovernodalin (elemanolide type STLs), and vernocinerascolide (germacrolide type STL), obtained in the dichloromethane extract of the *V. cinerascens* leaves for the first time. These components revealed strong response against *Trypanosoma brucei rhodesiense* bloodstream forms tested in vitro, with vernodalin showing the highest antitrypanosomal activity (Kimani et al., 2018). The STLs vernolide,

11β,13-dihydroovernolide, and vernodalin also showed antibacterial activity against certain Gram-positive species including *Bacillus subtilis* and *S. aureus* and Gram-negative species including *E. coli* and *Klebsiella pneumoniae* (Chaturvedi, 2011).

37.4.4 Antimalarial Activity

Artemisinin is an oxygenated sesquiterpene lactone that constitutes of a 1,2,4-trioxane ring structure, responsible for the antimalarial activity of this component. Clinical trials have shown the huge effectiveness of artemisinin in curing malaria as well as other infections caused by *Plasmodium falciparum.* A series of semi-synthetic analogues for artemisinin have also been reported such as arteether, artemether, artesunate, and dihydroartemisinin, with remarkable activity in response to *Plasmodium* species (Cui & Su, 2009). Quick responses in clinical trials have been obtained with the use of artimisinins as they kill and reduce around 10,000 parasites per erythrocytic cycle within minutes (White, 2008). A number of artemisinin-based combinatory therapies (ACTs) involving combined drug treatment area employed in many malaria-endemic regions and accepted as leading method for treatment of uncomplicated *falciparum* malaria (Kokwaro et al., 2007). Besides artimisinin, about 14 sesquiterpene lactones were isolated and characterized from *A. gorgonum.* Amongst these, many possessed antiplasmodial activities with hanphyllin and ridentin showing the fine IC_{50} values and structurally constituting of an exomethylene group crucial for the biological affairs of STLs (Ortet et al., 2008).

Lactucin and lactucopicrin, isolated from *Cichorium intybus* using their root extracts, have been recognized for their antimalarial properties as the light sensitive STLs. The root extract treatment of these two STLs was used against *P. falciparum* (the HB3 clone of strain *Honduras-1*) and revealed significant properties of the crude extract (Bischoff et al., 2004).

37.4.5 Antiulcer Activity

The improvement in gastric ulcers induced by ethanol as a result of anti-inflammatory activity of costunolide was observed in mice by suppressing induction of NF-κB, iNOS, NO, COX-2, and TNF-α. Likewise, dehydrocostus lactone also showed defense against the ethanol-induced ulcer based on the inhibition of malondialdehyde (MDA) overproduction and inflammatory cytokines (Zheng et al., 2016). The acetone extract of costunolide resulted in a significant cholagogic effect and antiulcer response in mice. The added concentration of costunolide prevented the gastric ulcer generation in a dose-dependent manner (Zahara et al., 2014).

Dehydroleucodine, a guaianolide type sesquiterpene lactone isolated from *Artemisia douglasiana*, revealed anti-inflammatory activity in rats in the acute and chronic phases of paw inflammation by adjuvant carrageenan-induced and cotton pellet-induced granuloma. These results support the property of dehydroleucodine as a fine anti-inflammatory agent and hence its usage in traditional medicine systems, while suggesting its cytoprotective properties against gastric ulcers (Guardia et al., 2003).

Some important STLs obtained from *Artemisia annua* including deoxyartemisinin and dihydro-epideoxyarteannuin B were tested in indomethacin- and ethanol-induced ulcers models in rats and showed a suppressed ulcerative lesion index for both indomethacin and ethanol. The suggested mode of the action for the antiulcerogenic activity of these compounds is an increased synthesis of prostaglandin (Foglio et al., 2002).

37.4.6 Antifungal Activity

Vulgarone B is obtained in the steam-distilled oil extracts of *A. douglasiana* as an active antifungal compound and shows high activity against plant pathogenic fungi such as *Botrytis cinerea, Colletotrichum acutatum, Colletotrichum gloesporioides,* and *Colletotrichum fragariae* (Meepagala et al., 2003). The postulated mode of action for vulgarone B is its function as a Michael-type acceptor for biological nucleophiles as the α,β-unsaturated carbonyl group of the compound is crucial for its antifungal response.

Costunolide and eremanthin, the two guaianolides type STLs, have been reported to significantly inhibit various pathogenic fungi such as *Trichophyton mentagrophytes, Epidermophyton floccosum,*

Magnaporthe grisea, and *T. rubrum,* while the growth of *Aspergillus niger, Candida albicans,* and *T. simmi* were moderately inhibited. Both the compounds presented almost similar response against most of the pathogenic fungi, inhibiting the fungal growth at minimum concentrations, while costunolide had better response against few as compared to eremanthin (Duraipandiyan et al., 2012).

Chicory roots are a rich source of many STLs and two of the guaianolide types with different chemical structures have been isolated and characterized. These include 8-deoxylactucin and 11b,13-dihydrolactucin, which indicated an inhibitory response of 28.7% and 18.5%, respectively, towards *Trichophyton tonsurans var. sulfureum,* the most sensitive fungus (Mares et al., 2005).

37.5 Concluding Remarks

STLs are considered as biologically significant plant secondary metabolites, most prevalent in the *Asteraceae* family. The diverse biological and physiological applications of STLs are governed by the existence of various structural types. Thus, these important plant secondary metabolites present themselves as attractive and efficient alternatives to be used in medicinal systems to existing chemical drug formulations.

REFERENCES

Abad Martínez, M. J., Del Olmo, L. M. B., Ticona, L. A., and Benito, P. B. 2012. The Artemisia L. Genus: a review of bioactive sesquiterpene lactones. *Studies in Natural Products* Chemistry, 37:43–65. https://doi.org/10.1016/B978-0-444-59514-0.00002-X

Adekenov, S. M. 2017. Sesquiterpene lactones with unusual structure. Their biogenesis and biological activity. *Fitoterapia*, 121:16–30.

Adio, A. M. 2009a. (−)-trans-β-Elemene and related compounds: occurrence, synthesis, and anticancer activity. *Tetrahedron*, 27(65):5145–5159.

Aldieri, E., Atragene, D., Bergandi, L., Riganti, C., Costamagna, C., Bosia, A., and Ghigo, D. 2003. Artemisinin inhibits inducible nitric oxide synthase and nuclear factor NF-kB activation. *FEBS Letters*, 552(2–3):141–144. https://doi.org/10.1016/s0014-5793(03)00905-0.

Alves, J. C. 2011. A review on the chemistry of eremanthine: A sesquiterpene lactone with relevant biological activity. *Organic Chemistry International*, 2011.

Barbero, M., and Prandi, C. 2018. Pseudoguaianolides: Recent Advances in Synthesis and Applications. *Natural Product Communications*, 13(3), p.1934578X1801300303.

Ben Salem, M., Affes, H., Ksouda, K., Dhouibi, R., Sahnoun, Z., Hammami, S., and Zeghal, K. M. 2015. Pharmacological studies of artichoke leaf extract and their health benefits. *Plant Foods for Human Nutrition*, 70(4):441–453. https://doi.org/10.1007/s11130-015-0503-8.

Bennett, M. 2002. Cloning and expression of sesquiterpene synthase genes from lettuce (Lactucasativa L.). *Phytochemistry*, 60(3):255–261.

Bischoff, T. A., Kelley, C. J., Karchesy, Y., Laurantos, M., Nguyen-Dinh, P., and Arefi, A. G. 2004. Antimalarial activity of Lactucin and Lactucopicrin: Sesquiterpene lactones isolated from Cichorium intybus L. *Journal of Ethnopharmacology*, 95(2–3):455–457. https://doi.org/10.1016/j.jep.2004.06.031.

Bohm, B. A., and Stuessy, T. F. 2001. *Flavonoids of the sunflower family (Asteraceae).* Springer Science & Business Media.

Bouwmeester, H. J., Kodde, J., Verstappen, F. W., Altug, I. G., De Kraker, J. W., and Wallaart, T. E. 2002. Isolation and characterization of two germacrene A synthase cDNA clones from chicory. *Plant Physiology*, 129(1):134–144.

Brown, E. D., Sutherland, J. K. and Sam, T. W. 1975. Medium-ring 1, 5-dienes. Part III. Cyclisation of germacra-1 (10), 4, 7-(11)-triene oxides. *Journal of the Chemical Society, Perkin Transactions*, 1. (22):2332–2336.

Bruno, M., Bancheva, S., Rosselli, S., and Maggio, A. 2013. Sesquiterpenoids in subtribe Centaureinae (Cass.) Dumort (tribe Cardueae, Asteraceae): Distribution, 13C NMR spectral data and biological properties. Phytochemistry, 95:19–93. https://doi.org/10.1016/j.phytochem.2013.07.002.

Cai, H., He, X., and Yang, C. 2018. Costunolide promotes imatinib-induced apoptosis in chronic myeloid leukemia cells via the Bcr/Abl-Stat5 pathway. *Phytotherapy Research*, 32(9):1764–1769. https://doi.org/10.1002/ptr.6106.

Canales, M., Hernández, T., Caballero, J., Romo de Vivar, A., Avila, G., Duran, A., and Lira, R. 2005. Informant consensus factor and antibacterial activity of the medicinal plants used by the people of San Rafael Coxcatlán, Puebla, México. *Journal of Ethnopharmacology*, 97(3):429–439. https://doi.org/10.1016/j.jep.2004.11.013.

Chadwick, M., Trewin, H., Gawthrop, F., and Wagstaff, C. 2013. Sesquiterpenoids lactones: benefits to plants and people. *International Journal of Molecular* Sciences, 14(6): 12780–12805.

Chaturvedi, D. 2011. Sesquiterpene lactones: structural diversity and their biological activities, In *Opportunity, Challanges and Scope of Natural Products in Medicinal Chemistry. Research Signpost*, Trivandrum. pp. 313-334.

Chen, J., Chen, B., Zou, Z., Li, W., Zhang, Y., Xie, J., and Liu, C. 2017. Costunolide enhances doxorubicin-induced apoptosis in prostate cancer cells via activated mitogen-activated protein kinases and generation of reactive oxygen species. *Oncotarget*, 8(64):107701–107715. https://doi.org/10.18632/oncotarget.22592.

Chen, Y., Zheng, H., Zhang, J., Wang, L., Jin, Z., and Gao, W. 2016. Reparative activity of costunolide and dehydrocostus in a mouse model of 5-fluorouracil-induced intestinal mucositis. *RSC Advances*, 6(7):5249–5258. https://doi.org/10.1039/C5RA22371G.

Cho, J. Y., Kim, A. R., Jung, J. H., Chun, T., Rhee, M. H., and Yoo, E. S. 2004. Cytotoxic and pro-apoptotic activities of cynaropicrin, a sesquiterpene lactone, on the viability of leukocyte cancer cell lines. *European Journal of Pharmacology*, 492(2–3):85–94. https://doi.org/10.1016/j.ejphar.2004.03.027.

Cho, S. H., Na, Y. E., and Ahn, Y. J. 2003. Growth-inhibiting effects of seco-tanapartholides identified in Artemisia princeps var. Orientalis whole plant on human intestinal bacteria. *Journal of Applied Microbiology*, 95(1):7–12. https://doi.org/10.1046/j.1365-2672.2003.01998.x.

Choi, H. G., Lee, D. S., Li, B., Choi, Y. H., Lee, S. H., and Kim, Y. C. 2012. Santamarin, a sesquiterpene lactone isolated from Saussurea lappa, represses LPS-induced inflammatory responses via expression of heme oxygenase-1 in murine macrophage cells. *International Immunopharmacology*, 13(3):271–279. https://doi.org/10.1016/j.intimp.2012.04.016.

Chung, E. Y., Byun, Y. H., Shin, E. J., Chung, H. S., Lee, Y. H., and Shin, S. 2009. Antibacterial effects of vulgarone B from Artemisia iwayomogi alone and in combination with oxacillin. *Archives of Pharmacal Research*, 32(12):1711–1719. https://doi.org/10.1007/s12272-009-2208-8.

Cui, L. and Su, X. Z. 2009. Discovery, mechanisms of action and combination therapy of artemisinin. *Expert Review of Anti-Infective Therapy*, 7(8):999–1013. https://doi.org/10.1586/eri.09.68.

De Kraker, J. W., Franssen, M. C., Dalm, M. C., de Groot, A., and Bouwmeester, H. J. 2001. Biosynthesis of germacrene A carboxylic acid in chicory roots. Demonstration of a cytochrome P450 (+)-germacrene A hydroxylase and NADP+-dependent sesquiterpenoid dehydrogenase (s) involved in sesquiterpene lactone biosynthesis. *Plant Physiology*, 125(4):1930–1940.

De Kraker, J. W., Franssen, M. C., Joerink, M., De Groot, A., and Bouwmeester, H. J. 2002. Biosynthesis of costunolide, dihydrocostunolide, and leucodin. Demonstration of cytochrome P450-catalyzed formation of the lactone ring present in sesquiterpene lactones of chicory. *Plant Physiology*, 129(1):257–268.

De Kraker, J. W., Franssen, M. C. R., de Groot, A., König, W. A., and Bouwmeester, H. J. 1998. (+)-Germacrene A Biosynthesis: The Committed Step in the Biosynthesis of Bitter Sesquiterpene Lactones in Chicory. *Plant Physiology*, 117(4):1381–1392. https://doi.org/10.1104/pp.117.4.1381.

Duke, J. A., and Duke, J. A. 2002. *Handbook of Medicinal Herbs (2nd ed)*. CRC Press.

Duraipandiyan, V., Al-Harbi, N. A., Ignacimuthu, S., and Muthukumar, C. 2012. Antimicrobial activity of sesquiterpene lactones isolated from traditional medicinal plant, Costus speciosus (Koen ex.Retz.) Sm. *BMC Complementary and Alternative Medicine*, 12(1):1–6. https://doi.org/10.1186/1472-6882-12-13.

Eisenreich, W., Schwarz, M., Cartayrade, A., Arigoni, D., Zenk, M. H., and Bacher, A. 1998. The deoxyxylulose phosphate pathway of terpenoid biosynthesis in plants and microorganisms. *Chemistry & Biology*, 5(9): 221–233.

Eljounaidi, K., Cankar, K., Comino, C., Moglia, A., Hehn, A., Bourgaud, F., et al. 2014. Cytochrome P450s from Cynara cardunculus L. CYP71AV9 and CYP71BL5, catalyze distinct hydroxylations in the sesquiterpene lactone biosynthetic pathway. *Plant Science*, 223:59–68. https://doi.org/10.1016/j.plantsci.2014.03.007.

Elsebai, M. F., Mocan, A., and Atanasov, A. G. 2016. Cynaropicrin: a comprehensive research review and therapeutic potential as an anti-hepatitis C virus agent. *Frontiers in Pharmacology*, 7:472. https://doi.org/10.3389/fphar.2016.00472.

Fischer, N. H., Olivier, E. J., and Fischer, H. D. 1979. The biogenesis and chemistry of sesquiterpene lactones. *In Fortschritte der Chemie organischer Naturstoffe (Progress in the Chemistry of Organic Natural Products).* pp. 47–320.

Fischer, N. H. 1990. Sesquiterpene lactones: biogenesis and biomimetic transformations. *Biochemistry of the Mevalonic Acid Pathway to Terpenoids.* pp. 161–201.

Foglio, M. A., Dias, P. C., Antônio, M. A., Possenti, A., Rodrigues, R. A. F., da Silva, E. F., et al. 2002. Antiulcerogenic activity of some sesquiterpene lactones isolated from Artemisia annua. *Planta Medica,* 68(6):515–518. https://doi.org/10.1055/s-2002-32570.

Garcia, D. E. and Keasling, J. D. 2014. Kinetics of phosphomevalonate kinase from Saccharomyces cerevisiae. *PloS One,* 9(1), e87112.

Geissman, T. A. 1973. The biogenesis of sesquiterpene lactones of the compositae. *Recent Advances in Phytochemistry,* 6:65–95.

Ghantous, A., Gali-Muhtasib, H., Vuorela, H., Saliba, N. A., and Darwiche, N. 2010. What made sesquiterpene lactones reach cancer clinical trials? *Drug Discovery Today,* 15(15–16):668–678. https://doi.org/10.1016/j.drudis.2010.06.002.

Ghosh, S. and Hayden, M. S. 2008. New regulators of NF-kappaB in inflammation. *Nature Reviews Immunology,* 8(11):837–848. https://doi.org/10.1038/nri2423.

Gopfert, J. C., MacNevin, G., Ro, D. K., and Spring, O. 2009. Identification, functional characterization and developmental regulation of sesquiterpene synthases from sunflower capitate glandular trichomes. *BMC Plant Biology,* 9(1):86.

Guardia, T., Juarez, A. O., Guerreiro, E., Guzmán, J. A., and Pelzer, L. 2003. Anti-inflammatory activity and effect on gastric acid secretion of dehydroleucodine isolated from Artemisia douglasiana. *Journal of Ethnopharmacology,* 88(2–3):195–198. https://doi.org/10.1016/S0378-8741(03)00211-3.

Gutensohn, M., Orlova, I., Nguyen, T. T., Davidovich-Rikanati, R., Ferruzzi, M. G., Sitrit, Y., et al. 2013. Cytosolic monoterpene biosynthesis is supported by plastid-generated geranyl diphosphate substrate in transgenic tomato fruits. *The Plant Journal,* 75(3):351–363.

Ha, T. J., Jang, D. S., Lee, J. R., Lee, K. D., Lee, J., Hwang, S. W., et al. 2003. Cytotoxic effects of sesquiterpene lactones from the flowers ofHemisteptia lyrata B. *Archives of Pharmacal Research,* 26(11):925–928. https://doi.org/10.1007/BF02980201.

Herz, W. 1977. Biogenetic aspects of sesquiterpene lactone chemistry. *Israel Journal of Chemistry,* 16(1):32–44.

Hua, P., Sun, M., Zhang, G., Zhang, Y., Song, G., Liu, Z., et al. 2016. costunolide induces apoptosis through generation of ros and activation of p53 in human esophageal cancer eca-109 cells. *Journal of Biochemical and Molecular Toxicology,* 30(9):462–469. https://doi.org/10.1002/jbt.21810.

Hua, P., Zhang, G., Zhang, Y., Sun, M., Cui, R., Li, X., et al. 2016. Costunolide induces G1/S phase arrest and activates mitochondrial-mediated apoptotic pathways in SK-MES 1 human lung squamous carcinoma cells. *Oncology Letters,* 11(4):2780–2786. https://doi.org/10.3892/ol.2016.4295.

Ikezawa, N., Göpfert, J.C., Nguyen, D.T., Kim, S.U., O'Maille, P.E., Spring, O. and Ro, D.K. 2011. Lettuce costunolide synthase (CYP71BL2) and its homolog (CYP71BL1) from sunflower catalyze distinct regio-and stereoselective hydroxylations in sesquiterpene lactone metabolism. *Journal of Biological Chemistry,* 286(24):21601–21611.

Kang, J. S., Yoon, Y. D., Lee, K. H., Park, S.K., and Kim, H. M. 2004. Costunolide inhibits interleukin-1β expression by down-regulation of AP-1 and MAPK activity in LPS-stimulated RAW 264.7 cells. *Biochemical and Biophysical Research Communications,* 313(1):171–177. https://doi.org/10.1016/j.bbrc.2003.11.109.

Kim, B. H., Lee, J.Y., Seo, J. H., Lee, H. Y., Ryu, S. Y., Ahn, B. W., et al. Artemisolide is a typical inhibitor of IκB kinase β targeting cysteine-179 residue and down-regulates NF-κB-dependent TNF-α expression in LPS-activated macrophages. *Biochemical and Biophysical Research Communications,* 361(3):593–598. https://doi.org/10.1016/j.bbrc.2007.07.069.

Kimani, N. M., Matasyoh, J., Kaiser, M., Brun, R., and Schmidt, T. 2018. Sesquiterpene lactones from Vernonia cinerascens Sch. Bip. and their in vitro antitrypanosomal activity. *Molecules,* 23(2):248. https://doi.org/10.3390/molecules23020248.

Kokwaro, G., Mwai, L., and Nzila, A. 2007. Artemether/lumefantrine in the treatment of uncomplicated falciparum malaria. *Expert Opinion on Pharmacotherapy,* 8(1):75–94. https://doi.org/10.1517/14656566.8.1.75.

Koo, T. H., Lee, J.H., Park, Y. J., Hong, Y.S., Kim, H. S., Kim, K.W., and Lee, J. J. 2001. A Sesquiterpene Lactone, Costunolide, from Magnolia grandiflora Inhibits NF-κB by Targeting IκB Phosphorylation. *Planta Medica*, 67(2):103–107. https://doi.org/10.1055/s-2001-11503.

Kwok, B. H. B., Koh, B., Ndubuisi, M. I., Elofsson, M., and Crews, C. M. 2001. The anti-inflammatory natural product parthenolide from the medicinal herb Feverfew directly binds to and inhibits IκB kinase. *Chemistry & Biology*, 8(8):759–766. https://doi.org/10.1016/S1074-5521(01)00049-7.

Li, H. J., Wang, W., and Liang, Y. S. 2011. Advances in research of dihydroartemisinin against parasitic diseases. *Chinese Journal of Schistosomiasis Control*, 23(4):460–464.

Lichtenthaler, H. K. 1999. The 1-deoxy-D-xylulose-5-phosphate pathway of isoprenoid biosynthesis in plants. *Annual Review of Plant Biology*, 50(1):47–65.

Ludwiczuk, A., Skalicka-Woźniak, K. and Georgiev, M. I. 2017. *Pharmacognosy: Fundamentals, Applications and Strategies*. pp. 233-266.

Manzano, P., Miranda, M., Orellana, T., and Quijano, M. 2014. Studies of the volatile compounds present in leaves, stems and flowers of Vernonanthura patens (Kunth) H. Rob. *International Journal of Organic Chemistry*, 04(05):314–318. https://doi.org/10.4236/ijoc.2014.45034.

Mares, D., Romagnoli, C., Tosi, B., Andreotti, E., Chillemi, G., and Poli, F. 2005. Chicory extracts from Cichorium intybus L. as potential antifungals. *Mycopathologia*, 160(1):85–91. https://doi.org/10.1007/s11046-004-6635-2.

Matejić, J., Šarac, Z., and Ranđelović, V. 2010. Pharmacological activity of sesquiterpene lactones. *Biotechnology & Biotechnological Equipment*, 24(sup1), 95–100. https://doi.org/10.1080/13102818.2010.10817819.

McGarvey, D. J. and Croteau, R. 1995. Terpenoid metabolism. *The Plant Cell*, 7(7):1015.

Medzhitov, R. 2008. Origin and physiological roles of inflammation. *Nature*, 454(7203):428–435. https://doi.org/10.1038/nature07201.

Meepagala, K. M., Kuhajek, J. M., Sturtz, G. D. and Wedge, D. E. 2003. Vulgarone B, the antifungal constituent in the steam-distilled fraction of Artemisia douglasiana. *Journal of Chemical Ecology*, 29(8):1771–1780. https://doi.org/10.1023/A:1024842009802.

Merfort, I. 2011. Perspectives on sesquiterpene lactones in inflammation and cancer. *Current Drug Targets*, 12(11):1560–1573. https://doi.org/10.2174/138945011798109437.

Mu, D., Qi, H., Chen, W., Yu, B., Zhang, C., and Zhang, Y. 2007. Calcium and survivin are involved in the induction of apoptosis by dihydroartemisinin in human lung cancer SPC-A-1 cells. *Methods and Findings in Experimental and Clinical Pharmacology*, 29(1):33–38. https://doi.org/10.1358/mf.2007.29.1.1063493.

Nakshatri, H., Rice, S. E., and Bhat-Nakshatri, P. 2004. Antitumor agent parthenolide reverses resistance of breast cancer cells to tumor necrosis factor-related apoptosis-inducing ligand through sustained activation of c-Jun N-terminal kinase. *Oncogene*, 23(44):7330–7344. https://doi.org/10.1038/sj.onc.1207995.

Nam, W., Tak, J., Ryu, J. K., Jung, M., Yook, J. I., Kim, H. J., and Cha, I. H. 2007. Effects of artemisinin and its derivatives on growth inhibition and apoptosis of oral cancer cells. *Head & Neck*, 29(4):335–340. https://doi.org/10.1002/hed.20524.

Newman, J. D., and Chappell, J. 1999. Isoprenoid biosynthesis in plants: carbon partitioning within the cytoplasmic pathway. *Critical Reviews in Biochemistry and Molecular Biology*, 34(2):95–106.

Nguyen, D. T., Göpfert, J. C., Ikezawa, N., MacNevin, G., Kathiresan, M., Conrad, J., et al. 2010. Biochemical conservation and evolution of germacrene A oxidase in Asteraceae. *Journal of Biological Chemistry*, 285(22):16588–16598.

Ortet, R., Prado, S., Mouray, E., and Thomas, O. P. 2008. Sesquiterpene lactones from the endemic Cape Verdean Artemisia gorgonum. *Phytochemistry*, 69(17):2961–2965. https://doi.org/10.1016/j.phytochem.2008.09.022.

Padilla-Gonzalez, G. F., dos Santos, F. A., and Da Costa, F. B. 2016. Sesquiterpene lactones: more than protective plant compounds with high toxicity. *Critical Reviews in Plant Sciences*, 35(1):18–37. https://doi.org/10.1080/07352689.2016.1145956.

Piet, D. P., Schrijvers, R., Franssen, M. C. and de Groot, A. 1995. Biotransformation of germacrane epoxides by Cichorium intybus. *Tetrahedron*, 51(22):6303–6314.

Rao, A. S., Kelkar, G. R. and Bhattacharyya, S. C. 1960. Terpenoids—XXI: the structure of costunolide, a new sesquiterpene lactone from costus root oil. *Tetrahedron*, 9(3-4): 275–283.

Rateb, M. E., El-Gendy, A. N. A., El-Hawary, S. S. and El-Shamy, A. M. 2007. Phytochemical and biological investigation of Tanacetum parthenium (L.) cultivated in Egypt. *Journal of Medicinal Plants Research*, 1(1):18–26.

Reddy, A. M., Lee, J. Y., Seo, J. H., Kim, B. H., Chung, E. Y., Ryu, S. Y., et al. 2006. Artemisolide from Artemisia asiatica: Nuclear Factor-κB (NF-κB) inhibitor suppressing prostaglandin E2 and nitric oxide production in macrophages. *Archives of Pharmacal Research*, 29(7):591–597. https://doi.org/10.1007/BF02969271.

Rodriguez E, Towers G. H. N., and Mitchell J. C. 1976. Biological activies of sesquiterpene lactones. *Phytochemistry* 15(11):1573–1580.

Rustaiyan, A., Faridchehr, A., and Bakhtiyar, M. 2017. Sesquiterpene lactones of iranian compositae family (astraceae); their chemical constituents and anti-plasmodial properties of tehranolide (A review). *Oriental Journal of Chemistry*, 33(5):2188–2197.

Seaman, F. C. 1982. Sesquiterpene lactones as taxonomic characters in the Asteraceae. *The Botanical Review*, 48(2):121–594.

Sen, S., and Chakraborty, R. (Eds.). 2019. Herbal Medicine in India: Indigenous Knowledge, Practice, Innovation and its Value. *Springer Nature*.

Shin, H. J., Kim, S. J., and Youn, H. S. 2012. Costunolide inhibits interferon regulatory factor 3 activation induced by lipopolysaccharide and polyinosinic-polycytidylic acid. *Food Science and Biotechnology*, 21(5):1343–1348. https://doi.org/10.1007/s10068-012-0177-z.

Simonsen, H. T., Weitzel, C. and Christensen, S. B. 2013. Guaianolide sesquiterpenoids: pharmacology and biosynthesis. In *Natural Products: Phytochemistry, Botany and Metabolism of Alkaloids, Phenolics and Terpenes, Springer*, pp. 3069–3098.

Sur, R., Martin, K., Liebel, F., Lyte, P., Shapiro, S., and Southall, M. 2009. Anti-inflammatory activity of parthenolide-depleted Feverfew (Tanacetum parthenium). *Inflammopharmacology*, 17(1):42–49. https://doi.org/10.1007/s10787-008-8040-9.

Tabernero, L., Bochar, D. A., Rodwell, V. W. and Stauffacher, C. V. 1999. Substrate-induced closure of the flap domain in the ternary complex structures provides insights into the mechanism of catalysis by 3-hydroxy-3-methylglutaryl–CoA reductase. *Proceedings of the National Academy of Sciences*, 96(13):7167–7171.

Tamokou, J. D. D., Mbaveng, A. T., and Kuete, V. 2017. Antimicrobial activities of African medicinal spices and vegetables. In medicinal spices and vegetables from Africa (207–237). Academic Press.

Tchen, T. T. 1958. Mevalonic kinase: purification and properties. *Journal of Biological Chemistry*, 233(5):1100–1103.

Tiuman, T. S., Ueda-Nakamura, T., Garcia Cortez, D. A., Dias Filho, B. P., Morgado-Díaz, J. A., de Souza, W., and Nakamura, C. V. 2005. Antileishmanial activity of parthenolide, a sesquiterpene lactone isolated from Tanacetum parthenium. *Antimicrobial Agents and Chemotherapy*, 49(1):176–182. https://doi.org/10.1128/AAC.49.11.176-182.2005.

Vega, A. E., Wendel, G. H., Maria, A. O. M., and Pelzer, L. 2009. Antimicrobial activity of Artemisia douglasiana and dehydroleucodine against Helicobacter pylori. *Journal of Ethnopharmacology*, 124(3):653–655. https://doi.org/10.1016/j.jep.2009.04.051.

Wang, J., Yu, Z., Wang, C., Tian, X., Huo, X., Wang, Y., et al. 2017. Dehydrocostus lactone, a natural sesquiter-pene lactone, suppresses the biological characteristics of glioma, through inhibition of the NF-κB/COX-2 signaling pathway by targeting IKKβ. *American Journal of Cancer Research*, 7(6):1270–1284.

White, N. J. 2008. Qinghaosu (artemisinin): The price of success. *Science*, 320(5874):330–334. https://doi.org/10.1126/science.1155165.

Willoughby, J. A., Sundar, S. N., Cheung, M., Tin, A. S., Modiano, J., and Firestone, G. L. 2009. Artemisinin blocks prostate cancer growth and cell cycle progression by disrupting Sp1 interactions with the cyclin-dependent kinase-4 (CDK4) promoter and inhibiting CDK4 gene expression. *The Journal of Biological Chemistry*, 284(4): 2203–2213. https://doi.org/10.1074/jbc.M804491200.

Wu, Q. X., Shi, Y. P. and Jia, Z. J. 2006. Eudesmane sesquiterpenoids from the Asteraceae family. *Natural product reports*, 23(5):699–734.

Zahara, K., Tabassum, S., Sabir, S., Arshad, M., Qureshi, R., Amjad, M. S., and Chaudhari, S. K. 2014. A review of therapeutic potential of Saussurea lappa – An endangered plant from Himalaya. *Asian Pacific Journal of Tropical Medicine*, 7:60–69. https://doi.org/10.1016/S1995-7645(14)60204-2.

Zhang, S., Won, Y. K., Ong, C. N., and Shen, H. M. 2005. Anti-cancer potential of sesquiterpene lactones: bio-activity and molecularmechanisms. *Current Medicinal Chemical – Anti-Cancer Agents,* 5(3): 239–249.

Zhang, S. 2004. Suppressed NF-B and sustained JNK activation contribute to the sensitization effect of parthenolide to TNF--induced apoptosis in human cancer cells. Carcinogenesis, 25(11):2191–2199. https://doi.org/10.1093/carcin/bgh234.

Zheng, H., Chen, Y., Zhang, J., Wang, L., Jin, Z., Huang, H., et al. 2016. Evaluation of protective effects of costunolide and dehydrocostuslactone on ethanol-induced gastric ulcer in mice based on multi-pathway regulation. *Chemico-Biological Interactions*, 250:68–77. https://doi.org/10.1016/j.cbi.2016.03.003.

Zunino, S. J., Ducore, J. M., and Storms, D. H. 2007. Parthenolide induces significant apoptosis and production of reactive oxygen species in high-risk pre-B leukemia cells. *Cancer Letters*, 254(1):119–127. https://doi.org/10.1016/j.canlet.2007.03.002.

38

Multiple Therapeutic Applications of Pomegranate Fruit and its Bioactive Phytochemicals in Health and Disease

Mostafa Gouda
Department of Nutrition & Food Science, National Research Centre, Giza, Egypt
College of Biosystems Engineering and Food Science, Zhejiang University, Hangzhou, China

Laila Hussein
Department of Nutrition & Food Science, National Research Centre, Giza, Egypt

Douglas W. Wilson
School of Medicine, Pharmacy and Health, Durham University, Durham, UK
Centre for Ageing & Dementia Research, Swansea University, Swansea, UK

Harpal S. Buttar
Department of Pathology & Laboratory Medicine, University of Ottawa, Ottawa, Canada

38.1 Introduction

Plants and plant-derived phytochemicals provide useful sources of food nutrients and therapeutic preparations for managing several health conditions in many parts of the world. Many modern drugs have been isolated from the plants (Gouda, et al., 2021a; Gouda et al., 2021b). The vast majority of people who use plant extracts or herbal remedies consider them safer than synthetic drugs (Ekor, 2014). Phytochemicals have been traditionally used for treating a wide array of chronic ailments like cardiovascular and neurological diseases, osteoarthritis, and cancer. Pg fruit and juice have shown bactericidal and virucidal effects against a number of highly pathogenic and drug-resistant strains of pathogens (Khorrami et al., 2020). Pomegranate (*Punica granatum* L.) is one of the most important non-pharmacological interventions that may be used as an adjunct therapy for the management of non-communicable diseases in patients with high oxidative burden (Wang et al., 2018a). Pg is one of the richest sources of polyphenolic ellagitannins and anthocyanins (Asgary et al., 2021). It has been observed that regular intake of Pg juice (PJ) lowers blood pressure (Asgary et al., 2017) and produces hypocholesterolremic effects (Asgary, et al., 2014), which are attributed to its inhibitory actions on the activities of two key enzymes involved in cholesterol metabolism such as 3-hydroxy-3-methylglutaryl-CoA reductase and sterol O-acyltransferase (Hussein et al., 2019). Pg is a member of the *Lythraceae* family whose derivatives have depicted potential cytotoxic activities and inhibition of cell proliferation, markers of migration, induction of apoptosis, and cell adhesion in prostate cancer cell lines (Yuan et al., 2018). There is growing interest among researchers and consumers in the fact that the bioactive compounds present in Pg can play a significant therapeutic role in disease prevention in humans. Recently, the consumption of Pg fruit and PJ either alone or in combination with other flavonoid-containing juices has shown increased trends in Western countries. However, not all that glitters is gold. Pg is not a panacea for every arterial or cardiac problem, but it could be an effective treatment for some related diseases, such as atherosclerosis (Kahramanoglu, 2019; Al-Jarallah et al., 2013).

There is a tremendous interest in research on the potential therapeutic applications of phytochemicals present in Pg as anticancer, cardioprotective, and neuroprotective agents as well as nutritional benefits for promoting health and well-being in humans (Gouda et al., 2016; Hussein et al., 2021). The focus of clinical and nutraceutical research related to Pg-derived phytochemicals is justified based on the historical usefulness of Pg as a nutritional agent and alternative therapy for treating a wide range of human maladies and disorders (Ismail et al., 2016).

Wilson et al. (2017) reported on the important role of antioxidants present in functional foods and their impact in the prevention of neurodegenerative diseases like Alzheimer's disease. They mentioned the relationship of brain functions with dietary choices, mainly in older humans. This included food color, flavor, and aroma, as they relate to dietary sufficiency or the association of antioxidants with neurodegenerative diseases. For instance, the antioxidants present in functional foods have the potential to inhibit the enzyme acetylcholinesterase, which is one of the risk factors for Alzheimer's diseas eand Parkinson's disease (Griffiths et al., 2016; King et al., 2021).

A number of studies have suggested that Pg juice and derivatives have the potential for the prevention of neurodegenerative disorders and can serve as antiaging adjuvants (Braidy et al., 2016). It has been reported that consumption of Pg juice can prevent dementia in adults > 50 years old, and its mechanism of action seems to be mediated through the essential amino acid tryptophan and its metabolites (i.e., serotonin, melatonin, niacin, etc.), which are important neurochemicals for brain function (Bookheimer et al., 2013; Yang et al., 2020). According to these authors, regular consumption of Pg juice significantly increased the plasma concentration of tryptophan metabolite indolepropionate, and decreased *Shigella* and *Catenibacterium* bacteria in the gut. *Shigella* is a well-known pathogenic Gram-negative bacterium that causes inflammatory bowel disease (IBD) and destruction of the intestinal epithelial barrier leading to leaky gut syndrome. Furthermore, the antimicrobial metabolite of Pg, urolithin A (UA), activates mitophagy and the recycling of defective cellular mitochondria, and consequently improved mitochondrial health in preclinical *Caenorhabditis elegans* models of aging and neuroscience (Andreux et al., 2019). UA benefits have also been observed in preclinical *C. elegans* including neurodegenerative disorders (Fang et al., 2019). After human participants drank a glass of Pg juice (contains 500 mg of UA), the gut microbiota produced urolithin metabolites, which were excreted in the feces and urine, but with interindividual variability due to the frequency and extent of people's natural ability to convert ellagitannins (ET) and ellagic acid (EA) into UA (Singh et al., 2021). Urolithins have shown, neuroprotective, cardioprotective, antidiabetic, antiobesity, anticancer, antioxidant, and antiinflammatory activities, as well as enhancement of muscular performance in athletes (Tomas-Barberan et al., 2017).

This chapter emphasizes the importance of Pg juice as a healthy food and the multiple benefits of biologically active ingredients present in different parts of Pg. We will also describe recent in vitro and in vivo studies reporting on the cellular and molecular mechanisms of various ingredients present in Pg. Based on the antioxidant, antiinflammation, and antimicrobial properties, the phytochemicals of Pg may be used for curing chronic diseases like some cancers, cardiovascular and neurodegenerative disorders, male erectile dysfunction, IBD, etc. Well-designed, randomized, and placebo-controlled clinical studies are needed to determine the dose-schedules as well as the long-term safety and efficacy of Pg-derived phytochemicals.

38.2 History of Pomegranate

The curative actions of Pg go back to Biblical times and beyond (Kahramanoglu, 2019). It was utilized as a traditional remedy for thousands of years under the Indian Ayurvedic and Unani systems of medicine. Extracts from the rind of Pg fruit and bark of the Pg tree were found to be effective against diarrhoea and dysentery in humans. Hippocrates (459–370 BC), the Greek physician and father of modern medicine, classified 300 medicinal plants by their pharmacological actions, where Pg was mentioned with astringent effects (Nigam, 2020). Also, the beneficial effects of Pg have been mentioned in several ancient religious scriptures like the Holy Bible and Holy Quran (Pourghayoumi et al., 2017). According to the

TABLE 38.1

Quantitative Analyses of Pomegranate Organic Acids, Sugar, and Individual Phenolics of Aril Juices. (Modified from (Kalaycioglu et al., 2017. Reproduced with Copyright Permission: 5092940464028.)

Cultivars/ Country	Organic Acid Content	Sugar Content	Individual Phenolics Content	Reference

Six cultivars/ Turkey	g/100 mL
	Citric acid: 0.2-3.2
	mg/mL
	Malic acid: 0.9-1.5
	Ascorbic acid: 0.14-0.69
		g/100 mL
		Fructose:
		  5.8-7.06
		Glucose:5.8-7.62
		Sucrose:
		  0.02-0.04
			-	(Ozgen et al., 2008)

Eight cultivars/ Iran	-	-	mg/L Ellagic acid: 7-160 Anthocyanins Delphinidin 3,5-diglucoside: 372-5301 Cyanidin 3,5-diglucoside: 242-2361 Delphinidin 3-glucoside: 49-1042 Pelargonidin 3,5-diglucoside:7-90 Cyanidin 3-glucoside: 2-358	(Mousavinejad et al., 2009)
Fiften cultivars/ Spain	g/L Citric acid: 0.60-18.54 Malic acid: 0.89-1.63 Tartaric acid: 0.17-0.41	g/L Fructose: 76-96 Glucose: 67-89	mg/L Ellagic acid glucoside: 2.1-17.9 Ellagic acid:1.1-142.0 Punicalagin α: 0.3-12.8 Punicalagin β: 1.0-31.4 Anthocyanins Delphinidin 3,5- diglucoside: 13.0-200.2 Cyanidin 3,5-diglucoside: 11.6-311.0 Pelargonidin 3,5 diglucoside: 0.4-14.5 Delphinidin-3-glucoside: 2.9-257.6 Cyanidin 3-glucoside: 4.0-354.2 Pelargonidin 3-glucoside: 0.1-23.8	(Mena et al., 2011)

Thirteen cultivars/ Tunisia	-	-	mg/L
			Delphinidin-3,5-
			  diglucoside: 33.16-406.72
			Cyanidin-3,5-diglucoside:2.02-9.80
			Pelargonidin-3,5-
			  diglucoside: 0.24-0.86
			Delphinidin-3-glucoside: 10.85-84.69
			Cyanidin-3-glucoside: 1.16-26.76
			Pelargonidin-3-glucoside: 0.19-1.31
				(Zaouay et al., 2012)

Eleven cultivars, 5 genotypes/ Turkey	g/L Oxalic acid: 0.0313-1.0167 Malic acid: 0.1175-2.2302 Citric acid: 0.6130-2.1823 Succinic acid: 0.0390-0.3293 Tartaric acid: 0.0330-0.1266 mg/L Lactic acid: 4.516-33.115 Fumaric acid: 0.0119-0.2990	-	g/L Gallic acid: 0.190-6.361 Catechin: 0.533-3.176 Chlorogenic acid: 0.0375-0.5473 Caffeic acid: 0.0162-0.0960 Syringic acid: 0.0214-0.0609 *p*-Coumaric acid: 0.0200-0.2456 Ferulic acid: 0.0446-0.2326 *o*-Coumaric acid: 0.0325-0.5514 Phloridzin: 0.0414-1.2155 Protocatechuic acid: 0.0169-0.4489	(Gundogdu et al., 2012)

(continued)

TABLE 38.1 (Continuied)

Quantitative Analyses of Pomegranate Organic Acids, Sugar, and Individual Phenolics of Aril Juices. (Modified from (Kalaycioglu et al., 2017. Reproduced with Copyright Permission: 5092940464028.)

Cultivars/ Country	Organic Acid Content	Sugar Content	Individual Phenolics Content	Reference
Seven cultivars, one wild genotype/ Crotia	-	-	Vanillic acid: 0.0106-0.1708 Rutin: 0.1306-1.3283 Quercetin: 0.1928-1.2473 mg/100 g Delphinidin 3,5-diglucoside: 0.43-8.58 Cyanidin 3,5-diglucoside: 0.45-8.7 Delphinidin 3-glucoside: 0.48-16.43 Cyanidin 3-glucoside: 0.64-19.14 Pelargonidin 3-glucoside: 0.13-1.25	(Radunic et al., 2015)
Six clones/Spain	g/100 g Malic acid: 0.43-0.73 Citric acid: 0.08-1.40 Ascorbic acid: 0.02-0.08 Succinic acid: 0.14-0.21	g/100 g Glucose: 4.83-6.03 Fructose: 8.43-10.07	-	(Melgarejo-Sanchez et al., 2015)
Nine cultivars/ Spain	-	-	mg/100 g* Punicalagin isomer: 20.8-2899 HHDP-gallagyl-hexoside: 17.5-5296 Granatin A: 11.4-372 Ellagic acid derivative: 28.4-320 Ellagitannin: 11.0-775 Granatin B: 11.0-2967 Ellagic acid derivative: 4.83-159	(Nuncio-Jauregui et al., 2015)
Ten cultivars/ China	-	-	μg/mL Punicalagin: 149.85-1042.93 Gallic acid: 0.70-17.19 Catechin: 4.88-41.23 Chlorogenic acid: 9.48-44.21 Caffeic acid: 1.11-2.56 Epicatechin: 9.28-35.65 Ferulic acid: 0.23-1.72 Ellagic acid: 0.25-1.02 Kaempferol: 0.25-17.79	(Li et al., 2015)
Eighteen different commercial samples of pomegranate juice	g/L Citric acid: 2.3-2.8 L-Malic acid: 1.3-1.4 Isocitric acid: <20 mg/L	g/L Glucose: 61.4-65.0 Fructose: 65.3-68.0	mg/L Punicalagin α: 230.9–359.40 Punicalagin β: 190.40–413.45 Punicalin α: 125.85–211.60 Punicalin β: 98.90–187.34 Ellagic acid: 268.67–389.64 Anthocyanins Delphinidin 3,5-diglucoside: 12.22-71.00 Cyanidin 3,5-diglucoside:15.54-67.00 Pelargonidin 3,5-diglucoside:1.00–5.00 Delphinidin 3-glucoside:2.89-46.00 Cyanidin 3-glucoside:5.00-81.00 Pelargonidin 3-glucoside: 0.79-20.00	(Vegara et al., 2014)

*: A total of 35 major derivatives of ellagic acid were identified.

Holy Quran, Pg grows in the Paradise Gardens and is considered one of the many delicious rewards in the Paradise (Akhtar et al., 2015). Thus, Pg and its components have a long history of benefits in health and disease, and the scientists and physicians are still discovering its therapeutic usages as alternative and complementary medicine. Recently, the biochemical analyses of pomegranate juices from different cultivars (Iran, Spain, Turkey, Croatia, Tunisia) have shown widely different bioactive macro- and micro-molecules like organic acids, sugars, and individual phenolic contents as summarized in Table 38.1 (Kalaycioglu et al., 2017).

38.3 Phytochemicals Present in Different Pomegranate Parts

The beneficial actions of Pg juices and bioactive phytochemicals are attributed to the irremarkably high antioxidant and antiinflammation capacities, which are correlated with their polyphenol contents (Gouda et al., 2016). According to Fouad et al. (2015), the antioxidant ability of Pg juices is three times greater than that of grape and tomato juices. The strong antioxidant activity is based on the reducing power assay of different parts of Pg. For example, the EC_{50} value of juice extract was 0.56–0.83 mg/mL, leaf extract was 0.55–0.71 mg/mL, peel extract was 0.66–105 mg/mL, and flower extract was 0.34–0.48 mg/mL based on the Pg cultivars (Amri et al., 2017). It has been reported that Pg juice is an important source of anthocyanins (cyanidin, delphinidin, pelargonidin), which give the fruit and aril red colors, and phenolics and tannins (punicalin, pedunculagin, punicalagin, ellagic acid) as shown in Figures 38.1 and 38.2 (Bar-Ya'akov et al., 2019). Using high-performance liquid chromatography (HPLC), Akyıldız et al. (2020) found seven different anthocyanins in eleven Pg cultivars of different countries (cyanidin-3,5-diglucoside; cyanidin-3-glucoside; delphinidin-3-glucoside; delphinidin-3,5-diglucoside; pelargonidin-3.5-diglucoside; pelargonidin-3-glucoside; malvidin-3,5-diglucoside) compared with Pg flower, which

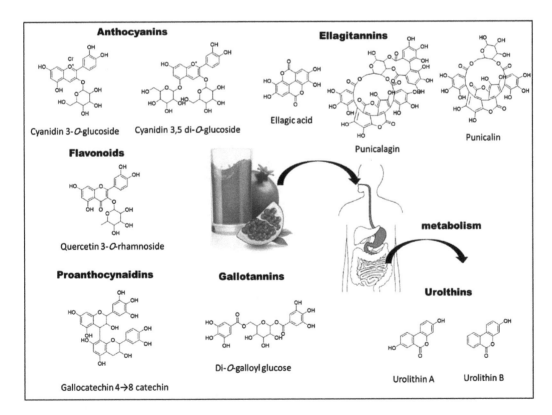

FIGURE 38.1 Representative examples of the major polyphenol classes reported in pomegranate juice. (Hegazi et al., 2021. Reproduced with copyright permission: 5092910207000.)

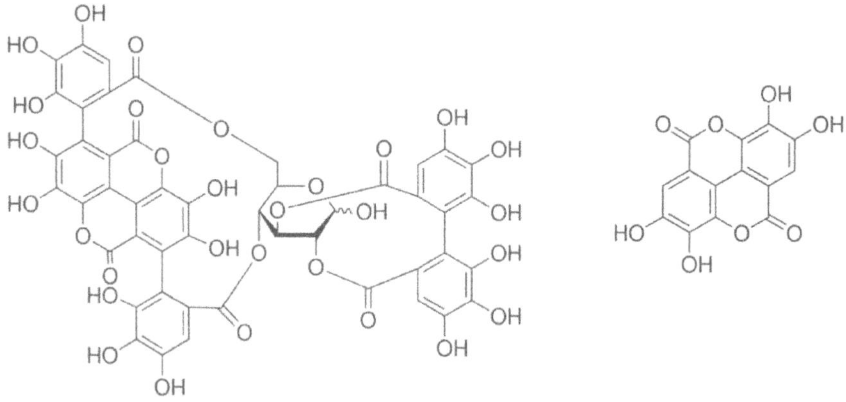

Punicalagin Ellagic acid

FIGURE 38.2 Chemical structures of punicalagin (IUPAC Name: (1R,35R,38R,55S)-6,7,8,11,12,23,24,27,28,29,37, 43,44,45,48,49,50-heptadecahydroxy-2,14,21,33,36,39,54-heptaoxaundecacyclo[33.20.0.04,9.010,19.013,18.016,25.0 17,22.026,31.038,55.041,46.047,52]pentapentaconta-4,6,8,10,12,16,18,22,24,26,28,30,41,43,45,47,49,51-octadecaene-3,15,20,32,40,53-hexone) and ellagic acid (IUPAC Name: 6,7,13,14-tetrahydroxy-2,9-dioxatetracyclo[6.6.2.04,16.011,15] hexadeca-1(15),4,6,8(16),11,13-hexaene-3,10-dione), which are the most abundant biologically active phytochemicals present in pomegranate fruit and juice.

has two anthocyanins (pelargonidin 3,5-diglucoside and pelargonidin 3-glucoside) (Zhang et al., 2011). Table 38.2 shows the phytochemical compositions of different parts of Pg.

The basic structure of Pg flavonoids is two aromatic rings linked through three carbon atoms that frequently form an oxygenated heterocyclic structure. Mass spectrometry data showed that Pg juice contains ellagitannins as the most abundant oligomeric phytochemicals. The chemical structures of the pomegranate ETs oligomers were elucidated by nuclear magnetic resonance (NMR), spectroscopic analyses, and other chemical analytical methods, which showed that the most abundant tetrameric form of ETs consists of a chemical formula, $C_{170}H_{122}O_{110}$, with Mol.Wt.3924-7360 (Hussein et al., 2018). Punicalagin (Figure 38.2), as a part of ETs, is a unique compound of pomegranate, and its concentration in the juice ranges from 4–565 mg/L, while its respective concentration in the pericarp and the peel may reach up to 20 g/kg (Gouda et al., 2016; Hussein et al., 2018).

Methanol extracts of Pg are rich in hydrolyzable tannins (punicalins and punicalagins), ellagic acid, a component of ETs, and gallic acid, a component of gallotannins (Akhtar et al., 2015). The analysis of different parts of Pg crude proteins showed that Pg seeds contain different concentrations of protein depending on the original source, such as Tunisia (16.8%), Egypt (13.2%), and Saudi Arabia (4.06%) (Bar-Ya'akov et al., 2019). Globulins (62.4 mg/g) and albumins (54.1 mg/g) make major fractions, followed by glutelin (33.2 mg/g) and prolamin (18.1 mg/g) in which it could be used as a novel sources of bioactive peptides that could be used in drug delivery (Elfalleh et al., 2011).

38.4 Cardioprotective and Antiosteoarthritis Effects of Pomegranate

Pg juice (PJ) has shown antihypersensitive, antiinflammatory, and antiatherosclerotic effects in healthy humans, along with other nutritional and health advantages. Razani et al. (2017) studied the cardioprotective potential of 220 mL/day PJ in 50 ischemic heart disease patients during 5 days of hospitalization. Their results suggested that PJ caused significant reductions in the intensity, occurrence, and duration of angina pectoris in patients with unstable angina. Also, it significantly lowered the levels of serum troponin and malondialdehyde, which are among factors responsible for CVDs (Gouda et al., 2016; Hussein et al., 2018). Haghighian et al. (2020) studied the effects of Pg peel extract (PPE) supplementation on the serum lipid profile and oxidative stress of 66 obese women aged 38–60 years with

TABLE 38.2

Major Bioactive Phytochemicals Present in Pomegranate Fruit, Juice, Seeds, Peel, and Flower

Part	Phytochemical	Unit	Amount	Reference
Juice				
	Total phenolics	mg/L	(4387-8460)	(Akyıldız et al., 2020)
	Total anthocyanins	mg/L	(135-1030)	
	Ellagitannins	mg/L	(1849-2991)	
	Flavanols	mg/L	(1136-4424)	
	Flavonols	mg/L	(0.51-2.08)	
	Flavones	mg/L	(3.89-6.88)	
	Ellagic acid	mg/L	(66-156)	
	Quercetin	mg/L	(8-30)	
	Gallic acid	mg/L	(60-109)	
	Catechin	mg/L	(11-46)	
	Caffeic acid	mg/L	(0.9-1.81)	
Seeds				
	Total phenolics	mg/100 g	(0.28-16.8)	(Costa et al., 2019)
	Tocopherols	mg/100 g	(524-1172)	
	Quercetin	mg/100 g	(0.13-1.86)	
	Vanillic	mg/100 g	(0.14-2.56)	
	Punicic acid	mg/g oil	(552-627)	
	β-carotene	mg/100 g	(0.95-1.49)	
Peel				
	Total phenolics	mg/g dw	(0.82-191)	(Živković et al., 2018)
	Ellagic	mg/g dw	(4.09-12.54)	
	Gallic	mg/g dw	(1.13-3.23)	
	Punicalin	mg/g dw	(28.38-65.67)	
	Punicalagins	mg/g dw	(7.04-35.05)	
Flower				
	Total phenolics	mg/g dw	(281-331)	(Bekir et al., 2016)
	Total flavonoids	mg/g dw	(13.7-29.5)	
	Anthocyanins	mg/g dw	(0.30-0.70)	
	Tannins	mg/g dw	(14.1-30.6)	
dw = dry weight				

knee osteoarthritis (OA). The subjects received 1000 mgPg extract/day for 8 weeks. They concluded that PPE significantly reduced the serum levels of total cholesterol and triglycerides in patients with knee OA (Haghighian et al., 2020).

Forest et al. (2007) reported that daily consumption of 8 ounces of Pg juice (1.5 mmol of total polyphenols) for 4 weeks improved erectile dysfunction (ED) in male patients with mild-to-moderate ED. This randomized, placebo-controlled, and cross-over design study enrolled 53 volunteers (21–70 years-old) with mild-to-moderate ED. The efficacy of Pg juice was assessed using International Index of Erectile Function (IIEF) and Global Assessment Questionnaires (GAQ). A beneficial trend was observed with Pg juice in men with mild and mild-to-moderate ED. Forty-two subjects demonstrated improvement in GAQ scores after Pg consumption, while 25 men reported marked improvement ($p = 0.058$) after drinking Pg juice daily for 4 weeks. Further well-designed, placebo-controlled, and randomized clinical trials with a large number of subjects are required to establish the effectiveness of Pg juice in ED patients. This may be a cost-effective, affordable, and safe way to treat ED, especially by men using nitrates for angina pectoris. Nitrates are contraindicated in patients using PDE-5 inhibitors like Viagra, Cialis, and Levitra.

38.5 Neuroprotective Effects of Pomegranate

The neuroprotective effects of pomegranate have been evaluated in different animal models of neurodegenerative diseases, such as Alzheimer's disease (Giménez-Bastida et al., 2021). The results these studiesshowed that PJ and its other contents have neuroprotection actions based on the biological activity of its ellagic antioxidants and their derived metabolites like urolithins in humans (Ahmed et al., 2014). Further, Kujawska et al. (2019) reported that the neuroprotective effects of PJ are mediated through ET-derived metabolites-urolithins. In that study, the authors examined the capability of PJ for protection against Parkinson's disease in a rat model through the improvement of several biomarkers: namely postural stability, inflammation reduction, enhancement of neuronal survival, reduction in lipid and α-synuclein oxidative damage, increase in mitochondrial aldehyde dehydrogenase activity, and maintenance of antiapoptotic Bcl-xL protein.

Urolithins and ellagic acid were detected in the animal brains after intravenous and oral administration. These results align with urolithins' capacity to cross the blood-brain barrier described by in silico studies (Yuan et al., 2016), setting the basis to perform an in-depth investigation into the cellular and molecular mechanisms of neuroprotection. Some in vitro and in vivo studies have described the antiinflammatory and antioxidant mechanisms of action for urolithins and their conjugated metabolites (Dasilva et al., 2019). It was reported that these molecules can cross the blood-brain-barrier to exhibit high potential for the neuroprotective benefits associated with pomegranate consumption. Another study by Bellone et al. (2019) described the neurophysiological improvements and shorter hospital stays in post-stroke patients under rehabilitation due to Pg consumption for one week. The preliminary findings of these studies provide novel insights regarding the Pg's therapeutic potential in the management of serious neurodegenerative diseases like Parkinson's disease and Alzheimer's disease. Well-designed, randomized, and double-blind studies are needed to establish the long-term safety, efficacy, and dose schedules for orally deliverable pomegranate formulations.

38.6 Pomegranate Bioactive Constituents Target Multiple Oncogenic Signaling and Molecular Mechanisms for the Prevention and Management of Cancer

Cancer is a multifactorial disease and over 200 types of cancers have been reported globally. It is well recognized that primary prevention is an effective way to fight cancers by using natural polyphenolic anticancer foods, vegetables and fruits, avoiding exposure to carcinogenic environment, smoking cessation, and lifestyle modifications. Cancer cells proliferate very rapidly and rely on high metabolic activities (Wang et al., 2018b). Several in vitro and in vivo studies have shown that Pg phytochemicals exert their anticancer effects partially by modulating NF-kB (nuclear factor kappa-light-chain-enhancer of activated B cells) activity (Sharma et al., 2017). PJ has been reported to have preventive as well as therapeutic properties against several important cancer types (Hussein et al., 2021). Induction of apoptosis, inhibition of metastasis, and proliferation are some of the main mechanisms by which PJ acts as an anticancer agent (Kandylis et al., 2020). The antiinflammatory, antiproliferative, and apoptotic effects of pgpunicalaginellagic acid (50 mg/L) were demonstrated after incubation with HT-29 human colon cancer cell line, with a reduction in the phosphorylation of the p65 subunit of NFκB, and its binding to the NFκB showed 79% inhibition in TNF-α protein expression (Liberal et al., 2017). As shown in Figure 38.3, the urolithin metabolites (which are produced from ET hydrolyzation by colon microbiota) inhibit cell proliferation by arresting cell cycle at G2/M and S-phase, and induce apoptosis by regulating caspases 3 and 9, cytochrome P450, p-ERK1/2 ratio, and cyclins A and B1 (Liberal et al., 2017).

One PJ study used 88 human cancers micro-RNA genes to investigate the effects of PJ on gene expression. The results showed that PJ significantly ($P < 0.05$) downregulated the expression of the cancer genes (such as miR-184, miR-203, miR-373, miR-124, miR-96, miR-373, and miR-301) compared to the control group (Ahmed et al., 2017). Resveratrol (3,5,4-trihydroxy-*trans*-stilbene) present in Pg promotes autophagy by suppressing Wnt/β-catenin signaling pathway, while Pgquercetin inhibits murine mammary cancer cell growth by targeting the Wnt pathway through upregulating of Dickkopf (DKK) 1, 2, 3,

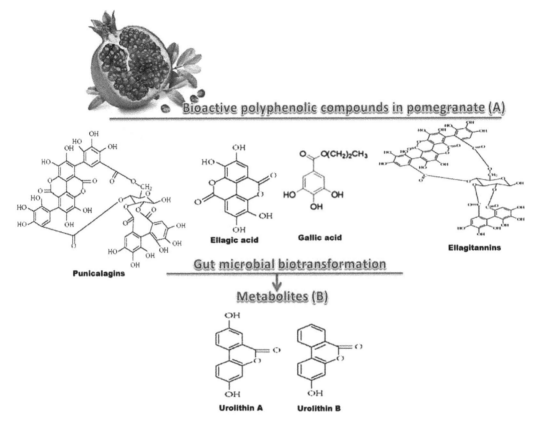

FIGURE 38.3 Bioactive polyphenolic compounds present in pomegranate and their metabolites detected in human urine. (Adapted from Hussein et al. (2021). Reproduced with copyright permission: 1096648.)

and 4 Wnt antagonists (Mukherjee et al., 2020). Overall, the health-promoting benefits and disease prevention effects of Pg phytochemicals have been attributed to their broad range of synergistic actions. It has been suggested that there is a synergy among pomegranate compounds that enhances their anticancer activity. For example, the combination of quercetin and ellagic acid produce greater inhibition of cancer cell growth in comparison with each of the substances used alone (Kandylis et al., 2020). Li et al al. (2016) mentioned that human lung carcinoma cells when treated with Pg leaves extract (200 mg/mL) for 48 h showed a significant decrease in lung cancer cell viability.

According to Wong et al. (2021), Pg-derived phytochemicals have enormous potential for cancer prevention and management. These authors suggested that flavonoids and ellagitannins present in Pg fruit and juice possess powerful antiproliferative, antiinflammatory, antioxidant, anticancer, and antimetastatic effects without significant toxicity. In breast cancer cells, fermented PJ showed a marked suppressive activity compared to fresh PJ. The plausible reason was attributed to the superior activity of aglycon forms of phenolic compounds compared to the glycosides in which the fermentation process is supposed to release sugar units from the phenolic structures (Çam et al., 2013). It has been estimated that nearly 30% of prostate cancer patients use commercial Pg extract as complementary alternative medicine in addition to standard treatments for prostate cancer prevention and treatment (Paller et al., 2017). PPE was found to act as cell cycle arrestor or apoptosis inducer against chronic myeloid leukaemia (CML) cell line, K562, in a dose-dependent manner. The fermented PJ and seed oil regulated the nuclear transcription factor-B (NF-B) in aggressive breast cellular cancer cell lines, which regulates cell survival, proliferation, tumorigenesis, and inflammation (Mandal et al., 2017). According to Wang et al. (2020), supplementation with Pg products can inhibit the levels of tumor necrosis factor alpha (TNF-α) and interleukin-6 (IL-6) and reduce the high-sensitivity C-reactive protein (hs-CRP) levels in the body. This

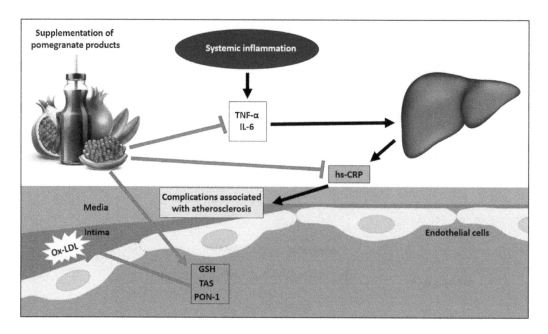

FIGURE 38.4 Completed pathway based on the positive findings of this meta-analysis and long-term studies. Tumor necrosis factor alpha (TNF-α), interleukin-6 (IL-6), reduced glutathione (GSH), total antioxidant status (TAS), paraoxonase-1 (PON-1), low-density lipoprotein (LDL), high-sensitivity C-reactive protein (hs-CRP), oxidized low-density lipoprotein (Ox-LDL), and vascular cell adhesion protein-1 (VCAM-1). (Reproduced with copyright permission: 5092900526825.)

could be due to the increase of glutathione (GSH) concentration and augmented activity of paraoxonase-1 (PON-1), which collectively play a crucial role by inhibiting the oxidation of low-density lipoprotein (LDL), high sensitivity to C-reactive protein (hs-CRP), oxidized low-density lipoprotein (Ox-LDL), and vascular cell adhesion protein-1 (VCAM-1) (Figure 38.4).Selma et al. (2018) reported that fermented Pg polyphenols, fresh Pg polyphenols, and pericarp polyphenols (derived from aqueous extract) can significantly inhibit cell proliferation. Pg juice-derived ellaginatinns like gallic acid and Pg seed oil can induce upregulation of migration-inhibitory factor (MIF) in MDA-MB-231 cancer cells (Costa et al., 2019). To maximize the chemotherapeutic efficacy of Pg extract, it was incorporated into an optimized solid lipid nanoparticle (NP). Poly(D,L-lactic-*co*-glycolic acid)-poly(ethylene glycol) (PLGA-PEG) formulation was loaded with Pg extract or individual polyphenols, such as punicalagin, and this loaded formulation exerted 2- to 12-fold higher effects on cell growth inhibition compared to their free counterparts (Priya Dharshini et al., 2020).

38.7 Antibacterial and Antiviral Activities of Pomegranate Fruit and Juice

Studies from different regions of the world have shown the bactericidal and virucidal effects of Pg in a number of highly pathogenic and drug-resistant strains of microorganisms (Khorrami et al., 2020). These studies were designed to determine the bactericidal potency of different extracts of the pomegranate plant against a wide range of different bacteria, utilizing disc diffusion assays or minimum inhibitory concentration (MIC). The antibacterial activity of freshly prepared and commercial PJ was tested using the in vitro agar diffusion method and the antimicrobial activity was expressed as the diameter of the zone of inhibition (ZOI). Freshly prepared PJ at a concentration of 3.6 mg/well inhibited the growth of seven types of pathogenic bacterial strains, including *Escherichia coli* 0157: H7 ATCC 6933, *Bacillus cereus* ATCC 33018, *Staphylococcus aureus* ATCC 20231, *Salmonella typhimurium* ATCC 14028, *Pseudomonas aeruginosa* ATCC 9027, *Listeria monocytogenes* ATCC 7644, and *Yersinia enterocolitica* ATCC 9610, while the commercial PJ revealed antibacterial activities against three out of the seven types tested pathogenic microorganisms: *E. coli, Listeria,* and *Pseudomonas* (Fouad et al., 2015). These findings suggested the antibacterial effect of PJ regarding the thermal treatment during industrial processing on the structural configuration of bioactive flavonoid molecules and partially explains the conflicting results obtained from some clinical studies on the biopotency of different brands of commercial Pg components on cancer cells. The virucidal activity of PJ extracts was also reported against human immunodeficiency virus (HIV) (Houston et al., 2017). Pgpunicalagin treatment of mice challenged with a lethal dose of enterovirus 71 resulted in a reduction of mortality and relieved clinical symptoms by inhibiting viral replication. The results showed that punicalagin reduced the viral cytopathic effect on rhabdomyosarcoma cells to $IC_{50} = 15$ µg/ml. The authors suggested that punicalagin had the potential for further development as antiviral agent (Yang et al., 2012). It may be worthwhile to investigate the antiviral effects of punicalagin against the SARS-CoV-2 or the novel coronavirus COVID-19 that is responsible for the current pandemic.

38.8 The Prebiotic Properties of Edible and Non-Edible Parts of Pomegranate

It has been estimated that the gastrointestinal (GI) tract of healthy adults contains microbial flora in the range of 1000 bacterial species and 100-fold more genes than are present in the human genome. The GI tract microbial flora provide beneficial effects in the development of immune system, prevent pathogenic infections, help in nutrient acquisition, and also assist in maintaining the gut-brain interaction (Zheng et al., 2020). Gut microbiota can transform intact phenolic compounds into their bioactive metabolites and the accumulation of these microbial metabolites play a key role in promoting changes in the gut ecosystem, including the promotion of healthy microbial population. Dietary polyphenols preserve the gut microbial balance by stimulating the growth of beneficial bacteria and the inhibition of pathogenic bacteria, and consequently exert prebiotic-like effects (Rodriguez-Daza et al., 2021). The non-edible parts of pomegranate are reported to be rich in polyphenolic compounds with beneficial properties, thereby suggesting that pericarp phytochemicals may be useful for developing novel prebiotic products capable of restoring the normal composition of the gut microbiota (Lavoro et al., 2021).

38.9 Future Opportunities, Challenges, and Conclusion

There are many promising aspects of developing nutraceuticals and alternate remedies from Pg and its constituents. The current difficulties surrounding the manufacture of Pg-derived products is the lack of reliable and consistent processing techniques and the proper investments in promoting the health benefits and therapeutic effectiveness of Pg phytochemicals by the food and drug industries. For instance, the pasteurization process and the preservation techniques may produce biochemical changes in the physicochemical composition of Pg's bioactive components, resulting in the reduction of its antioxidant, antiinflammation, and antibacterial activities (Fouad et al., 2015). Therefore, more suitable and easier-to-manufacture Pg formulations should be investigated. Good manufacturing practices and quality control methods should be used in making Pg-derived nutraceuticals. Also, standardization of bioactive Pg compounds obtained from different cultivars should be done to ensure benefits in health and disease.

More physicochemical studies should also be done with Pg combinations with other novel sources like microalgae to evaluate their industrial applications for securing a clean label for future needs of these high protein-valued sources as suggested by our recently published study (Gouda et al., 2021c). The future prospective will be to combine Pg phytochemicals with other drug delivery process like nano-emulsions and nano-encapsulations to enhance the gut absorption and bioavailability of Pg products. Well-controlled, randomized, and double-blind studies are warranted to establish the long-term safety, efficacy, and dose schedules for orally deliverable pomegranate formulations.

Acknowledgments

The author (MG) gratefully acknowledges Elsevier and Bentham Science Publishers for granting the copyright permissions.

REFERENCES

Ahmed A, Subaiea M, Eid A, Li L, Seeram P, & Zawia H. (2014). Pomegranate extract modulates processing of amyloid-β precursor proteinin an aged Alzheimer's disease animal model. Current Alzheimer Research, 11(999): 1–1. https://doi.org/10.2174/1567205011666141001115348

Ahmed FE, Gouda MM, Hussein LA, Ahmed NC, Vos PW, & Mohammad MA. (2017). Role of melt curve analysis in interpretation of nutrigenomics' microRNA expression data. Cancer Genomics & Proteomics, 14(6): 469–481. https://doi.org/10.21873/cgp.20057

Akhtar S, Ismail T, Fraternale D, & Sestili P. (2015). Pomegranate peel and peel extracts: Chemistry and food features. Food Chem, 174: 417–425. https://doi.org/10.1016/j.foodchem.2014.11.035

Akyıldız A, Karaca E, Ağçam E, Dündar B, & Çınkır Nİ. (2020). Changes in quality attributes during production steps and frozen-storage of pomegranate juice concentrate. Journal of Food Composition and Analysis, 92: 103548. https://doi.org/10.1016/j.jfca.2020.103548

Al-Jarallah A, Igdoura F, Zhang Y, Tenedero C, White E, MacDonald M, et al. (2013) The effect of pomegranate extract on coronary artery atherosclerosis in SR-BI/APOE double knockout mice. Atherosclerosis 2013;228(1):80–89. https://doi.org/10.1016/j.atherosclerosis.2013.02.025

Amri Z, Zaouay F, Lazreg-Aref H, Soltana H, Mneri A, Mars M, & Hammami M. (2017). Phytochemical content, Fatty acids composition and antioxidant potential of different pomegranate parts: Comparison between edible and non edible varieties grown in Tunisia. Int J Biol Macromol, 104(Pt A): 274–280. https://doi.org/10.1016/j.ijbiomac.2017.06.022

Andreux PA, Blanco-Bose W, Ryu D, Burdet F, Ibberson M, Aebischer P, et al. (2019). The mitophagy activator urolithin A is safe and induces a molecular signature of improved mitochondrial and cellular health in humans. Nature Metabolism, 1(6): 595–603. https://doi.org/10.1038/s42255-019-0073-4

Asgary S, Karimi R, Joshi T, Kilpatrick KL, Moradi S, Samimi Z, et al. (2021). Effect of pomegranate juice on vascular adhesion factors: A systematic review and meta-analysis. Phytomedicine, 80: 153359. https://doi.org/10.1016/j.phymed.2020.153359

Asgary S, Keshvari M, Sahebkar A, & Sarrafzadegan N. (2017). Pomegranate consumption and blood pressure: A review. Curr Pharm Des, 23(7): 1042–1050. https://doi.org/10.2174/1381612822666161010103339

Asgary S, Sahebkar A, Afshani MR, Keshvari M, Haghjooyjavanmard S, & Rafieian-Kopaei M. (2014). Clinical evaluation of blood pressure lowering, endothelial function improving, hypolipidemic and anti-inflammatory effects of pomegranate juice in hypertensive subjects. Phytother Res, 28(2): 193–199. https://doi.org/10.1002/ptr.4977

Bar-Ya'akov I, Tian L, Amir R, & Holland D. (2019). Primary metabolites, anthocyanins, and hydrolyzable tannins in the pomegranate fruit. Front Plant Sci, 10: 620. https://doi.org/10.3389/fpls.2019.00620

Bellone JA, Murray JR, Jorge P, Fogel TG, Kim M, Wallace DR, & Hartman RE. (2019). Pomegranate supplementation improves cognitive and functional recovery following ischemic stroke: A randomized trial. Nutr Neurosci, 22(10): 738–743. https://doi.org/10.1080/1028415X.2018.1436413

Bookheimer SY, Renner BA, Ekstrom A, Li Z, Henning SM, Brown JA, et al. (2013). Pomegranate juice augments memory and FMRI activity in middle-aged and older adults with mild memory complaints. Evid Based Complement Alternat Med, 2013: 946298. https://doi.org/10.1155/2013/946298

Braidy N, Essa MM, Poljak A, Selvaraju S, Al-Adawi S, Manivasagm T, et al. (2016). Consumption of pomegranates improves synaptic function in a transgenic mice model of Alzheimer's disease. Oncotarget, 7(40): 64589-64604. https://doi.org/10.18632/oncotarget.10905

Çam M, Durmaz G, Çetin A, & Yetim H. (2013). Antioxidant capacity of pomegranate juice and its role in biological activities. 499–511. https://doi.org/10.1016/b978-0-12-397154-8.00008-7

Costa AMM, Silva LO, & Torres AG. (2019). Chemical composition of commercial cold-pressed pomegranate (Punica granatum) seed oil from Turkey and Israel, and the use of bioactive compounds for samples' origin preliminary discrimination. Journal of Food Composition and Analysis, 75: 8–16. https://doi.org/10.1016/j.jfca.2018.09.004

DaSilva NA, Nahar PP, Ma H, Eid A, Wei Z, Meschwitz S, et al. (2019). Pomegranate ellagitannin-gut microbial-derived metabolites, urolithins, inhibit neuroinflammation in vitro. Nutr Neurosci, 22(3): 185–195. https://doi.org/10.1080/1028415X.2017.1360558

Ekor M. (2014). The growing use of herbal medicines: Issues relating to adverse reactions and challenges in monitoring safety. Front Pharmacol, 4: 177. https://doi.org/10.3389/fphar.2013.00177

Elfalleh W, Tlili N, Ying M, Sheng-Hua H, Ferchichi A, & Nasri N. (2011). Organoleptic quality, minerals, proteins and amino acids from two tunisian commercial pomegranate fruits. International Journal of Food Engineering, 7(4). https://doi.org/Artn 1210.2202/1556-3758.2057

Fang EF, Hou YJ, Palikaras K, Adriaanse BA, Kerr JS, Yang BM, et al. (2019). Mitophagy inhibits amyloid-beta and tau pathology and reverses cognitive deficits in models of Alzheimer's disease. Nature Neuroscience, 22(3): 401-+. https://doi.org/10.1038/s41593-018-0332-9

Forest CP, Padma-Nathan H, & Liker HR. (2007). Efficacy and safety of pomegranate juice on improvement of erectile dysfunction in male patients with mild to moderate erectile dysfunction: a randomized, placebo-controlled, double-blind, crossover study. Int J Impot Res, 19(6): 564–567. https://doi.org/10.1038/sj.ijir.3901570

Fouad MT, Moustafa A, Hussein L, Romeilah R, & Gouda M. (2015). In-vitro antioxidant and antimicrobial activities of selected fruit and vegetable juices and fermented dairy products commonly consumed in Egypt. Research Journal of Pharmaceutical Biological and Chemical Sciences, 6(2): 541–550.

Giménez-Bastida JA, Ávila-Gálvez MÁ, Espín JC, & González-Sarrías A. (2021). Evidence for health properties of pomegranate juices and extracts beyond nutrition: A critical systematic review of human studies. Trends in Food Science & Technology, 114: 410–423. https://doi.org/10.1016/j.tifs.2021.06.014

Gouda M, Chen K, Li X, Liu Y, & He Y. (2021a). Detection of microalgae single-cell antioxidant and electro-chemical potentials by gold microelectrode and Raman micro-spectroscopy combined with chemometrics. Sensors and Actuators B: Chemical, 329: 129229. https://doi.org/10.1016/j.snb.2020.129229

Gouda M, El-Din Bekhit A, Tang Y, Huang Y, Huang L, He Y, & Li X. (2021b). Recent innovations of ultrasound green technology in herbal phytochemistry: A review. Ultrason Sonochem, 73: 105538. https://doi.org/10.1016/j.ultsonch.2021.105538

Gouda M, Huang Z, Liu Y, He Y, & Li X. (2021c). Physicochemical impact of bioactive terpenes on the microalgae biomass structural characteristics. Bioresour Technol, 334: 125232. https://doi.org/10.1016/j.biortech.2021.125232

Gouda M, Moustafa A, Hussein L, & Hamza M. (2016). Three week dietary intervention using apricots, pomegranate juice or/and fermented sour sobya and impact on biomarkers of antioxidative activity, oxidative stress and erythrocytic glutathione transferase activity among adults. Nutr J, 15(1): 52. https://doi.org/10.1186/s12937-016-0173-x

Griffiths K, Aggarwal BB, Singh RB, Buttar HS, Wilson D, & De Meester F. (2016). Food antioxidants and their anti-inflammatory properties: A potential role in cardiovascular diseases and cancer prevention. Diseases, 4(3). https://doi.org/10.3390/diseases4030028

Gundogdu M, & Yilmaz H. (2012). Organic acid, phenolic profile and antioxidant capacities of pomegranate (Punica granatum L.) cultivars and selected genotypes. Scientia Horticulturae, 143: 38–42. https://doi.org/10.1016/j.scienta.2012.05.029

Haghighian MK, Rafraf M, Hemmati S, Haghravan S, & Asghari-Jafarabadi M. (2020). Effects of pomegranate (Punica granatum L.) peel extract supplementation on serum lipid profile and oxidative stress in obese women with knee osteoarthritis: A double blind, randomized, placebo controlled study. Advances in Integrative Medicine. https://doi.org/10.1016/j.aimed.2020.05.001

Hegazi NM, El-Shamy S, Fahmy H, & Farag MA. (2021). Pomegranate juice as a super-food: A comprehensive review of its extraction, analysis, and quality assessment approaches. Journal of Food Composition and Analysis, 97: 103773. https://doi.org/10.1016/j.jfca.2020.103773

Houston DMJ, Bugert JJ, Denyer SP, & Heard CM. (2017). Correction: Potentiated virucidal activity of pomegranate rind extract (PRE) and punicalagin against Herpes simplex virus (HSV) when co-administered with zinc (II) ions, and antiviral activity of PRE against HSV and aciclovir-resistant HSV. PLoS One, 12(11): e0188609. https://doi.org/10.1371/journal.pone.0188609

Hussein L, Gouda M, & Buttar HS. (2021). Pomegranate, its components and modern deliverable formulations as potential botanicals in the prevention and treatment of various cancers. Curr Drug Deliv, 18(0): 1–15. https://doi.org/10.2174/1567201818666210203180853

Hussein L, Gouda M, & Labib E. (2018). Pomegranate cultivation, pomological properties, processing,global market and health benefits. In S. R.A. & A. M. (Eds.), *Pomegranate* (pp. 267–302). NY, USA: Novo Publisher.

Hussein L, & Singh RB. (2019). Developments on the applications and the suitability of functional fermented sour sobya as a viable source of novel probiotics in the managements of gastrointestinal disorders and blood lipid profiles. The Role of Functional Food Security in Global Health, 2019: 579–602. https://doi.org/10.1016/b978-0-12-813148-0.00035-9

Ismail T, Calcabrini C, Diaz AR, Fimognari C, Turrini E, Catanzaro E, et al. (2016). Ellagitannins in cancer chemoprevention and therapy. Toxins (Basel), 8(5). https://doi.org/10.3390/toxins8050151

Kahramanoglu I. (2019). Trends in pomegranate sector: production, postharvest handling and marketing. Int J Agric For Life Sci, 3(2): 239–246.

Kalaycioglu Z, & Erim FB. (2017). Total phenolic contents, antioxidant activities, and bioactive ingredients of juices from pomegranate cultivars worldwide. Food Chem, 221: 496–507. https://doi.org/10.1016/j.foodchem.2016.10.084

Kandylis P, & Kokkinomagoulos E. (2020). Food applications and potential health benefits of pomegranate and its derivatives. Foods, 9(2). https://doi.org/10.3390/foods9020122

Khorrami S, Kamali F, & Zarrabi A. (2020). Bacteriostatic activity of aquatic extract of black peel pomegranate and silver nanoparticles biosynthesized by using the extract. Biocatalysis and Agricultural Biotechnology, 25: 101620. https://doi.org/10.1016/j.bcab.2020.101620

King RS, Peacock-Chambers E, Wilson D, Shimer J, Foss S, Visintainer P, & Singh R. (2021). Impact of maternal medication for opioid use disorder on neurodevelopmental outcomes of infants treated for neonatal opioid withdrawal syndrome. J Neonatal Perinatal Med. https://doi.org/10.3233/NPM-200615

Kujawska M, Jourdes M, Kurpik M, Szulc M, Szaefer H, Chmielarz P, et al. (2019). Neuroprotective effects of pomegranate juice against Parkinson's disease and presence of ellagitannins-derived metabolite-urolithin a in the brain. Int J Mol Sci, 21(1). https://doi.org/10.3390/ijms21010202

Lavoro A, Falzone L, Gattuso G, Salemi R, Cultrera G, Leone G, et al. (2021). Pomegranate: A promising avenue against the most common chronic diseases and their associated risk factors (Review). International Journal of Functional Nutrition, 2(2). https://doi.org/10.3892/ijfn.2021.16

Li X, Wasila H, Liu L, Yuan T, Gao Z, Zhao B, & Ahmad I. (2015). Physicochemical characteristics, polyphenol compositions and antioxidant potential of pomegranate juices from 10 Chinese cultivars and the environmental factors analysis. Food Chem, 175: 575–584. https://doi.org/10.1016/j.foodchem.2014.12.003

Li Y, Yang F, Zheng W, Hu M, Wang J, Ma S, et al. (2016). Punica granatum (pomegranate) leaves extract induces apoptosis through mitochondrial intrinsic pathway and inhibits migration and invasion in non-small cell lung cancer in vitro. Biomed Pharmacother, 80: 227–235. https://doi.org/10.1016/j.biopha.2016.03.023

Liberal J, Carmo A, Gomes C, Cruz MT, & Batista MT. (2017). Urolithins impair cell proliferation, arrest the cell cycle and induce apoptosis in UMUC3 bladder cancer cells. Invest New Drugs, 35(6): 671–681. https://doi.org/10.1007/s10637-017-0483-7

Mandal A, Bhatia D, & Bishayee A. (2017). Anti-Inflammatory mechanism involved in pomegranate-mediated prevention of breast cancer: The role of NF-kappaB and Nrf2 signaling pathways. Nutrients, 9(5). https://doi.org/10.3390/nu9050436

Melgarejo-Sanchez P, Martinez JJ, Legua P, Martinez R, Hernandez F, & Melgarejo P. (2015). Quality, antioxidant activity and total phenols of six Spanish pomegranates clones. Scientia Horticulturae, 182: 65–72. https://doi.org/10.1016/j.scienta.2014.11.020

Mena P, Garcia-Viguera C, Navarro-Rico J, Moreno DA, Bartual J, Saura D, & Marti N. (2011). Phytochemical characterisation for industrial use of pomegranate (Punica granatum L.) cultivars grown in Spain. Journal of the Science of Food and Agriculture, 91(10): 1893–1906. https://doi.org/10.1002/jsfa.4411

Mousavinejad G, Emam-Djomeh Z, Rezaei K, & Khodaparast MHH. (2009). Identification and quantification of phenolic compounds and their effects on antioxidant activity in pomegranate juices of eight Iranian cultivars. Food Chem, 115(4): 1274–1278. https://doi.org/10.1016/j.foodchem.2009.01.044

Mukherjee N, & Panda CK. (2020). Wnt/beta-Catenin Signaling Pathway as Chemotherapeutic Target in Breast Cancer: An Update on Pros and Cons. Clin Breast Cancer, 20(5): 361–370. https://doi.org/10.1016/j.clbc.2020.04.004

Nigam M. (2020). Chapter 3 – Phytomedicine: Scope and current highlights. In *Preparation of Phytopharmaceuticals for the Management of Disorders* (pp. 39–54): Elsevier Inc. https://doi.org/10.1016/b978-0-12-820284-5.00013-7

Nuncio-Jauregui N, Nowicka P, Munera-Picazo S, Hernandez F, Carbonell-Barrachina AA, & Wojdylo A. (2015). Identification and quantification of major derivatives of ellagic acid and antioxidant properties of thinning and ripe Spanish pomegranates. Journal of Functional Foods, 12: 354–364. https://doi.org/10.1016/j.jff.2014.11.007

Ozgen M, Durgac C, Serce S, & Kaya C. (2008). Chemical and antioxidant properties of pomegranate cultivars grown in the Mediterranean region of Turkey. Food Chem, 111(3): 703–706. https://doi.org/10.1016/j.foodchem.2008.04.043

Paller CJ, Pantuck A, & Carducci MA. (2017). A review of pomegranate in prostate cancer. Prostate Cancer Prostatic Dis, 20(3): 265–270. https://doi.org/10.1038/pcan.2017.19

Pourghayoumi M, Bakhshi D, Rahemi M, Kamgar-Haghighi AA, & Aalami A. (2017). The physiological responses of various pomegranate cultivars to drought stress and recovery in order to screen for drought tolerance. Scientia Horticulturae, 217: 164–172. https://doi.org/10.1016/j.scienta.2017.01.044

Priya Dharshini LC, Vishnupriya S, Sakthivel KM, & Rasmi RR. (2020). Oxidative stress responsive transcription factors in cellular signalling transduction mechanisms. Cell Signal, 72: 109670. https://doi.org/10.1016/j.cellsig.2020.109670

Radunic M, Jukic Spika M, Goreta Ban S, Gadze J, Diaz-Perez JC, & MacLean D. (2015). Physical and chemical properties of pomegranate fruit accessions from Croatia. Food Chem, 177: 53–60. https://doi.org/10.1016/j.foodchem.2014.12.102

Razani Z, Dastani M, & Kazerani HR. (2017). Cardioprotective Effects of Pomegranate (Punica granatum) Juice in Patients with Ischemic Heart Disease. Phytother Res, 31(11): 1731–1738. https://doi.org/10.1002/ptr.5901

Rodriguez-Daza MC, Pulido-Mateos EC, Lupien-Meilleur J, Guyonnet D, Desjardins Y, & Roy D. (2021). Polyphenol-mediated gut microbiota modulation: Toward prebiotics and further. Frontiers in Nutrition, 8. https://doi.org/Artn 68945610.3389/Fnut.2021.689456

Selma MV, Gonzalez-Sarrias A, Salas-Salvado J, Andres-Lacueva C, Alasalvar C, Orem A, et al. (2018). The gut microbiota metabolism of pomegranate or walnut ellagitannins yields two urolithin-metabotypes that correlate with cardiometabolic risk biomarkers: Comparison between normoweight, overweight-obesity and metabolic syndrome. Clinical Nutrition, 37(3): 897–905. https://doi.org/10.1016/j.clnu.2017.03.012

Sharma P, McClees SF, & Afaq F. (2017). Pomegranate for prevention and treatment of cancer: An update. Molecules, 22(1). https://doi.org/10.3390/molecules22010177

Singh A, D'Amico D, Andreux PA, Dunngalvin G, Kern T, Blanco-Bose W, et al. (2021). Direct supplementation with Urolithin A overcomes limitations of dietary exposure and gut microbiome variability in healthy adults to achieve consistent levels across the population. Eur J Clin Nutr. https://doi.org/10.1038/s41430-021-00950-1

Tomas-Barberan FA, Gonzalez-Sarrias A, Garcia-Villalba R, Nunez-Sanchez MA, Selma MV, Garcia-Conesa MT, & Espin JC. (2017). Urolithins, the rescue of "old" metabolites to understand a "new" concept: Metabotypes as a nexus among phenolic metabolism, microbiota dysbiosis, and host health status. Mol Nutr Food Res, 61(1). https://doi.org/Artn 150090110.1002/Mnfr.201500901

Vegara S, Marti N, Lorente J, Coll L, Streitenberger S, Valero M, & Saura D. (2014). Chemical guide parameters for Punica granatum cv. 'Mollar' fruit juices processed at industrial scale. Food Chem, 147: 203–208. https://doi.org/10.1016/j.foodchem.2013.09.122

Wang D, Ozen C, Abu-Reidah IM, Chigurupati S, Patra JK, Horbanczuk JO, et al. (2018a). Vasculoprotective effects of pomegranate (Punica granatum L.). Front Pharmacol, 9: 544. https://doi.org/10.3389/fphar.2018.00544

Wang P, Zhang Q, Hou H, Liu Z, Wang L, Rasekhmagham R, et al. (2020). The effects of pomegranate supplementation on biomarkers of inflammation and endothelial dysfunction: A meta-analysis and systematic review. Complement Ther Med, 49: 102358. https://doi.org/10.1016/j.ctim.2020.102358

Wang Y, Xia Y, & Lu Z. (2018b). Metabolic features of cancer cells. Cancer Commun (Lond), 38(1): 65. https://doi.org/10.1186/s40880-018-0335-7

Wilson DW, Nash P, Buttar HS, Griffiths K, Singh R, De Meester F, et al. (2017). The role of food antioxidants, benefits of functional foods, and influence of feeding habits on the health of the older person: An overview. Antioxidants (Basel), 6(4). https://doi.org/10.3390/antiox6040081

Wong TL, Strandberg KR, Croley CR, Fraser SE, Nagulapalli Venkata KC, Fimognari C, et al. (2021). Pomegranate bioactive constituents target multiple oncogenic and oncosuppressive signaling for cancer prevention and intervention. Semin Cancer Biol, 73: 265–293. https://doi.org/10.1016/j.semcancer.2021.01.006

Yang J, Guo Y, Lee R, Henning SM, Wang J, Pan Y, et al. (2020). Pomegranate metabolites impact tryptophan metabolism in humans and mice. Curr Dev Nutr, 4(11): nzaa165. https://doi.org/10.1093/cdn/nzaa165

Yang Y, Xiu J, Zhang L, Qin C, & Liu J. (2012). Antiviral activity of punicalagin toward human enterovirus 71 in vitro and in vivo. Phytomedicine, 20(1): 67–70. https://doi.org/10.1016/j.phymed.2012.08.012

Yuan T, Ma H, Liu W, Niesen DB, Shah N, Crews R, et al. (2016). Pomegranate's neuroprotective effects against Alzheimer's disease are mediated by urolithins, its ellagitannin-gut microbial derived metabolites. ACS Chem Neurosci, 7(1): 26–33. https://doi.org/10.1021/acschemneuro.5b00260

Yuan Z, Fang Y, Zhang T, Fei Z, Han F, Liu C, et al. (2018). The pomegranate (Punica granatum L.) genome provides insights into fruit quality and ovule developmental biology. Plant Biotechnol J, 16(7): 1363–1374. https://doi.org/10.1111/pbi.12875

Zaouay F, Mena P, Garcia-Viguera C, & Mars M. (2012). Antioxidant activity and physico-chemical properties of Tunisian grown pomegranate (Punica granatum L.) cultivars. Industrial Crops and Products, 40: 81–89. https://doi.org/10.1016/j.indcrop.2012.02.045

Zhang L, Fu Q, & Zhang Y. (2011). Composition of anthocyanins in pomegranate flowers and their antioxidant activity. Food Chem, 127(4): 1444–1449. https://doi.org/10.1016/j.foodchem.2011.01.077

Zheng DP, Liwinski T, & Elinav E. (2020). Interaction between microbiota and immunity in health and disease. Cell Res, 30(6): 492–506. https://doi.org/10.1038/s41422-020-0332-7

Index

A

Acetaldehyde 239
Acetyl co-a 268, 269
Acetylation 149, 366
Activating transcription factor 3 (ATF3) 405
Acupuncture 159
Adenovirus 137
Adenylcyclase 180
Adipocytes 61, 62, 134, 135, 403, 418, 425
Adiponectin 87, 211, 212
Adipose cells 134, 136
Adipose-derived stem cells 61, 509
Adrenal cortex 177
β-Adrenergic receptor 147, 179
β-Adrenergic signaling pathway 179
β1-Adrenoceptor 179, 180, 181
β2-Adrenoceptor 180
Adrenocorticotropic hormone (ACTH) 147, 148
Aedes 255
Aerobic glycolysis 264–266, 268–270
Agaricales 80
Agaricomycetes 80
Alanine aminotransferase (ALT) 86
Albendazole 255
Alcohol 101, 239, 243, 590, 594
Aldolase 266
Aldose reductase 208, 294
Aldosterone 177, 179
Alexa 35, 36, 40
Alkaloids 90, 437, 472, 473, 589
Alleviate 136, 157, 331, 378, 511, 576, 577
Alum-based immunoadjuvants 331
Alveolar bone 135, 136, 138
Alzheimer's diseases 104, 107, 128, 511, 612
Amastigote 255, 257–259, 470–475
Amblyopia 111, 118, 120
Amikacin 365, 366, 370
Aminoglycoside acetyltransferase 366
Aminoglycoside phosphoryltransferase 366
Aminoglycosides 364, 366, 367
Aminophospholipid 103, 104
Amitriptyline 295
Amniotic membrane 58, 60, 62, 63
Amniotic membrane transplantation 59
Amorphous aluminum hydroxyphosphate sulphate 352, 353
Amoxicillin 365, 487
Amphipathic 101
Amplified fragment length polymorphism (AFLP) 224
Anaesthesia 57, 117, 140
Anamorphic prism 22
Anatomy 128, 161, 301

Anca-associated vasculitis 322
Androgens 234
Angiogenesis-related genes 211
Angiotensin II (ANG II) 105, 176, 178
Angiotensin type 1 (AT1) 177
Angiotensinogen 176, 177
Aniridia 57, 114
Anopheles 255
Antagonist 107, 147, 160, 209, 323, 378, 457, 473, 613
Anthelminthic medicines 255
Anthocyanins 301, 605, 609, 610
Antiangiogenic 59, 82, 400
Antiatherosclerotic 82, 610
Antibodies 11, 17, 26, 33, 39, 42, 233, 317, 318, 325, 328, 344, 351, 408, 537, 548, 554
Antibody titration 39
Anti-inflammatory 91, 138, 168, 211, 258, 299, 301–308, 484, 511, 606, 610, 612–613
Anti-inflammatory cytokines 138, 258, 299, 306, 430
Antimicrobial resistance (AMR) 363–364, 369–371
Aphakia 118
Aphasia 158
Apical papilla 60, 134–136, 509, 513
Applied behavior analysis (ABA) 157
Aquaporin 1 56
Argon-ion lasers 21
Articulation disorder 158
Artificial intelligence 3, 7, 46, 111
Asialoglycoprotein receptor (ASGPR) 552
Aspartate aminotransferase (AST) 86, 88, 511
Asteraceae 589–599
Asymptomatic microfilaremic 256
ATP dependent flippases 103
ATP synthase (complex V) 105, 268
ATP-binding cassette (ABC) 234, 369, 443
Atrial natriuretic peptide 280, 281
Attention deficit hyperactivity disorder (ADHD) 163
Attenuated microbe 138
Attenuated virus 137
Attenuation 148, 388, 510
Autism spectrum disorder (ASD) 155, 156
Autofluorescence 26, 35, 36
Autoimmune diseases 60, 138, 319–324, 597
Autologous 59–62, 64–65, 135, 136, 510
Azoospermia 224, 225

B

B cell lymphoma 330
Balovaptan 160
Bandpass filters 17, 18, 22, 25, 26
Basidiomycetes 80, 91, 92

621

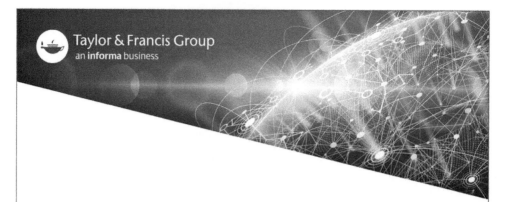
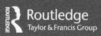
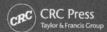